ABNORMAL PSYCHOLOGY

ABNORMAL PSYCHOLOGY

Florence Schumer

Independent Practice, New York City

D.C. Heath and Company

Lexington, Massachusetts Toronto

Credits:

Cover illustration by Edward Hallstrom, from *Schizophrenia Bulletin,* Volume 5, No. 3, 1979. The artist, who was a mental patient at the time, says that he painted it "to symbolize all the fears of a young woman I knew while I was working in New York years ago, and her withdrawal into herself."

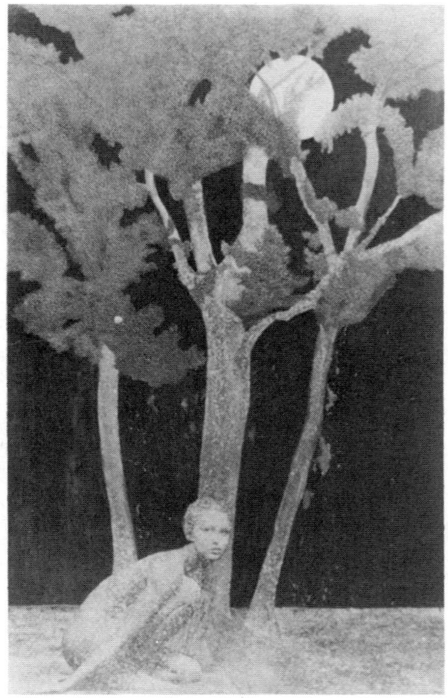

Chapter-opening photographs:

1 Culver Pictures
2 David Maybury-Lewis
3 Cary Wolinsky/Stock, Boston
4 Mark Antman
5 Ellis Herwig/Stock, Boston
6 University of Wisconsin Primate Laboratory
7 J. M. Richardson/Black Star
8 Robert V. Eckert, Jr./The Picture Cube
9 Sepp Seitz/Woodfin Camp
10 Arthur Tress
11 Mary Ellen Mark
12 T. Simon/Liaison
13 Jim Harrison/Stock, Boston
14 Bruce Roberts
15 Peter Simon/Black Star
16 Ed Lettau/Photo Researchers
17 T. C. Fitzgerald/The Picture Cube
18 Tex Fuller/Woodfin Camp
19 Paul Fusco/Magnum
20 Michael Weisbrot/Stock, Boston
21 Jean-Claude Lejeune/Stock, Boston

Published simultaneously in Canada.

Printed in the United States of America.

International Standard Book Number: 0-669-95695-3

Library of Congress Catalog Card Number: 82-82587

For Leo, my husband of many years, who not so patiently,
but always admiringly, put up with my writing of books
but did not live to see this one finally brought to completion

and

For my patients, all of them—past, present, and future—who
are not only my true teachers but who also never fail to
impress me with the strength and persistence of their
wills to make better lives for themselves

About the Author

Florence Schumer holds a Ph.D. from Yale University, where she was a Yale Fellow for four years, Clinical Psychologist in the Department of Psychiatry, and an externe in the Department of Pediatrics at the Yale-New Haven Hospital. She was Senior Psychologist at counseling centers at New York University and Cornell University Medical College, Research Associate in the Research Center for Human Relations, and Assistant Professor in the Department of Psychology at New York University and at Barnard College, where she was also Adjunct Associate Professor. In these and other academic settings, both undergraduate and graduate, Dr. Schumer supervised, trained, and taught students in abnormal and clinical psychology. She was also Senior Research Scientist in the Family Research Unit at the Wiltwyck School for Boys; Biometrics, at Columbia University; and at the Institute for Developmental Studies, New York University.

Dr. Schumer is a Fellow of the American Psychological Association and has been serving on the editorial board of the *Journal of Abnormal Psychology* since 1974. She has coauthored several books, including one with Salvador Minuchin on family treatment, another with Joseph Zubin and Leonard Eron on projective techniques, and a third, on brain-damaged children, with Cynthia Deutsch. Among her numerous articles and research activities are those in connection with gender and schizophrenia, projective techniques, and the personalities and family organization of ghetto, minority-group children.

In addition to her writing, reviewing of books and articles, and consulting activities, Dr. Schumer is currently in full-time private practice (with adults and children) that includes diagnostic and assessment activities, psychotherapy, and couple and family counseling.

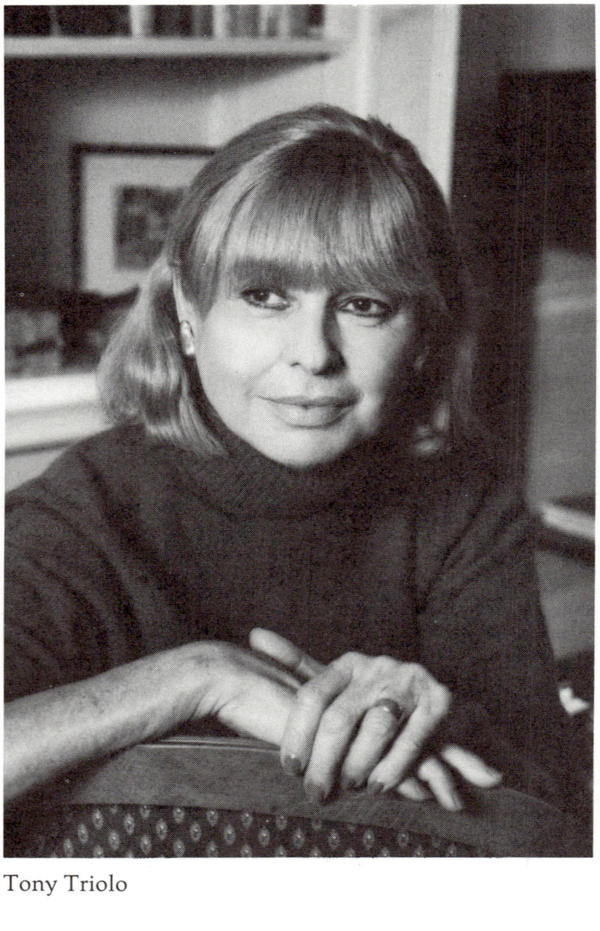

Tony Triolo

Foreword

There was a time when textbooks on abnormal psychology could be counted on one's fingers, and the only numbers to be found in them were page numbers. During the last decade, a plethora of abnormal texts have been written and their contents have varied along the entire continuum from phenomenology to quantitative objectivity. Why do we need another?

I have examined this text with this question in mind and have become convinced that this text does not fit into the general mold. It breaks it. Its avowed purpose is to integrate the variety of schools of thought that plague (if you are a pessimist) or enrich (if you are an optimist) the field of psychopathology.

The chapters are not separate entities, each dealing with a different point of view alien to its neighbor. Instead, each chapter tries, and more often succeeds, in integrating its theme across the various schools of thought. With the individual patient as its focus, it presents an integrated view of his problems, assets, and liabilities against the background of the options contending for explanation. Despite our ignorance of etiology, several plausible causal models are presented, leading the reader to at least hopeful working toward, if not to arriving at, a solution to the age-old enigma of psychopathology. The primary source of this salutary approach is the author's history of combining a research career with the life of an active clinician in private practice. The book draws on live patients in real-life clinical situations and community settings and displays their problems, assets, and liabilities against the web of potential explanatory models of etiology without the dogmatism trends often perceived in the single-minded clinicians or scientists limited to a specific school of thought. In addition, she has, in the course of an active writing career, developed a felicitous style that makes for exciting reading.

This excitement largely results from her ability to exploit the fact that, despite the progress made in our knowledge, our understanding of the causes of mental disorders is still extremely limited. To be sure, there are some who feel that they know where the answers are to be found and, like ground hogs, dig deeper and deeper into their particular areas of expertise. Others, with a wide, sweeping eclecticism, ignore the facts that do not fit their point of view. To recognize that today's facts are fragmented and do not fit our theories, and yet to retain the optimistic attitude that somehow we can eventually make sense of mental disorders is the spirit of this book and is the reason that I, for one, wish that I had written it myself.

The perspective provided in the epilogue epitomizes the various chapters and leaves the reader with the feeling that, despite the apparent ignorance now permeating the field, there are signs of emerging understanding that bid well to remove some of the mystery that enshrouds the mental disorders. This feeling of wonderment, puzzlement, and hopefulness is what makes this book different.

Joseph Zubin, Ph.D.
Research Career Scientist, VA
and
Distinguished Research Professor of Psychiatry
University of Pittsburgh
School of Medicine

Preface

I'm often asked three questions about *Abnormal Psychology:* Why did you write it? For whom was it written? And how is it different from the other books in the field? Let me answer these questions one at a time.

Why Was this Book Written?

When I was approached to write this book, I welcomed the opportunity to try my hand at writing a textbook. I thought it would be fun, and provide a much-needed vacation from the rigors and demands of the professional and academic books I had coauthored. I was completely mistaken. I had looked forward to a breather but instead became immersed in an arduous challenge that was to become one of the most intellectually and physically draining commitments that I had ever undertaken. Further, I was forced to scrutinize and evaluate some very comfortable preconceptions about psychopathology that I had carried for some time.

In accepting this challenge I also wanted to write a textbook that would be lively and interesting, one that would generate a sense of excitement and wonderment about scientific discovery in the field of abnormal behavior. I was determined not to shy away from the harsh objectivity of empirical evidence and to present psychology as a discipline with contours and controversy. I resolved to describe people and their problems as they really are: with symptoms that are not clearcut, perhaps treated by clinicians who do not treat them "as advertised" or who subscribe to theories about behavior that may not be valid or even open to tests of validity. I also wanted to present the field as it really is, in a state of flux, with many gaps in our knowledge but with a future that holds great promise, laced with exciting possibilities that link it with previously unrelated disciplines, such as biochemistry and neurophysiology. I felt a strong commitment to objectivity, to scientific method, and to flexibility in permitting research evidence a fair hearing.

For Whom Was this Book Written?

Abnormal Psychology was written for the abnormal psychology course offered in most undergraduate psychology departments, and although a previous introductory course is appropriate, it is not necessary. For psychology majors who have already had several courses in psychology, Part I (Chapters 1–7) could be assigned for reading in the early weeks of the course, with the major share of the semester devoted to Parts II and III. For beginning students, with or without an introductory course, Part I could be assigned over a longer period of time. Part I includes not only an introduction to the field but also an exposition of cultural variables, science and scientific methods, diagnosis, psychological testing, and various theories, both psychological and "physical," of abnormal behavior. Part II contains the clinical chapters. They cover an extremely wide range of abnormal behaviors and are filled with case illustrations, clinical examples, and descriptive materials, as well as vignettes and sidelights of general and academic interest. Yet, the material is experimentally and theoretically oriented, with meticulous coverage and evaluation of the research literature and with an emphasis on up-to-date content. Part III contains the chapters on interventions and treatment methods and is similarly extensive in coverage; these chapters are also heavily laced with illustrative and case material but continue to be stringently evaluative in the light of empirical outcome data. This book, thus, is comparable to others used for abnormal psychology courses, but in most areas it has a wider scope of coverage and goes deeper and more critically into its substance, chapter for chapter, than is usual.

How Is this Book Different from Others in the Field?

Abnormal Psychology reflects my deep conviction about the significance of learning and of sociocultural and environmental variables in the incidence, expression, and course of clinical problems; in each of the chapters, I have consistently focused on and highlighted these themes. At the same time, I felt committed to examining, weighing, and sifting emerging research findings from the neurosciences relevant to causal and/or associated variables in psychopathology. I discovered intriguing possibilities along these lines—in alcoholism, substance abuse, and additional clinical areas above and beyond the major depressive disorders and schizophrenia—and felt obliged to report these possibilities, even if they were only promising, as long as the empirical evidence was beginning to trickle in.

This book gives more than lip service to cultural variables and to epidemiological considerations. Although an early chapter emphasizes these themes, throughout all of the other chapters there are separate sections on the incidence of the syndromes to age, gender, social class, and ethnicity—relationships that are considered again and again in the search for causal variables.

I have tried to take the student with me on an exciting excursion that explores the causes and treatments of abnormal behavior, and in this journey I have deliberately focused on covering as much ground—the relevant literature—as possible. At the same time, I was determined to be rigorous, even "hardnosed," in evaluating the empirical evidence that I was accumulating along the way. I extended this general frame of reference, also, to the evaluation of treatment and therapy outcome and attempted to cover, in some detail, the methodological problems involved in doing this kind of research.

Abnormal Psychology is a cross-disciplinary, rather than eclectic, book that does not fear to cross borders, leap from one paradigm or model to another, and evaluate the new territories that come into view as a result. My goal was to ferret out the underpinnings of aberrant behavior and to present the various possible paths to modifying such behaviors, even if, in this search, unpopular or unfashionable steps had to be taken. To illustrate, I believe that the cognitive models offer the most promise for effective treatment; but because my allegiance is to science and the evidence that accumulates under the umbrella of scientific procedures, it became easy for me to acknowledge, for example, the significance of some of the psychopharmacological advances in the treatment of certain types of depression or schizophrenia.

To aid the student in this exploration, I have introduced some specific features, too numerous to list in their entirety. One example: specific treatment and interventive methods are touched on again and again in Part II in the context of the clinical content of these substantive chapters. Because interventions are not dealt with in detail until the final chapters of the book, I have written a short foreword to Part II that briefly describes the major therapeutic approaches. Thus the student is not left "hanging" until these therapies are discussed in detail in Part III (Chapters 19–21).

This book is liberally interlaced with clinical illustrations, derived primarily from my own files and experiences. Yet these clinical summaries appear in "strong," experimentally oriented contexts in which the experimental and theoretical literature plays a crucial role. The clinical and research material on substance abuse is divided into two chapters, with one chapter entirely devoted to alcohol abuse. I decided to write two chapters on schizophrenia; Chapter 11 provides the student with extensive clinical and descriptive coverage of schizophrenia and its subtypes, and outlines in detail some of the diagnostic and research models that help us to understand schizophrenia. This content is more than ample for an undergraduate course that may or may not be followed by other courses. Chapter 12, an optional chapter, presents high-level theoretical and experimental material in this complex area for advanced students and psychology majors. The book is designed, however, so that Chapter 13 can be assigned immediately following Chapter 11 with no loss in continuity.

I made several other decisions about the substance of this book. For example, because I do not feel that there are dichotomous "laws" about behavior that apply to either children or adults exclusively, I decided not to deal with children in a separate chapter. I chose instead to cover childhood pathology in as many relevant chapters as I could. Thus in the clinical chapters, as well as those focusing on theory and therapy, the discussion is very much concerned with children, including adolescents. In addition, high-risk strategies, the search for predictive variables, and preventive approaches in our field are emphasized throughout the book—content that very much concerns children.

Similarly, I decided not to separate the complex moral, ethical, and subjective issues in our field from their relevant applications. For example, questions of consent, voluntariness of participation in experiments, the determination of dangerousness, decisions about who gets treated or not, confidentiality of records, sexism in treatment, and the damaging nature of diagnostic labels are dealt with both within and at the ends of all chapters.

In the same vein, the DSM-III is interwoven throughout the book, in addition to formal presentations in Chapter 4 and the Appendixes, which compare the DSM-II and the DSM-III on specific diagnoses. The DSM-III is viewed critically, and alternate systems are discussed. Yet so much of the research literature employs the DSM-III's nomenclature that to avoid a detailed description of it, because of dissatisfaction with it methodologically, is to rob students of background and familiarity with terms they will have to read and talk about again and again in this and other books.

Abnormal Psychology is a big book. There are many dozens of formal case illustrations and capsule case summaries and examples. There are over 100 Spotlights (each intrinsically related to and extensions of the text, yet lively and focused for "spicy" reading) and about 175 photographs, not to mention dozens of cartoons, drawings, charts, and graphs. Well over 100 detailed capsule summaries of suggested readings appear at the ends of chapters, as do about 100 specific issues for individual consideration. There are approximately 1,600 entries in the reference list and a 1,000-word glossary at the end of the book, in which I was directly involved, so that consistency of definition and usage within the book is guaranteed.

The challenge for me—and I think I met this challenge—was to make this "big" book palpable, human, and people oriented, and to present a wealth of hard-edged material simply and with a liveliness that will excite interest in the student.

Finally, My Thanks

The careful and objective reviews (at that time, anonymous) of various drafts of my manuscript were immeasurably helpful, indeed influential, in shaping revisions in early versions of this book. The reviewers were Linda Baskett, Jim Eison, Mervin B. Freedman, Ray Hawkins, Steven D. Hollon, and Michael W. O'Hara.

Paul Mussen deserves special thanks for his guidance, critical reading of various drafts of the manuscript, and editorial assistance. He was, in addition, reassuring and supportive when morale, energy, and motivation to complete this formidable task were beginning to waver. Joseph Zubin's scientific and personal integrity and friendship served as a model to inspire me to think about and to evaluate phenomena in ways that need not subscribe to prevailing paradigms, despite the "fashion." I also warmly acknowledge a few friends who were so supportive and understanding during the years I was working on this book; they will not be mentioned by name, but they know who they are.

Sonya Guterman, who read and evaluated parts of my manuscript, and Irving Kosow, who helped me to get started, deserve special mention, as does Jean Johnson, without whom this text could not have appeared in this form. She patiently and intelligently deciphered and retyped, many times over, all versions and stages of the manuscript. I am also deeply grateful to Jill Charlton, Kathryn M. Adorney, and Karen M. Simon for their important contributions to this book and for their diligence, persistence, and scholarship in helping me with thousands of daily details. Karen Simon also collaborated with me in the writing of Chapter 20.

I sincerely appreciate and acknowledge the efforts of the many people at D. C. Heath who painstakingly brought *Abnormal Psychology* to publication, notably Barbara Piercecchi, Nancy Osman, Elizabeth Van de Kerkhove, and especially Bryan Woodhouse, with whom I have had much contact, sometimes even daily, in these past months. D. C. Heath's involvement also reflects the work of Mary Stuart Lang and Martha Johnson.

Finally, I gratefully acknowledge my son Robert Schumer for his critical and scholarly reading of many sections of the manuscript, his enthusiasm and interest in science, especially the neurosciences, his contagious sense of fun in intellectual inquiry, and his overall support and encouragement when confidence lagged. He gets my buoyant thanks.

F. S.

Brief Table of Contents

Contents

ABNORMAL PSYCHOLOGY

Part I

Introduction

Chapters 1–7

1

Abnormal Behavior: Definitions, Causes, and Historical Perspectives

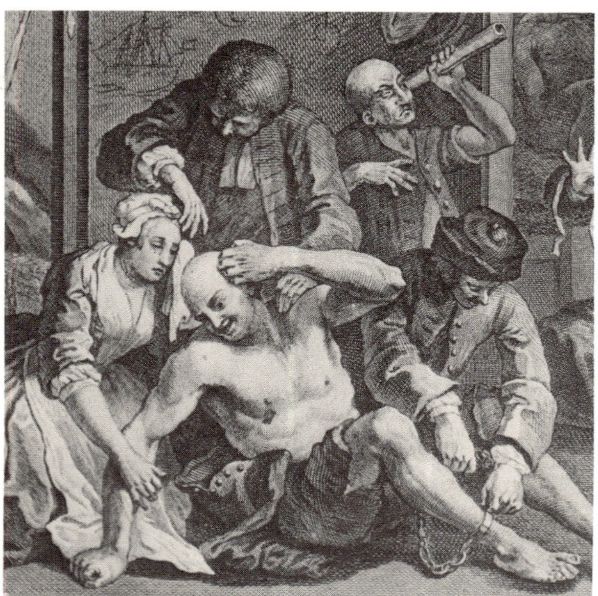

This is a book about abnormal behavior. But what does the term *abnormal behavior* mean?

The first section of this chapter surveys different views and perspectives about abnormal behavior in an attempt to define its characteristics. To begin with, we will look at everyday words that people use to call someone's behavior "abnormal." Then we will describe more formal attempts to define abnormal behavior (and some problems in connection with these attempts). Another section illustrates what it feels like to suffer the distress sometimes associated with abnormal behavior. Finally, we present some general characteristics of abnormal behavior that form a working frame of reference for this book.

The chapter continues with a simple presentation of possible underlying causes of abnormal behavior and concludes with a survey of how people through the ages perceived and treated people whom they designated as "crazy."

Words For Abnormal Behavior

Spotlight 1.1 presents a list of everyday words that refer to "abnormal" people or "abnormal" behavior. Spotlight 1.1 also contains a much smaller list of words used to characterize *normal* behavior. A glance at Spotlight 1.1 yields some obvious differences between the lists. The words for abnormal behavior are more colorful, come more easily to mind, and comprise a fairly lengthy list. Almost all of the words in the "abnormal" list have a harsh, judgmental, or derisive quality, while most of the

Spotlight 1.1 Words, Words, Words

Immediately below is a long list of words that people use to refer to "abnormal" behavior, followed by a much smaller list of words that refer to "normal" behavior. Can you add to these lists? Why is the first list so much longer than the second?

Words That Refer to "Abnormal" Behavior

mentally ill
crazy
sick
insane
mad
abnormal
deranged
demented
deviant
aberrant
disordered
pathological
psychopathic
loco
screwball
bats in the belfry
wacky
out of one's skull
mad as a hatter
not having all one's marbles
emotionally ill
off one's rocker
freaked out
batty
cracked
running amuck
being tetched
going haywire
gaga
spooky
spacey
meshugah
maniacal
off the wall
non compos mentis
unbalanced
has personality problems
monomaniacal
schizy
stark-mad
loony
off one's nut
flipped out
flaky
psychotic
neurotic
psychoneurotic
manic
eccentric
odd
weird
bizarre
queer
lunatic
mentally diseased
unstable
nutty as a fruitcake
nut
crackpot
freak
kooky
goofball
a screw loose
going beserk
becoming unhinged
buggy
psycho
dotty
irrational
spaced out
taking leave of one's senses

Words That Refer to "Normal" Behavior

sane, sanity
reasoning
balanced
emotionally healthy
mentally healthy
in possession of one's faculties
soundminded
rational
stable
emotionally mature
compos mentis
in possession of one's senses
well adjusted
normal
soberhead
in one's right mind
all there
have it all together
being all together

words in the "normal" list connote self-control, level-headedness, even-keeled control of oneself by one's mind, and other "sober" qualities which some of us admire or wish we possessed.

Why are there so many more words for abnormal than normal behavior? Apparently our language is abundantly expressive when it comes to words that mean "crazy" or insane. As a matter of fact, Roget's *International Thesaurus* (1962) contains about ten times as many synonyms and equivalent expressions for insanity than for sanity. Even words that describe facilities for the *treatment* of abnormal behavior have an expressive, often derisive, quality. When people are admitted to a mental institution they find themselves in an asylum, sanitorium, madhouse, bedlam, home, nuthouse, funny farm, loonybin, booby hatch, or padded cell. When people have babies, an appendix removed, or a slipped disk, they simply go to a hospital. It is of interest that most of our words for *medical* problems are without the negative or harsh quality that words for emotional problems carry.

The quantity and quality of words alluding to abnormal behavior suggest that people may become anxious, uncertain, even frightened about behavior different from their own and that they may deal with such feelings by resorting to a rich variety of judgmental labels that have a derisive and derogatory quality. It may be that the harsh quality of such words also reflects a cultural tradition: nonconformity and "deviant" behavior have frequently been associated with "bad," punishable personality qualities. Nonconforming behavior may also arouse fear and suspicion because of its unfamiliarity or unpredictability.

In any event, it should be obvious that the domain of abnormal behavior is laced with a wide variety of harsh labels that may reflect a perception of deviance from cultural and societal standards. For example, we may make fun of people who talk to themselves in public, have a childish temper tantrum in a social situation, or run naked through the streets. They may be objects of ridicule because of their nonconforming behavior and not because they are doing anything that is intrinsically comical.

Some social scientists believe that the labeling process—by which one person categorizes another as "crazy"—produces special problems for the labeled person as a result of the negative personal interactions and judgments that accompany the label (Farina and Ring, 1965; Murphy, 1976; Scheff, 1966). *Labeling theory* is the general term applied to the study of this labeling process. Studies of labeling behavior attempt to understand the reasons why and in what ways people apply labels to others and the effects that different labels have on the labeler as well as on the labeled person's interpersonal relationships and judgments (for example, Cox, Costanzo, and Coie, 1976).

Some people believe that the words for abnormal behavior should be eliminated from our language. Then we would be forced to describe behavior that is different from our own with such words as unexpected, unconventional, or unpredictable. Our words might even take a turn for the positive: creative, unique, exceptional, extraordinary, rare, individual, imaginative, fanciful. Do you agree?

The words commonly used to refer to abnormal behavior have not helped us to define abnormal behavior. Are the experts of any help?

DEFINING ABNORMAL BEHAVIOR

Is there some professional agreement as to what constitutes abnormal behavior? There is, in fact, little agreement about definitions of abnormal behavior, nor is there uniformity of opinion as to the characteristics of *mental illness*, a term that is troublesome and controversial, as we shall see later. Yet we have all seen or heard of people who behave in "abnormal" ways that we think could be reflections of mental illness (sometimes called mental disease or psychopathology): they threaten to kill us or themselves; they express extreme, unrelieved fear or unhappiness; they stop eating or moving about or caring for themselves; they are afraid to go outdoors or to mingle with people; or they hear and see things the rest of us do not.

Can we construct a working model to guide us in our survey of abnormal behavior? Let us examine the possibilities.

The Statistical Model: Mental Illness as Deviation from the Norm

According to the statistical (or normative) approach to defining abnormality, behavior that adheres or conforms to the norm or to what the majority of a group does is equated with mental health while behavior that is deviant or does not conform to this rough "average" is considered abnormal, an indication of mental illness. In designating what is average or "normal" behavior, the statistical model assumes that most human traits and behaviors vary over a wide range and can be represented graphically in what is called the normal curve.

The normal curve or normal frequency curve, is a curve representing the frequency with which the values of a variable are obtained or observed an "infinite" number of times when the variation is subject to the "law of chance" (English and English, 1958). The curve is bell-shaped, with the highest frequency in the middle, and a gradual, symmetrical tapering toward the extremes.

Figure 1.1, which illustrates a normal frequency curve, shows the distribution of heights of 761 soldiers in the Army of the Potomac during the Civil

Figure 1.1 A bell-shaped curve showing the distribution of the heights of 761 Civil War soldiers, as depicted on an old chart.

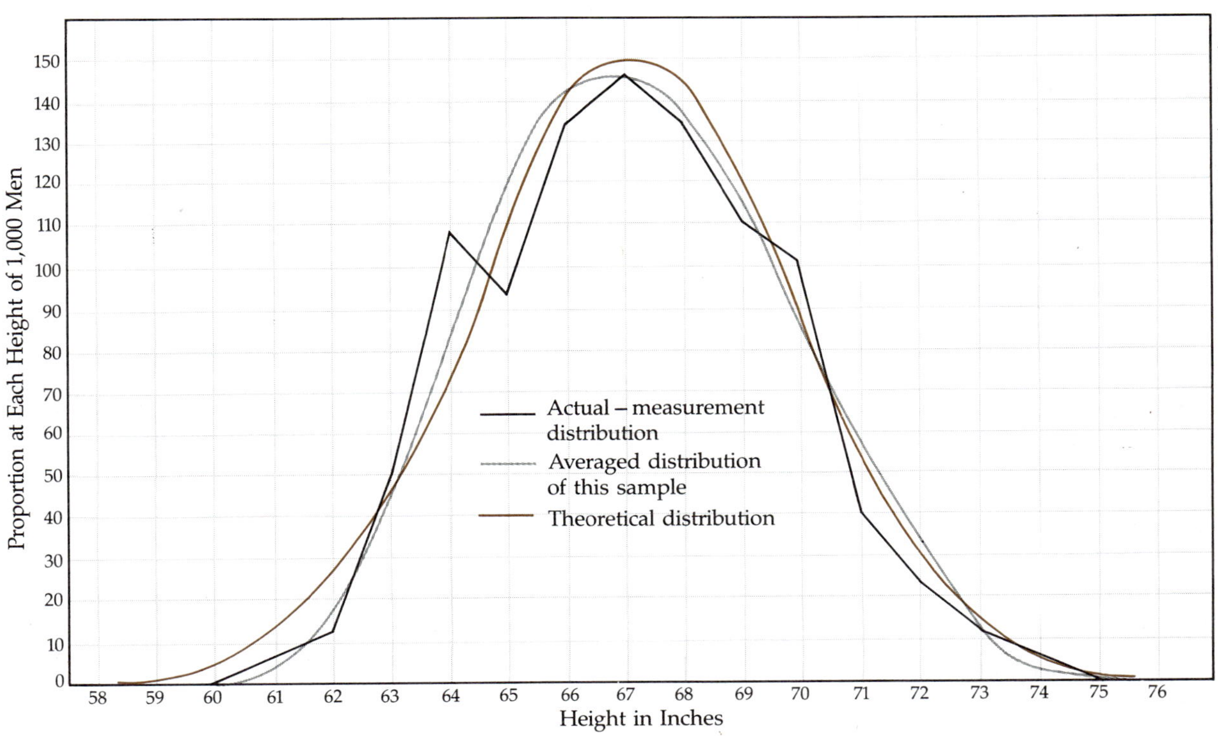

War (see Griffin, 1962, p. 79). According to this curve, the vast majority of these men were between 62 and 73 inches tall; relatively few were shorter than 62 inches or taller than 73 inches. One might say, then, that normal height is between 62 and 73 inches and abnormal height is anything greater or less than heights within this normal range.

Although heights of the Civil War soldiers were indeed normally "distributed" (as seen in Figure 1.1), many human qualities, characteristcs, or traits do not fall on a perfect, bell-shaped curve, nor are they normally distributed. Is the trait of honesty normally distributed? Is mental health? How about creativity?

To assume that mental health is equated with some norm has serious problems. First, the statistical definition of abnormality lacks "directionality," in that infrequent behavior in either direction from the central tendency would be regarded as abnormal (Buss, 1966; Sabshin, 1967). Thus an uncommon yet desirable trait—for example, outstanding musical ability, or outstanding physical or intellectual endowment (such as great strength or genius)—would also be regarded as abnormal, as would unusually productive, perceptive, empathic, happy, contented, or satisfied people.

To deal with this problem, we could say that being unusually productive and empathic is good, while being unusually underproductive and lacking in empathy is bad or not good and that an unusual amount of a valued, socially desirable characteristic would not be regarded as abnormal. Falling back on values about good, bad, desirable, and undesirable, however, goes beyond a purely statistical approach.

Consider still another problem with the normative approach. Each family, subgroup, society, and culture has its own set of norms and standards. When we talk of adherence to some norm, what is the reference group?

In our culture, we might regard certain behaviors as indications of disturbance; the same behaviors might not only be acceptable but actually required in other cultures (for example, keeping one's face covered in public). Even within our own

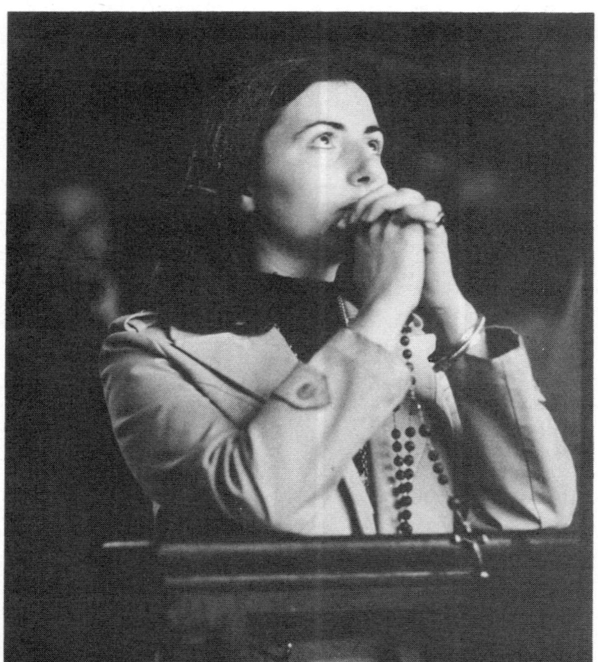

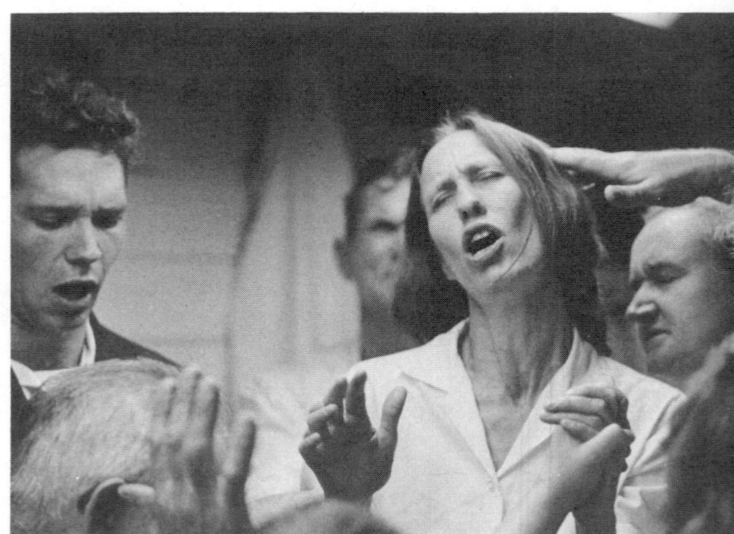

The overt expression of religious feelings can take many forms, depending on one's upbringing and social and cultural group membership. (Left: Owen Franken/Stock, Boston. Above: J. R. Holland/Stock, Boston)

Spotlight 1.2 What's the Name of The Frame?

Historical and cultural frames of reference are of great significance in judging abnormal behavior. Without further information, how would you perceive the following behaviors?

- A 58-year-old man regards anyone who touches him with acute terror.
  —He is mentally disturbed: he has an intense, irrational fear of being touched (haphephobia; *défense de toucher*).
  —He is a perfectly "normal" nineteenth century tribal king in a society that has strict taboos against anyone touching him.
- A rich, 50-year-old man suddenly gives to his enemies all of his wealth and possessions.
  —He is in an acute period of intense mental disturbance characterized by impulsivity, extreme depression, and guilt.
  —He is a nineteenth century Kwakiutl Indian going through a "normal" cultural rite to best his rivals.
- A young girl actively hallucinates (she sees the devil) and seems terrified by her enemies.
  —She is experiencing an acute, toxic reaction to drugs, with extreme fear and paranoid thoughts—that is, ideas characterized by delusions of persecution.
  —She is an eighteenth century Italian peasant girl having a religious vision; revered by her kinspeople throughout her lifetime, she was later sainted.

society, many subgroups and subcultures have their own distinct "flavors" or lifestyles, exemplified by food tastes, childrearing practices, male-female roles, sexual patterns, and almost any other area of human social activity. What is normal and what is abnormal? Does the majority culture determine mainstream normality? Spotlight 1.2 illustrates how cultural frames of reference can modify our designations of normality and abnormality.

The "Ideal State" Model: Mental Illness as Failure to Meet Mental Health Criteria

To avoid some of the problems of statistical definitions of mental health or illness, is it possible to construct objective criteria of "good" or "ideal" mental health and then watch for deviations from such standards as indicators of underlying pathology? For example, the following is a "composite picture of the normal person":

. . . a steady individual who deals with situations in a task-oriented fashion, and maintains a proper balance and integration between himself and his environment. His involvement is measured and appropriate to the situation. He performs reasonably close to his capacity level and is much less burdened by irrelevant factors (Shakow, 1967, p. 317).

Other frequently expressed views define mental health specifically in terms of problem-solving ability or "efficiency in meeting task requirements" (Wishner, 1955), or propose that mentally healthy individuals are in charge of themselves and aware of inner drives and motivations (Kubie, 1954); still other views emphasize personal and social responsibility and "democratic social interest" factors (Shoben, 1957).

Several objections arise in using "ideal" models of mental health to define mental illness. One is that many frequently expressed ideals are bound up with beliefs, values, and goals that are embedded within the culture or subculture rather than based on objectively defined criteria that can be universally applied across many groups of people. For example, must the normal or healthy personality always show social responsibility or democratic social interest? Or is the dedicated artist who works in isolation not normal?

Approaches based on definitions of ideal mental health would probably exclude most people from the "healthy" category. Very few people, for example, function close to capacity or are aware of all of their inner motivations. Although ideal concepts of normality may represent a striving toward a Utopian ideal, and even though they influence our thinking about abnormal behavior, they have little practical usefulness and may even misrepresent mental health by overstating the case (Offer and Sabshin, 1974; Sabshin, 1967).

Despite some of the foregoing objections, what does a survey of the writing on abnormal psychology yield regarding definitions of ideal mental health? Perhaps gross departures from these criteria would help us to shed a little light on the nature of psychopathology. This was the motivation behind one such survey (Jahoda, 1958), which yielded the following categories of definitions of mental health:

1. attitudes of the individual toward himself/herself—self-awareness; acceptance of self; correctness or reality of self-concept
2. personal development, growth, and self-actualization of the individual—realization of one's potential and resources
3. integration and coherence of the individual's personality—the way in which psychological parts fit together and are balanced, coordinated, and unified
4. the autonomy of the individual—degree of independence and self-sufficiency; ability to stand on his or her own feet without making unreasonable demands on others; resistance to or at least ability to stand apart from social influences
5. the individual's orientation to reality—degree to which perceptions of the world are free from distortions and influences based on personal needs
6. environmental mastery—including many aspects of the individual's relationship to the people and situations around him or her, such as ability to love, work, have friends, play, solve problems, and adjust to situational requirements

Do departures from the foregoing ideals constitute psychopathology? There is little agreement among the experts about the answer to this question.

The Disease or Medical Model

The disease model of mental illness* rests on an analogy to the medical model of *physical* illness. The medical model for physical illness assumes that pathological (diseased) states can be traced to concrete causes such as trauma (injury), germs, biochemical defects, viruses, infections, or abnormal conditions of the tissue, hormones, organs, or brain.

In the actual face-to-face clinical situation in the medical doctor's office, the disease or medical model generally involves the following steps: diagnosis of the causes of pathology (etiology), based on inquiry and examination—a step generally producing a name or a label for the disease; treatment recommendations based on diagnostic considerations—a step aimed at the arrest, reversal, or cure of the pathological condition; and prognosis, or prediction of the ultimate course of the disease toward recovery or degeneration—a step frequently based on past experience.

The disease model of mental illness similarly assumes that there are identifiable causes of the pathology, and that therefore a diagnosis of the pathological process can be made, from which recommendations for treatment and predictions about the most likely course and outcome of the disease will logically flow. Above all, this model assumes that mental and emotional disturbances reflect disease

* Legal designations of insanity, based on such considerations as competence to stand trial, knowing right from wrong if accused of a crime, being able to participate in one's own defense, as well as being competent to make decisions about one's finances (as in making a will) are often required by the courts and by some of our other institutions. Most often, the criteria to make such designations are unclear, vary from state to state, and require expert testimony that may turn out to be inconsistent. In addition, since legal definitions do not necessarily overlap with psychological ones, we will not address ourselves to the question of legal "sanity" or "insanity" in this chapter. However, Chapter 18 (pp. 557–58) returns to this extremely important theme.

processes. Many clinicians—for example, Adams (1964), Albee (1977), and Szasz (1960, 1973a)—have challenged this model. Some of their arguments are:

Mental illness and physical disease cannot be equated. Most people with mental problems have difficulty with social and interpersonal relationships, manifested by loneliness, poor self-confidence, or sexual dysfunctions. A medical or disease model implies that a single cause or group of causes can account for such problems. The one-to-one cause-and-effect relationship in the arena of human behavior is rarely found, however. What is called mental illness is often simply a collection of different behaviors about which society passes judgment—for example, juvenile delinquency or certain types of sexual preferences. Because many words in the field of abnormal psychology *appear* to be medical—for example, mental *hygiene,* mental

Spotlight 1.3 Of Mind and Medicine

Here are three physicians' views of the medical model, representing the range of opinion from actively promoting it to demolishing it. We begin first with Kraepelin (1865–1926), often considered to be the father of modern psychiatry (a medical specialty that focuses on the study and treatment of mental disorders), and generally credited with establishing the precedent for the disease approach to abnormal behavior. At about the turn of the century, Kraepelin introduced the first of a series of lectures to a group of physicians who were untrained in psychiatry as follows:

Gentlemen: The subject of the following course of lectures will be the Science of Psychiatry, which, as its name implies, is that of the treatment of mental disease. It is true that, in the strictest terms, we cannot speak of the mind as becoming diseased, whether we regard it as a separate entity or as the sum total of our subjective experience. And, indeed, from the medical point of view, it is disturbances in the physical foundations *of mental life which should occupy most of our attention. But the incidents of such diseases are generally seen in the sphere of psychical events, a department with which the art of medicine has dealt very little as yet. Here we are not so much concerned with physical changes in size, shape, firmness, and chemical composition, as with disturbances of comprehension, memory and judgment, illusions, hallucinations, depression, and morbid changes in the activity of the will. With the help of the ideas you have derived from general pathology, you will usually be able to find your way in a new department of medicine without any serious difficulty (Kraepelin, 1913, p. 1).*

Some physicians, however, even though they adhered to the medical model, came to realize the inadequacy of a strictly medical approach to mental illness. Gregory Zilboorg, for example, wrote over forty years ago:

Mental diseases are apparently the only diseases which deserve the appellation of social diseases, not because they are caused by social factors alone but because a mentally sick individual functions with the totality of his endowments. A psychological conflict leading to a disease cannot but use as its vehicle the sum total of the cultural problems which are characteristic of the individual's age (Zilboorg and Henry, 1941, p. 523).

And finally, here is an even more extreme position about the medical model:

Disease means bodily disease. Gould's Medical Dictionary *defines disease as a disturbance of the function or structure of an organ or a part of the* body. *The mind (whatever it is) is not an organ or part of the body. Hence, it cannot be diseased in the same sense as the body can. When we speak of mental illness, then, we speak metaphorically. To say that a person's mind is sick is like saying that the economy is sick or that a joke is sick. When metaphor is mistaken for reality and is used for social purposes, then we have the makings of myth. The concepts of mental health and mental illness are mythological concepts, used strategically to advance some social interests and to retard others, much as national and religious myths have been used in the past (Szasz, 1973a, p. 97).*

health, mental *illness, diagnosis, pathology, cure, sickness*—we are left with the false impression that the behaviors to which they refer are diseases.

Another criticism of the disease model is that it involves labels and diagnoses that negatively affect the attitudes people have about emotional problems, a view expressed earlier in this chapter. In addition, an implicit theme of the disease model is that the afflicted individual has no personal control over his or her problems (Farina, et al., 1978). This view reinforces the sense of helplessness that characterizes many people with emotional problems: "I cannot master my problems since I am mentally ill ("sick"). Therefore, somebody is going to have to take care of me." Such attitudes on the part of the mentally ill person mean that they are less likely to work at resolving their problems. On the other hand, people who think that their problems are the result of learned habits make more of an effort to understand and to change those behaviors (Farina, et al., 1978).

Finally, we must mention Thomas Szasz again. Szasz has launched a particularly violent attack on the medical model (see Spotlight 1.3) by denying the existence of mental illness altogether. He believes that problems of living and of belief and value systems are at the core of what people call mental illness, which is really a deviation from some norm definable in social, ethical, and legal, but never *medical,* terms. Further, some person or institution is defining that deviance. Why should we choose a *disease* approach, he asks, to cure a social, legal, or ethical deviance? Mental illness, he continues, is basically a question of conduct—the struggle of an individual with the problem of how he or she should live. Since the traditional notion of mental illness as disease is inadequate, he concludes that the term *mental illness* should be eliminated from our vocabulary.

Subjective Reports of Anguish: An Additional Parameter

Most psychologists agree that neither casebook illustrations nor rigidly defined "objective" criteria adequately portray the inner anguish and suffering that firsthand, oral, or written personal accounts convey. Many descriptions of personal experiences during a "breakdown" and recovery have been published. Written by people who could look within themselves and then find the words to describe what they felt, such reports provide some flavor of the pain, suffering, and terror that mental patients experience. These accounts are clearly not representative of those who have experienced mental anguish, since only a few disturbed people are articulate enough to express their inner feelings with such fine detail.

Spotlight 1.4 presents several descriptions of emotional turmoil. Although the reports would not be regarded as objective data, even the most hardheaded scientist will admit that mental illness cannot be adequately described unless the inner language of the suffering person is also acknowledged.

MENTAL ILLNESS: A WORKING FRAME OF REFERENCE

Our approach recognizes the existence of patterns of "abnormality"—dysfunctional and maladaptive behaviors—regardless of labels. These patterns are often accompanied by subjectively experienced emotional distress, anxiety, irrational fear, paralyzing indecisiveness, or great hopelessness and depression, as well as more objectively observable behaviors. Most clinicians are familiar with these indications of emotional distress, which may reflect the presence of deep, underlying pathology. This section attempts to characterize the possible earmarks of such pathology.

Some Characteristics of Mental Illness

We frequently find in people whom we will designate as abnormal or as mentally ill, some or many of the following characteristics. (The presence of any of these behaviors and states in an individual, however, *does not automatically signify mental illness.*)

1. *Inability to make decisions and plans or to have control*

Spotlight 1.4 Varieties of Psychopathological Experience

Landis and Mettler (1964) have compiled an impressive group of direct, firsthand subjective reports of what it was like to suffer an acute emotional "breakdown." These reports were culled from many sources, some anonymous. The exquisite detail of this personal material—notes, diaries, memoirs, letters—provides a rich reservoir for the researcher and student of abnormal behavior alike. Even the novelist and poet can be led to a closer understanding of human behavior when he or she reads of the pain, anguish, and personal suffering experienced during such states as hallucinations, relapses into illness, periods of sudden lucidity, disorders of thinking, disorders of perception, *petit mal* seizures (see Chapter 13, p. 345), maniacal excitement and elation, the pain involved in opium withdrawal, deep depression, intense states of agitation or anxiety, delusional feelings of confusion, suicidal urges, and many more states of personal suffering.

Here are some excerpts from such reports:

[Disorders of thought, delusions]:
Something has happened to bring my mind into the wrong way of thinking—The trouble is I didn't control myself when I could and now I can't. . . . It isn't sickness—it's wickedness—I've been thinking wrong and acting wrong. . . . I know that affects the mind—I am under a cloud—I blame nobody but myself. . . . Satan got hold of me. . . . I think I must be insane—the possession of my soul and body by the devil—I can't grasp this thing of my being here—I have lost my identity (p. 164)

[Mania]:
I [began by having] an indescribable nervous feeling. . . . My nights were sleepless. . . . The blood seemed to be carried to my brain in such quantities that the skull was too small to contain the brain enclosed therein. . . . The muscles which heretofore (during the period of depression) had refused to respond to stimuli now refused to remain at rest. To keep physically quiet was an utter impossibility. The strain of trying to keep still was fast wearing me out. I would lie in bed and jump up and down on the springs; I would make numerous excuses to go for a drink and to the toilet, simply to be doing something. . . . Thoughts crowded into my mind too rapidly for expression. Talking was the greatest relief imaginable. . . . (p. 49)

[Hallucinations]:
The evening of the day that I became ill, I was astounded and amused to see appear, on a kind of ledge going the round of the room formed by beams situated at some distance from the ceiling, about one hundred little men and women about six inches in height. They wore yellow, red or blue trousers and skirts. . . . Certain of them were mounted on small bay-colored horses proportionate in size. . . . These personages gradually disappeared and departed in columns at the end of half an hour (p. 118)

[Petit mal *"attacks"*]:
[This sort of seizure] caused no pain, it lasted a few seconds, I saw and heard and moved while it happened. I have often crossed a room, and, while not losing sight or bearings, not know how *I crossed it. The sequence of consciousness was so little broken by it, that after it had happened it seemed not an atom of time or myself had been missing, and I only knew it had happened again by the numb sensation in the centre of the brain which followed it. . . . It seemed like a tiny wheel—the wheel say, of a watch, whirring at blurring speed. . . . in my head while I went on with whatever I was doing, guided by* the consciousness left over *rather than the consciousness of the moment. . . . (p. 225)*

Source: Landis and Mettler, 1964.

over one's life. The person may feel paralyzed, powerless, helpless, and at the mercy of outside forces.

2. *Disturbing feelings of agitation, depression, fear, or panic* (sudden, intense, overwhelming fear). Often these feelings engender such discomfort that they drive people to seek help. Inner discomfort, however, is not always present in people with emotional problems.
3. *Disturbing and distressing thoughts, feelings, and*

compulsions (irresistible urge to perform an act despite one's wishes). These may be accompanied by feelings of panic, especially when the inner urge violates the individual's sense of "what is right" (such as impulses to murder someone, or to set fire to, or destroy, something). Such powerful recurrent thoughts or obsessions (sometimes called *idées fixes*) are extremely disturbing to people who have them.

4. *The presence of hallucinations (perceptions that have no basis in reality) and/or delusions (persistent, false beliefs).* Although some may report that they know such experiences are distortions, most people who hallucinate or who have delusions are unaware that they are misperceiving or distorting reality.
5. *Distorted perceptions, problems in spatial orientation, impairment in thinking and judgment (cognition), and speech and language difficulties.*
6. *Conversion symptoms (physical dysfunctions for which there appears to be no organic—i.e., physical—cause),* such as some types of fainting spells, sudden loss of voice, or paralysis of limbs.
7. *Impaired or lowered performance in one or more areas of day-to-day functioning, with little or no organic explanation.* Examples are reduced ability to work, loss of interest in sex or food, or diminished capacity to enjoy things.
8. *Psychosomatic or psychophysiological disorders.* These disorders, such as some types of ulcers or chronic diarrhea, are demonstrable physical or bodily dysfunctions with origins that have a large emotional or psychological component.
9. *Loss of ability to care for oneself or to be concerned with one's survival.* Examples include self-mutilation, such as burning or cutting one's flesh, starving one's self to death, or eating the neighbor's garbage.
10. *Abuse of substances such as drugs and alcohol, with extremely disruptive consequences to the person's life and relationships.*
11. *Problems in development.* As the child develops and matures, he or she might show problems in language, motor coordination, thinking processes, perception, or social skills that may reflect psychopathology.
12. *Difficulties in maintaining minimum standards for "acceptable" behavior,* as determined by one's social group. Examples are flagrant and repeated lying, repeated failure to keep promises, not paying debts, failure to adhere to culturally expected behavior, or persistent violation of social standards (such as walking naked in the streets).
13. *Repeated acts that infringe upon the rights of others.* This includes violence toward others or encroachment on their rights for survival—for example, parents who torture or even murder their children.

Some of the foregoing characteristics tend to go together, forming "clusters"; this clustering is called a syndrome. For example, in certain forms of severe depression, the clinical syndrome is characterized by inability to make decisions, deep despair and hopelessness, frequent preoccupation with body problems, impaired and lowered performance in many areas of day-to-day functioning, and, on occasion, disturbing and distressing thoughts.

Students reading clinical descriptions for the first time often have a tendency to recognize a friend, relative, or themselves as fitting the clinical category or diagnosis under consideration. Although making these analogies is a temptation difficult to resist, there is no valid basis for doing so. The preceding clinical descriptions and those that follow in the pages ahead are presented for descriptive and illustrative purposes only and not for use in clinical diagnosis, a complex procedure that requires years of professional training and experience.

THE CAUSAL ARRAY

Is it valid to assume that a single cause underlies psychopathology and shapes its progress? In recent years, the "single cause" approach has been abandoned by many behavioral scientists, who now believe that disturbed behaviors may arise from a multiplicity of causes. For example, one hyperactive (characterized by excessive motor activity) 10-year-old boy was depressed and moody, was doing poorly at school, and was occasionally violent toward his younger brother. These reactions were shown to be very much related to a recent divorce of the parents and to a new school situation. In addition, however, a history of childhood seizures (convulsions; see Chapter 13), poor coordination, and oxygen-deprivation at birth suggested that organic factors may also have underlain some of the behavioral pathology.

The following paragraphs briefly discuss some of the causal clusters to which we will be alluding in the chapters ahead. These clusters are not presented in any order of importance. Furthermore, it is their interactions, rather than any single thrust, that probably represent the most realistic model for understanding pathology, a position underscored by Zubin (1972), whose six general clusters—ecological (that is, relationship of individuals to their environment) developmental, learning and conditioning, hereditary, internal environment, and neurophysiologic—are implicit in this longer list.

Sociocultural factors. Characteristics of an individual's social and cultural environment, such as poverty, poor education, migration, unemployment, and powerlessness may be influential in the development or "shaping" of some emotional problems and clinical syndromes—for example, some types of mental retardation.

Learning and conditioning. Many psychologists believe that most emotional disorders are learned or acquired in response to certain conditions in the environment in much the same way that normal behaviors, such as table manners, are learned. For example, some studies have shown that an individual may learn to feel helpless if he or she is repeatedly exposed to situations in which there is no way out, or may develop irrational fears as a consequence of specific life experiences. Peer interaction, early training to behave like others in one's social group (socialization), and models in the child's surroundings, such as parents, teachers, and television heros and heroines, are all influential factors in this learning process.

Family interactions. Relationships among family members and specific parental attitudes and behaviors have long been recognized as important influences in the development of abnormal behavior. Harsh and abusive child-rearing practices, deep-seated conflicts between parents, parental overprotectiveness or negligence, and unwritten family codes and standards are recognized as powerful causative ingredients in disturbed behavior.

Genetic factors. There may be some genetic (inherited) predisposition for certain types of pathology. For example, research indicates that genetic or inherited factors may contribute to the etiology of schizophrenia and some disorders of mood (see Chapters 10–12).

Developmental factors. Several important factors may profoundly influence the maturing process of the developing child in such areas as motor coordination, speech and language skills, and learning ability. These include circumstances during the mother's pregnancy and before, during, and immediately after childbirth, as well as in the early childhood years—for example, deficiencies in nutrition and acute, infectious diseases. Impaired development in areas crucial to maturation may make a singularly important contribution to later pathology.

Biochemical, metabolic, and physiological factors. Certain biological processes have been shown to be of great significance in the production of emotional and behavioral disturbances. For example, hypoglycemia, a physical condition in which the glucose (sugar) level of the blood drops below a critical point, may lead to listlessness, irritability, and depression. The body's biochemical response to stress or to being chronically angry may also play a significant role in the "wear and tear" on tissues and organs, possibly even to the extent of contributing to psychosomatic dysfunctions such as ulcers. In addition, recent evidence indicates the crucial role played by brain chemicals in inducing or modifying fluctuations of mood, deep depressions, and even irrational and illogical thinking patterns, as in schizophrenia.

Organic diseases and infectious states. Brain tumors, disorders of the nervous system, such as meningitis, or cerebrovascular problems (for example, reduced blood supply to the brain) may contribute to some types of disturbed behavior, such as impaired judgment, memory loss, and spatial disorientation.

Stress and life events. Some people undergo more intense or stressful life events (for example, airplane crashes, wartime bombings, rape, murder of a parent, or continuous physical abuse) than do others. Not all people who undergo such events, however, later show emotional problems (for example, see Spotlight 12.2). Apparently, there are vast individual differences in ability to withstand the impact of these powerful experiences, as we shall see in the pages ahead. The study of the relationship between stressors (stressful life events) and psychological and psychophysiological disorders (physical disorders that may arise, in part, from emotional causes) and of individual differences in reaction to stressful events is of great current interest among behavioral scientists (see Chapter 8).

Personality. At any point in time, people respond in unique ways to their worlds. They are perceiving, reacting to, and judging events around them in the light of their own special histories, background, and developmental circumstances. Some people are shy, others are aggressive or competitive. They can be moody, controlling, comical, well organized, sluggish, "hyper," or somewhat depressed. Psychologists refer to these distinctive and enduring sets of traits and qualities that are parts of each one of us as temperament, or personality. People have gone to great lengths to construct theories about how our personalities develop. Chapter 6 will have a great deal more to say about theories of personality, especially in connection with the origins of poorly adjusted or "unhealthy" personalities.

One aspect of personality that will be discussed more fully later on concerns adequacy or competence to cope with stressful situations as they arise in day-to-day living, even before the onset of pathology. Evidence points to the importance of the premorbid (preceding the disturbance) personality in determining important aspects of certain disorders, such as the chronicity (persistence over time) of a schizophrenic episode.

The Field Approach

The causal model assumed by this book can be called a field approach. This model assumes that many forces both within and outside of the organism affect the organism at any given time. Thus, to understand the cause of a particular behavior, one must look at the interaction of those forces.

A field approach suggests, for example, that genetic predispositions for a particular pathological condition may require the occurrence of certain environmental events before the possible pathology becomes a certainty. For example, genetic factors may make an individual particularly prone to intense anxiety reactions in stressful situations. This predisposition toward anxiety, however, will not become evident without the occurrence of certain stressful conditions in the environment.

A field approach thus stresses the interaction of various factors in the causation of particular abnormal behaviors. Sometimes, however, we can trace the most probable origin of some type of pathology to one particular factor. This is particularly true for diseases and states traceable to organic and physiological conditions, such as brain tumors, oxygen deprivation, or certain kinds of drug states. It does not necessarily follow, however, that because we can sometimes trace the most probable origin of some abnormal state, we therefore know how to change or modify it. On the other hand, we can sometimes modify abnormal behavior even when we do not know its source or origin.

The causal array, in sum, may be said to include: the culture, subculture, and family in which one lives; the specific nature of the learning that has taken place; the individual's genetic predispositions, capacities, and limitations; the developmental events that have occurred; neurophysiological and biochemical events and processes; the current physiological state of the organism, including nutritional factors and health; how the individual has been taught to view the surrounding world of things, people, and events; the stressful life events the person has experienced; and his or her self-perceptions, goals, strivings, aspirations, and personality. It is most likely that the influences of such variables co-exist at any point in time, even though sometimes the discussions that follow will suggest that one or another of them might be especially important in attempts to understand and control a particular pathological state.

ABNORMAL PSYCHOLOGY THROUGH THE AGES

The Pre-Christian Era

Demonological period. Primitive people thought that aberrant behavior, such as inexplicable aggression and violence, convulsive attacks, and delirious or hallucinatory episodes, was caused by evil spirits, demons, or other powers emanating from the gods or certain people; even the *wishes* of ordinary people could accomplish the malevolent work of the bad spirits. The Bible makes several references to this explanation for madness. The Old Testament, for example, describes King Saul as being influenced by an evil spirit of the Lord.

In many ancient societies, placating, pleasing, punishing, or driving the bad spirits out were all employed in attempts to modify unacceptable behavior. *Trepanation* or *trephination* (drilling a small, circular hole in the skull of a person) was a frequent practice designed to allow the evil spirits to escape from entrapment in the body. It was thought that shamans (medicine men) and priest-doctors, who used artifacts, totems, charms, objects, and "magical" articles such as amulets and talismans, as well as rituals of various kinds, could become possessed by evil spirits themselves while attempting to treat their patients.

Classical period. In ancient Greece, the foremost thinkers and philosophers dwelled at length on how to classify the varieties of unusual behavior they perceived and in conjecturing and speculating about the best methods of treatment. Greek poetry and mythology contains descriptions of epilepsy (a disease characterized by convulsions and seizures), depression, and episodes of "frenzy." Although gods and goddesses were felt to be responsible for insanity, there was concern with control, treatment, and cure by humans. The methods covered a wide range, including chains for violent people, flogging and beating, mystical and religious rites, medicinal herbs and potions, and purging. More humane approaches included recreational activities such as music, sports, walking, gymnastics, being read to, and simple custodial care.

Hippocrates (460–355 B. C.) was among the first to suggest specific, rational causes for madness. He believed that the brain was the seat of the mind and that brain pathology was the reason for various disorders. He suggested, for example, that epilepsy was not a "sacred" disease, but, like other diseases, had clearly defined characteristics and causes. Hippocrates classified mental disorders into mania (uncontrollable excitement), melancholia (severe depression), and dementia (general decline in or loss of intellectual abilities). He described in great detail certain states, such as brain infections, epilepsy, and postpartum (following childbirth) psychosis. He ruled out the gods as causes of human ailments, and he advocated special legal consideration for the insane in the courts.

People were aware of the connection between the senses and the brain several centuries before Christ. Yet dualism—a philosophic view that there were two separate and distinct entities in the universe and in people, the spiritual-mental and the physical-material—still held sway. In this model, the mind and mental activities were generally associated with rational activity and the pure and the good. The body, on the other hand, was associated with irrational activity and pleasure, which was regarded as evil and base. Even Plato (427–347 B.C.), in his description of the soul, distinguished rational from libidinous elements (instinctual drives that are pleasure seeking and sexually oriented).

The Dark and Middle Ages—The Psyche as a Battleground for Good Versus Evil

Although in ancient Roman times after the birth of Christ, men like Galen (130–200 A.D.) developed many insights about symptoms (a behavioral sign that suggests pathology), brain functions, and sensory systems (having to do with the senses), many of these advances, as well as the humane methods for treating people, were repressed in the Dark and Middle Ages (from roughly the middle of the fifth century to 1350 A.D. These times were characterized by demonology and an ideology about life, people, good, and evil that contained one major polarized conflict: God versus the devil. Deviant or unusual behavior was viewed as "bad"—an action against God; it was associated with the devil and with the evil spirits and forces emanating from him. Good, during these times, was associated with the soul, the church, and Christianity.

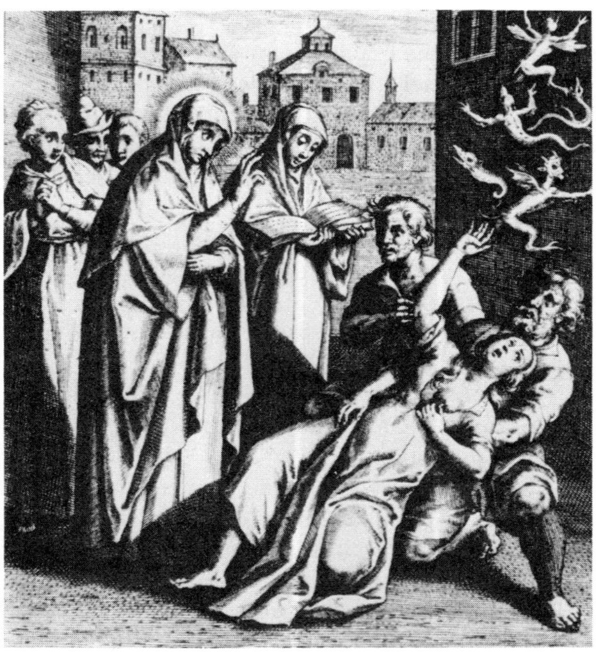

For many centuries, madness was thought to be produced by evil spirits, demons, or the devil, with exorcism the major method of treatment. (The Bettman Archive, Inc.)

Rigid religious dogma, and an unyielding, binding fear of the devil held sway. The terrifying possibility that one could be invaded by the devil or be placed in his powers was an overwhelming factor in shaping human behavior. Many historians believe that there was never more madness and illness than during these centuries. The pervasive mood was one of great individual guilt. But group guilt was also common, judging by the mass terror or mass frenzy of large groups of people in monasteries, nunneries, or schools. In such group "madness," visions and delusions were simultaneously shared by large numbers of people. These "psychic epidemics" were prevalent throughout the Middle Ages, reaching their peak in frequency in the fifteenth and sixteenth centuries. Today, although we may find occasional evidences of "group hysteria," its occurrence is so unusual as to be newsworthy.

Treatment of the mentally ill assumed that a battleground existed within the disordered individual for a vicious struggle between God and the devil. When God won, the soul took over and was in charge of the body. But if the devil won, the body was in charge. Methods for individual treatment (and occasionally for large groups) were aimed at exorcising the devil. Coaxing or cursing him out, insulting, even embarrassing him, as well as incantations, were tried to begin with; if these methods did not work, more drastic and painful methods of physical torture—anguishing to the "host"—were employed. These included blood-letting, immersion in scalding hot water, or repeated, forced vomiting.

Thus theology, rather than empiricism or even the rudimentary science of the pre-Christian Greeks and Egyptians, was the dominant force of the times. All human behavior and the workings of the universe, stars, planets, organisms, and tissues, were explained as God-given. To question or to explore the laws of nature was heresy and evil. To pursue, teach, and find ways of further confirming such total cosmology was considered true scholarship. The social and intellectual climate, was, thus, one of extreme control and suspicion.

If certain people were thought to make contact or were in league with the devil, any neighbor could point an accusing finger. The possibility of witchcraft was on everyone's mind. The ruthless persecution of "witches" here and abroad reached a frenzy in the fifteenth to seventeenth centuries. Even as late as the end of the eighteenth century, there was a legal witchcraft trial in the United States—with a burning at the stake.

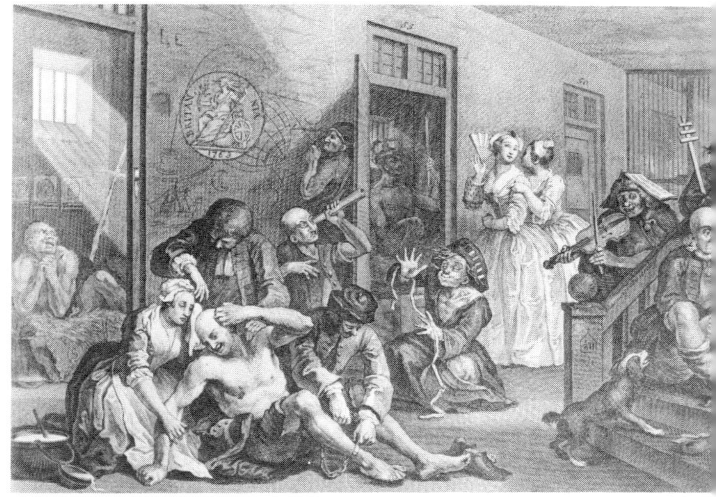

Mental hospitals were (and some still are) large repositories for the insane, who received little attention from the authorities, as shown in this eighteenth-century Hogarth engraving of a scene in the famous London asylum known as Bedlam. (Culver Pictures)

Reform and Humanitarianism

By the beginning of the eighteenth century, the church was struggling with and at times even losing hold of its total cosmological notions. Metaphysics (a branch of philosophy that attempts to explain the origin and structure of the universe) was being attacked by Voltaire and many other French writers and philosophers. The rise of capitalism, the bourgeois revolution, the industrial revolution, and a spirit of scientific interest and inquiry resulted in the questioning of rigid church dogma.

Thus while incarceration or chaining were still being practiced as methods of treating the insane, exorcism was becoming a less frequent practice, and many large institutions and hospitals were adopting more humane attitudes toward the insane. During this period certain crusaders passionately advocated wide reforms, based on a change in cultural attitudes. The mentally ill were now being regarded as poor, unfortunate people whose suffering required compassion, not punishment. At the time of the French Revolution, Pinel (1745–1826) transformed Salpêtrière, the prison for the mentally disturbed, into a hospital in which chains, rags, and the general filth were reduced or eliminated altogether. Esquirol (1772–1840) continued this practice. In other countries, humanitarian reforms were sought by William Tuke in England (1827–1895), Benjamin Rush (1745–1813) and Dorothea Dix (1802–1887) in America, and Chiaruggi (1759–1820) in Italy.

The Modern Era

Several trends developed and flowered in the last two centuries:

1. A physical and organic orientation to the understanding of mental abnormality was once again stressed, initially as an antidote to the demonic point of view. Insanity came to be regarded by many as a disease process; and it was thought that brain pathology could account for all types of mental diseases.

Thus the development and introduction of phrenology by Gall (1758–1828) was in its day a "modern" attempt to link the brain, as the organ of the mind, to separate mental faculties (Boring, 1929). Phrenologists believed that particular sections of the surface of the brain corresponded to different human abilities and functions. They also believed that the relative strength or weaknesses of those sections could be discerned by examining the external shape of the skull covering the relevant part of the brain. By mapping the areas of the brain and their corresponding functions, they attempted to provide a diagnostic guide for the examination of skulls.

2. About the middle of the nineteenth century, Griesinger (1817–1868) wrote a classic textbook on mental disease and brain pathology which greatly influenced Kraepelin, the founder of modern psychiatry. Kraepelin's classic textbook (1883) introduced the celebrated classification scheme (nosology) of psychopathology. In this classificatory system, still in wide use today, groups of symptoms that tend to cluster together as syndromes were thought to form a disease entity or a single disease itself, such as schizophrenia or depression. This classificatory approach has much in common with a medical approach and, as already noted, placed mental illness squarely into the hands of the physician.

Kraepelin was very much influenced by what was happening in the sciences during his century and the preceding one: concern with classification and order, as evidenced in the work of Linnaeus (1707–1778) in botany. Another classifier was Hughlings Jackson (1835–1911) in England, who developed an evolutionary approach to the nervous system, in which complex, higher-order functions of the mind, such as thinking, memory, judgment, speech, and the ability to abstract, were localized in higher levels of the nervous system, while less complex functions, such as involuntary responses, were localized in lower levels. This distinction plays an important role in diagnosing some kinds of mental illness, particularly those caused by organic factors, such as brain tumor.

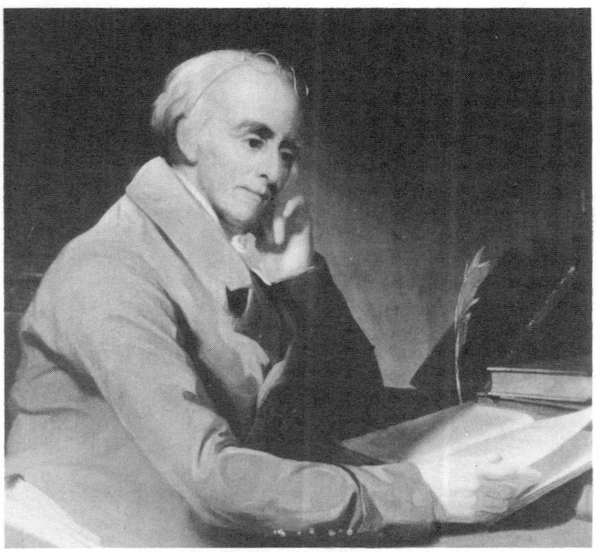

Phillipe Pinel (1745–1826) (below, left), Benjamin Rush (1745–1813), and Dorothea Dix (1802–1887) were reformers who helped to change social and cultural attitudes toward the mentally ill. (The Bettman Archive, Inc.)

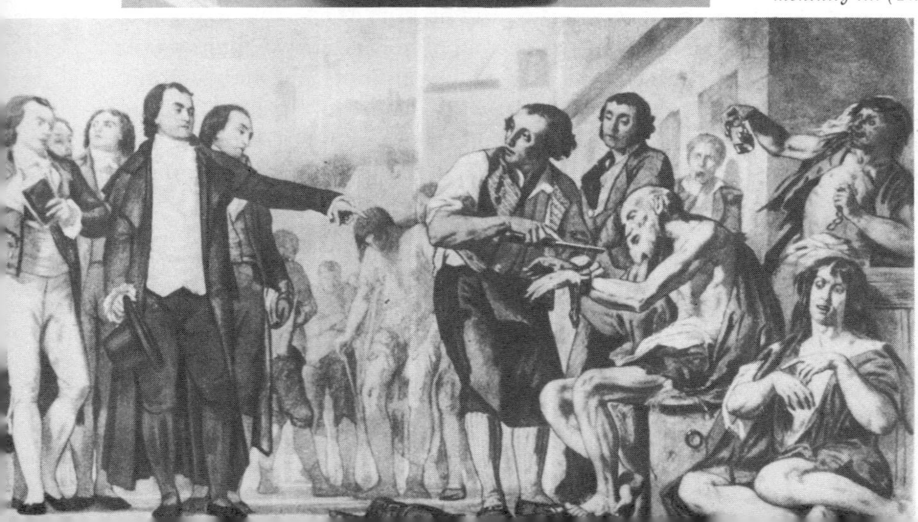

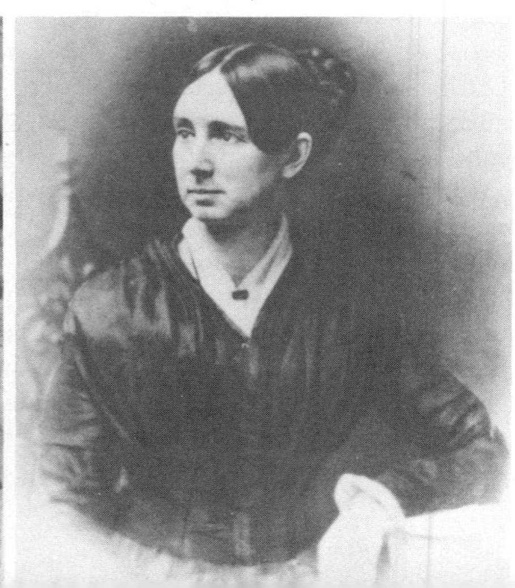

3. In this so-called modern era of thought about abnormal behavior, mental illness was viewed by some people as bearing a relationship to a person's physical type. Such attempts to associate abnormal behavior with body type have a long history; ancients like Hippocrates and Galen were fascinated by the easy simplicities of such a typological system. In this century, Kretschmer (1925), Sheldon and Stevens (1942), and the Gluecks (1956) tried to demonstrate that the physical constitution one inherits—one's body type—is associated with certain kinds of emotional entities, personality types, and psychological syndromes.

Kretschmer, for example, delineated various physiques—pyknic (short and tending toward roundness and heaviness), asthenic (tall and lean), athletic (muscular), and dysplastic (not fitting any category) which he believed were associated with certain types of mental illness. The pyknic type, he thought, will more likely develop a manic-depressive disorder (characterized by marked fluctuations in mood from manic to depressed—now called bipolar affective disorder), while schizophrenia occurs more frequently in people with other body builds.

Such systems of relating constitution to personality and temperament have not endured because of scientific criticism—perhaps because, like phrenology and some of the other strictly physical systems, they ignored the influence of learning, interpersonal behavior, family interactions, culture, and the kinds of factors other people in the field were beginning to stress. However, few will deny that physical variables, even preconceptions about beauty, do affect the development of personality and temperament. People's reactions to each other depend to some extent on their appearances, which, in turn, tend to elicit certain kinds of responses from them. Those of us with certain physical attributes (excessive height or shortness or weight, for example) will, in turn, come to think, perceive, and feel about ourselves in special ways as a reflection of the social learning that takes place as we develop and grow. It is the inevitability of the relationship of constitutional (inherited) type to temperament or to

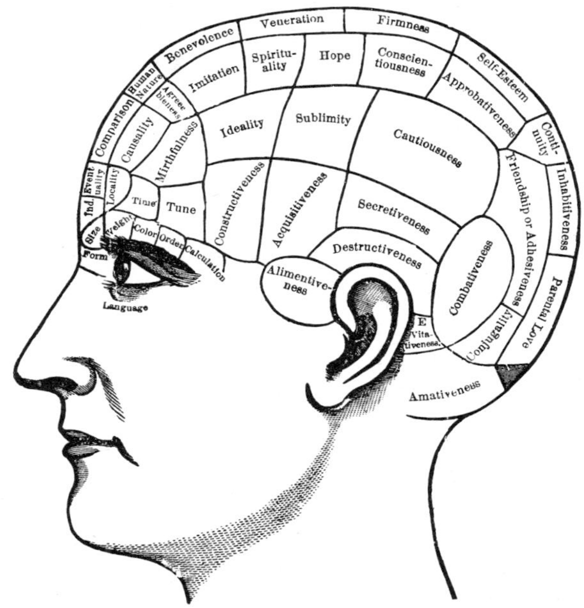

A phrenologist's concept of human abilities and traits, as represented on areas of the skull. (Culver Pictures)

mental illness that is regarded as simplistic and overgeneralized, not the more general view just expressed.

4. Early in the nineteenth century, another historical development was taking place, culminating in the work of Freud at the beginning of the twentieth century, specifically his remarkable contributions to the understanding of the emotions and of unconscious forces (not conscious, not in immediate awareness) in the origin of the neuroses (mild emotional disorders). Many people do not realize that this development had its roots in the complex story of hysteria, (a syndrome that includes symptoms now referred to as conversion disorders), in which the individual loses the use of a body part or sense organ although it is physically intact.

Functional disturbances (those with no known physical origins) such as hysterical blindness, hysterical anesthesia (loss of feeling), hysterical loss of ability to speak (aphonia), hysterical paralysis, and countless other losses of function in which no organic or physical cause for impairment could be found, fascinated many physicians and healers as early as the beginning of the nineteenth century. Especially fascinating were demonstrations that in hysterical blindness, for example, the retina and optic nerve were transmitting messages to the brain, or that in the case of hysterical deafness or paralysis, the relevant body organ or part was actually quite healthy—in excellent working order.

Thus, generations before Freud, people had come to realize that psychological or emotional elements were involved in functional disturbances. These nonphysical elements were thought to be related to suggestion or self-suggestion (the process of influencing a person or oneself to accept an idea or belief without criticism or personal evaluation). But it did not matter what the reasons were, because various "healers" were beginning to have great success in treating and curing functional disorders through a variety of nonmedical methods, generally through some form of suggestion, persuasion, or hypnosis (see Chapter 21, pp. 642–48).

In this history of success with the so-called hysterias, certain people played significant roles: Mesmer (1734–1815), for example, a Viennese working in Paris, cured many of the functional disorders through a version of hypnosis called "mesmerism," attributing his success to "animal magnetism." Braid (1795–1860), an English surgeon, performed mesmerism with his patients, but called it hypnotism. Liebault (1823–1904), a French physician who used hypnotism extensively in his practice, taught his methods to Charcot, a French neurologist (1825–1893). Freud (1856–1939) and Janet (1859–1947) were students of Charcot; they were very impressed with the possibilities that hypnotic methods contained for the cure of nonphysical illnesses.

During the early years of his work with patients, Freud employed adaptations of hypnotic methods. He soon began to develop a complex theory about the origins of mental disturbance, focusing on the structure of the mind, unconscious drives, and early infantile conflicts. He was to devote his entire life to the development of his theories and a complex method for treating emotional problems (see pp. 110–18 and pp. 569–72). His work had far-reaching impact, especially because it was a purely psychological theory, in which psychic energies rather than physical forces were of central importance.

5. At about the same time that Freud was introducing his revolutionary theories, another equally far-reaching approach to the understanding of behavior was germinating. This approach gave rise to the conditioning theories and methods of Pavlov in Russia. As a result of Pavlov's seminal work, many experimental psychologists now believe that fears, maladaptive ways of solving problems, and, as a matter of fact, most of the symptoms of neuroses, such as anxiety, can be explained by principles of learning.

The profound influence of Pavlov's work in Russia on American thinking and research in psychology is seen in the work of Watson in the early twenties, and in the later achievements of other experimental psychologists, such as Clark Hull, B. F. Skinner, and Neal Miller.

If most of our behavior, adaptive or otherwise, is learned, it stands to reason, it was thought, that the same learning principles could be employed to

A photograph, taken in the 1890s, of a group of French physicians watching a colleague hypnotize his patient. (The Bettman Archive, Inc.)

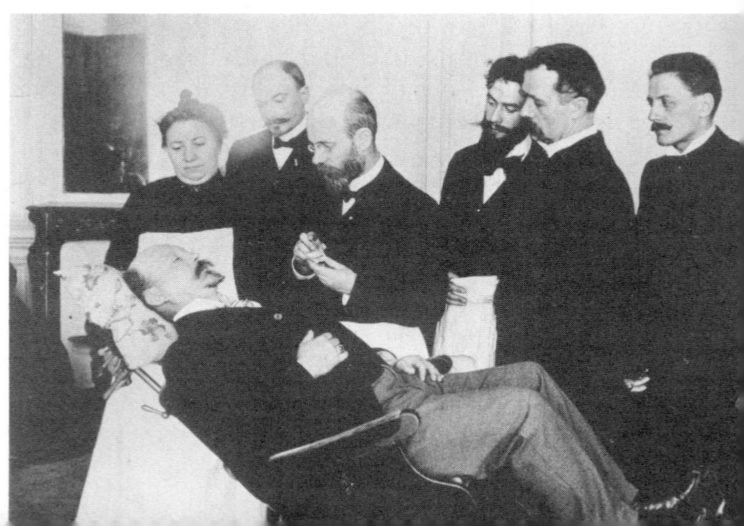

help people "unlearn" or change their habits. This line of thinking had profound significance on the field of abnormal psychology. Chapters 6 and 20 return to these themes.

6. Another approach to understanding abnormal behavior has been gathering strength: a physically oriented, "inside-the-skin" model, which once again attempts to link organic processes to abnormal behavior. Although this approach has held sway throughout the centuries, there is now an entirely new look, made possible by the availability of sophisticated tools, techniques, and experimental methods. These may help researchers understand the relationships between abnormal behavior and neurophysiological processes, brain functions, genetic predispositions, and various physiological and biochemical states in ways unknown to the scientists of yesterday.

This new model has had great influence on treating certain types of disorders as a result of pharmacological interventions (drug therapy; see Chapter 21).

Overview

When we delve into the far reaches of history and examine the available recorded or prerecorded evidence—which includes archaeological and anthropological findings, as well as pre-Christian literature—we learn that people have always scrutinized, categorized, and evaluated the behavior of others. If that behavior seemed deviant—that is, seemed to differ from their own behavior or from their expectations of others' behavior—some special action or, at the very least, attention, seemed appropriate.

At such times designations of madness or insanity were frequently made. Through the ages the numerous and diverse attempts to deal with such deviance anticipated many methods currently in use, such as drugs and herbs. Although there have been universal attempts to control or at best to modify deviant behavior, uniformity as to what is regarded as aberrant is not generally found. As we have already suggested, no one set pattern of behavior then or now has consistently been regarded as constituting insanity.

Further, history teaches us that the particular ways in which so-called abnormal people have been perceived and treated were very much reflections of the social and religious views of the times. For example, we learn that in some societies, if the behavior and speech of a "peculiar" person seemed to have "favorable" political or religious coloration or significance, rather than receiving the usual flogging and punishment, that individual was held in high esteem (Menninger, 1944). Even the intellectual giants were products of their times. For example, although they disagreed about many issues, the eminent philosophers Socrates, Plato, and Aristotle shared a commonly accepted view about human behavior: since the human psyche (mind-soul) had something divine about it, any deviation from the expected and the acceptable had to be treated through some sort of appeal to the divine. In dealing with deviant behavior, the stress on gods, demons, temples, prayers, and incantations during the classical Greek period was thus both logical and understandable in its time.

The next chapter examines these and related cultural considerations in greater detail.

SUMMARY

This chapter described various problems in connection with defining abnormal behavior. It listed numerous popular labels for "madness" but found them not helpful in defining the properties of abnormal behavior. In addition, it pointed out that these labels are harsh, judgmental, and injurious to the people thus designated. The chapter then reviewed different approaches to defining abnormal behavior including the statistical, "ideal state," and medical or disease models. We found each approach to have serious drawbacks. Chapter 1 also presented a loose framework for defining abnormal behavior. This consisted primarily of several major objective and subjective qualities, feelings, and behaviors that seemed to best characterize people regarded as mentally disturbed. Just as there is no single definition of abnormality, there is no single cause of it. This book uses a multicausal, "field" approach, which acknowledges many internal and external factors that could produce abnormal behavior. Finally, the chapter presented views about "madness" as perceived through the ages, including the perspectives and approaches that dominate the field today.

Highlights

1. There are many more labels for abnormal than normal behavior, and most of the former have a derogatory, judgmental quality, possibly because of the fear aroused in many people in the face of nonconformity.
2. "Labeling theory" considers some of the consequences of designating individuals as mentally ill.
3. The statistical, "ideal state," and medical models are the three main theoretical frameworks for describing abnormal behavior. These models are not entirely satisfactory, because they each make several unwarranted assumptions.
4. Subjective descriptions of emotional distress are frequently helpful in attempts to understand abnormal behavior.
5. A multifaceted model of abnormal behavior includes such factors as being unable to make decisions, the presence of hallucinations, impairment in thinking and judgment, conversion symptoms, and loss of abilty to care for oneself, among several other criteria.
6. The question of what causes abnormal behavior is probably best answered by a "field" approach, which views disordered behavior as arising from many variables, probably in interaction with one another. These include: sociocultural variables; learning and conditioning; family interactions; genetic, developmental, biochemical, metabolic, and physiological factors; organic diseases and infectious states; stress and life events; and personality variables.
7. Attitudes toward and treatment of madness today are generally dominated by Freudian, Pavlovian (learning and conditioning), and "inside the skin" models.

ISSUES AND QUESTIONS

1. Can you think of ways in which your personal values and beliefs enter into your judgments about what is normal and what is abnormal? Do you tend to avoid or distrust others if their behavior differs unpredictably from yours?
2. Can you think of instances in which you had to explain somebody's behavior to yourself? Was it important to you to "understand" this behavior? When you found you could not "understand" the other's responses, were you bewildered? frightened? angry? Did you feel the need to control the other person?
3. How do you feel about nonconformity *within* your immediate circle of friends? How do you feel about nonconformity *outside* your circle of friends? Do you have two sets of standards?
4. Spotlight 1.1 presented a list of words alluding to abnormal behavior. Can you add to this list? Can you find neutral words to use instead? Can you find positive or favorable words?
5. Do you think there is a difference between assigning a name to somebody's behavior or symptom and calling him or her a name? Example from medicine: Is there a difference in attitude toward the labeled person when one says, "Her skin shows signs of leprosy," in contrast to, "She is a leper."? When someone is called a schizophrenic, even though he or she no longer shows symptoms—that is, is asymptomatic—does it imply that once a schizophrenic, always a schizophrenic?
6. Chapter 4 will contain more material on Dr. Thomas Szasz and his controversial views. This chapter described his position on mental illness (there is no such thing) and on labeling people

as mentally ill (metaphor and myth). Dr. Szasz tends to place responsibility for human conduct directly on the shoulders of the person responding or behaving (whether illegally, in a nonconformist way, or even in an incomprehensible way). This is a view of human conduct that represents a personal system of ethics. Do you share this view?

SUGGESTIONS FOR FURTHER READING

Beers, C. W. *A mind that found itself: An autobiography.* Garden City, N. J.: Doubleday, Doran, 1933. Also in paperback. This book, originally published in 1907, was instrumental in awakening early twentieth-century American society to the need for preventing and treating mental illness. The first part of the book is Beers's vivid account of his thoughts, feelings, and anguish during an eight-year period of mental illness and of the abusive treatment he received while incarcerated in sanatoriums. Beers and his autobiography became the inspiration for the development of the sweeping mental hygiene movement in America.

Deutsch, A. *The mentally ill in America: A history of their care and treatment from colonial times.* New York: Columbia University Press, 1949. This book surveys the history of the mental health movement in the United States, from the demons and witches of colonial times to the mental health movement that began after World War II. Here we find a history of the laws of commitment and of changing attitudes toward deviant behavior. We see also the trend toward state care (discernible in the years following the Civil War, with Massachusetts leading the way in 1863).

Green, H. *I never promised you a rose garden.* New York: Signet, 1964. Paperback. Although this book is fiction, it vividly portrays, within the context of a compelling story, the hallucinations and delusions of a 16-year-old, schizophrenic girl. As a subjective account of mental illness, it poignantly brings home to the reader the suffering of a person experiencing severe emotional and cognitive disturbance.

Jahoda, M. *Current concepts of positive mental health.* New York: Basic Books, 1958. This slim, well-written book is now a classic. It surveys the literature and then categorizes and evaluates various conceptualizations as to what mental health is. In so doing, it communicates the difficulties and differences of opinion in, and implications of, the various attempts to define this elusive concept.

Offer, D., and Sabshin, M. *Normality: Theoretical and clinical concepts of mental health. Rev. ed.* New York: Basic Books, 1974. This book was written for the purpose of clarifying the assumptions made by researchers, theorists, and clinicians regarding normality and abnormality. It explains various definitions of normality and synthesizes these definitions into four perspectives. In a lengthy appendix, the authors compiled detailed definitions and opinions from selected writings of various persons mentioned in their book. This is an excellent reference book on normality.

Scheff, T. J. (Ed.) *Labeling madness.* Englewood Cliffs, N. J.: Prentice-Hall, 1975. Scheff's presentation of issues concerning labeling and mental illness—labeling theory—is clear, readable, and thought-provoking. This book contains Scheff's own views as well as reports by other authors on labeling theory.

Szasz, T. S. *The myth of mental illness: Foundations of a theory of personal conduct.* New York: Hoeber-Harper, 1961. Also in paperback, rev. ed, 1974. This significant, controversial book presents Szasz's early, dramatic statements concerning his views that mental illness is a myth, a fiction—that it is not at all similar to physical disease. In this book Szasz depicts the conduct of individuals as the consequence of the struggle to deal with the rules imposed upon them by society. Whether or not a person follows these rules or deviates from them is the personal responsibility of the individual and does not reflect the presence or absence of illness or disease, according to Szasz. Clinicians therefore cannot diagnose or treat individuals for illnesses they do not have; they can only deal with their social behavior, values, and ethics.

Zilboorg, C., and Henry, G. W. *A history of medical psychology.* New York: Norton, 1941. This is a well-documented, scholarly, yet highly readable history of mental disorders and their treatment, and the accompanying cultural, religious, and philosophical attitudes from the ancients to the recent past (pre-World War II). This volume has become a standard reference work.

2

Epidemiology, Culture, and Psychopathology

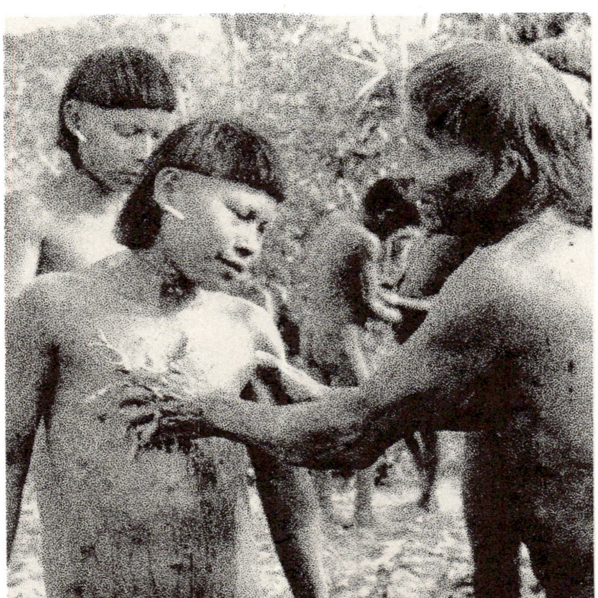

The Extent of Mental Illness

Mental illness is the most frequent type of illness in this country. It is estimated that one in every ten Americans will be mentally ill or mentally incapacitated at least once in his or her life. According to a 1977 report by the President's Commission on Mental Health, between 20 and 32 million Americans require mental health care at any point in time, over 50 million Americans have experienced severe emotional stress, and over 30 million Americans have actually received some sort of treatment for mental problems in 1976 (Lyons, 1977). These figures suggest that over 15 percent of Americans have some kind of mental disorder, a percentage that researchers think holds for the rest of North America and Europe, as well. Mental illness is obviously a major health problem.

These figures outline only a segment of the picture. Many people may be mentally ill but do not come to the attention of the authorities or researchers and therefore go unreported—for example, the many accidents and suicides associated with alcoholism or the severe depressions hidden at home.

The despair of divorce, the anguish of senility, and the loneliness of enforced retirement are data not usually tabulated, nor are the minor, everyday emotional problems that do not qualify as mental illness: anxiety before an examination, the frustration and humiliation of a personal rejection or a sexual failure, and the ways we deal with and defend against the feelings these painful experiences engender. Further, mental anguish is also experienced by those who live with or who in some way are close to people who commit murder or suicide or who waste their lives in a miasma of drugs. Mental illness and emotional disorders are more widespread than many of us care to admit, and the nature of these disorders is extremely varied. Chapter 2 and many other portions of the book attempt to describe and explore the staggering scope of this problem.

THE EPIDEMIOLOGY OF MENTAL ILLNESS

One method of examining the scope or prevalence of an illness in different societies or among different segments of the same society is through the gathering and analysis of epidemiological data. Epidemiology is the study of the types of diseases and the frequency of their occurrence in large groups of people. Data yielded by epidemiological studies are indispensable for public planning of the location and type of health-care facilities. Epidemiological data can also often shed light on the possible causes and treatment of a disease process, or at least point to promising areas for further investigation. For example, the higher incidence of lung disease among coal miners than in the rest of the population is an indication that something peculiar to the life and environment of the coal miner (such as the coal dust itself) may have caused, or contributed to, this disease.

In abnormal psychology, epidemiology is the study of the incidence and distribution of abnormal psychological states in defined populations. For example, one might tabulate the numbers of people at different age levels who are patients in mental institutions, then further categorize these data in order to compare persons living in or near urban areas with those living in rural areas. Or one might tabulate the age of first admissions (people admitted for the first time) to state mental institutions and categorize them according to the psychological disorders, such as schizophrenia or manic-depressive psychosis, for which they were admitted.

Epidemiological data can also be used to evaluate the mental health care needs of various groups of people and, in some cases, to increase knowledge of the factors that might be causing or aggravating a particular pathology. For example, Table 2.1, an epidemiological chart comparing the numbers of people from different demographic groups admitted to mental hospitals with their numbers in the population as a whole, shows that in Chicago, the proportion of nonmarried people (single, separated, widowed, and divorced) who were admitted to mental hospitals (61.7 percent) is larger than the proportion of nonmarried persons in the Chicago population as a whole (40.2 percent). These data, it might be concluded, suggest that there is a correlation between being nonmarried and mental illness.

However, correlations (variables or trends related to or associated with each other) do not necessarily indicate causal connections. From the data in Table 2.1, we cannot, with assurance, conclude that marital status (single, separated, divorced or widowed) *causes* mental illness. Nevertheless, awareness of the correlation between marital status and admission to mental hospitals is useful because it may lead to increased understanding of possible causes of mental illness.

Complexities in Interpreting Epidemiological Data

Subjectivity. When studying epidemiological data, one must proceed carefully. The interpretation of such data is often a subjective process in which perception and judgment are based on a personal frame of reference rather than on more objective

Table 2.1 Comparison of Chicagoans Admitted to Mental Hospitals to the Chicago Population as a Whole (July 1, 1960, to June 30, 1961)

	Patient Population		City of Chicago Population	
Demographic Variable	*Number*	*Percentage*	*Number*	*Percentage*
Sex				
Total	10,653	100.0	3,550,404	100.0
Males	5,495	51.6	1,726,986	48.6
Females	5,158	48.4	1,823,418	51.4
Race				
Total	10,653	100.0	3,550,404	100.0
White	8,698	81.6	2,712,748	76.4
Nonwhite	1,955	18.4	837,656	23.6
Age				
Total	10,653	100.0	3,550,404	100.0
Under 25	879	8.2	1,412,277	39.7
25–44	4,187	39.3	956,920	27.0
45–64	3,994	37.5	834,632	23.5
65 and over	1,593	15.0	346,575	9.8
Marital Status				
Total	10,653	100.0	2,630,047[a]	100.0
Single	2,957	27.8	630,051	24.0
Married	3,945	37.1	1,572,559	59.8
Separated	1,196	11.2	86,521	3.3
Widowed	1,354	12.7	251,164	9.5
Divorced	1,068	10.0	89,752	3.4
Unknown	133	1.2	—	—
Nativity				
Total	10,653	100.0	3,550,404	100.0
Foreign born	817	7.7	438,392	12.3
US born	5,691	53.4	3,112,012	87.7
Unknown	4,145	38.9	—	—

Source: From L. Levy and L. Rowitz, *The ecology of mental disorder* (New York: Human Sciences Press, 1973), p. 27. [a]Population 14 years of age and over.

criteria. Spotlight 2.1 illustrates how easy it is to draw biased, subjective conclusions from epidemiological charts.

Genetic versus sociocultural explanations. In drawing conclusions from epidemiological data, some interpretations as to causes may seem obvious. Closer examination reveals that other interpretations of the same data may be equally plausible.

For example, one classic epidemiological survey studied the incidence of various kinds of mental disorders among the Hutterites, an English-speaking North American religious sect with German origins (Eaton and Weil, 1955). This information about the Hutterites was compared to data for other societies in a procedure known as a crosscultural survey. Compared to the other cultures studied, the Hutterites had the highest proportion of manic-

Spotlight 2.1 Over A Century Ago: Biased Interpretations?

The following Table from the U.S. Census of 1840, and a letter from an anonymous reader to the *New York Observer* both appeared in the August 1851 issue of *The American Journal of Insanity:*

Statistical Table From The U.S. Census of 1840

States	*Total White Population*	*Insane and Idiots*	*Proportion*	*Total Color'd Population*	*Insane and Idiots*	*Proportion*
Maine	500,438	537	1 in 950	1,355	94	1 in 14
New Hampshire	284,036	486	1 in 584	538	19	1 in 28
Massachusetts	729,030	1,071	1 in 662	8,669	200	1 in 43
Vermont	291,213	398	1 in 731	730	13	1 in 56
Connecticut	301,856	498	1 in 606	8,159	44	1 in 185
Rhode Island	105,587	203	1 in 520	3,243	13	1 in 249
New York	2,378,890	2,110	1 in 1,108	50,031	194	1 in 257
New Jersey	351,588	369	1 in 952	21,718	73	1 in 293
Pennsylvania	1,676,115	1,946	1 in 861	37,952	187	1 in 256
Delaware	58,561	52	1 in 1,126	19,524	28	1 in 697
Maryland	317,717	387	1 in 821	151,515	141	1 in 1,074
Virginia	740,968	1,052	1 in 704	498,829	381	1 in 1,309
North Carolina	484,370	580	1 in 835	268,549	221	1 in 1,215
South Carolina	259,084	376	1 in 689	335,314	137	1 in 2,440
Georgia	407,695	294	1 in 1,387	283,697	134	1 in 2,117
Ohio	1,502,022	1,195	1 in 1,257	17,345	165	1 in 105
Kentucky	590,253	795	1 in 742	189,575	180	1 in 1,053
Louisiana	158,457	55	1 in 2,873	193,954	45	1 in 4,310

It is obvious . . . from the . . . schedule, that there is an awful prevalence of idiocy and insanity among the free blacks over the whites, and especially over the slaves. Who would believe, without the fact, in black and white, before his eyes, that every fourteenth colored person in the State of Maine is an idiot or lunatic? *And though there is a gradual improvement in their condition, as we proceed west and south yet it is evident that the free States are the principal abodes of idiocy and lunacy among the colored race. (As quoted in Szasz, 1973b, pp. 44–45)*

The anonymous interpreter, obviously pro-slavery, stated that freed blacks in the Northern states were more subject to lunacy and idiocy than the slaves in the South. He or she felt that the table provided irrefutable evidence for the superiority of slavery over freedom. Drawing this conclusion from this material shows how statistics can be misleading. First, there is the critical question of what constitutes lunacy and idiocy. Definitions differ from place to place. Other basic questions include: Who provided the state figures? Did slaves die earlier than freedmen? Were slaves part of an untreated population that never came to the attention of public facilities and census-takers? That is, in the Northern states, runaway slaves might have become public charges, whereas their peers in the slave population did not. Would the social dislocation experienced by runaway slaves enter into these figures?

depressive patients. The explanation could easily be a genetic one (that is, that manic-depressive disease is inherited) in the light of the social isolation and generations of intermarriage among the Hutterites.

However, a *cultural* explanation might also be used for these findings. The Hutterites are characterized by intense communal cohesiveness and a strict adherence to religious ritual stressing duty to God and society. The guilt, self-punitive attitudes, and fear and tension associated with this upbringing might be regarded as compatible with depression. But, of course, this would apply only to the depressive aspects of the manic-depressive syndrome.

An epidemiological finding from another study revealed the extremely high proportion of cases of schizophrenia in certain areas of northern Sweden (Eaton and Weil, 1955). This finding could be attributed to genetic factors, for reasons similar to those relevant to the Hutterite case. On the other hand, the high proportion of schizophrenia in the Swedish communities studied can also be explained by social and cultural factors: these communities had a preponderance of single males and geographically isolated farmers and were found to have a low degree of social cohesiveness. Such social seclusiveness might thus be compatible with schizophrenia and actually might be conducive to the development of schizophrenia in people who have difficulty coping with their daily lives.

The chicken or the egg? Here is another example of the difficulties encountered in drawing conclusions about the causes of mental illness from epidemiological studies. In one large-scale population study, the characteristics of all but 1 percent of 2,550 inhabitants of a small rural area in southern Sweden were studied (Essen-Möller, 1961). Ten years later, in a followup study, they were reexamined. One finding of this study was that among the unmarried of the original population, an extremely large proportion (compared to the married people from the original population) suffered from psychosis, feeblemindedness, and major personality deviations. How can these data be interpreted? Does single status produce subsequent problems? Or does having problems make it less likely that people will marry?

The researchers also found that more of the alcoholics, "asocials," and abnormal personalities moved away from the area than did the other groups in the study population. Does the community exert pressure for its deviants to leave? Does abnormality induce a desire to leave? Or does residential stability cause peace of mind? Simply looking at the facts will not provide answers to these questions. Knowing that a greater incidence of mental illness occurs among unmarried persons in a society, or that the social deviants tend to leave their society more frequently than nondeviants, does not explain why those facts are as they are. We can only infer possible explanations and then look for additional evidence in support of our inferences.

Culture and epidemiology. Sometimes interpreting epidemiological data requires a good deal of knowledge about the culture of the people studied—their style of life, knowledge, beliefs, values, and kinship patterns. For example, we generally find that the lower the social class, the greater the number of first admissions to mental hospitals. However, the rate of increase with declining social class varies among different ethnic groups (for the results of studies of French-Canadian, Polish, British, and German populations, see Murphy, 1965). In addition, as people get older, admission rates tend to increase. But here again, striking differences occur among ethnic groups. Murphy explains these differences in the light of the cultural attitudes and practices of the groups studied. For example, he found a consistent trend among the Chinese of Singapore: although, as expected, the rate of admissions *increased* with declining social class, it *decreased*, regardless of social class, with increasing age. This finding was not duplicated among other ethnic groups in Singapore, such as the Malaysians. The significance of these data is that among the Chinese—even in the lower classes—strong family ties that include respect, tolerance, and concern for the elderly are deeply embedded in cultural tradition. The Chinese aged, regardless of class, have always had a place in the homes of their families, with a resulting decrease, rather than increase, of first-admission rates.

Culture and diagnostic labeling. A pervasive difficulty in crosscultural surveys of mental illness is that the same classifications and labels may be used in reference to different sets of behaviors. Unless the criteria employed for a specific diagnosis, such as schizophrenia, are the same in different cultures, then we may be comparing apples with oranges rather than with apples. Different cultures tend to "prefer" different diagnostic labels; that is, given an individual with a particular set of symptoms, one culture will label it in one way and another culture in another way. This is regarded as a deep, underlying difficulty in comparing epidemiological mental-illness data across cultures (Dohrenwend and Dohrenwend, 1969, 1973; Zubin, 1969).

Diagnoses and designations of mental illness used in crosscultural epidemiological studies are sometimes arrived at through interviews and questionnaires. Words and language can be interpreted in different ways by members of different social and cultural groups (Leff, 1973). Therefore, interviewer's judgments about the respondent may be biased unless he or she is familiar with the interviewee's social and cultural background (Al-Issa, 1977).

One way to handle this issue may be to investigate thoroughly the cultural context of a specific society or subgroup of that society, and then define psychopathology in terms of whether or not a set of behaviors is predictable within the culture and under what circumstances (Hammer and Zubin, 1968). For example, an Eskimo who crawls on the floor and barks like a dog is respected as a shaman if that behavior occurs within the context of a séance. However, the same behavior exhibited in ordinary, everyday circumstances without apparent control of onset is evidence of insanity within the same Eskimo culture (Murphy, 1976).

Another possible solution to the problem of diagnostic inconsistency across cultures and societies is being met by the development of straightforward, objective procedures such as questionnaires and controlled interviews that could be used appropriately in many types of diverse societies (Hare and Wing, 1970; and Spitzer and Endicott, 1973).

Who appears in epidemiological charts? An additional problem in interpreting epidemiological data is that many people with emotional problems do not appear in statistical tables. Some mentally ill people are in private treatment. Others seek help in ways that mainstream researchers usually do not acknowledge in their formal data-collecting methods. These may include assistance from gypsies, faith healers, astrologists, palmists, and so forth.

Moreover, large numbers of individuals who may be in need of treatment do not seek it. People in treatment, contrasted with people not in treatment, may differ in important ways that may not necessarily reflect the presence, or the severity, of the disorder. For example, whether or not an individual seeks treatment, receives treatment, or even *knows* about treatment is often related to educational level, social class, and income. Using data based on individuals undergoing some kind of treatment or in some kind of treatment facility is therefore misleading. Thus "true" prevalence rates of emotional disorders are extremely difficult to ascertain (Dohrenwend and Dohrenwend, 1973; Zubin, 1969). It may be that depression, schizophrenia, and other disorders are more prevalent than our data suggest.

Another problem in epidemiological data collection concerns the criteria chosen to indicate pathology. These criteria cover a broad range and include hospital first admissions, length or duration of hospitalization, and speed of recovery. Obviously some consensus is required before groups, cultures, or even different periods of time can be compared regarding incidence of mental illness.

Despite the foregoing drawbacks, epidemiologists can sometimes draw extremely useful inferences from their data. In certain instances, a continuing series of researches can systematically explore hypotheses (tentative explanations for certain data) in ways that produce socially and scientifically significant results. Spotlight 2.2 presents such a series of researches. In these investigations, the socioeconomic characteristics of the individuals studied played an important role. By general convention, studies that explore the relationship of an individual's class or economic status employ a rating or classification that identifies that individual along income, educational, or social-class levels. This SES rating (socioeconomic status) is an index of the social class and economic level of an individual or group of individuals. The SES index is generally derived from such information as employment or occupational level of the household head, family income, educational level of household head, geographical location of dwelling, and self-reports of social position or class identification. The lower the income, education, or class, the lower the status of the person being studied.

Spotlight 2.2 A Continuum of Reproductive Casualty

Pasamanick (1961), an eminent epidemiologist, and his colleagues explored the relationship between various prenatal factors and later neuropsychiatric disorders (behavioral abnormalities related to organic disturbance of the nervous system, primarily the brain). They developed various hypotheses as they went along, exploring these again and again in as many ways as possible.

In these studies, which began in New Haven, continued in Baltimore, and were further extended to New York City, it was first noted that prematurity and various complications of pregnancy increase at a dramatic rate as one descends the SES scale. As a result of detailed data examination, Pasamanick hypothesized and later confirmed:

Inasmuch as prematurity and complications of pregnancy are associated with fetal and neonatal death, usually on the basis of injury to the brain, there must remain a fraction so injured who do not die; depending upon the degree and location of trauma they do go on to develop a series of disorders extending from cerebral palsy, epilepsy, and mental deficiency through all types of behavioral and learning disabilities which are a result of lesser degrees of damage sufficient to disorganize behavioral development and lower thresholds to stress; and further, these abnormalities of pregnancy are associated with certain life experiences, usually socioeconomically determined with the consequence that they themselves and their resulting neuropsychiatric disorders find greater aggregation in the lower strata of our society (pp. 260–261).

Pasamanick concluded that the severity of pregnancy and birth complications varies along a continuum that is partially associated with SES. These complications, in turn, result in damage to the fetus and baby that ranges along a continuum from various degrees of neuropsychiatric disability to death, and is, at least in part, socioeconomically determined. There is much evidence to support the thrust of Pasamanick's conclusions. For example, a study of infant mortality rates in New York City showed that 42.8 of every 1,000 babies born alive in New York's Harlem (a ghetto area in which there is high incidence of poverty) die in infancy, compared to 19.0 per 1,000 babies, citywide (Sterne, 1978).

Pasamanick does indeed indicate the serious possibility that social environment and socioeconomic status are related to life itself and to the kinds of survival possible within that life. As life (and normality) unfold, poverty can make dramatic incursions. Threats—in the form of various degrees of neuropsychiatric involvements, learning disabilities, and related malfunctions—occur on a continuum of seriousness, according to Pasamanick, with death on the one end and relatively minor problems on the other. An important social implication of Pasamanick's work is that slums, poverty, and social deprivation require serious preventive social attention if we are to make any progress in curtailing the incidence of mental illness and related disabilities.

CULTURE AND ABNORMAL PSYCHOLOGY

Most researchers and practitioners in the field of human behavior agree that cultures and subcultures have powerful impacts on individuals in many subtle ways not always within conscious awareness. Dress styles, tastes in food, courtship patterns, goals, and values—all these modes of doing and thinking are learned from the immediate social environment. Thus, too, tastes in sex, even the ways in which individuals rebel, express difficulties and conflicts, fail to solve problems, or attempt to reduce anxiety are culturally determined. Culture provides the manner and the style in which we live and the choices and decisions we make about our goals. Cultures are transmitted from family to family, generation to generation. Although many subcultures exist in a heterogeneous society such as ours, a considerable common culture remains at its core.

Systematic comparisons of cultures throughout the world—crosscultural studies—demonstrate that the incidence and prevalence of mental illness vary from culture to culture. Even the degree and kinds of symptoms found, types of treatments used, and responses to treatment are strikingly diverse (de Reuck and Porter, 1965; Dohrenwend and Dohrenwend, 1973; Opler, 1959). How does this come about?

How Culture Influences the Development of Mental Illness

It is commonly believed that as we grow up, certain tensions, anxieties, conflicts and fears are engendered by cultural pressures. The general nature of some of these pressures, rather than their specific content, can be described, even though the cultural context may differ from society to society (Leighton and Murphy, 1965; Wittkower and Dubreuil, 1968). Thus some or many of the following factors may be powerful shapers of mental illness or psychopathology within any given culture:

1. Certain cultural taboos within some societies may be extreme, relentless, and harsh. For example, during earlier times in our own culture many young women who engaged in sexual relations before marriage experienced intense shame and guilt, and such feelings may have adversely affected their later sexual functioning and sense of self-worth.

2. The belief systems of a particular culture and the group support connected with those beliefs may be of great importance in creating abnormal behavior among some individuals. For example, Australian aborigines believe that if ritually placed bones point in a particular direction, thought to symbolize death, the person to whom they point is to be ignored—treated as if dead. This may arouse enormous fear and aberrant behavior in the ostracized victim, and may even eventually lead to adrenal exhaustion and death (Kiev, 1976).

3. Some cultures produce common personality types as a result of specific childrearing practices. Eventually certain of these types may be poorly prepared to handle stress or to adapt to life crises. For example, children who are authoritatively directed and supervised in their every activity may develop passive, acquiescent personalities that, in adulthood, may hinder their ability to assertively satisfy their own needs and to cope with the stresses of adult responsibilities.

4. The social values of a culture may conflict with the religious tenets within that culture, engendering conflicting drives that can never be resolved. For example, the religious creed (for example, "Love thy neighbor") conflicts with the drive for power and acquisition of wealth—two sets of values that characterize our own culture.

5. The sentiments, beliefs, and values of a culture sometimes produce damaging emotional states. Cultural beliefs in black magic, evil spirits, the devil, and witches, for example, often result in intense fears and anxieties. Similarly, the emphasis our culture places upon achievement is anxiety-producing for many individuals, especially those who do not reach a stated or implied level of competence or have available to them the kinds of opportunities necessary to fulfill their aspirations (Kiev, 1976).

6. In some societies, expectations and roles for its members (worker, mother, wage earner, achiever) are suddenly and irrationally withdrawn or changed. For example, in our own society, the retired and elderly are expected to relinquish some of the interests and activities that had provided structure and meaning to their lives for many years.

7. The style, expression, or even subjective labeling of a particular mental illness or emotional experience may differ from culture to culture (Leff, 1973). For example, although guilt and suicidal ideas and acts are uncommon among African depressed patients, these symptoms are typical of European depressives (King, 1978).

8. Cultural characteristics have been shown to affect the incidence of particular pathological syndromes. For example, the high incidence of schizophrenia in some Oriental countries has been ascribed to cultural practices of meditation and social withdrawal—particular cultural behavior patterns that are thought to foster a loss of reality testing (Wittkower and Rin, 1965). In addition, cultural factors have been employed to explain the wide variation in suicide rates, drug addiction, and alcoholism found in different societies.

9. Certain cultural roles may produce stress, engendering mental illness in the people who are expected to fulfill these roles. Our expectations of sexual prowess and occupational achievement in males, for example, may be extremely frustrating for many males in our society who are unable, for various reasons, to fulfill this "macho" image.

10. Some cultures assign a culturally prestigious function or role to individuals with certain disorders, thus perpetuating their incidence. For example, the outstanding characteristic of a shaman or witch doctor in Eskimo culture is "thinness," a presumed ability to tell the future and to see things that others are unable to see (Murphy, 1976).

11. Cultures may go through dramatic social changes and upheavals too quickly for the adequate adjustment of their members. Industrialization, urbanization, and wartime conditions are often associated with increases in alcoholism, suicide rates, or excessive drug use. Similarly, members of one culture who have emigrated to another culture frequently experience increased emotional disturbance during the long period of assimilation to the new culture. For example, upon their arrival in Israel, poor Arabic and Yemenite Jews were reported to have great difficulty adjusting to mainstream Israeli culture; their subsequent maladjustment was characterized by school dropout, delinquency and crime, and various kinds of social and educational pathology (Cohen, 1964). In similar fashion, when high-altitude Peruvian Indians descended from their mountains to coastal urban areas where they could earn a better living, the impact of the social upheaval they experienced was reflected in a variety of physical symptoms, paranoid symptoms, anxiety, and a striking increase of alcoholism and psychotic states (Fried, 1959).

12. Cultures, to varying degrees, engender specific fertility and breeding patterns that influence the distribution and incidence of certain kinds of disorders, especially those that may have a genetic component. Socially isolated cultures, for example, are more likely to result in frequent intermarriages among limited numbers of families. Thus the high incidence of manic-depressive psychosis among the Hutterites, mentioned earlier in this chapter, might be explained by inherited characteristics shared by members of that society.

13. Cultures may also modify and influence the distribution and incidence of some disorders by factors such as poor hygiene, nutritional deficiencies, childbirth rituals, and other conditions or practices engendered within the culture that may have a powerful influence on producing certain kinds of mental disorders or in increasing the risks for them (see Spotlight 2.2).

The different pressures a culture places on its members will thus affect the amount and type of mental illness within that culture. Spotlight 2.3 lists several findings demonstrating differences in incidence of psychopathology among various cultures. Can the specific conditions or factors in these societies be successfully linked to the epidemiology of mental illness within their boundaries?

Since not all people within a given culture de-

Spotlight 2.3 Behavioral Aberrations Around the World

Behavioral aberrations and disturbances are found in varying degrees throughout the world. Social psychiatrists, anthropologists, and psychologists relate many of these variations to cultural influences. Here are some incidence patterns. Can these patterns be explained by cultural factors?

1. Certain kinds of infectious psychoses (mental disturbances that may follow an infection of the central nervous system), characterized by delirium, hallucinations, and confusion, are frequent in some locales, infrequent in others.
2. High incidences of manic-depressive illness occur in underdeveloped nations.
3. Unusually high suicide rates occur in Japan, Sweden, Denmark, and Switzerland.
4. "Hysterical" symptoms, or conversion disorders (such as blindness, paralysis, or deafness without physical cause), have virtually disappeared in the past several generations in American and European countries, but have become more common in other nations, such as India, Lebanon, Egypt, and Tunisia.
5. Although obsessive-compulsive syndromes (neuroses characterized by repeated unwanted thoughts or an excessively rigid need for order, perfectionism, and neatness) are not uncommon in large cities, they are rarely found in the rural areas of Asia and Africa.
6. Psychosomatic ailments such as ulcers and high blood pressure are commonly thought to be associated with urban living and the tensions and competitions found therein. They also occur frequently among the people of the African bush, however.
7. Presenile and senile psychoses (loss of mental faculties accompanied by mental disturbances such as delusions or ideas of persecution associated with the aging process) are less common in the developing nations than in the developed nations.
8. Sexual deviations are less common—but probably more socially tolerated—in the developing nations than in the more advanced societies of the world. (from Wittkower and Dubreuil, 1968)

velop mental illness, we must still explain why only some people fall prey to the cultural pressures described. In addition, explanations must be sought for the converse phenomenon; that is, why, despite wide cultural differences throughout the world (in childrearing practices for example), do certain diseases such as schizophrenia appear in virtually all cultures?*

* Later chapters will explore how biochemical and related factors play an extremely important role in the development of some types of mental illness. The material in this chapter should not be interpreted as suggesting that sociocultural factors *alone* can account for all forms of pathology.

The Shifting Scene: Fads and Fashions in Symptoms and Treatment

Symptoms. The incidence and prevalence of various symptoms and syndromes (patterns of symptoms that characterize a particular disease) differ not only from culture to culture, but also within a particular culture over time. For example, a shift from "medieval acedia" (apathy) to "Protestant melancholia" (depression) occurred in Western Europe during the fourteenth through seventeenth centuries. Also, in the past one hundred years, a dramatic decrease in the symptoms of mania (excitement, frenzy) occurred in Western culture, while an increase in depressive symptoms has been found in many parts of Africa and Asia. Further, there has been a marked decrease in so-called hysterical (conversion) symptoms in the developed nations since the early 1900s (Murphy, 1973).

More detailed study of why such shifts take place is needed. From preliminary work, however, it seems likely that the extent to which people who display particular symptoms develop further pathology is in part a function of the social context: how their culture views, accepts, or rejects the behavior in question (Murphy, 1973).

Sorting out these social and cultural factors is a very complex task. A closer look at one group of symptoms, hallucinations, illustrates this point (see Spotlight 2.4).

Treatment. Fads and fashions in treatment methods exist among and within cultures, regardless of the culture's level of sophistication. This problem is in part due to difficulties in defining and understanding abnormal behavior.

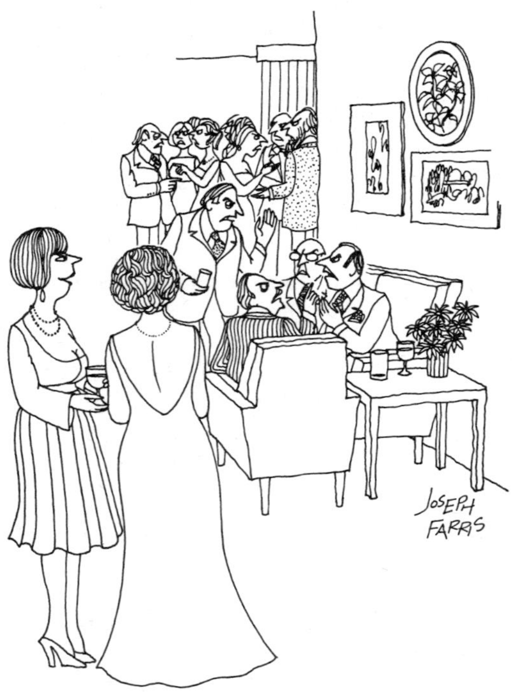

DRAWING BY JOSEPH FARRIS, © 1981 THE NEW YORKER MAGAZINE, INC.

"The era of self-doubt is certainly over."

Many of the fads in treatment methods blossom through the centuries, only to fade ingloriously; some, however, may return again and again, usually with different names. Treatment methods range from dream interpretation, exorcism, catharsis (the talking out of emotions with a consequent release of tension), electroconvulsive treatment, or ECT (administration of electrical impulses to the brain to induce seizures), herbal potions and medicines, flogging and other corporal punishment, isolation and incarceration, prayers and incantations, and musical and recreational therapies, to lectures and inducements.

Modern society continues to be characterized by a proliferation of treatment methods, most of which display a familiar life cycle: they are introduced; they receive enthusiastic reception; there are reports of remarkable results following their use; and there is a period of critical evaluation. The cycle ends, unfortunately, with a dismal picture:

> *Often such therapeutic developments have more of the qualities of certain political and religious movements, rather than scientific developments, and they strongly become identified with a particular leader, as seen in psychoanalysis with Freud or insulin therapy with Sakel. As techniques are rejected, they are often reintroduced in new guises with new names and new theoretical foundations. This type of circular movement has been seen in the application of moral therapy, hospital treatment, psychotherapy, drugs, and physical therapies. (Tourney, 1967, p. 785)*

Even today, differences in treatment methods among the various cultures and subcultures are extensive. Some of these methods—the methods of folk medicine—such as magic, faith healing, witchcraft, and shamanism are regarded by many as bizarre, prescientific, or irrational and are therefore not accepted as legitimate therapeutic practices.

Folk medicine for the treatment of mental disorders is practiced all over the world. Not relegated to "less developed" societies and hidden corners of our own society, folk medicine is alive and well in some of our own neighborhoods, especially in urban and rural areas where large ethnic populations reside. In many of our subcultures, large numbers of people do not turn to the middle-class verbal psychotherapies, that consist, primarily, of talking

Spotlight 2.4 A Symptom Is A Symptom—Or Is It?

Specifying the cultural and social factors that influence the expression, incidence, diagnosis, and effects of a particular symptom or pattern of symptoms is a very complicated business. Cultural studies of hallucinations, for example, indicate that the definition of hallucinatory experiences and their frequency vary from culture to culture, as do the attitudes and feelings of individuals toward their hallucinations.

1. American and British clinicians have different criteria for identifying hallucinations. Americans are less likely to differentiate among hallucinations, pseudohallucinations (the patient is aware that his or her hallucinatory perceptions are not "real"), and other types of vivid mental imagery than are their British counterparts. Americans, thus, are more likely to diagnose a patient as experiencing hallucinations than the British.

2. Nonwestern societies tend to make few distinctions among schizophrenic hallucinations, pseudohallucinations, dreams, and other fantasies. In addition, these subjective experiences, rather than being considered pathological, are considered to be evidence of possession by or contact with spirits, often a socially acceptable, and, in some places, socially desirable, occurrence.

3. The labeling of an experience as hallucinatory may depend upon linguistic factors. An individual who says "I see . . . I hear . . . " rather than "I thought I saw . . . It is as if I hear . . . " is more likely to be regarded as having hallucinations. However, the expression of the concept "as if" requires a certain level of linguistic skill. Labeling someone's experience as hallucinatory based on his or her "I-see" or "I-hear" description may thus actually be a diagnosis of that individual's lack of skill in linguistic expression (Sarbin, 1967).

4. Individuals in different cultures who ingest the same hallucination-inducing drug may experience totally different sorts of hallucinations. Western subjects report "meaningless" hallucinations and frequent mood shifts, whereas members of some Indian tribes who take drugs in a socially defined context report meaningful visions followed by a calm feeling of personal satisfaction (Wallace, 1959).

5. Although studies have shown that as many as 10 to 25 percent of all normal persons in rationally-oriented cultures such as ours experience hallucinations, hallucinatory experiences are considered to be negative and are frequently accompanied by a great deal of anxiety. On the other hand, cultures that value other modes of explaining experience encourage their members to observe, note, and report their hallucinations and fantasies. Thus the stigma of having a hallucinatory experience in a culture that does not accord such experience an accepted status may actually contribute to the development of further pathology. (from Al-Issa, 1977)

with a professionally trained person, for help. They often turn, instead, to authorities in their own culture whom they understand and trust. For example, a poor Chicano residing in a large city who still lives by the old country values of emotionalism may consult the *curandero* (faith healer) in the barrio (neighborhood), rather than an Anglo therapist, when he seeks help.

Spotlight 2.5 presents examples of folk practices around the world. Some of these may seem strange or bizarre. Rather than simply reacting to them, however, consider the fact that your judgment may be ethnocentric (belief in the superiority of one's own group)—an attitude shaped by the particular values and perspectives of one's own culture. However, if the judgments (or judges) were reversed, how would a South American Indian raised in the Brazilian jungle, for example, respond to astrological advice tossed about at a San Francisco cocktail party, or to the various kinds of screaming

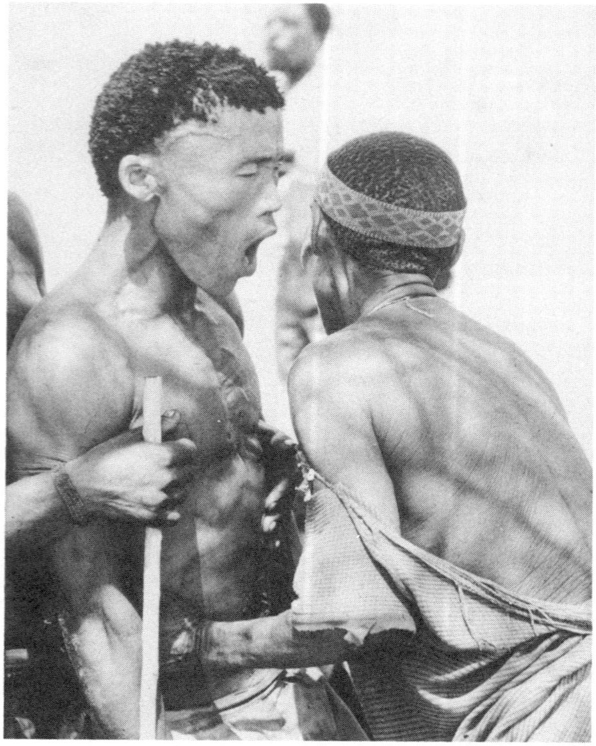

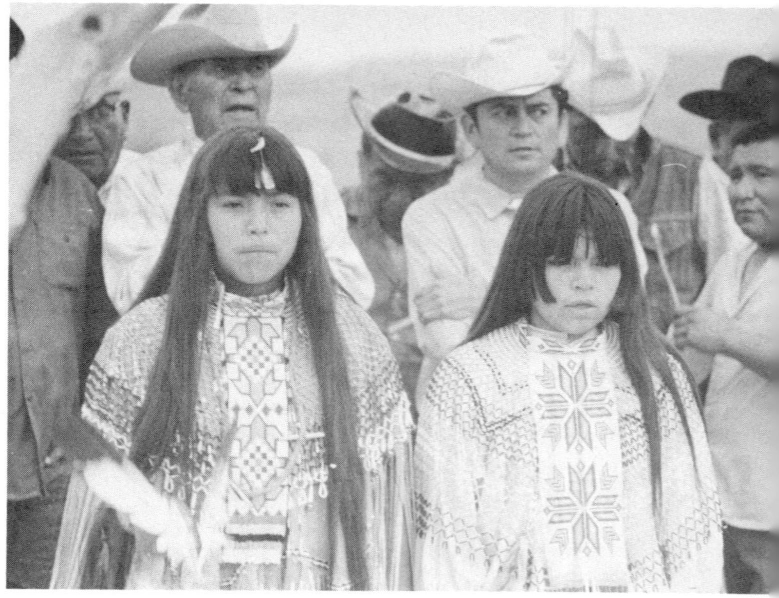

"Folk" treatments? An African shaman and North and South American Indians in activities designed to modify, control, or shape the behavior of others according to cultural standards. (Anthro-Photo/Left: Marjorie Shostak. Above: Martin Etter. Below left: David Maybury-Lewis.)

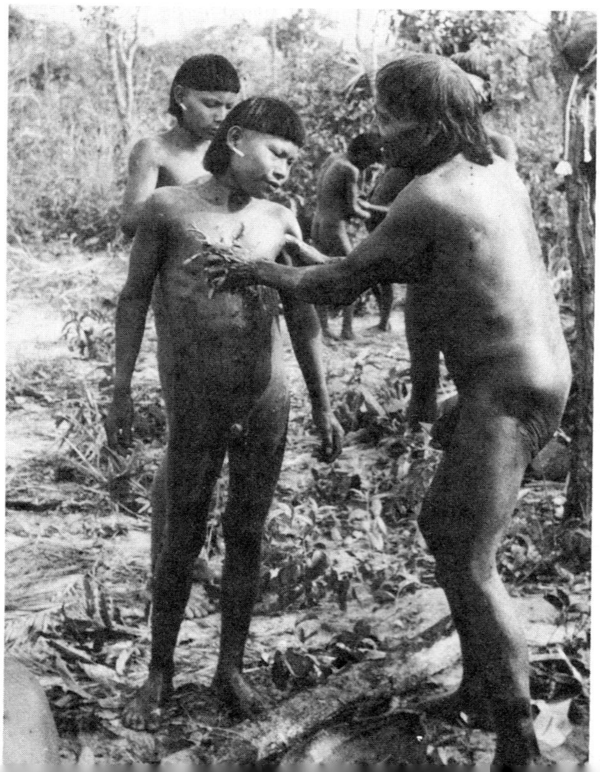

and touching in some contemporary American therapies, or to the ritual of lying on a couch in still other kinds of therapies?

American Culture and Mental Health

Within most complex cultures, substantial subcultural variations exist in habits, moral codes and values, standards for behavior, and general styles of living. Further, there are often differences between men and women and among social and economic levels and ethnic groups regarding incidence of psychopathology.*

* The chapters that follow will explore this theme in greater detail in the context of specific clinical syndromes and treatment methods.

Spotlight 2.5 Folk Therapy: Would the AMA Approve?

Here are some practices used to modify aberrant behavior in different societies around the world.

1. According to the customs of certain Eskimo groups the utterances of an insane person are actually communications from a supernatural being residing in that person. Thus a psychotic Aivilik Eskimo woman diagnosed as having stolen a fox eventually came to believe that a fox was living inside of her. Treatment of abnormal behaviors in these cases usually involve exorcism of the spirit (Murphy, 1964).

2. The Nigerian Yoruba often use the practice of cutting the skin of a mentally disturbed person to introduce curative substances into the blood. One such medicine is made of "certain roots, the filings of a human tooth, and a small quantity of fluid collected from a putrifying human corpse." The substances are introduced through cuts made at the location of the trouble: for example, for visual hallucinations they are made under the eyes, for auditory hallucinations in front of the ears, and for general psychosis the cuts are made in the head (Prince, 1964).

3. Exorcism is frequently used by Shona witch doctors to drive out the evil spirits that they believe are the cause of mental illness. Usually the witch doctor will wave an animal tail over the afflicted person while sprinkling medicine on him or her. Another cure involves forcing the evil spirit into an animal and then driving the animal into the woods (Gelfand, 1964).

4. After losing her second baby, an African woman began wailing, shouting, and screaming. She also became physically violent. A native doctor was called and he accused the mother of having caused the death of her baby herself through witchcraft. As treatment, he urged that she confess this fact, which she did. After the woman's "confession" the doctor pronounced her cleansed, after which her symptoms subsided completely (Dawson, 1964).

5. Anxiety and nervous conditions are thought by the Jews of Yemen to be caused by the evil eye. Treatment of such disorders include cutting three parallel scratches to draw blood and then throwing cold water onto the patient from behind, applying a hot nail to the supposed seat of the ailment (head, stomach, back) to enable the evil spirit to leave through the burn, and feeding a burned fertile egg to the patient (Hes, 1964).

6. In Turkey, relatives of a mentally ill person may pray and sacrifice the life of an animal at an *odjak* or magical place or site where evil spirits are thought to be warded off. After the ceremony, the relatives tie a piece of cloth to the *odjak* before leaving it, and then distribute the meat of the sacrificed animal among the poor (Oztürk, 1964). (from Kiev, 1964).

Poverty, SES, and psychopathology. In the early 1960s, a confluence of many political and social forces suddenly focused the spotlight on the millions of impoverished Americans who were not only poor, but appeared to have developed a lifestyle in response to their economic condition—a so-called culture of poverty that characterized people who lived within a world of chronic poverty (Harrington, 1962).

More often than not, the impoverished are prevalent among the minority groups of our nation. The mountain people in Appalachia, the Anglo and Mexican migrant workers, blacks living in inner city areas, the aged, the rural migrants to large cities, the skid-row alcoholics—these groups have all experienced poverty. They are bound by a common denominator of apathy, poor physical health, joblessness, fear, alienation from dominant middle-class values, and despair.

Sociologists point out that the culture of poverty is inherited, not by way of the genes, but through family styles transmitted in each generation from parent to child. This heritage includes hopelessness, the street styles of the children, fear, and patterns of family disorganization.

Many disadvantaged children have lifestyles and linguistic habits that are in conflict with the dominant culture of the schoolroom—its formal language, and requirements to sit still, pay attention, and respect authority. These demands may clash with the inclinations, characterized by an action orientation (an emphasis on movement and motility) observed in many low-SES children. Perhaps the seeds for emotional stress are sown very early, for many such children find the school experience difficult and stressful (Bernstein, 1964; C. Deutsch, 1973; M. Deutsch, 1963; and Riessman, 1962).

That there may be an association between extreme poverty and mental illness, therefore, does not come as a surprise. What are the actual findings? Researchers working in this area agree that the lower the social class the more evidence there is for psychopathology of various kinds, especially when number of symptoms (anxiety or depression, for example) is used as a criterion (Derogatis, Yevzeroff, and Wittelsberger, 1975). The evidence is so overwhelming, as a matter of fact, that the association between poverty and psychopathology is no longer questioned. Why this association occurs, however, is still open to investigation (Dohrenwend and Dohrenwend, 1969, 1974; King, 1978).

Here are some of the findings most often referred to:

1. In a classic study of the New Haven community in which the population was categorized on a SES scale from I through V, not only was there greater prevalence of psychological disorder among the lowest of the social classes, but there was a striking relationship between social class levels and kinds of treatment administered (Hollingshead and Redlich, 1958). For example, lower-class patients tended to be administered somatic treatments, such as electroconvulsive therapy, more frequently than verbal treatment. Diagnostic labels also differed for the same complaints: upper-class groups would be more likely to be diagnosed with a psychological label than the lower-class groups, in which physical diagnoses (and physical treatments) prevailed.

These investigators not only demonstrated that incidence and types of pathology differed from class to class, but also that there were sharp, dramatic differences in incidence between the two groups at the lowest end—the lower-class group (IV) and the group consisting of the most marginal and disorganized (perhaps classless) workers of the population (V).

2. Another classic study, based on a random sample (a number of persons selected without bias from a population in such a manner that they will represent the larger population) of over 1,500 adults, was the Midtown Manhattan study (Srole et al., 1962), which tended to confirm the general findings of Hollingshead and Redlich. Subjects were interviewed and later rated as to degree of mental health. Dramatic correlations were found between social class and ratings of degree of impairment (from "well" to "incapacitated"), with, as might be expected, sharp increases of frequency of the "impaired" ratings as one goes down the social scale and increases of "well" ratings as one goes to upper levels.

3. Still another study of mental disorders of childhood was based on a random sample of 1,034 households with a wide range of ethnic, economic, and social class characteristics (Langner et al., 1970). The children studied were chosen from families of one or more children ranging in age from six to eighteen. The methods used for data gathering included interviews with mothers, direct examination of children, and various questionnaires and ratings. We will note only one of the major findings: as one went down the income scale there was a dramatic rise in ratings of emotional impairment of the children.

The association between poverty and psychopathology is clear. Do the pressures and frustrations of lower-class membership produce mental illness, or is there a "downward drift" to bottom levels by people who are ill (or becoming ill) be-

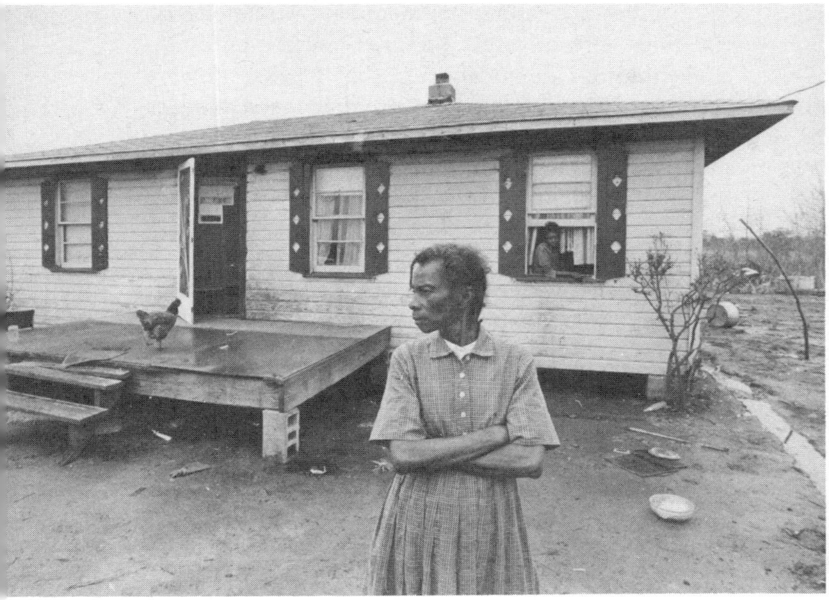

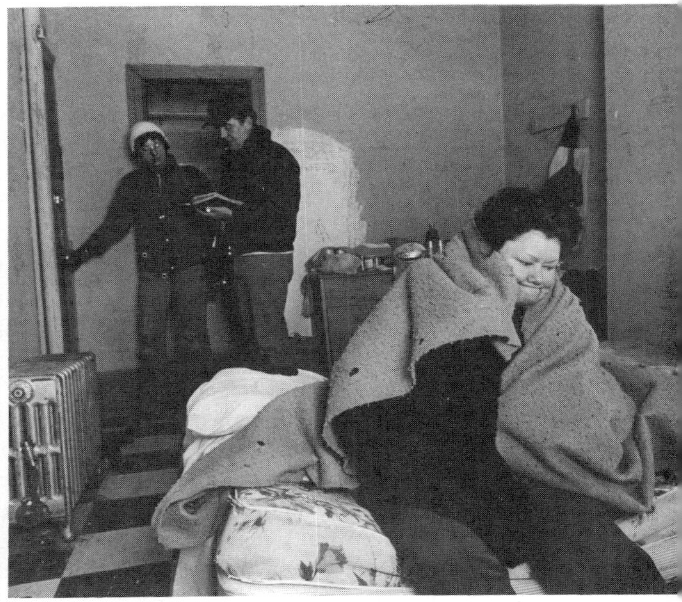

The association between poverty, whether rural or urban, and mental illness is a strong one. (Left: Nick Sapieha/Stock, Boston. Right: Diego Goldberg/Sygma)

cause they can no longer adapt to or function in the mainstream? The "downward drift" hypothesis tends to be preferred by those who are proponents of a genetic basis for mental illness but does not rule out social and cultural explanations for downward mobility. In any event, extensive reviews of relevant data have not resolved this issue (Dohrenwend and Dohrenwend, 1974).

Social class and psychotherapy. As suggested earlier, the kinds of treatment offered, the availability of treatment, who is seeing whom, even the length of the treatment session, vary considerably with social and economic class.

In addition, many of the traditional (usually verbal) treatment procedures (see Chapter 19) are inappropriate for large segments of our population. Of great importance may be the difference in values, goals, and orientation between a middle-class therapist and a lower-class patient. Even overall orientation regarding approach—"things will get better if you come every week"—may seem pointless to a jobless worker whose delinquent child, let us say, is in trouble with the police. Practical considerations, such as time, travel expenses, babysitters for working-class mothers, have all been obstacles and problems in the effective application of traditional therapeutic methods to the poor.

Race and mental illness. Frequently, in our society, racial minority status is associated with lower-class status. One might expect, then, a relationship between race and mental illness. This is not as clear-cut as the relationship between social class and mental illness, however. As a matter of fact, race alone does not predict or account for prevalence of psychopathology (Dohrenwend and Dohrenwend, 1969, 1974; King, 1978; Levy and Rowitz, 1973). However, other factors, such as poverty or residence in ghetto areas or areas undergoing rapid social change, are related to both high risk of mental disorder and race (Levy and Rowitz, 1973).

Being black—both in the North and the South—has its own special effects on emotional development. Growing up in a black lower-class family is more closely associated with emotional disability than growing up in a white lower-class family (King, 1978).

Not only blacks, but other minority groups—Hispanics, for example—who may be raised in poverty may experience apathy and despair, lowered self-esteem, self-hatred, and role confusion. Negative self-image and despair result not only from social prejudice but also from possible conflicts engendered by comparing "success" models, represented by the pimp, prostitute, or sports or entertainment celebrity, to "failure" models provided by parents who may hold menial jobs or be unemployed (Pettigrew, 1964; Sexton, 1965). With this pattern of stress, confusion, and despair, it is small wonder that mental and emotional disability flourish among minorities in the ghetto.

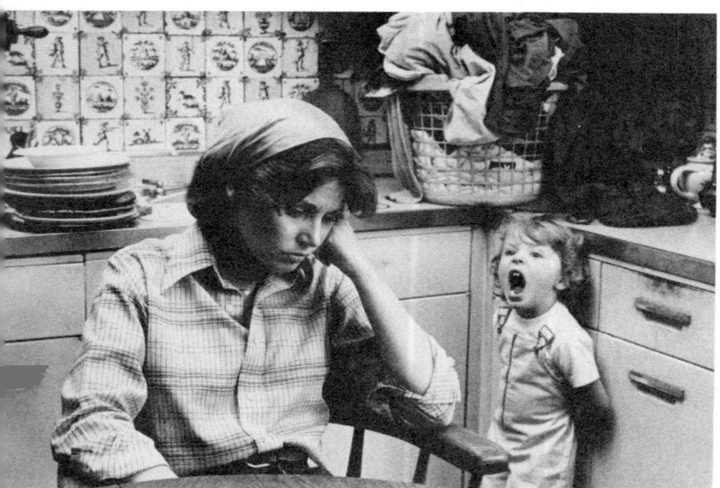

In our culture, women tend to show more psychological symptoms—for example, depression—than do men. (© 1981 Ed Lettau/Photo Researchers, Inc.)

Studies indicating that diagnoses vary along racial lines intensify this picture. These studies include findings demonstrating that blacks showing the same behavior as whites are diagnosed as more disturbed; that the same behavior labeled as schizophrenic for black women is diagnosed as neurotic for white women; and that hospital admission rates for blacks are much higher than those for whites (King, 1978).

Thus the evidence suggests that racial minorities are not only exposed to greater pressure in our society, but even with all other factors held constant, diagnostic labels are more severe for blacks and other minorities.

Who gets treated—and where—and who does not get treated are also associated with ethnic status (Dohrenwend and Dohrenwend, 1969). And in some specialized types of treatment, such as psychoanalysis (see Chapter 19), there is a strikingly low percentage of black patients (Thomas and Sillen, 1972).

In inner-city medical and psychiatric private services, blacks are less likely to receive treatment early in their illness and are more likely to be required to display dramatic symptomatology before receiving treatment. The implication that there is failure to meet the treatment needs of large portions of our population is clear. But there is also another implication: blacks must show more acute pathology and be more severely disabled before receiving help.

Other population groups and mental health: women, the aged, and homosexuals.

1. *Women.* Throughout the ages, women have been perceived and treated as the second sex and cast into an inferior role. Even some psychological theories, such as those of Freud, in which the concept of penis envy (the female's unconscious desire for a penis) plays a dominant role, assumed that women are inferior to and jealous of men.

Because many women have negative feelings about being female, their self-images, self-esteem, standards for behavior, and attitudes toward their own achievement have suffered. There is also little doubt that in addition to difficulties of lowered self-esteem, conflict about achievement, or the use of intellectual abilities, women have also suffered in the economic arena (Study finds female Ph.D's . . . , 1975).

In this society, women have had to struggle to maintain high standards of beauty and youth while coping with simultaneous household, childbearing, childrearing, and employment responsibilities. They have had to suppress intellectual expression of ideas and opinions for fear of being called "castrating." In addition, as dependents of their husbands or other men, some women have suffered even more specifically in terms of deprivation of civil rights. For example, as late as the nineteenth century, in Illinois a man could have his wife committed to a mental institution if he wished, for whatever reasons, without her having recourse to appeal or representation by any outside source (Deutsch, 1949).

The sense of powerlessness and conflict about role and self-image thus engendered could certainly be associated with emotional and mental disorders, especially depression. What is the evidence? Female gender alone apparently does not cause mental illness. Nor are rates of mental illness associated with being male or female. At best, there is only inconclusive evidence for a gender relationship, since true prevalence data are difficult to obtain (King, 1978; Dohrenwend and Dohrenwend, 1969, 1974).

However, because of many sociocultural factors, it is easy to demonstrate many male-female differences in the epidemiology of certain disorders and symptoms. Women, it is thought, are more vulnerable to becoming mentally ill (Chesler, 1972; Gove and Tudor, 1973; Nathan and Harris, 1975). They report more symptoms than men, more depression and unhappiness, more anxiety, more physical complaints, and more concern about interpersonal relationships (Garai, 1970; Phillips and Segal, 1969; Warheit, Holzer, and Arey, 1975). Further, as will be discussed in a later chapter, women are often subject to biases and prejudices in how they are perceived and treated in the therapeutic situation (see Chapter 19, pp. 596–98).

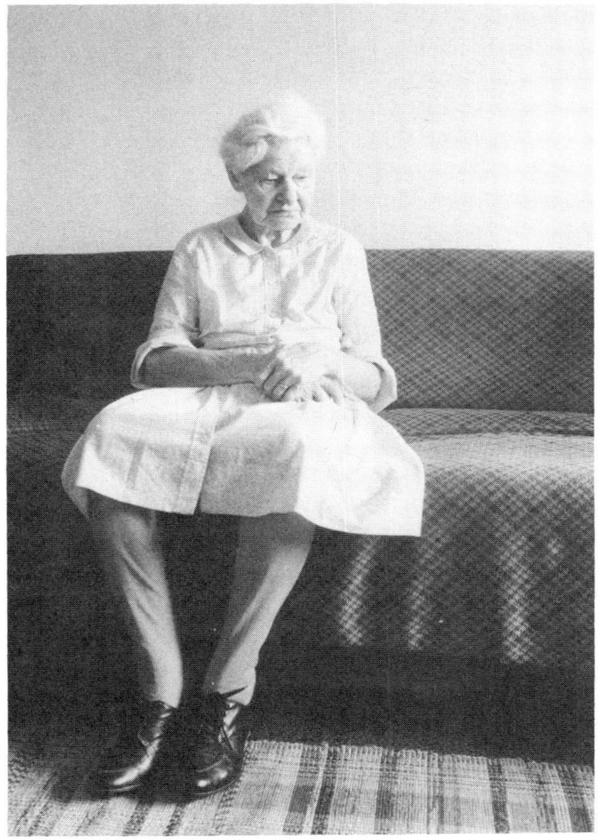

Because of youth-oriented themes in our society, elderly people have too much time on their hands and feel isolated and worthless. (Paul Conklin)

2. *The aged.* In 1975 over 22 million people in the United States were 65 years of age or older. It is estimated that in the year 2000 this figure will increase to 30 million, representing about 10 to 12 percent of the population. With our increased knowledge and skills in extending the lives of the elderly, there has not been a parallel increase in knowledge about their emotional, social, and psychological needs. Further, we have not yet made in-

roads into the youth-oriented themes that prevail in our interpersonal interactions and mass media. As a result, many of the aged in our society are outcasts, near-to-be-discarded people for whom society has no room. They are often hospitalized or institutionalized because they cause us pain, anguish, embarrassment, and fear. Our nursing homes are filled with elderly people who are no longer cared for at home. Many of those who struggle to "make it" in the community live under marginal, near-starvation conditions.

That the aged have special problems in many societies is an accepted fact. But vast cultural variations in the treatment of the aged is also an accepted fact. A World Health Organization report went so far as to suggest that the status of the elderly in backward nations is much better than that in the wealthier nations (Aged live better . . . , 1974). This probably results from our tendency to induce feelings of helplessness, powerlessness, dependence, fear, and depression in the elderly, whether they are hospitalized or not.

Chapter 13 will describe several clinical syndromes associated with organic and physical deterioration of the aging brain. When these special pathologies are ruled out, however, it has been found that the aged suffer from no greater incidence of mental illness than younger people (Dohrenwend and Dohrenwend, 1969). The majority of elderly people are not senile, continue to have sexual and romantic interests and activities, and, although often lacking in sexual partners, have the same needs for intimacy and closeness as younger people. And they continue to have the same needs for attention and a sense of doing something useful and productive.

Nevertheless, normal aging may be accompanied by changes in personality as the body declines, vision and hearing fail, and the older individual feels cast aside as a "nobody." Children and grandchildren go their own ways and spouses and friends die; sometimes disease and physical weakness occur. The body becomes less attractive: the skin wrinkles, there is a stooped carriage, and knuckles become gnarled. But the emotional consequences of undervaluing the elderly may take a far more devastating toll than does actual physical decline.

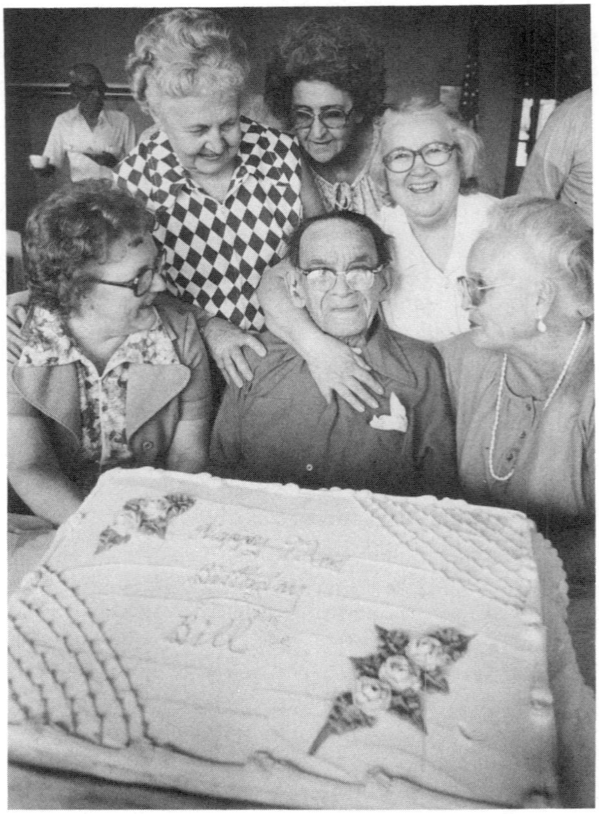

Elderly people have the same needs for affection, intimacy, and attention as do younger people. (Michael Hayman/Stock, Boston)

3. *Homosexuals.* For generations, homosexuals, both male and female, have been victimized in social, interpersonal, economic, and political arenas. Until fairly recently, guilt, shame, fear of discovery, and lowered self-esteem characterized many, if not most, homosexuals. Much of this picture is changing, however, as a result of the gay rights movement and its effects on inducing changes in atti-

tudes toward variations in sexual preference and orientation.

Although homosexuals are no longer regarded as mentally ill by the professional community, there are some people who claim that homosexuals should be assisted to change their sexual preferences, if they wish to do so. Whether or not psychotherapy should be offered at all to homosexuals, even if they intensely desire to change their sexual preferences, has elicited some controversy. Chapter 15 returns to this theme in greater detail.

SUMMARY

Chapter 2 described the extent of mental illness and introduced some epidemiological methods as well as some of the difficulties in interpreting epidemiological data. The influence of cultural forces on psychopathology was examined, especially the different ways sociocultural factors can induce conflict. Fads and fashions in symptoms and treatment practices were illustrated and the point made that these have varied not only throughout the ages but also from culture to culture. Finally, within our own society, the relationship between several sociocultural variables and mental health was examined. These variables included poverty and SES, gender, age, and sexual orientation. These relationships will be examined in greater detail in the chapters that follow.

Highlights

1. Mental illness characterizes about 15 percent of our population and is probably the most frequent type of health problem extant.
2. Epidemiology, the study of the incidence and prevalence of diseases in different demographic and cultural groups, in addition to having many practical public policy applications, is frequently helpful to scientists studying the origins of psychopathology by suggesting causal hypotheses. Yet epidemiological correlations do not definitively confirm one or another hypothesis because of the many problems in interpreting epidemiological data. One of these problems concerns the question of the true incidence of a pathological process in a given population, since many instances of pathology are not recorded and are therefore not included in the statistical data from which conclusions are drawn.
3. Different cultures can shape the development of psychopathology within their domains through a variety of cultural forces and pressures such as taboos, belief systems, values, conflicting roles, common personality types, social change and upheavals, and related sociocultural variables.
4. Symptoms of mental illness and various treatment practices vary from culture to culture and era to era. The acceptability or nonacceptability of deviant behavior—hallucinatory experiences, for example—also varies, depending on the cultural context. Some treatment practices may be effective because of belief in their power to heal, which may explain the apparent fading of effectiveness of many treatments with the waning of positive beliefs in them after an initial flurry of popularity.
5. In our own culture, study after study indicates the strong relationship between poverty or socioeconomic status (SES) and mental illness. Although there is an empirically established relationship between racial minority status and mental illness, it is not clear whether or not this is due to the complex relationship between this status and low SES.
6. This chapter also examined the relationship between other types of group membership and incidence of mental illness. Women are not more prone to psychopathology because of gender alone, but there is some evidence that they show more symptoms, more depression, and greater sense of helplessness—states that

may well be engendered by social factors. Although no greater incidence of mental illness among the aged than among younger groups has been found, the amount of loneliness, unhappiness, and even despair that exists among the elderly is probably also engendered by cultural factors. With regard to homosexuals, most professionals no longer regard homosexuality per se as relevant to considerations concerning the incidence of mental illness.

ISSUES AND QUESTIONS

1. As you look at your own culture, subculture, and family, can you specify some of the cultural elements that might influence your mental health? Can you isolate instances when you were made to feel so ashamed or guilty that you can still experience traces of these feelings today? Do you think you were deprived of some roles as a consequence of familial attitudes (so-called "feminine" ones, for example, among males)?
2. Do you know of older men and women in our culture who are made to feel ashamed and guilty because they continue to want to be attractive or because they seem to have sexual drives? Do you know of women who have been made to feel guilty (called "masculine," "aggressive," "castrating") because they are intelligent, have something to say, are smarter than some of their male peers, or speak out before they are spoken to?
3. Two equally trained and competent people, one twenty-five years old and another sixty-five, are employees of your firm. One of them must be let go because of economic reasons. As their employer, how would you choose between them and why?
4. Are you aware of any commonsense (folk) practices for curing or treating emotional problems that your own family members and relatives have used? Have the rituals of your religion influenced these practices?

   Have your relatives employed more accepted contemporary practices? Are these as rational as you originally thought they were? Can you describe specific methods your parents might have used to help you get over some problem, such as stuttering, school phobia, nightmares, enuresis, nailbiting, drug abuse? Were these methods based on rational beliefs and knowledge, common sense, myth and folklore, or perhaps some combination of these?

SUGGESTIONS FOR FURTHER READING

Cooper, B., and Morgan, H.G. *Epidemiological psychiatry.* Springfield, Ill.: Thomas, 1973. The history, methodology, and application of epidemiological research are presented in this excellent book. The uses of epidemiological data for the planning of mental health services, for clinical diagnosis and treatment, and for the discovery of causal factors of an illness are discussed. Actual epidemiological data are presented throughout the book. For an advanced-level, thorough overview of the major basic theoretical and practical aspects of epidemiological approaches to mental health, this book is highly recommended.

Fanon, F. *Black skin, white masks.* New York: Grove Press, 1967. Paperback. Originally published in Paris as *Peau noire, masques blancs* (1952), by Editions de Seuil; translated by C. M. Markmann. Although this book was written over thirty years ago, it still provides a scholarly, subjective account of the influence of white culture on the black individual. The author, a black man from the French Antilles, writes beautifully and honestly of the social, cultural, and psychological factors that contribute to the development of feelings of inferiority, paranoia, and aggression among black persons living in a white, colonized society. This book is informative, highly readable and relevant, and profoundly thought-provoking.

Hollingshead, A.B., and Redlich, F.C. *Social class and mental illness: A community study.* New York: Wiley, 1958.

Paperback. This classic report, although criticized for some important methodological problems, is based on an early interdisciplinary attempt to discover whether social class is related to mental illness. The authors found that treatment, symptoms, and even expectations on the part of the therapist were very much related to social class variables.

Kiev, A. (Ed.) *Magic, faith and healing: Studies in primitive psychiatry today.* New York: Free Press, 1964. Paperback. This fascinating collection of anthropological studies of mental illness and its treatment in various cultures around the world provides an important perspective to abnormal behavior. Introductory and closing chapters written by the editor guide the reader through this dazzling array of superstitions, rituals, and values.

Levy, L., and Rowitz, L. *The ecology of mental disorder.* New York: Human Science Press, 1973. This is a clear, simple presentation and analysis of epidemiological data pertaining to the incidence and prevalence of mental disorder as a function of community characteristics. In addition to reviewing many previous studies, the authors present data from a study of mental hospital admissions in Chicago from July 1, 1960, to June 30, 1961. These data were analyzed according to demographic as well as geographic characteristics. The tables are straightforward, the discussion clearly organized, and the conclusions at the end of each chapter and at the end of the book facilitate quick referencing and provide clear summaries of the data.

3

Science and Abnormal Behavior

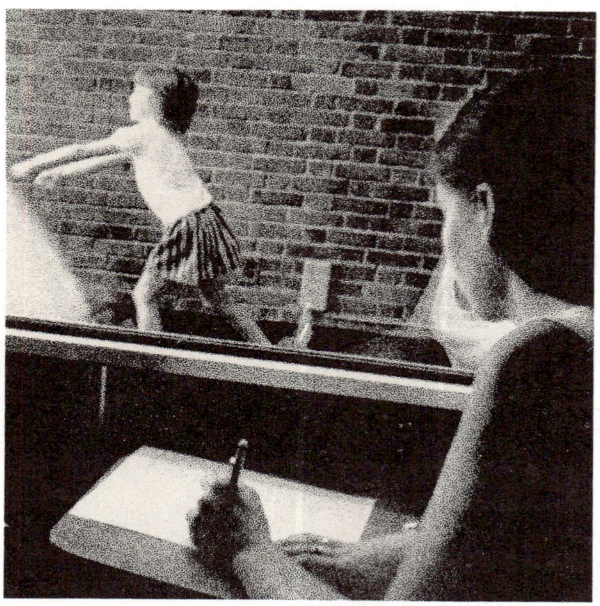

The causes of abnormal behavior have baffled thinkers throughout the ages. In many cultures, including our own, many myths and superstitions arose to explain behavior different from that of the mainstream. Modern western society, however, has realized the need for a more scientific approach to the problem of understanding behavioral deviances. How can science and scientific methods aid us in answering questions about abnormal behavior?

Stated simply, science offers us the means to seek explanations for how events or conditions occur and to explore the causes of events, phenomena, or behaviors. That is, science provides methods to help us make sense of and satisfy our curiosity about the world around us. Perhaps a more important, as well as a more practical, advantage offered by scientific methods is an opportunity to control, modify, even predict the events we are trying to understand—in this instance, aspects of abnormal behavior.

For example, one of the problems that has concerned people for centuries is the depression, relentless hopelessness, or apathy that can afflict some people. We can go to depressed persons themselves to find out what makes them become this way; or we can go to experts for their opinions. However, the answers to questions such as "What causes depression?" can vary widely, depending on the prevailing cultural view and on whether or not people recognize or understand the questions asked of them. In addition, experts, even within the same culture, disagree widely.

A recent hypothesis is that some depressions are caused by biochemical events within the brain of the depressed person. If this hypothesis is valid—that is, has been verified by empirical evidence and is therefore correct and "true"—then perhaps the problem of depression could be ameliorated by finding ways to alter or modify the biochemical components that have been implicated in its cause. Perhaps it would even be possible to predict, from early signs, who would be most likely to experience depression. Most important, finding the means for preventing a depressive episode might be possible.

Scientific methods provide us with a framework of logical or rational procedures to confirm or disconfirm hypotheses, such as the one above, through systematic explorations of real events, rather than through reliance on dogma, common folk concepts, or an expert's opinion. A scientific approach may be useful in our quest not only to understand human behavior, but also to alleviate aspects of functioning that cause distress—it can both increase knowledge and provide social benefits. In fact, the scientific approach may be the best method available in our search for meaningful and accurate explanations in order to understand, predict, and control abnormal behaviors.

This chapter will describe some aspects of the scientific method and their application to the study of abnormal behavior.

THE SCIENTIFIC APPROACH: ATTITUDES AND ASSUMPTIONS

Science is based on a complex set of attitudes that underlie methods of inquiry into the nature of reality. Whereas physical reality is the subject matter of many sciences—physics, chemistry, biology, and physiology—the social sciences, the science of abnormal behavior among them, involve inquiry into the realities of social behavior. Although the content of the two types of sciences differ—physical reality, on the one hand, and social reality, on the other—scientific methodology based on the scientific attitudes that guide inquiry is basically the same for all the sciences.

The basic assumption underlying scientific inquiry is that events in nature are orderly, obey particular laws, and occur with regularity—that is, occurrences are not random or chance events.* Scientists are dedicated to attempts to reveal and to understand this order, to piece together the structure of events by isolating their causes, and to articulate the rules that determine the relationships of events to each other.

Science assumes that the underlying order in the universe can be made plain by the application of certain general methods. These scientific methods and tools, it is claimed, offer the best opportunities for making valid statements about reality, since these statements can be checked, confirmed, disconfirmed, and altered through constant reapplication of scientific method. Scientists differ from philosophers, logicians, or theologians who may

* It is true that when considering the very smallest, most basic particles of matter, physicists say that there is an authentic element of uncertainty or unpredictability. Put on more global levels, most scientists proceed on an assumption of predictable and orderly causality in nature and matter (like day following night) and hold that events are caused by other events; that is, events do not occur spontaneously and randomly without a prior cause or set of preceding conditions.

also believe in the lawfulness and regularity in the universe, but who attempt to understand this order through systematic thought or speculation, rather than by systematic references to the real world.

Another feature of science is its attitude that dogma, private opinion, and authority are always to be questioned; personal opinions and beliefs, although frequently useful in the construction of scientific hypotheses and theories are not the means by which scientific explanation is verified. Thus we accept that the speed of light is 186,000 miles per second not because of Einstein's claim, but because the observable, concrete evidence supports Einstein's hypothesis. Empirical verification of scientific statements based on observation or actual experience rather than private or personal dogma, then, is a key characteristic of science.

Another aspect of the scientific viewpoint is that although the focus and content of scientific inquiries might vary with different disciplines, scientific methods cut across all disciplines. Thus the systematic study of behavior, abnormal or otherwise, can follow the same scientific rules as the study of biochemistry or astronomy.

The social sciences seem less open to scientific understanding than physics or chemistry for a number of reasons. We may lack the tools, devices, and know-how relevant to the measurement of human behavior; or the causal components of human behavior may be more numerous than is the case with nonhuman phenomena; or, human interactions may be more complex and the human organism's mental and emotional responses less understood and less predictable. Human behavior may never be understood or predicted with the precision with which physical events can be understood and predicted, but attempts to do so will certainly continue. Underlying these efforts is the belief that a scientific approach is the best available one.

Thus far we have discussed the attitudes which scientists have toward inquiry into the nature of reality. But where do we go from there? Where do we start, and what does the scientific method consist of?

THE SCIENTIFIC METHOD: STARTING POINTS AND PROCEDURES

Classification and Categorization

One of the first steps a scientist must take toward understanding a particular phenomenon is to observe the events of interest and attempt to classify and categorize what he or she observes. Thus scientists studying abnormal behavior must first attempt to find general categories of abnormal behaviors. For example, some abnormal behaviors involve hallucinations and others do not; some involve mood changes or "swings," whereas mood is not involved in others. Still other unusual behaviors may be characterized by relentless, paralyzing anxiety or great distortions in judgment and thinking. Classifying abnormal behaviors according to such differences constitutes a beginning step in trying to uncover the orderliness and lawfulness that can be assumed to underlie abnormal behavior in general.

However, the lack of consensus among researchers in this field as to the proper criteria for classification of abnormal behaviors has already been introduced. This remains an important issue in abnormal psychology that will be discussed in the next chapter.

Hypotheses, Theories, and Laws

Once behaviors, phenomena, or events have been categorized and classified, the next task in scientific procedure is to generate ideas or hypotheses to account for the various facts and their interrelationships. For example, one might observe and identify the peculiar logic and thinking that characterize the problem-solving behavior of some schizophrenics. The next step would then be to form hypotheses about, and theories to explain, the causes of such irrationality.

Theories are a critical component of scientific endeavor. Sound theories provide a perspective for relating seemingly isolated events, perhaps even facts, hitherto thought to be irrelevant and unrelated to each other. A sound theory also permits empirically verifiable hypotheses to follow from its tenets and content. Thus, for example, according to the double bind theory, people who become schizophrenic (see Chapters 11 and 12) were forced to develop ways to accommodate to and cope with contradictory demands in their environments. An illustrative example is seen in the instance of a mother exhorting her son to "be independent," and when he is, she exhibits her hurt and neglected feelings, or she punishes him severely; in either case, the child has received contradictory messages. One empirically verifiable hypothesis following from this theory is that significant double-bind events and messages could be uncovered in the life history of most, if not all, individuals diagnosed as schizophrenic. Before this theory can be said to be valid, however, the hypotheses it generates must be tested repeatedly with many kinds of schizophrenic people at different ages and stages of their illness.

Occam's Razor. Theories that are simple but that can predict a broad base of events and occurrences are regarded as "elegant" theories by scientists. The more complex a theory is—the more exceptions, deviations, and convolutions its proponents must make to adjust it to what is actually found in reality—the less elegant it is. Consider the double bind theory, for example: if empirical observation and testing demonstrates that all persons who have experienced double bind communications do not become schizophrenic, then the double bind theory would have to be adjusted to account for this finding. If still later, findings reveal that many schizophrenic people have not experienced double bind communications, still further adjustments in the theory are required to fit the facts. The simple theory would by now have many ifs, ands, and buts—perhaps with regard to variables such as age, intelligence, SES level, early history, number of close relatives with a history of schizophrenia, and so on. These qualifying factors however, would weaken the explanatory and predictive value of the basic theory. Simplicity—"parsimony"—then, is an important aspect of any theory. William Occam, a fourteenth-century philosopher, pointed out the value of this rule of thumb for theory making; this maxim has come down to us through the centuries with a name—Occam's Razor.

Paradigms and paradigm shifts. When one theory seems to account for the various available facts, it often becomes a "paradigm," or system for thinking about those facts. For example, Freud's instinctual, biologically oriented theory of human psychology was accepted by many psychologists early in this century as the framework within which to think about human behavior: it was the prevailing paradigm of its time.

According to Kuhn (1962), typical, or what he refers to as "normal," scientific activity consists of refining and perfecting the beliefs and conceptualizations of the prevailing paradigm until some entirely revolutionary change of paradigm—paradigm shift—takes place. "Normal" science is peaceful, with traditional areas defined and carved out and with scientists busily trying to solve "puzzles" within the paradigm. A revolution or paradigm shift occurs when facts generated from hypotheses based on a theory prove to be inconsistent with the theory. When this first occurs, scientists will try to alter the existing theory to fit the new evidence. Too many alterations, however, result in a lack of parsimony, an indication that the theory is not adequate. Eventually, often on the basis of a brilliant intuition on the part of a scientist, a totally new theory will be presented that will deal more parsimoniously with the existing evidence. The new theory then becomes the new paradigm and will, in turn, generate its own hypotheses to be verified. Within Kuhn's framework, the cycle of scientific change is characterized by: a prevailing "paradigm," followed by a "crisis" (when the new facts no longer fit the old paradigm), which leads to "revolution," whereby a new theory is accepted as the paradigm in the field.

Today the field of abnormal psychology may be experiencing such a paradigm shift. Just as Freud's instinctual theory of abnormal psychology shifted, in the view of many behaviorists, to a learning paradigm, which held that abnormal behaviors are learned, some contemporary scientists are turning to a biological paradigm that views many abnormal behaviors as behavioral symptoms caused by genetic, biochemical, and neurophysiological factors.

Laws and theories. Natural laws are simple truths about the universe that have great scope and generality. The law of gravity, Einstein's general and special theories of relativity, and Newton's laws of motion are examples. These laws are simple in their statement but so far-reaching as to account for the motions and travels of all the heavenly bodies, the orbits of the planets around the sun, and the motions of objects on the surfaces of the earth or in the air around us. There are as yet few wide and universal laws in the behavioral sciences—and still fewer in regard to abnormal behavior.

Many theories have been proposed concerning how abnormal behavior develops. Some of these are more testable, more open to public inquiry and scientific investigation, and therefore sounder theories—whether they are eventually demonstrated to be "right" or "wrong." As more and more evidence verifying a particular theory accumulates, the validity of that theory acquires more certainty; it includes more data, it has greater predictive value, and it is more practically useful. Evaluations of particular theories will be discussed in greater detail in Chapters 6 and 7 and throughout this book.

SCIENTIFIC "TOOLS"

The "tools" used in scientific endeavors refer not only to the instruments used to sharpen direct observations (such as telescopes or electrical devices that record brain waves) but also to *methods* that do not belong to the same class as the telescope or electroencephalograph device—for example, quantification, statistics, and the experiment.

Measurement

In most scientific disciplines, including psychology and the study of abnormal behavior, modes of quantification and measurements—are also tools. Although measurements are not in themselves scientific, their use permits comparisons and contrasts intrinsic to scientific explanations for questions such as: What is the relationship of SES and the occurrence of schizophrenia? Does one particular kind of treatment reduce depression more than another? Are levels of certain biochemicals in the brain reduced in clinical depression?

Spotlight 3.1 elaborates on the use of numbers and another tool for using numbers in the pursuit of science—statistics.

Other important methods in abnormal psychology aid in diagnosis, permit comparison of groups, and help to sharpen observations or to make inferences about individuals and their behavior. These aids include interviews, ratings, questionnaires, and various types of assessment methods that will be described and illustrated throughout this book.

The Experiment

A powerful method that does more than enhance conjecture about the causes of events is the experiment. Experiments are controlled observations of the effects that the manipulation or deliberate changing of one variable has on another. The independent variable is the variable for which effects are to be studied. This variable is manipulated by the experimenter and its effects on another variable, the dependent variable, are measured. These terms make sense, since what happens to the dependent variable depends upon what effect the independent variable has on it.

For example, if an hypothesis states that marijuana smoking impairs intellectual functioning, then the experimenter might have some individuals smoke marijuana (the independent variable) and then measure their performance on various tests or

Spotlight 3.1 Numbers and Statistics: Tools in the Aid of Knowledge

In the field of abnormal behavior, discussion focuses on such entities as anxiety, depression, sexual dysfunctions, phobias, conflicts, aggression—variables concerned with the emotional life of the person being studied. Research in this field often raises questions about how much or how little a particular process, event, or trait has changed as a result of some intervention; or how much or how little one process, event, or trait seems to be associated with others; or whether or not groups of people differ in some way when compared, let us say, for the nature or extent of pathology.

A convenient, clear, unambiguous way of framing questions, getting information, making comparisons, and expressing findings is through the use of numbers. Let us, for example, explore the hypotheses that many more disturbed children come from broken families than from intact families; or that the more intense the depression in adults, the greater the likelihood that these persons had experienced guilt as children.

In attempting to understand the association between disturbed children and intact homes, the first step is to "count heads." In the group of children to be studied, who are the disturbed children? Are some children more disturbed than others? What kinds of measures are appropriate? Observing the children and rating them as to disturbance? Or giving them a test to measure the degree of disturbance? Whatever the approach, some numerical system would be useful, especially for obtaining an estimate of the relative intensity (size, strength, degree) of the variable—the disturbance—for each subject.

To illustrate: If the study population consists of thirty children, each one receives a score or number based on the measurement of disturbance (by means of observations, tests, or ratings). The next question is then: Do the high scorers (above the average score on the particular measure) tend to come from broken homes? And do those who are low scorers on the disturbance measure tend not to come from broken homes? In actual research, of course, one would probably want to know a good deal more about the lives of these children. For example, because duration of exposure to the broken home situation might be of significance in determining extent of disturbance, how early in the life of the child did divorce or separation take place?

One of the first steps, then, in answering a question scientifically is to decide on a means of measuring the data and a system for assigning values, or numbers, to these measurements. Numbers make it possible to make abstractions and to summarize the data of research investigations. Further, they facilitate comparing procedures and communicating results.

Scientists gather data to draw conclusions about their hypotheses. They wish to make generalizations from their data. On the test of disturbance, for example, say that scores could extend, or range, from 1 (no disturbance) to 20 (highly disturbed) and that a question is raised as to whether John and Mary with scores of 10 are more disturbed than Frank and Jane, with scores of 8. Is a 2-point difference on this test meaningful? Is a 10-point difference?

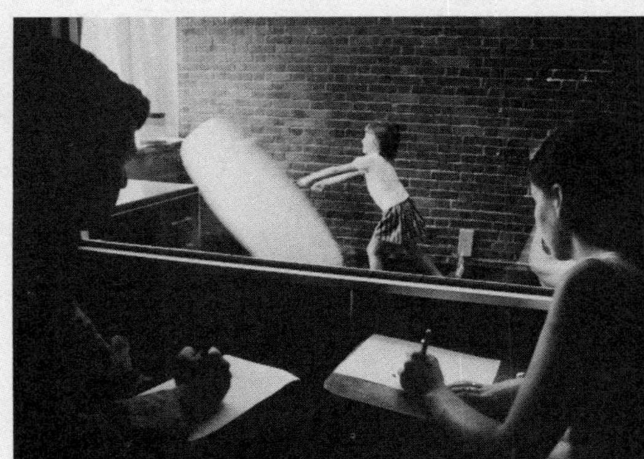

Systematic and objective observation, leading to quantifiable data, is one step in the experimental method. (Cary Wolinsky/Stock, Boston)

To make these sorts of decisions, researchers use certain statistical procedures to estimate the probability that a particular result occurred simply by chance. In this way, it could be learned that the 2-point difference could have easily happened by chance and that John, Mary, Frank, and Jane are not actually different in degree of disturbance. In similar fashion, the statistical procedure could determine that Richard's score of 18 and Eliza's score of 8 on this test was not likely due to chance. This difference, in statistical terms, is called significant.

Statistics are also helpful in making comparisons between groups. For example, if we wanted to compare the school performance of students who use drugs to those who do not use drugs, we might first want to compute the students' grade point averages (GPA) as a measure of their school performance. We could then compare the average GPA of students who do not use drugs to the average GPA of the drug users. Any difference we might find would presumably tell us about the differences in school performance of the two types of students.

But how would we know whether or not the difference is a difference worth noting? One method is to determine whether or not the observed or measured difference could have happened by chance. That is, the students selected for one group might, by chance, have had a higher GPA than those in the other group. Statistical methods enable us to estimate the probability that a difference between the two groups could not have happened by chance. In scientific reports, the phrases "significant difference," or "significant finding," or "statistically significant," indicate small likelihood that the result was obtained simply by chance.

Statistical methods also enable measurement of the degree of correlation, or association, of the two factors. For example, the hypothesis that the more intense the depressive symptoms in adults, the greater the likelihood that they experienced childhood guilt might be put another way: Are childhood feelings of guilt correlated with depression in adulthood?

Correlations may be strong or weak and are expressed numerically; they can be positive or negative. An example of a negative (inverse) correlation would be *low* self-image and *high* anxiety before tests. An example of a positive correlation would be *low* scores on a test of adjustment in adolescence and *low* scores on a test of marital adjustment ten years later.

Correlations do not imply causation. For example, if we indeed found that disturbed children tend to come from broken homes, we would not know whether or not having a disturbed child strained the marriage and precipitated divorce, or whether the separation of the parents caused the emotional disturbance, or whether disturbance in children and marital discord both stem from other causes.

Correlations thus permit many types of interpretations that must often be tested further. For example, the tendency to be overweight and to feel depressed may be correlated. But does being overweight cause depression? Or is the direction of causality reversed—that is, does the depression cause the overeating? Or, are overeating and depression caused by *other* factors?

There are many findings in the research domain of abnormal behavior that are correlational, as we shall see. For example, poverty and low SES are often associated with or correlated with schizophrenia, alcoholism, and other disorders. The precise nature of the *causes* of schizophrenia, alcoholism, and many other disorders, however, are yet to be determined.

measurements of intellectual functioning (dependent variable). However, whether or not marijuana smoking impairs intellectual functioning could not be ascertained unless a sound comparison is obtained. A control group of subjects who do not smoke marijuana and are given the same tests of intellectual functioning as the experimental group of subjects would provide the necessary comparison.

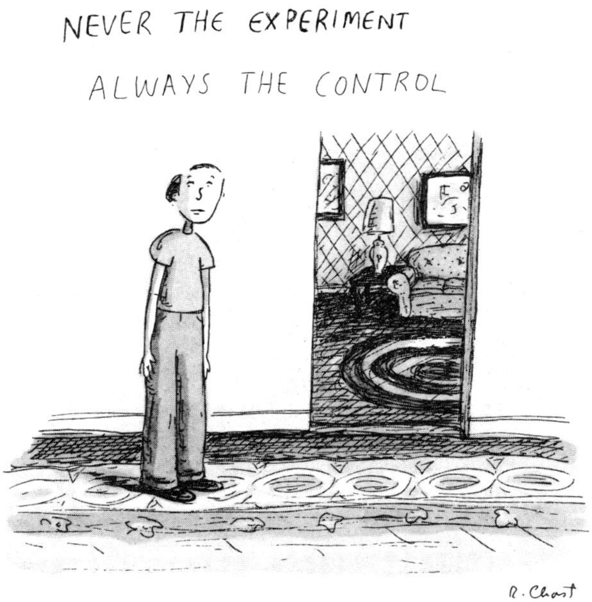

DRAWING BY R. CHAST; © 1981 THE NEW YORKER MAGAZINE, INC.

In this case, the experimental group would smoke marijuana and then take the tests and the control group might smoke regular cigarettes (made to look and taste like those made from marijuana) and also take the tests. If the control group performs better than the experimental group, we can assume that marijuana smoking did indeed impair the intellectual functioning of subjects in the experimental group. Subjects in each group would, of course, not know the purpose of the experiment nor whether they were smoking marijuana or tobacco.

It is common to assign subjects to either the experimental or control groups randomly (without bias). This makes it unlikely that the subjects' behavior in the experimental group changed because the subjects' characteristics were different to begin with from the characteristics of subjects in the control group. The goal is that the control and experimental groups be exactly alike in all ways (subject characteristics, expectations, treatment, time of exposure to experimental situation, experimental attitudes), *except* for the introduction of the independent variable. In this way, on a strictly logical basis, the results of the experiment can be attributed to the manipulation of the independent variable.

To return to the discussion of causality: because of the high degree of control over the observations derived from an experiment, experiments are often—though not always—used to test hypotheses about causal relationships among events. In the example just presented, we would be in a better position to say that marijuana smoking causes impairment of intellectual functioning if we obtained positive results from our experiment than if we were simply to ask several marijuana smokers whether or not they thought that their functioning is impaired by smoking marijuana or if we asked some experts.

It is rare to find a crucial experiment in psychology, a test of a theory so striking and dramatic that it results in either invalidating or totally confirming a theoretical system. Scientists deal primarily in probabilities, not absolutes.

More often than not, a series of experimental findings point the way toward confirming a given explanation or disconfirming another. Sometimes the evidence is reorganized by a scientist so that totally new implications emerge from the same accumulation of data.

The experiment is by no means the only tool for testing the validity—the accuracy or truth—of our hypotheses. Careful observations or the prediction of certain events are also powerful tools. Correlation coefficients, graphic representations of data, and epidemiological reports also suggest interpretations as to what is happening by organizing the data in systematic ways. But experimental methods have certain advantages over other methods when it comes to testing out a particular hypothesis; an experiment also allows the investigator to make some statement about the probability that the findings are correct. Further, an experiment is repeatable and its results are reportable. In addition, if the rules are followed, an experiment forces the experimenter to make public to the world at large the operations and measurements employed in the experiment. But above all, the logic upon which the experimental method is based controls the way an investigator formulates questions so that appropriate answers can be obtained. When properly conducted, an experiment can indicate that causal relationships exist, it can indicate the direction of causality, and it can rule out third-variable causality.

Other Research Methods

The experiment may be the most powerful tool in the sciences, but in most types of researches in abnormal psychology it is not the most frequent method employed. Other, less precise methods are used because of some very important, even obvious, reasons. One reason concerns the inaccessibility of many different types of clinical subjects. For example, a homicidal rapist or a schizophrenic in an acute delusional state will not be readily available for an experiment. An additional consideration, even if some subjects *are* available—such as addicts in a detoxification center or prisoners in a state facility—is the ethical issue of enforcing experimental conditions on unwilling subjects. Also, some events and behaviors occur infrequently; and when they do, an experimenter may not be present. Examples are explosive rages, acute delusional states touched off by excessive use of illicit drugs, or attempted suicide.

One of the most troublesome—perhaps insurmountable—problems is that some types of experiments are not possible with human subjects. These are the experiments that pose danger or threat, psychologically or physically. Examples include surgical probing of the brain (in the absence of medical necessity), the withholding of a medication with known beneficial effects from patients who need it, the introduction of dangerous chemicals and drugs to alter behavior, and the inducing of overwhelming stress. Despite these limitations, there are many other ways to explore hypotheses and to test ideas concerning abnormal behavior, although, admittedly, conclusions from these nonexperimental methods are less precise and tend to permit fewer generalizations.

The chapters that follow provide descriptions of many fascinating experimental explorations. However, much of the material in this book is based on other types of observations and research methods, some of which are now briefly described.

1. *The clinical case study.* Intensive, judicious review of clinical case material, especially material that is carefully compiled and from which the effects of the subject's memory are carefully weighed, can yield many speculations, hypotheses, and insights about abnormal behavior, and may even rule out some misconceptions. Many of Freud's hypotheses, for example, were developed from the careful study of single cases. A word of caution, however: generalizations from case studies cannot only be misleading but also can seriously misrepresent cause-and-effect relationships. One would not wish to generalize, for example, about the causes of homicidal behavior from a detailed case history of one murderer. Yet much can be learned from case material, as the chapters that follow will document.

2. *Single-subject experiments.* In contrast to the individual case study are experiments that, unlike those thus far described, employ only one subject to test an hypothesis. Many of the principles described in Chapter 20, which discusses behavioral approaches to helping people to change, are based on studies of a single subject. Typically, the subject's behavior is measured, some procedure for retraining the subject is introduced to demonstrate the change in behavior, and the behavior is shown to resume its original level when the change agent is removed. If, in addition, it can be shown that when the change agent or independent variable is *re*introduced, the behavior changes once again in the expected direction, a strong case can be made for drawing some causal connections between the two variables. However, what if there is no return to initial levels after the change variable has been removed? Can we conclude that the experimental effect is not valid? Not necessarily, for like mercury in some types of thermometers, return to an initial level may not be possible. In any event, single-subject experiments suffer from many of the disadvantages of case studies, including lack of control subjects, an extremely limited and possibly un-

representative sample for study, and the possibility that chance or other unknown factors could influence the results.

3. *Contrasted-groups method.* Many investigations in abnormal psychology focus on a group of subjects who share some clinical characteristic—teenagers who are alcoholics, for example. It might be of considerable interest to compare psychological data about these subjects to similar data obtained from matched groups of teenagers who are *not* alcoholics, but are, let us say, heroin users. Perhaps differences between these subjects could be found in emotional makeup (dependency, for example) or in level of experienced anxiety. From these findings many interesting hypotheses for further exploration could emerge; yet we could not be completely sure that our results could be applied to other similar groups, such as adult drug and alcohol abusers or to samples of subjects that did not share exactly the set of characteristics in our research sample.

4. *Retrospective studies.* If various types of accumulated data on the subjects described above were available to the researchers—data such as presence or absence of birth difficulties, history of hospitalizations, school records of truancy, parental arrest records, and so on—a retrospective study would be possible. The task of the researchers might be to look for relationships between one or more of these early variables and later status: for example, whether or not the subject shows a propensity for alcoholism, drug addiction, or neither (provided a control group of normal subjects is also available). It would not be enough to show that some significant relationships were indeed found between early variables and current status (for example, a history of alcoholism in the father might be associated with alcoholism in the teenage son but not in the daughter). Retrospective studies often yield interesting hypotheses and speculations that must be confirmed in new samples before valid generalizations can be made. However, causal connections could not be made between the father's and the offspring's alcoholism until more refined research is conducted.

5. *Longitudinal and follow-up research.* In contrast to retrospective research investigation is longitudinal research, in which subjects are followed over a period of years to test one or more hypotheses about the origins and development of a pathological process. Do families in which a parent has severely abused a child produce adults who abuse *their* children? Only follow-up research can provide the answer. (To evaluate incidence data on child abuse in the next generation, it would also be necessary to follow matched control families in which there is *no* history of child abuse.) Follow-up research of this nature often yields strikingly rich, sometimes crucial data, but, unfortunately, is extremely expensive and time consuming. In later chapters, a special application of longitudinal research will be discussed. This approach, known as the high-risk strategy, tests hypotheses about children or other subjects who are thought to be particularly vulnerable for the later development of a mental illness, such as schizophrenia. High-risk research, whether focused on schizophrenia, mental retardation, alcoholism, or any other area, has recently become quite popular. It not only tests hypotheses about etiology, but also offers the opportunity to learn more about early characteristics of high-risk individuals so that preventive efforts can be applied. This opens up additional research questions: for example, what constitutes the most effective program for preventing certain identified high-risk children from developing into, for example, seriously destructive and anguished alcoholics?

6. *Analogue experiments.* Because some experimental manipulations are not easily accomplished, researchers may at times construct an experimental situation that attempts to represent, or be analogous to, the actual situation. These researches, referred to as analogue experiments, often yield hypotheses, insights, and directions for further research, despite the fact that they do not necessarily provide definitive answers. For example, how may we learn more about clinically depressed children who have made suicide attempts without subjecting them to the stress of an experimental situation? We might induce a depressed mood in one group of children by showing them a sad film and a happy mood in a different (matched) group of children by showing them a happy film. Differences between these two

groups of children with regard to how anger is expressed after a frustrating experience would then be observed. Is anger directed toward the frustrating agent or turned against the self? Analogue experiments provide artificial glimpses into real circumstances. This research, for example, would not yield data specific to clinical depression and attempted suicides of these children. Yet a good deal would undoubtedly be learned about mood and aggression from explorations of this nature.

7. *Animal studies.* As the study of abnormal behavior becomes increasingly interested in the brain, the body's biochemistry, and in patterns of response to extreme stress or conflict, it has become increasingly necessary to test certain hypotheses or to explore particular avenues through work with animals. Much of what has been learned about the mechanisms of the brain, the biochemistry of mood and emotions, behavior under conditions of extreme conflict, principles of learning and conditioning, and even the effects of maternal deprivation has been directly or indirectly derived from experimental work with animals, especially cats, rats, and monkeys. Generalizations from this kind of research must necessarily be carefully evaluated before relevance to human behavior is assumed.

In experimental procedures, as well as those in the preceding descriptions, observations and measurements of various types are obtained to assess the behavior under scrutiny. Many different kinds of data will be described in the pages that follow—all of which are presented to explore differences between groups, relationships of variables to each other, and so on. Psychologists work with many different types of data. These include self-reports in the form of questionnaire responses or interviews, personal documents, school, hospital, and other institutional records, ratings by experts, and psychological test responses. Additional data to be considered also consist of brain wave recordings, family history records, and biochemical findings such as those obtained from urinanalysis. Many of these data sources will be described in detail; traditional types of psychological tests, for example, are illustrated in Chapter 5. In typical research explorations in the field of abnormal psychology, data are handled statistically to specify various aspects of the findings and the degree of confidence that can be placed in them. Correlational methods are the most frequently used of these statistical methods. (Spotlight 3.1 described correlational methods in greater detail.)

Some Rules of the Scientific "Game"

Public enterprises have sets of rules so that participants can communicate with each other and understand what each is talking about. For example, in the field of international games and sports, what if individual nations or clubs were made to compete without prior definition of the penalties, wins, and various standards for proper play? National boundaries or personal whim notwithstanding, if a game is to be entered and the winner determined, an individual competitor must know the preset rules, definitions, and methods of determining wins, losses, and ways of scoring. Because science is a public enterprise, preset rules are also necessary. It differs from games in many respects, however, especially regarding the requirement in science of empirically referenced rules, as opposed to arbitrary ones.

One of the foundations of the scientific method is the communication of scientific procedures and findings so that others—colleagues and peers—understand them without ambiguity. Other rules of the scientific "game" include:

Objectivity and ethics. Scientific findings must be reported in a nonbiased, impersonal manner understandable to others. The procedures must be reported exactly as they were carried out and the results must not be misrepresented to make a point.

Operational definitions. Describing a behavior or trait in terms of the procedures by which it is observed or measured enables scientists to objectify and repeat the way they define the event under study. For example, a psychologist studying anxiety might ask subjects to rate the amount of anxiety they feel on a scale of 1 to 7, with 1 meaning "very anxious" and 7 meaning "not at all anxious." The operational definition of anxiety in this case would be the person's self-rating on the anxiety scale. Operational definitions of this sort permit scientists to make public the definitions they are using when they report their particular research. Not all operational definitions of anxiety must be of this self-report nature. Experimenters could make their own observations of a subject's anxiety or they could use a formal test of anxiety. Whatever the procedure, it would have to be made public so that conclusions drawn are meaningful to other scientists. In addition to understanding the procedures and conclusions, other scientists may wish to repeat or duplicate the experiment or research investigation to see whether or not the reported findings reappear in the new investigation. Operational definitions facilitate such attempts at replication.

PROBLEMS IN CONDUCTING THE EXPERIMENT

There are many factors—not necessarily planned and often unplanned—that affect outcome of an experiment. Some of these apply to situations in which experimenter or examiner and subject are in a controlled situation such as an experiment, psychological testing session, or a therapeutic situation. We shall refer to situations in which the experimenter or examiner interacts with a subject as E-S interactions.

Demand Characteristics

Most experimental and testing situations provide hidden and sometimes not-so-hidden cues that convey the purpose of the experiment (Orne, 1962). Because many people want to perform well, to be good subjects, they will often respond in a manner that they hope will help the experimenter. If they are able to pick up on any of the cues regarding the experimenter's hypothesis, they might respond in ways that will confirm the experimenter's expectations.

For example, imagine that an investigator is interested in knowing whether schizophrenics will make more bizarre stories in response to pictures than normal persons. The schizophrenic subjects may guess the hypothesis and deliberately give their imaginations free rein. Their responses might then, indeed, look more bizarre than those of the normals, but it would not be clear whether this would be due to their schizophrenic condition or to the demand characteristics of the study.

Biasing can occur, of course, in the other direction as well. Subjects may discern the experimenter's hypothesis and attempt to disconfirm it by responding in a manner contrary to that predicted by the experimenter. Even control subjects might know that they are controls by observing differences between themselves and the experimental subjects in the experimental conditions. They might modify their behavior in unknown ways—in ways, perhaps, of which both they and the experimenter are unaware.

One way of offsetting some of these problems in the experimental situation is referred to as the double blind procedure, in which neither the experimenter nor the subject knows the nature of the group—experimental or control—to which the subject has been assigned. For example, to evaluate the effects of certain medications on patients, some subjects are administered the actual medication and some are administered a placebo (a preparation containing no active ingredient). If neither the subject nor the experimenter knows beforehand which group is given what substance, there could be no influence on experimental outcome of this prior knowledge.

In abnormal psychology, problems inherent in the context of the experiment are of particular significance. They arise particularly in the treatment and psychological testing situations in which the clients or patients might attempt to modify their responses in accordance with what they think the clinician wants or does not want rather than in accordance with what is actually needed for the experiment—their own feelings, attitudes, and spontaneous wishes.

The Self-Fulfilling Prophecy

A self-fulfilling prophecy is ". . . a *false* definition of the situation evoking a behavior which makes the originally false conception come *true*" (Merton, 1948, p. 195). In other words, if one perceives a situation in a particular way, or erroneously expects a certain consequence in that situation, the likelihood is that the outcome will actually occur. Many anticipated fears, for example, may actually occur because the individual *expects* the situation to be fear producing. For example, a mother who is overprotective of, or lacks confidence in, her child—"Be careful, you will fall," or "You're sure to fail the test tomorrow because you haven't studied enough"—may indeed prove justified in her predictions because of how she structured the situation.

Self-fulfilling-prophecy effects are easily demonstrated in the laboratory in a variety of experimental contexts (Kintz, et al, 1965; Rosenthal, 1963, 1978; Rosenthal and Fode, 1963) in which it has been shown that the experimenter can unconsciously manipulate outcome in ways that are favorable to him or her. Teachers can also influence their students' achievement by encouraging them to meet their (the teachers') unconscious or conscious expectations for them: favorable expectations yield favorable results (Rosenthal and Jacobson, 1966, 1968), as well as the converse.

Similarly, in the treatment or testing of subjects, ample evidence exists to indicate that clinicians can influence the verbalizations, behavior, kinds of insights, and dreams their patients bring to the situation. These may be ways that are not necessarily planned or conscious on the part of either the clinician or client, but may play an important role in determining the outcome of the therapy or testing.

Some patients, for example, may adopt the mannerisms, style, and even goals and values of their therapists to please them—and be totally unaware of this process. What is even more surprising is that some therapists may be unaware of this possibility, stating only that their patients "seem to be progressing" or are becoming "better adjusted." Thus, although there is some question about the consistency of the empirical findings of the Rosenthal studies (see Cronbach, 1975; Wilkins, 1977) as applied to experimental and classroom situations, there seems to be striking evidence that such effects are quite prominent in the clinical situation. Later chapters will pursue this subject in greater detail.

Other Hidden Variables: The Scene, E-S Interactions, and Examiner Effects

In addition to the subjects' perceptions of the experiment and the presence of prophecies and wishes on the part of the experimenter or clinician, other variables have been shown to affect outcome and results of the experimental situation. These include: how the experimenter presents the task to the subject, the hidden hierarchical relationship of experimenter to subject, and various other E-S interactions that emerge on the basis of sex, race, age, or official status.

A subject being evaluated by a classroom volunteer will undoubtedly behave differently than if examined by the professor, for example. Differences in physical behavior (leaning across the desk or coffee table) and differences in protectiveness (female subjects are treated more protectively) have been demonstrated; and anxiety levels of experimenters have been shown to diminish with increased familiarity with their own experimental situations (Rosenthal, 1966, 1967). All of these might easily affect experimental outcomes.

The context of the situation—the scene—is also of some significance in determining outcome. Is the experiment taking place in a school? a prison? a hospital? an employment office? For example, a psychological evaluation of a troublesome child made in the principal's office might result in entirely different findings than a similar evaluation made in the after-school playgroup setting.

Subject Variables

Whether or not subjects are institutionalized against their will—in a prison or hospital, for example—also present variables that affect outcome of an experiment. On the other side of the coin are volunteer subjects who often provide the reservoir from which experimenters draw for study. Such studies yield conclusions frequently applied to subjects in general. The specific problems that arise when volunteer subjects are used in experiments have been described at length (Rosenthal and Rosnow, 1975). Spotlight 3.2 describes some of these problems.

Educational level and verbal productivity—factors related to SES—also influence a subject's response in the experimental, testing, and therapeutic situation. This inference has already been drawn from material presented in Chapter 2. Although many experimental situations can control for the influence of some of these factors—for example, by assigning subjects and experimenters to experimental groups in such ways as to minimize effects of intelligence, education, or various E-S interactions—most individual testing and therapy situations cannot build in such controls as readily.

Spotlight 3.2 The Volunteer as Subject: Just An "Average" Person?

In studying abnormal behavior, the focus is on increasing our understanding of why dysfunctions in human behavior come about, as well as in developing an understanding of the most effective ways of modifying these dysfunctions. For example, why are some people always angry? Was the behavior learned? Can the behavior be unlearned? Or, are those who suffer from anguishing headaches without apparent physical (organic) cause similar to one another in some way—in background, personality, or even in approach to solving problems?

To answer these questions, studying particular individuals in actual situations is the optimal research condition. But will these clinical cases come forward? Will they volunteer for a psychological study? And if some of them do, will they differ from those who did not? For example, would a group of substance abusers who volunteered for a study differ in important ways from the larger group of substance abusers (with unknown qualities) who did *not* volunteer?

Here is another illustration: How convinced would you be if someone told you that a careful study of twenty college seniors—all volunteers—disclosed that 90 percent of them had had homosexual experiences by the time they were fifteen years old? Wouldn't you wonder whether or not the volunteers represented the seniors in general?

Studies have demonstrated that people who volunteer for psychological studies have characteristics that distinguish them from nonvolunteers (Rosenthal and Rosnow, 1975). For example, this research found that volunteers, compared to nonvolunteers, tend to be better educated, more intelligent, more sociable, more in need of social approval, and generally of higher SES. According to Rosenthal and Rosnow, volunteers also tend to be more unconventional and more interested in "arousal-seeking" than nonvolunteers. In addition, males are less likely than females to volunteer for various studies, unless the research is "emotionally stressful," in which case the opposite is true.

These and other volunteer characteristics not mentioned here can affect research in several ways. One problem concerns making generalizations on the basis of research conducted with volunteers. To the extent that the characteristics of volunteers are not those of the population at large, such research results may be biased. For example,

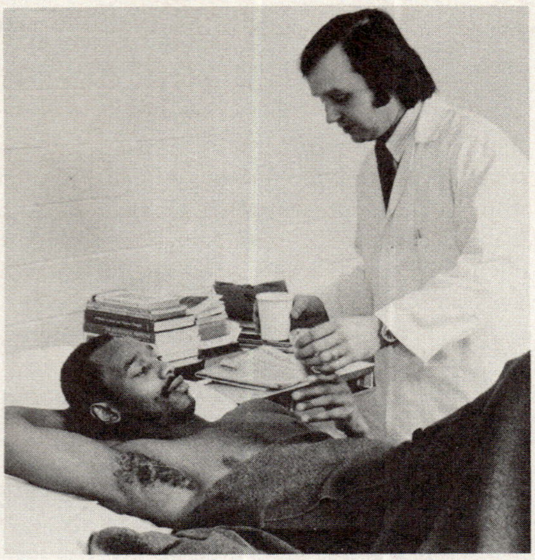

How representative a subject is this prison volunteer—and for what population of experimental subjects? (J. P. Laffont/Sygma)

research designed to study the influence of therapists on the verbal output of clients might be affected by volunteers' need for social approval. Also, volunteers may be particularly cooperative and thus more likely to be influenced by the experimenters' unconscious communications as to the response they (the experimenters) hope to find.

Still another problem, somewhat related to the first, is the problem of motivation of volunteers. Since personal motivation can affect performance on many tasks, volunteers who are motivated to participate in research will tend to perform in ways characteristic of highly motivated persons—with particular diligence and concentration, for example. This is not, however, the usual state of affairs; most people do not act on high levels of motivation all of the time.

All of this is not to say that research using volunteer subjects is without value. It simply means that consideration must always be given to the possibility that the known or unknown characteristics of volunteer subjects might have influenced research results.

SUMMARY

This chapter explained the importance of scientific inquiry—specifically, scientific method—in the pursuit of knowledge about the origins of abnormal behavior, and posited the scientific mode of inquiry as the best available method of examining the validity of various explanations. It also presented some of the assumptions, methods, and tools of science, including techniques for measuring and comparing data, and the experiment—a particularly powerful tool. The chapter also described other research methods, especially some of those used in abnormal psychology. Finally, it discussed problems in conducting the experiments and in interpreting their results as possible pitfalls in generalizing from specific findings.

Highlights

1. Scientific methods—a set of procedures and tools—offer the most powerful and rational approach to discovering "truths" about the world around us, including the "world" of abnormal behavior. An important assumption made by scientists is that there is an underlying orderliness and regularity in nature that one day can be made plain to investigators through systematic exploration and direct or indirect observation. Another assumption that scientists make is that empirical tests and proofs are superior to dogma, private opinion, and "expert" testimony in the pursuit of truths about the world around us.
2. Scientific methods, attitudes, and assumptions

cut across all disciplines and are not intrinsic to, let us say, the biological or physical sciences only. The rules of science are generally universally applicable.
3. "Good" theories are parsimonious, relate events previously considered to be unrelated, and lead to empirically verifiable hypotheses.
4. Scientific tools include measurement and statistics as well as the experiment. The latter consists of controlled observations of the consequences on one variable of manipulating another variable. The independent variable is the manipulated variable in the experiment, while its effects are measured in relation to the dependent variable. The experiment lets us examine causal connections between variables.
5. Most research in the field of abnormal behavior employs nonexperimental methods that are not precise enough to permit confidence in generalizing from the results. Yet innovative and ingenious explorations can yield many insights about pathological behavior and impart much about the degree of promise contained in a line of inquiry. Methods touched on include the clinical case study, single-subject experiments, contrasted groups method, retrospective studies, longitudinal and follow-up research, analogue experiments, and animal studies.
6. Statistics aid research by providing the means for comparing results of observations and experiments. They allow researchers to evaluate whether or not differences between groups could have been due to chance, and to assess the degree to which variables are correlated with each other.
7. Although many of the findings in abnormal psychology are of a correlational nature, the fact that two variables are correlated—overweight and depression, for example—does not imply causality. Further, correlations do not demonstrate the *direction* of causality—which causes what—or whether, perhaps, *both* variables are due to another cause.
8. Other rules and conventions of science relate to objectivity of methods of data collection, ethics in conducting inquiries, the use of operational definitions of terms, and reporting results of experiments accurately, without changing the data or their analysis to obtain a desired outcome.
9. There are many other factors that can affect the outcome of observations and experiments. These include demand characteristics, self-fulfilling prophecies, various subject and experimenter characteristics and interactions, and the use of volunteers as subjects.

ISSUES AND QUESTIONS

1. Often clinicians, such as therapists, depend on the scientist working behind the scenes to point the way toward diagnosis, treatment, cure, and the understanding of pathology. But the latest information in medication, advances in genetics, or treatment of depression may already be old by the time it filters down to the practitioner. Similarly, news articles in magazines such as *Time* or *Newsweek* about advances in the sciences, medicine, and abnormal psychology are usually outdated. A researcher or scientist may spend years in a line of research before his or her work is reported by the popular magazines. But by this time, the scientist has moved on in the particular endeavor or has taken a different research direction. Perhaps this is the reason many people think of the sciences as unconcerned with the everyday, real world. Have you ever thought about this researcher-practitioner-consumer lag?

   Popular magazines and the press often focus on some scientific discovery that may contain sensational overtones, playing it up for purposes other than imparting information. Sometimes these reports are premature, deceptive, and irresponsible in their simplistic presentation. Should there be some control over the media? Should control be left in the hands of the researcher? Think of the expenditure of money and the heartache that can result from a promise exaggerated in the media that is never fulfilled, let us say, with regard to a vitamin cure for schizophrenia or mental retardation.

2. Do you feel in awe and fearful of statistical methods? Does it help to regard statistical procedures as only a tool, a method, in the sciences rather than a scientific goal in itself?
3. You are studying anger in children as expressed toward each other and toward an authority, such as a teacher. You are now faced with the problem of measuring anger to test the hypothesis that excessively stern parents rear angry children. You have time, money, experimenters, and a classroom of eight-to-nine-year-old children. How will you operationally define (measure) anger or excessive sternness? Will you look at the child's overt behavior, such as hitting or shouting? Or will you look at excessive disciplinary measures on the part of parents, such as spanking? How will you account for the child who is sullenly and quietly angry, or the disapproving parent who never spanks his or her child?
4. Ethical research principles involve the obtaining of informed consent from the subject before research procedures begin. When consent is voluntarily obtained, the researcher might be lulled into thinking that the research about which the subject has been informed can then be conducted ethically. Further issues remain, however. For example, what does voluntary consent mean to a prisoner who wants to be viewed favorably by a parole board? What about psychology students who are required to participate in research for course credit and who give "voluntary" informed consent? In the discussion of different clinical subgroups (such as the mentally retarded) in subsequent chapters of this book, the questionable meaning of "voluntary" consent will be examined in greater detail.

   We can also point to special problems that concern scientists regarding the ethics of certain research procedures, even when informed consent has been obtained. One of these problems involves research that uses deception. Research in abnormal psychology involves people, and people have ways of guessing, modifying, distorting, and controlling their thinking and behavior as they interact with others and in various situations. Therefore, some psychological research procedures attempt to minimize these uncontrolled variations by deceiving the subject. For example, in research about effects of alcohol on sexual arousal, the control subjects would be given nonalcoholic beverages but told they are drinking alcoholic beverages. For the experiment to be effective, they could not be told to behave *as if* they were drinking alcohol. Some people argue strongly against research that uses deception. How do you feel about this?
5. The ethical issue over the use of deception in research is only one of several that are currently being debated in the scientific community. Not all of these issues have been resolved. Many principles have emerged from this debate, however, encouraged by the efforts of the National Commission for the Protection of Human Subjects of Biomedical and Behavioral Research, mandated by Congress in 1974. Here are some of those issues and principles:
   a. Children, the mentally infirm, and the mentally retarded are frequent subjects for research study. Neither a court of law, a guardian, nor a parent should offer these subjects to a research team if the subject refuses, especially if there is even minimum risk of hurt or injury. This principle is to be safeguarded unless participation in the research is essential for the life or health of the child. But who is to decide the latter?
   b. Another principle is one that establishes the routine procedure of imparting the results of the research to all participants, possibly

even during the study (as long as the research would not be spoiled) but certainly after the research is terminated.

c. Researchers should seriously question the use of prisoners and other institutionalized populations for drug research.

d. Researchers should inform subjects about the possible side effects, risks, and dangers before their participation in a study. The United States Army violated this principle when it gave various hallucinatory drugs to hundreds of soldiers without informing them of possible risks. Further, the Army conducted only minimal follow-up on the eventual outcome and consequences of the research for each of the subjects.

e. One common ethical research practice is for the investigator to ingest a sample of any chemical or medicine he or she plans to administer to subjects before the actual investigation. This try-it-yourself-first policy is not always of scientific value, however. Since the medication is usually designed to control pathology or symptoms (to reduce anxiety or counteract heroin addiction, for example), how would it help to know that the "normal" investigator was not affected adversely by the chemical substance?

f. How can adherence to the foregoing principles be safeguarded? What kinds of controls can be instituted to insure the protection of subjects in research projects that are not funded by public moneys? Should there be a "scientific court" to rule on these issues?

6. Can socially useful, even imperative, research ever be justified if it violates some of the above principles? For example, the Army justified its research with the mind-altering drug LSD on unsuspecting soldiers on the basis of its relevance to the national security. Because this substance could be used against us, the Army claimed, we need to know how to diagnose its use and counteract its effects. The Army claimed that if subjects had been informed of the purposes of the LSD experiments, the findings would have been invalidated. How does one attempt to solve this and related problems?

7. Sometimes the experimental treatment is useful in its potential to control disturbing, anguishing, abnormal behavior—intractable pain or anxiety, overwhelming or paralyzing fear, or an acute schizophrenic episode, for example. If individuals in some clinical groups (the acute schizophrenics, for instance) are randomly assigned to a medication group and others to a control group, are not members of the control group being deprived of a useful, beneficial medication? On the other hand, scientists owe society *repeated* demonstrations of clinical and experimental effectiveness of treatments before approving commercial production and sales. How is this dilemma resolved?

   Some scientists support a policy of stringent research that sometimes overlooks the immediate health needs of the subjects. The long-range benefits of research to society, they claim, is a broad, humanitarian goal involving the increase of knowledge, the enhancement of human dignity, and the eventual reduction of human pathology. What do you think? Does this represent an overriding ethic that can stand on its own?

8. Concerns also arise regarding the use of animals in research that investigate the effects of drugs, electrical stimulation, alcohol ingestion, and various brain interventions on behavior in order to shed light on human pathology. In 1976, for example, The American Museum of Natural History in New York City was the object of militant, angry protests involving many public figures when some aspects of research conducted by two staff members became known; the research concerned the sexual behavior of cats, which were being studied physiologically through surgical removal of some of their glands, nerves, or brain tissue. It was argued that such research was trivial, irrelevant,

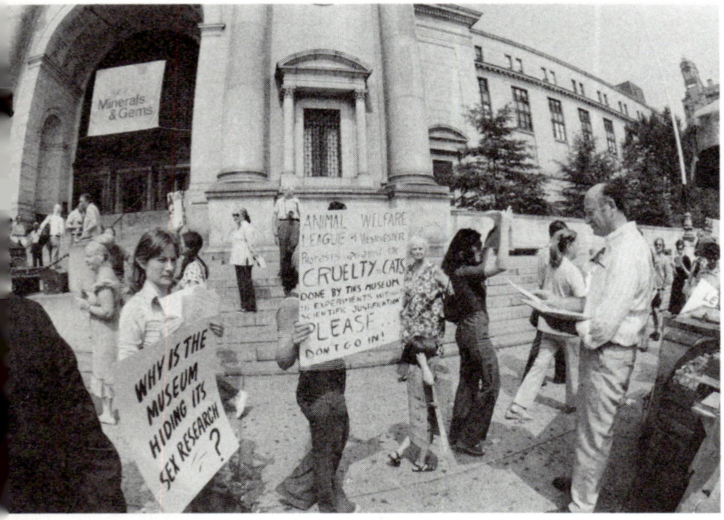

Demonstrators at the Museum of Natural History in New York City in 1976. In recent years many people have raised issues in connection with conducting scientific research using animals. Would you join these demonstrators? (United Press International Photo)

and useless. Who should decide the ultimate significance of a series of researches—the public or other scientists? Some animal research has shed great light on human health problems with regard to cancer-producing substances, the effects of alcohol and nicotine on the body, the origins of aggressive behavior, and the effectiveness of drugs in controlling certain symptoms.

Much of what we know about the human brain and its functions also comes from work with animals. Should there be rules that apply especially to household pets like dogs and cats and higher animals like monkeys and apes? Where do you stand on this issue of animal rights?

SUGGESTIONS FOR FURTHER READING

Agnew, N. M., and Pyke, S. W. *The science game: An introduction to research in the behavioral sciences.* 2nd ed. Englewood Cliffs, N. J.: Prentice-Hall, 1978. This engaging book presents the basics of science in a way that highlights its human content. It provides the fundamentals of experimental and quasi-experimental design, statistics, and theory testing. Clear and interesting examples illustrate the major points. The student who wants to learn more about the practice of science will find this book enjoyable.

American Psychological Association. *Ethical principles in the conduct of research with human participants.* Washington, D. C.: American Psychological Association, 1973. This little booklet describes in clear, direct language, with many illustrations from actual incidents and researches, ten ethical principles that experimenters should adhere to when conducting research with human subjects. For example, Principle 3 states that ethical practice requires the investigator to inform the participant of all features of the research that reasonably might be expected to influence willingness to participate and to explain all other aspects of the research about which the participant inquires. Failure to comply with this principle of "informed consent" greatly increases the investigator's responsibility to protect the welfare and dignity of the research participant. Principle 9 states that where research procedures may result in undesirable consequences for the participant, the investigator has the responsibility to detect and remove or correct these consequences, including, where relevant, long-term after-effects. This booklet is highly recommended—almost a must—for those who wish to do research in abnormal psychology.

Barber, T. X. *Pitfalls in human research: Ten pivotal points.* New York: Pergamon, 1976. Paperback. In this book, the author concisely and briefly (in 90 pages) presents ten major factors that may bias the outcome of research with human subjects. Each factor is simply described, examples demonstrating how that factor has affected research results are given, and finally, procedures for controlling those factors are suggested. This straightforward, readable book can serve both as an introduction to experimenter effects for students and as an efficient handbook for researchers.

Deese, J. *Psychology as science and art.* New York: Harcourt Brace Jovanovich, 1972. Paperback. This little book is for those interested in pursuing certain issues regarding scientific method. The author questions the value of applying strict scientific methods, especially the experiment, to the study of behavior. He states that we assume that independent variables influence dependent variables because experimental situations are controlled and do not therefore allow for the myriad hidden possibilities that might account for the actual research findings. Further, placing natural phenomena into a laboratory situation is itself questionable—yet we do it all the time. For example, it is probably of little value to generalize from subjects' anxiety levels during an experiment to the anxiety a schizophrenic patient, in acute panic, experiences in a real-life situation. Our experiments, Deese says, often provide us only with limited, sometimes artificial, glimpses into the laws of nature.

Kuhn, T. S. *The structure of scientific revolutions.* Chicago: University of Chicago Press, 1962. Paperback available. Referred to by many as a classic, this short work contains Kuhn's analysis of the history and progress of science and is important reading for anyone interested in taking a close look at the scientific process. Drawing largely upon literature related to the physical sciences, this book is not easy reading, but well worth the effort. While Kuhn's analysis is convincing, it is nonetheless only one view of how science proceeds.

Rosenthal, R. *Experimenter effects in behavioral research.* Enlarged ed. New York: Irvington, 1976. This author was among the first of a group of scientists concerned with identifying and studying the biasing effect experimenters can have on the outcomes of their research. In this book, Rosenthal explains what experimenter effects are, reviews the numerous studies of those effects, and finally offers suggestions for controlling them. As a detailed and thorough account of an important aspect of research methodology, this book is a useful reference for further study in this area.

4

Diagnosis of Abnormal Behavior

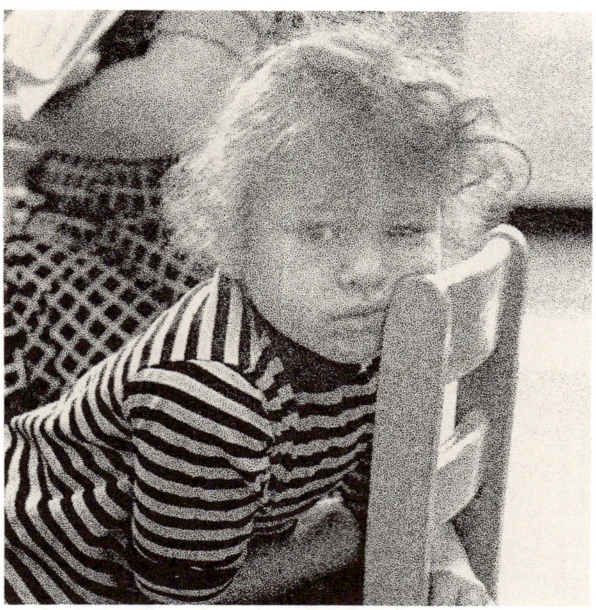

Peter, a college sophomore, complained of frequent dizziness, fainting spells, headaches, and periods of forgetfulness. The college health officer made a tentative diagnosis of some kind of brain dysfunction and had him hospitalized for further medical tests.

A middle-aged couple was referred to a specialized service for marriage counseling. The woman, after twenty-five years of marriage, was preparing to leave her husband who during the previous six months had become increasingly abusive and assaultive, apparently with little provocation. She thought he was becoming "psychotic."

Margie, a pretty, high-school senior who had had a moderately good academic record and had been a popular cheerleader was referred to the guidance counselor. She had been cutting classes, failing to bring in homework assignments, and lying to her teachers. She was described as listless, moody, and "not with it" most of the time. The teacher who referred her thought that Margie was having a "nervous breakdown."

An excitable, abusive, hyperactive child was doing so poorly at school and was so disruptive in the classroom that he was placed in a special class. He was tentatively labeled by the school principal as having "minimal brain damage" in conjunction with a "learning disability."

These individuals were referred for further study through interviewing, examination, or testing of one sort or another. They were fortunate. In each instance, a sensitive and discerning clinician picked up on cues derived from the patients' responses in a special clinical situation that employs various methods and techniques in order to arrive at an accurate evaluation of their pathology. Certain diagnoses—explanations for the unexpected or disordered behavior—were ruled out by these methods and others became more likely. These procedures—often called differential diagnoses—led in each instance to suggestions for treatment, contained some implications for the kind of recovery that could be expected, and resulted in arresting or reversing the difficulty.

It was determined that Peter, the college sophomore, was suffering from an acute anxiety condition, not a brain tumor, that was affecting his physical and bodily well-being in dramatic ways and was disrupting his ability to remember, solve problems, and concentrate. Several months of psychotherapy alleviated these symptoms.

The middle-aged man's irritability, chronic anger, and occasional violent outbursts were found to result from a malignancy in the brain. The tumor was surgically removed, his behavior changed dramatically, and he and his wife are now preparing to celebrate their thirtieth wedding anniversary in Hawaii.

Margie, the pretty, high-school senior, was found to be an alcoholic. She is undergoing specialized treatment with a group of other teenage alcoholics and is on the road to recovery.

The boy with minimal brain damage and a learning disability was actually suffering from his extremely disorganized, slum background. His mother, a prostitute and drug abuser was rarely home, and when she was, her "johns" were with her. She beat the child mercilessly when he asked for food, and he was always hungry, depressed, and lonely—overwhelmed and bewildered by his world. Now in a foster home, he is doing at least average work in school, and his teachers claim that his above-average intelligence will one day allow him to do even better. He shows no evidence of brain damage.

Making a diagnosis does not necessarily involve typical procedures that all clinicians follow. However, some system or scheme for classifying and categorizing abnormal behavior is generally employed. There are many advantages to having an objective system for classifying abnormal behavior. For the clinician, the hope is to organize or categorize information in order to provide the most effective treatment and the most accurate prognosis. For the researcher, if subjects are properly classified, a search for common factors leading to knowledge about causes and treatment is made possible. These are ideal states, however, and deviations from these ideal conditions are the rule rather than the exception.

Because different societies have different standards by which to judge behaviors, differing views of the nature of a disorder may be derived from the same symptoms. Pathology may be expressed in a

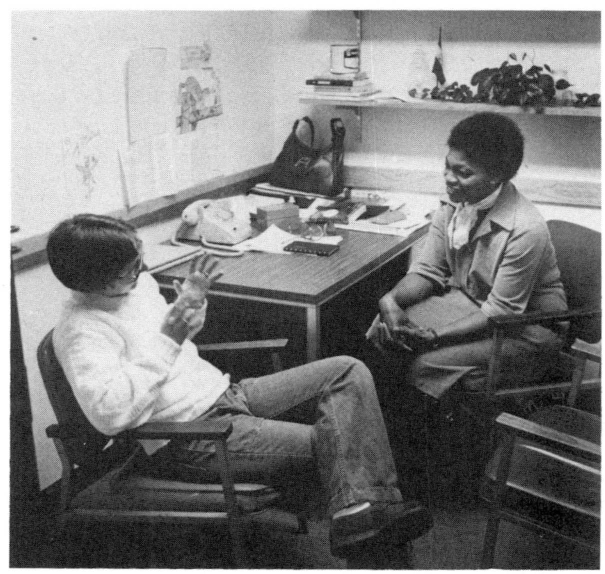

Diagnostic procedures, if reliable and valid, can be extremely important in determining the appropriate treatment. (© 1979 Eric A. Roth/The Picture Cube)

variety of ways, depending on the times and the cultures; and fashions and fads are not unusual.

Even within the same cultural contexts, wide shifts occur from decade to decade in the kinds of diagnoses regarded as popular. For example, from 1954 to 1974, the diagnosis of affective (mood) disorders—such as some forms of depression—increased threefold in one large mental hospital (Blum, 1978).

In general, then, the social context often determines whether or not someone is regarded as sane or insane, an issue emphasized in Chapters 1 and 2.

Dissatisfaction with Diagnostic Systems: Validity and Reliability

The use of diagnoses in dealing with patients—that is, classifying or grouping them according to some scheme (such as psychoneurotic or psychotic), with appropriate subtypes—has been the subject of considerable controversy. Diagnostic systems are said to be crude and unstable, subjectively interpreted, and there is often wide disagreement among the experts as to their use. Even when agreement exists, the ultimate accuracy of the diagnosis may be difficult to determine. These dissatisfactions and criticisms generally revolve around questions of reliability and validity.

Reliability. Do clinicians and experts agree on the diagnosis of a particular patient? Is there a consensus about how certain symptoms are viewed; that is, do they always specify a particular diagnosis? For example, do experts always diagnose schizophrenia if there are hallucinations, or depression if there is apathy, weight loss, and a depletion of energy? These considerations—the degree of agreement among or between diagnosticians—are questions that concern reliability. Stated another way, reliability may be regarded as the consistency with which patients are classified.

Many reviews of empirical agreement and disagreement in the diagnostic statements of different experts (for example, Arthur, 1969; Spitzer and Fleiss, 1974; Zigler and Phillips, 1961; and Zubin, 1967) demonstrate that there is generally poor agreement between and among them. This type of estimate of diagnostic agreement (inter-rater reliability), however, tends to vary from diagnostic category to category. For example, there tend to be higher agreement for organic diagnoses (those that indicate a physical basis for the disturbance) and lower agreement for diagnoses of nonorganic conditions. When all diagnostic categories are combined, the evidence suggests that the percentage agreement varies from about 40 to 85 percent, depending on the particular investigator.

Many factors determine the reliability of diagnoses. The less complex the dimension being judged (for example, depth of depression) or the closer the rated trait is to actual behavior (for example, restlessness and breathing difficulties), or the more severe the disturbance (for example major convulsions daily), the greater the likelihood of high reliability. On the other hand, although very broad categories of differential diagnosis elicit high agreement (for example, psychotic versus general personality problems), very poor agreement is found when specific diagnostic subtypes are rated (Schmidt and Fonda, 1956). That is, clinicians might show high agreement when designating one patient as flagrantly psychotic and another as not, but may disagree regarding the particular type of psychosis the patient is showing; or, if there is agreement that the pathology is schizophrenic, the type of schizophrenia displayed may be in question. In other words, complex problems, subtypes within diagnostic categories, and what is referred to as middle-range (not extreme or flagrant) diagnoses—a range that probably applies to the vast number of people who come for help—are not rated reliably, even by experts.

Thus the level of agreement among the experts with regard to rating or classifying disturbed behavior or people according to some diagnostic system, is not high. Researchers have thus painted a complex and many-faceted picture of reliability. Some additional features of this portrait of reliability are presented in Spotlight 4.1.

Spotlight 4.1 Reliability of Diagnosis: Not a Rosy Picture

The general picture of reliability of diagnostic statements, we have noted, has not been very promising. For example, the severity of the pathology, the type of diagnosis being made, and the simplicity or narrowness of the dimension being rated are all related to the reliability obtained when the experts are compared. Agreement among experts employing the conventional classification systems has not only been disappointingly low but has also been shown to fluctuate with certain conditions and situations. Some of these conditions, and some additional problems that enter into the assessment of reliability, follow.

1. Agreement among diagnosticians tends to vary with the setting—whether, for example, it is an extremely busy clinical outpatient facility or a research center with nonemergency cases and plenty of time for training and study.

2. Agreement also tends to vary with the orientation of the rater—whether, for example, he or she is a diagnostician only or a therapist only, and the particular views he or she might have about the origin of the pathology. The more rigorously trained or older experts yield higher agreement, for example.

3. The confidence with which the diagnosis is made is also related to the amount of the agreement. High-confidence ratings tend to be associated with moderate to extremely high agreement, whereas the opposite is true when there is low confidence.

4. Regional and geographical variations also occur with regard to diagnostic agreement—not only from country to country but also within a particular country.

5. Another consideration concerning how to evaluate findings of agreement or disagreement is the problem of base rates—the frequency of diagnoses made within a hospital, community, or country. Fluctuation of base rates should come as no surprise, since we have already described the fact that diagnostic fads, styles, and preferences exist, depending on which group of diagnosticians one is considering.

By ascertaining the base rates of a particular setting, we can make a diagnosis that has fairly high agreement with the experts in that setting. For example, by sheer knowledge of base rates alone—that a hospital staff, let us say, uses a diagnosis of schizophrenia in 70 percent of its cases—a rater who classified all patients (even without seeing them) as schizophrenic would be in agreement with the clinicians at the hospital 70 percent of the time. The high reliability (or agreement) figures thus obtained would tell us little about the actual reliability of the diagnosis of schizophrenia.

6. There is generally poor agreement about the significance of many symptoms. Although a fairly high degree of agreement exists concerning the presence or absence of certain simple symptoms, such as headaches, the universality of such symptoms lessens their usefulness in distinguishing different diagnostic groups.

7. Consistency of diagnoses for a patient over a period of time also falls on a fairly low level. However, consistency is generally regarded as a poor criterion of reliability, since assessing the nature of the problem is difficult: patients may change over a period of time, their disease process may alter without treatment over time, or the patient may change as a result of medication or other forms of treatment.

Validity. Since validity concerns the accuracy, "truth," and predictive usefulness of a diagnosis, it is even more difficult to assess than reliability. There is ample evidence demonstrating that many diagnoses do not accomplish the purposes for which they are intended—that is, suggest the etiology or cause, indicate the course of the disease, and lead directly to a program for treatment. In any event, critics claim that diagnoses reveal little about the whole person and his or her problems and what to do about them.

This book is concerned with the validity of diagnoses—how close we are to approximating actual knowledge about the nature of a particular category such as drug addiction or depression or mental retardation. Reliability in relation to diagnoses has been the subject of more empirical exploration than validity because, despite many problems, reliability is easier to measure or assess. It is important to note that if a diagnosis has low reliability it automatically must have low validity. On the other hand, if a diagnosis has high reliability, this does not automatically signify high validity; it might even have *low* validity. If, for example, all blue-eyed people were diagnosed as schizophrenic, this procedure would have extremely high reliability, but very low validity.

Overview of diagnosis. Most experts agree that serious problems exist regarding the use of diagnoses and diagnostic statements and that their reliability and validity are open to further question and exploration.

The issue of clinical diagnosis is such a complex, controversial, and yet crucial issue. . . . It is readily apparent that any research on diagnostic groups, for example, schizophrenia or manic-depressive psychosis, can be no better than the validity or meaningfulness of the diagnoses secured and used. This problem has plagued research in this area for many years. On the one hand, systematic and reliable classification of subjects facilitates research and the accumulation of potentially meaningful data about types of psychopathology. On the other hand, if the classification scheme used for such research is beset with problems of clarity, reliability, and validity, the results based on such classification are bound to be limited in their usefulness. An unreliable and loose scheme is bound to produce unreliable and variable results. The most highly quantified data and the most exacting statistical analyses cannot provide worthwhile conclusions if the assumptions or foundation on which they are based are weak (Garfield, 1978, p. 606).

Many practitioners, however, feel the need for *some* diagnostic system as do many researchers, although they deplore adherence to diagnostic methods that have been shown to be subjective, unreliable, and frequently of little value in helping people to solve their problems (Garmezy, 1978; Spitzer and Fleiss, 1974; Zubin, 1967; Zubin, et al., 1975; and Zubin, 1977–1978).

THE DSM-III

In order to improve the poor record of earlier diagnostic systems, intensive efforts have been directed toward developing classification schemes that are open to empirical study and validation. To aid in this goal, elaborate attempts have been made to specify in great detail the characteristics that comprise each of the diagnostic categories and subcategories. One such diagnostic system is the Third Edition of The *Diagnostic and Statistical Manual* (DSM-III) of the American Psychiatric Association (1980). Whether these efforts will in the long run demonstrate improvement over earlier systems is yet to be seen.

Description

The DSM-III was developed over a period of years by a special committee of the American Psychiatric Association to improve upon the classification of mental disorders in the DMS-II (1968). Dissatisfaction with the use of DSM-II was apparent; major criticisms concerned its unreliability and its failure to provide, except in vague detail, the specific characteristics and objective criteria of its diagnostic types and subtypes.

The DSM-III was developed in conjunction with a system used by the World Health Organization and their categories overlap to some extent. Detailed specification in the DSM-III of objective criteria for making a diagnosis represents a distinct advance over earlier versions. As a result, however, it is extremely long and detailed. Listing 4.1 presents the major categories of the DSM-III and Appendixes A and B list the complete DSM-III and DSM-II diagnostic codes. The major differences between the DSM-II and DSM-III will be touched on

Listing 4.1 General Diagnostic Categories in the DSM-III: Axes I and II*

Axis I

Disorders Usually First Evident in Infancy, Childhood, or Adolescence
- Mental retardation
- Attention deficit disorder
- Conduct disorder
- Anxiety disorders of childhood or adolescence
- Other disorders of infancy, childhood, or adolescence
- Eating disorders
- Stereotyped movement disorders
- Other disorders with physical manifestations
- Pervasive developmental disorders

Organic Mental Disorders
- Dementias arising in the senium and presenium
- Substance-induced

Substance Use Disorders

Schizophrenic Disorders

Paranoid Disorders

Psychotic Disorders Not Elsewhere Classified

Neurotic Disorders are now included in Affective, Anxiety, Somatoform, Dissociative, and Psychosexual disorders below

Affective Disorders

Anxiety Disorders

Somatoform Disorders

Dissociative Disorders (or Hysterical Neuroses, Dissociative Type)

Psychosexual Disorders

Factitious Disorder

Disorders of Impulse Control

Adjustment Disorder

Axis II

In Children (Primarily)

Specific Developmental Disorders
- Developmental reading disorder
- Developmental arithmetic disorder
- Developmental language disorder
- Developmental articulation disorder
- Mixed specific developmental disorder
- Atypical specific developmental disorder

In Adults (Primarily)

Personality Disorders
- Paranoid
- Schizoid
- Schizotypal
- Histrionic
- Narcissistic
- Antisocial
- Borderline
- Avoidant
- Dependent
- Compulsive
- Passive-Aggressive
- Atypical, mixed or other personality disorder

* *Note:* A detailed listing of the diagnostic categories of the DSM-III is presented in Appendix A. Appendix B presents the DSM-II (1968) diagnostic categories. Appendix C presents the major differences between the DSM-II and the DSM-III. Almost all of the categories listed in Listing 4.1 (DSM-III) are described in detail in the chapters that follow.

in the chapters that follow, and Appendix C presents a detailed description of the differences in each diagnostic area.

The DSM-III was evaluated in over one hundred clinical facilities with regard to its practical use. The ultimate validity and reliability of these categories, however, remains an unanswered research question.

According to its developers (see Spitzer, Sheehy, and Endicott, 1977), one of the chief advantages of the DSM-III is that it requires its users to rate any particular patient along several dimensions. The DSM-III, it is claimed, thus acknowledges the complexities of people and their behavior; the system also acknowledges that people interact with their social environments as well as the fact that many processes can be occurring simultaneously. A person with ulcers, for example, can also manifest depression and may be suffering from great anxiety because of joblessness and marital problems.

The diagnostic use of the DSM-III requires that patients be rated on each of five "axes". Axes I and II include the formal clinical syndromes. Axis I covers all the usual categories (such as schizophrenic disorders or organic mental disorders) and Axis II covers the personality disorders (adults) and specific developmental disorders (children). It is assumed that ratings on Axis I refer to the *principal* diagnosis, unless otherwise indicated; that is, if the principal diagnosis is made on Axis II, this must be specifically stated. When there is *no* diagnosis on Axis II, this must also be made explicit. Axis III requires a statement about the presence of any physical disorder or condition. Axis IV requires a rating of the severity of psychosocial stressors. And Axis V requires a rating for the highest level of adaptive functioning during the past year. These ratings require that the clinician consider stressful events in the patient's life as well as the level of performance the patient had previously shown in meeting the demands of his or her world. In this way, the clinician has more information for the determination of appropriate treatment goals.

How is the DSM-III used? A twenty-year-old student, for example, might be classified on Axis I as having a specific type of schizophrenic disorder as determined by several pages of objective description. This patient, however, also shows some compulsive traits, such as need for perfectionism and neatness, and is reserved and tends to establish formal relationships with others. The patient is therefore classified on Axis II as showing a compulsive personality disorder. A minor cardiac condition and anemia are physical conditions noted on Axis III.

Axes IV and V are the most relevant for our purposes, but they are presented with very little detail and illustration. This remains one of the criticisms leveled against DSM-III. Tables 4.1 and 4.2 present Axes IV and V.

Our patient receives a rating of 7 on Axis IV: catastrophic. His mother, father, and little sister were killed in an automobile accident. He was given a rating of 2 (very good), however, on Axis V because his performance as a student was excellent during the months before the accident; he received good grades, led a student organization, and achieved financial independence through part-time work and a scholarship.

The knowledge of the castastrophic event in the patient's life, together with an appraisal indicating how well he functioned prior to the catastrophe, permitted the therapist to set up an intensive treatment plan for this bewildered student that had as a goal reinstating his previous level of good functioning. This was accomplished by daily, brief contacts with an understanding, warm counselor over a period of months. These contacts provided him with an opportunity to express his grief openly and without shame, to make immediate daily plans for study and free time, and gradually to re-enter his busy world of academic and social activities without guilt.

Evaluation

While it is too soon to review the validity, reliability, and practical usefulness of the DSM-III as a classificatory system, it has nonetheless provoked a flurry of criticism from psychologists everywhere (Achenbach and Edelbrock, 1978; Garmezy, 1978; Salzinger, 1977; Schact and Nathan, 1977; and Zubin, 1977–1978). Here are some of the highlights of these criticisms:

1. Inclusion or lack of inclusion of any particular diagnostic category in this system was not based on assessing its reliability, nor are there built-in techniques for assessing reliability.

2. The relationship of culture and SES to dis-

Table 4.1 Axis IV of the DSM-III: Severity of Psychosocial Stressors*

Code	*Term*	*Adult Examples*	*Child or Adolescent Examples*
1	None	No apparent psychosocial stressor	No apparent psychosocial stressor
2	Minimal	Minor violation of the law; small bank loan	Vacation with family
3	Mild	Argument with neighbor; change in work hours	Change in school teacher; new school year
4	Moderate	New career; death of close friend; pregnancy	Chronic parental fighting; change to new school; birth of sibling
5	Severe	Serious illness in self or family; major financial loss; marital separation; birth of a child	Death of peer; divorce of parents; arrest; hospitalization; persistent and harsh parental discipline
6	Extreme	Death of a close relative; divorce	Death of parent or sibling; repeated physical or sexual abuse
7	Catastrophic	Concentration camp experience; natural disaster	Multiple family deaths
0	Unspecified	No information, or not applicable	No information, or not applicable

**Axis III, not presented, requires a code for any physical condition the subject manifests. Axis IV, according to the DSM-III "provides a coding of the overall severity of a stressor judged to have been a significant contributor to the development or exacerbation of the current disorder. An individual's prognosis may be better when a disorder develops as a consequence of a severe stressor than when it develops after no stressor or a minimal stressor."*

turbed behavior is not even considered in this system, nor is the list of the psychosocial stressors in the patient's history concerned with actual research findings in this area that might shed light on the relationship of environmental stress and pathology.

3. The criteria for diagnosing a particular subtype are too simple, too inclusive, and not necessarily representative of the reservoir of empirical knowledge available.

4. Practitioners who use the system are given no instruction, no special understanding of the general problems in making a diagnosis. The DSM-III thus perpetuates the myth about the accuracy of the medical model of diagnosis.

5. An incorrect assumption is that this system is "true" or valid, rather than simply a practical and convenient working model for the practitioner. One criticism notes the definitive aura surrounding the DSM-III, which implies that this system can accurately classify all non-normal behavior. In fact, many exceptions have been found. The categories for schizophrenia, for example, have been especially singled out as appearing to be more precise, objective, and reliable than is warranted by empirical evidence (Morey and Blashfield, 1981). In addition, some of the descriptive criteria for schizophrenia have been found to apply to *other* psychotic states as well, and therefore cannot be used with confidence in defining schizophrenia.

6. An important dimension that is omitted is response to treatment (often a crucial test of diagnostic validity), especially in regard to some of the chemical treatments of the major psychoses and some forms of depression (see Chapters 10–12 and 21).

7. The DSM-III does not confront the question of what is abnormal and what is normal—an issue raised in Chapter 1. On what grounds does this system clearly delineate abnormal from normal? What is actually being classified?

8. Another criticism holds that the inclusion of several axes by which to judge patients provides an

Table 4.2 Axis V of the DSM-III: Highest Level of Adaptive Functioning Past Year*

Levels	*Adult Examples*	*Child or Adolescent Examples*
1 Superior Unusually effective functioning in social relations, occupational functioning, and use of leisure time	Single parent living in deteriorating neighborhood takes excellent care of children and home, has warm relations with friends, and finds time for pursuit of hobby	12-year-old girl gets superior grades in school, is extremely popular among her peers, and excels in many sports. She does all of this with apparent ease and comfort
2 Very good Better-than-average functioning in social relations, occupational functioning, and use of leisure time	A 65-year-old retired widower does some volunteer work, often sees old friends, and pursues hobbies	An adolescent boy gets excellent grades, works part time, has several close friends, and plays banjo in the jazz band. He admits to some distress in "keeping up with everything"
3 Good No more than slight impairment in either social or occupational functioning	A woman with many friends functions extremely well at a difficult job, but says "the strain is too much"	An 8-year-old boy does well in school, has several friends, but bullies younger children.
4 Fair Moderate impairment in either social relations or occupational functioning, or some impairment in both	A lawyer has trouble carrying out assignments, has several acquaintances, but hardly any close friends	A 10-year-old girl does poorly in school, but has adequate peer and family relations
5 Poor Marked impairment in either social relations or occupational functioning, or moderate impairment in both	A man with one or two friends has trouble keeping a job for more than a few weeks	A 14-year-old boy almost fails in school and has trouble getting along with his peers
6 Very poor Marked impairment in both social relations and occupational functioning	A woman is unable to do any of her housework and has violent outbursts toward family and neighbors	A 6-year-old girl needs special help in all subjects and has virtually no peer relationships
7 Grossly impaired Gross impairment in virtually all areas of functioning	An elderly man needs supervision to maintain minimal personal hygiene and is usually incoherent	A 4-year-old boy needs constant restraint to avoid hurting himself and is almost totally lacking in language skills
0 Unspecified	No information	No information

**According to the DSM-III, coding on Axis V "permits the clinician to indicate his or her judgment of an individual's highest level of adaptive functioning (for at least a few months) during the past year. This information frequently has prognostic significance, because usually an individual returns to his or her previous level of adaptive functioning after an episode of illness."*

erroneous impression that the complexities of human behavior are being successfully handled and judged, when in actuality, the axes comprise overlapping, simplified ratings of extremely complex aspects of human behavior. They ignore, for example, the influential impact of poverty and slum life on an individual's behavior or on level of adaptive functioning.

9. Another criticism has been leveled at the inclusion of specific developmental disorders (for example, arithmetic or reading disorder) in the list of diagnostic categories. Are these in fact mental disorders? The DSM-III has been regarded as particularly inadequate in its categories of childhood and adolescent disorders (Foltz, 1980; Achenbach and Edelbrock, 1978). Some of the problems raised concern the limited consideration of reliability evidence as well as inadequate attention to a large body of empirical data about childhood problems.

10. And finally, the DSM-III has become exhaustively long—a nonparsimonious classification scheme that may have lost its original purpose. For example, there are now 230 categories for mental disorder (compared to 145 in the DSM-II). Almost every possible deviance or difference appears in the current listing, including many that critics claim are hardly mental disorders at all. The difficulty in establishing nonartificial lines between normal and abnormal is clearly seen in the differing nature of what was included in the DSM-II and what now appears in DSM-III. Artificial distinctions between and among categories have thus arisen.

This artificiality may have crept in because of practical needs rather than scientific interests. . . . Entrenched clinical practice and such considerations as utility, ease of application, acceptability to practitioners, third-party payments, professional considerations, and other extraneous influences . . . threaten to thwart the original scientific thrust (Zubin, 1977–1978, p. 5).

LABELING AND THE MEDICAL MODEL REVISITED

Diagnostic practices, even if reliable, are under attack for reasons that go beyond the sorts of criticisms noted above. Opponents of the medical model state that the very process of diagnosing individuals,—that is, labeling them as if emotional conflicts and problems are reflections of disease—locks people into categories that stigmatize them. This point of view notes that labels tend to persist for long periods of time, even when the emotional conflict or deviant behavior diminishes or disappears entirely. For example, labeling a child as having a "conduct disorder" or "learning disability" implies a disease process that affects the child even when that child is symptom-free. Labeling individuals, rather than behavior, is thus a serious problem in most diagnostic systems.

Some problematic aspects of the labeling process were touched on in Chapter 1. Spotlight 4.2 returns to these considerations by focusing on the work of two active opponents of labeling and diagnosis, Thomas Szasz and David Rosenhan.

Spotlight 4.2 Thomas Szasz and David Rosenhan: Articulate Opponents of Diagnosis and Labeling

1. Thomas Szasz, a psychiatrist and social philosopher, has been a relentless opponent of the medical model for several decades (1960, 1961, 1963, 1964, 1965). In his view, mental illness is a metaphor; behavior cannot be called sick; and there is no such thing as mental illness.

Szasz has been severely critical of the concept of viewing emotional problems as *disease*. He also was among the first ranks of those opposed to the incarceration of the so-called mentally ill and, in many instances, of their consequent loss of civil rights.

Szasz's view of symptoms is that they reflect interpersonal and social reactions—that is, problems of communication rather than disease processes. Symptoms are simply feelings, ideas, behaviors, and inclinations that are considered undesirable or alien by others—relatives or experts, for example (who may or may not be in sympathy with the patient).

Szasz's original thesis, which he developed as a philosophy of behavior, states that the "mental" difficulties people may experience are concerned with difficulties in following the rules imposed by one's culture. Personal deviations from such rules, he continues, should be handled (if the culture so wishes) by legal or other standards, but not by the use of a psychiatric label or by hospitalization. Terms like sanity, insanity, and mental illness are pejorative; they victimize the labeled people who then become society's scapegoats.

Rather than advocating that the rights of the mentally ill should be protected and that the laws of commitment should be humanized, Szasz feels that *all* individuals should be protected against the possibility of being diagnosed and labeled.

2. Although many observers of the mental health scene share Szasz's general views, a dramatic demonstration of his position received a flurry of attention in the scientific community. This was a study by Rosenhan (1973), who sought to confirm empirically the notion that the differentiation of sane from insane and any specific diagnosis of an individual not only depends on the context of the situation, but also is a subjective, biased process rather than one based on the characteristics of the individual judged.

In this study, eight normal subjects gained admission to several mental hospitals by presenting phony symptoms (hearing voices). Upon admission to the hospital, the symptoms were dropped entirely, and the "pseudopatients" behaved normally from then on. They were never detected as phony by any of the hospital staff, and, in all but one case, were diagnosed as schizophrenic. Eventually, they were discharged with a diagnosis of schizophrenia in remission (temporarily symptom-free).

Rosenhan's classic article described the many ways in which the diagnosis and label determined how staff members on all levels regarded the normal subjects: no matter how they behaved, their schizophrenic label stuck with them. This was the case even though the subjects' normal behavior was observable for adequate time periods (the average length of hospitalization was 19 days, ranging from 7 to 52 days for each of the subjects). Of interest is that most of the other patients tended to detect the normalcy of the pseudopatients, while none of the staff members did.

Rosenhan not only confirmed Scheff's view (1966) that psychiatric labels have a "life of their own" (once labeled a schizophrenic the label persists: the individual *is* a schizophrenic even though he or she is not *behaving* accordingly) but also suggests that hospitals and their staff members cannot distinguish the sane from the insane.

Since the publication of this study there has been considerable controversy regarding its implicit but sweeping generalization that diagnoses and labels and designations of sanity vs. insanity are meaningless activities (see, for example, Millon, 1975; Spitzer, 1975; and Weiner, 1975).

Some of the criticisms of Rosenhan's work stem from the following considerations: no control group was used; errors in diagnosis also occur with physical illness (as in inaccurate designation of or failure to designate early symptons of cancer; the study was not a true test of whether it is possible to distinguish the sane from the insane in ordinary circumstances; since the diagnoses were made in a mental hospital, it was logical to assume that they had emotional problems; further, the issue of base rates should be considered (most diagnoses of patients *are* schizophrenic, after all); and finally, the question of the validity of the diagnostic judgments was never really tested, since "pseudo," rather than actual, patients were the subjects of the studies.

These are all reasonable criticisms of Rosenhan's work. Yet there is probably great significance in the implications of his study, even though a valid test of his thesis was not made. Rosenhan's plea for examining the methods of assigning labels to people, especially the tendency to call healthy people sick, should, in any event, be heeded.

OTHER CLASSIFICATION SYSTEMS: A LOOK TOWARD THE FUTURE

Although the DSM-III has major faults (some of which have been mentioned) it is a frequently employed classification system. Nonetheless, concern with developing a more adequate diagnostic scheme has led some researchers to consider other models. Psychologists interested in abnormal behavior are not alone in their quest for the most reasonable, reliable, and valid classificatory scheme. For example, in the biological sciences, the classificatory tradition laid down by the botanist Carolus Linnaeus in the eighteenth century, which created a system based on forms and appearances (morphology), is currently being challenged by taxonomists (classifiers). It may be more important, some claim, to classify plants and animals on the basis of molecular, genetic, or biochemical makeup than by morphological characteristics, or to classify on the basis of similarity or number of common factors (Webster, 1982). Similarly, many psychologists are proposing newer ways of viewing the diagnostic process.

The prototype model. A recently proposed approach to the diagnostic process attempts to approximate how clinicians actually categorize a patient. The prototype is the ideal model or standard of a category that contains all or most of the features (for example, feelings, behaviors, thoughts) that experts attribute to a diagnosis. The construction of prototypes has been demonstrated for such categories as aggressive-impulsive, depressed-withdrawn, and borderline-disorganized (in which the subjects were children) and for such categories as schizophrenia (Cantor, Smith, French, and Mezzich, 1980; Horowitz, Post, French, Wallis, and Siegelman, 1981; Horowitz, Wright, Lowenstein, and Parad, 1981). Although no one person possesses *all* the characteristics of a prototype, some have more than others. Thus a clinician can diagnose an individual as depressed if he or she manifests many of the characteristics of the prototype. Other individuals, however, might display only a limited number of the features of the prototype but still be regarded as depressed. It is therefore claimed that the unreliability of many diagnostic decisions may arise from the possibility that categorizations of people are based on different degrees of overlap or approximation of the features of the prototype.

Prototypes are constructed on the basis of judgments by experts. As a result, they reflect only the experts' views or perceptions of pathology, rather than the pathology itself: they may not, therefore, be valid representations of what is actually occurring. On the other hand, the prototype approach offers a model for understanding some of the problems encountered in making a diagnosis. For example, such a model may clarify why different experts disagree in the diagnosis of the same person—that is, why the presence of a particular characteristic may elicit a prototype diagnosis by one expert but not another; it may also aid in systematizing what clinicians do and think when they make a diagnosis.

Classification of childhood pathology. Most experts agree that the classification of childhood disorders is woefully unreliable and inadequate (Achenbach and Edelbrock, 1978). In the past decade or so, there has been a flurry of attempts to amend this situation by rooting out the common factors in childhood disorders that appear again and again in case records of disturbed children or in the statements of the clinicians who work with them.

Empirical efforts of this sort have yielded many common variables found to represent the typical disorders that children display. One large-scale study (Achenbach, 1966), which analyzed the case records of 300 children of both sexes, ages four to 15, through the statistical method of factor analysis, found that the disorders could be broadly classified in terms of internalizing versus externalizing factors—that is, showing problems, such as fears, on the one hand, as opposed to acting out, on the other—or by degree of disturbance. In addition to these "broad-band" categories, disorders could also be classified by "narrow-band" categories—for example, aggressive behavior; obsessions, compulsions, and phobias; somatic complaints; and schizoid thinking and behavior. Empirical efforts of

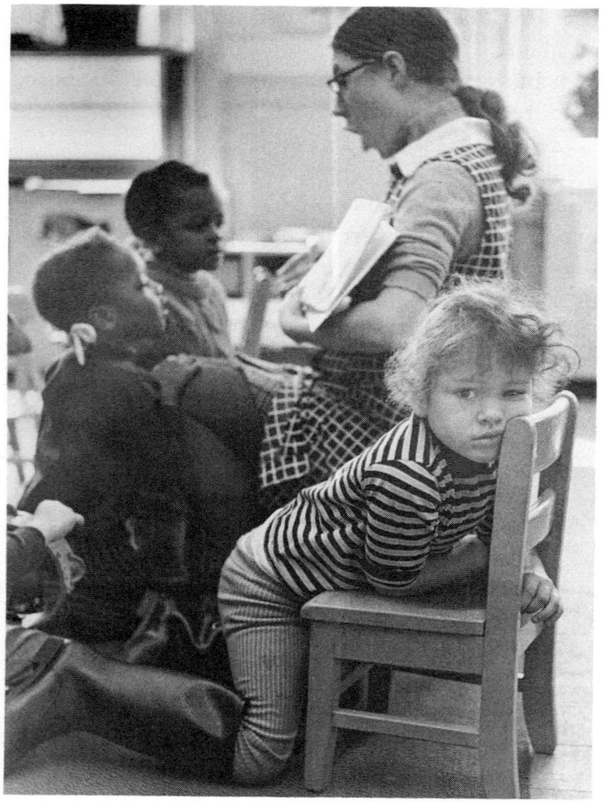

Johnny seems listless and depressed and is unable to focus on and attend to the teacher's interesting picture-story. What is his problem? (Mark Antman)

this sort may one day yield a reliable classificatory system that will replace the more traditional, less refined models in use today.

Trends toward specification. In recent years, certain specific and narrow models for classifying types of pathologies have been proposed. These models are characterized by attempts to distinguish among individuals who fall *within* a clinical subtype. Such diagnostic models are less concerned with broadly identifying a person as a "depressive," for example, than with specifying the particular kind of "depressive" that person may be. These systems tend to be moving away from the broad categories of the typological Kraepelinian approach (currently exemplified by the DSM-III) by searching for fine differences within subtypes that might point, among many possibilities, not only to etiological underpinnings but also to treatment strategies.

Throughout this book, your attention will be drawn to the rich possibilities of this approach. Some examples include classifying people as to whether or not they are prone to certain types of drug addiction, or prone to developing physical symptoms (asthma, for example) in response to psychological stress. Or, one day it may be possible to classify people by the nature of their *sleep* patterns, a diagnostic vista with many potential uses.

Examples of such classificatory models are:

1. Classification of schizophrenic pathology on the basis of paranoid versus nonparanoid criteria or on the basis of premorbid adjustment or "intactness" of cognitive variables (see Chapter 11).

2. Classification of mental patients on the basis of their adjustment to, and behaviors in, their social worlds, rather than according to the more traditional diagnostic criteria. For example, one determination might concern the question of dangerousness to self and others (see Chapter 18). Although this kind of classificatory scheme would obviously have much practical value, its possibilities are a long way from being realized.

3. Classification of people with depression on the basis of biochemical, psychological, and familial factors that could lead directly to selection of the appropriate treatment strategy (see Chapter 10).

4. Classification of children according to their potential learning ability and/or the degree to which familial and cultural factors might hold them back from achieving the level to which they could aspire (see Chapter 14).

5. Classification of people not by the usual Kraepelinian categories but by the most effective treatment mode for their specific problem—for example, pharmacological methods or methods that stress new learning.

Classifications based on assessment procedures. Other classification trends are based on the development of special testing procedures that permit public scrutiny of validity and reliability. Many of the traditional psychological tests described in the next chapter do not yield the kinds of objective, reliable data needed to support a good diagnostic system, despite their important clinical uses. Others, like the Minnesota Multiphasic Personality Inventory (MMPI), however, have already proven to be of considerable usefulness for both clinical and research purposes (see pp. 97–99).

The specific advantages of classifying people according to their behavior in the troublesome area (behavioral assessment) will be noted from time to time and elaborated upon in special detail when behavioral approaches to treatment are described in Chapter 20. Similarly, classification of people who have sustained some type of injury to their central nervous systems through neuropsychological assessment procedures is particularly helpful in specifying areas of deficit that require retraining. Chapter 13 discusses such classificatory approaches when it describes the organic mental disorders.

The foregoing are only a few of the possibilities that lie ahead. You will note that one of the qualities of many of these newer methods is the lack of dogmatic commitment to a single discipline and a willingness to cross borders, let us say, from psychology to neurophysiology or biochemistry. This makes sense, as you will see demonstrated in many chapters of this book.

THE POSITION OF THIS BOOK REGARDING DIAGNOSIS

Despite thorny problems in the use of a diagnostic system such as the DSM-III, this and similar schemes are so widespread that they serve a useful, practical way to summarize or at least organize the vast amount of data from research and from case studies in the domain of abnormal behavior.

Criticisms of the DSM-III and of diagnostic labeling systems are cogent in that they reflect specific ethical as well as methodological problems regarding our ability to understand the nature of mental and emotional disorders. Yet, along with other clinicians, the writer continues to feel the need for a diagnostic system that would provide a structure, however rudimentary, around which knowledge that is rapidly accumulating could coalesce.

This book is organized principally, but not entirely, around the DSM-III categories, with full attention to systems that will refine and may even replace it. One practical consideration in the decision to adhere roughly to the traditional clinical entities is that in this country, as well as many others, most clinicians and researchers from different disciplines employ these designations in their practical work and in their reports of scientific investigations. You will be better prepared to understand their communications, many of which are described in this book, if you are familiar with their language.

Thus most of the clinical groups in the DSM-III are described in this book, with special emphasis on affective, organic, anxiety, psychosexual, and substance-induced disorders. Mental retardation and antisocial behavior patterns are also described. The material covered is very much concerned with the serious issues raised by the critics of diagnostic systems. Social and cultural factors, reliability, validity, and empirical evidence, as well as the ethical dilemmas raised by many of the professional practices of people in the mental health field will receive particular attention.

SUMMARY

This chapter discussed many of the problems of traditional diagnostic systems that attempt to classify abnormal behavior, with special attention to issues of reliability and validity. One widely used, recently revised classificatory scheme is the DSM-III of the American Psychiatric Association (1980). Chapter 4 also presented the diagnostic categories and multiaxial schemes employed in this detailed nosological system and listed Axes IV and V, ratings for severity of psychosocial stressors (Axis IV) and for highest level of adaptive functioning during the past year (Axis V). It also reviewed several criticisms of the DSM-III as well as some problems in connection with the medical model. Finally, it was pointed out that although the chapters ahead roughly employ many (but not all) aspects of the DSM-III classification, many other classification schemes are also possible. Some of these will undoubtedly supplement or refine the DSM-III, while others may replace it entirely.

Highlights

1. For the clinician, as well as the researcher, there are several advantages in classifying emotional disturbance. These include providing possible "leads" for treatment and prognosis, as well as a framework for finding common denominators that might shed light on the origins of psychopathology. However, serious problems of objectivity, reliability, and validity of traditional systems have prompted many clinicians and researchers to seek improved classification systems. It is hoped that such refined systems will not only be open to objective empirical evaluation but also be constructed so that reliability and validity considerations are given serious attention.
2. The DSM-III purports to be an improvement over earlier systems by (a) providing detailed, objective criteria and illustrations as aids in making diagnoses; and (b) requiring the use of ratings on axes that acknowledge the significance of psychosocial stressors in producing pathology as well as the previous level of functioning in determining the outcome of the "disease" process.
3. Although it is still too early to draw definitive conclusions about the validity, reliability, and practical usefulness of the DSM-III, its content has thus far received considerable criticism along some of the following lines: the diagnostic categories were not evaluated for reliability; cultural variations in the expression of symptoms were not considered; and the system, because of its arbitrary and dogmatic presentation and exhaustive length, has an unwarranted aura of validity and definitiveness.
4. An extremely important criticism is the failure of the DSM-III to confront the sorts of questions raised in Chapter 1 regarding distinctions between normality and abnormality. As a consequence, serious objections have been raised about the inclusion of many behaviors—for example, certain types of sexual dysfunctions or reading disorders.
5. Another form of criticism emphasizes that the diagnostic labeling employed by the general medical or disease model is perpetuated by this and similar diagnostic systems, thus creating serious ethical as well as substantive problems.
6. Finally, although this book is organized generally, but not entirely, around the DSM-III categories, other newer and more refined approaches to diagnosis may one day supplement or replace this system. These will be described in appropriate sections of the chapters that follow. Some of these approaches include the prototype model, modes of classifying childhood pathology, the use of narrower and more specific subtypes *within* diagnostic categories, and classifications based on assessment procedures—for example, in the behavioral and neuropsychological areas.

ISSUES AND QUESTIONS

1. This chapter delineated some of the pros and cons of diagnostic systems and discussed some of the general issues involved in diagnosing and labeling emotional or behavioral difficulties. Where do you stand on these questions? Is it possible to adhere to a classificatory

approach and, at the same time, remain concerned about its impact on those classified and its need for validation and refinement?

2. One aspect of Szasz's view is that he is directly opposed to any kind of referral of an individual for diagnosis or treatment. Szasz points out that when schools, courts, or corporations make recommendations for diagnosis (or treatment), the individual concerned is virtually coerced into abiding by the recommendation because he or she is dependent on these institutions in significant ways. "Blackmail" is implicit, and people go along with the process, despite invasion of their privacy and decision-making options, because they are aware of the benefits or punishments involved. Szasz noted that many parents of "troublesome" children are exactly in this position when they are asked to have their child tested or treated. The implicit threat is that the child will be deprived of schooling unless there is compliance with the request. As long as anyone other than the individual himself or herself requests professional help, Szasz thinks that help should not be available, offered, or recommended.

   Do you agree with this position? Consider an assaultive child in the classroom; the child's parents are abusive, refusing to discuss the problem or to seek professional help. Should the teacher respect the wishes of these parents? What about the welfare of the child? What about the rights and safety of the other children?

SUGGESTIONS FOR FURTHER READING

American Psychiatric Association. *DSM-III. Diagnostic and statistical manual of mental disorders.* 3rd ed. Washington, D. C.: American Psychiatric Association, 1980. Whether or not you agree with this system, the DSM-III is in wide use in the mental health field. If you wish to continue in this field, having this manual handy for reference, research, and clarification is not a bad idea.

Garfield, S. L. Research problems in clinical diagnosis. *Journal of Consulting and Clinical Psychology,* 1978, *46,* 596–607. This brief, lucid article summarizes some of the problems raised in Chapter 4 concerning diagnoses. Special attention is given to problems of sampling, control groups, base rates, and the general deficiencies of classification systems. Garfield's article appears in an issue of this journal which is devoted entirely to general clinical research problems in the field of abnormal psychology, as well as to specific areas such as depession, obesity, and smoking. This article (and several in this issue written by other researchers) is highly recommended for those who plan to continue studying in this field.

Szasz, T. S. *The myth of mental illness: Foundations of a theory of personal conduct.* New York: Hoeber-Harper, 1961. This significant, controversial book represents Szasz's early, dramatic statements concerning his views that mental illness is a myth, a fiction, and in no way similar to a physical disease. Szasz depicts human conduct as a struggle focused on attempts to deal with the rules imposed by society. Szasz holds that whether or not a person follows these rules or deviates from them is the personal responsibility of the individual and does not reflect the presence or absence of illness or disease; clinicians therefore cannot diagnose or treat individuals for illnesses they cannot have. They can only deal with their clients' social behavior and their systems of values and ethics.

Szasz, T. S. *The manufacture of madness: A comparative study of the inquisition and the mental health movement.* New York: Harper & Row, 1977. Paperback. Once again Szasz presents his radical ideas about psychiatry. In this book he makes the case that so-called modern, psychodynamic psychiatry does not represent an advance over the medieval superstitions and practices of the witch-hunts. In fact, Szasz lucidly argues that psychiatry is a continuation of the Inquisition and that the concept of mental illness has been misused by psychiatrists in order to gain and exercise power. This is a fascinating book—about both the mentally ill and witches.

5

Interviewing, Observing, and Psychological Testing–Some Traditional Methods

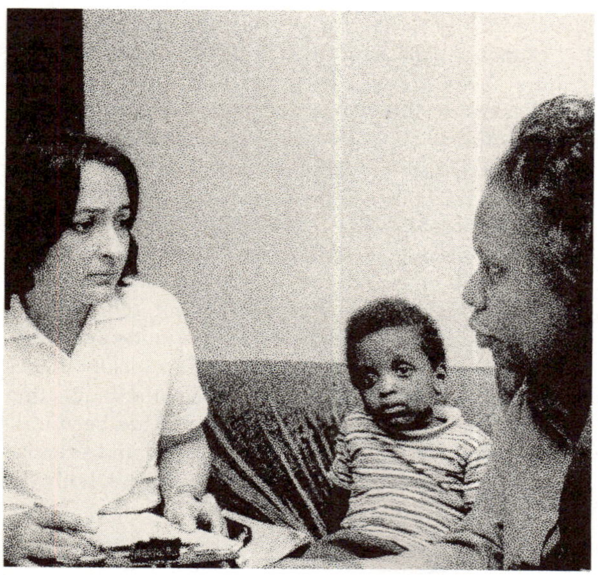

This chapter surveys some of the most frequently used, traditional methods in psychological observation and measurement that have been developed over a period of decades.

At the end of the preceding chapter, some of the newer directions in diagnosis were described and it was noted that these emerged, in part, from dissatisfaction with the older classification models. Some of these newer approaches were developed as the need to delineate the patient's problems more narrowly became apparent. These considerations, as well as new and innovative approaches to treatment, have changed the nature of psychological testing to a considerable degree.

For example, one approach that represents a departure from the more traditional approach is generally called behavioral assessment. Behavioral assessment methods were developed to find ways to isolate certain behaviors so that they could be understood sufficiently well to be changed. In this approach, the complex personality pictures provided by some of the methods to be described in this chapter (for example, see projective methods, pp. 100–104) or the fitting of the patient into a diagnostic category is thought to be less relevant than a method which disclosed, let us say, the precise nature of the patient's fear, when the fear is most intense, and what he or she does to avoid the fear-producing situation. These assessment methods are described in Chapter 20, when procedures for modifying maladaptive behavior through various behavioral interventions are discussed.

Behavioral assessment methods as well as other types of assessment procedures, for example, neuropsychological assessment, can be understood essentially only in the context of relevant clinical chapters. For example, Chapter 13 and Chapter 14 describe neuropsychological assessment and discuss methods for assessing the learning potential of so-called mentally retarded children. Chapter 10 covers tests for exploring the content of certain types of depression. This chapter is designed only to familiarize you with the more general, traditional field of psychological assessment procedures as widely practiced in this country and abroad. You are reminded that many additional types of assessment procedures are presented throughout this book.

INTRODUCTION

How do we arrive at a diagnosis—an assessment or evaluation of a patient's problem—so that treatment recommendations about how to deal with his or her problem can be made?

In the field of abnormal psychology, there are many sources of information about patients that include observations, interviews, test scores, neurological and medical findings, introspective statements, reports by the patient's family, and records from schools, courts, and hospitals. How do we know that diagnostic statements about personality and emotions reflect the actual situation? The answer is simple: we do not know, unless relevant evidence is presented.

Research on diagnostic methods is continually challenging the methods that psychologists use, and these efforts involve a search for evidence that our ways of diagnosing people do indeed "work." It is not sufficient to claim, for example, that an individual's drawings of figures reveal the key to his or her gender identity or self-image. You would be correct in asking: What is the evidence for this claim? This question concerns *validity,* a concept already introduced and about which more will be said later in this chapter.

THE CLINICAL INTERVIEW

Most clinicians would agree with the statement that the interview is the backbone of the clinical interaction. However, there is considerable disagreement about the degree of formality or structure an interview should contain. Some clinicians tend not to pose questions directly; other clinicians indirectly solicit certain kinds of information thought to be significant. Still others conduct a formal interview in a highly structured manner.

Many corporations, hospitals, clinics, and psychological and psychiatric facilities use their own interview forms and questionnaires. In this way, uniform material is obtained for subjects seen in those settings.

What content is covered in these interviews? In addition to such demographic data as birthdate, place of birth, address, education, employment history, number and age of siblings, and birthplace of parents, interviews generally also include inquiry into: history of physical and psychological symptoms; sexual background; social and personal development; hobbies and interests; current physical and emotional status; history of medication and drug and alcohol intake; family history of physical and emotional status; and history of hospitalizations and/or treatment of subject or members of the family.

Many clinicians have their own special interests

and approach. Whereas some inquire specifically about early childhood events, others may stress only current interpersonal interactions. Still other clinicians, concerned with modifying the specific behaviors about which the patient is dissatisfied, may look for the factors in the patient's life that sustain the undesirable behavior.

Interviews are not necessarily conducted on a one-to-one basis. Many interviews are conducted with all members of the family present. Some clinicians, when working with a child, will not see the parents alone, ever. To do so, they claim, is to violate the trust of the child. Other clinicians will interview one, then the other, of a married couple, before seeing them together. In any event, format, content, "facts" covered, and general style of interviews are not consistent or uniform.

Despite this variation, almost all clinicians agree that conducting a good interview involves special skill. Trained clinicians differ from those who are untrained in many ways. Chiefly, however, experienced clinicians know that appearances do not always reveal meaningful information; as long as self-report and verbal methods are used, there is always room for doubt as to the veracity of the content that emerges. Some clinicians, of course, are less concerned with the so-called facts than with the interaction and the interrelationship of patient and clinician and his or her actual behavior as observed.

Interviews are not always on a one-to-one basis; many are conducted with all members of the family present. (Ellis Herwig/ Stock, Boston)

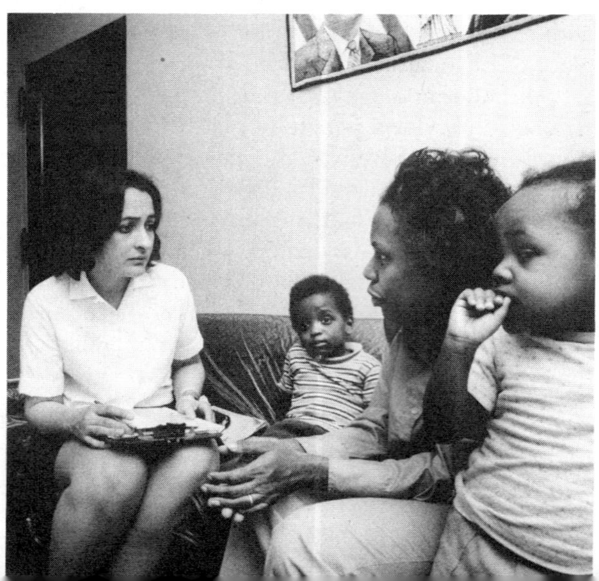

One constantly surprising event in the professional life of a clinician is that what is learned from interviewing separately two members of a dyad (a close pair in a social system like mother and child, husband and wife, or lovers) is that reports about each other can differ extensively. For example, a man was referred for therapy by his family physician with complaints of chronic, persistent impotence, lack of sexual interest, and little or no opportunity to "try out" rewarding, positive sexual behavior. A few weeks later, his wife was interviewed at the husband's request. She spoke of incident after incident of surprising her husband in sexual encounters, in a succession of "one-night stands." Did the husband want his wife to discover his extramarital activities in this way? Or was the wife reporting wished-for fantasy material about her husband—that is, material she had invented? Sometimes close members of a dyad unconsciously share myths and reinforce each other's pathology and symptoms. The unfolding of the "truth" may be painstakingly slow, may not even be necessary, or may take on a completely different light as additional material emerges. In this instance, it was later learned that the woman was permitting, even encouraging, her husband's sexual encounters and their interruption by hiring, and then firing in a rage, a succession of young household helpers.

Interviewers vary considerably in the kinds of content they elicit from subjects. In addition, it has been easily demonstrated that they can be influenced in their judgments about the interviewee if certain labels are applied to the subjects beforehand—if for example, "patient" as opposed to "job applicant" (Langer and Abelson, 1974). Also, the behavior, verbal and other, of the subject has, in turn, been shown to influence the way in which the interviewer conducts the interview (Salzinger, 1978). The point is, interviews do not necessarily produce objective, standard material that can be relied on as accurate indications of the "true" status of the subject.

Objectifying the Subjective: Structured Interviews and Computer Diagnoses

The preceding chapter described the poor reliability of diagnosis. This state of affairs, plus problems concerning the clinician's subjectivity and the lack of reliability of many psychological tests has led to the development of other, more objective, approaches. These include: systematic ways of obtaining objective information about the symptoms and background of patients through the use of structured interviewing methods; and the development of computer programs using objective data that can lead to a diagnosis.

The structured interview may employ a certain number of loose, ambiguous, open-ended questions. But it primarily uses direct, straightforward queries and often requires the rating of certain behaviors of the subject, such as attention span, rate of speech, or posture.

Structured interviews have many advantages. Since the same ground is covered for all patients, responses of groups of patients (including those from different cultures) can be compared. In addition, responses of a patient can be compared to his or her responses at a later time. All responses from this type of interview can be fed into a computer to obtain or refine diagnostic information. Spitzer, Endicott, and their colleagues have worked extensively in the development of structured interviews and inventories (Burdock and Hardesty, 1962; Spitzer, Burdock, and Hardesty, 1963; Spitzer and Endicott, 1973; Spitzer, Endicott and Fleiss, 1967; Spitzer, Endicott, Fleiss, and Cohen, 1970; and Spitzer, Fleiss, Burdock and Hardesty, 1964). The schedules they developed have been shown to be reliable and to differentiate various kinds of diagnostic groups. Spotlight 5.1 presents selected items from one of these structured interview schedules,

The use of computers in diagnosing patients has some advantages over the use of clinicians, but also some disadvantages. Computer programs for diagnosing patients generally involve input of observations, interview data, ratings, and background information by which the diagnostic category is formulated—processed—and printed out. One advantage a computer possesses is that it is completely reliable: given the same information twice, it will produce the same diagnosis. Another advantage is that the rules by which a diagnosis is made by a computer—its program—can be based on large-scale research and evidence that most clinicians are either not aware of or do not have immediately available to them. A computer program is based on empirical evidence of the relationship between certain indicators, signs, and symptoms, and a diagnostic category; for example, a combination of loss of appetite, sleeplessness, worries about the future, and an increased desire to die might yield a diagnosis of depression. These relationships can then not only be made public but are also subject to further scrutiny and investigation.

Computer diagnosis suffers from some limitations, however. These include the same problems clinicians have regarding the imperfect relationship of symptoms to diagnosis, the unreliability of diagnoses and classificatory schemes themselves, and, most important of all: computerized diagnoses are valid essentially only for populations similar to the ones from which the program was derived.

Clinicians versus computers in diagnosis. Many people have questioned whether or not a clinician actually does "better"—is more consistent and valid than a computer. That is, given certain symptoms, interview content, responses to tests, and certain kinds of background situations, how would assessment by clinician and computer compare? An important consideration in favor of computers is their lack of subjectivity. Clinicians might unconsciously modify perceptions about patients as a result of extraneous variables. For example, some studies have shown that therapists tend to rate patients as more improved when their patients express values similar to those they themselves hold (Welkowitz, Cohen, and Ortmeyer, 1967). Computers would not be influenced toward or against patients in this way, unless specifically programmed to do so.

This kind of argument was put forth years ago—even before the popular use of computers—by

Spotlight 5.1 Selected Items from the Mental Status Schedule

Here are some items from the beginning of a structured interview. After first obtaining standard data such as age, marital status, nature of work, and inquiring about the patient's problems or difficulties (Items 1–8, not presented here), the interviewer then probes certain symptomatic areas, checking T for true or NT for not true on a standard list of questions. The interviewer is also required to indicate such behavioral and physical features of the subject as refusing to shake hands or perspiring profusely.

	Interview Schedule	Inventory of Content and Behavior
Mood	What kind of moods have you been in recently?	9. Indicates he has alternating periods of elation and depression (extreme ups and downs) ___ 10. Says he feels nothing, has no feelings or feelings have dried up ___
Worries	What kind of things do you worry about? *If patient indicates worries:* (How much do you worry?)	11. Says he has no worries or that nothing bothers him ___ 12. Mentions that he worries a lot or that he can't stop worrying ___
Fears	What kind of fears do you have? Some people have fears they know don't make sense—like crowds or certain activities. What kind of fears do you have like this? *If patient indicates a fear:* Does this fear of ______ prevent you from doing something you want to do?	13. Indicates that he has lots of fears or that he keeps feeling afraid of different things ___ 14. Mentions a fear of being abandoned or left all alone ___ 15. Indicates that he is fearful of losing his mind or losing control of his emotions ___ 16. Indicates that he had an irrational fear of a particular object or situation (e.g., crowds, heights) ___ 17. Says he gets attacks of sudden fear or panic ___ 18. Indicates that his fear prevents him from participating in some activity ___
Anxiety	How often do you feel anxious or tense? (How much of the time do you feel this way?)	19. Admits that he is bothered by feelings of anxiety ___ 20. Admits that he feels anxious all the time ___
Restlessness	What about feeling restless?	21. Complains of feeling restless or unable to stay still ___
Depression	How often do you feel depressed or blue? (How much of the time do you feel this way?)	22. Admits that he is bothered by feelings of sadness or depression ___ 23. Admits that he feels depressed or despondent all the time ___
Crying	When was the last time you felt like crying?	24. Admits that he feels like crying ___

	Interview Schedule	Inventory of Content and Behavior	
Self-Appraisal, Guilt	How do you feel about yourself? Do you like yourself? (When you compare yourself with other people, how do you come out?)	25. Mentions that he loves himself or that he thinks he is perfect	___
		26. Accuses himself of being unworthy, sinful or evil	___
		27. Indicates he is bothered by feelings of inadequacy or says he doesn't like himself	___
		28. Indicates that he is bothered by feelings of guilt	___
Response to Criticism	How do you feel when people criticize you? What do you do when people offer advice?	29. Indicates that he feels hurt or overwhelmed when criticized	___
		30. Indicates that he gets angry when criticized or that he customarily rejects advice	___
Inter-personal Relations	How are you getting along with people? What kinds of trouble do you have with people? Whom do you feel you can trust the most? Who bothers or upsets you the most? (Why?)	31. Complains about the way peers or strangers treat him	___
		32. Complains extensively about the way people in positions of authority or power treat him (e.g., staff members, police, employer)	___
		33. Complains extensively about member of family, friend or associate	___
		34. Indicates that he cannot trust other people	___
		35. Mentions that he feels people take advantage of him or push him around	___
		36. Expresses jealousy, rivalry, or bitter envy toward member of family, friend or associate	___
	How do you feel when you are with people?	37. Mentions that he feels inhibited or uncomfortable with people	___
		38. Indicates that he feels distant or isolated from people	___
		39. Says he stays by himself or likes to be alone	___
	How do people seem to feel about you? What about your friends? (How do they feel about you?)	40. Says that he feels people avoid, reject or dislike him	___
		41. Says he is in love with or loved by everybody or some person he does not know (e.g., interviewer)	___
		42. Indicates he feels he has no friends	___

Source: From Spitzer, Burdock, and Hardesty, 1963.

Meehl (1954), as a problem of clinical versus statistical (actuarial) prediction. Clinicians themselves have past records of "hits" and "misses" and this information, the clinician's credibility, is a bit of actuarial information that can help to evaluate the merit of the clinician. By and large, most people agree that clinicians have something "extra"—judgment, intuition, wisdom, and experience—that computers do not possess. An up-to-date, wise clinician can probably fare better, in terms of hits and misses, than a computer program; average clinicians would probably fare worse. But even this argument is open to empirical exploration (Zubin, et al., 1975).

Computer-patient interviews are now possible, though they are still in the formative stages of development. They, too, possess both advantages and disadvantages. They can be programmed to pursue certain lines of inquiry in depth, if required; several interviews can be conducted simultaneously; and they can obtain standard, objective content in a neutral, nonjudgmental way. On the other hand, the inflexibility of a computer, its failure to respond to verbal, postural, emotional, interpersonal, and visual nuances, cues, and its inability to exercise intuition, have insights, or show compassion, empathy, and warmth render this type of interview less than optimal at least for the present.

RATING SCALES AND OBSERVATIONS

An essential aspect of the clinical interaction between the examiner and subject is the quality of that interaction—the behaviors that are not tested but that nevertheless emerge—and the general mood and "tone" of the subject.

A keen observer will, thus, note such features of E-S (examiner-subject) interaction and general behavior as: mood, overt display of anxiety, awkwardness, negativism, compliance, hostility, attention and concentration, speech quality, smoking habits, handedness, fluency and articulateness, level of self-insight, cooperativeness, and dozens of other characteristics of behavior.

One way of systematizing some of these observations is through the use of rating scales, which not only forces the examiner to look for certain dimensions but also requires determination of the intensity or strength of that characteristic; even the confidence with which the rating is made can be recorded. The use of rating scales has the additional advantage of yielding quantifiable data so that further explorations of reliability, validity, correlations, and other research manipulations are possible. Rating scales have the added advantage of permitting the comparison of subjects along the dimension rated. For example, in a longitudinal study that explored the relationship of family processes and achievement and behavior of children at school, it was necessary to measure various aspects of the families' modes of communication, (Schumer and Deutsch, 1970). To obtain this information, two trained interviewers were asked to independently observe and then rate—along several dimensions—the family members in interaction with one another at home.

An illustration of one of the rating scales employed follows:

Mother's, father's or parental figure's role in maintaining the "rules" of effective communication

Illustration of behavior reflected in this rating: Mother or family "leader" does not seem to expect members to follow the "rules" of communication, that is, listening, expecting a response, not shifting content, not interrupting; family leader fails to redirect or refocus subject matter of family discussion to the relevant topic, the subject matter at hand.

Ratings (encircle one):

4	3	2	1	X
fails to enforce rules of effective communication			*enforces* rules of effective communication	can't rate

Note that ratings (4) and (1) are extreme anchor points, with ratings of (2) and (3) more moderate ratings that "belong" in the direction of either extreme.

The use of these and many other ratings made it possible to correlate various aspects of family background and style with a wide array of educational data without having to rely on self-reports, questionnaires, and nonquantifiable observations. It should also be noted that the ratings employed in this study were highly reliable—that is, a high level of agreement was achieved between the two independently obtained ratings.

PSYCHOLOGICAL TESTS

Another method clinicians use for arriving at a diagnosis involves the use of psychological tests. Referred to as "devices" or "instruments," they are designed to tell us about individual differences. They specifically tell us the way in which an individual compares to others with regard to the dimension, quality, or trait being measured. In abnormal psychology, the tests used are special tests of personality and emotions. But intelligence tests, tests of perception, tests of thinking, and many other tests assist the clinician in making diagnostic decisions.

All of us are familiar with tests of various sorts for evaluation of aptitude, job training, or college entrance. Tests that are used for diagnosis and for assessing the conflicts and emotions an individual may be experiencing are probably less familiar. Regardless of the purpose of the test, however, to be a "good" one—that is, to be able to predict the behavior of, or categorize, the individual accurately—it must possess some important qualities. One of these is validity. This is the same quality expected of a diagnostic system; it should do what it sets out to do. Its results or scores or ratings about a person should possess some truth.

Another quality of a good test is reliability, again a familiar concept discussed in connection with agreement among judges or raters is making a diagnosis. Validity and reliability as applied especially to psychological tests have some special meanings. Spotlight 5.2 describes these in a little more detail.

Spotlight 5.2 Validity and Reliability of Tests

Validity

A good psychological test is valid to the degree that it measures what it claims it is measuring, just in the way an instrument that is supposed to measure blood pressure is expected to actually measure blood pressure rather than body temperature or some other body function. Those who construct psychological tests are expected to show that they have explored in various ways the degree to which their test is valid and to make this information public to potential users of tests.

Imagine, for example, a test designed to predict whether or not high school students are likely to become alcoholics as adults. Without information as to how often high scores on this test actually make accurate predictions, or how often scores from this test agree with an *established* test of alcoholism-proneness (the validity of which is known), we would not want to trust the results of this test. Just because a test *appears* to be valid does not make it so: appearances are inadequate for establishing validity.

Face validity—appearances—may seem to make sense, but is generally not of crucial value in regard to validity. It may, for example, appear logical and sensible to think that posture is a clear indication of a person's mood: droopy shoulders indicate depression while the chin held high indicates a good mood. On the face of it, it would seem that posture is a valid measure of mood. However, other factors, such as inherited skeletal structure, may also affect posture so that some people with droopy shoulders may not actually be depressed. Other evidence must be accumulated in addition to appearances to validate the posture-mood test.

Test developers establish the validity of a test—does it measure what we say it measures—in many different ways. These techniques all involve some attempt to show how much the scores from the new test correlate with other kinds of information, such as scores from an already established test or with actual data that evaluates the accuracy of the prediction.

In the case of the test for proneness for alcoholism, the test developer may wish to show how highly Johnny's score (and that of others in his class) is associated with his score on an accepted, valid test of proneness for alcoholism. Are high scores on the first test associated with high scores on the second? Or the test developer might wish to show that the scores on the alcoholism proneness test are associated with information about the actual drinking patterns of the subjects. High scores are obtained by drinkers, low scores by nondrinkers. These methods of establishing validity are examples of concurrent validity, which has to do with correlating scores for subjects with other information obtained about them during the same general period of time.

If we gave Johnny and his classmates the test for alcohol-proneness during their senior year in high school and then checked up on their drinking patterns ten years later, could we show that high scores on the test were obtained by those who are now drinking heavily or are alcoholics, whereas low scores predicted those who are moderate drinkers or nondrinkers? This approach to establishing validity is called predictive validity. In any event, these methods of demonstrating test validity rely on actual empirical explorations rather than on appearances.

Reliability

As with diagnoses, reliability concerns consistency and repeatability. Although validity of a test is perhaps its most important quality, it cannot be valid unless it is reliable. For example, a tape measure that yields different inches each time for your height is not a reliable measure and therefore cannot be valid. That is why test developers concern themselves initially with making sure a test is reliable.

One way to measure the reliability of a test is to see if it yields the same results in a second administration. This is called test-retest reliability. A test that measures the intensity of a subject's conflicts in the sexual area should yield the same score, generally speaking, if repeated a week later. If the score on such a test varied considerably over a fairly brief period of time, then it would not be a very reliable test.

Test-retest methods have certain disadvantages and drawbacks. Subjects may remember their previous responses and repeat them, resulting in an inflated picture of reliability. In addition, the trait or behavior being measured might actually change over time so that fluctuations in scores are reflections of real change rather than of poor reliability. Regarding the test of sexual conflicts, the subject may have solved some of his or her problems between testing sessions, resulting in score changes that reflect good validity rather than poor reliability.

Another method of estimating reliability that has fewer of the foregoing problems is called alternate-form reliability. For any subject, scores on two tests— the original one and a parallel or equivalent form which shares the same characteristics as its model—would be compared. If the test is reliable, an individual should score similarly on both the original and the alternate forms. Memory factors would not be a problem, and if the tests are given with a short interval between administrations, neither are changes over time.

There are still other ways of assessing the reliability of a test—for example, by correlating scores on the odd-numbered items of a test with the scores on the even-numbered ones (split-half-method). Theoretically, a perfectly reliable test should yield a perfect correlation of scores from the two halves.

The important thing to remember is that a test is a poor one, perhaps even useless, if it has low reliability.

If we know, then, that a test is valid and reliable, we can feel confident about its use. Certainly, the accuracy of any measuring instrument, whether it is a yardstick or a test of emotional maturity, is of vital interest to anyone interested in its use. A good test will openly document its validity and reliability so that its users or potential users will know, with reasonable certainty, how accurately and consistently it is measuring whatever it claims to be measuring.

In addition to being valid and reliable, a good test should be standardized. That is, it should permit the subjects' responses or scores to be compared to the performance of other (comparable) subjects, thus providing a standard for interpreting their "meaning." Spotlight 5.3 explores this aspect of tests in greater detail.

A good test has many additional qualities including some obvious ones, such as clarity of questions or parts so that it will be understood by those taking it, or adequate, representative sampling of the area it is covering. Many additional technical characteristics of tests exist but are outside of the domain of this discussion. It becomes obvious that

Spotlight 5.3 Norms and Standardization

Fred, a college student, obtained a score of 23 on a test designed to measure level of anxiety. What does Fred's score tell us about Fred? Practically nothing, since we do not know what that score means. A score of 23 out of a possible 50 would tell us something different than would a score of 23 out of 24. Even so, is a score of 23 out of 50 a high score or low score?

One way to approach these questions would be to compare Fred's score to the scores of other students. Is his score average? below average? above average? A set of norms for the test given Fred would provide answers to these questions.

Test norms are essentially summaries of the test performances of a group of subjects regarded as representative of the population in which we are interested. This group of subjects is called the standardization sample since it provides a common standard against which individual scores can be compared.

Norms can provide the average score and the range of scores of the standardization sample. Since the standardization sample is chosen to represent a certain population—in the case of Fred it might be male college students—its scores also provide an estimate of the average and range of scores of this college population as a whole.

Norms can also be expressed as percentiles. Percentile scores express what percent of the sample fell below a particular score. Using the example of Fred and the anxiety test, if the average score on this test was 30 and a score of 23 corresponded to the 25th percentile, we would know that Fred is below average in level of anxiety but exceeds 25 percent of his peers in this regard.

There are still other ways to express norms, such as grade levels or mental ages. Regardless of how they are expressed, standardized norms provide a means for interpreting particular test results.

It is of vital importance that norms accurately reflect the population of interest; otherwise, interpretations based on those norms will be incorrect. For example, what could be learned about the aggressiveness of a corporation executive from a score on a test for which the standardization sample was a group of prison inmates? Obviously inferences about the executive based on the prison norms would be questionable.

The issue of the representativeness of standardization samples is an extremely important one. Some of the furor surrounding the relevance of intelligence tests for ethnic minority children, for example, is based on the fact that several of the most widely used intelligence tests did not contain sufficient numbers (if any) of minority group children in their standardization sample.

Good or sound psychological tests, then, establish their norms by using large standardization samples that represent the population for which the test will be used. Characteristics of the standardization sample are made available for the test user so that informed and relevant comparisons can be made.

many of the "tests" appearing in magazines or newspapers—to assess emotional stability or level of anxiety, for example—are not good psychological tests.

While generally much more sophisticated than the typical newspaper variety, psychological tests are rarely perfect instruments—certainly not as accurate or reliable as a thermometer or a ruler or other precision measuring device. Since there is much room for error, some clinicians prefer to use many of their instruments loosely, rather than strictly and inflexibly, in order to arrive at impressions about their clients.

The clinical "battery." Clinicians often use tests to obtain a detailed picture of their clients' personal and emotional functioning. They, or the clinician referring the client for testing, may wish an evaluation at the beginning or ending phases of treatment or counseling. Sometimes the referring clinician has doubts about diagnosis and/or treatment and requests a differential diagnosis. This may involve distinguishing psychotic from nonpsychotic functioning or organic from nonorganic origins of symptoms.

A sophisticated clinician rarely uses a single score or test for surveys, relying rather, on his or her clinical judgment, experience, observations of the patient, a clinical interview, reasons for referral, and statements from other clinicians (such as neurologists, teachers, and physicians) or from members of the patient's family. In addition, the wise clinician is likely to use a battery of tests—a group of several tests designed to survey as broad a spectrum of the patient's functioning as possible. Results of this clinical assessment are usually written in the form of a clinical report, which is generally sent to the clinician who made the referral.

INTELLIGENCE TESTS AND CLINICAL DIAGNOSIS

Most of you are familiar with the word *intelligence* and the concept of *intelligence testing.* But what is intelligence? What do intelligence tests claim to do? And why are clinicians interested in intelligence testing?

What is intelligence? Intelligence or intellectual capacity refers to an individual's capacity to learn and to solve problems. Various cognitive capacities, such as memory, judgment, and numerical skills are assumed to fall within the domain of intelligence. Intelligence tests presumably measure several of these capacities rather than any unitary function.

An individual's intelligence, or capacity to solve problems, is not an inflexible, inborn, inherited, fixed quantity. On the contrary, the cognitive skills that are usually thought to comprise "intelligence" seem very much influenced by schooling, cultural background, motivation, and the kinds of experiences a person has had in life. In general, a strict genetic hypothesis about intelligence—that it is already set by the time a child is born—is held in serious doubt by most psychologists (Dorfman, 1978; Kamin, 1974).

What are intelligence tests? Intelligence tests measure performance: they do not measure something that "exists" in the brain. The tasks selected to indicate performance that represents intellectual ability on any given test are chosen or invented by the test developer. These tasks presumably sample the domain thought to reflect intellectual capacity; vocal beauty, thus, would not be part of this domain. By convention, vocabulary knowledge, arithmetic skill, and similar cognitive functions belong in this domain. Performance in these areas is easily affected by such factors as education, cultural environment, and various personality and emotional variables of the individual such as motivation or level of anxiety. Even the attitudes of the subject toward the examiner and the test situation affect the level of performance.

Intelligence tests yield individual scores based on performance norms derived from a standardization sample. To the extent that such a sample is not representative of the individual or individuals tested, the intelligence score will be biased.

Use of intelligence test scores to reflect fixed, invariant qualities is highly questionable, especially if that score locks an individual into a stereotyped view of his or her potential for change, achievement, or occupation. Some children from the slums and ghettoes might do poorly on intelligence tests early in life. But they would be severely handicapped if their scores were used to fix their futures.*

Why do clinicians use intelligence tests? Clinicians use scores from and responses to intelligence tests to aid in differential diagnosis, to classify level of mental retardation, and to assess the quality of intellectual functioning an individual possesses as a possible indication or reflection of pathology. Here are some examples of how intelligence tests, usually administered as part of a battery of tests, are used.

A young child was referred for testing because her teacher thought she was of extremely low level intelligence—possibly retarded—and should be in a special class. As a result of a skillfully administered test battery, the child was shown to be of at least average intelligence, but suffering from such high anxiety, fear, and tension, that she was unable to learn anything in the classroom, much less relate to any of the other children or the teacher. The child did very poorly on all items on the test that had to do with school—items that required reading, facility with numbers, or vocabulary knowledge—and rather well on all of the items that did not—such as recognition of missing elements in everyday, pictorial scenes.

One eleven-year-old boy was thought to be psychotic, and he was about to be hospitalized when an intelligence test disclosed that he possessed extremely low intelligence. In this instance, the intellectual parents—both scientists—would have preferred emotional illness rather than low intelligence.

Another patient—a middle-aged man—showed such uneven, spotty, unpredictable performance on an intelligence test that the clinician recommended a neurological examination to assess the possibility of some brain dysfunction. The neurological examination did indeed indicate a brain tumor.

Intelligence and other kinds of testing disclosed that suspected mental retardation in a mute, withdrawn, youngster was unwarranted and that the youngster was highly intelligent, but suffering from emotional disturbance. In addition, she was found to have considerable hearing impairment that contributed to her emotional, social, and educational isolation.

The Binet and Wechsler Scales. Intelligence tests were first developed in France by Binet and Simon (1905) to classify children for the school system. The early Binet scales consisted of tasks—such as stringing beads or counting blocks—classified by age levels. Tests passed by a large majority of normal children of a particular age were included at a particular level (the five-year level, for example); all tests passed by normal six-years-olds were included within the six-year level, and so on. A child taking

Noverbal tests, such as the one being administered here, attempt to assess important aspects of intellectual functioning. (Copyright Sepp Seitz 1982)

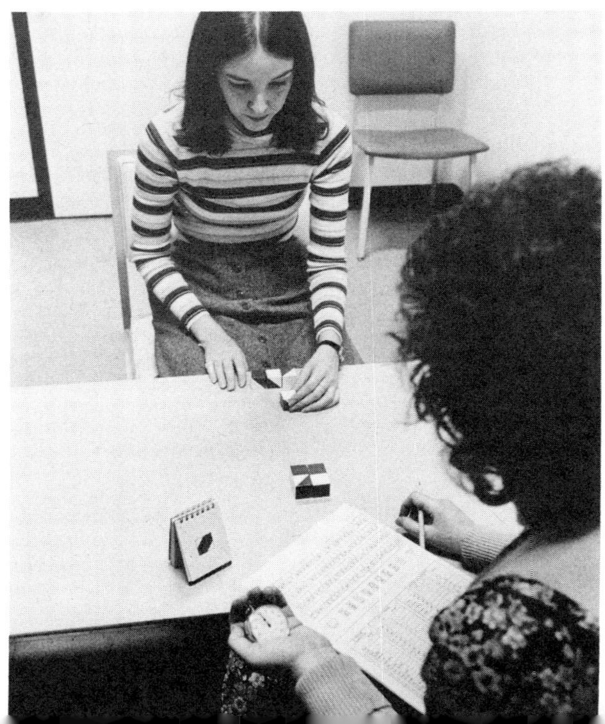

* See Chapter 14, pp. 379–82, for further discussion of these points.

the test could be placed within the most appropriate age level as determined by the level at which he or she passed all tests but failed all those on a more difficult level. Thus, the concept of mental age was born.

By dividing the child's mental age by his or her actual age, and multiplying this quotient by 100, the IQ score, or intelligence quotient, was obtained. For example, a child whose performance was equivalent to that of a five-year-old on the Binet scale but whose actual age was four years would have an IQ of 5/4 × 100 = 125 (actually, in months, 60/48 × 100 = 125). A child of eight years who receives a mental age of eight on this scale would have an IQ of 96/96 (months) × 100 or 100, an average IQ score.

The Binet intelligence test was revised and introduced to this country by Terman in 1916. Since that time, this test, which has come to be known as the Stanford-Binet scales, has been revised several times. The most recent revision (Terman and Merrill, 1973) attempted to deal with criticisms of the previous scales regarding their limitations and bias in standardization samples: the revision now includes minority groups, whereas the previous samples did not.

The Wechsler Intelligence Scales are among the most widely used intelligence tests and have been adapted for preschool childre, school-age children, and adults. Spotlight 5.4 describes some of the items from the revised Wechsler Intelligence Scale for Children (1974).

Spotlight 5.4 Wechsler Intelligence Scales

The Wechsler Scales of Intelligence, developed for adults of about ages sixteen to seventy-five (WAIS—Wechsler Adult Intelligence Scale, 1955), school-age children of about ages six to sixteen (WISC-R—Wechsler Intelligence Scale for Children, Revised, 1974), and preschool children about four and one-half to six and one-half years of age, or for older mentally retarded children (Wechsler Preschool and Primary Scale of Intelligence—WPPSI, 1967) are among the most widely used intelligence tests today. The WAIS and WISC have Spanish editions. For convenience, the Wechsler Scales retain the IQ when a final score is computed, but this is arbitrary, since these scales do not make use of a quotient to obtain the IQ as do the Binet scales.

All of the Wechsler scales contain several subtests or sections; generally there are five verbal tests and five nonverbal tests. The verbal tests yield a Verbal IQ, the performance tests a Performance IQ, and there is also a score based on both, the Full Scale IQ.

Illustrated below are paraphrased items from the verbal subtests of the WISC-R, the revised children's scale, and typical instructions from the performance scale. All of the Wechsler scales generally contain the same kinds of subtests, although the difficulty of the items varies considerably, depending on the test—adult, school-age, or preschool.

The tasks in the Wechsler scales are attractive and interesting to most subjects and they cover a

Verbal Scale	*Typical Item (Paraphrased)*
General Information	How many nickels make a dime?
General Comprehension	What should you do when you see a man forget his hat when he leaves his seat in a restaurant?

Arithmetic	Sue had two pieces of candy and Joe gave her four more. How many pieces of candy did she have altogether?
Similarities	In what way are a lion and tiger alike?
Vocabulary	What does pencil mean?
Digit Span (optional)	
digits forward:	I am going to say some numbers. Listen carefully, and when I am through say them right after me. 5 9 8 3
digits backward:	Now I am going to say some more numbers, but this time when I stop I want you to say them backwards. 6 3 9 2

Performance Scale

Picture Completion	What important part is missing? 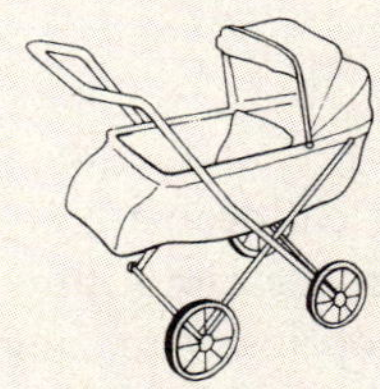 The Psychological Corporation
Picture Arrangement	Arrange these in their right order so as to make a sensible story.
Block Design	Now make one like this, using nine blocks.
Object Assembly	These pieces, if put together correctly, will make a duck. Go ahead and put them together. 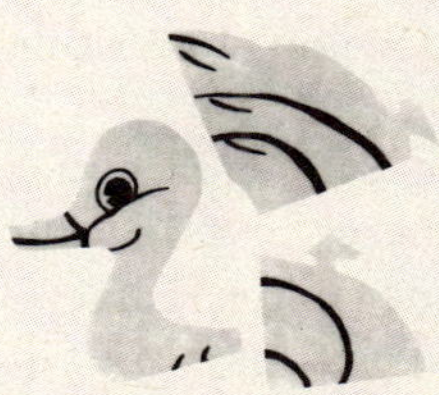 The Psychological Corporation
Coding	I want you to put in each of these squares the marks that should go there, like this.

Source: Items listed are similar to those on the Wechsler Intelligence Scale for Children–Revised.

wide age range. They permit the clinician to make inferences about the functioning of the subject by an examination of differences in the level of performance between and among sections of the test and between Verbal and Performance IQs.

For example, a patient showed extremely poor "recent" memory for numbers, as reflected by a relatively low Digit Span subtest score, and extremely good "old" memory, as reflected by a relatively high Vocabulary subtest score. Is he suffering from some organic brain dysfunction that sometimes produces this discrepancy? This is of course only a tentative inference that must be checked against many other criteria before its validity can be established; such discrepancies may also appear in very anxious people.

In this instance, however, the middle-aged patient showing this discrepancy also obtained a relatively high Verbal IQ of 130 and a rather low Performance IQ of 90. The poor performance on visual, motor, and spatial tasks of the performance scale, poor immediate memory, and a consistent pattern on some additional clinical tests administered as part of the battery resulted in a referral for a neurological examination. This examination did, indeed, yield positive findings: the patient was suffering from an early malignancy in the brain that was surgically removed.

DEVELOPMENTAL SCALES

Clinicians working with very young children are often called upon to classify them for various purposes, such as hospitalization or adoption. Are they neurologically impaired? mentally retarded? Are they developing normally in physical, perceptual, and language skills? For example, a two-year-old considered for adoption was examined and found to be so severely retarded that placement within a normal home would have been highly damaging, for both the adoptive parents and the child, who required special, professional placement that could give him an opportunity to develop his skills maximally.

Developmental scales make use of the fact that many functions and behaviors emerge and develop gradually, with age. These include motor, perceptual, numerical, and language functions, for example the ability to creep, stand, walk, hop, talk, walk backward, bounce a ball, repeat tapping on a drum, recognize color and size differences, locate parts of one's own body, tie shoe laces, copy simple designs such as circles, squares, and triangles, follow simple directions, place blocks in a tower, count, read and the like. These scales employ norms, so that the behavior of any particular six-month-old baby, for example, can be compared to that of normal six-month-old babies.

An important aspect of development concerns the establishment of lateral dominance, that is consistent right-left preference in use of hands, eyes, and feet. Mixed lateral dominance, that is, absence of consistent right or left preference, may be troublesome when skills such as reading and writing are introduced. For this reason, to complete the diagnostic picture, tests of lateral dominance are generally included in various developmental scales and one test is devoted entirely to exploring this question (Harris, 1956).

The Draw-A-Man test (Goodenough, 1926) was based on the early recognition that ability to draw a human figure developed with age. For years, this test was used as a simple method for roughly ascertaining developmental levels. Today most developmental scales incorporate some variation of this task (see p. 103 for illustrations).

PERSONALITY INVENTORIES

Because of the need for a speedy screening method for spotting possible mental disturbance among World War I recruits, rapid methods for obtaining personal data were introduced. The first of these, the Woodworth Personal Data Sheet, established a precedent for a parcel of subsequent inventories (such as the Bell Adjustment Inventory [1938] and the Bernreuter series [1935]). These tests consist of a series of printed statements to which the subject responds in some way—generally by checking "yes" or "no." For obvious reasons, these instruments are referred to as self-report methods.

The items in the early Woodworth inventory consisted of 116 questions about obsessions, nightmares, phobias, excessive headaches, fear of crossing streets, worry about bodily health, and other symptoms. Here are some examples: Do you bite your nails? Do you wet your bed? Do your palms get sweaty when you meet new people? Do you suffer from insomnia? These are typical of most self-report inventory questions, and although they seem to possess a certain amount of obvious ("face") validity and are easily and objectively scored and administered, such inventories have many problems.

Self-report inventories require that a subject report personal material truthfully, without malingering or faking—an assumption not always warranted. In addition, responses are meaningful only if the subject possesses some reading ability, introspective skill, and awareness of his or her symptoms.

Further, a powerful criticism of these early inventories was that subjects tended to report information about themselves or check items that reflected socially desirable responses—that is, that projected a favorable rather than an unfavorable image of themselves. The forced choice method is one solution to this problem. In this method, the subject is forced to choose between one of two paired items that is most (or least) characteristic of him or her. Each item in the pair has equal social acceptability or unacceptability. The social desirability of the item is established beforehand, through empirical research, but the subject does not know this. For example, here are items of equal social desirability from one personality inventory (Edwards Personal Preference Schedule, 1953):

- I feel depressed when I fail at something.
- I feel nervous when giving a talk before a group.

Since the desirability of an item and the positive or negative self-image it portrays are equated, the subject is forced to choose items on the basis of content rather than social acceptability.

Another criticism of early inventories is that they yielded one score presumably reflecting either a single dimension of personality or the totality of an individual's personal functioning; this reflected a naive and mechanical view of emotions that was becoming increasingly obsolete. The development of certain technical methods of treating scores made it possible to "extract" from the items in the inventories those clusters or factors that went together so that several independent scores could be obtained from the subjects' responses. Inventories could now be scored for several traits simultaneously, representing for many psychologists a more meaningful way of assessing the complexity of personality. One such inventory, for example, yields scores for the following traits: general activity, ascendance-submission, masculinity-femininity, inferiority, and nervousness (Guilford-Martin Inventory, 1948).

The Minnesota Multiphasic Personality Inventory (MMPI). In contrast to the more rudimentary inventories of the early years, the Minnesota Multiphasic Personality Inventory (MMPI) (Hathaway and McKinley, 1943) is a methodologically more sophisticated approach. The MMPI consists of 550 statements, printed on cards or in booklet form (for group administration), such as:

- I believe I am being plotted against.
- I am afraid of losing my mind.
- My neck spots with red often.
- I sweat very easily even on cool days.
- I can sleep during the day but not at night.

The subject is asked to classify the statements into categories of true, false, and cannot say. The content of items covers an extremely wide range, including: neurological problems, religious and political attitudes, health and psychosomatic concerns, sexual disturbances, and a range of classical symptoms such as delusions, hallucinations, obsessions, and phobias.

The subject receives a score on each of several

clinical scales. These, with an interpretation of what high scores on each of these scales mean, are:

1 Hs—Hypochondriasis: undue concern with health and bodily symptoms
2 D—Depression: depression and despondency
3 Hy—Hysteria: infantile, impulsive emotions and frequent physical symptoms with no organic basis
4 Pd—Psychopathic Deviation: antisocial, impulsive, guiltless acting out, sometimes with criminal intent
5 M-F—Masculinity-Femininity: either "masculine" interests for females or "feminine" interests for males
6 Pa—Paranoia: suspicious, overvigilant perception of the world; feelings of persecution
7 Pt—Psychasthenia: excessive compulsiveness or complusive indecision; worrisome thoughts; high anxiety level
8 Sc—Schizophrenia: retreat from others; odd or unusual behavior
9 Ma—Hypomania: active, impulsive, socially oriented; excitement or elation if scores are very high
10 Si—Social Introversion: shy, and introverted

The method (called criterion keying) used to determine which of the 550 items constitute each scale is based on actual empirical investigations. The items that distinguish the responses of normals from those of a particular clinical or pathological group are included in the scale for that group. For example, if it is found that normals do not say yes to a query about whether they hallucinate while schizophrenics *do* say yes, that question is included in the scale for schizophrenia.

The MMPI has received extensive research attention; it is a quick, reliable, easy-to-administer instrument that is objectively scored and interpreted. Most psychologists send their subjects' responses to services that provide automated computer interpretation. The computer's diagnostic statements are of course only as sound or valid as the programmer's formulations or rules for making diagnostic decisions. Spotlight 5.5 presents a typical MMPI printout.

Spotlight 5.5 *MMPI Profile of Betty, A Thirty-Three Year-Old Woman*

Betty sought psychotherapy when she was thirty years old, having just moved from a middle-class Dallas suburb to New York City and finding herself to be lonely, frightened, and depressed. She described herself as a reasonably talented actress with no professional experience or training but with a background of many successful amateur appearances in high school and community drama groups. She further claimed to be "hooked" on uppers, downers, alcohol, and, if she could get it, cocaine; also, she said that she was constantly battling a tendency to be at least thirty pounds heavier than she wished to be. Indeed, during the first months of therapy, she was heavy, listless, depressed, and confused about her future plans. She described her childhood and adolescence as a lonely, unhappy period, noting that her pattern of substance abuse began during adolescence and continued, on and off, for about fifteen years. She had always felt that she was different from her peers: bigger, more ungainly, less pretty, less socially skilled.

Her goals in seeking treatment were in these areas: she wanted to lose weight, feel more attractive, and fall in love, with marriage as an ultimate goal. Also, it was important, she felt, to control her depressions and improve the quality of her life while, at the same time, going off all substances. Finally, whether or not she ever married, she wanted to be financially self-supporting—as an actress, she hoped.

Today, some of these goals have been met. She is off drugs, has maintained a long period (two years) of weight control, is subject to fewer and less intense periods of depression, and is self-supporting as a free-lance "bit" player on daytime television "soaps" and commercials. She is, and feels, extremely attractive, has many friends, and is enjoying her life, although she has not fulfilled what she describes as her most important goal: to fall in love and marry.

Betty took the MMPI recently at the age of thirty-three, when she had a few consultative sessions with the therapist. The profile, scores, and computer statements that follow agree with her self-description that today, she is reasonably untroubled, emotionally speaking, and her life is productive and satisfying.

Scale	T SCORE WITH K	RAW SCORE WITH K	T SCORE WITH-OUT K	RAW SCORE WITH-OUT K
?				0
L			46	3
F			58	6
K			46	10
1 Hs +.5K	46	11	48	6
2 D			57	23
3 Hy			47	17
4 Pd +.4K	64	25	68	21
5 Mf			51	36
6 Pa			38	4
7 Pt +1K	43	21	47	11
8 Sc +1K	44	19	48	9
9 Ma +.2K	48	16	50	14
0 Si			52	27

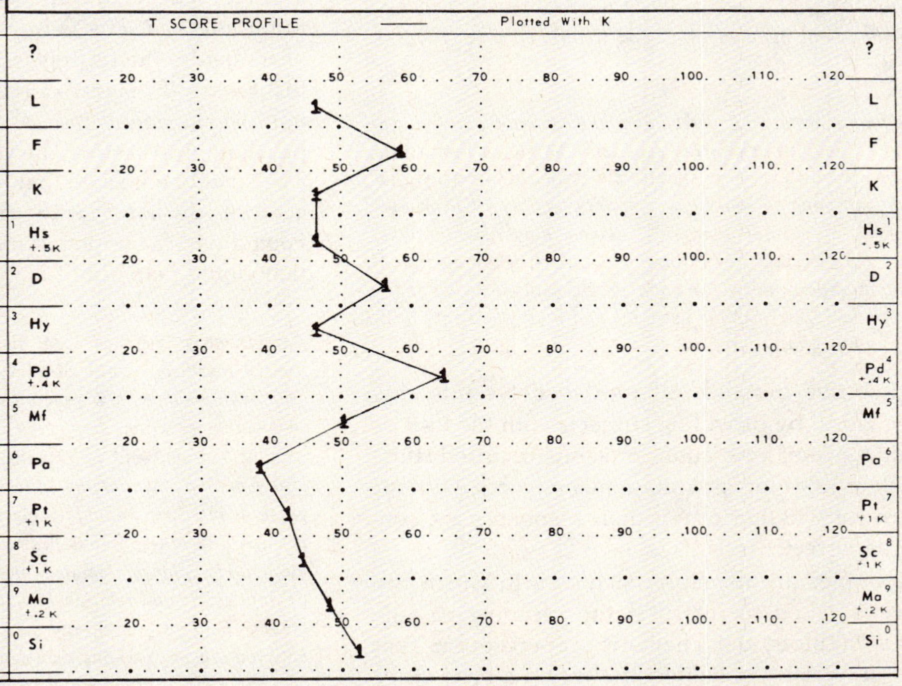

-INDEPENDENT OR MILDLY NONCONFORMIST.
-VIEWS LIFE WITH AVERAGE MIXTURE OF OPTIMISM AND PESSIMISM.
-HAS CAPACITY TO MAINTAIN ADEQUATE SOCIAL RELATIONSHIPS.
-NORMAL FEMALE INTEREST PATTERN FOR WORK, HOBBIES, ETC.
-NORMAL ENERGY AND ACTIVITY LEVEL.
-TOUGH MINDED.
-MAY HAVE POOR SELF-CONCEPT. PROBABLY WOULD LIKE TO DISCUSS EMOTIONAL PROBLEMS.
-FEW SOMATIC COMPLAINTS. LITTLE CONCERN ABOUT BODILY HEALTH.
-STRONG INTERESTS IN PEOPLE AND IN PRACTICAL MATTERS.
-PROBABLY NOT A WORRIER. TENDS TO BE RELAXED REGARDING RESPONSIBILITIES.

Source: Minnesota Multiphasic Personality Inventory. Copyright 1943, renewed 1970. All rights reserved. Distributed by NCS Interpretive Scoring Systems, P.O. Box 1416, Minneapolis, MN, under license from The University of Minnesota. Reproduced with permission.

PROJECTIVE TECHNIQUES: PRIVATE WORDS

What is of major significance for understanding the individual personality is that the individual organizes experience as he warps, twists, distorts and otherwise fits every situation, event and person into the framework of his private world, giving them the affective significance which they must have for him in his private world. Moreover, the individual may attempt to impose his personal beliefs and feelings upon the world of people and events or carefully guard his private world from any public disclosure that might reveal his own ideas and feelings. (Frank, 1948, p. 15).

. . . we may approach the personality and induce the individual to reveal his way of organizing experience by giving him a field (objects, materials, experiences) with relatively little structure and cultural patterning so that the personality can project upon that plastic field his way of seeing life, his meanings, significances, patterns, and especially his feelings. Thus we elicit a projection of the individual personality's private world *because he has to organize the field, interpret the material and react affectively to it. (Frank, 1939, pp. 402–403).*

Projective methods attempt to delve into this private world by providing subjects with the task of making sense of ambiguous or semistructured stimuli such as ink blots or ambiguous pictures, without concern for whether or not their responses are correct or incorrect.

Examples are the Rorschach test, in which the subject is asked to interpret the meaning of ambiguous inkblots, the Thematic Apperception Test (TAT), in which the subject makes up a brief story about a pictorial situation, or handwriting analysis, in which the idiosyncratic or unique attributes of an individual's personality are examined through specimens of his or her handwriting. Many projective methods have been developed (puppet play, for example), but only several of the most frequently used methods will be described here.

Projective methods emerged as a revolt against the objective, more narrowly defined personality tests just described. These methods were thought to be better designed for unraveling deep, underlying personality processes and motivations because they provided an opportunity for subjects to project inner feelings, conflicts, fantasies, and self-attitudes by allowing them to choose their own personal method of responding, in contrast to other tests that specified the type of response required.

Rorschach technique. Following are excerpts from a clinical report based principally on the Rorschach technique. The subject was an extremely intelligent fifty-year-old substance-abuser who used drugs to "get by" in life rather than for "kicks" (see Chapter 17). He had been, but was no longer, a successful brain surgeon. His wife had divorced him several years before the testing session and he had not seen his twenty-five-year-old daughter (*their* decision, not his) since that time. A year after he was seen for psychological testing, he died of a drug overdose. The suicide note said that he had never been able to achieve closeness with others or to become involved with a support system, in or out of therapy, that would help him.

. . . patient is concerned about his future integrity, ability to pull himself together, sexual adequacy, and lack of a close intimate relationship. This is a psychoneurotic personality with an obsessional orientation, deep needs for close attachments, great anxiety, depression, and continuous, troublesome thoughts (mostly guilty ones) regarding his failures in life. . . . this is an anguished, insecure, uncomfortably shy person who is extremely ill at ease with others unless heavily supported through drugs and alcohol. He is lonely, isolated, unable to achieve in work, at play, or in interpersonal relationships, any enduring satisfactions. His tenuous hold on himself and on a lifeline to others forces him to look toward medications and drugs—legal or otherwise—to bolster him. He is filled with self-pitying, alienated fantasies in which punishment, fears about the future, and fears about his emotional integrity and wholeness are enmeshed, creating an extremely unhappy inner life. . . . This is a tormented person—cautious, fearful, and sensitive who does not trust his ability to cope with his life. . . . note that cognitive pathology is not present, but past history and obsessive doubts pull him in ways that should be watched, lest the poor social supports in his life, in interaction with inner anguish and torment, cause him to "act out" . . . It is difficult to evaluate the tremulousness, anxiety, and general state of motoric agitation he is experiencing, since the drug picture here is so complex. On the other hand, sudden withdrawal of ingested substances is not recommended. . . . This highly intelligent, resourceful, person feels he is going nowhere. He is reaching out for help—mostly in terms of support just now—in a therapeutic relationship in which he does not feel threatened.

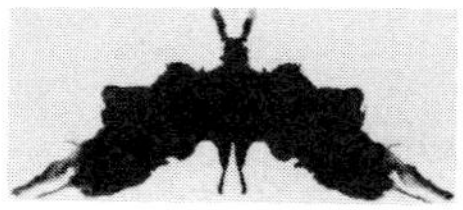

Figure 5.1 Plate V of the Rorschach Inkblot Test. (Copyright 1942 by Hermann Rorschach. Reproduced by permission of Verlag Hans Huber, Publishers.)

Hermann Rorschach's work with inkblots over sixty years ago changed the face of personality testing (Rorschach, 1942). He made blots by dropping a blob of ink on a sheet of paper, folding the sheet to spread the ink, then unfolding the sheet. He found that different diagnostic groups, such as schizophrenics or depressives, could be identified by the kinds of responses they gave when asked to say what the blots looked like, what they could be.

The Rorschach test consists of ten inkblots, five made with achromatic ink, two with red and achromatic ink, and three with many colors. The examiner hands the cards to the subject one at a time and asks him or her to say all the things the blot looks like, what it seems to be. There is no right or wrong way of proceeding, the examiner explains, stating that this is not a speed test. If the subject wishes, he or she is allowed to turn the cards in any direction. The subject is also informed that when through with each card, it can be put down.

The examiner records all of the subject's responses, the position in which the card is held (whether upside down or sideways) and the time it takes for a response to be given for each card (reaction time). The subject is encouraged to give more than just one response per card. After each card has been shown, there is an inquiry, in which the clinician makes sure of the exact location of the response, what in the response influenced or determined the particular response (such as shading, color, or a combination of shading and shape), and whether the subject saw human or animal motion in the response (such as someone dancing; bears dancing; a tug-of-war between people, a person soaring in space).

Each response is then scored for its location, determinant, and whether or not it is a popular response (there are empirically determined lists for the latter (for example, "bat" for Card I) and the frequency of tallies in each of these categories is ascertained. The relative frequencies within the categories, the context of the responses, as well as several other considerations constitute the raw material that goes into a Rorschach interpretation.

Hermann Rorschach, and clinicians and researchers after him, discovered the varied characteristics, especially among diagnostic groups, of responses to inkblot stimuli. For example, depressives tend to give very few responses to the inkblots. In contrast, schizophrenics tend to give peculiar or unusual responses, or to see themselves in the blots ("this is a bat that is going to get me and tear me from limb to limb"), or to give responses highly tinged with bizarre and violent content (for example, dismemberment, penises being electrocuted, fecal matter being smeared). To illustrate, the following responses were given to the same colored card.

From a twenty-nine-year-old woman, preoccupied with her body and obsessed with her inability to have an orgasm:

1 pelvis
2 vagina
3 skeleton
4 symbolic face
5 penis, arteries coming out of it
6 sunnyside egg
7 kidneys and intestine
8 wishbone

From a depressed man with suicidal ideation:

1 I can't see anything . . . it doesn't look like anything . . . looks like a colored design
2 just some smears of paint

From a schizophrenic man in his twenties:

1 an accident . . . a bullet wound because fighting over the same heart
2 God versus evil tearing it up
3 split in the middle and the ooze is coming through . . . very sick
4 boy with a broken heart who wants to bite this all off

Rorschach diagnoses and interpretations of personality are based on empirical evidence of how different groups of people respond to the blots and on an elaborate theory concerning the "meaning" of the determinants (color, shape or form, or shading or texture). The relative frequencies of these determinants are of great importance. For example, an excessive number of shading or texture responses (such as bearskin rugs or satiny surfaces) suggests, according to many Rorschach experts, a cautious, watchful personality. Or, an excessive number of color responses (blood, flower, sunset) with little or no movement responses suggests an explosive, impulsive personality.

Despite the fact that it is a very popular instrument, use of the Rorschach test presents many problems (Schumer and Zubin, 1972; Zubin, Eron, and Schumer, 1965). Chief among these is the failure to establish precise validity for the scoring components (and the interpretations based upon relationships among them). Other problems include: difficulties in ascertaining the reliability of scores; the great variation and subjectivity of interpretation that occurs from one clinician to the next; the extensive time required for administration, scoring, interpretation and write-up; and the fact that responses of subjects have been shown to be very much affected by intelligence and educational level—a poor characteristic for an instrument designed to measure emotions and personality.

Nevertheless the richness of interpretative material, the move away from a single-score approach, the stress on the complex emotional make-up of the individual that the Rorschach permits, and the possibility of delving into the inner depths of the individual (the Rorschach has been likened to an X-ray of the personality) have made this instrument an extremely important member of the clinical battery.

Thematic Apperception Test (TAT). This pictorial technique, like the Rorschach, is one of the most widely used methods in clinical testing (Morgan and Murray, 1935; Murray, 1943). The TAT aims to plumb the subject's inner fantasies. It consists of twenty cards, some of which are designated for boys, some for girls, and some for men or women. Most of the pictures contain a person or people in varied situtions that are open to different interpretations; about half of the pictures are unusual or bizarre. The subject is told:

> *I am going to show you some pictures, one at a time; and your task will be to make up as dramatic a story as you can for each. Tell what has led up to the event shown in the picture, describe what is happening at the moment, what the characters are feeling and thinking; and then give the outcome. Speak your thoughts as they come to your mind. Do you understand? . . . Here is the first picture (Murray, 1943, p. 3, Manual).*

The tester records in longhand or on tape the verbatim stories of the subject. Usually the stimuli are presented in one session, rather than two (as Murray had originally intended), and the examiner chooses those judged most relevant to the patient's problems. Interpretation is generally based on the content of the subject's responses, but many differ-

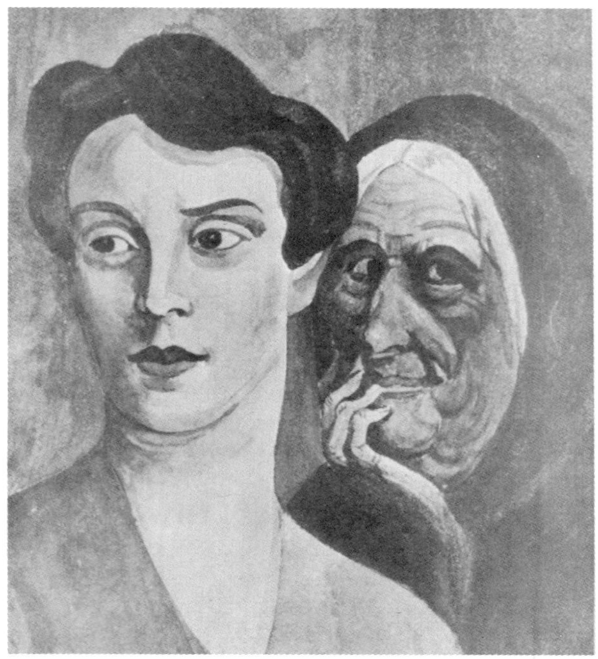

Figure 5.2 Card 12F of the Thematic Apperception Test. (Reprinted by permission of the publishers from Henry A. Murray, *Thematic Apperception Test,* Cambridge, Mass.: Harvard University Press, Copyright © 1943 by the President and Fellows of Harvard College, © 1971 by Henry A. Murray)

ent scoring systems are available (such as the one in Zubin, Eron, and Schumer [1965]). Reliability of scoring systems is generally quite good, but reliability of the instrument as a whole is less well established.

Three different stories for one of the TAT pictures (which depicts a partially nude woman lying on a cot and a fully dressed man standing facing away from her with his head partially covered by his arm) follow. The first is from an intelligent man with a paranoid personality (see Chapter 9) who also shows much obsessional indecision:

The woman is lying limp and the arm is not held firmly and she's sleeping . . . no she's dead or ill . . . and the man is very upset . . . It couldn't be after sex because how come he's dressed and she's not . . . But it could be that she's sick and he came to see her . . . but he also appears upset . . . On the other hand, he could have just gotten up and she's still sleeping and for some strange reason he was lying next to her fully dressed . . . but he's too dressed for that . . . He's upset and maybe there are tears . . . if that's so, he's lost something or someone . . . I don't know . . . There are other possibilities. . . .

From another intelligent man, described as showing extreme depression (see Chapter 9):

The woman is dead or ill, very ill and young man either having caused her death or she just died . . . But he's showing remorse or grief even if he did not cause it . . . all I can say . . . or just had intercourse . . . ashamed of what has done . . . her figure seems much too inert and too limp . . . She's probably dead . . . and husband is grief-stricken. . . .

And finally, from still another intelligent man with psychosomatic symptoms (see Chapter 8), sexual dysfunctions, and a history of alcohol and drug abuse:

She seems ready for him . . . that's what I thought of first . . . My second impression is that he has a headache and that she has overdosed and that he just discovered her and maybe feels guilty . . . If he had been there earlier, instead of the bar he was drinking at and had shown her more compassion, she would not have been dead . . . He forever carries the guilt with him . . . goes out and has another drink to relieve his headache. . . .

Overall, the TAT is an easy-to-administer test that possesses face validity, especially if it is assumed that the subjects identify with heros or heroines and that the plights, conflicts, moods, outcomes, and ways of dealing with anxiety ascribed to these story characters are actually valid characterizations of the subject. These assumptions, however, have not been empirically validated. Yet, many clinicians claim that the TAT generates much insight into the subject's inner emotions, conflicts, and fantasies, especially if used in a clinical battery. In addition, the TAT is interesting to people, can be modified for many groups (children, for example,) and seems natural and unstilted in the clinical setting. Although many methods based on the TAT model have been developed in the past few decades, none is as widely used as the TAT.

Figure drawings. Ever since the introduction of the Goodenough Draw-A-Man test for the assessment of the intellectual development of children, clini-

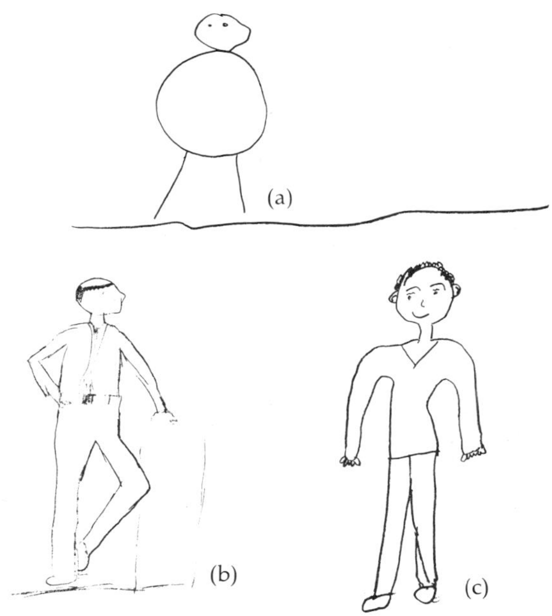

Figure 5.3 Drawings of male figures by three different subjects. (a) Drawn by a depressed, prematurely senile 65-year-old male of extremely high intelligence. (b) Drawn by an extremely intelligent, normal 11-year-old female. (c) Drawn by a depressed 40-year-old male of above-average intelligence who also shows some obsessional symptoms. (a) (b) (c)

cians have been fascinated by the possibilities of using a subject's drawing of a man or a woman as a projective device. Drawings also provide an opportunity for the clinician to ask questions about the figures the subject has drawn on the assumption that the subject is actually identifying with them.

Clinical interpretations of the subjects' figure drawings are based not only on the content of responses to such queries as "What gets him angry?" but also on such structural characteristics as the solidity of the pencil line, placement on page, size of figure, presence or absence of certain features, and emphasis on facial characteristics such as eyes or ears (Machover, 1949).

The reliability and validity of available scoring and interpretative systems for drawings have not been clearly established; the figure drawing test therefore does not entirely qualify as a sound test. Yet many clinicians find this method quite useful when administered as part of a test battery.

Expressive movements. The way an individual moves through life—his or her style of body movements has often been thought to provide a rich observable reservoir for interpretation. Thus handwriting, walking style, posture, bodily movements (Spiegel and Machotka, 1974), and spontaneous doodles and drawings have all been presented as reflecting an individual's emotional make-up.

In varying degrees, these methods possess face validity—that is, they seem to make interpretative sense. Often a kind of analogous reasoning is used: a person who walks or stands in a tight, controlled, rigid way is said to possess these qualities in personal characteristics. Although such interpretive possibilities are fascinating to the layman, many of these methods offer little more than armchair psychology if they do not go beyond the descriptive level to a level that involves the test development procedures described earlier.

According to one hypothesis (Berg, 1959, 1967), any behavior that deviates from some norm (test content itself is unimportant) can be the proper context of a personality test. However, whether reading facial expressions or handwriting, we cannot judge the merit—validity or reliability—of the interpretations we assign without providing empirical evidence.

SPECIAL CLINICAL TESTS

Certain tests yield useful clues as to the nature of the subject's thinking processes, such as ability to form abstractions. Other tests measure such functions as memory, visual-motor coordination, spatial perception, and reasoning. These special clinical instruments are useful because sometimes, in conjunction with other tests and observations, they point to the possibility of impairment in central nervous system functions (organicity) or to the presence of certain types of thinking disorders associated with schizophrenia. Only one such clinical test—a widely used one—is described below.

Bender Visual Motor Gestalt Test This test, introduced by Bender (1938), requires the subject to copy as best as he or she can, without a time limit, the nine simple designs, which are presented one at a time. The execution of this seemingly simple task involves a complex interaction of visual and motor skills—skills that are often extremely vulnerable to brain damage and various kinds of central nervous system (CNS) pathologies. This test is also quite useful in the assessment of possible developmental difficulties in children.

The methods described in this chapter are among the most frequently used techniques in assessing patients. These include observations, interviews, and tests. It should be emphasized once again that most clinicians use these methods as frameworks on which to add their own intuition and judgment; a wise and experienced clinician contributes something extra when he or she appraises a patient.

The psychological tests described in this chapter are not the only methods for appraising patients. You are reminded of the discussion at the end of Chapter 4 and at the beginning of this chapter that

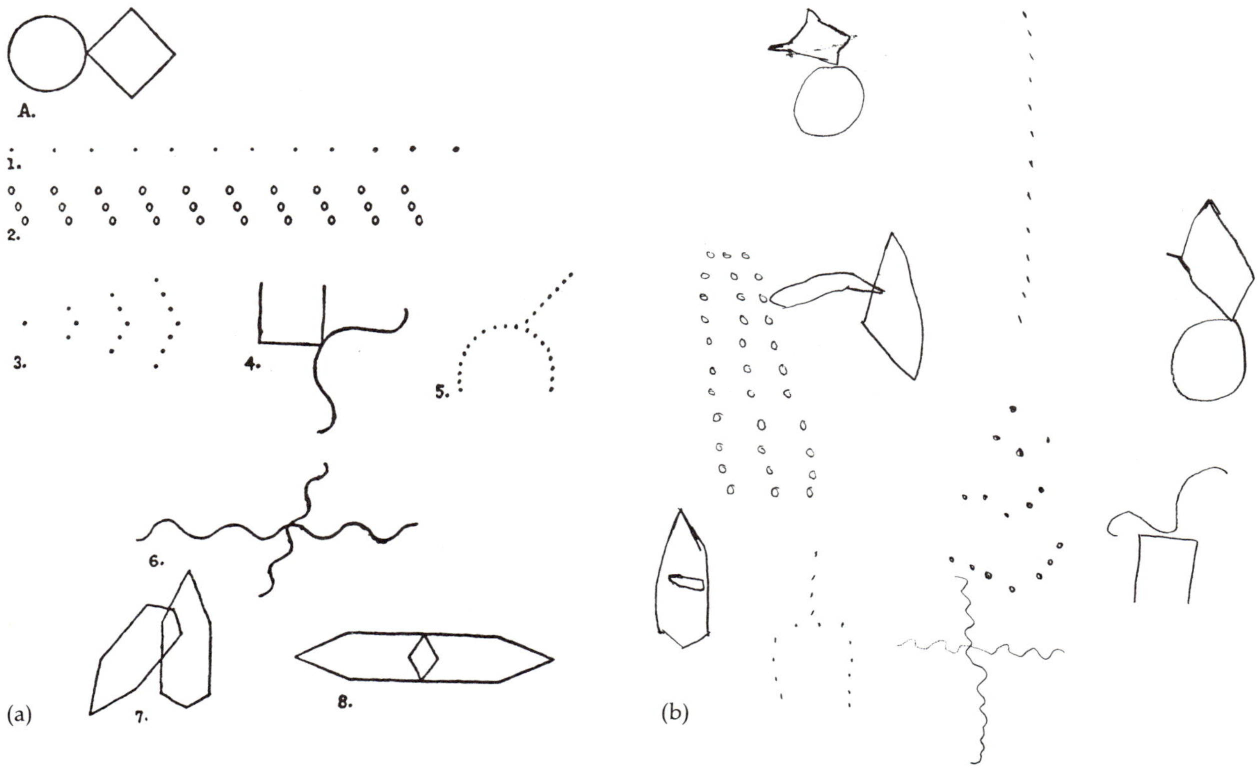

Figure 5.4 The Visual Motor Gestalt Test. (a) Designs 1–8 and A (introductory design) appear on separate cards. They are presented one at a time to the subject, with the simple instruction to copy them "the way you see them." (Taken from the Bender™ Visual Motor Gestalt Test, published by the American Orthopsychiatric Association) (b) Copies of the designs in (a) made by a neurologically impaired, intelligent, adult woman.

many new methods and approaches to diagnoses and assessment have emerged and will be described in relevant chapters throughout this book.

SUMMARY

This chapter surveyed some special methods that psychologists use to obtain data about people for purposes of assessing their emotional status or making a diagnosis. These methods include diverse types of interviews, ratings and observations, and psychological tests. The chapter discussed various aspects of the construction and use of psychological tests, including norms, standardization, and considerations concerning their validity and reliability. Finally, it presented and illustrated some of these tests, including intelligence tests, developmental scales, personality inventories, projective methods, and special clinical tests.

Highlights

1. Interviews are the backbone of the clinical interaction. Yet, they do not always yield objective, reliable information about the status of the subject. Although structured interviews, rating

scales, and computer diagnoses may solve some of the problems of the clinical interview, they, also, have disadvantages.

2. A sound psychological test should be standardized and its validity and reliability empirically established and made public. The face validity of many popular tests tells us little about its validity.
3. Although intelligence tests such as the Binet and Wechsler scales often serve a useful function in the clinical battery, the IQs yielded by these instruments do not reflect inborn, fixed, invariant structures, functions, or capacities.
4. Although many personality inventories are objective and easily scored, and some of them are fairly reliable, they suffer from the same problems as do many other self-report techniques. For example, subjects may not be inclined to respond truthfully about traits they consider to be undesirable, also, early inventories tended to reflect only single dimensions of personality. Forced-choice items and tests constructed so that they yield scores that reflect several distinct personality dimensions solve some of these problems. The Minnesota Multiphasic Personality Inventory (MMPI), one of the most widely used personality instruments, can handle many problems that less sophisticated personality inventories cannot deal with.
5. The development of projective methods provided more of an opportunity to delve into the complex, subjective world of inner emotions and processes than did the personality inventories, by presenting test situations in which subjects are required to interpret or assign meaning to semistructured or ambiguous stimuli with little awareness of what they are revealing. However, despite the claims made for instruments like the Rorschach and Thematic Apperception Test and the richness of the interpretations they made possible, serious questions about the reliability and validity of these and many other projective techniques continue to be raised. By and large, these instruments have not fulfilled their promise.

ISSUES AND QUESTIONS

1. Psychological tests have been criticized on many grounds. For example, they often permit the questionable practice of labeling individuals, "locking" them into diagnostic categories that follow them through their school, job, or military careers. Test results, in the form of reports, scores, and interpretations are often accessible to institutional staff members, nurses, teachers, doctors, and aides, thus representing an invasion of privacy. The use of tests is also questioned in connection with determining promotions, raises, and the hiring and firing of employees. Tests have also been singled out as providing unfair and inappropriate assessments of populations with educational limitations, reading difficulties, and ethnic minority backgrounds.

   Because of these problems, some suggest that the kinds of testing described in this chapter be discarded entirely. Others holding more moderate views suggest that psychological testing be employed only at the request of the client and that the report be sent only to the client. Do you agree? Consider the many beneficial uses of tests before taking a position on this matter. Remember, for example, the children who were incorrectly thought to be psychotic or mentally retarded before testing cleared up the misdiagnosis.
2. The persistent use of the term *IQ* as if it represented something real that existed in the brain rather than being the name for a ratio score derived from a human-made instrument, is a phenomenon worthy of exploration. It is rather a remarkable observation that although many tests do not yield such scores (because they are not age scales and do not permit a ratio score to be calculated), developers of some tests are forced to translate their natural scores to IQ scores because of public, even professional, demand. Because the myth of the stability and possible inheritability of the IQ, has been perpetuated, clamor has arisen in some quarters

for the elimination of the phrase from professional and lay terminology. Do you agree?

3. The unreliability, vulnerability to misinterpretation, and incomprehensibility of many clinical reports (to all but those familiar with the style of the person writing them) are well known. Should patients or subjects be sent copies of reports written about them? Would the possible damage to their self-esteem be too great a risk? Might an unstable person become extremely agitated as a result? Should such reports be written at all?

SUGGESTIONS FOR FURTHER READING

American Psychological Association. *Standards for educational and psychological tests.* Paperback. Washington, D. C.: American Psychological Association, 1974. This little booklet—soon to be updated—was prepared by a special committee of professionals who use and understand psychological tests. It sets guidelines and standards for the proper use of tests in the light of their potentially abusive aspects. Guidelines for establishing reliability, validity, and making public the norms on which tests are based are clearly outlined. It also addresses itself to the limitations and dangers of generalizing from test scores to many subgroups in the population, such as those with reading difficulties, foreign language backgrounds, or limited educational backgrounds. This manual is essential for the developer of tests, the user of tests, and students who wish to know more about these psychological tools.

Anastasi, A. *Psychological testing.* 5th ed. New York: MacMillan, 1982. This basic text provides an introduction to psychological testing. General issues such as reliability, validity, standardization, and ethics of test administration and application are thoroughly discussed. More than half the book is devoted to a description of various tests of intelligence, vocational aptitude and interest, educational aptitude and achievement, and personality. Diagnostic use of various tests for clinical purposes is also discussed. For those who plan to continue studies in psychology, this book is a must for the reference shelf.

Cronbach, L. J. *Essentials of psychological testing.* 3rd ed. New York: Harper & Row, 1970. This is an excellent, detailed, formal survey not only of tests and their use, but also of methodological issues and problems. This book is for students who want to know more about the technical aspects of test development and test construction and are looking for a sober evaluation of general methods in this area.

Zubin, J., Eron, L. D., and Schumer, F. *An experimental approach to projective techniques.* New York: Wiley, 1965. This book is recommended for students who wish to continue their work in psychology. The authors pay special attention to the complex methodological problems of establishing the validity and reliability of the Rorschach and Thematic Apperception Test (TAT).

6

Psychological Theories of Abnormal Behavior

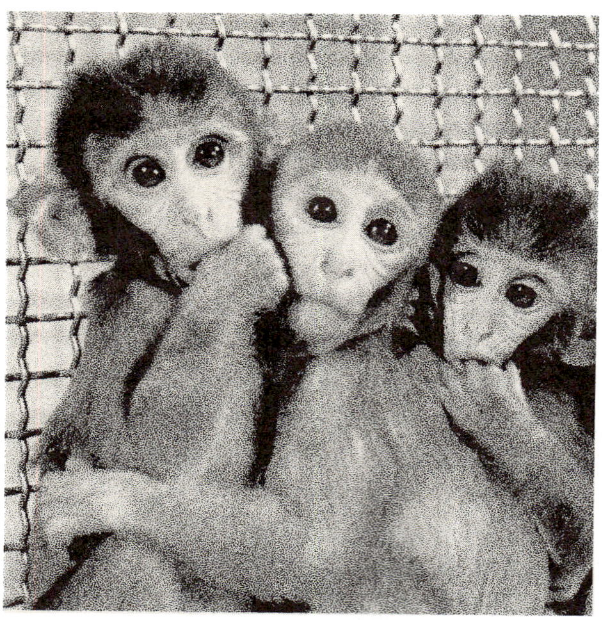

Chapter 1, which described the causal array, noted that many different kinds of variables could produce abnormal behavior. These variables include sociocultural factors, learning and conditioning, family interactions, stress responses and life events, and genetic and biochemical factors, among others. Chapter 1 also noted that the most useful etiological model is probably one that acknowledges an interaction of several factors—a model called a field approach.

This chapter describes in greater detail several psychological theories and models—viewed separately—that attempt to account for the etiology of abnormal behavior. The sociocultural explanations for abnormal behavior have already been described in earlier chapters. The present material continues to present and evaluate the different theoretical positions held by scientists in this field.

Why are there such a variety of theories of abnormal behavior? Diverse attempts to explain human mental pathology persist because no one theory or set of explanations answers all the questions concerning aberrant human behavior. The search continues for the key to the overall understanding that could predict, control, and modify pathological behavior. For eventually, if the scientific effort is successful, one theory would emerge as having accumulated more validity than others, the other approaches, less fortunate, would fade away.

At the present time, we are far from this ideal state. For there is no one accepted theory of abnormal behavior. Various theories that attempt to explain why certain people display abnormal behavior each yields its own characteristic type of research investigations; and each suggests different methods for controlling or treating mental illness. For example, if one subscribes to the notion that the biochemistry of the individual's inner make-up is related to whether pathology will develop under certain conditions of stress, then a biochemical approach to treating that pathology might be appropriate. On the other hand, if one believes that hidden, repressed, unconscious motives are responsible, then uncovering and exploring some of these motives might be the solution.

Some of the theories described in this chapter are less scientific than others, since they may go nowhere—are dead ends—with regard to verifiability. Yet, even these less objective approaches may be helpful in providing insights into the complex, mysterious forces that underlie behavior.

Spotlight 6.1 describes a theory of mental illness that has little current status, but which once had intrigued many people as possibly having some worth.

Spotlight 6.1 Theory or Myth? The Debunking of a Superstition

How does one decide whether an explanation for mental disturbance constitutes a scientific theory or is simply an example of folk psychiatry rooted in superstition and false beliefs? This is a difficult question. One generally accepted answer is that if the explanation is scientific it must be verifiable: it must generate predictions which will support or undermine its validity.

That mental illness is caused directly by phases of the moon is an example of a long-standing superstition that finally, it is hoped, has been laid to rest by scientific evidence. Over the centuries, various cultures have attributed mental disturbances to the moon; the English word "lunacy" is derived from the Latin word *luna*, meaning moon. A recent review of sixteen studies attempting to document lunar effects on human behavior and mental disturbance has shown, however, that such effects are rarely found (Campbell and Beets, 1978). Even when positive results are obtained, they can generally be dismissed as resulting from research errors or confounding factors.

1. Several studies attempted to correlate psychiatric hospital admissions to phases of the moon. Four of the studies showed no significant relationships, and the two studies that yielded positive results were not successfully replicated.
2. Studies that attempted to correlate suicide and suicide attempts with lunar phases also yielded insubstantial results. Some studies reported significant results one year but not another. Other studies showed correlations in opposite directions in various years: that is, one year the suicide rate was significantly higher during certain lunar phases and another year it was significantly lower. Most studies, however, yielded insignificant correlations.

3. Attempts to find an association between homicides and lunar phases have also yielded contradictory results. Although two studies yielded positive findings, three found no relationship whatsoever.

One factor that may account for the results of the few studies that found correlations between moon phases and abnormal behavior is the calendar weekly cycle—the days of the week on which full moons tend to fall. Since there are generally fewer hospital admissions on weekends, years during which the full moon tends to fall on weekdays would artificially show a higher incidence of mental hospital admissions during the full-moon phases than, for example, during the ten days prior to the full moon. One study, which initially showed positive results, later yielded no full-moon effect when day of the week was controlled statistically.

Thus although for centuries people have been noting a correspondence between lunar phases and various abnormal behaviors, there does not, in fact, seem to be scientific support for these inferences. The possibility nonetheless exists that if people subscribe to a superstition, expect certain occurrences, and believe in the power of particular natural events to influence behavior, then behavior can be influenced accordingly. These beliefs and expectations may well inflate, in some cultures, the relationship between lunar phases and certain behaviors—for example, bizarre responses of one sort or another, and even suicide attempts. Beliefs and expectations are indeed powerful determinants of behavior.

PSYCHODYNAMIC* APPROACHES: FREUD AND HIS FOLLOWERS

Freudian Theory

Sigmund Freud (1856–1939) lived and worked most of his life in Vienna. He was remarkably advanced in his thinking and in his attempts to question the mores and taboos of the repressive Victorian era in which he lived. The double standard, repression of sexuality, and little public acknowledgement that people had emotions, bodies, and biological urges was the order of the day.

Freud's writings (1904; 1924; 1933; 1940; see also Jones, 1953–1957) articulated and brought out into the open the hidden motivating forces that underlie human behavior. Outer appearances and inner lives do indeed differ, and it was Freud who helped us to take a closer look at our inner worlds.

Chapter 1 noted that the origins of Freud's revolutionary approach to psychopathology can be found in the nineteenth-century work of practioners such as Charcot and Janet. These physicians, with whom Freud studied, were intrigued with certain kinds of symptoms—hysterical (conversion) symptoms—which, although involving some loss of physical function, could not be accounted for by physical causes. They discovered that symptoms such as loss of speech (aphonia) or inability to see or walk could be dramatically eliminated by nonphysical methods such as hypnosis or suggestion—and this despite the fact that patients with these symptoms had no awareness that they were not suffering from actual physical disabilities.

When using hypnosis in the treatment of hysterical symptoms, Freud found that some of his patients could relive early, vivid, frightening or traumatic experiences (extremely stressful early childhood events that inflict great psychological damage on the individual). After coming out of their hypnotic states, these persons experienced considerable relief from their symptoms and sometimes even a permanent cure.

* This is a general term with several meanings; most often, however, it is used to denote approaches that explain behavior, especially pathological behavior, on the basis of (usually unconscious) motives and drives.

Freud found that not all patients could be hypnotized, however. He discovered that some patients could be encouraged through "talking out"—catharsis or abreaction—to search for, find, and sometimes relive the original painful event that caused the symptom. Thus, without hypnosis, Freud could achieve dramatic symptom reduction with some of his patients. To facilitate the talking-out process, he developed the technique of free association, which involved having patients say whatever came to their minds. This technique enabled him to examine the inner workings of the mind more closely while simultaneously helping the patient uncover forgotten, painful experiences and conflicts.

From his work with patients' free associations, Freud developed theories about how the human mind develops and functions. However, the sample from which Freud derived his theories consisted primarily of affluent female patients who came to him for help with regard to mental disturbances. Many scientists have argued that a view of mental development based upon data from such a biased sample must be limited.

Descriptions of some of the key concepts of Freud's theories follow. It should be noted that Freud did not believe in a strictly mechanical approach to the emotional life of the individual. Rather, he spoke of interactions, complex forces, and a rich embroidery of drives and feelings.

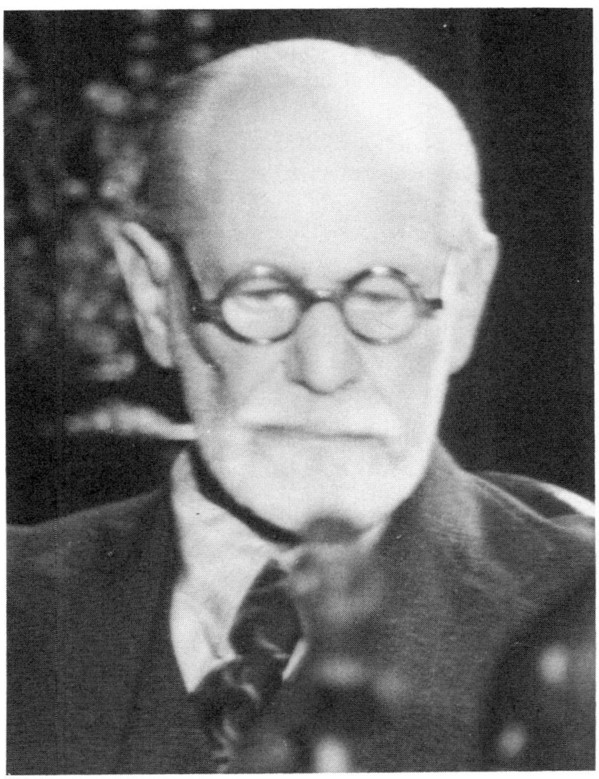

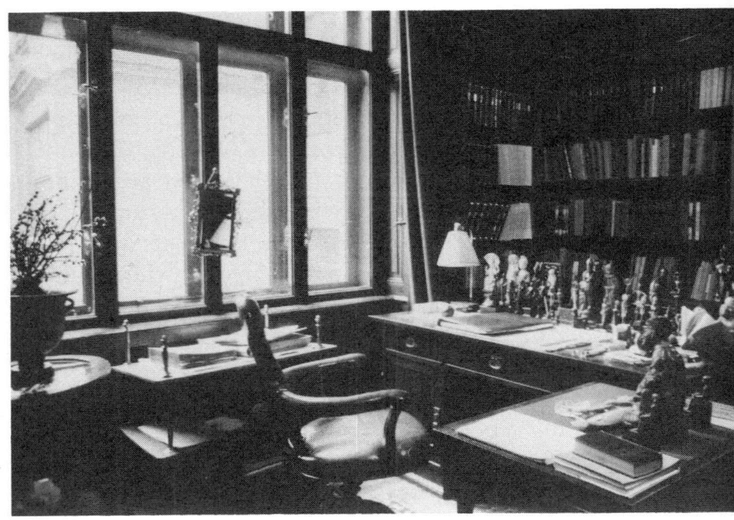

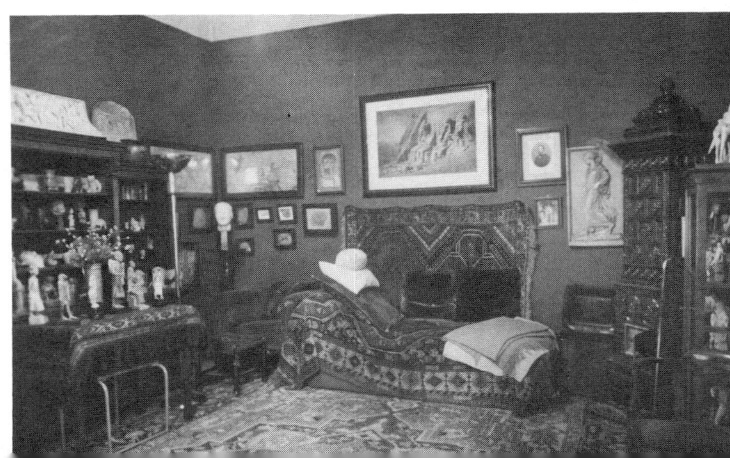

Sigmund Freud—in 1938, just before he fled Vienna because of its social and political climate—and his den where he saw patients. (Photographs by Edmund Engelman)

Structure of the mind. Freud stated that the human mind is composed of three major structures: the id, ego, and superego.

The id consists of the mass of innate drives and bodily instincts characterized as heightened states of tension that are released when the instinct or drive is satisfied. The instinctual impulses that comprise the id, are thus constantly pushing for satisfaction, which results in tension release. Sucking or defecating are examples of id drives. Since the release of tension is pleasurable, the id functions in accordance with the pleasure principle; that is, it seeks pleasure in the form of release of tension through the expending of instinctual drive energy. Drives or instincts are thwarted, modified, twisted, or buried by many forces. Freud was a pioneer in attempting to understand systematically the impact of these forces.

Over time, as the organism has increasing contact with reality, the ego develops. The ego enables the individual to find satisfaction for id impulses and drives in the world of reality while, at the same time, inhibiting those id impulses that come into conflict with reality. For example, the id impulse to defecate when the need arises becomes inhibited and redirected by the ego as the young child learns to control the frequency of bowel movements and also learns that toilets are the appropriate places for satisfying this particular urge.

The ego, then, functions according to the reality principle. As social and family pressures take hold, the pleasure principle must be discarded or modified so that the growing child can function socially in the larger world. Many people, however, are unwilling or unable to control their impulses. Freudians sometimes explain the behaviors of certain kinds of impulsive, infantile adults as resulting from an inability or unwillingness to function on the basis of the reality principle.

The superego incorporates the social values and moral tenets of the society in which the individual lives. Originally formed through the child's identification with his or her parents, the superego is the conscience of the self and is responsible for the shame, guilt, remorse, and sense of wrongdoing that is felt by many individuals when they flaunt the mores they have internalized.

Some people are said to have poor or faulty superego development. Freudians describe the personalities of many criminal and antisocial types in this way: although their sense of reality may be intact, their sense of right and wrong is askew. At the other extreme are those individuals who have such a sense of righteousness, conscience, and need to live up to moral principles that they do not seem to be "human." These people are regarded as having excessive superego development.

In actuality, all three parts of the mind (or personality or emotional makeup)—the id, ego, and superego—are in constant interaction with one another, pushing, pulling, winning out, being overcome. Explained in Freudian terms, much of the pathology and many of the symptoms described in chapters of this book that follow arise from conflicts in the mind's battlefield.

Processes of the mind. Although Freud did not discover unconscious mechanisms, his emphasis on and systematic exploration of the nonconscious aspects of human behavior was a key contribution to the understanding of emotional conflicts. Until Freud, many people thought that the only wishes and desires that motivated people were those which were in conscious awareness. By suggesting the existence of an unconscious reservoir of instincts, drives and wishes, Freud made it possible to explain hitherto unexplainable emotions and behaviors.

According to Freud, the masses of unconscious material, with its pushes, strivings, conflicts, hidden and forbidden wishes and fantasies, loves, and hates are primary processes. As in dreams, this inner content is not bound by logic, rational processes, and the limits of reality. Two mutually exclusive wishes—wishes which by their very nature cannot both be satisfied—can exist side by side in the unconscious. This is possible because they are of a primary nature, unaffected by demands of reality.

Secondary processes are reality-based thinking processes. They modify primary-process material so that it becomes more compatible with the demands of reality. A wish for food becomes a search for food through using secondary-process thinking.

When secondary, reality-based processes are dysfunctional, primary processes break through. Incestual drives and fantasies, for example, are primary-process impulses that sometimes appear in the behavior of disturbed people whose reality-testing or secondary-process thinking and control are impaired.

Defense mechanisms employed by the ego also serve to inhibit and modify primary process material. Painful or shameful material, memories of forbidden desires and experiences, and primal-scene memories (memories or fantasies of witnessing the sexual intercourse of one's parents) would be too disruptive to the functioning of the ego if allowed to remain on conscious levels. They are therefore repressed—buried in the unconscious—where they will be out of conscious thought, although in Freudian terms, not out of mind. For example, intensely destructive, aggressive wishes toward one's parents may cause intense anxiety if allowed expression or even conscious awareness. According to psychoanalytic theory, these wishes are forced into the unconscious by various defenses, the chief of which is repression.

If not well disposed of or well defended against, these painful thoughts and forbidden wishes will break through as abnormal behaviors and symptoms. Although symptoms such as severe depression may be uncomfortable, even anguishing, actually impeding or obstructing an individual's daily life, they are, according to Freud, a more socially acceptable means of expression of a forbidden wish than the direct expression of the wish itself.

Sometimes the defenses against painful, unacceptable wishes and the powerful need to retreat from the anxiety and shame they engender produce dramatic negative results. They seem to backfire in the form of symptomatic behavior that may be bizarre and unhealthy. For example, denial of aggressive, homicidal impulses toward a frustrating, harsh parent may result in the individual turning the anger and hostility toward himself or herself, saying, in effect, "I am no good; I hate myself; I am worthless; I deserve to be severely punished." This inverted anger is regarded by many Freudians as one explanation of depression.

Not all defenses against unacceptable impulses produce severe symptoms. As a matter of fact, many different kinds of defense mechanisms are used by all of us at one time or another. Spotlight 6.2 describes some of these. Do you recognize any of these mechanisms in yourself?

Freud believed that if the repressed wishes and memories, which he held were the cause of painful symptoms, could be articulated and rendered conscious, the symptoms would no longer be needed as disguises for the wishes, and would simply disappear.

Spotlight 6.2 Anna Freud and Some Mechanisms of Defense

Anna Freud, Sigmund Freud's daughter, dedicated a lifetime to the application of psychoanalytic principles to the study of children and adolescents. She was among several clinicians to elaborate on the significance of the ego in the structure of the psyche as the component that helps the individual to get along in the world (1946a). She was particularly interested in studying the ways in which the ego handles painful, shameful, and undesirable mental material, maintaining that repression is not the only such mechanism.

The descriptions that follow are of some universal mechanisms—defense mechanisms—that people use to handle or deal with certain kinds of experiences that cause anxiety or embarrassment. Highly disturbed people also use some of the mechanisms. In Freudian language, these spontaneous mechanisms are used to deal with pushes from the id or the strictures of the superego to obtain psychic equilibrium or balance; we are not consciously aware of bringing them into play. In this way, anxiety and awareness of humiliation, fear, guilt or other painful experiences are avoided.

Rationalization: assigning some rational or plausible explanation to a motive, behavior, or activity to cover the true reason or motive. There are two favorite kinds: "sweet lemon"—it could have been more worse; or "sour grapes"—I didn't want it anyway.

Reaction formation: the transformation of a forbidden, shameful wish into its opposite; displaying excessive aggression or anger toward someone on whom one is unusually dependent (such as a parent), is an example.

Denial: this can involve simple, normal forgetfulness, repression, amnesia, or detachment from the act, emotion, or memory of a painful event.

Sublimation: the repression or suppression of a sexually desired object, activity, or wish with the substitution of a nonsexual, usually socially desirable activity, such as daydreaming and fantasy activity; violence, aggression, or sexual wishes can be sublimated into wrestling or similar socially acceptable encounters.

Intellectualization: denying or covering a strong drive or unacceptable impulse or drive with intellectual, cognitive activity; by this means, affective experiences and strong emotions are avoided.

Displacement: transferring an unacceptable drive, wish, or emotion from one person to another where it becomes more acceptable and less painful; for example, latent homosexual impulses of men toward boys could be displaced onto group work with boys' organizations, or excessive anger toward one's father could be displaced toward the boss or professor.

Compensation: excessive or exaggerated development of an area to avoid a sense of inferiority or pain associated with awareness of certain personal limitations.

Isolation: withdrawal or retreat, mostly from emotional expression, emotional experience, or emotional memory concerning an unacceptable impulse or drive.

Undoing: repetition of a wish, fantasy, or impulse—as if by magic—through the use of rituals, acts, and ceremonies, thus removing the painful thought's magical power to create pain or anxiety.

Projection: attribution to others of one's own unacceptable wishes, desires, thoughts, drives, or impulses.

Introjection: incorporation of characteristics, qualities, and traits of the loved object to avoid the painful, anxiety-producing effects of loss, separation, or removal from that loved one.

Identification: avoidance of harmful, punitive, or anxiety-producing effects of another on oneself by identifying with the other, more powerful figure; identifying with the aggressor if one is a victim, is an example.

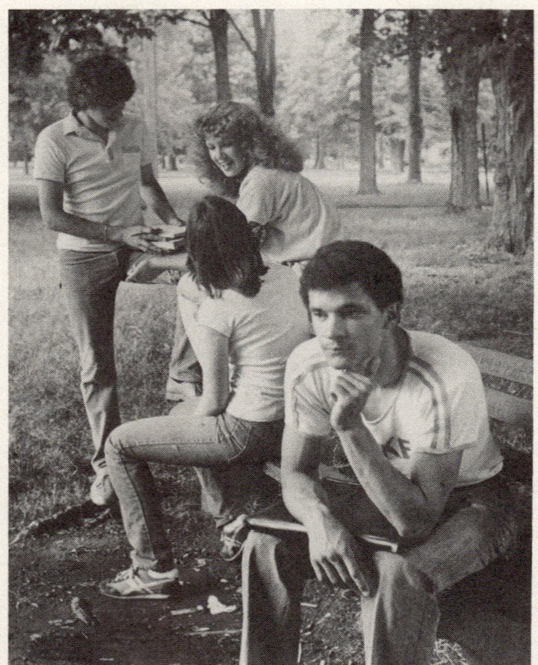

Is this young man displaying the defense mechanism of isolation? (Sybil Shelton/Peter Arnold, Inc.)

Instincts, sexuality, and sexual development. All babies are born with instincts, which comprise the inner core of energy and drive in adults as well. According to Freud, they fall into two major categories: the sexual, life instincts, or libido, and the death instinct. Libidinal drives are the primary and basic forces within the individual. They consist of energies and tensions that are sexual, pleasurable, and erotic in nature and they are concerned with living and with growth.

Stunned by the scope and destructiveness of World War I, Freud added aggression and the death instinct to his theory as a separate, autonomous, basic drive. Along with the striving for life there is a push toward death, with a return to an inanimate state as the ultimate goal of living.

The history of what happens to these drives in any individual is the history of that individual's developing personality. Since libido is seen as a basic drive, Freud's theories of infantile sexuality and of psychosexual development occupy a key place in his schema of individual personality formation—or deformation.

Psychosexual stages are developmental phases that all individuals pass through. The human organism is born into a world dominated by a need for survival: eating, breathing, urinating, and defecating are essential. The primary concern of the infant in the earliest stages, up to the second year of life, is on sucking and feeding. This earliest period of sexual development is called the oral phase, in which the primary love object is the mother or mother surrogate. In the anal phase, emphasis is placed on bowel control; erotic activity and pleasure seeking focus on defecation and bowel retention. This period occurs roughly from two to four years of age. In the phallic phase, from about three to five years, the child focuses on the genital area, which through autoerotic (masturbatory) activities, yields pleasurable body sensations,. That is, the child experiences erotic, sexual pleasure in these areas. During the latency stage, from approximately six to eleven years, the sexual drives are inactive. At puberty, at around the twelfth or thirteenth year, a reawakening of sexual interest and drive occurs.

According to Freudian theory, the quality of the child's experiences during these stages will determine the personality characteristics he or she develops. In addition, various symptoms can become fixed, attached to, or associated with early psychosexual stages and the relationships formed at those stages, leading to fixation at one or another of these stages. A strong need for continual oral nourishment are aspects of being fixated at the oral stage, and a typical Freudian view of the adult alcoholic is that the alcoholic is fixated at an oral stage in which there is strong dependency on the mother. Fixation at the anal phase (particularly the "anal-sadistic" phase, which would involve hurting others) is manifested by retention of feces (constipation), often accompanied by an excessive preoccupation with cleanliness and orderliness.

Sometimes a defensive maneuver against the deep, harsh, and overpowering demands of reality may force an adult to regress to an early, infantile psychosexual level in which primary-process strivings guided by the pleasure principle are the dominant forces in the person's behavior. Freudians believe that many psychotics are regressed. To confirm this view, they point, for example, to chronic schizophrenics, who play with their feces, or urinate in bed, or babble like babies.

The most critical psychosexual stage, according to Freud, is the phallic or Oedipal stage—the period during which the child must deal with Oedipal issues, the resolution of which can result in normalcy or neurosis. During the phallic stage, the boy becomes attracted and attached to his mother in a romantic sexual way, referred to by Freud as the Oedipus complex. The son is competing with his father, and wishes the father would die so that he could have his mother to himself. The boy feels very guilty about these feelings and develops a fear of brutal retaliation. For his shameful thoughts and desires, he fears that his penis will be cut off, and he may then develop a castration anxiety, or castration complex.

If the boy is unable successfully to repress his desires for his mother and to identify with his father, he will live with an unconscious fear of castration, according to Freud, which can result in symptoms of extreme passivity or homosexuality.

At around three to five years of age, girls shift from their attachment and dependency on their mothers to favoring their fathers. Sexual attraction to the father is an aspect of the female counterpart of the Oedipus complex (sometimes referred to as the Electra complex). Another characteristic feeling of little girls at this age, according to Freud, is anger and frustration at the lack of a penis. Because very young girls feel that the penis is powerful and superior, they develop penis envy, which becomes a significant aspect of psychosexual development. For example, Freud held that little girls wish for babies by their fathers as a substitute for their lack of penises. According to this view, unless penis envy is resolved, little girls will compete with little boys, and as they grow into womanhood, with men—a competitive striving that arises out of a sense of injury, inferiority, and failure to accept the feminine role of childbearer and homemaker. This particular Freudian principle is especially controversial because it assumes female inadequacy, male supremacy, and biologically simplistic views about the rigidity of social roles and gender identity.

The Freudian legacy. The contribution of Freud to the understanding of the complexities of human behavior, especially abnormal behavior, can never be

Spotlight 6.3 Unconscious Wishes and Psychopathology

Defending against unacceptable wishes—experienced as intensely uncomfortable, sometimes unbearable, if allowed to remain on the conscious level—sometimes produces maladaptive behavior and symptoms. The power of these totally unacceptable, unconscious wishes to "seep through" in distorted fashion can be illustrated by some of the classic psychoanalytic case descriptions found in Fenichel (1945).

For example, an interpretation of agoraphobia (fear of open streets, being in public, being in crowds) in a young woman was interpreted as a defense against hostile exhibitionism directed toward her mother—a wish that was unacceptable to the patient:

The anxiety attacks of a female patient with agoraphobia and crowd phobia had the unconscious definite purpose of making her appear weak and helpless to all passers-by. Analysis showed that the unconscious motive of her exhibitionism was a deep hostility, originally directed toward her mother, then deflected onto herself. "Everybody, look!" her anxiety seemed to proclaim, "my mother let me come into the world in this helpless condition, without a penis." Originally the attack represented an attempt to exhibit a fantasied penis (p. 200).

Irrational, excessive concern over the health or well being of a relative, such as a child or a spouse, actually reflects a defense against hostile wishes toward that person:

Analysis shows that the person who has to be protected represents an unconsciously hated person, who, therefore, actually needs protection not from external dangers but rather from inner death wishes. Often what has been repressed returns from the repression, and continuous caretaking or reassuring affection may become objectively a torture (p. 207).

And with regard to the ritualistic, compulsive pressure to count that some children display:

Counting may . . . represent a counting of seconds, that is, a measuring of time . . . The basic connections between time measuring and anal eroticism have been mentioned. The time measuring, being originally a measurement of the interval between two occasions of being placed on the toilet, may then be used as a defense against the temptation toward anal masturbation, and may eventually become a substitute for anal masturbation (pp. 288–89).

Source: Fenichel, O. *The psychoanalytic theory of neurosis* (New York: Norton, 1945). Reprinted by permission of the publisher.

overestimated. His attempts to bring together the unfolding of a human life with needs and drives and social forces impinging on it, were grand in scale, as befits the wonder and richness of a life. More important, for Freud, the complex interaction of drives, motivations, and inner processes spans a lifetime, beginning with the baby and ending only at death. He emphasized motivational elements, especially unconscious motivational elements, and the privacy and secrecy of an individual's unconscious, accessible to both patient and doctor only by a process of long, often painful, exploration.

The fact that people experience conflicting feelings simultaneously—that emotions can be ambivalent, ambiguous, and contradictory—is an observation made repeatedly by Freud: things can be other than what they seem to be or what we say they are. "I love you" does not always mean the same thing for all people. People can love *and* hate those closest to them—mother, father, or children—at the same time.

And human lives were regarded as embodied, as having tissue and flesh. For the first time, psychologists could consider and describe with professional dignity, previously unacceptable, aspects of human biology in relation to human motives and behavior. Sexual matters, feces, body fluids (menstrual blood, mucus, vomit), anal sensations, infantile sexuality, pregnancy fears or fantasies, aggressive impulses, love-hate relationships, incestuous, bisexual, and homosexual strivings—the very aspects of human life never acknowledged by Victorian society were now out in the open. It became possible to speak freely about "unspoken" drives, repressed memories, inner feelings, and "shameful" conflicts. It was also now possible to entertain the notion that even children could have erotic and sexual impulses. And it was possible to acknowledge the powerful impact of unconscious pushes within individuals and of the guilts they might harbor over failure to meet the social standards and expectations of others. Freud also opened up new vistas for the treatment of mental disorders; Chapter 19 will describe Freudian treatment methods in some detail.

The Freudian heritage is still strongly felt today. Abnormal behavior is generally viewed as a psychological rather than a medical phenomenon. Talking things out, verbal therapies in general, and the training of nonmedical professionals were all made possible by Freud's innovations. By attempting to place explanations for a wide range of abnormal behavior within one grand scheme, the psychoanalytical framework represents an extremely ambitious project, the impact of which is still being felt throughout the world.

The critics' voices. Freud's contributions were met by many theorists and clinicians with uncritical acceptance. Even staid experimentalists were so taken with the logic and grandness of Freud's views that some dropped their rigorous adherence to parsimonious explanations to search for experimental verification of Freudian principles (for example, Dollard and Miller, 1950). Many began ingenious laboratory experimentation with animals to search for experimental analogues of Freudian concepts. For example, it was demonstrated that learned aggressive behavior among rats could be "displaced" to celluloid dolls (Miller, 1948). Rats were experimentally shown to "regress" to a former mode of behavior when frustrated (provided the former mode had already been learned); even "reaction-formation" had been demonstrated with rats in the laboratory (Mowrer, 1940).

Critics of Freudian theory point out that most studies presumably supporting psychoanalytic theory were poorly executed. Repetitions of such experiments often failed to yield the same positive results. In addition, many of Freud's theoretical concepts, such as the death instinct, cannot be scientifically verified. Many critics believe that the scientific status of Freudian theory can neither be proved, disproved, or explored in systematic ways—that many Freudian principles are simply inaccessible to experimental verification. Freud's verifications came from his own evaluations and case illustrations rather than from replicated, empirical evidence.

Another difficulty with the Freudian framework

is that because it attempts to explain so much of human thought, emotion and behavior, simple tests of some of its assumptions have little impact on the scope and complexity of the theory as a whole. When contradictions are discovered, the introduction of additional principles to account for the exception to the rule seems to be the usual solution. Elegant theories are simply not constructed this way.

As for the actual content of Freud's views, many feel that the biological and instinctual orientation of the Freudian approach overlooks the significance of social and environmental factors as determinants of psychopathology. Similarly, the universality of sexual explanations in accounting for most pathology is also questioned.

Critics also claim that Freud's theories were heavily biased by the prevailing viewpoints of his times, and that he did not see the immediacy of his own social milieu as it affected his thinking. For example, Freud proposed that male and female roles within the family unit—that is, the male as the head of the family and the female as housewife and mother—were biologically determined, healthy, and normal. His hypotheses about penis envy and the nature of emotionally healthy female sexuality as represented by the capacity to achieve vaginal orgasm are today considered to be outmoded concepts.

Overall, extensive reviews of evidence in support of Freudian hypotheses suggest that there may be some evidence for such aspects of Freudian theory as the anal character (character traits of meticulousness, orderliness, excessive neatness, and stubbornness tend to go together) and the oral character (persons preoccupied with oral satisfactions tend to be talkative, dependent, submissive, and childish). However, most of the studies reviewed fail to produce evidence in support of Freudian hypotheses (Fisher and Greenberg, 1977; Kline, 1972). For example, support was not found for principles having to do with psychosexual development, structure of the mind (ego, id, and superego), and instinctual wishes. Nor was Freud's theory of infantile experiences as the source of various character types confirmed. Evidence for the validity of specific explanations of some of the neuroses or psychoses was also not found, including, among others, Oedipal conflicts for conversion hysteria, anal-sadistic regression for obsessional neuroses, and repressed or projected homosexuality for paranoid schizophrenia.

Nonetheless, the debate over the validity of Freudian theory goes on as part of a larger struggle to provide scientific explanations for the bewilderingly complex array of human experience and behavior.

Freud's Disciples and Followers

Freud was surrounded in Vienna by students, colleagues, admirers, and followers. Some of these adherents broke away from the inner circle to form psychoanalytic schools of their own. The more prolific of these theorists, such as Carl Jung, eventually established their own status, support, adulation, and fame.

In actuality, the differences among analytic schools essentially reflected refinements in approach that were magnified in the minds of the analysts themselves. The point is that in actual treatment methods (for example, the one-to-one patient-doctor approach, the use of talking methods that relied on introspection, and the reliance on unconscious motivation as a theoretical base) were all shared by most of the "deviant disciples" (for example, Jung, 1916; Rank, 1936; and Reich, 1960).

Carl Jung, who attracted to his fold powerful, wealthy people, illustrated perhaps more than anyone else how Freud's attempts to understand the individual and his or her problems could be expanded, modified, and reconstructed. Jung believed in the racial inheritance of mental content, the collective unconscious, and universally inherited belief systems. He elaborated his views by a far-reaching, impressive study of the occult, fairy tales, folklore, mystical beliefs, religious systems, universal symbols, the arts and tribal rites of primitive peoples, and the cultural and social universals through the ages. His emphasis on dream content as reflections of racial instincts and memories of the ancestral past, and his strong beliefs in mysticism made for appealing and provocative reading. Yet in contemporary psychology, Jung's approach seems to have little direct usefulness for understanding, predicting, or treating abnormal behavior.

The New Freudians: Recognition of Social Forces

Dissatisfaction with the instinctual and biological aspects of Freudian theory resulted in the development of several psychoanalytic approaches to understanding abnormal behavior that tended to acknowledge, more than Freud did, the role of social conditions, culture, and socially induced conflicts in the neurotic individual's experiences.

The psychoanalysts that fell within this group are sometimes called neo-Freudians (for example) Alfred Adler [1927]—known for his work on the inferiority complex and for the striving toward superiority that human beings possess; Erich Fromm [1941, 1947]; Karen Horney [1937, 1945, 1950]; and Harry Stack Sullivan [1953, 1962]).

In some of these neo-Freudian approaches, society is regarded as the culprit in producing pathology. In others, the view is stressed that individuals need to relate to each other in a productive, supportive way. If this is not possible, or if the individual has few opportunities to do so, a condition of alienation and despair can result.

Social forces that can induce conflict can come from the family setting, such as the quality of the mother-child relationship. But conflicts can also arise from opposing social values—for example: be kind, compassionate, and considerate but at the same time be competitive, become successful, and be a winner.

The roles of the unconscious and of sexual conflicts and repression are generally deemphasized by the neo-Freudians. Instead, basic anxiety, interpersonal relationships and conflicts, and the fear of being alone are stressed. Problems in the real world such as war, violence, and economic insecurity are acknowledged as important factors in attempts to understand how anxiety, insecurity, inferiority complexes, and other kinds of neurotic conditions arise. In therapy, learning to modify actual behavior is given increased importance. Also, the therapist is permitted to be more active in the treatment situation.

Yet the treatment approaches of the neo-Freudians still employ verbal methods, a one-to-one patient-doctor situation, and a frame of reference in which the therapist is the authority regarding what constitutes normality. However, despite adherence to older, more conventional methods, the neo-Freudians, in their recognition of social frames of reference, made immeasurable contributions to the understanding of abnormal behavior by placing it in the context of the patient's real world.

Erik Erikson

Erikson has become a popular figure among students through his compassionate and extensive writings concerning crises in adolescence that occur in the attempts to discover one's own ego identity (1968). Erikson suffered his own identity crises. Growing up in Germany, he was the son of Danish parents—a non-Jewish father and a Jewish mother whose background included a rabbi and a minister. When his mother remarried a Jew, he was a "goy" [a non-Jewish outsider] to his mother's husband's family but was scapegoated as a "Yid" at school.

Erikson's contribution to psychological theory lies in his views concerning individual development throughout the life cycle, from birth to death. He conceptualized this development as a series of stages, each with age-appropriate crises and conflicts that must be resolved so that the individual can proceed to the next stage. In many ways, Erikson's early stages are similar to Freud's conceptualizations of the childhood psychosexual stages. Erikson's extensions of these stages to the middle years and old age represent a significant step toward the recognition of middle-aged adults and the elderly as real people, with real crises, conflicts, and problems.

The changes required of an individual as different needs and interests, expectations, views, and outlooks develop at various significant phases of his or her life are emphasized throughout Erikson's ego psychology. When an individual, through parental, social, or inner blocking is unable to adapt to the conflicts and solutions appropriate to the life crisis of those particular years, a sense of growth, development, inner unity, and personal contentment is stymied, and growth toward the next stage is made difficult or impossible. This picture of ego development has been popularized in a variety of magazines and books because it makes sense; a popular audience can identify with the stages that Erikson outlines. For example, one elderly patient, extremely depressed and isolated, was able to understand, to relate to, the ego stage of late adulthood Erikson describes by deliberately exploring for himself the ways he could come to terms with the eventual death he (and all other people) face.

Spotlight 6.4 summarizes Erikson's life stages.

Spotlight 6.4 Erikson's Life Cycle: The Psychosocial Crises

The psychosocial stages of life, as delineated in Erikson's scheme, are developmental phases most of us must confront and deal with. Note how relative to our own culture these stages are—and how much they relate to the mainstream elements of our culture.

Infancy: the oral-sensory stage. The infant focuses on the lips, fingers, and nourishment—the taking in of food. It is at this time that the child builds up basic trust and security in his or her world, provided the relationship between the mother and child is mutually gratifying. If not, the seeds for mistrust, anger, suspicion, and various other pathologies later in life are sown.

Second and third years: the muscular-anal stage. Young children learn to walk, to master their environments, and to control their bowel movements. At this time, they develop confidence, assurance, and autonomy. If frustrated, opportunities to feel a sense of mastery become limited. If made to feel foolish or ashamed, the child learns to feel inadequate and to develop self-doubt.

About four to five years: the locomotor-genital stage. During these years the child shows curiosity, emulates adults, and develops sexual or romantic attachments to the parents of the opposite sex. If thwarted in these impulses, the child can develop a guilt complex, castration complex, and become confused in role identification.

Ages six to eleven: latency state. During this period the child is actively learning about the world, is busy at school, and develops interests and skills outside the home. If the child is unable to feel that he or she can have an impact on the environment, feelings of inferiority and incompetence may develop at this time.

Ages twelve to twenty: puberty and adolescence. The finding and establishing of one's ego identity (who one is), ideological values, sexual interests, and a sense of independence from one's parents take place during these years. Failures to achieve these goals may result in role confusion, bisexual orientation, value confusion, and conflicts about dependence-independence.

Young adulthood: love, work, and intimacy. The young adult becomes committed to work and to love, and develops interest in the mutuality of a marriage. If this does not take place, the young adult becomes isolated, self-indulgent, and eventually unable to establish stable, enduring relationships.

Middle adulthood: generativity. The middle years are characterized by a desire to guide the younger generation and to help shape society. The middle-aged adult would otherwise live only for himself or herself in stagnation, self-absorption, and personal gratification.

Late adulthood: ego integrity. Winning the battle over the despair that is faced when one faces death is a question of ego integrity. By this is meant an acceptance of self, one's past, and the life cycle, which includes death.

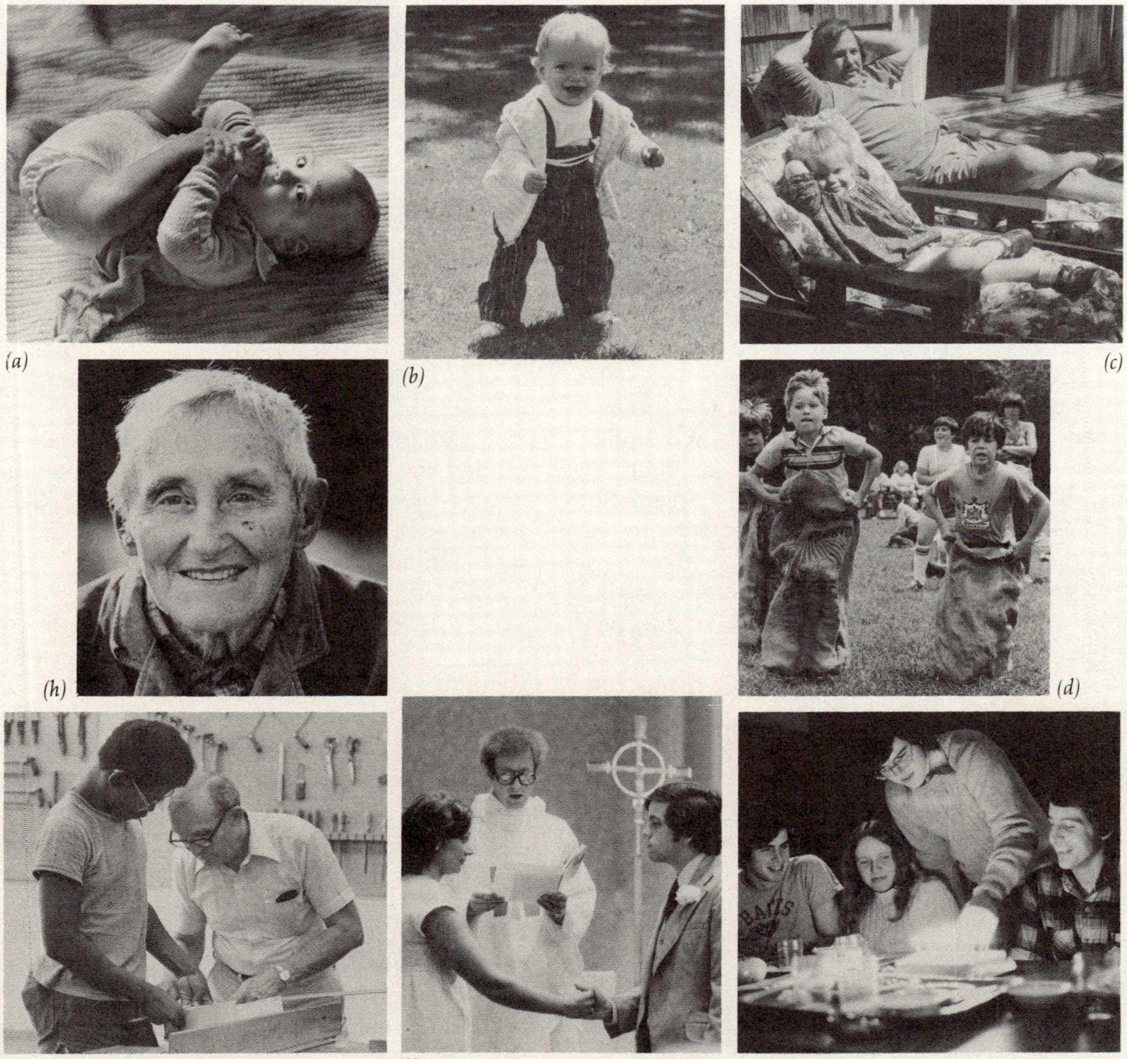

(a) (b) (c) (h) (d) (g) (f) (e)

According to Erikson's theory, a person, in order to develop normally and achieve a satisfying life, must successfully resolve a crisis in each stage of his or her life. They are: (a) infancy: trust versus mistrust; (b) age 2–3: autonomy versus shame and doubt; (c) age 4–5: initiative versus guilt; (d) age 6–12: industry versus inferiority; (e) puberty and adolescence: identity versus role confusion; (f) young adulthood: intimacy versus isolation; (g) adulthood: generativity versus stagnation; (h) maturity: ego integrity versus despair. (Clockwise, beginning at upper left: Alan Carey; Gabor Demjen/Stock, Boston; George Gardner; Phyllis Graber Jensen/Stock, Boston; Frank Siteman/Stock, Boston; Owen Franken/Stock, Boston; Thomas England/Photo Researchers; Michael Hayman/Photo Researchers)

HUMANISTIC APPROACHES

Maslow and Others

Several approaches to personality development reflect an understanding about people and their emotions that share a common humanistic thread (Angyal, 1941; Goldstein, 1939; and Maslow, 1954). Although differing in actual substance, these approaches generate an optimistic, forward-looking acceptance of individuals and their conflicts. These views stress each individual's potential for change, growth, and self-actualization. Self-actualization—freedom from anxiety, growth of the individual toward fulfilment, self-acceptance, and full use of one's capacities and inner resources—is a guiding principle in defining a healthy, well-adjusted person. These humanistic approaches talk of the "whole" person in a "dynamic, environmental field."

Humanistic psychology views people as essentially good—as possessing innately positive natural characteristics. However, favorable social conditions and environments are necessary for optimal growth.

Humanistic views of mental health are highly valued by many and have influenced the development of special techniques for changing behavior—helping individuals to grow—including various encounter and human potential methods (see Chapter 19).

Carl Rogers

Rogers' views (1951, 1961) are based on a phenomenological approach to understanding the personality—a view holding that an individual's experiences can be known only to that individual. His thinking grew out of many years of therapeutic experience, during which time he confirmed his impression that counseling had more to do with each person's unique perception of reality and self (the "me," the feelings and conceptions and inner thoughts about one's self known only to one's self) than with the real, objective world. Therefore, any attempt to understand or modify a person's behavior involves seeing the world as that person sees it.

When one's concept of one's self and one's desires, goals, and ambitions (the ideal self) and the world of reality are in accord—have achieved congruence, according to Rogers—then that person is free of tensions and anxiety. However, when the ideal self and reality are not congruent, pathology will result.

Like other humanistic approaches, Rogerian therapy (see Chapter 19) assumes that the individual carries within the self the potential for change, problem solving, and self-fulfilment. This means that minimal activity or direct intervention and guidance on the part of the counselor is essential to allow the individual's potential for change within the self to flower. A nonjudgmental, permissive therapeutic climate is necessary to allow growth to take place.

THE HERE-AND-NOW AND FAMILY FORCES

Existentialism and R. D. Laing

"Truth is not formulated but lived." This motto seems to be the common thread running through a treatment approach generally referred to as existential (Galdston, 1961). The existential approach to treating individuals in need of help for emotional problems emphasizes the actions people take in the solutions to their problems rather than their words, conceptions, and intellectual formulations. The here-and-now is of key importance. Patients are to be understood only in *their* terms, not in terms of the values, theories, moral judgments, language, and meanings assigned by the clinician.

Within this view, each person is responsible for facing his or her problems and making his or her own decisions about the future. Basic anxiety exists, but this emerges from each individual's having to deal with death, alienation from others, or helplessness and powerlessness to solve one's own problems rather than from infantile sexual conflicts or innate biological determinants. In treating people, emphasis is placed on getting them to assume a sense of involvement and action *today* rather than on reviewing the past (Boss, 1963; Buber, 1958; Jaspers, 1963; May, 1961; and May, Angel, and Ellenberger, 1958).

R. D. Laing, a Scottish clinician, whose extensive writings have explored many topics concerning mental disturbance, including the myth of mental illness, the dehumanization of mental patients, and the political and social aspects of diagnostic labels, is especially eloquent in his discussions of schizophrenia (1960; 1967; and Laing and Esterson, 1964).

According to Laing, the incomprehensibility of many schizophrenics results from failure to understand the patient from the point of view of his or her personal struggle—the need to baffle and mystify the doctors, parents, and agents of society who have baffled him or her. Most people who attempt to treat so-called sick individuals, Laing says, do not listen to, and therefore do not understand them.

Laing assumes that there is a constant power struggle among members of a family (see next section), and, as if by prior agreement, families tend to victimize certain of their members. So-called schizophrenic family members "choose" to behave, think, and talk in certain ways as part of their attempts to engage in battle with their opponents—the family members who are victimizing them. They are caught up in the games that people around them are playing. Schizophrenics are not "sick." Rather, they are different in their ways of handling overwhelming anxieties and in dealing with losing struggles.

Family Forces

One of the enduring interests of social scientists is in the primary family unit—the nuclear family—as the chief instrument for the socialization of the child. Socialization is the process by which the child learns to live with and become like other members of his or her group, culture, and society. Although the giants in psychology, such as Freud, have always acknowledged the significance of the family in the development of neuroses (as in weaning, toilet training, or the Oedipal situation), they stressed the one-to-one relationship—mother and son or father and daughter or mother and daughter, rather than the more complex climate of the whole family group and the interactions of its members. However, students, teachers, researchers, and clinicians interested in personality development have come to appreciate the effects of family forces which can not only socialize a child into its new culture, but also can maintain a pathology that traps all members and stifles individual growth. For it is now known that family forces can create and sustain illness in one or more of its members to maintain the family as a whole.

Some families scapegoat one member—frequently a child—who willingly fills this role for the sake of family harmony. In such families, when an emergency, such as a fire or automobile accident (not to mention lesser crises such as lateness), occurs, the scapegoated child is blamed. He or she might protest, but in the long run permits the scapegoating, allowing the family to continue on its way.

An impressive portion of family theory developed from observations of families with a schizo-

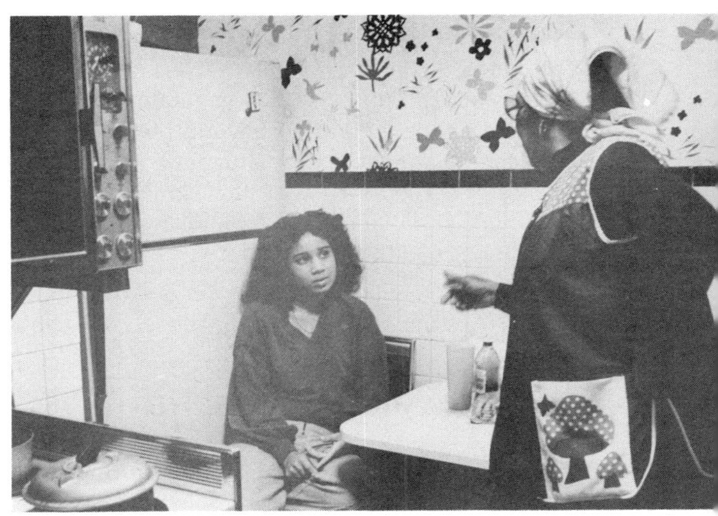

Some family members are consistently scapegoated. (Sybil Shelton/© Peter Arnold, Inc.)

phrenic patient. These observations have yielded special methods for studying families that include, for example, classifying their "atmosphere" or ways of communicating (Bateson, Jackson, Haley, and Weakland, 1956, 1963).

One contribution made by investigators in this field is the double bind theory, described in Chapter 3, which is concerned with the communication of two inconsistent messages "accompanied by a prohibition against noting their inconsistency" (Jackson, 1959, p. 139). One of the messages could be on a verbal level and the other on a nonverbal level; regardless of the mode, however, these "double messages" create a strong conflict for the receiver of the message—often a child who wishes to please the parent sending the messages.

For example: A mother verbally encourages her young son to be close to and to interact actively with his father. But she whines, looks tearful, accuses him of disloyalty, and feels generally hurt and rejected when he attempts to follow her verbal suggestions. He becomes confused, and is unable to respond to her wishes, to point out the inconsistency, or even to escape from the situation because their relationship and interdependency is of extreme importance to him and he dare not risk destroying their mutual need. In some views, these "double bind" situations, characterized by incompatible messages, set the stage for later schizophrenic disturbance.

The family approach has generated methods for treating patients that go beyond the traditional one-to-one patient-doctor situation. These approaches entail working with the family members, as a group, simultaneously. Family therapy methods are described in Chapter 19.

TRAITS AND FACTORS: "NONDYNAMIC" APPROACHES

A trait is commonly regarded as an enduring characteristic of an individual. Examples of traits are honesty, passivity, independence, aggressiveness, "nervousness," irritability, stubbornness. The list is virtually inexhaustible. Most people can be characterized by these traits along some dimension of intensity or frequency of manifestation. For example, John is an extremely honest, dependent, passive and compliant individual who is rarely nervous or irritable. Mary is an extremely honest, aggressive, dependent, and stubborn individual who is sometimes irritable and usually extremely nervous.

The set of traits and their strengths (or frequency of manifestation) that an individual possesses makes that individual different or unique. According to the trait psychologist, this is the key to understanding abnormal behavior.

In Allport's approach (1961), functional autonomy refers to the continuation of an enduring trait without reward or reinforcement from the environment. In this sense, Allport's approach is in sharp contrast to learning approaches as well as to Freudian approaches. For Allport, the study of childhood events and the history of the individual is simply not necessary to understand that individual. Instead, he stressed the study of the individual through personal documents such as letters and autobiography, and through his or her own special case background. This is referred to as the idiographic method—the study of the individual event or case, as opposed to the study of groups of individuals as would be required in setting up norms for tests. The latter is called the nomothetic method—designed to discover general laws.

In stressing the here-and-now of an individual and his or her situation, as well as underscoring the self and conscious determinants of behavior, Allport thus stands in contrast to those who offer theories of abnormal behavior that emphasize hidden, unconscious elements or the history of a person and his or her conflicts.

Another approach to traits is shared by a group of theories derived from testing large groups of disturbed and nondisturbed people. This empirical research yields theories of abnormal behavior that claim that disturbed individuals could be characterized by the strength of their scores on certain common factors (Cattell and Kline, 1977; Eysenck,

Spotlight 6.5 Attachment and Mothering

Observations of animal and human infants have indicated that attachment—closeness in an actual physical sense—is necessary for normal emotional, physical, and social development. For example, observations of human infants raised in institutions, such as foundling homes and hospitals, show that even with maximally conscientious attention to their physical needs and care, infants without adequate mothering, in the form of handling, cuddling, caressing, and stroking, gradually show loss of initiative, blandness, constriction in emotional and social response, diffidence, depression, retardation in verbal areas, and rigidity and awkwardness in physical response (Provence and Lipton, 1962).

Harry Harlow (Harlow and Harlow, 1962; 1966; Harlow and Zimmerman, 1959) demonstrated that when infant monkeys were raised with wire-mesh, mother-surrogate monkeys, one of which was covered with soft terry cloth, they tended to spend more time clinging to and cuddling the terry cloth "mother." This was true even if the wire-mesh monkey offered the milk for feeding. The monkeys simply spent more time in the area of the terry-cloth monkey when satiated, no matter which of the effigies offered the milk—they clung to it when frightened; they cuddled, held, and maintained contact with it when not feeding; and they played near it. In short, attachment behavior, even when not feeding, occupied a significant portion of the infant monkey's behavior.

Harlow also demonstrated that monkeys raised in isolation, without any contact with other monkeys, later showed abnormal behavior—socially, sexually, and physically. They seemed frightened and avoided contact with other monkeys, displaying aggression toward them. If early isolation lasted longer than six months, the monkeys were likely never to recover from this initial social deprivation.

On the other hand, even without mothering, monkeys raised with adequate peer contacts and opportunities for playing and for physical and social interaction with other monkeys appeared to

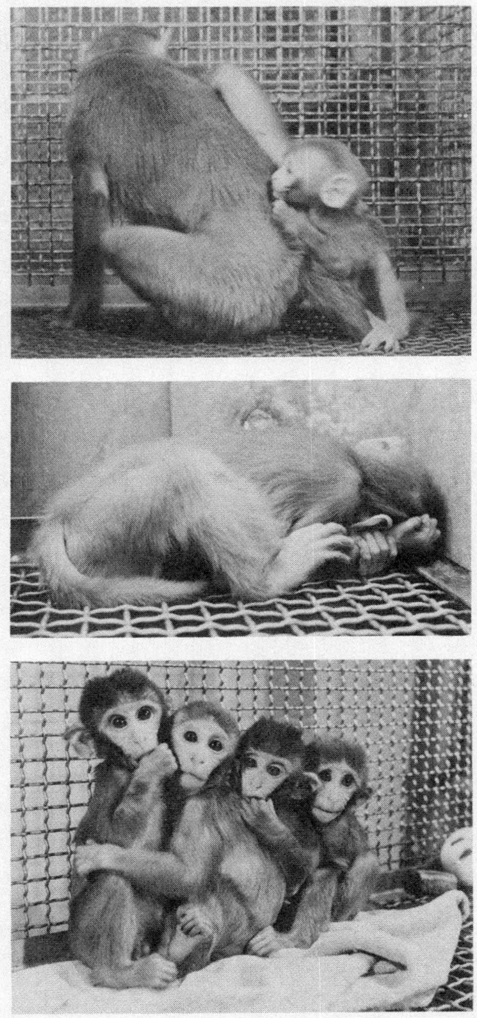

These fearful, clinging monkeys, raised in total or partial isolation, without physical contact with peers or mothers, display abnormal behavior. The adult monkey, raised with only a cloth mother-surrogate, refuses to nurse her infant. Some monkeys show self-biting or aggressive behavior as the photographer approaches, while others crouch next to each other in fear. Some of this behavior, Harlow discovered, can be modified or reversed if peer physical or social contacts are introduced early enough. (University of Wisconsin Primate Laboratory)

develop normally. Things that moved, even if not living, were apparently better for normal development than no moving things at all. It would seem that peer contacts at an early age, at least with monkeys, are essential. This is the case even when there is adequate mothering.

Adult rhesus monkeys who were themselves raised without mothers ("motherless mothers") were found to be abusive, incompetent mothers (Ruppenthal, et al., 1976). On the other hand, if given an opportunity to play with peers as they were growing up, or later with their own children, they were less likely to be incompetent mothers.

In some of their investigations, Harlow and Harlow (1962) carefully observed monkeys raised in isolation, partial isolation, and with normal mothers, motherless mothers, and peers. Figure 6.1 is a graphic summary of some of the results of their studies.

Although studies of "nonhuman animals, even monkeys, will never resolve the baffling complex roles of various kinds of early experience in the development of the human personality" (Harlow and Harlow, 1962), more and more evidence is accumulating, even with humans, that early interpersonal deprivations, especially limited opportunities for social and physical contacts, might be the groundwork for the development of a disordered, fearful, aggressive, and incompetent personality later on in life.

Figure 6.1 Summary of the Harlows' results. The Harlows' experimental studies indicated that monkeys isolated for six months are aberrant in every respect. Play with peers seems even more necessary than mothering to the development of effective social relations. (From "Social deprivation in monkeys" by Harry F. Harlow and Margaret Kuenne Harlow. Copyright © 1962 by Scientific American, Inc. All rights reserved.)

Experimental Condition	Present Age	Behavior				
		None	*Low*	*Almost Normal*	*Probably Normal*	*Normal*
Raised in isolation						
Total						
Cage-raised for 2 years	4 years	Play, Defense, Sex				
Cage-raised for 6 months	14 months	Defense, Sex	Play			
Cage-raised for 80 days	10½ months			Play, Defense, Sex		
Partial						
Cage-raised for 6 months	5 to 8 years		Play, Sex	Defense		
Surrogate-raised for 6 months	3 to 5 years		Play, Sex	Defense		
Raised with mother						
Normal mother; no play with peers	1 year	Sex	Play			Defense
Motherless mother; play in playpen	14 months			Defense	Sex	Play
Normal mother; play in playpen	2 years					Play, Defense, Sex
Raised with peers						
Four raised in one cage; play in playroom	1 year				Play	Defense, Sex
Surrogate-raised; play in playpen	2 years				Sex	Play, Defense
Surrogate-raised; play in playroom	21 months					Play, Defense, Sex

■ Play □ Defense ■ Sex

1952a, 1967*; Guilford, 1959). (The technique, called factor analysis, is a technical, statistical method for deriving common components that could account for the wide variations that people show in their responses to some personality inventories [Chapter 5].) Some of the criticisms of the trait and factor approaches have ascribed to them a mechanical, nondynamic view of behavior that overlooks the complex interlocking of needs, conflicts, past history, learning, and unconscious motivation in the characterization of behavior, abnormal or otherwise.

A different issue in connection with the trait and factor approaches arises from the person-situation views of Mischel and his associates (Bem and Allen, 1974; Bem and Funder, 1978; Mischel, 1973, 1976). The foregoing discussion of personality traits has proceeded as if these traits represent enduring, consistent features of personality that are demonstrable in a variety of different situations. Situations have been ignored—especially their influence on behavior and traits. Actually, the correlations among traits across situations is very low. Certain kinds of expressive features such as writing style or posture might be consistently evident across situations for each individual, but there is reason to believe that this is not the case for most traits. As a matter of fact, individuals even differ in the degree to which they are consistent from situation to situation. This is why psychologists can predict traits consistently better for some individuals than for others. In any event, there is some question regarding the validity of assigning all people some value as to the degree or intensity of a trait, as if everyone has the same number and same types of traits that differ only in their strength (high, moderate, or low).

In short, behaviors are often situation-specific. Personalities cannot be characterized by permanent attributes and traits they carry around with them. This view holds that psychologists interested in assessing people should be concerned with the interactions between the person and the situations and conditions in which the behavior emerges (Mischel,

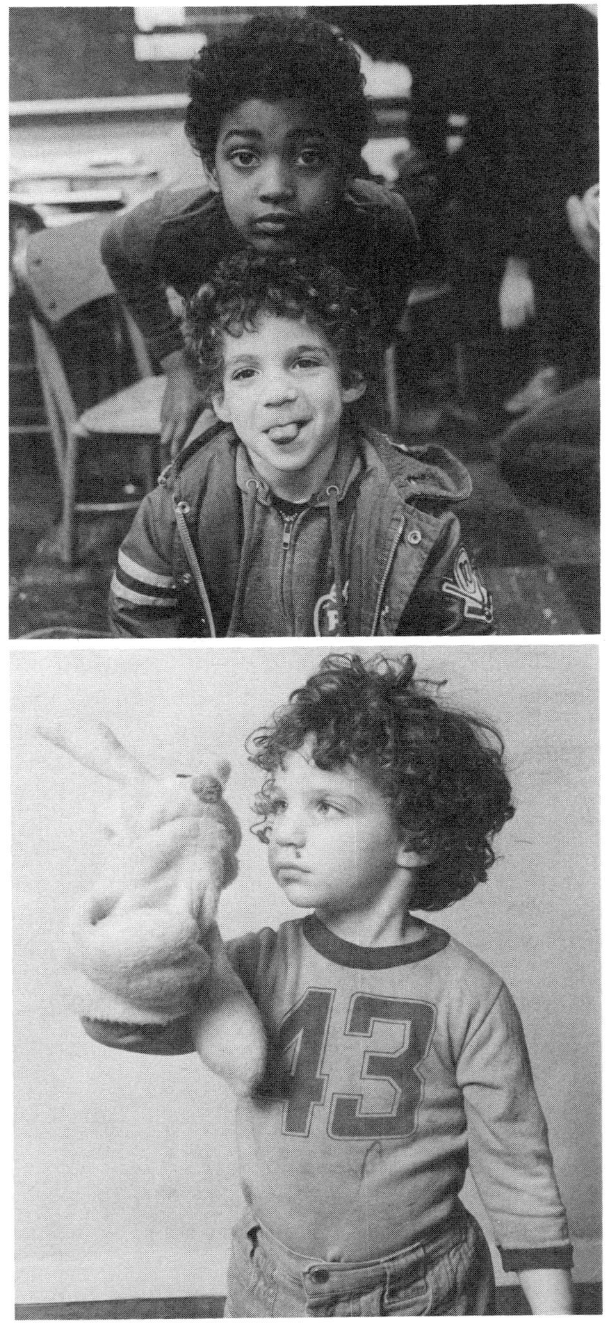

The same person may show different personal and social behaviors, depending on the situation. Stepehen Shames/Woodfin Camp)

* Eysenck's views are described in Chapter 9.

1973). Neither the situation alone (a hostile, competitive, stress-producing environment, for example), nor the personality alone (an extremely passive person, for example,) is the best predictor of behavior. It is more likely that person-situation interactions, in which each pole assumes importance, is the most valid predictor of behavior. This approach challenges the more traditional testing approach (outlined in Chapter 5), in which it is assumed that emotions, conflicts, personalities, and potential for certain kinds of behaviors are carried within the individual regardless of the situation the individual is in.

BEHAVIOR THEORY AND ABNORMAL PSYCHOLOGY

Behavior theory refers to a large number of theories of abnormal and normal personality. The most influential of these are Pavlov's classical conditioning theory, Skinner's operant learning theory, and Bandura's social learning theory. All behavior theories share a common assumption, however. They take the standpoint that much human psychopathology is acquired through learning. Thus the same principles by which we understand normal behavior can help us to explain and to treat abnormal behavior. The discussion of the most influential behavior theories that follows will provide a background for discussion of the behavioral interventions described in Chapter 20.

Classical Conditioning

The first widely known experimental study of abnormal behavior was performed by Ivan Pavlov. He experimentally produced "neuroses" in his dogs by training them to respond in two entirely contradictory ways in the same situation. For example, he might ring a bell and then, on randomly determined occasions, shock the animal; on other randomly determined occasions, he might ring the same bell and then feed the animal. Under such conflict circumstances, some dogs showed extreme fear and refused to eat even when hungry, while others became extremely apathetic.

Classical conditioning (Pavlov, 1927) is the type of learning in which a natural response, an unlearned, biologically controlled, reflex response, such as salivation, is elicited by an unnatural stimulus such as a bell after pairing the unnatural stimulus with a natural one such as food. In this example, the food is called the unconditioned stimulus (UCS). It elicits the unconditioned response (UCR), salivation, without any prior training by the experimenter. If the food is presented immediately after the conditioned stimulus (CS), the sound of the bell, the bell will eventually elicit salivation when it is presented without the food. Salivation has become the conditioned response (CR) because it is now a natural response to an unnatural stimulus. A summary of this process is:

1. UCS (food) ⟶ UCR (salivation)
2. CS (bell) + UCS (food) ⟶ UCR (salivation)
3. CS (bell) ⟶ CR (salivation)

Sometimes the pairing of the conditioned stimulus and the conditioned response must be strengthened (reinforced) by reintroducing the food. For if the bell is sounded again and again without occasional pairing with food, the conditioned response will disappear. This is called extinction: the CS no longer elicits the CR. However, spontaneous recovery often occurs after extinction: under certain circumstances, a conditioned response will reoccur spontaneously at a later time.

Another important process is that of generalization. When another sound is substituted for the original bell (CS)—for example, one that is louder or one with a different frequency—the new sound will also elicit salivation, but less of it, than the original bell. The greater the similarity of the new stimulus to the conditioned stimulus, the more similar the response will be to the original conditioned response. Thus the response generalizes to the new stimuli.

The complementary process to generalization is called discrimination. If the old and new bells are rung alternately, and if the old bell is always paired with food, and the new bell never paired with food, salivation will extinguish to the new bell but not the old one. Thus the animal will discriminate between the two sounds; it has learned that only one of them "predicts" food.

In addition to laying the groundwork for behavioral therapies, classical conditioning principles have been useful in helping to understand some kinds of abnormal behavior. It has been suggested that individuals with certain types of psychological problems can be more quickly conditioned than others. For example, it has been claimed that introverts are much more conditionable than psychopaths, and that phobias may extinguish very slowly and generalize easily to many different kinds of situations. And sometimes, even after a response is extinguished, spontaneous recovery may occur. This can be seen when the "cured" heroin addict returns to his old neighborhood and experiences anguished cravings for a "fix".

Operant Learning

In the course of investigating the role of learning in behavior, B. F. Skinner (1938, 1969) noticed that many types of behavior did not seem to be acquired through classical conditioning. In Pavlov's model, the learned response (CR) is elicited by the CS in much the same way that a knee jerk is elicited by a tap to the knee: it is a reflexive action. Skinner noticed, however, that much behavior operates upon the environment, rather than being a reflexive response to the environment. Such behavior is called operant or instrumental because is serves a function for the individual who emits it. Skinner's model of operant learning is:

$$S^D \rightarrow R \leftarrow S^R$$

In this model, a stimulus (S^D) signals the individual that the occurrence of some response (R) is likely to be followed by a second stimulus (S^R). If the S^R has the effect of increasing the rate, intensity, or likelihood of the behavior it follows, it is called a reinforcing stimulus. On the other hand, if the S^R has the effect of decreasing the rate, intensity, or likelihood of the behavior, it is called a punishing stimulus. Thus an individual learns that in a particular setting (S^D), a particular behavior (R) is likely to produce pleasant or unpleasant results (S^R).

Notice some of the differences between operant learning and classical conditioning: An operant response *precedes* its reinforcer (S^R), whereas a classically conditioned response *follows* its reinforcer (UCS). Furthermore, operant responses are typically overt, skeletal behaviors, such as eating or hand-washing, whereas classically conditioned responses are typically emotional reactions, such as fear or anxiety. Both, however, are presumed to be learned without cognitive mediation. The relationship between the stimuli and the responses automatically results in learning; the person does not need to be aware of the relationship. In order to understand why a person acts in a particular way—for example, engaging in self-mutilation or compulsive handwashing—a Skinnerian would seek therefore to identify the antecedents (S^Ds) and the consequences (s^Rs) of that behavior. This is called a functional analysis.

Reinforcement control refers to the relationship between a behavior and its consequence: $R \leftarrow S^R$. This is thought to be the most important part of a functional analysis because operant psychologists consider present behavior to be determined by the S^Rs that have followed that behavior in the past. Therapies based upon reinforcement control of behavior are called contingency management techniques—techniques that alter the problem behavior by altering the consequences of that behavior.

Stimulus control refers to the relationship between a behavior and its antecedents: $S^D \rightarrow R$. Determination of stimulus control is also necessary for a complete functional analysis. According to the operant view, S^Ds take on reinforcing or punishing characteristics through their association with S^Rs. Thus they can influence the subsequent behavior.

Both stimuli and responses can show generalization and discrimination. For example, if a child learns that she will be punished if she hits her brother, she may generalize this learning to her sister. She may thus be less inclined to hit her sister than she was before, even though she had not been punished for this (stimulus generalization). On the other hand, if she does hit her sister and is not punished, she will discriminate the consequences of this action under the two stimulus conditions:

(1) brother → hit ← punishment, so probability of hitting decreases
(S^D_1) (R) (S^R_1)

(2) sister → hit ← no punishment, so probability of hitting does not decrease
(S^D_2) (R)(S^R_2)

Furthermore, the response—hitting her sister—may generalize to other aggressive behaviors: the child may not only hit her sister, but may pinch and scratch her as well if she is not punished (response generalization). However, if she is punished for one form of aggression but not another, she will discriminate between the two responses: she will only use the unpunished form.

Response generalization is an important process for understanding behavior therapies. To illustrate, let us say that you wish to train a retarded child to urinate in the toilet rather than on the floor. If you wait for the desired behavior to occur so that you can reinforce it, you may wait forever. A better strategy would be to *shape* the desired response by reinforcing successively more exact approximations to it. In the case of the retarded child, it is relatively simple to toilet train him by reinforcing behaviors that move toward the final goal: walking in the direction of the bathroom, going into it, removing his pants, and so on. Thus therapists can take advantage of the tendency of reinforcement to increase the likelihood of a whole range of similar behaviors. They can subsequently reinforce a slightly different behavior that is a close approximation to the desired result.

Skinner's learning paradigm has been an extremely useful model for work in psychopathology. His conceptualizations and methods have probably been as influential in the field of abnormal psychology as Freud's were at an earlier time. Understanding behaviors—normal or abnormal—in terms of their reinforcement histories makes sense to many psychologists, especially those concerned with modifying undesirable behavior. And it is in the domain of modifying behavior that the logic and simplicity of Skinner's operant methods produced results—perhaps more than most theoretical views—in terms of symptom reduction and the learning of more favorable behavior patterns.

Skinner's theory contains an elegance in the parsimony of its explanatory concepts. Skinner and his followers are not concerned with drives—the internal motivating states that so many earlier theorists alluded to—and such constructs as the unconscious, instincts, mechanisms of defense, intent, feelings, ego, conflict, repression, and cognitions are also eliminated. Skinner refers to these as "explanatory fictions."

The demonstrable success in treating many kinds of problems offered by Skinnerian principles and the ease with which they can be understood and applied has led proponents, especially Skinner himself, to extend these principles into a belief system about a better world in which societies can be "shaped" by technicians who know how to wield learning principles (Skinner, 1971). Such generalizations have elicited a storm of critical opinion.

Critics of Skinner's approach claim that it is too simplistic, elementary, and mechanical: it does not take will, motives, inclination, and conscious desire into account. Nor does it go under the skin of the organism and consider measurable biochemical substances (hormonal imbalances, for example), and physical structures (brain lesion, for example).

Many critics also raise questions about the behavior control aspects of Skinner's approach, suggesting the relevance of ethical issues in considering a "technician's" attempts to "control" the behavior of another person or groups of people. We will raise these issues again later in the book.

Finally, some specific inadequacies of the Skinnerian approach have been increasingly clear to psychologists interested in understanding both normal and abnormal behavior as well as methods of behavior change. One is the failure in Skinner's model to accord any role to cognition. Another is the fact that the operant paradigm accounts for the development of new behaviors only through shaping: it cannot account for the *first* occurrence of a response; reinforcement can influence a response only if it has occurred at least once before. The sections that follow describe some approaches that have emerged from such considerations.

Cognitions and Abnormal Behavior

A view that has gained momentum in recent years stresses cognitive processes as a significant determinant of abnormal behavior. That is, the way one thinks, perceives, interprets, and judges—and the view one has about his or her world—is at least as important, if not more so, in the shaping of abnormal behavior as are the inner conflicts, unconscious wishes, hidden traits, forbidden strivings, and early childhood traumas implicated by the more traditional theorists. Further, this view would generally hold that the characterization of abnormal behavior as an end product of a person's reinforcement history (as the Skinnerians would hold) is a vast oversimplification. For people have brains—with thoughts, expectations, beliefs, goals, aspirations, and concepts of what is rewarding or not rewarding. This cognitive content is being accorded considerable weight as both an explanatory or etiological variable for some disorders, such as depression, and as a key aspect of certain treatment approaches.

There is no one "school" that characterizes the cognitive orientation. Diverse influences arising from different sources have contributed to the development of these views. For example, one early hypothesis proposed that emotion is experienced as a response to cognitive processes (rather than the other way around). That is, when a person feels aroused at a given moment, he or she will label that experience of arousal as one emotion or another, depending on the way that person evaluates the immediate situation. If on the basis of past experience, their immediate situation is viewed as "fun" (attending a party, for example), then being excited in that "fun" situation will be interpreted as "happiness" or "joy." However, for an individual who views parties as "scary," the excitement might be interpreted as "fear" (Schacter and Singer, 1962).

Another series of researches suggests that, rather than immediate rewards, expectations and thoughts about future goals can be powerful determinants of behavior (Mischel, 1973)—a simple formulation but a rather significant departure from the mechanistic reward-reinforcement contingencies of the strict behaviorists. Another view holds that the egocentric, magical, prelogical thinking of very young children—thinking that circumvents or ignores entirely the usual cause-and-effect relationships—may persist into adulthood and account for some of the symptoms of the psychoneuroses (Serban, 1974; 1978). Still another cognitive view is that depression emerges as a result of the distorted thoughts the patient has about his or her blame and responsibility for things that go wrong: I am to blame; I am worthless—that's why things will always go wrong (Beck, 1974).

These views all share a common thread: cognitions exert a powerful influence on behavior and emotions. The chapters that follow will pick up this thread again.

Bandura's Social Learning Theory

Many of the principles of social learning theory were clarified in Albert Bandura's work on psychological modeling, which refers to the human ability to learn by watching someone else (a "model") perform the activity. This may not seem to be a significant improvement on operant theory; however, if everything had to be learned through personal experience—the premise of operant learning—it is doubtful that many of us would have survived childhood. For example, one would have to be hit by a car before learning to look both ways before crossing the street. While personal experience is clearly important, it probably accounts for only a fraction of what we know.

Modeling has several important functions, some of which will be discussed in Chapter 20. One of its most significant functions is to teach new cognitions, based on the assumption that we acquire standards for our behavior, attitudes, goals, and expectations for the future by observing the actions of others, especially our parents.

Because people have standards of adequacy regarding their behavior, they can set goals for themselves and can alter their own behavior—they can self-regulate. They are thus able to reinforce themselves for accomplishments that meet or exceed their goals and to punish themselves when they fall short of their goals.

Unlike classical conditioning and operant learning theory, social learning theory does not presume that individuals are automatically influenced by their environment; the ability to self-regulate their own behavior permits some measure of autonomy from the environment. However, in Bandura's view (1978), it is as much a mistake to say that cognition causes behavior as it is to say that the environment causes behavior. Instead, behaviors, environments, and cognitions can be seen as interlocking, continuous determinants of each other. This idea is called reciprocal determinism, which may be diagramed as follows:

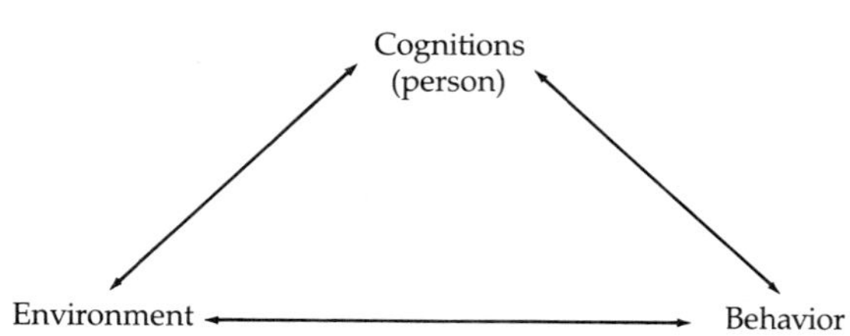

In this theory, people alter their environments through the use of symbols, such as language, by selecting what they will respond to, by developing their own goals and values, and by altering their own behavior. The environment alters a person's cognitions by providing models and by reinforcing and punishing certain behaviors. And behavior alters cognitions by providing a person with information about what he or she can and cannot accomplish, and with information about the probable consequences of behavior.

In this view of learning, it is easy to see why "awareness" is extremely necessary. Response outcomes are interpreted, understood, processed in diverse ways. For example, a past reinforcer can only influence a person if that person *expects* to be reinforced in the same way in the future. If, on the other hand, a person believes that the reinforcement was just a lucky occurrence, it will not influence the expectation of future reinforcement, and will not, therefore, influence future behavior. Outcome expectations are thus an important determinant of people's actions.

Another very important type of cognition is one's self-efficacy expectation—a person's expectation of how "efficaciously" he or she can perform a certain behavior (Bandura, 1977b). Research has shown that the single best predictor of a person's level of performance on a task, such as how close a phobic person can get to a snake, is the person's self-efficacy expectation. Not even the person's past achievements on the same task predict as well as this cognition.

Although personal experience is the best source of efficacy expectations, they can arise from several sources. These include modeling, verbal persuasion, and physiological arousal. However, information from all sources must be cognitively appraised in order to be learned. In therapy, these sources of information can be used as powerful tools for changing people's cognitions and behaviors.

In fact, Bandura (1977b) has proposed that *all* improvements made in the course of psychotherapy—regardless of the orientation of the therapist—are the result of altering the client's self-efficacy expectations. And, although the truth of this hypothesis has not been definitely validated, some very compelling data exist in support of this and other aspects of Bandura's theory.

This brief review demonstrates the degree to which learning theories have changed since the time of Pavlov. As they have become more complex, more cognitive, and more person-oriented, theories and approaches have emphasized that outcomes of a response do not all have the same influence on people. The consequences of one's acts are interpreted and understood ("processed") by different people in different ways. People are not passive agents, shaped mechanically by the environments around them but can, in good part, exert power and control over their own environments by self-rewards and self-punishments.

As we shall see, these views are beginning to have considerable influence on the nature of therapeutic interventions, especially those which emphasize self-control and self-determination, in addition to offering explanatory principles for understanding human behavior. Later chapters discuss treatment methods and explore this influence more fully.

SUMMARY

Theories concerning the origins of abnormal behavior not only determine the types of inquiries conducted but also the general thrust of the findings that emerge, and these theories differ widely. This chapter surveyed a wide range of psychological theories about the nature and origins of disordered behavior in some detail, including the following psychodynamic and nonpsychodynamic approaches: Freudian theory; the neo-Freudian modifications; eclectic views; humanistic, family, and trait approaches; and various types of learning models, including classical and operant conditioning, social learning, and cognitive approaches. No one theory or set of models accounts for all of the "facts" about psychopathology, but some theories lend themselves more readily to empirical exploration and are thus more easily subject to verification. By these criteria, the strictly traditional psychoanalytic model is less "acceptable" than the behaviorally oriented approaches.

Highlights

1. Freudian theory has had a very significant impact on twentieth-century thought through its implicating and exploring the inner workings of the mind—emotions, conflict, the unconscious, and defenses against painful mental content—in the development of the neuroses. Freud constructed a complex model of the psyche and its structure—id, ego, and superego—and processes—repression, symptom-formation and defense mechanisms. His theoretical formulations of normal and pathological development included infantile sexuality and psychosexual levels of development, Oedipus and castration complexes, penis envy, libido, and the death instinct. These constructs were radically innovative when first developed by Freud but have since been integrated and modified within the fabric of twentieth-century thought, though seldom without serious criticism and reservations. Overall, Freud was influenced by the availability for study of a restricted sample of patients as well as by the prevailing views in his own culture. The vast superstructure of Freudian theory is not entirely accessible to empirical, objective exploration and confirmation and the little that has been done along these lines has not been too promising.
2. The essentially biologically and instinctually oriented views of Freud were modified somewhat by many of his followers, such as Adler, Fromm, Horney, and Sullivan. These theorists acknowledged the importance of culture, interpersonal and social conditions, and socially induced conflict and deemphasized the unconscious and infantile sexuality in their views of the development of the neuroses.
3. Humanistic approaches, such as those of Maslow and Rogers, stress an optimistic view of human development and of conflict by underscoring the individual's potential for growth and change. These approaches are less concerned with infantile conflicts and sexual strivings than they are with each individual's self-

appraisal, ideals, personal strivings, and goals. In this approach, even conflicted, disturbed people are completely accepted and respected rather than viewed as tormented by deep, ugly, shameful and distorted fantasies that reflect taboo, forbidden impulses and strivings.

4. Family models of pathology emphasize both the interactions among family members and the general climate of pushes, pulls, and strains within the family as a unit rather than the early history and unconscious conflicts of a disturbed family member. Although the family model was developed in an attempt to understand the genesis of schizophrenia, family theory is now employed to explain the development of other types of pathology as well.
5. Trait approaches are less concerned with the past history of the individual and his or her unconscious mechanisms than they are with the set of traits and their strengths that make an individual unique, and in some instances abnormal. Trait psychology and the development of methods to measure traits have relied heavily on the statistical technique known as factor analysis to characterize the unique qualities of different individuals. Recently, the views of Mischel and his associates have pointed up the significance of evaluating a personality in the context of person-situation interactions rather than by personal traits alone.
6. The researches of Harlow and his associates with monkeys have suggested the possibility that the absence of mothering contacts and peer interactions early in the life of the human baby may subsequently produce a variety of disturbed behaviors, including excessive fear responses, anxiety, withdrawal, and aggressiveness.
7. Behavior theory is the general name applied to various approaches sharing the view that psychopathology is acquired through learning. Classical conditioning, operant learning theory, and social learning theory each provides a framework for understanding and modifying various types of abnormal behavior. Social learning theory in particular attempts to account for some of the difficulties in operant learning by introducing such concepts as modeling and self-regulation—processes that are of great importance in understanding the development and modification of behavior. The view that people perceive, judge, and can evaluate their own behavior, rather than being passively shaped by events and circumstances, plays a crucial role in newer approaches that emphasize cognitions, self-control, and self-determination in the understanding of personal development and its modification.

ISSUES AND QUESTIONS

1. Have you ever discovered that your motives for wanting to do something were not what you originally thought they were? That is, were you unconsciously motivated by drives of which you were unaware? Think of examples of this in your life. Does knowledge of your unconscious motivation change your attitudes toward the desirability of your original goal?
2. Think of socially unacceptable wishes, fantasies, and desires that you have. Some of these probably were concerned with aggression or sex; perhaps hostility, jealousy, or anger toward someone in your family has been involved. Did you feel anxious when you experienced such feelings? Anxiety is uncomfortable. How did you deal with the anxiety? Did you busy yourself with other things? Did you rationalize your impulses? Did you drink, eat, or go to sleep? What defense mechanisms did you use to allay or reduce this discomfort?
3. Can you conceptualize an aspect of poor adjustment you see in yourself in terms of learning theory? For example, if you become argumentative and angry when criticized, or extremely withdrawn in competitive situations, are you able to trace the learning history of such responses or groups of responses by using Pav-

lov's, Skinner's, or Bandura's models? Or is it easier for you to conceptualize these behavior patterns in the Freudian language of unconscious conflict and defenses against forbidden wishes? Perhaps it is easiest to think of them as enduring traits that are characteristic of you in most situations.

4. Think again about the problem you considered in answering question 3., viewing it in terms of Bandura's ideas of reciprocal determinism. Can you describe the relationships among your cognitions, behaviors, and environments that serve to perpetuate this problem? Are some of these elements in competition? For example, does your roommate encourage you to do something that deviates from your own goals?

SUGGESTIONS FOR FURTHER READING

Bandura, A. *Social learning theory.* Englewood Cliffs, New Jersey: Prentice-Hall, 1977. Paperback available. This book provides a concise, understandable overview of Bandura's social learning theory. As such, it emphasizes the prominent roles played by vicarious, symbolic, and self-regulatory processes in psychological functioning. Any student who is intrigued by Bandura's ideas will find this book both interesting and informative.

Freud, S. *New introductory lectures on psychoanalysis* (1933). New York: Norton, 1965. Paperback available. This brief outline of psychoanalytic theory, written by the master himself, is a classic.

Hall, C. S. *A primer of Freudian psychology* (1954). New York: New American Library, 1973. Paperback available. For a simple, accurate, and brief account of the main elements of Freud's psychoanalytic theory, this book is an excellent resource. It is especially useful for those reading about psychoanalytic theory for the first time.

Hall, C. S., and Lindzey, G. *Theories of personality.* 3rd ed. New York: Wiley, 1978. This comprehensive book covers in a direct way a variety of approaches to the understanding of personality, emotions, and abnormal behavior. The critical evaluations—both positive and negative—are thoughtful and are based on a sound respect for science as well as people.

Kline, P. *Fact and fantasy in Freudian theory.* London: Methuen, 1972. This book summarizes the experimental and nonexperimental findings confirming or disconfirming Freudian theory over a thirty-year period, going beyond Sear's attempt to do the same job in 1943. In this survey, Kline provides a concise presentation of Freudian concepts and sorts them into those than can be subjected to empirical investigation and those that cannot.

Skinner, B. F. *Walden two.* New York: Macmillan, 1948. Paperback available. This is probably Skinner's most famous book. In it he provides a fictional account of a modern Utopia in which human problems are solved through operant learning. It also demonstrates the author's conviction that such values as personal freedom and dignity are obsolete. As you might guess, this book has been quite controversial, inducing extreme reactions in its readers. This novel nonetheless raises many thought-provoking ideas.

Skinner, B. F. *About behaviorism.* New York: Random House, 1976. Paperback. In this book, Skinner refutes many of his critics' arguments against behaviorism and operant learning. In doing so, he provides functional analyses of such seemingly abstract concepts as perception, language, thought, knowledge, motivation, and free will. The student will find this book to be an interesting, readable overview of many of Skinner's revolutionary ideas.

7

Biological Approaches: Going "Underneath the Skin" to Understand Abnormal Behavior

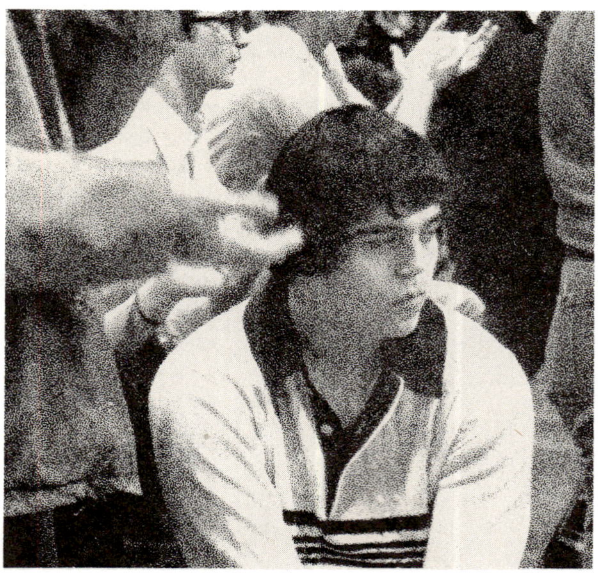

Johnny wakes up with feelings of terror. His pajamas and sheets are drenched with perspiration. He can barely breathe, thinks he is dying, feels a dreadful pounding in his ears, and thinks that his heart is beating so loudly that his neighbors will be awakened. He is experiencing an acute anxiety attack.

Jane's moods are so dramatically changeable that she is bewildering to herself, her husband, and her coworkers. She shifts from anguishing despair and insistent thoughts of suicide to infectious elation and "highs"—switching back and forth between these extremes every few months. She is probably suffering from bipolar affective disorder (see Chapter 10).

Christopher, a ten-year-old, has frequent fainting "spells" and, on rare occasions, convulsions. He is being examined for a brain malignancy.

Melanie is six years old. She cannot tie her shoelaces, hop on one foot, or count. She is probably mentally retarded.

Brian suffers from terrifying hallucinations, bizarre thoughts, and a constant fear that his landlord is slowly killing him by sending gamma rays through the plumbing into his faucets in the kitchen and bathroom. Doing dishes, showering, and toileting are horrifying experiences for him. During most of his waking hours he dwells on how to survive at home without being slowly murdered. At the clinic, he was diagnosed as suffering from paranoid schizophrenia, a psychosis with delusions of persecution.

Frances has dangerously high blood pressure for which there is no apparent physical cause. Her pressure shoots up and remains so during and after any situation that she interprets as an evaluative one, when she feels she is being "sized up." She suffers from essential hypertension, a physical disease that may have strong emotional components.

Perry, a four-year-old, behaves as if he does not see people. He seems to be looking right through them and makes no attempt to communicate with them. He frequently bangs his head against the walls in his room. He is fascinated by bright lights and stares at bulbs and shiny surfaces with hypnotic fascination. He sometimes has terrible (presumably unprovoked) rages. He is an autistic child (see pp. 392–96).

Frank has recurrent, frightening thoughts that he will murder someone. He has been suffering from this profound fear for thirty years but has never hurt a fly. Roy, on the other hand, suffers from periodic rages of such intensity and violence that his wife and children, at different times, had to be hospitalized for broken limbs.

Joe has repeatedly tried to shake his heroin habit but each time cannot tolerate the physical and psychological anguish of withdrawal and so falls back on his habit. His girlfriend Betty has had so many bad acid trips that all who know her regard her as a vegetable, a "zombie."

Clarice understands everything anyone might say to her and can communicate most of her ideas fairly well. She cannot, however, say *names* for things. She has had specific injury to her brain (a "stroke") and is suffering from aphasia (see pp. 347–49).

Dan has had brain surgery, and although he seems to be able to do everything he was able to do formerly, his wife and family are concerned that his behavior and general temperament have changed. But they are unable to specify exactly how.

What do these people have in common? They all suffer from some dysfunction that impairs the quality of their lives. Although they have diverse emotional and psychological problems, it is apparent that their physical selves are also very much involved. Johnny's anxiety attacks are experienced as intense physical discomfort. Jane's illness may have a strong biochemical component (see Chapter 10). Christopher is eventually diagnosed as having a brain tumor. Brian's terrifying thoughts take place somewhere in his mind (brain). Joe's severe intestinal withdrawal symptoms of diarrhea accompanied by vomiting are acutely distressing bodily reactions. And so on for the others.

People who demonstrate abnormal behavior have skin, bones, muscles, bodily organs, nervous systems, brains, biochemical make-ups, and genetic predispositions. How is this biological complexity associated with the subjective events and observable behavior that comprise psychopathology? Many psychologists are beginning to suspect that some very powerful possibilities in these areas for understanding, modifying, and perhaps even curing and preventing many forms of psychopathology have been too long overlooked. This chapter continues the presentation of theories and models for abnormal behavior by looking underneath the skin, so to speak, for causes and correlations.

THE CENTRAL NERVOUS SYSTEM (CNS): THE BRAIN AND ITS SUBPARTS

The central nervous system (CNS) is comprised of the brain and its various subparts and connecting sections, such as the brain stem and the spinal cord. The basic unit of the CNS is the nerve cell or neuron. Neurons are microscopic structures, often smaller than a millimeter, sometimes considerably larger. To provide an idea of how small a neuron is, consider that the human brain has ten to fourteen billion nerve cells. Neurons also appear in other areas of the nervous system—specifically in the peripheral nervous system, which is outside of the brain and spinal cord and includes nerves going to and from muscles and skin.

The function of the neuron is to receive, process, and transmit information. Neurons are part of a staggeringly complex system of communications, the primary function of which is the transmitting of messages to the brain from energy (light or sound, for example) falling on the receptors and conversely, from the brain to effectors that activate muscles or glands so that walking, talking, secreting, digesting, breathing, or crying can occur. Neurons also transmit messages within the brain itself: dreaming, thinking, inner language, ideas, insights, judgments, feelings, bodily sensations, pain, nausea, hunger, dizziness. Although most neurons are not physically linked, that is, not in direct contact with one another, they form a complex maze of surfaces that display an enormous capacity for interrelatedness. Each neuron has a branchlike or weblike structure of dendrites (see illustration) that maximizes its surface for receiving and transmitting messages from other neurons; for any particular neuron, therefore, thousands upon thousands of communication possibilities exist. Most neurons also have a single axon, which may project a great distance through the body to send messages to other neurons; some axons actually are several feet long.

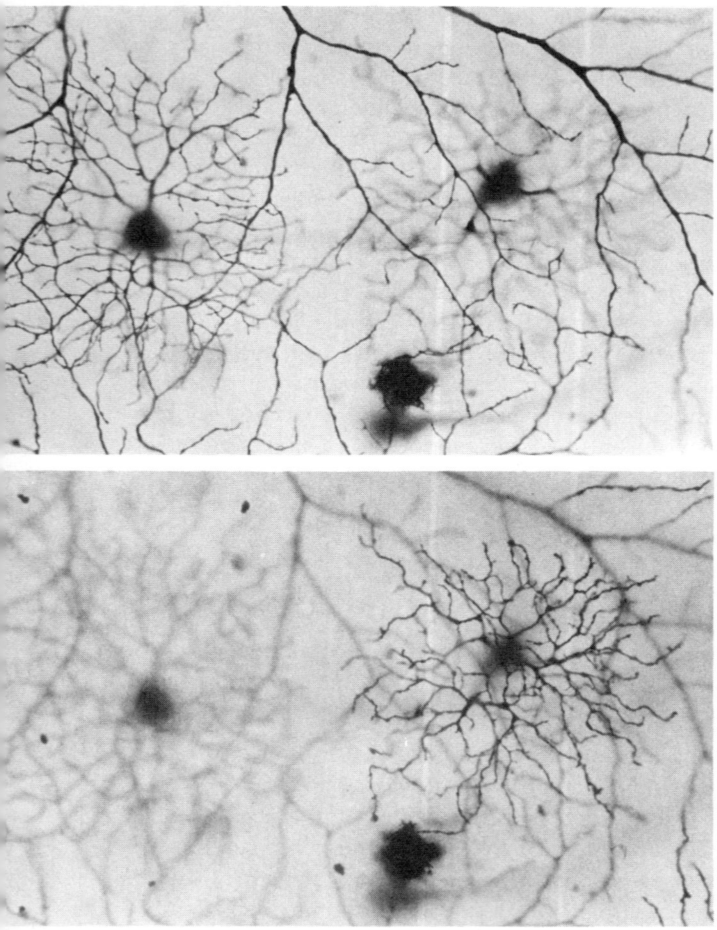

Figure 7.1 Photomicrographs of neurons in the cat retina. Both views are of the same area, but the focal planes of the views differ, bringing some of the dendritic trees into sharper focus. (Courtesy of Dr. R.-B. Illing, Department of Psychology and Brain Science, M.I.T.)

Once activated, neurons return to their normal or "resting" state in about one/thousandth of a second (millisecond). A neuron is activated entirely or not at all, and when it is activated it cannot be stimulated to become even more active. This activation is called an impulse. But neurons can be activated again and again, some as frequently as 1,000 times per second. The rate of impulses is the nervous system's code for the intensity of a message.

How do neurons transmit messages? They become electrochemically activated, and in the process, can activate other neurons across a gap or functional connection called a synapse. Activity at the synapses is now thought to be the primary determinant of the electrochemical messages that are carried by the neuron. This synaptic action takes place through the properties of certain chemicals generally called neurotransmitters. (There are also other neurochemicals called neuroregulators and neuromodulators.) Interestingly, the activity at the synapse itself was thought at one time to be primarily electrical, but evidence overwhelmingly now implicates chemical rather than electrical action across these functional junctures. The role of neurotransmitters in the regulation of neuronal activity and in the transmission of neuronal impulses is especially relevant, it appears, in some forms of pathology—a consideration that will be discussed in greater detail in subsequent sections of this chapter.

Certain neural groupings and pathways consist of a dense clustering of specialized neurons; these pathways, called nerves, have distinct functions. The optic nerve, for example, which contains about half a million neurons, transmits impulses from the retina (the specialized sensory receptors in the eyes) to the brain.

The brain, the CNS organ within the skull, is the most complex organ of the human body. Tightly packed together, its billions of cells permit an unbelievably large number of possible interconnections—trillions, perhaps.

The human brain, comprising about 2 percent of body weight in humans, is separated, when seen from above, into two hemispheres, the left and the right. Oddly, most sensory messages and input from the left side of the body go to the *right* hemisphere of the brain and the right hemisphere, in turn, regulates, controls, and transmits messages having to do with motor activity of the *left* side of the body. Conversely, the *right* side of the body and the *left* hemisphere are functionally connected: the left hemisphere is in charge of motor activities of, and receives sensory messages from, the right side of the body. These hemispheres are separated by a long gap, the longitudinal fissure, but are connected by a group of fibers called the corpus callosum.

The fact of two hemispheres, each with different duties and functions, it appears, yet connected to each other, is of great interest to researchers investigating human behavior, especially abnormal behavior. Spotlight 7.1 describes some left-right hemisphere findings.

Spotlight 7.1 Right-Left Hemisphere Functions

Recent evidence suggests that the left hemisphere of the brain is largely responsible for verbal, abstract, symbolic, and cognitive functions and skills while the right hemisphere is largely responsible for artistic, musical, spatial, mechanical, and imaginative skills and abilities. In addition, in intact humans, the right hemisphere apparently regulates and moderates emotions and feelings (Schwartz, Davidson, and Maer, 1975). Interestingly, strong right-left dominance and preferences generally do not appear in the other species.

The corpus callosum, the group of nerve tissues that connects the hemispheres, must at times be surgically severed for life-sustaining purposes, as in the occurrence of uncontrollable seizures (convulsions). Such surgery often reduces, or even eliminates the seizures. Patients who have undergone this procedure generally demonstrate little or no change in temperament, personality, or general intelligence. More striking are observations that confirm inferences about left- and right-hemisphere functions, the study of which is referred to as split-brain research.

When the corpus callosum is intact, information is shared by both hemispheres. When, however, it is severed in higher organisms, two independently functioning brains emerge, each with special skills and abilities. This was discovered in the 1950s by Roger W. Sperry, who received a Nobel Prize in 1981 for his innovative research efforts in this area. Subsequent experimentation with split brains confirmed the expected differences in hemispheric skills (Gazzaniga, 1967). For example, patients could not identify verbally a picture of a spoon presented only to the right hemisphere; they could, however, identify a spoon presented to the right hemisphere by picking it out from among various objects presented to the left hand. Apparently the right hemisphere was "intelligent"—it knew what the object was, even though it could not name it.

When subjects were told to copy a simple picture using the left (nonpreferred) hand (regulated by right hemisphere function), performance was better with this hand than when the preferred *right* hand (regulated by left hemisphere function) did the copying (see Figure 7.2). The division of labor between right and left hemispheres thus receives ample confirmation. But is this division clearcut and rigid?

It seems that through the preschool years, both hemispheres are linguistically capable—both can understand the rules of grammar, for example. In the fifth year, however, the left hemisphere seems to take over most of the language functions, whereas the right hemisphere develops superior skills in visual and spatial manipulations and perceptions and in responsiveness to emotions. A person may have a vocabulary of a fourteen-year-old but the syntactical ability of a five-year-old, due to right hemisphere function. Striking technical improvements in the devices that study how messages are sent to the appropriate hemisphere of the brain have permitted this research, indicating that the right hemisphere is not as deficient in language ability as had once been thought (Rensberger, 1975).

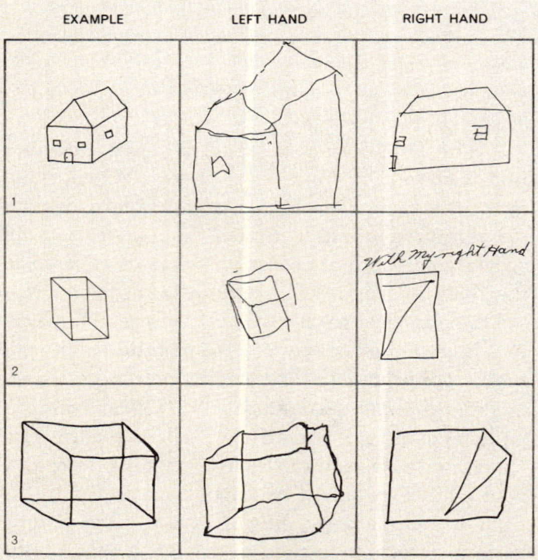

Figure 7.2 A right-handed "split brain" patient's copies of simple examples executed by left and right hands. Note how much better the left-hand drawings are. (From Gazzaniga, 1967, p. 28. Reprinted by permission of the author.)

As more evidence accumulates, researchers are beginning to think that the earlier, simple associations put forth by the right-left hemisphere investigators might have to be modified. Nevertheless it seems that not only can most people be classified according to the dominance of the right or left hemisphere, but also, they can be shown to differ in some important ways, depending on this dominance.

Several findings from right-left hemisphere research follow (Bakan, 1969; Gur and Gur, 1974; Gur and Gur, 1975; Gur and Reyher, 1973; Sackeim, Gur, and Saucy, 1978; and Schwartz, Davidson, and Maer, 1975):

1. Eye movements to the right or left experienced during problem-solving activity are related to the preferred cerebral hemisphere an individual relies on when thinking. Those whose eyes move to the left presumably prefer the *right* hemisphere, whereas those whose eyes move to the right prefer the *left* hemisphere. Right movers, because of left-hemisphere dominance, can be classified according to their *manner* of solving problems: they show greater analytic skills and rationality. Left movers (with right-hemisphere dominance), on the other hand, tend to use more creative, intuitive, and wholistic problem-solving methods.
2. Although some correlation was found between hypnotic susceptibility (hypnotizability) and right-hemisphere dominance, further exploration of this relationship showed that the earlier formulation was too simple. Additional findings showed that sex, handedness, and eyedness variables were also important. For example, the predicted relationships seem to hold for left-handed females—that is, that they are more hypnotizable—and right-handed males—that they are less hypnotizable—but not for right-handed females or left-handed males.
3. Right and left lookers may also differ in personality, as evidenced by the difference in de-

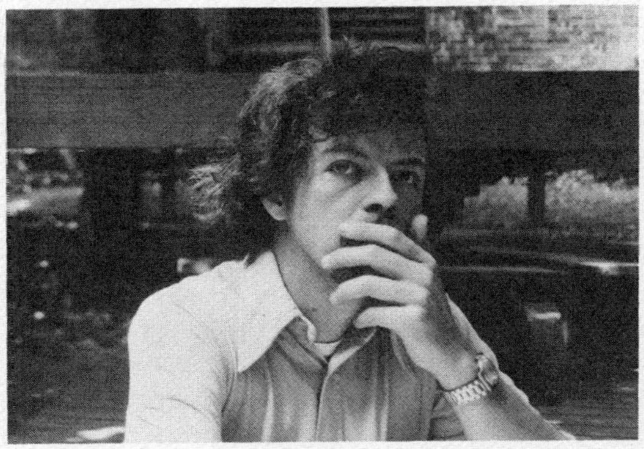

People tend to move their eyes to the left or right while thinking, depending on their preferred cerebral hemisphere. (© 1979 Eric A. Roth/The Picture Cube)

fense mechanisms they are more prone to use. Left lookers (with right cerebral dominance) tend to use repression and denial, whereas right lookers (with left cerebral dominance) tend to use such mechanisms as projection or turning against others. There are some indications, too, that left lookers report more psychosomatic symptoms (physical illnesses due largely to emotional factors) than do the right lookers.

4. A period of dominance of right hemisphere over the usually dominant left hemisphere may be responsible for certain levels of consciousness reported by people as transcendental, mystical, and ecstatically or exultantly spiritual or religious. It has been suggested that this neurophysiological state can be achieved by extreme attentional focus, sensory deprivation (an absence or monotony of stimulation), or even by certain life crises (Ruskin, 1975).
5. Right-handed subjects, who normally look to the right (left cerebral dominance) when answering questions, tend to shift their gaze to the left, showing a cerebral shift, when answering questons having affective, emotional overtones or spatial content. (Example of a spatial/emotional question: "When you visualize your father's face, what emotion first strikes you?" or "Picture and describe the last situation in which you cried" [Schwartz, Davidson, and Maer, 1975, p. 287]).
6. It is possible to split photographs of faces to create composites made up of two left or two right halves. When facial composites of posers expressing the emotions of happiness, surprise, fear, sadness, anger, and disgust were judged as to intensity of emotional expression, it was found that left-side composites were rather consistently found to be more expressive than right-side composites, indicating apparent asymmetries in hemispheric control over facial expression, also.

What is responsible for right-left hemisphere differences? The answer to this question is not clear. Some evidence indicates that there are many structural, inborn asymmetries (differences) between the hemispheres—some of such large magnitude that they are even visible to the naked eye in post-mortem examination (Galaburda, LeMay, Kemper, and Geschwind, 1978). It is too early to tell whether and how these are specifically related to the differences in hemispheric function that have been observed.

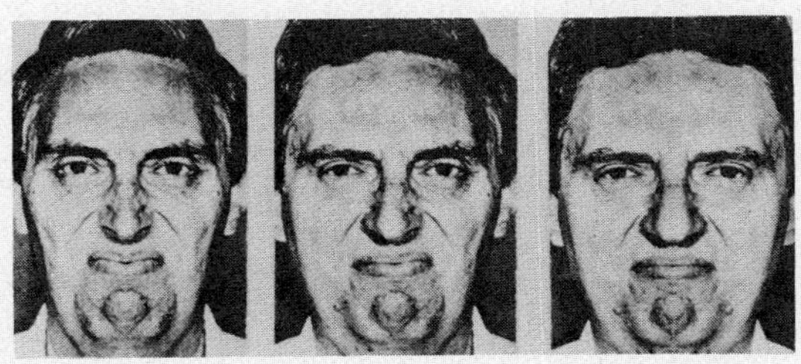

Figure 7.3 The photograph in the center is the original; those to either side are composites, showing what the face would look like if both halves were exactly the same. Note the differences. (From H. A. Sackheim, R. C. Gur, and M. C. Saucy, Emotions are expressed more intensely on the left side of the face, *Science* 202: 434–36, 1978. Copyright 1978 by the American Association for the Advancement of Science)

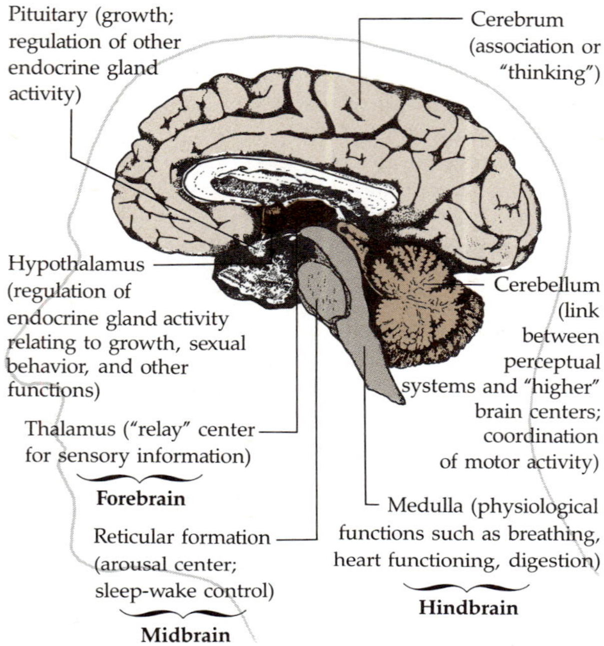

Figure 7.4 A medial (bisected front to back) view of the human brain, showing the major structures and some of their principal functions.

Figure 7.4 indicates that a large portion of the brain is the cerebrum. The cerebrum differentiates humans from other animals because of its relatively larger size and complexity and its domination of other parts of the brain. The outer layer or bark of the cerebrum is called the cerebral cortex ("gray matter"). It is folded and convoluted on its own layers. If stretched out to lie flat it would cover a surface many, many times its seeming surface area. The cerebral cortex is responsible for speech, thinking, memory, judgment, reasoning, and related cognitions. It also carries and interprets visual, auditory, olfactory, and gustatory input, controls voluntary motor activity, and is the seat of the will and consciousness, the controller, interpreter, and "experiencer" of emotions, the regulator of sexual activity, and the general interpreter of the world around the organism.

Each cerebral hemisphere, as seen in Figure 7.5, is divided into four parts or lobes: the frontal lobe, the parietal lobe, at the top and back of the brain, the occipital lobe, at the bottom half of the brain, and the temporal lobe, near the ear area of the head. These lobes, generally speaking, specialize in different functions. Chapter 13, pp. 349–51, describes some of these specialized functions. In general, gross injury to these lobes, such as that sustained in gunshot wounds and brain tumors, has demonstrable effects on behavior that are fairly predictable, depending on which lobe is affected.

Within each of the lobes, researchers have been able to identify many subparts—structures that can sometimes be identified when injured through a lesion or trauma, on the basis of the patient's specific symptom or difficulty. The relationship between a lesion and its effects is not always fixed, however, and some brain structures have the capacity to assume functions not always associated with them.

Lying in the center of the brain, underneath the cortex, are many small, phylogenetically older (that is, in an evolutionary sense) groups of functionally

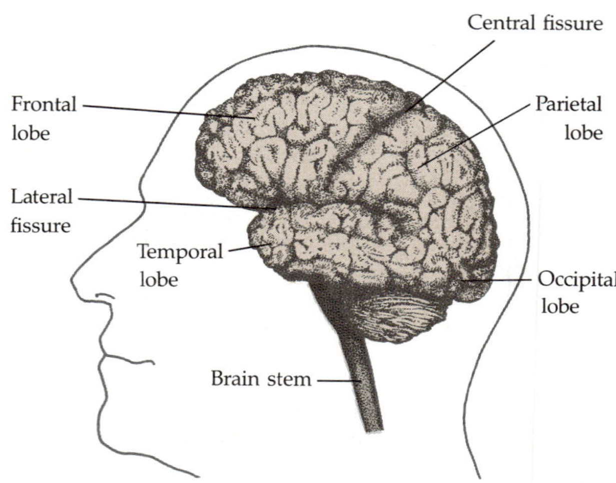

Figure 7.5 The cerebral lobes. These lobes, generally speaking, specialize in different functions. The temporal lobes are associated with language, speech, and hearing; the frontal lobes, with control of voluntary muscles and the higher thought processes; the parietal lobe, with body sensation; and the occipital lobe, with vision.

related neurons known as nuclei, all richly connected to one another, to the cortex, and to other neurons outside the brain. These groups of neurons are organized into a few structures consisting of several nuclei.

The diencephalon consists of the thalamus and hypothalamus (see Figure 7.4). The thalamic structure is the relay center for the sensory (afferent) pathways that send incoming messages to higher (cortical) nerve centers or to lower nerve centers for interpretation and integration.

The hypothalamus controls visceral functions and is very much involved with the autonomic system and, indirectly, with the endocrine system. The hypothalamus thus, together with other systems, regulates the various internal processes responsible for life itself, such as cardiovascular and respiratory activities. The hypothalamus is also involved in the expression of emotional activities through the various organs and glands it regulates, directly or indirectly.

These structures and several others comprise a functional network known as the limbic system. This is sometimes thought of as the "old" cortex (it is, among mammals, a much older series of structures in contrast to the more "recently" developed neocortex of human beings) and is in charge of the organism's internal world. The limbic system is the regulator of the individual's behavior concerned with basic survival: fighting, fleeing, sexual behavior, mobilization of motivation and energy, and temperature control; it is also the seat of such emotions as fear and rage.

In the back of the head, behind the cerebral cortex, lies the cerebellum which consists of a mass of nerve tissues responsible for maintaining the skeletal system, balance, posture, gait, and general equilibrium. Injury to the cerebellum can be detected by the difficulties an individual displays in these motor areas.

The brain continues down into the spinal cord with no separation. The brainstem, which connects the brain with the spinal cord, contains several important systems, including the network of neural structures that concerns attention and arousal, called the reticular activating system (RAS) or reticular formation. Spotlight 7.2 describes some aspects of attention and arousal.

Spotlight 7.2 Attention and Arousal

One afternoon in my office, I saw in consultation a seven-year-old brain-damaged girl. She was distractible and unable to focus on or attend to the questions I asked. Also, she was so hyperactive that progress in the session was almost impossible. That same day I had a therapy session with a "vigilant" man: he was oversensitive and overalert to any and all stimuli. He seemed to be constantly watchful and exuded a heightened awareness of the world around him; the doorbell upstairs, my own motions, and some smudges on the wall seemed to get equal attention from him. The next morning, again in consultation, I was face to face with a dejected, immobile woman who did not seem responsive to any but the most dramatic question, salient stimuli, or abrupt happening. She seemed to be truly underaroused by the world around her. Although these people were suffering from different problems and experiencing different feelings, they shared something in common: they were all showing attentional dysfunctions.

What is attention?

Attention is the responsiveness of an organism to a portion of the stimuli impinging on it, accompanied by a decrease or absence of responsiveness to other (wider) portions of that stimulus array. Attention is the contact point between the organism and the world around it. Moreover, it often reflects or is vulnerable to various kinds of mental, emotional, and CNS difficulties, as illustrated by the three capsule observations just presented.

Attentional dysfunctions can create problems

in learning at school, in productivity on the job, and with any task or activity that requires sustained interest or ability to follow directions along a single line or purpose toward a goal. Attentional problems of brain-damaged and schizophrenic persons are well known to clinicians and some have observed that teaching attentional skills to individuals with such pathological conditions (in order to reduce disorganized and scattered attention, for example) goes a long way toward facilitating learning (Buss and Lang, 1965; Deutsch and Schumer, 1970; Lang and Buss, 1965).

Distractible, inattentive, overaroused, or underaroused states may have many causes, including the learning history, cultural training, and level of motivation of the individual. However, some attentional difficulties can be linked directly to dysfunctions in the reticular activating system (RAS), which involves some of the neural structures and cells in the core of the brainstem. The RAS is essential for maintaining the organism in an aroused, wakeful state with a high level of awareness that permits, directs, and holds attention on specific sensory inputs (Jaspers, 1963).

The limiting and controlling of an overaroused or overattentive state—reticular inhibition—is an equally important mechanism, limiting the range of attention and perception so that everything in the stimulus array is not attended to. Reticular inhibition thus permits increased focus on limited aspects of the stimulus array (Hernández-Péon, 1966). For example, when you are solving a problem, studying, or listening carefully to a record, you would not want to be attentive to or aroused by all the other stimuli around you: street noises, the ticking of a clock, your neighbor's plumbing problems, or your noisy refrigerator. People with some abnormal conditions show just this pattern: they are over-responsive to extraneous or irrelevant cues. On the other hand, other kinds of abnormal conditions can be characterized by a different attentional pattern. Some people seem incapable of being aroused by the stimuli that ordinarily capture our attention. This condition characterizes autistic children, for example, and some types of schizophrenics.

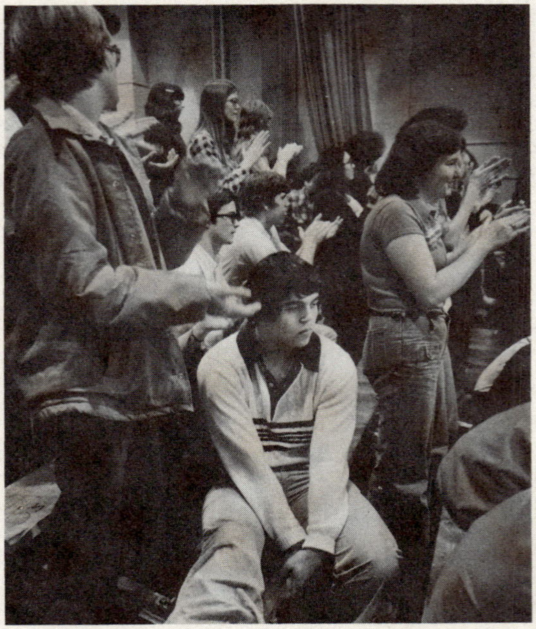

Attentional difficulties often reflect emotional problems. (© 1979 J. M. Richardson/Black Star)

Attention is central to an understanding of many types of pathological behavior. Descriptions of additional kinds of attentional difficulties will be presented in the chapters that follow.

THE AUTONOMIC NERVOUS SYSTEM (ANS)

Imagine that you are in a hot, crowded movie theater sitting in the middle of a long row of seats. Someone shouts "Fire!" What happens to you? If you tend to respond the way most other people do, you probably will find, as you sense a rising confusion, desperation, and panic, that you begin to perspire profusely; your breathing becomes irregular and shallow; your heart starts to beat furiously; soon you may feel a pounding within your head.

And you would probably become aware of an overwhelming impulse to flee.

The system of the body that is "energizing" you in this way is helping you to prepare for handling danger or attack; later, the same system will help to quiet you after the stress period is over. This system is called the autonomic nervous system (ANS). It is comprised of many structures that send messages to organs and glands throughout the body. These include the stomach, rectum, bladder, sweat glands, lungs, and heart. Figure 7.6 shows how extensive the ANS is.

The autonomic nervous system keeps us going—keeps us alive—by regulating the internal systems of the body, such as breathing and heart rate, without our conscious awareness. It is essentially an involuntary system. There is evidence, however, that some aspects of this system can be brought under voluntary control. Thought at one time to be a system entirely separate from the CNS, today researchers are acknowledging the possibility that control over parts of the ANS may also reside in the brain and spinal cord.

The ANS consists of two subsystems—the sympathetic and the parasympathetic systems.

The sympathetic system prepares the organism for an emergency by releasing a variety of energizers and initiating various physiological events so that the organism can protect itself. For example, the heart beats faster, there is a flow of adrenalin for energy, sugar is released from the liver, perspiration is increased, the pupils of the eyes dilate,

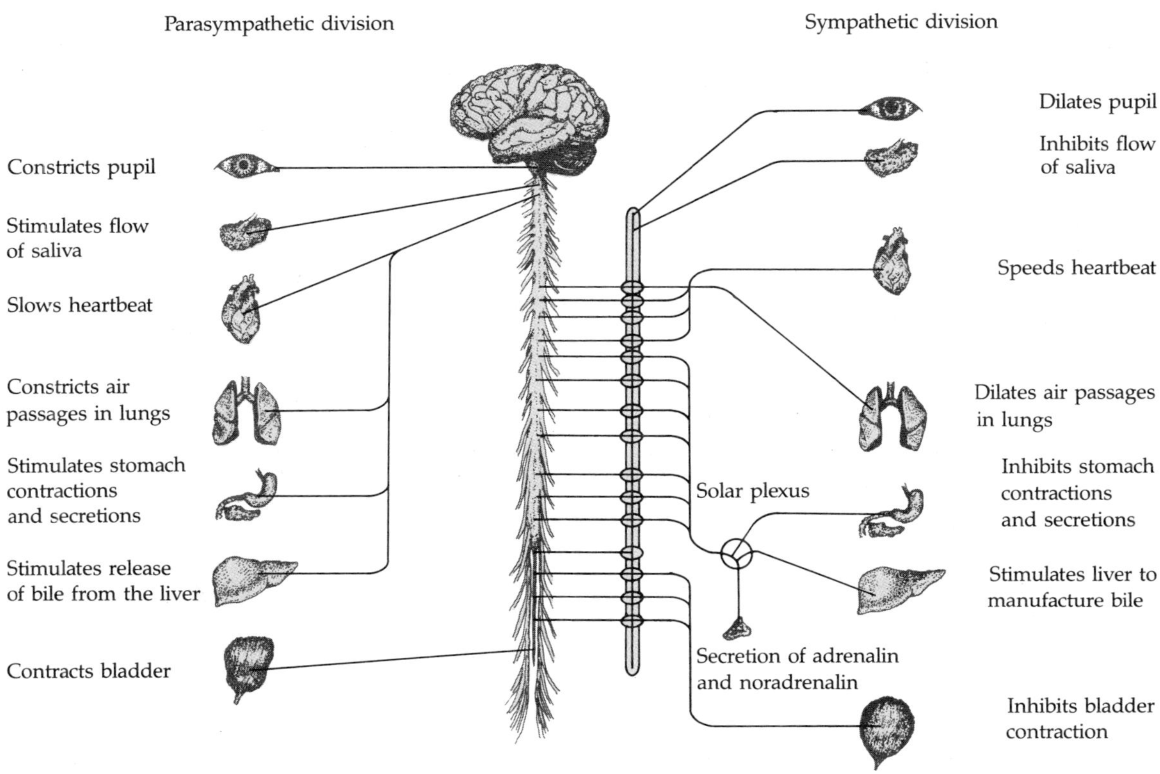

Figure 7.6 A schematic representation of the two divisions of the autonomic nervous system (ANS), showing the functions of each.

Spotlight 7.3 Monitoring the "Insides": Indicators of Emotions and Abnormal Behavior

Researchers of behavior pathology are increasingly mindful of the importance of reliable methods for measuring the activities of various systems and organs of the body, such as the brain or the autonomic nervous system, so that they can learn more about the relationship of physiological functions to specific symptoms, disordered behaviors, and emotional states such as anxiety, stress, anger, and conflict. These methods attempt to reflect, through the body's overt actions, what is actually going on under the skin—covert behaviors, so to speak. If such measurements are recorded continuously (and many measurements can be recorded simultaneously), we can obtain not only a "glimpse" into such internal states as sleep, arousal, dreaming, conflict, excitement, and sexual behavior but also, a permanent record for later study.

One widely used method, electroencephalography (EEG), measures and records the continuous electrical and chemical activity of the brain. If electrodes are placed on various parts of the scalp and the electrical output is charted graphically during changes of stimulation (for example, during various waking and sleeping states), the typical patterns of brain waves that emerge during each of these periods can be recorded. Because various types of brain and behavior pathologies generally produce characteristic patterns, the EEG has become an important diagnostic tool, together with other methods, in the study and detection of different types of brain abnormalities (see Chapter 13).

Another group of measures often used to reveal the relation between overt and covert physiological processes is based on the fact that changes in electrical potential are produced by movements of various parts of the body. In addition to the electrocardiogram (EKG), which records the electrical activity produced by the muscular contractions of the beating heart through electrodes placed near the heart and a limb, there is the electromyogram (EMG), which records electrical changes produced by activation of a muscle. Changes in blood pressure can also be recorded on a continuous basis through use of the sphygmomanometer.

One of the most frequently used indicators of autonomic activity is the galvanic skin response (GSR), which measures changes in electrical resistance on the skin. This measure is especially useful in studying people in anxiety-producing, conflictful, or stressful situations, since it is well known that these situations (such as great fear) result in increased perspiration. Because sweating reduces electrical resistance of the skin, measures of electrodermal changes taken from the palm, for example, if recorded graphically and continuously, can yield information concerning the subjects' internal autonomic responses as they are being questioned or evaluated or while they are dreaming, fantasizing, and so on.

When continuous records of GSR, blood pressure, and respiratory activities are recorded simultaneously, sudden changes from a preestablished baseline have been regarded as indicators of autonomic disturbance. Such a record, called the polygraph (lie detector), has often been introduced during pretrial hearings and even as evidence to a jury to establish or demolish the credibility of a witness. Many representatives of government, business, and the criminal justice system (the police, for example) have relied for years on this autonomic "mirror" and there is a rather flourishing commercial polygraph industry in this country.

In the light of many questions concerning the reliability and validity of the polygraph as a measure of deception, considerable controversy exists regarding the ethics of using such records for or against witnesses and defendants. As a matter of fact, in deception tests, the use of a control question to serve as the autonomic baseline for veracity entails many problems because autonomic changes can occur even when the subject is not lying. Although there is argument against the use of the polygraph as valid testimony or evidence for or against deception (Lykken, 1979), some reputable investigators continue to hold that its proper use is of enormous benefit to "innocent defendants, the judicial process, and society in general" (e.g., Raskin and Podlesny, 1979). What is your opinion about using the polygraph to establish or weaken a person's credibility?

the hairs of the skin are raised, and the salivary glands and digestive, bladder, and rectal functions are inhibited. The body is prepared for action, for an emergency—for fleeing or for fighting.

The parasympathetic system is in many ways reciprocal to the sympathetic system. It slows the body down and seems to serve a restorative function for bodily processes so that greater passivity and relaxation are induced. For example, the pupils of the eyes become constricted, heart rate slows down, there is a relaxation of rectal muscles and bladder controls so that defecation and urination occur, and there is preparation for the digestive system to work effectively.

The autonomic nervous system is deeply involved in—as a major bodily accompaniment to—strong emotions such as fear, anxiety, terror, and panic. Because these strong emotions are often significant aspects of disordered or dysfunctional behavior, psychologists studying abnormal behavior are especially intrigued by attempts to measure autonomic responses so that the emotions accompanying them can be better understood. As a matter of fact, the monitoring and measuring of various activities of the autonomic nervous system have its counterparts in other areas. For researchers are also interested in studying the biochemical makeup of body fluids (blood or urine, for example) or electrical brain waves as well as many other indicators of biological and CNS activity as part of a broad attempt to explore the relationship of these internal systems to various abnormal states. Spotlight 7.3 highlights this area.

THE ENDOCRINE SYSTEM

The endocrine system, an extremely complex system of glands, sends hormones (chemicals that have various regulatory functions) into the blood stream. These hormones control, regulate, and stimulate the organs of the body in ways that sustain normal and appropriate growth, sexual structures and functions, emotional tone, and mood. Imbalances in and among glandular functions, under or over secretion of individual glands, and other dysfunctions of this system can result in an extraordinarily wide range of disorders in mood, feelings, growth, and sexual development and behaviors (Sachar, 1976).

Much is known about the functions of the endocrine system—for example, the pituitary system (sometimes called the master gland) controls the other glands, while the adrenal medulla releases hormones that prepare the body for action and for emergency with a great mobilization of energy by releasing epinephrine and norepinephrine. However, there is still a great deal to learn about the complex workings of this system and its relationship to disordered behavior.

Spotlight 7.4 presents a list of glands and their functions, and Figure 7.7 is a diagram of their general location in the body.

NEUROCHEMISTRY AND ABNORMAL STATES

Most of the physiological events described thus far seem to rest on the action of some chemical. Neuronal discharges, synaptic transmissions, the actions of the sympathetic and parasympathetic system, the endocrinological system, and the brain itself are all dependent on the chemicals within the blood, within the cells, or at the synapses. Some of the chemicals produced by the endocrine system, such as adrenalin (epinephrine) and noradrenalin (norepinephrine), have been known for some time to be related to fear and anger.

These chemicals, as well as many others, have been specifically studied in regard to their actions in the brain and the CNS. Implications of this relatively recent research with regard to mood, emotions, mental illness, mental retardation, drives, and the modification or treatment of all these conditions are far reaching (McGeer and McGeer, 1980). The specific focus of research in this area is on the chemical substances referred to as neuroregulators; these consist of neurotransmitters, which allow information to be conveyed from nerve cell to nerve cell, and neuromodulators which increase or decrease nerve cell activity (Barchas, Akil, Elliott, Holman, and Watson, 1978; Holman, Barchas, and Elliott, 1976; Iversen, 1979). The list of known or hypothesized chemicals in the brain that may be neuroregulators is becoming larger and larger, with new substances still being discovered. For example, in the past several years chemicals called endorphins and enkephalins have been discovered to resemble opiate-like substances with many pain-reducing qualities. These natural, physiologically produced chemicals, found in great concentration in the area of the hypothalamus, may be responsible for easing the pain of narcotics withdrawal in some people or helping others to cope with disorganizing panic and pain in the face of danger. The chapters that follow will describe these natural chemicals in greater detail.

In addition to those already mentioned, several other neurotransmitters have gained wide attention. One of these is serotonin, found in unusually large or small amounts in the brain, especially in the limbic system (the brain structures closely associated with emotions). Serotonin has been found in relatively more than usual or less than usual quantities in various pathological states. As a result, the hypothesis implicating excessive serotonin in the etiology of schizophrenia has held sway in some circles, whereas the hypothesis of serotonin deficiency has been implicated in the etiology of some forms of depression.

A deficiency of dopamine, another neurotransmitter, has been implicated in Parkinson's disease, a neurological disorder. Some of the antipsychotic chemicals used in the treatment of schizophrenic patients (see Chapter 21) are held to be effective because they block the actions of dopamine in the CNS. The dopamine hypothesis of schizophrenia, which posits an excess of dopaminergic activity in the brain, has become another widely held theory. These theories and related biochemical approaches to the puzzle of schizophrenia will be elaborated in Chapter 12.

The effectiveness of drugs in treating certain kinds of disorders is probably due to the fact that these drugs replace, inhibit, "mimic," or in some way interact with chemicals already found in the body. Many drugs resemble natural substances found in the body, even though they are manufactured in the laboratory.

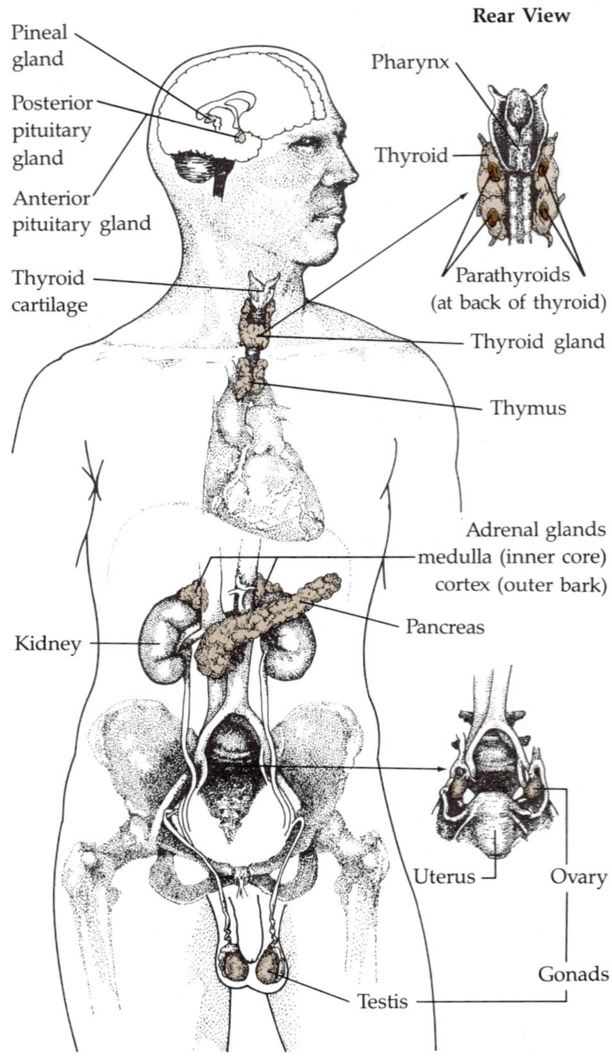

Figure 7.7 The locations and functions of the major endocrine glands.

In the pages that follow and in much of the literature on abnormal psychology, the important role that various neuroregulators (neurotransmitters and neuromodulators) may play in the etiology of many abnormal states is emphasized. Several significant

Spotlight 7.4 The Endocrine System: The Glands and What They Do

Below is a list of the major glands. Some hormones are released through the triggering action of other hormones, some by neural impulses, and still others by chemicals introduced into the body from the outside. Hormonal output can also be triggered by environmental events, whether it is tears caused by excessive wind or increase of sugar level because of a startling noise. Hormones act in combination, in antagonism, or in reinforcement of each other. The list of hormones secreted by these glands is not a complete one, nor is the description of their functions.

Gland	Hormone	Effect
Anterior pituitary ("master gland")	GH—growth hormone	Stimulates growth
	TSH—thyroid stimulating hormone	Stimulates thyroid secretion
	ACTH—adrenocorticotropic hormone	Stimulates adrenal cortex secretion
	FSH—follicle-stimulating hormone LH—luteinizing hormone	Promotes secretion of sex hormones and Development of germ cell
	PL—prolactin	Develops corpus luteum and increases milk production
Posterior pituitary	Vasopressin	Smaller arteries constrict
	Oxytocin	Uterus contracts Milk production increases Kidney water reabsorption
Thyroid	Thyroxin	Increases metabolism
Parathyroids	Parathormone	Increases blood calcium Lowers blood phosphate
	(Vitamin D)	Prevents loss of calcium and phosphate
Adrenal cortex	Corticoids	Sodium retention Potassium loss Liver glycogen formation Increases carbohydrate metabolism Male sex hormone
Adrenal medulla	Norepinephrine	Mimics sympathetic nervous system
	Epinephrine	Raises blood pressure Stimulates ACTH release
Pancreas		
Alpha cells	Glucagon	Increases blood glucose
Beta cells	Insulin	Lowers blood glucose
Gonads	♂ Androgen ♀ Estrogen	Fertility and secondary sex characteristics
Pineal gland	Melatonin	Suppresses sex behavior

Source: Slightly modified from Leukel, *Introduction to physiological psychology*, 3rd ed. (St. Louis: The C. V. Mosby Co., 1976), p. 41.

models based on neuroregulators, such as the enkephalins, the endorphins, dopamine, and serotonin will be noted repeatedly in this context. There are dozens of neurochemicals produced in the brain about which our ignorance is sizable. We do know, however, that these substances are of fundamental importance to the working network of neurons, organs, and glands that underlie all behavior and mental and emotional states. At the present time, we not only know little about how most of these chemicals act on neurons, but even less about their interactions and their effects on behavior.

In the meantime, you should be cautioned against oversimplified statements in this new and exciting area of understanding, for neurotransmitters, like hormones, work in complex interaction—blocking, enhancing, or inhibiting the effects of other neurotransmitters (Antelman and Caggiula, 1977; Holman, Barchas, and Elliott, 1976). These neurochemical interactions are extremely complex and it does not yet seem possible to posit a one-to-one relationship between a deficiency or abundance of a particular neurotransmitter, such as dopamine, and a behavioral pathology.

Moreover, no one particular ideal neurochemical level within the body may exist; some individuals might need a special type of chemical balance for normal behavior, whereas others do not. Further, learning may also influence the biochemical properties and mechanisms of the body. It may therefore not be possible to speak of inherited biochemical levels that rigidly unfold for any particular individual. For certain psychological states and life events may modify neurochemical activity, which may then stabilize and only later result in disordered behavior. The implication is that disastrous life events or environmental deprivations early in life may alter neurochemical activities in ways that may produce behavioral pathology later in life (Barchas, et al., 1978).

The richness of this field lies not only in its possibilities for increasing our understanding of the brain and its functions, but also in its potential for yielding methods for modifying many different disorders that may be determined, entirely or in part, by imbalances and dysfunctions in the body's complex neurochemical system. These may range from chronic and unrelieved states of anxiety, fear, and anger, attentional dysfunctions, mood and affective disorders, and schizophrenia, to a variety of neurological disorders, such as Huntington's, Parkinson's, or Alzheimer's disease (see Chapter 13).

GENETIC DETERMINANTS OF ABNORMAL STATES

In the chapters that follow, many references will be made to the possibility that some abnormal conditions are influenced, in large part, by the individual's genetic characteristics. Some kinds of mental retardation, neurological disorders, atypical sexual structures (morphological sexual aberrations such as underdeveloped sexual organs), and hormonal malfunctions—all of which have profound effects on behavior—may have a genetic basis. Relevant literature on the significance of genetic factors in the development of bipolar affective disorders (manic-depressive illness) and schizophrenia will also be summarized. However, because most pathological conditions concern behaviors that arise in a social context in which there is a strong learning component, it is difficult to imagine, except in rare instances, a one-to-one relationship between genetic factors and abnormal behavior.

Genes are the basic, most simple functioning unit in heredity. In humans, genes number in the tens of thousands—estimates are more than 50,000 (McKusick and Ruddle, 1977)—and they appear in regular, predictable positions on a chromosome. There are twenty-three pairs of chromosomes within the nucleus of each human cell. When a sperm cell and an ovum unite, a set of twenty-three chromosomes from the father unites with a set of twenty-three chromosomes from the mother to form a new set of forty-six chromosomes in the cell that develops into the baby. The new combinations are random and the possibilities for kinds of pairings are amazingly high. But offspring get half of their hereditary programming or information from their fathers and half from their mothers and therefore have two copies of each gene.

The twenty-third pair of chromosomes—the sex chromosomes—within each cell determines the sex of the organism; the others are called autosomes. Females carry an XX pair of sex chromosomes, and males, an XY pair. An offspring thus receives an X chromosome from his or her mother, but either an X or Y chromosome, based only on chance, from his or her father.

The discovery of a method for photographing stained chromosomes (karyotyping) and an international agreement for numbering the positions of each pair of chromosomes opened up a new vista

Spotlight 7.5 A Limited Genetics Glossary

In this and subsequent chapters, occasional reference will be made to genetic factors and their possible relationship to pathology. A basic glossary of terms frequently used in genetics follows.

autosome any chromosome other than a sex chromosome

chromosome one of the threadlike, deep-staining nucleoprotein bodies that carry the genes

concordant similarity of a characteristic or trait in individuals of groups

discordant dissimilarity between sets of individuals or groups in that one has one form of a trait or characteristic and the other has another form

dizygotic type of twins produced by the fertilization of two different eggs by two different sperm; commonly referred to as fraternal twins

dominant that trait displayed when an individual carries two different forms of a gene; the dominant form of the gene masks other possible forms

DNA abbreviation for deoxyribonucleic acid, in which the genetic information is coded

expressivity degree or severity of expression of a trait controlled by a particular gene

gamete mature germ cell (sperm or egg)

gene unit particle of DNA or a unit of heredity with a fixed location on a given chromosome; about 250 human genes, of about 50,000, have been mapped

genotype genetic constitution or make-up of an individual

heritability degree to which the trait or characteristic is controlled by genetic factors

karyotype chromosome set of an individual as shown by a photomicrograph of a cell in which the number, size, and shape of the chromosomes are displayed

locus the position or site of a gene on a chromosome

monozygotic type of twins derived from a single, fertilized ovum; commonly referred to as identical (MZ) twins

mutation a sudden change in the genetic material of an organism, usually of a single gene; a gametic mutation is inherited, a mutation in other kinds of cells (somatic) is not inherited

phenocopy an environmentally caused trait or characteristic that resembles one that is genetically caused

phenotype the appearance of an individual arising from his or her genotype in interaction with his or her environment

recessive a trait, strictly speaking; less precisely, a form of gene; a recessive trait remains undisplayed if an individual carries the dominant form of that trait; it is expressed only when another identical gene copy exists

RNA abbreviation for ribonucleic acid, synthesized by copying one strand of a DNA template

sex linkage trait specified by a gene located on the sex chromosome, usually the X chromosome

zygote cell resulting from the union of a maternal and a paternal gamete

Source: Adapted from Rosenthal, 1971, pp. 160–64.

for the study of aberrations in genetic structures. For example, it was discovered in 1959 that children with Down's syndrome (mongolism—see Chapter 14) have an extra copy of a small chromosome. Chromosomal aberrations can consist of an especially small chromosome, an extra sex chromosome, or an especially long chromosome. Chromosomal aberrations can be observed through the karyotyping of cell composition even when the offspring is still in the uterus through a method called amniocentesis (see Spotlight 14.3, pp. 375–76). This is a procedure generally used after the fourth month of pregnancy. It consists of inserting a long, thin needle into the mother's abdomen to obtain some of the cells in the fluid that surrounds the fetus, permitting subsequent examination for defects.

Certain alternate forms of genes are not expressed (recessive) if paired with other forms (dominant). Such genes are commonly called recessive genes. Some abnormal conditions occur only if both maternal and paternal genes are of the recessive type. If an abnormal condition is associated with a dominant gene, it will be expressed no matter whether its "mate" is dominant or recessive. If an abnormality is caused by a gene that appears in a sex chromosome, it is described as sex-linked when referring to its genetic characteristics. Genes causing abnormality may occur in the autosomes, as well. A few abnormal conditions have been traced to gene mutations, or sudden changes in genetic material. If such changes occur in the egg or sperm cell, they are transmitted along with other inherited material to the offspring.

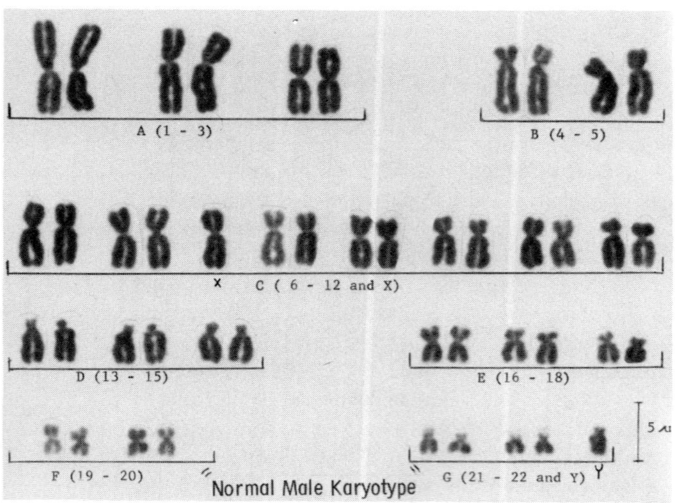

Figure 7.8 A normal male karyotype: photographs of stained chromosomes. (L. F. Meisner, State Hygiene Laboratory, Madison, Wisconsin)

Whereas chromosomal or biochemical aberrations can often be objectively observed, genetic determinants as the basis of abnormal behavior are much more difficult to ascertain. Further, the common assumption that there is complete dominance or recessiveness of a gene, and that this characteristic determines whether or not a trait is expressed or developed, is not entirely warranted:

> *As a matter of fact, complete dominance or recessiveness is much more the exception than the rule. Many factors influence phenotypic expression. A gene is essentially a chemical unit. Although any given gene probably has only a single primary action, each step of the biochemical processes in which it is involved may have many effects on the developing organism. . . . It is probable, then, that the effects of the action of one gene are likely to be influenced in turn by the actions of other genes, and it would be unlikely to find many instances in which a single gene is solely responsible for the development of a given trait. Similarly, since each step in the chemical progression influences what happens next, it is clear that any single gene may ultimately influence many characteristics rather than one (Rosenthal, 1971, p. 30).*

The methods generally used in attempts to discover whether or not genetic determinants are involved in an abnormal condition (see Schulsinger, 1980) are:

1. *Incidence in successive generations.* The course of a disease can be traced through several generations for incidence. By inference, a condition could be regarded as hereditary if it emerges in successive generations according to a predictable pattern.

2. *Expectancy rates.* Rates of a disease in the general population can be compared with the rates of the disease or condition in the relatives of a given family. An important consideration before jumping to genetic conclusions is that families share a culture as well as genes. The influence of learned values, beliefs, and rituals would have to be ruled out

as possible factors in the etiology of a disease before a definite genetic inference could be made.

3. *Twin method (raised together).* Twins raised together can be identical (monozygotic) or fraternal (dizygotic). The fraternal twins share 50 percent of genetic material, while the identical twins, since they developed from the same cell, share 100 percent of this genetic material. The frequency of a condition or disorder in the identical twins compared to that for the fraternal twins—who are not more closely related genetically than any pair of nontwin siblings—is an excellent way to study the genetic influence on certain pathological conditions.

4. *Twin method (raised apart).* The difficult search for identical twins raised apart may yield rewarding results. The difference in commonality (similarity) between identical twins raised apart compared to that for twins raised together can shed light on the possibility of genetic determinants of a disease or condition. If identical twins with totally different environmental backgrounds have the same pathological condition to the same extent as those raised together, one would have to seriously consider the possibility of genetic influences on the condition.

5. *Degree of concordance.* Concordance means similarity. If a trait is entirely determined by heredity, we would find perfect concordance in identical twins. Between fraternal twins, parent-child, and nontwin siblings pairs, we would find 50 percent concordance rates; and between other relatives, such as an individual and his or her grandparents, aunt, uncle, and first cousins, a concordance rate of 25 percent and so on, would be found.

6. *Adoptee method.* Some adopted children are raised by abnormal or pathological parents. Some adopted children are not. If there is a greater incidence of pathology in the former situation, then a good case can be made for environmental rather than genetic factors. If some adopted children become schizophrenic and others do not, and their biological parents can be found, then if there is greater incidence of pathology in the parents of the disturbed children, then a good case can be made out for genetic, rather than environmental, factors.

In all genetic studies of behavior, there are things to watch out for that could lead to an erroneous interpretation of the influence of heredity. An increase of concordance rates with closeness of family relationships (consanguinity) does not necessarily validate a genetic interpretation, because there is generally also an increase of environmental similarity under such circumstances. Also, even if siblings or identical twins tend to show similarity of traits (say, 30 percent concordance), unless the concordance in the general population is known, no interpretation—genetic or environmental—is possible.

A third problem arises from the general finding that pathology in one or both parents is usually accompanied by greater frequency of pathology in their offspring than among offspring of normal parents. But offspring raised in a sick family setting are subject to various kinds of stress, unpredictable familial behavior, and the expression of pathology on the part of the parents—environmental, rather than genetic, influences.

The chapters that follow will explore the possibility that genetic factors are implicated in some abnormal mental states. As already suggested, however, except for the most obvious instances of neurological or hormonal disorders, or in the case of objective chromosomal or biochemical aberration, a one-to-one relationship between heredity and pathology is difficult to establish. This is so not only because of the problems in conducting research in this area, such as those noted above, but also because genetic unfoldings always take place within an environment—be it social or biological.

PREVIEW AND OVERVIEW

In this chapter, various internal structures and events were shown to bear an important relationship to emotions and to many pathological states. With an eye to subsequent chapters, some of the implications of this material are highlighted below:

1. *Emotional responses and the body.* The total involvement of the body in an emotional response, from the higher centers of the brain, to the limbic system, to peripheral nerve endings, reflects a wondrous, complex network.

Almost immediately after receiving and acting upon the proper sensory or intellectual signals, these areas of the brain send their own meticulously coded instructions to another very complex portion of the brain, the hypothalamus. . . . It is the prime function of your hypothalamus to supply a "body" to any emotion perceived higher up in the brain, but it also has something to do with the quality of an emotion, too. For example, if all connections between an animal's hypothalamus and the higher areas of the brain are severed, thus freeing the hypothalamus from all constraint, the animal becomes hopelessly maniacal and deadly dangerous.

As a rule, the stimulated hypothalamus sends out . . . coded signals whose precise character depends upon the particular emotion perceived. For example, if you are suddenly confronted with a sorrow-inducing situation, the hypothalamus will send signals to your tear glands, to the blood vessels in your face, and to nerve complexes governing your lungs and heart. You will turn pale, burst into tears, begin to sob, and your heart probably will slow down.

On the other hand, if you become intensely angered by some phenomenon, your hypothalamus will almost instantaneously send signals to all or almost all the nerve endings of your sympathetic nervous system . . . causing them to secrete relatively large amounts of epinephrine and norepinephrine (otherwise known as adrenalin and nonadrenalin, or as a group, as catecholamines). In addition, this same fit of anger will probably also induce the hypothalamus to send additional messages to the pituitary gland, the master of all endocrine glands, urging it to discharge some of its own exclusively manufactured hormones (such as growth hormone) and also to send out chemical signals to the adrenal, sex, and thyroid glands and the pancreas as well, so that they in turn may secrete excess amounts of their *exclusively manufactured hormones.*

(M. Friedman and R.H. Rosenman, Type A behavior and your heart *(New York: Alfred A. Knopf, 1974), pp. 173–74.)*

The point is that any strong emotional response is accompanied by, and is often experienced as, an intense, sometimes global involvement of one's "insides." If certain emotions, such as anger, are chronic, it is a reasonable assumption that this affects the body. The wear and tear on particular organs of the body result from the body's stress response—much in the way that a bridge might begin to show a weak girder or other structural difficulty after years of use. It is believed that some physical ailments—ulcers or high blood pressure, for example—might arise in some people because of their body's stress response. These ailments have been traditionally called psychosomatic (or psychophysiological); they are explored in Chapter 8 in greater detail.

2. *Anxiety.* We have already described heightened autonomic responses during periods of fear. You have all experienced these feelings in situations that realistically *should* elicit fear. For example, in approaching a "blind" curve in your car—with a steep drop on your side of the road—you suddenly see a car coming from the opposite direction swerving into your lane at high speed. But some people seem to show unrelieved, extreme levels, or occasionally increased levels, of autonomic activity *without* a discernible cause. These chronically or intermittently fearful people experience anxiety, terror, or panic with their usual accompaniments: breathing difficulties, increased heart rate or palpitations, dryness of mouth, dizziness or lightheadedness, excessive perspiration, and an overwhelming urge to flee.

Are these anxiety-prone people different from the rest of us? Most of the abnormal states that will be described—including even only moderately dysfunctional states as in some of the neuroses—are accompanied by anxiety, can be characterized by anxiety as its most dominant symptom, or are thought to be generated by anxiety. As a matter of fact, the pervasive role of anxiety in psychopathology is so striking that it will be explored in greater detail later (Chapter 9), along with the clinical grouping that is especially relevant—the anxiety disorders.

3. *Stressors, life events, and psychopathology.* This chapter has deliberately focused on the internal systems, events, and structures within the body that bear a strong relationship to emotions and to various abnormal conditions. It should be obvious that these physiological structures and processes do not exist or unfold arbitrarily or in a vacuum. The surrounding environmental events play a crucial role in eliciting these processes and even in determining whether or not they will play a role in behavior.

Of what significance is a life event in the unfolding of an abnormal state? Are intense events and circumstances, such as nuclear accidents, mutilating surgery, death of a spouse or a child through accident or war, or persistent poverty, sufficient in and of themselves to provoke psychopathology? Are similar happenings equally catastrophic or stressful to different people? What is the interaction between these events and biological, biochemical, and genetic factors in the etiology of a disease? Many of the chapters that follow will return to these important issues, particularly in discussions of psychosomatic ailments, depression, and schizophrenia.

A related question concerns the specific relationship of genetic structures to environmental events in the expression of certain diseases. We shall see again and again, especially in discussions of certain kinds of depression or schizophrenia, that biological determinants are crucial in, yet do not bear a one-to-one relationship to the unfolding of the disease process. The diathesis-stress approach, especially in regard to schizophrenia, holds that the genetic contribution to the expression of such pathological states arises from an interaction of predisposition—based on biochemical, inherited propensities—with certain kinds of environmental conditions or persistently stressful events, such as relentless poverty. In other words, although genetic predisposition might provide the basis for poor coping skills, marginal adjustment, and vulnerability, such predisposition does not necessarily lead to schizophrenia, unless the "right" environmental conditions are present. Chapter 12 explores this approach again when the schizophrenias are discussed.

SUMMARY

Chapter 7 continued the survey of theories of abnormal behavior with a consideration of approaches that looked at "under-the-skin" variables. It briefly reviewed the possible role of the brain and central and autonomic nervous systems, as well as endocrinological and neurochemical variables in relation to disordered behavior. The discussion also evaluated the role of genetic factors in determining abnormal behavior and reviewed the methods by which scientists evaluate the contribution of the genes to the expression of psychopathology. It was generally concluded that the kinds of variables described in this chapter could not alone account for abnormal behavior, because such processes and mechanisms operate in an environment, be it organismic, familial, or cultural. Yet the body's responses cannot be ignored in the study of abnormal behavior, for internal events play an important if not crucial role in producing and sustaining disordered cognitive and emotional states, anxiety, and various psychosomatic and psychophysiological ailments.

Highlights

1. The study of people with various types of psychopathological symptoms may have too long overlooked physiological variables. Psychologists are currently interested in determining the extent to which such variables, and especially their interactions, underlie, determine, or are indirectly associated with abnormal behaviors. If indeed such associations are found, they may suggest powerful opportunities to modify, even "cure," certain types of psychopathology.
2. The basic unit of the central nervous system (CNS) is the neuron. The basic function of the neuron is to receive, process, and transmit information from energy falling on the receptors, to send messages to effectors to activate muscles and glands, and to transmit messages within the brain itself, as in dreaming, thinking, feeling emotion and pain, and so on. For most neurons, there are thousands upon thousands of communication possibilities. Neurons are electrochemically activated and in this process activate other neurons across a "gap" called a synapse. Synaptic activities are determined chiefly by the properties and interactions of chemicals called neurotransmitters. This gen-

eral class of neurochemicals apparently plays an extremely important role in the regulation of mood, emotions, and the organization of thinking processes and has become a focus of intense study among many scientists interested in certain types of psychopathology—for example, schizophrenia.

3. The human brain, whose billions of cells may have trillions of interconnections, is separated into two hemispheres. Most sensory messages from the left side of the body go to the *right* hemisphere, which in turn, regulates and transmits messages having to do with the left side of the body. Conversely, the right side of the body and the *left* hemisphere are functionally connected. The left and right hemispheres, although connected to each other, seem to specialize in certain functions, and these "right-left" differences apparently are related to behaviors relevant to abnormal psychology.
4. The text briefly described the cerebral cortex and the four lobes of each cerebral hemisphere—the frontal lobe, the parietal lobe, the occipital lobe, and the temporal lobe. In addition, other structures, such as the diencephalon (which consists of the thalamus and hypothalamus) were also noted. These structures play an important role in regulating such systems as the autonomic nervous system and the endocrine system, which in turn regulate and control life functions such as cardiovascular and respiratory responses as well as responses having to do with anxiety, mood, and emotions. These and several other structures form a close network called the limbic system, which is the seat and regulator of basic survival functions, such as fighting, fleeing, sexual behavior, motivation and the mobilization of energy, and the control of temperature. Emotions such as rage and fear are apparently also seated in the limbic system. Also briefly noted was the cerebellum, a mass of nerves responsible for balance, gait, posture, and equilibrium. Injury to the cerebellum and to other brain sites can often be detected by the nature of the disordered behavior the injured individual displays—for example, with regard to gait or equilibrium or to certain types of cognitive functions.
5. The importance of attentional levels in some forms of disordered behavior—for example, extreme distractibility, inattentiveness, or various types of excessive under- or overarousal—was noted. Some of these difficulties can be attributed to dysfunctions in one of the CNS systems—the reticular activating system (RAS), or reticular formation.
6. The autonomic nervous system (ANS) is comprised of many nerve structures that control organs and glands all over the body. The ANS, which regulates the internal systems of our bodies (such as the respiratory and cardiovascular systems), consists of two subparts: the sympathetic system, which prepares the individual for emergency and stress by increasing heart rate, enhancing adrenalin flow, releasing sugar, and inhibiting bladder and rectal functions, and the parasympathetic system (in many ways the converse of the sympathetic system) which acts by producing a general slowing down of the functions just noted. The ANS is responsible for producing the strong bodily correlates of anxiety, terror, and panic—emotions that are very much involved in disordered behavior. For this reason, many people who are interested in controlling aspects of psychopathology are also interested in learning more about the ANS and in finding ways to monitor and control some of its specific functions.
7. The endocrine system produces various hormones—chemicals that are intricately involved in the control of human responses in a variety of areas: mood, feelings, sexual responses, for example. Hormonal dysfunctions are thus of great significance in producing many types of abnormal behaviors.
8. It has become clear that many, if not most, of the foregoing functions are achieved by different types of neurochemical events. Certain

types of chemical interactions may be the most important physiological substrate of disordered behavior. Researchers have known for some time that some chemicals—the hormones epinephrine and norepinephrine, for example—are related to fear and anger. We are only beginning to learn about other types of chemicals—for example, the broad class of neuroregulators that control activity in and around nerve cells. Even incomplete knowledge about the action of certain neurochemicals (for example, serotonin and dopamine) has already proved to be of enormous significance in understanding the development and control of some of the major types of psychopathology.

9. Abnormalities in basic genetic structures and processes may cause, or at least contribute, to some pathological behaviors. Nevertheless, it is difficult to establish a one-to-one relationship between heredity and most abnormal conditions, since genetic "unfoldings" always take place within an environment that, even on a biological level, can be shaped by "outside" factors.
10. Several research avenues can help to sort out the role of genetic determinants in abnormal conditions. These include, in addition to the following of successive generations to record the course of a disease among relatives, several more sophisticated methods: studying expectancy rates of a disease in the general population compared to rates among different groups (and degrees) of relatives; comparing the degree of concordance among monozygotic (identical) twins, compared to dizygotic (fraternal) twins raised apart and together; and utilizing adoptee methods. Certain precautions, it was pointed out, must be taken in interpreting data from such investigations. For example, although offspring raised by schizophrenic parents may tend to show greater pathology than offspring raised by healthy parents, it is not altogether clear that the higher incidence of pathology is entirely due to genetic factors.

ISSUES AND QUESTIONS: NATURE VERSUS NURTURE

1. Sometimes philosophical and scientific questions are phrased in oversimplified ways, resulting in misleading and simplistic answers. An example of such a question is whether behavior is due to *nature* or *nurture*—heredity or environment. Many observers and researchers in the field of human behavior and development do not accept this simple dichotomy. Rather, they hold that from the very moment of conception, the genetic development of the individual involves a series of events that take place not in a vacuum but in the immediately surrounding environment of cells, structures, and biochemical events. Thus environment plays a role even in prenatal development, according to this point of view, and the developing fetus can be influenced by many complex, interacting, environmental variables that may be biochemical, social, or cultural. Precisely where heredity stops and environment begins is therefore an artificial, unanswerable question. What are your thoughts on the nature-versus-nurture issue?
2. A great controversy has arisen over a new branch of genetics that attempts to explore the biological and genetic bases of social behavior. This discipline is called sociobiology and its chief founder, O. W. Wilson (1975, 1978), proposes that a much larger sphere of human social behavior is genetically determined than was previously thought. Such instances of social behavior include altruism, mating, marriage, incest taboos, even warfare. According to Wilson, species that displayed certain kinds of altruistic behaviors tended to survive through the ages because "built-in" behaviors, which protected one's own kin, helped to continue the species by permitting the birth of future generations. For example, the disadvantages of not being protected by one's neighbors when attacked by a predatory stranger are obvious;

without such protection, future generations would have fewer and fewer opportunities to be born. Thus through natural selection, species that were more altruistic than others survived, whereas the others did not.

Sociobiology even claims that biochemistry and brain functions may be responsible for our propensity for hope, optimism, and for dealing with despair (Tiger, 1979). The human need for religious beliefs, spiritual values, "something to look forward to," and for a better life, it is thought, may have roots in natural biochemical substances within our bodies—substances that fight spiritual as well as physical injury.

The sociobiological position has received severe criticisms, some of which include:

- sociobiology developed its principles from the world of animals—principles that may therefore be inapplicable to the world of humans with its complex social and cultural networks.
- sociobiology tends to overlook the constant flux and interaction between genes and environment so that attempts to assess the relative contribution of each to behavior are pointless.
- the biological determinism of the sociobiological framework is really an excuse for maintaining the social order with all of its ills; if social behavior is biologically determined, changing it becomes impossible.

What is your opinion on these matters?

SUGGESTIONS FOR FURTHER READING

Leshner, A. I. *An introduction to behavioral endocrinology.* New York: Oxford University Press, 1978. Those interested in the role that hormones play in human and animal behavior will find this readable review of the literature most informative. Eating, aggression, sex, parenting, and emotional reactions are some of the behaviors discussed. In addition, there is a short review of basic endocrinology in the appendix that provides a concise and handy summary of the material discussed in the text.

Wittrock, M. C., Beatty, J., Bogen, J. E., Gazzaniga, M. S., Jerison, H. J., Krashen, S. D., Nebes, R. D., Teyler, T. J. *The human brain.* Englewood Cliffs, N. J.: Prentice-Hall, 1977. This book, written for persons unfamiliar with the technical jargon of the neurosciences, consists of a collection of articles by renowned researchers in that field. The first part of the book presents a simple overview of the structure, evolution, and basic processes of the brain; the second part presents recent findings regarding the hemispheric processes of the brain; and the third part presents educational implications of recent brain research. If split-brain studies fascinate you, the second section of this book presents that literature in a clear, concise manner. This book is recommended as an introduction to neuroscientific understanding of human behavior and experience.

Part II

The Clinical Syndromes

Chapters 8–18

Foreword to Part II

Part II of this book introduces you to clinical illustrations and case studies. You will read about various people as if they were perfect "prototypes"—the classic depressive or classic alcoholic. In reality, these "cases" are people with *mixtures* of problems and symptoms. Depression, anxiety, and interpersonal problems, for example, often accompany most pathologies, so that even though each of the illustrations is used to exemplify a specific diagnostic category, you can assume that many other symptoms are also present.

You will be reading about people who actually exist. Although I have modified their ages and other identifying characteristics (occupation, for example) to protect their privacy, the details of their disorders as to symptoms, intensity of despair, or life difficulties are not fictions.

Most of these people were seen because they sought help for their problems. And indeed, most of them were treated by the referring clinicians, by staff members in public or private facilities or by myself, employing one, another, or a combination of methods. Although detailed descriptions of these methods are presented in Chapters 19 through 21, capsule summaries of the major treatment approaches are presented here to aid you as you read the clinical chapters that follow. But you may also wish to read about some of these methods in greater detail. If so, the chapters and pages to which you can turn are also presented. Just as real clinical cases are often mixtures of symptoms and therefore departures from the standard diagnostic categories, so are treatment methods departures from the standard when used by practicing clinicians. Many of the methods described below, for example, are used in conjunction with one another; and within most of these treatment categories, many variations of technique are employed.

Psychoanalysis. (Chapter 19, pp. 569–72.) Psychoanalytic treatment is a formal application of principles developed by Sigmund Freud on the basis of his extensive study of the neuroses and other pathological conditions (see Chapter 6). Psychoanalytic treatment involves one-to-one analyst-patient sessions several times weekly and can extend over a period of several years. During this time, the patient does most of the talking; the analyst becomes more verbally active in interpreting the meaning of this material in later phases of the treatment. The goal is to explore or analyze deep layers of repressed, unconscious material, especially memories of early, painful, childhood experiences. To do so, various aids are used, such as free association, wherein the patient is encouraged to say whatever comes into his or her mind without censorship, and dream interpretation, wherein the analyst relies for interpretation on a rich lore of Freudian symbolic meanings of dream content.

Psychotherapy. (Chapter 19, pp. 572–79.) Psychotherapy refers to a large class of different methods that are less rule-bound than formal psychoanalysis. These methods or techniques range from psychoanalytically oriented approaches to counseling and direct persuasion of the patient or client. Generally speaking, psychotheraputic methods are used by a trained person to help another person modify his or her behavior, feelings, symptoms, and/or interpersonal relationships. Psychotherapy sessions are held once or twice weekly and extend over a shorter time span—say, six months to a year or two—than psychoanalysis. Hypnosis, medication, biofeedback, and behavioral approaches are generally not regarded as psychotherapy. Psychotherapy generally tends to employ one-to-one verbal methods—hence the appellation "talking therapies."

Group therapy. (Chapter 19, pp. 582–84.) Group therapy refers to several different methods that attempt to help people modify their behavior, attitudes toward themselves and others, and feelings through group sessions that meet once or twice weekly (or more). Composition of the groups can be homogeneous (teenagers, alcoholics, obese adults, or married couples, for example) or heterogenous, with many different age groups and problems represented. The groups can be led by a clinician who may be extremely active or extremely passive. Some groups are leaderless, but a therapist might have individual sessions with a group's members. Although methods vary considerably—some groups, for example, have tasks and exercises to perform while others are completely unstructured—the assumption of most group approaches is that the interpersonal interactions that unfold in a group are analogous to and often reflect interactions in real-life situations. Individuals may consequently learn more about themselves in this treatment situation than in a one-to-one patient-doctor relationship.

Family therapy. (Chapter 19, pp. 584–85.) In this method of treating people, the entire family, rather than the individual, meets with the family therapist once or twice weekly, on the assumption that some families create and sustain "sickness" in one or more of their individual members. Although there are many kinds of family approaches, most of them assume that usual or typical family patterns—such as who talks to whom, who is the scapegoat, how messages are communicated, and the general nature of family interactions—are the elements to be confronted and changed, rather than any one individual's symptoms (even those of the so-called sick family member). Since the family system engenders and then helps to maintain the problems and conflicts of the individual members, only when that system changes can an individual member change.

Behavioral treatments. (Chapter 20.) Principles derived from the experimental psychology of learning have been applied to the task of teaching people how to act, think, and respond emotionally in ways that give them more satisfaction. Many psychologists have claimed success using classical and operant learning techniques to treat a wide variety of pathological conditions, including unrealistic fears and phobias, chronic anger, mutism and defective speech, drug and alcohol abuse, compulsions and obsessions, and autism and hallucinations. Unlike psychodynamically oriented therapies, behavioral treatments are applied without addressing presumed inner conflicts or unconscious motivations. Rather, they aim to directly alleviate or eliminate maladaptive behaviors and thoughts through explicit, objective procedures.

Psychopharmacological interventions. (Chapter 21, pp. 650–55.) It is possible to control, modify, and even eliminate some abnormal conditions and behaviors through medications containing chemicals that interact with or replace substances already in the body (such as neurotransmitters and hormones). Psychoactive medications are often used in conjunction with some of the other treatments, such as psychotherapy, group therapy, or behavior methods. The effectiveness of many of these medications with some kind of patients seems reasonable in the light of the large role played by biochemical events in many aspects of human behavior (see Chapter 7). The psychoactive drugs in widespread use are generally grouped into three classes: the antianxiety drugs (minor tranquilizers), the antidepressants, and the antipsychotic drugs (major tranquilizers).

Biofeedback. (Chapter 21, pp. 639–42.) Autonomic responses, such as heart rate, blood pressure, muscle tension, and skin temperature are generally not under voluntary control. Sometimes these bodily functions are abnormally high, fast, or slow, and consequently out of the range that is healthy for normal functioning. We can now measure these physiological events and record them on a continuous record as they are happening. If the subject can view his or her record of the particular process being monitored, and if some signal is provided when internal responses deviate from the normal or healthy range, he or she may be able to control (without conscious awareness) such responses so that they remain within the desired range. The voluntary control of a biological function in this way is called biofeedback.

Hypnosis. (Chapter 21, pp. 642–48.) This treatment method is neither sleep nor a trance but, rather, a heightened, intense, focused attentional response to suggestion of two kinds—first, a willingness to accept the notion of becoming hypnotized (hypnotic induction) and, second, a willingness to accept the suggestions of the hypnotist (an example of which might be not to feel anxiety on airplanes). The range of hypnotizability varies among individuals—from those who can be easily hypnotized to those who cannot be hypnotized at all.

8

Life Events, Stress, and Disorders of the Body

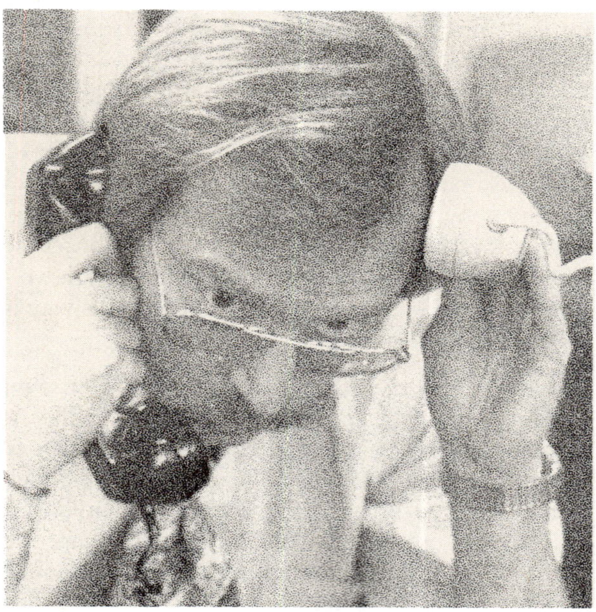

Last year I saw two twenty-year-old college juniors for psychotherapy and counseling. Susan began psychological treatment after a series of physicians were unsuccessful in decreasing her obesity, frequent headaches, and attacks of asthma. She began to gain weight when she was about eleven years old. As a child she had frequent asthma attacks, but these disappeared in her early 'teens. When she went to college, these attacks suddenly resumed, and she also began to complain of many aches and pains, especially discomforting headaches for which there seemed to be no physical basis. Susan's parents were divorced when she was ten years old. From about that time until she left for college, she and her alcoholic mother moved from state to state.

Betty, the other twenty-year-old, also had an alcoholic, divorced mother, and experienced a series of geographical relocations. However, she was lean and healthy and had no bodily aches and pains. She has many friends and is successfully completing her tenure as assistant editor of her college paper. Betty had sought psychological counseling for educational and career planning.

In Chapter 7, some of the physiological bases for emotional responses were described. It seems evident that chronic and persistent arousal has significant impact on the body. Both Susan and Betty described acutely stressful experiences as they were growing up. Yet, physiologically, each responded in different ways. Perhaps their life events and stressful circumstances were perceived in different ways by each of them.

This chapter probes the mystery of the body's response to stressful events. Why is there variation among people regarding the development of bodily symptoms in response to persistent stress? Although these physical symptoms—sometimes referred to as psychosomatic (from the Greek "psyche"—soul or mind—and "soma"—body) or psychophysiological—are real enough, it is frequently held that their origins are largely psychogenic—psychological or emotional, rather than physical.

LIFE EVENTS AND THE CONCEPT OF STRESS

Prior discussions of the body and its responses—its biochemical processes and genetic predispositions—may have presented these responses as if they existed in a vacuum. Actual people, however, function in the real world of situations and events, some good, some bad. Do such events bear a relationship to disease or health? Many researchers believe that important life changes, such as the birth of a child, marriage, divorce, loss of a job, or the death of a spouse have a cumulative effect on later onset of diseases in that the greater the number of such events, the more likely the occurrence of a disease (Dohrenwend and Dohrenwend, 1974; Holmes and Rahe, 1967; Rabkin and Struening, 1976; Selye, 1978). In other words, a succession of responses to important life changes—whether desirable or undesirable—may predispose the body to later illness, presumably by requiring adaptation, accommodation, and adjustment.

To explore the relationship of life events to disease, it is first necessary to find some way of quantifying the life events (and their impacts) an individual has experienced. Spotlight 8.1 describes one of the most widely used scales developed for this purpose. A considerable amount of research with this instrument has indeed disclosed moderate relationships of number of social stressors and later onset of various diseases.

Soon other questions were raised regarding the relation between stressful life events and onset of illness. For example, is it change alone, if cumulative, that creates the kind of wear and tear that could lead to disease, or is it the desirability or undesirability of a series of events (Gersten, Langner, Eisenberg, and Orzeck, 1974)? Is an individual's subjective definition or perception of an event significant? (What one individual may perceive as desirable, others may not.) For example, a move into a low-rent, sunny apartment near campus may come as a bonanza, a stroke of luck, for you; however, a similar move forced on an arthritic, partially blind, eighty-year-old woman may be experienced as a major blow—one that might even precipitate an acute emotional disorder. Thus the assessment of life events and their relationship to later illness must take into account, it was thought, the interaction between the individual's characteristics and perceptions and the event itself (Redfield and Stone, 1979; Sarason, Johnson, and Siegel, 1978).

The Life Experience Survey (LES), a self-report questionnaire, was developed to assess the impact of both desirable and undesirable life changes (Sarason, Johnson, and Siegel, 1978). This questionnaire asks respondents to check various life events that have occurred in the past year and to rate their personal impact—from extremely negative to extremely positive—at the time of their occurrence. Such events as marriage, detention in jail, or death

Spotlight 8.1 Surveying Life Events: The Social Readjustment Rating Scale

Early investigators assumed that life changes, regardless of whether they are desirable or undesirable, require mobilization of energies to deal with accompanying changes in living patterns. These changes were called social stressors. A succession of life changes could be associated with later onset of illness, it was thought (Holmes & Rahe, 1967). These researchers did not assume that such events actually caused illness. Rather, they held that exposure to many social stressors, if accompanied by faulty adaptive responses, could contribute to or even precipitate later illness by increasing the individual's susceptibility to negative environmental agents, such as contagious or infectious diseases.

A widely used systematic method for ascertaining the number of changes in a person's life was developed by Holmes and Rahe (1967). On the basis of data gathered from about 5,000 patients, a pool of 43 items was collected over a period of years. These items were then presented to a smaller sample of subjects who were asked to rate their relative degree of "necessary readjustment" using their own as well as others' experience. They were asked: "Is this event indicative of more or less readjustment than marriage? Would the readjustment take longer or shorter to accomplish?" Their task was to rate the different events as higher or lower in regard to necessary readjustment than the arbitrarily established number of 500 for marriage. The Social Readjustment Rating Scale (SRRS) is the result of this research. Its items are arranged in rank order with the mean value for each item (divided by 10) appearing after it. Those items requiring the most intense and/or protracted period of readjustment are at the top; most of these items reflect "ordinary" rather than catastrophic life events.

As you read the following list, think of how you would have ranked the events in relation to their possible impact on you.

Rank	Life Event	Value
1	Death of spouse	100
2	Divorce	73
3	Marital separation from mate	65
4	Detention in jail or other institution	63
5	Death of a close family member	63
6	Major personal injury or illness	53
7	Marriage	50
8	Being fired at work	47
9	Marital reconciliation with mate	45
10	Retirement from work	45
11	Major change in the health or behavior of a family member	44
12	Pregnancy	40
13	Sexual difficulties	39
14	Gaining a new family member (e.g., through birth, adoption, oldster moving in, etc.)	39
15	Major business readjustment (e.g., merger, reorganization, bankruptcy, etc.)	39
16	Major change in financial state (e.g., a lot worse off or a lot better off than usual)	38
17	Death of a close friend	37

Rank	Life Event	Value
18	Changing to a different line of work	36
19	Major change in the number of arguments with spouse (e.g., either a lot more or a lot less than usual regarding childrearing, personal habits, etc.)	35
20	Taking out a mortgage or loan for a major purchase (e.g., for a home, business, etc.)	31
21	Foreclosure on a mortgage or loan	30
22	Major change in responsibilities at work (e.g., promotion, demotion, lateral transfer)	29
23	Son or daughter leaving home (e.g., marriage, attending college, etc.)	29
24	In-law troubles	29
25	Outstanding personal achievement	28
26	Wife beginning or ceasing work outside the home	26
27	Beginning or ceasing formal schooling	26
28	Major change in living conditions (e.g., building a new home, remodeling, deterioration of home or neighborhood)	25
29	Revision of personal habits (dress, manners, association, etc.)	24
30	Troubles with the boss	23
31	Major change in working hours of conditions	20
32	Change in residence	20
33	Changing to a new school	20
34	Major change in usual type and/or amount of recreation	19
35	Major change in church activities (e.g., a lot more or a lot less than usual)	19
36	Major change in social activities (e.g., clubs, dancing, movies, visiting, etc.)	18
37	Taking out a mortgage or loan for a lesser purchase (e.g., for a car, TV, freezer, etc.)	17
38	Major change in sleeping habits (a lot more or a lot less sleep, or change in part of day when asleep)	16
39	Major change in number of family get-togethers (e.g., a lot more or a lot less than usual)	15
40	Major change in eating habits (a lot more or a lot less food intake, or very different meal hours or surroundings)	15
41	Vacation	13
42	Christmas	12
43	Minor violations of the law (e.g., traffic tickets, jaywalking, disturbing the peace, etc.)	11

Source: Reprinted with permission from the *Journal of Psychosomatic Research* II: 213–18, T. H. Holmes and R. H. Rahe, The social readjustment rating scale, Copyright 1967, Pergamon Press, Ltd.

of a spouse are listed among a group of sixty items that include ten special events for students only, such as failing a course or developing financial problems concerning school.

A review of research with this instrument (Sarason, et al., 1978) does indeed indicate that negative or undesirable life events (negative life change scores) were associated with various measures of anxiety, depression, discomfort, and social nonconformity. In addition, students who sought psychological counseling reported significantly more negative life changes than did students who

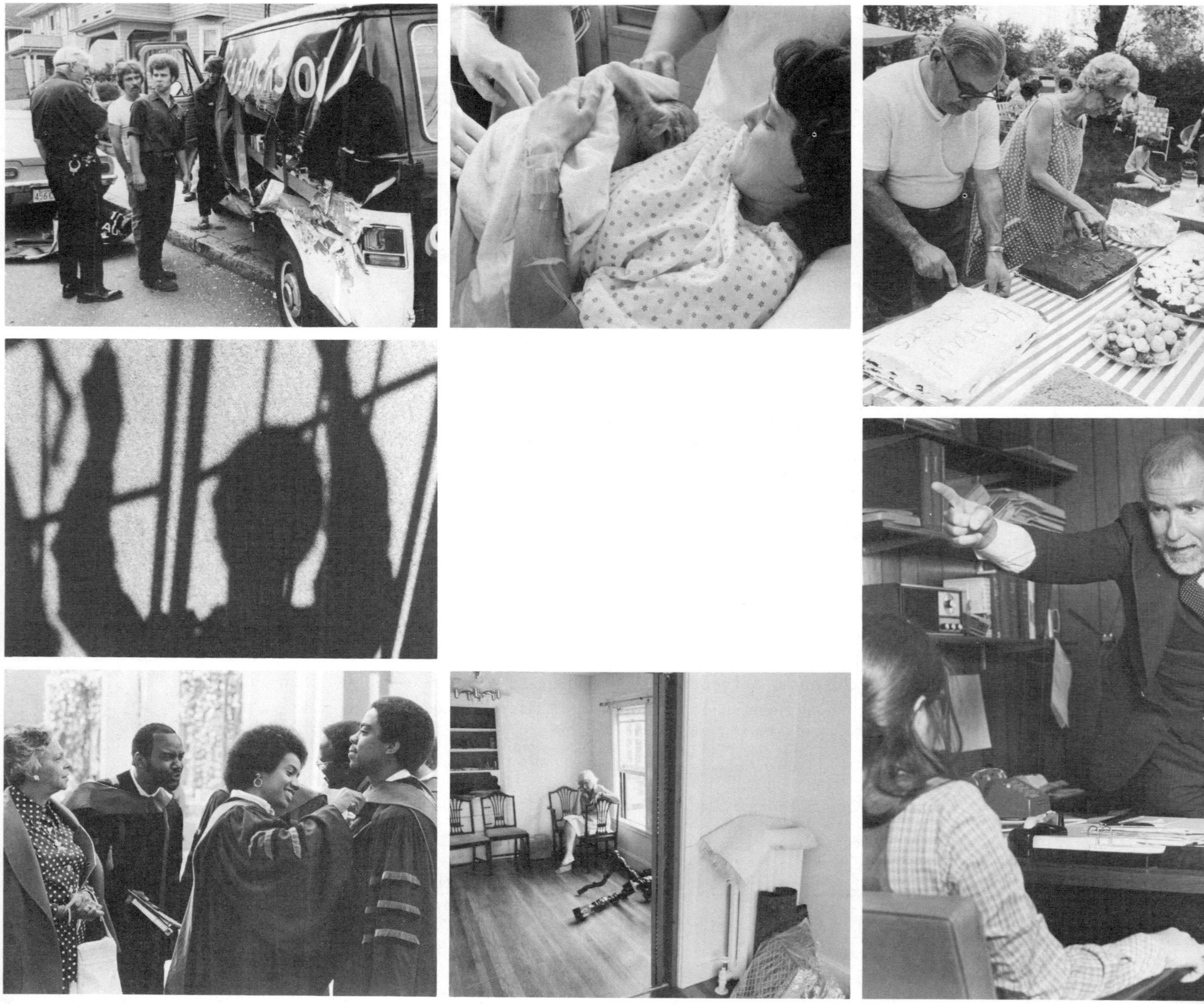

Are important life events—such as a traffic accident, birth of a baby, retirement, being fired, moving, graduation, and going to jail—related to the subsequent development of disease? (Clockwise, from top left: Pamela Price/The Picture Cube; J. D. Sloan/The Picture Cube; Michael Weisbrot/Stock, Boston; Eric Roth/The Picture Cube; Gabor Demjen/Stock, Boston; Frank Siteman/The Picture Cube; Andrew Brilliant/The Picture Cube)

did not. Positive change scores, however, were not associated with various measures used in several of the studies, lending support to the hypothesis that only negative or undesirable life changes or events are associated with stress—in these instances as reflected in psychological difficulties.

What can we learn from life events research over the past several decades? Summaries of this material (Dohrenwend and Dohrenwend, 1970, 1974; Hinkle, 1974; Hudgens, 1974; Rabkin and Struening, 1976; and Sundberg, Snowden, and Reynolds, 1978) indicate that:

1. Some demonstrations (for example, Holmes and Masuda, 1974) that all life changes, whether positive or negative, are significantly associated with the onset of disease are currently being questioned, with greater emphasis being placed on undesirable life events and how an individual perceives these events.

2. Negative life changes, however, do not account for all the variation among people in propensity for developing problems. Some empirical evidence suggests that a preexisting susceptibility or resistance to the impact of life changes exists. That is, given the same number of negative life experiences, some people may be at greater risk for illness or disease; they apparently do not weather life's storms as easily as other people.

3. What factors contribute to amount of risk? Susceptibility or resistance to disease and illness most likely result from a number of factors that include: an individual's genetic and biochemical predisposition; current coping ability and competence to solve problems; existing habits and patterns of response; and the availability of social support systems.

4. Personal competence reduces risk. People who are more competent, more able to cope with serious or undesirable changes, fall into a lower-risk group. Some of the literature suggests that personal competence to face severely stressful events may be related to intelligence, personality type, past experiences and habits, a feeling that one is in charge of one's own fate, biological predisposition, skills, assets, and availability of choices and options in life.

5. Social support systems reduce risk. Social supports refer to family, friends, community facilities and clinics, spouse, enduring ties, and the social groups to which an individual belongs.

6. Low socioeconomic class and the stress-producing aspects of poverty and ghetto-living are apparently associated with greater severity of stressful life events, but not necessarily a greater *number* of such events.

7. Life events cannot cause mental illness such as depression or schizophrenia, but they can exacerbate (increase the severity of, aggravate) preexisting conditions or cause the overt expression of certain predispositions, depending on the individual's coping ability.

Stress and Bodily Adaptation: Hans Selye

We have seen that life events and the way they are perceived can affect an individual's vulnerability to disease. Cumulative events have shown modest relationships, for example, to sudden cardiac deaths, accidents, athletic injuries, tuberculosis, leukemia, multiple sclerosis, and diabetes, as well as to many minor medical complaints (Rabkin and Struening, 1976).

How does this association come about? You are already familiar with the notion that there is a strong and intense physiological response to emotional and stressful situations. Generations ago, Cannon noted

> *The strong emotions, as fear and anger, are rightly interpreted as the concomitants of bodily changes which may be of utmost service in subsequent action. These bodily changes are so much like those which occur in pain and fierce struggle that, as early writers on evolution suggested, the emotions may be considered as foreshadowing the suffering and intensity of actual strife. On this general basis, therefore, the bodily alterations attending violent emotional states would, as organic preparation for fighting and possible injury, naturally involve the effects which pain itself would produce. . . . increased blood sugar, a larger output of adrenalin, an adapted circulation, a greater number of red corpuscles and rapid clotting (Cannon, 1929, pp. 219–220).*

Cannon pointed out the significance of homeostasis, the body's striving to maintain physiological "normalcy"—a steady state—despite internal or external changes. The physiological responses to strong emotions, pain, and danger involve acute body changes. Because the body "wants to return to normal" and will "fight" to do so, homeostatic mechanisms are brought into play.

These general observations fascinated Hans Selye, an endocrinologist, who observed that the body, especially the glands, respond in predictable ways to any demand made upon it—be it an infection, physical injury, poison, exposure to cold or heat, X-rays, pain, grief, anxiety, or conflict. Selye calls the body's response *stress* and the agent or event creating the demand the *stressor*.

Selye's view concerning the body's special stress responses, first articulated in 1936, attempted to explain an extremely wide range of diseases as the body's "fight to maintain the homeostatic balance of our tissue, despite damage" (1978, p. 13). Selye's view is not the usual view of disease. Instead of perceiving disease as direct damage by germs, poisons, or traumatic events on the body, he regarded disease as the result of the body's ways of dealing with attempts to injure it. In other words, diseases such as high blood pressure, gastric ulcers, or rheumatoid arthritis can result from the body's attempt to adapt to noxious demands made upon it by some stressor, such as a germ, a strong emotion, excessive exposure to the elements, or cancer. The body's attempt to defend itself against such assaults involve a series of steps Selye calls the general adaptation syndrome (GAS).

The GAS tends to deal with different kinds of aggression against the body with the same sequential set of responses. According to Selye's description, during the first stage, a general alarm reaction occurs. The second stage of adaptation to or resistance to the stressor brings into play very strong responses such as the flooding of the body with powerful hormones (the corticoids, for example). The second stage thus employs strong body responses that defend against, help to destroy, or facilitate coexistence with an injury, germ, or noxious event. The body's response to injury, for example, can incapsulate the germ or injury with tissue, thus preventing invasions of the rest of the body. The third stage is characterized by exhaustion in which the body surrenders to the aggression by reducing excessive defensive maneuvers; in this way the body attempts to return to normal.

In other words, the GAS works hard to keep the body safe by defending it against many different kinds of aggressions through powerful bodily responses that involves the pituitary and adrenal systems (see Chapter 7) and almost all organs and biochemicals of the body. The stress response is thus a necessary coping response that deals with the changes and demands made upon us daily.

Sometimes, however, the GAS does not do its work successfully. Selye believes that many of the diseases we are familiar with are actually results of unsuccessful attempts to deal with an assault or stressor, a point noted earlier. These diseases, the diseases of adaptation or maladaptation, generally result from an excess of or hypersensitivity to the hormones released by the body in its stress response. They result, in other words, from the body's own ways of dealing with a stressor unsuccessfully.

Hormones released during the GAS may contribute to the possibility of sudden death due to cardiac arrest. This could be precipitated by severe emotional stress resulting from events such as the death of a close relative, a sudden loss of status, or threat of danger. Selye suggests that the alarm caused by the "evil eye" or other magical and supernatural practices and rites performed by shamans (medicine men) or voodoo priests could also cause sudden death in the targeted victim for the same reason.

But not all individuals show chronic patterns of disease; not everyone is a coronary candidate or sufferers from rheumatoid arthritis. What accounts for the differences in proclivity to develop "diseases of adaptation"? The next sections consider this question. But first, it may be of interest to point out possible danger signs that may be warnings that the GAS is not working successfully (Spotlight 8.2).

Spotlight 8.2 Selye's Warnings of Undue Body Stress

Are there danger signs to inform you when your body's response to stress is not working to protect you from danger? That is, are there warnings that suggest the possibility that you are at risk for "diseases of adaptation"? Yes, according to Selye. But in reading this list, it is important to remember that all of us experience these signs at one time or another, and they most often disappear without outside help. If sudden changes in your behavior persist and become chronic patterns of response in daily living, then you should probably begin to question the stressful elements in your life and do something about them—for example, obtain some diversion.

1. General irritability, hyperexcitation, or depression
2. Pounding of the heart
3. Dryness of the throat and mouth
4. Impulsive behavior
5. The overpowering urge to cry or run and hide
6. Inability to concentrate, flight of thoughts, and general disorientation
7. Feelings of unreality, weakness, or dizziness
8. Predilection to become fatigued
9. "Free floating anxiety" (nonspecific fear or anxiety)
10. Emotional tension, feeling "keyed up"
11. Trembling and nervous tics
12. Tendency to be easily startled by small sounds
13. High-pitched, nervous laughter
14. Stuttering and other speech difficulties
15. Bruxism (grinding of the teeth)
16. Insomnia, which is usually a consequence of being "keyed up"
17. Hypermotility (increased tendency to move about without any reason; an inability to take a physically relaxed attitude, such as sitting quietly in a chair or lying on a sofa)
18. Sweating
19. The frequent need to urinate
20. Diarrhea, indigestion, queasiness in the stomach, or vomiting
21. Migraine headaches
22. Premenstrual tension or missed menstrual cycles
23. Pain in the neck or lower back
24. Loss of or excessive appetite
25. Increased smoking
26. Increased use of drugs, such as tranquilizers or amphetamines
27. Alcohol and drug addiction
28. Nightmares
29. Accident proneness

Source: Adapted from *The stress of life* by Hans Selye. Copyright © 1978, and used with the permission of, McGraw-Hill Book Company.

ORGANIC DISEASES AND SYMPTOMS WITH PROBABLE OR PROMINENT EMOTIONAL ORIGINS

It has been clear for many years that some people are more vulnerable to certain kinds of somatic disorders, such as headache or high blood pressure, without specific physical etiology. Spotlight 8.3 presents several capsule summaries of patients whom I saw in consultation, and who can be characterized as having psychophysiological disorders.

These disorders tend to have some common characteristics. They often involve body organs innervated by the autonomic nervous system, such as the heart, stomach, or lungs. There is actual and demonstrable physiological change or damage in the system that may require immediate medical treatment, such as an acute condition of ulcers or a life-threatening asthma attack. Sometimes, these physiological responses are normal occurrences in certain emotional states, such as in acute fear conditions when an increased heart rate occurs. To

Spotlight 8.3 Capsule Case Summaries of Some Psychophysiological Disorders

A list of psychophysiological involvements would need to be exhaustive and would include many conditions in addition to those described below and in the pages that follow. A comprehensive list would include skin, respiratory, sleep, eating, cardiovascular, endocrinological, gastrointestinal, genitourinary, muscular, and pain disorders.

Described below are brief descriptions of several patients whom I saw in my office in the course of a year. In most instances, medical treatment was necessary. However, almost all of these patients were also helped by means of psychotherapy, hypnosis, biofeedback, or other methods that encouraged them to be more in charge of monitoring in situations potentially capable of producing the tension, anxiety, and stress found to exacerbate their bodily responses.

Many of these patients were not consciously aware of the tension-producing interactions that had precipitated the body's responses. For example, a young married woman developed vaginal constriction before going to bed at night and an older married woman had chronic vaginal infections. Each expressed great discomfort during sex with their husbands. In each case, there was a history of prepubertal sexual molestation by a relative and an underlying fear, long ago repressed, that this could happen again.

Case for case, fear, depression, anger, hostility or rage, deep-seated jealousy, impending sense of panic, or a great desire to flee seemed to be strongly associated with the symptom. Yet, there seemed to be something special about their biological and physical make-ups that differentiated them from patients who developed phobias, obsessional symptoms, or anxiety attacks.

1. A successful, forty-year-old woman with a long history of colitis (inflamation of the colon) and excruciating pain after eating also suffered from periods of constipation alternating with diarrhea. When she was a child, these symptoms disappeared during summer vacations; at the time she sought treatment, they diminished on weekends when she was away from the challenge of her competitive job as magazine newswriter with a weekly deadline. She sought help at the advice of her physician so that she could increase the duration of asymptomatic periods.

2. A thirty-year-old man could find no relief from a persistent, chronic neck distortion *(torticollus)* that twisted his head and neck sideways over his left shoulder ("wry neck"). His boss sympathized with his condition but his colleagues and clients did not. Eventually he had to take a leave of absence. His symptom cleared up during his enforced holiday, during which he also became separated from his wife.

3. A fifty-year-old executive suddenly developed embarrassing symptoms: severe reddening of the face and neck, excessive perspiration, and hand tremors whenever he had to talk to a group, small or large. His symptoms became incompatible with his position as sales manager of his firm, and he began to suffer from severe depression for which he sought help.

4. A tense twenty-five-year old man, entering his medical internship at a city hospital, sought assistance in learning how to handle his extreme stress responses in any pressured situation. At those times, his periods of disturbing sleeplessness, restlessness, and jitteriness would often be accompanied by severe chest pains. He feared that he would die from coronary disease at an early age, just like his father and grandfather. Actually, this patient fit the so-called coronary candidate category (as well as Friedman and Rosenman's [1974] Type A personality; see pp. 176–77).

5. A fifty-year-old woman complained of severe backache. It was apparently intractable. She had seen many physicians—orthopedists and neurologists—to no avail. The onset of the pain parallelled the beginning of menopause.

6. The father of one of my patients does a great deal of traveling, during which he lectures for his corporation. Occasionally, the patient's mother travels with him. On those menstrual days that coincide with the beginning of a trip on which her mother accompanies her father, my patient be-

comes totally incapacitated and sometimes faints at school. No one in the family seemed to understand the sequence of circumstances that occasionally forced the patient's mother to give up her trips. These people are currently in family treatment.

7. John, an untenured assistant professor in a department of biochemistry in an urban college, participates in departmental committee meetings, senior honors' seminars, and a funded research project. Last year he developed the following symptom: If anyone of higher academic status than himself is present when he must speak in public, he becomes dizzy, weak, feels the blood rushing from his head, and thinks he will faint. He has actually fainted a few times. He now avoids all such situations. There is a new baby in the family, he has no savings, and he is panic-stricken over the possibility that he will be fired. He is in psychotherapy and has also begun a program of behavior therapy to help him return to meeting his responsibilties.

8. A forty-year-old rigid, perfectionistic, ambitious scientist was frequently forced to make arrangements for her assistant to take over her experiments. She began to worry about her professionalism and her merit as a scientist. She suffered from migraine headaches of such severe, debilitating pain that on many days she could not leave her apartment to go to work.

9. A twenty-five-year-old obese woman suffered from asthma since early childhood. Her attacks began at night on a vacation trip when she became aware that her mother and father slept together while she slept alone in the next room. Today the attacks resume each time she goes away on a trip with her husband. She expresses an association between fear of being abandoned, left alone in a strange place, and the anxiety associated with these attacks. She has learned that her obesity incapacitates her, making her into an invalid, so that she will always be taken care of as a dependent. To be thin, she says, is to "have to make it on your own . . . to grow up."

10. When Roger was a college senior—an honor student—he had to be hospitalized with bleeding ulcers just before final examinations, and did not graduate with his class. The same sequence of events had occurred when he was a high school senior. Now in law school, he sought psychotherapy to prevent a repetition of this scenario before his next graduation.

qualify as a psychophysiological or psychosomatic symptom, however, these states must be more severe and chronic. Generally, the psychological causes or factors in these disorders are unknown to the patient.

Later in this chapter, conversion disorders—physical symptoms which do not involve real physical damage but appear to simulate bodily diseases and dysfunctions of one sort and another—will be described. Psychophysiological symptoms are differentiated from conversion symptoms not only because they are associated with actual physical or tissue damage, but also, unlike conversion symptoms, they are not easily modified by suggestion.

Why are some people prone to psychophysiological disorders? And among these people, why are they prone to *specific* types of disorders?

Psychodynamic explanations first arose from early psychoanalytic formulations that were later discarded as too simplistic. Early psychoanalytic explanations placed great emphasis on the symbolic nature of symptoms. For example, ulcers in males might be explained as a repressed desire for a baby, with consequent severe guilt. The stomach in such patients was the symbolic substitute for the uterus but it was "punished" severely for the forbidden wish by developing ulcers.

These early formulations intrigued psychoanalysts like Franz Alexander and his colleagues in Chicago who in the 1930s became dedicated to the notion that specific emotional conflicts were associated with specific organic disorders (Alexander,

1939, 1950). Thus essential hypertension (high blood pressure with no physical etiology) was believed to arise from conflicts over the expression of great rage and anger. In similar fashion, menstrual cycle dysfunctions were seen as arising from conflicts regarding sex role and sexual feelings.

Other psychodynamic approaches attempt to explain specific physical disorders on the basis of personality types (Dunbar, 1954). For example, asthmatic symptoms are developed by oral personality types, who shows dependency, feelings of helplessness, and need for infantile nurturance. Ulcerative colitis appears in obsessive-compulsive personalities. And observations of people susceptible to various kinds of coronary disease suggest that they show distinctive personality traits and life styles.

On the whole, an invariant association between specific conflicts or personality type and specific diseases has not been confirmed by the empirical literature (Freedman, et al., 1972; Grinker, 1973).

Some opinions hold to the "weak link in the chain" approach. That is, organ vulnerability—constitutional or inborn predisposing factors—makes some people more susceptible to headache or high blood pressure, say, than colitis or diarrhea under conditions of chronic stress. The weak-link theory suggests that responses to stress are the same from individual to individual. What differs is the predisposition to breakdown of one organ in the system as opposed to others. Researchers who assign greater weight to learned factors in the origin of psychophysiological symptoms tend to hold that patterns of body response to stressors are more variable, more subject to modification as a result of the individual's history, than the organ-vulnerability approach implies (Lachman, 1972).

Most contemporary thinking about psychophysiological symptoms tends to reflect a complex view that combines several elements, beginning with the chain of events that arises from the body's response to stressors and to strong emotions such as anger, fear, and anxiety. Individual differences in the body's stress responses may arise from genetic and inherited predispositions that determine the nature and intensity of biochemical and hormonal responses. For example, some people may overreact autonomically to situations, and may even stay aroused longer than others (Malmo, 1975). However, because various types and patterns of autonomic reactions can be learned, and thus become associated to a variety of different types of external stimuli (Lachman, 1972), learning also plays an important role, since we respond in typical patterns depending on our learned tendencies or general personality factors. In addition, each of us perceives potentially threatening or stressful situations in different ways.

Some Psychophysiological Syndromes and Disorders

This section describes some special syndromes. These do not represent the range and variety of psychogenic symptoms that people display. Some, like psychogenic sexual dysfunctions will be described in Chapter 15. The syndromes below are typical in that they appear to demonstrate the complex interweaving of biochemistry, predisposition, and individual response to stressful events that might lead to physical symptoms.

Peptic ulcers. Peptic ulcers are erosions or lesions of the lining of the stomach or upper portion of the intestines (duodenum). They are sometimes referred to as gastric or duodenal ulcers, but there is some evidence that gastric and duodenal ulcers differ in etiology and physiological and psychological correlates (Rosenbaum, 1967). Gastric secretions of pepsin and hydrochloric acid, which aid in food digestion by breaking down food substances, would also digest the walls of the stomach or intestines, were they not protected by a layer of mucus. This "self-digestion" is indeed what occurs when an excessive amount of gastric secretions is present: high-level gastric activity erodes the mucus layer and attacks the walls of the stomach or duodenum. The results are attacks of extremely sharp pain occurring any time from one to four hours after eating; the pain is

Spotlight 8.4 Body Image and Psychophysiological Ailments

You all know that sometimes you feel one way and sometimes another way about your body—content with it and accepting, or the reverse. Some people feel ugly, awkward, ungainly—ashamed of their bodies—and expect that others will perceive them accordingly. Others may feel closed off, protected from anticipated onslaught by the world by what they feel to be the steely armor of their bodies; they are guarding themselves against a hostile world. The image one has of one's body probably bears some relationship to attitudes toward other people and to the world as well as to oneself.

A group of researchers has suggested that one way of classifying body image might be with regard to two descriptive characteristics: boundary—the degree to which the body is viewed as a barrier, a demarcation of one's self from the rest of the world; and penetration—the degree to which, according to the individual's view, the outside world can make impact, that is, how vulnerable the body is to outside forces (Fisher and Cleveland, 1958; Fisher, 1970). Some people might thus regard their bodies as a weak barrier, a flimsy boundary between themselves and others. They may also feel their bodies to be highly vulnerable, able to be easily penetrated, influenced, and affected by the outside world.

Are such distinctions actually found? Yes, according to these authors. Can they be measured? Yes, again. On the Rorschach test, for example, responses of "mummies," or "knights in armor" would receive high barrier (boundary) and low penetration scores. Responses of "people with flimsy clothes" or "people whose insides can be seen" or "X-ray photographs" would receive low barrier and high penetration scores.

The authors wondered whether body attitudes could be related to psychophysiological ailments. Modest evidence does exist suggesting a moderate association between these scores and certain kinds of physical involvements. For example, ulcer patients were found to have lower barrier scores and higher penetration scores than those found for a group of arthritic patients (Cleveland and Fisher, 1960). The important question, however, is whether or not such body images actually *cause* a particular physical complaint rather than simply accompany it.

A rather strong argument can be made for the emergence of these body attitudes as a result of the physical involvements. In any event, a longitudinal study exploring whether or not body image variables actually predict the emergence of later psychophysiological ailments would have to be conducted to test this hypothesis.

relieved by antacid medications or by eating once more.

Here are some facts about peptic ulcers. They occur more frequently in men than women, an imbalance that has become especially evident in the last several decades, and the disorder appears to run in families. The incidence of peptic ulcers is greatest in urban, industrialized centers and in upper income groups. The pain associated with ulcers is sharpest during the afternoon and night, especially after midnight. Ulcers tend to be chronic conditions, lasting over a period of ten to twenty-five years, but there are many remissions, during which symptoms of the disease diminish or disappear, and exacerbations, during which symptoms worsen—frequently associated with emotional crises and acutely painful life events. Its incidence has declined in the past several decades.

How is such an array of diverse characteristics explained? Empirical data suggest that certain people have biological predispositions to respond to stressful occurrences by excessive gastric secretions. Although the data attempting to link specific personality types with the development of ulcers are less impressive, they should not be brushed aside.

Stressful events and emotional situations are associated with increases in gastric secretions in most people—not just ulcer patients—through normal autonomic processes. Anxiety during premedical examinations, for example, increases this secretion (Mahl, 1950). Increased gastric secretion in response to stress has been amply demonstrated in animals. For example, "helpless" rats who could not avoid or escape from shock developed more ulceration than control rats who received the same amount of shock but could escape (Weiss, 1971).

Although both ulcer patients and nonulcer patients show increases in hydrochloric acid in highly stressful, emotionally loaded situations, ulcer patients show more intense bodily reactions lasting over a longer period of time (Mittelmann, Wolff, and Scharf, 1942). But whether under stress or not, ulcer patients secrete four to twenty times as much acid at night than nonulcer patients (Dragstedt, 1956).

Environmental events may trigger the disease. But current evidence also indicates a strong genetic and familial factor. As noted, ulcers run in families. Twin studies show a 50 percent concordance for duodenal ulcers in MZ (identical) twins and drop to 14 percent in DZ (fraternal) twins (Eberhard, 1968). The ulcer develops as a result of extraordinarily high levels of pepsinogen I in the blood of particular individuals, who are many times more prone to have ulcers than other people (Mirsky, 1958). Apparently a tendency to have high levels of this chemical is a genetic trait parents can pass on to children. Ulcers develop in 40 to 50 percent of people with this genetic trait, but are not found in those who do not possess the trait (A genetic link . . . , 1979).

People who develop ulcers may thus have strong biochemical predispositions causing them to respond physiologically in ways that differ from those who do not develop ulcers. These ulcer-prone persons may also perceive stressful events as more disturbing and emotionally upsetting. The increased incidence of ulcers among men and in urban settings—facts we already noted—supports this view. Thus from this perspective there may be some support for the view of Franz Alexander that ulcer patients have conflicts regarding the expression of aggression, independence, and ambition because of simultaneously existing dependency needs. However, most empirical evidence does not consistently support a specific emotional theory of ulcers independent of biochemical events (Weiner, 1977).

Since not all individuals with biochemical predispositions develop ulcers, delineation of the environmental factors and individual differences in personality, conflicts, and appraisal of stressful situations that trigger ulcer mechanisms awaits further research.

Cardiovascular disorders. Essential hypertension refers to a chronic condition of elevated levels of blood pressure in the arteries. These heightened levels are generally caused by vasoconstriction of the blood vessels without associated organic disease. Although drugs and/or diet (also biofeedback) can reduce elevated blood pressure levels, the etiology of 90 percent of these cases is not understood (Marx, 1977). Certain forms of hypertension can lead to dangerous pathology of other organ systems and can lead directly to arteriosclerotic heart disease. The incidence of hypertension seems to be higher among obese people, leading some researchers to implicate diet and high-salt intake as a contributing etiological factor.

Although it is easy experimentally to elevate blood pressure through inducing anxiety, preventing anger from being expressed, and creating situational stress in experimental subjects, psychoanalytic formulations, such as those of Franz Alexander, that associate chronic hypertension with repressed anger, rage, and a tendency to have one's feelings easily hurt have not been clinically or experimentally verified (Marx, 1977; Reiser, 1967). That is, evidence for a hypertensive personality is either inconsistent or lacking. One investigation that yielded findings in support of the hypertensive personality hypothesis is described in Spotlight 8.5.

Spotlight 8.5 Elevated Blood Pressure and Inhibited Power Drive

Many clinicians are of the opinion that hypertensive people share common personality characteristics. A frequently stated view is that hypertense people feel a great deal of anger but do not express it—that is, they inhibit their anger from overt expression. The "suppressed anger" hypothesis of essential hypertension was examined in a longitudinal study which attempted to evaluate whether people who control or inhibit their anger and hostility are predisposed to develop essential hypertension (McClelland, 1979).

Subjects were 78 males who were tested every five years for blood pressure from 1940 (junior year in college) until 1972–1974. The subjects were administered the TAT (a picture-story test; see Chapter 5) in 1950–1952. The important question was to determine whether psychological predisposition preceded or followed elevated blood pressure levels.

To measure "psychological predisposition"—controlled or inhibited anger— the subjects' imaginative stories in response to the TAT pictorial stimuli were scored according to several standard methods. For example, story content that referred to "impact on others" by aggression, persuasion, or any method that caused an emotional response in others comprised the Power score. TAT content was also scored for Affiliation—the need to be friendly with others. The researchers assumed that if Power scores were higher than Affiliation scores, more anger or aggression is present. There was also an Activity Inhibition score—the number of times the word *not* appears in the stories, and this was held to be an index of inhibition or control over one's actions. Blood pressure was measured by the usual sphygmomanometer method.

An examination of findings ruled out the possibility that blood pressure levels predetermined later personality scores. It was found on the other hand, that personality predisposition in the form of suppressed anger (as measured by TAT scores) did indeed predict elevated blood pressure levels twenty years later. Figure 8.1 illustrates this finding graphically.

Figure 8.1 graphically illustrates mean diastolic pressure in men aged fifty-one to fifty-three classified into four groups according to Power motive at age 30. The first two groups at the left showed higher Power drive than Affiliation drive, but the subjects in the group at the extreme left showed stronger need to control their actions. The two groups at the right showed greater need for Affiliation than Power and therefore were not characterized as having strong Power motives. Subjects with the highest inhibited Power drive at age 30 (at the extreme left) showed the highest diastolic pressure at ages fifty-one to fifty-three.

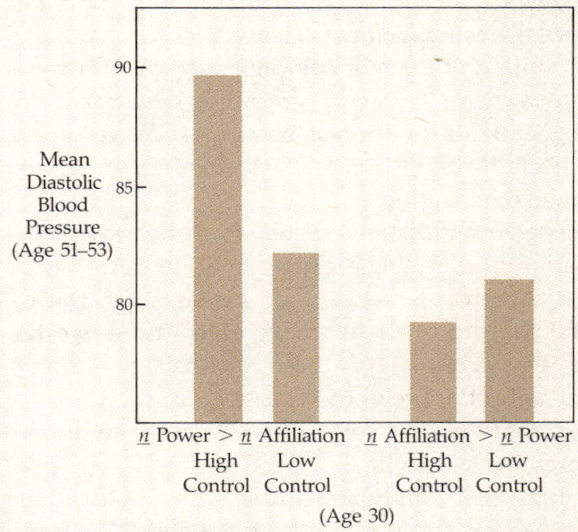

Figure 8.1 Mean diastolic blood pressure of men, aged 51–53, classified into four groups according to their TAT scores at the age of 30. (From D. C. McClelland, Inhibited power motivation and high blood pressure in men, *Journal of Abnormal Psychology,* 1979, *88,* 182–90. Copyright 1979 by the American Psychological Association. Reprinted by permission of the author.)

Some researchers are of the opinion that continued exposure to stressful situations may induce hypertension. They point to the greater incidence of essential hypertension as one goes down the SES scale and among blacks. On the other hand, other researchers believe that stressors do not *cause* essential hypertension, but may very much affect the course of the disease; that is, it may drive elevated levels even higher, perhaps precipitating a stroke.

The lack of specific etiology in essential hypertension is an intriguing problem, especially since its mystery presents a grave health hazard. But there is some agreement that essential hypertension can result from any number of dysfunctions of body systems that regulate blood pressure. And while genetic factors play some predisposing role in most instances of the illness, social and psychological factors also play an important role in several (but not all) types of the disease, primarily in interaction with predisposing factors (Weiner, 1977).

Despite unknown or complex etiology of essential hypertension, some progress has been made in helping patients to control or reduce dangerously high levels through biofeedback or other methods that induce relaxation.

More Americans die of coronary heart disease than of any other single cause. In 1975 one to two million Americans had heart disease. Of these, 675,000 will die or already have died, and it is estimated that 175,000 of these deaths are among people under the age of 65 (Glass, 1976).

Are there indeed coronary candidates—individuals predisposed to heart disorders. If so, who are these high-risk candidates? One view holds that evidence exists for a "coronary personality"—a personality type (Type A) more prone to coronary disease than others (Friedman and Rosenman, 1974; Glass, 1977). The characteristics of these high risk candidates include: feeling under constant pressure to achieve and to produce; feeling pressed for time; prone to set achievement quotas and deadlines for themselves; and in constant struggle to maintain competitive control over their worlds. When they lose control—through loss of a job, for example, or death of a spouse—they are overwhelmed and become candidates for a sudden heart attack. Type A personalities contrast sharply with Type B personalities, who handle stressful situations in less catastrophic ways.

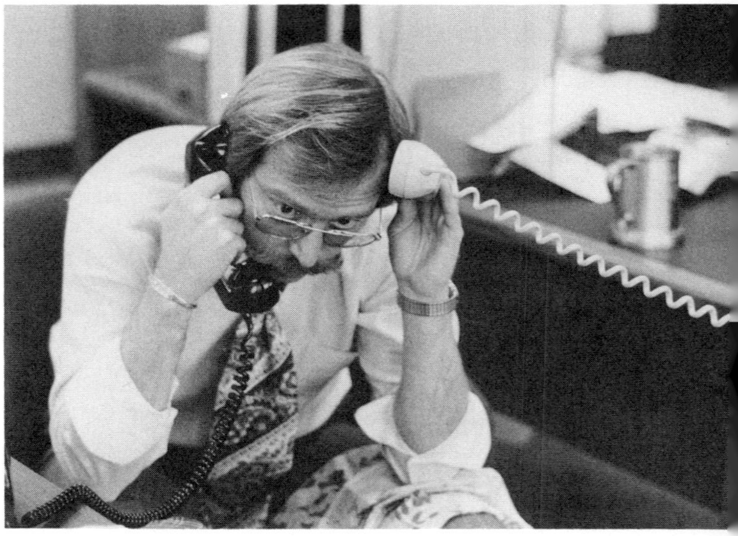

Type A personalities, with their constant pressures, worries, and deadlines, are thought to be high-risk coronary candidates. (Robert V. Eckert, Jr./The Picture Cube)

Those comprising the Type A group, it is conjectured, are characterized by chronic discharge of high levels of norepinephrine, epinephrine, and ACTH into their bloodstreams in a hypothalamic stress response that reflects an angry struggle with their worlds. These excessive biochemical imbalances result in increased levels of cholesterol and fat as well as dysfunctional bloodclotting mechanisms that can block the flow of blood to the arteries and force the heart to work harder, thus increasing coronary risk.

One hypothesis about individuals in the Type A personality group is that they are more hostile than those in the Type B group. This general observation was tested experimentally: Type A and Type B subjects were asked to shock other subjects as punishment in a learning task. In actuality, the shocks were not real and the subject was a "confederate." Type A subjects who had been teased and bullied by the confederate before the learning task administered significantly greater shock than the Type Bs, who had been similarly provoked. There was no difference between Types A and B subjects who had not been bullied prior to the learning session. This led to the conclusion that in situations in which hostility is provoked, Type A subjects indeed differ from Type Bs in expressing greater hostility toward the provoker (Glass, 1977). Figure 8.2 illustrates these findings graphically.

Still, not all Type A individuals have sudden heart dysfunctions or develop coronary disease. Moreover, it should be emphasized that there is some tendency for coronary disease to run in families. Although the one-to-one association of Type A personalities with heart disease is probably too simple, it does suggest, once again, that the precise mechanisms of biochemical predisposition, stress, and individual temperament offer a rich field for further research in understanding the elusive psychophysiology of coronary disease.

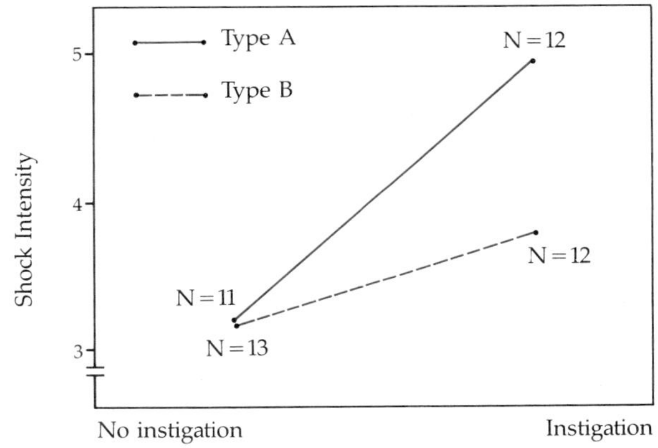

Figure 8.2 Personality type and hostility score. Type A subjects used higher mean "shock" intensities as punishment, in a learning situation, of a confederate who had previously provoked them than did Type B subjects under similar circumstances. (From D. C. Glass, *Behavior patterns, stress, and coronary disease;* Erlbaum, 1977, p. 69. Reprinted by permission.)

*Asthma.** It is commonly agreed that asthma, a respiratory dysfunction, is one of the major psychophysiological diseases. Bronchial asthma is an "obstructive disease of the bronchial airways characterized by a tendency of the bronchial tree to respond by bronchoconstriction, edema (swelling), and an excessive secretion to a variety of stimuli" (Weiner, 1977, p. 224). The symptoms of asthma generally appear in an attack of an acutely discomforting nature, lasting for several hours or longer. Attacks are characterized by enormous difficulty in breathing (dyspnea): gasping for air, wheezing, and shortness of breath. It is estimated that about 40 percent of these attacks occur during sleeping hours.

Although onset of asthma can be at any age, almost half of reported asthma cases appear before adolescence. In children, asthma is more frequent among boys than girls, but this distribution evens out during adulthood. Many people outgrow asthma—up to 45 percent, it is estimated—but many do not. Why this is so adds to a growing list of questions arising from many curious, still unexplained facts about asthma. For example, prevalence rates vary across nations—ranging roughly from 0.7 percent of the population in Sweden to over 5 percent in the United States; and, it has been found that suggestion may play a role in inducing some instances of asthma (Luparello, et al., 1971)

What causes asthma? Genetic and biological factors apparently play a small, predisposing role in onset, for unless there is a tendency for bronchial constriction to occur under certain conditions, there is no asthma. However, a vast literature on asthma indicates that allergic, infectious, and psychological variables play an extremely important role with regard to onset and maintenance of the disorder in both children and adults.* (See Weiner, 1977, p.

* Much of the content in this section is based on Weiner's extensive review on the psychobiology of asthma (1977).

* Studies include those by Munro Ford (1963), Graham, et al. (1967), Pearson (1968), Rees (1956), Rees, (1964), Williams, et al. (1958), and Wright (1965).

226, for a summary of these researches which, through observations, case histories, medical tests, and psychological tests, explored the relative contribution of physical and psychological factors in the first and repeated occurrence of asthma.) Psychological factors, it would seem, are of no small significance in accounting for instances of asthma.

What are some of these psychological factors?

1. Observations and self-reports of asthmatics indicate that great emotional tension frequently precedes an asthmatic attack.
2. Clinicians report intense familial conflicts within the asthmatic's family.
3. Asthmatic children seem to show strong dependency needs and separation fears (but this could *result from* rather than *precede* the asthmatic disease).
4. Persons who are predisposed to have asthma sometimes have difficulty in expressing emotion openly and directly.
5. In children, a stressful situation, such as death of a parent, may precipitate the first attack.

Apart from the foregoing generalizations, no single conflict can account for asthmatic disorders, contrary to the notions of Franz Alexander. Also, no one personality pattern characterizes all asthmatic patients (Stein and Schiavi, 1967). And if such factors as orality and denial of affect are associated with the asthmatic personality, these traits are said to characterize other syndromes, too, such as alcoholism. Finally, contrary to earlier reports, there is little evidence to confirm the notion that asthmatic attacks can be conditioned in animals or humans.

Even though the enigma of asthma remains, we do know enough about it to make the general statement that biological and physiological factors interact with the individual's perception of and response to stressful situations—especially in families that encourage dependency on the part of the patient—in determining the first occurrence of an attack, precipitating recurrent attacks, and sustaining the illness over a period of years.

SLEEP, DREAMS, AND SOME ASSOCIATED DISORDERS

Sleep and dreaming disorders are frequent complaints in the offices of most clinicians. For example, one of my patients suffered from such horrifying nightmares that she could not get herself to lie down at night. Another, at the insistence of her husband, sought help for the screaming, shouting, and wailing that characterized her sleep. Still another patient awakened for years at four A.M., unable to fall asleep again. Frequently, these complaints were symptoms of or associated with other problems, such as depression.

What is sleep? At nighttime, under ordinary circumstances, with the reduction of sensory input—that is, lowered lights and silence (no stereo, TV, or conversation)—a person can usually relax sufficiently to fall asleep. Sleep has been defined as a "readily reversible suspension of sensorimotor interaction with the environment, usually associated with recumbency and immobility. . . . it appears to interrupt wakefulness periodically. . . . it provides physiological background for experience of dreaming. . . . " (Dement, 1967, p. 77). Sleep is actually a complex set of neural events which is not the passive opposite of wakefulness. It is a highly active state now known, partially as a result of the researches of scientists such as Kleitman, Aserinsky, and Dement in the early 1950s, to consist of various stages (see Dement and Kleitman, 1957; Kleitman, 1963).

If you were to tape open the eyelids of a sleeping subject, you would discover, as sleep occurs, that his or her eyes drift slowly back and forth. As sleep progresses, there is a regular sequence of events. After about ten minutes ("point of no return"), sleepers go through four stages of sleep for about the next half hour. Each stage is characterized by its own EEG pattern (see Figure 8.3). Stage 4 is the deepest level of sleep, and sleepers during this stage can barely be roused. After about ten minutes of Stage 4 sleep, subjects gradually return to Stage 1 sleep over a forty-minute period. They do not

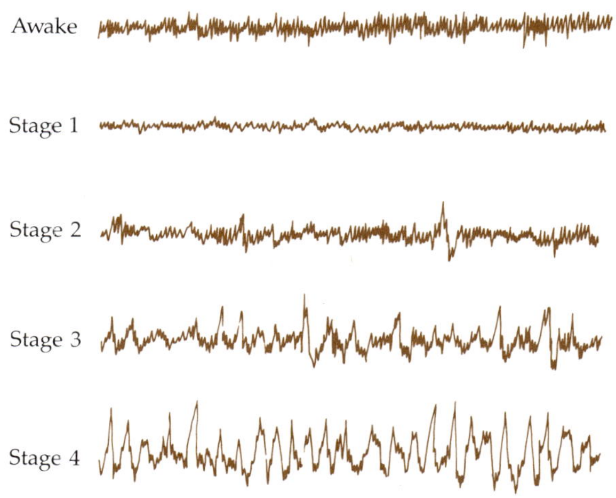

Figure 8.3 EEG tracings of sleep stages. These sample tracings of a subject's brain waves were made during a single night. The recording paper was moving under the pens at ⅓ the standard speed, which means that the waves are somewhat pushed together. (From W. C. Dement, An essay on dreams, in *New directions in psychology,* vol. II; © 1965 by Holt, Rinehart & Winston. Reprinted by permission of CBS College Publishing.)

awaken, however. They go into another kind of sleep, characterized by rapid eye movements (REM); REM sleep is dreaming sleep. REM sleep and the other kinds of sleep (NREM) have important differences, including whether or not dreaming takes place. These differences are described more fully in Spotlight 8.6.

Sleep disorders. The past decade has seen a rapid rise in research attention to sleep disorders, yielding not only information about their physiological and psychological origins, but also methods for their alleviation (Dement, 1967; Kales, Scharf, and Kales, 1978; Mitler, et al., 1975; Webb and Cartwright, 1978).

Although some researchers differentiate organic from nonorganic sleep disorders, this discussion will not make this distinction since there is some evidence suggesting the existence of underlying neurochemical regulatory mechanisms that induce *all* sleep and wakefulness cycles, whether normal or not (Holman, et al., 1975). It should be understood, however, that in some sleep disturbances—insomnia for example—emotional and psychological factors may be of great significance, whereas in other disorders—narcolepsy for example—specific neurochemical dysfunctions might be the cause.

One of the most frequent complaints in the clinician's office is insomnia. Approximately one out of every seven women over age 30 and one out of every sixteen men over age 30 complain of insomnia often or fairly often according to the results of a survey of over 700,000 people (Kripke and Simons, 1976). Temporary insomnia (short periods of extended wakefulness) might be an offshoot of situational tension or temporary emotional problems. These difficulties in falling or remaining asleep tend to disappear as the problem is solved. Persistent insomnia however, is not so easily resolved.

Curiously, many people who say they never sleep at all actually do quite a bit of sleeping, according to EEG monitoring. Moreover, we can all get by with less sleep than we think we need. The amount of NREM sleep we usually get can be greatly reduced without real harm, although we tend to need a certain amount of REM sleep. It is important to know that almost all of these insomnias, whether short-lived or persistent, will tend to increase in severity after a period of regular or even temporary use of sedatives.

Insomnia is often associated with depression. But many other disturbances in the sleep-wakefulness cycle are also associated with depression, suggesting that both depression and insomnia are associated with biochemical imbalances, even though the nature of this association is not easily understood.

Sleepwalking disorder (somnambulism) and sleep terror disorder (pavor nocturnus) are two dramatic disorders that generally begin in middle childhood—from about six to twelve years of age—and usually disappear by adulthood. Unlike nightmares (terrifying dreams), bruxism (grinding of the teeth), and

Spotlight 8.6 To Sleep: Perchance to Dream—REM and NREM Sleep

What are the differences between REM and NREM sleep?

REM Sleep	NREM Sleep
REM sleep occurs every 90 minutes and lasts about 20 minutes. These periods increase in duration as the night progresses.	There are four stages of NREM sleep, characterized by about 90 minutes of descent from Stage 1 to Stage 4—the deepest sleep—and ascent again to Stage 1.
REM sleep is characterized by dreaming. If awakened, subjects report vivid, bizarre, dramatic dreams, with a great deal of imagery and, frequently, emotional expenditure. All dreams are in color. Often, dream content is characterized by paralysis, immobility, being unable to flee, slow motion, or sensations of falling or flying. These, we have learned, are associated with the physiological state of the sleeper.	During these four stages, if subjects are awakened, they report everyday thoughts and ideas that do not have the vivid imagery of the REM dream.
The need for REM sleep decreases with age. In the uterus, almost all sleep is REM sleep. About 50 percent of the sleep of babies is REM sleep; about 20 to 25 percent of all sleep in normal young adults is REM sleep. REM sleep is characterized by Stage 1-type EEG patterns of relatively fast, mixed-frequency, low-voltage waves. All mammals have REM sleep. The normal progression is not directly from wakefulness to REM sleep (see text).	The four states or NREM sleep, reflecting different kinds of neural activity, are illustrated by characteristic EEG patterns as shown in Figure 8.3. These are generally slower, higher amplitude waves than those of REM sleep. Stage 4 sleep occurs mostly in earlier periods of sleep. NREM occurs *first* in the normal pattern, and is then interrupted by REM sleep.
In REM sleep, there is actual paralysis, an inability to move, which prevents sleepers from casting about, breaking limbs, or hurting others in the course of very active dreams.	In NREM sleep, although there is a decrease of motor activity, there is no actual inhibition of activity and there is some muscle tone.
Eye movements are rapid—as rapid as the shifts from fixation to fixation—as the sleeper focuses on one thing or another (try it and see how rapid these can be), but there is no particular pattern in their motion.	In NREM sleep, the eyeballs shows a slow, side-to-side movement. When one goes from wakefulness to sleep, these movements sometimes occur with hypnagogic imagery—visual images that occur while falling asleep or awakening.
During REM sleep, there is an increase of blood pressure, oxygen utilization, gastric secretion, heart rate, and neural activity. Respiration is irregular, and there is penile erection and vaginal engorgement. Just before REM sleep, biochemical changes apparently occur involving neurotransmitters, cortical stimulation, and cellular structures in	During NREM sleep there is a general slowing down of heart rate, blood pressure, and respiratory and urinary cycles, and a reduction of body temperature. These physiological events serve a restorative function and can also occur during a resting and reclining state when one is relaxed. The major difference between wakefulness and NREM

REM Sleep	NREM Sleep
the pontine reticular formation (mass of cells on the brain stem that give rise to fibers that have broad effects on the activity of large areas of the cerebral cortex).	sleep is an abrupt change in EEG pattern and an interruption of responsiveness to environment—an "involuntary suspension of interaction between organism and environment."

Source: Adapted from W.C. Dement, Sleep and dreams, in A. M. Freedman, H. I. Kaplan, and H. S. Kaplan (Eds.), *Comprehensive textbook of psychiatry,* copyright © 1967, the Williams & Wilkins Co., Baltimore.

rhythmic head banging, these disruptions in normal sleep patterns do not occur during REM sleep. Their onset is generally from about a half hour to a few hours after sleep has begun during periods of deepest sleep, usually Stage 4, and they can last from several minutes up to a half hour. Estimates of prevalence are as high as 6 percent among children, with greater incidence among males than females (according to the DSM-III). Of interest is that among children, there seems to be no association of these disorders with other kinds of pathology. Among adults, however, they may occur in association with personality or anxiety disorders (see Chapter 9).

Sleepingwalking disorders refer to recurrent episodes of rising from bed and walking about without bumping into furniture, usually with an expressionless face. Episodes may involve purposeless movements like picking on the blanket or mechanically getting dressed. There is resistance to being awakened, but after awakening, or the next morning, there is complete amnesia for the event.

Sleep terror disorders, not to be confused with nightmares, are repeated episodes of sudden awakenings from sleep, usually with a piercing, panicky scream. During the episode, which lasts several minutes, there is intense anxiety, dilated pupils, perspiration, and a quickened pulse. The individual cannot be comforted during this period of terror but often later describes an acutely uncomfortable sense of dread. No dream content is reported and generally there is complete amnesia for these events the next morning.

Narcolepsy, or "sleeping attacks" is a pathological state that reflects organic dysfunction. Unlike the normal sleep cycle, which takes the sleeper through several sleep stages before the REM stage, these attacks plunge the patient directly from wakefulness into REM sleep. Suddenly, the narcoleptic experiences vivid hallucinations, sleep paralysis, and muscle weakness as he or she is going about usual daytime activities.

Narcolepsy is treated with medications. However, many of the difficulties and disorders in sleeping patterns actually result from misuse and abuse of medications and drugs. For example, protracted alcohol ingestion leads to REM sleep deprivation in alcoholics. When chronic alcoholics go "on the wagon," the terrifying hallucinations and delirium (DTs) associated with abstinence are probably a manifestation of "REM rebound," the daytime REM activity that the body employs to make up for its loss.

Dreaming. During REM sleep, the brain is very actively dreaming. Since there is no sensory input, how do REM dreams evolve? Why does the brain supply its own vivid story line? What is the function of dreams? We do not know the answers to these questions, but there are some hypotheses.

1. According to the Freudians, dreams were thought to be pathways to the unconscious. Dream content contains repressed wishes and taboo fantasies, needs, and desires that are too shameful for conscious awareness. They gratify forbidden impulses. Dream interpretation is based on presumed

symbolism of much of their manifest (obvious, overt) content. For example, caves might be vaginas, and horses, snakes, or guns, phalluses. The universality of these meanings and the conviction that dreams reflect deep unconscious wishes have been questioned by many contemporary dream researchers.

2. Some researchers propose that dreams are right-hemisphere functions that serve to reduce anxiety, resolve conflicts, and piece together the emotional events of the day. The left hemisphere is too busy contending with day-to-day problem solving to perform these emotional functions. These hypotheses tend to emphasize the reduction of tension, the dealing with feelings, that dreams achieve for us (Cartwright, 1978ab; D. B. Cohen, 1979; McGrath and Cohen, 1978; Webb and Cartwright, 1978). One important researcher in this group of dream theorists (Cartwright) even suggests that dreams are so important in conflict resolution and emotional problem solving that we should actively seek *conscious* control over our dreams to increase their highly useful and adaptive functions.

It is too early to say how valid these intriguing hypotheses are. Although there is not yet substantial empirical evidence for the relationship between dreaming and emotional conflict resolution, most dream investigators are prepared to await the evidence before arriving at conclusions.

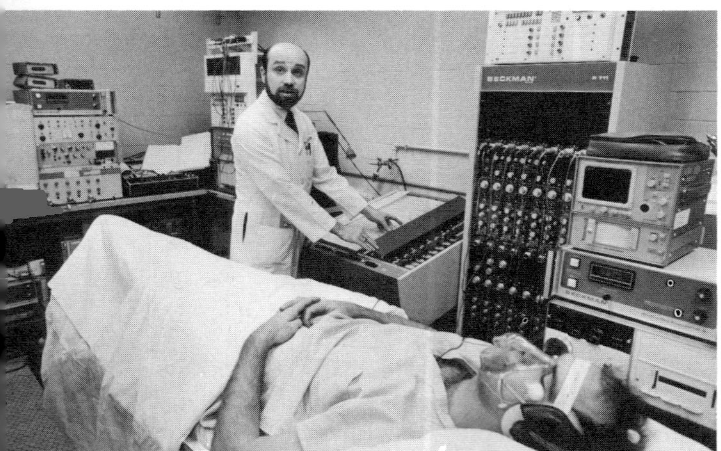

An experimental subject being monitored in a sleep laboratory. (Richard Younker/Click, Chicago)

3. Another intriguing theory proposes that dreams are nothing more than the cognitive content provided by neural activation of the brain in its attempt to make coherent sense of its intense activity by creating some kind of story. This theory is called the activation-synthesis theory (Hobson and McCarley, 1977; McCarley and Hobson, 1977).

More specifically, dreaming is caused by physiological events that include activation of giant nerve cells in the brain stem that send impulses to the cortex, creating an explosion of neural activity that activates memories, emotions, and feelings. The sleeping REM brain, especially its sensory system, that is being stimulated experiences variations in duration, intensity, sequence, and location of this neural activation. And these variations determine the content of the dream, with its flashes of color, shifts of scenes, sense of falling, immobility, and vivid, illogical, sometimes bizarre substance.

However, since each individual's emotions, memories, and cognitive content is unique, dreams can and *do* reflect each person's uniqueness—his or her personality, needs, and drives. Dreams, thus, after all, may be helpful in understanding that person, not necessarily through Freudian interpretations but through the simpler explanation based on the physiological activation of the brain during REM sleep. This interpretation of dreams starts from physiology. A dream about sex might be activated by penile erection or by neural centers that monitor erections. The memories and experiences of the dreaming individual are employed to make sense of the neural messages received, not the other way around.

The study of sleep cycles, dreams, and various disorders in these universal functions thus offers exciting possibilities for further understanding our brain and its complex functions during one third of our lives. For the psychopathologist, sleeping and dreaming disorders are of particular interest, since so many of the symptoms and complaints for which people seek help focus on this portion of their lives.

EATING DISORDERS: OBESITY, ANOREXIA NERVOSA, AND BULIMIA

Obesity

A young married woman, one-hundred and fifty pounds overweight, has been unable to control her binge-eating behavior and craving for sweets. Years of psychotherapy have not helped, nor have all the other special programs and groups to which she subscribed. Warnings by her physician, embarrassment at the beach, difficulty in climbing stairs, even in walking, have not helped either.

Why is it difficult for some people to lose weight despite the problems they encounter in their daily lives and their unhappiness with how they look and feel? To raise only a few possibilities, is obesity a symptom of emotional conflicts, of deep inner needs, or of depression? Do obese people share certain personality characteristics?

Definitions of obesity vary (20 percent above standard weight for a given age, sex, and body frame? 50 percent above?). People also differ with regard to preferred weight; cultural standards, group pressure, and concepts of good looks and beauty are components in such preferences. In our culture, overweight is correlated with *low* social status; in other cultures, however, obesity is a sign of prestige, of *high* social status (Goldblatt, Moore, and Stunkard, 1965), probably because of its association with better than average wealth. Even with these variations, there is some agreement that obesity is one of the major health problems in this country and that its prevalence seems to be increasing (Kolata, 1977). Some estimates are that there are thirty to eighty million obese Americans. In any event, there seems to be staggering numbers of people who are seeking help for weight problems.

What causes obesity? There is little agreement, but a plethora of hypothesis.

Psychodynamic approaches. Older—frequently psychoanalytic—views hold that obesity results from emotional conflict and repressed needs. Overeating and obesity thus reflect oral dependency, unresolved oral conflicts, or fixation at or regression to oral stages (see Chapter 6). Another approach subscribes to the notion that uncontrolled eating occurs in response to emotional arousal, such as heightened levels of anxiety, and that eating reduces anxiety levels. Still others hold that the eating behavior of obese people results from a confused response to various states of arousal or to uncomfortable or intolerable feelings, such as poor self-image. Finally, some views suggest that obese or overweight people share similar personality traits, such as tendency to be depressed or passivity.

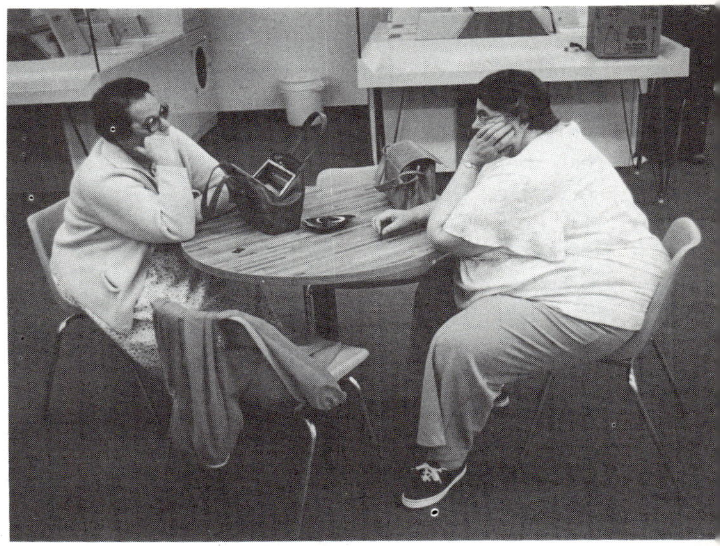

Psychologists are interested in studying the reasons some people are unable to lose weight, despite their apparent unhappiness and their claims of high motivation to do so. (Robert V. Eckert/The Picture Cube)

One interesting hypothesis is that obese people suffer from a failure to identify the cues that signal surfeit or satiety. This pattern is thought to arise from pathological closeness of mother and child (symbiosis) in early feeding interactions in which the mother stuffs the child and does not allow him or her to build up reality cues for satiety. The obese person thus misinterprets physiological cues of discomfort as cues for hunger. These perceptual confusions also reflect deficiencies in the way obese patients regard their own identity and worth, relying only minimally on self-cues or subjective standards. Such patients require external cues to establish their boundaries emotionally, as well as with regard to eating (Bruch, 1961; 1973).

In counseling or therapy sessions, many obese patients confirm some of these dynamics. They will describe anxiety-reduction after binge-eating, deep satisfaction while sneakily eating, compulsion to eat when depressed or anxious, or overprotective (yet hostile) mothers who fed them constantly. Some obese patients describe fantasies associated with their body image: they are pregnant, but virgins; or their weight is an effective barrier against sexual-encounters. They sometimes describe many distortions of body image, including beliefs that they are extremely attractive.

Reviews of the empirical literature, however (Leon and Roth, 1977), indicate that obese people show no consistent set of traits, needs, or pathological conditions, such as orality or depression. Further, while there is moderate evidence that obese people eat more when anxious, there is little evidence to suggest that eating reduces their anxiety (Herman and Polivy, 1975).

Schachter and the externality hypothesis. Obese individuals, according to a widely held view, are responsive to salient external rather than internal cues. That is, rather than responding to internal physiological states of hunger, the eating behavior of obese people is characterized as being under the control of environmental cues (Schachter and Rodin, 1974). Initially, this work arose from observations of obese rats who ate excessively because of a certain type of brain lesion (ventromedial). Eventually, these observations led to hypotheses about obese humans.

In a group of related studies, Schachter and his colleagues found that obese subjects were generally more responsive, frequently overreacting to certain external cues such as auditory tones, visual scenes, positive or negative emotional stimuli, and food-related stimuli, than subjects of normal weight. Obese subjects were also shown to be responsive to stimuli high in salience (prominence) and attractiveness, eating more *good*-tasting food than non-obese subjects. But when stimuli *low* in salience were introduced, differences between them and subjects of normal weight were not found. Obese subjects also differed from normal-weight subjects in being more finicky in eating habits and in expending less effort to get food, even when hungry.

Subsequent evaluations of this work have yielded some critical opinions (Cox, 1976; Leon and Roth, 1977; Milich, 1975; Rowland and Antelman, 1976; Rodin, 1974, 1981). These criticisms raise objections to parallels drawn between rats and humans and object to empirical work with overweight college students (mostly male) as being unrepresentative of the obese population (who are usually older and heavier). Above all, the "externality" of obese individuals is questioned, for whereas some obese people are shown to respond to food attractiveness, salience, and taste, others do not. Most studies, however, do support the hypothesis that obese people work less to get food than normal-weight subjects (Leon and Roth, 1977).

Overall when obese people (50 percent above ideal weight) were studied, they were shown to be *no more responsive to external cues* than those with normal body weight (Rodin, 1974).

Nisbett and "fat cells." According to Nisbett's theory, some individuals are biologically programmed to be fat (Nisbett, 1972). Obesity thus results from the body's craving to replenish stores of certain acids in specialized fat cells. The number of these cells in people, obese or thin, is relatively stable, but obese people have more of these fat cells than those of normal weight. The number of fat cells, according to Nisbett, has strong biological and genetic predetermination. However, the normal level of fat stores in these cells can be modified by early nutritional experiences and learning. These effects are irreversible. A young child, for example, with a certain number of fat cells and level of fat stores that are predetermined in this way will continue to eat, as an adult, until the normal level of fat stores is reached. In obese people, this level may be extremely high, compared to basically nonobese people. For an obese individual, weight reduction is likened to getting a person of normal weight to reduce: the drive to eat is controlled by the hypothalamus, which in obese people, controls food intake until it reaches its normal baseline for that particular person.

Overall there is evidence suggesting a strong biological component in some individuals that predetermines their obesity. This may be why there is no one emotional conflict or personality type that characterizes obese people. However, one aspect of Nisbett's theory that would be compatible with a psychogenic approach is that truly obese people, if underfed or below normal weight, become anxious, driven, and restless until gratified.

Not all obese babies develop into obese adults. And thin babies can develop into obese adults. Learning and emotions do enter into the total picture. Further, social and cultural factors are also associated with high or low weight (Kolata, 1977).

Chronic stress, overweight, and rats. Evidence with rats suggests that at least some types of obesity can be accounted for by chronic stress (Rowland and Antelman, 1976). Rats became considerably overweight under certain stressful conditions (mild tail pinch), leading the researchers to believe that at least some nongenetic obesity could be accounted for by chronic stress. But their work also lends support to Schachter's externality approach, for during the mild stress, rats showed "stress-related increase in responsiveness to environmental stimuli," actually becoming more goal-directed and more aware of stimuli around them.

What conclusions can be drawn from this diverse material? There is no one explanation for obesity that accounts for all the empirical data. One set of researches point to the significance of a large learning component in eating behavior; overeating can thus be conceptualized as a heavily reinforced set of behaviors. Other data indicate a high possibility that there are different groups of obese

Listing 8.1 DSM-III Categories and Additional Syndromes Described in Chapter 8

DSM-III Categories

Eating Disorders
- Anorexia nervosa
- Bulimia (episodic eating binges)

Somatoform Disorders
- Somatization disorder
- Conversion disorder (or hysterical neurosis, conversion type)
- Psychogenic pain disorder
- Hypochondriasis (or hypochondriacal disorder)

Factitious Disorders
- With psychological symptoms
- Chronic factitious disorder with physical symptoms

Sleepwalking Disorder; Sleep Terror Disorder

Additional Syndromes

Peptic ulcers

Cardiovascular disorders
- Essential hypertension

Asthma

Insomnia

Narcolepsy

Obesity

Headache

people—some being depressed or anxious, others having a biological need for eating until normal fat-cell level is reached, and still others showing a pattern of "externality" in their responsiveness to environmental cues.

It is generally agreed that treating obesity is enormously difficult. Even when there is immediate success, obese people tend to regain the weight they have lost; that is, although success has been noted with methods such as behavior therapy, psychotherapy, hypnosis, various nonprofessional methods (Weight Watchers, for example), and innovative techniques in groups or family settings, it has largely been in the short run rather than the long run. Follow-up research almost invariably yields findings of eventual weight gain and/or dropout from treatment (Hall, et al., 1974; Kolata, 1977; Leon, 1976; Yates, 1975).

Overall, although obesity may be associated with a variety of causative factors, the key to any treatment program is to change eating patterns by increasing energy expenditure and decreasing caloric intake. The "teeter-tottering" of weight loss and gain that so many obese people experience, however, often reduces self-confidence and increases feelings of depression, helplessness, and dependency. Some clinicians believe, therefore, that physical risks notwithstanding, obesity might be better left alone in some cases, provided a thoroughgoing assessment of each individual situation is made.

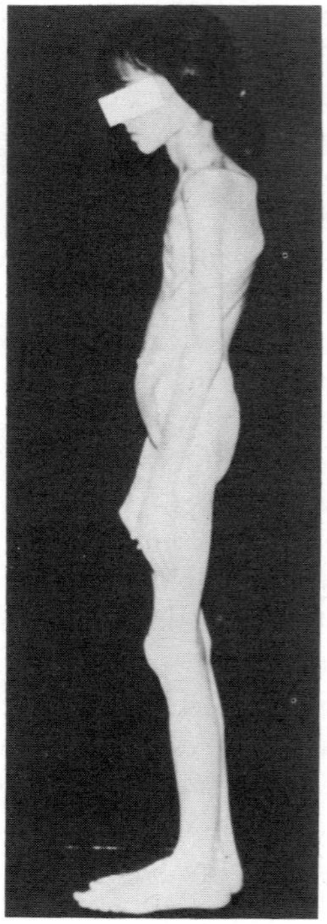

An anorexic patient. Anorexia nervosa most frequently appears in females in their 'teens, twenties, and thirties, and symptoms can be so extreme as to be life threatening. (Courtesy of Dr. W. Stewart Agras, Stanford University)

Anorexia Nervosa

Anorexia nervosa is a serious, life-threatening condition characterized by an intense avoidance of eating—so intense, in fact, that death is often a result. It is most common in adolescent girls and young women in their twenties and thirties (according to the DSM-III, it is predominantly a female disorder). Weight can sometimes voluntarily be reduced to as low as forty or fifty pounds. Since amenorrhea (cessation of menstruation) precedes weight loss in almost all if not all instances of anorexia nervosa, this and other observations of such patients suggest the possibility that some endocrinological dysfunction—along with other factors, such as cultural emphasis on thinness or particular temperament—contributes to the development of this bizarre behavior pattern (Bemis, 1978).

The DSM-III describes the following criteria for diagnosing anorexia nervosa:

1. Intense fear of becoming obese, which does not diminish, even with extreme weight loss
2. Body image disturbance, for example, claiming to "feel fat," even when emaciated
3. Weight loss of at least 25 percent of original body weight

4. Refusal to maintain body weight over a minimal normal weight for age and height
5. No known physical illness that would account for the weight loss

Anorexic patients are frequently active, energetic, and bright. They are generally ambitious, educationally and professionally. Although there is complete awareness of what is happening to them, most patients state they cannot help themselves. They know that they might look bizarre to others, but their own self-concept and idealized images of beauty "force" them to eliminate any possible fat on their bones, even though they know that they might die. They are depressed and often anxious, but frequently, these feelings emerge from concern that they will gain weight as a result of their excessive preoccupation with food—with eating, cooking, and hoarding food—rather than from concern over their grotesque symptoms.

Many anorexics are compulsive eaters, often devouring food secretively—for example, binge-eating late at night, after everyone else has gone to bed. They often engage in self-induced vomiting or use cathartics to rid themselves of any ingested food.

In the course of interviews with these patients, some common ground is evidenced. Often, there is a history of obesity in the family or there might have been stress on being thin and fit, meeting the popular standards of a diet-conscious teenager who can wear clothes well. As a matter of fact, reviews

Case 8.1 Anne: Anorexia Nervosa

Anne is a twenty-year-old junior in an Eastern woman's college. Six months ago, she weighed eighty-five pounds. Anne is five feet, eight inches tall, never goes to the beach, avoids tennis clothes, but looks stunning in sports clothes, and often wears bulky sweaters, achieving a modish "layered" look. She "knows" others will be repelled if her bodily contours were disclosed in any way. But secretly, she believes herself to be truly attractive. Anne has stopped menstruating and is worried about this. She occasionally enjoys sexual relations with a boyfriend who understands how severe her illness is.

Anne chronically craves food; it is an obsession with her. She eats between classes, cuts classes to eat, lives alone because of the full refrigerator she can keep, and steathily sneaks away from social situations or from group activities to eat. She is a familiar figure in every restaurant, grocery store, and diner near (but not *too* near) campus because she buys and eats in bulk. Five hamburgers and five milkshakes do not satisfy her; she walks as rapidly as she can to the next restaurant, where she orders several roast beef sandwiches and five desserts—pies and sundaes, mostly. She get back to her room, somehow, forces herself to vomit, falls into a drugged, stuperous state for about an hour, and then catches her next class. She has spaced her classes and activities to fit her obsessional pattern. She gets up at four in the morning to walk for four miles. She is tireless and energetic and fun to be with—if you can keep up with her—and is a straight A student. However, she is dying of starvation.

Anne has a rather common disturbance called anorexia nervosa. She also shows several other obsessional symptoms and is a compulsively neat and organized person. Anne has attempted suicide twice, not because of depression, she claims, but because she can see no way to break the pattern that dominates her life. She has been in and out of hospitals for intravenous feeding so many times that it is not clear whether she will make it. She feels trapped. Yet she is convinced, and will argue stubbornly, with a sense of impending panic, that she is heavy, any food intake tends to put weight on, weight is disgusting, and she would feel really sick even with a few pounds of added weight.

Anne was always a "good" child, in the conventional sense. She tried hard to please her parents, especially her father. In therapy, dreams of sexual encounters with her father and fears of pregnancy emerged, and she discovered that she would have rather been a boy, or a young child, at least in body. Yet, she would like to get married and have several babies. Anne wants to be a lawyer.

Anne's anorexic pattern apparently began when she was fourteen years old and was beginning to develop breasts and to gain weight. A few months earlier she had one menstrual period. About this time her father commented about her becoming a woman, having to watch out for boys "taking advantage" of her, and watching her weight—otherwise she'll get to be chubby like her mother. The next day, she undressed in front of the mirror, becoming increasingly disgusted with her rounding body. She immediately went on a stringent diet, and at the same time became increasingly obsessed with food, craving it constantly. Her anorexic symptoms were fully developed by the time she was a high school senior. She was popular nevertheless, and few people knew of her secret eating and self-induced vomiting. It became a family secret—the skeleton in the closet, both literally and figuratively.

A combination of psychotherapy which yielded much insight, medication to curb her appetite, and medication to relieve anxiety somewhat modified her death-course behavior. She now weighs one hundred pounds, but is still not menstruating. She is not dying, but feels that she is unable to gain the additional ten pounds that she needs. She would rather die, she claims. She has begun a program of rewards for each five-ounce weight-gain she shows, which, with the help of her therapist, may actually work.

of the clinical literature support the notion that there are probably some common early childhood factors that predispose girls to later anorexia. These include conscientious, conforming behavior in shy, anxious children who are orderly, neat, and planful. Generally, some factor such as onset of menstruation, college entrance, or marriage precipitates the shift from "normal" dieting and weight consciousness to pathological anorexia. Psychodynamic theories also implicate disturbed mother-daughter relationships, family pathology (Rosman, Minuchin, and Liebman, 1975), fear of becoming pregnant, and anxiety regarding becoming a grown, adult woman.

Although many anorexic patients confirm some of these familial factors and dynamics, it is quite likely, as already indicated, that some organic or endocrinological dysfunction interacts with cultural background and temperamental and familial factors to create this condition.

How is anorexia treated? With what success? Anorexic conditions may be so serious as to require hospitalization for some patients. Understandably, the "force-feeding" methods used are deeply resented by involuntarily hospitalized patients. Many return to their usual anorexic behavior when discharged.

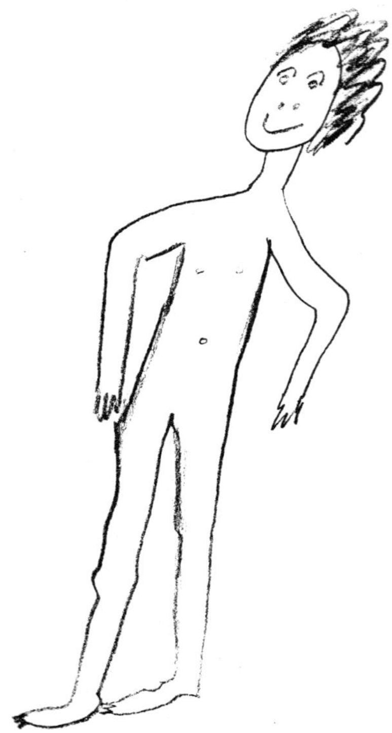

Figure 8.4 This drawing of a female body was made by an intelligent, twenty-year-old, eighty-pound, female anorexic patient. She called it a "fat" drawing. She regards her own starved, skeletal body as extremely attractive.

Patients who can be treated on an outpatient basis have more options open to them. These include traditional psychotherapy, psychoanalysis, behavioral methods, family methods (Minuchin, Rosman, and Baker, 1978), and medication. Often, combinations of all these are used.

No single treatment method has been shown to be most effective, even though each claims some success. There is the usual "successful" demonstration of *immediate* results, in this case, weight gain, followed by little or no maintenance of gain later on. The sad facts are that about one third of anorexic patients remain chronically ill or die, with estimates of death rates ranging from 10 to 25 percent (Bemis, 1978; DSM-III, Van Buskirk, 1977).

Bulimia

In the foregoing discussion, binge-eating was mentioned in the context of obesity and anorexia nervosa. Bulimia is the name assigned to a repeated, compulsive pattern of binge eating in which weight is neither excessively below or excessively above the normal range. Excessive ingestion of food may dominate the daily habits of the bulimic patient, often accompanied by repeated self-induced vomiting or use of cathartics; this is generally followed by self-disgust and depression, until the process is repeated, once more.

One of my patients, a 22-year-old college graduate, was aware of this obsessional pattern and sought help to change it, having unsuccessfully tried to do so with many other therapists. This time, she wished me to "convince" her family to hospitalize her so that she could be prevented from indulging in her "disgusting habit." The year before, as a matter of fact, she *had* been hospitalized for a month (her family thought it was for drug abuse). The day she was released, she proceeded immediately to the nearest cafeteria, then to a lunch counter, then to a roadside hamburger joint, then home for self-induced vomiting. Disgusted, but relieved, she repeated this pattern until midnight, when she went home, exhausted, to force vomit and sleep. Her family refused to have her hospitalized again, incidentally, and this patient dropped out of treatment, presumably to continue her bulimic pattern while at the same time, seeking help elsewhere. The patient never did permit a discussion of how she could be helped: a combination of cognitive and behavioral methods might have been effective.

The origins of this disorder are not known, nor are prevalence rates, which seem to be rising rapidly. Bulimia appears most often among females, generally first appearing during adolescence or young girlhood. Although there may be undue body preoccupation and concern with one's looks, bulimia, in contrast to anorexia nervosa, is not characterized by life-threatening, extremely severe weight loss. However, there are some similarities in patterns of behavior when the two types of eating disorders are compared, as the following DSM-III criteria for bulimia suggest:

1. Recurrent episodes of binge eating
2. at least three of the following:
   a. consumption of high-caloric, easily ingested food during a binge
   b. inconspicuous eating during a binge
   c. termination of binges by abdominal pain, sleep, social interruption, or self-induced vomiting
   d. repeated attempts to lose weight by extreme diets, self-induced vomiting, cathartics, or diuretics
   e. frequent weight fluctuations due to alternating binges and fasts
3. Awareness that the eating pattern is abnormal and fear of not being able to stop voluntarily
4. Depressed mood and self-deprecating thoughts following eating binges
5. Bulimic episodes not due to anorexia nervosa or any known physical disorder

HEADACHE

Headaches are common complaints in the clinician's office—so common, in fact, that their significance (irritability, absenteeism, avoidance of responsibilities, subjective anguish) is often overlooked.

Apart from an extremely small number of patients whose headaches are due to actual physical injury to or inflammation or other pathology of the brain (tumor, for example), most headaches probably arise from an individual's response, in the light of their psychological and physiological predisposition, to stressful situations (Bakal, 1975). Most headaches, thus, fall into our classification of psychosomatic or psychophysiological disorder.

Of these, the most common are the tension headache, the migraine headache, or some combination of both. The tension headache ("nervous headache") is produced by continued muscle contraction of the frontalis, a rectangular layer of muscle on the forehead. Biofeedback methods that signal patients when they are or are not contracting the frontalis can help many of them to control their pain (see Chapter 21).

Although migraine headaches are less common than tension headaches (Ogden, 1952), they are by far the more severe complaint. Migraine headaches, which can last from six to eight hours up to a few days, can be so excruciating that some sufferers are unable to attend school, go to work, or perform ordinary daily routines. Migraine symptoms are often accompanied by dizziness, nausea, vomiting, and blurred vision.

What is migraine? Patients describe their headaches as an intense aching or throbbing that is at first pulsing, then steady and unilateral (on one side). In some forms of migraine, there is a prodromal (before actual onset) stage, caused by a period of vasoconstriction (narrowing) of cranial blood vessels with its accompanying diminution of blood supply to tissues of the brain. This condition may provide some people with a premonition or aura that warns them of the migraine to follow. The aura is usually of a sensory nature. The actual headache itself occurs as a result of rather extensive vasodilation (opening, spreading) of the cranial blood vessels. Estimates of incidence run about five to ten percent in the general population, mostly among females (Adams, et al., 1980; Friar and Beatty, 1976).

There is some agreement that there may be an inherited predisposition for migraine (it tends to run in families), there may be some relationship to a history of vomiting or severe motion sickness (Selby and Lance, 1960), and that certain foods, alcohol, or bright lights can "trigger" an attack. Some clinicians also believe that there are common personality characteristics among migraine sufferers. These traits include high drive, rigidity, and perfectionism in people who are anxious and unable to express anger and resentment. Many migraine patients also report parental suppressive attitudes (Henryk-Gutt and Rees, 1973; Rees, 1974). Often, perceived psychological stress triggers or is in some way related to the migraine attack. Migraine attacks in children, for example, were found to be associated with school failure (Brown, 1977).

Generally, it would seem that for individuals with "appropriate" physiological predisposition, the most valid predictor of whether or not migraine will occur is some interaction of their personality with their perception of stressful situations. That is, even with predisposition, personality alone or stressor alone would not sufficiently explain or predict the migraine (Bakal, 1975). Overall, however, the etiology of migraine is still not clear (Adams, et al., 1980).

There is some success in treating migraine headache with medications that reduce the dilation of cranial blood vessels or through use of biofeedback methods that attempt to do the same through temperature regulation (Adams, et al., 1980; Friar and Beatty, 1976). Methods that generally induce relaxation are also moderately successful. There is little evidence for effectiveness of the "talking" therapies in treating this type of headache.

SOMATOFORM DISORDERS: DISORDERS THAT SUGGEST PHYSICAL ILLNESS

Individuals who complain of dizziness, headache, chest pains, or various other bodily aches and discomforts are familiar to all of us. They are as bewildered by what is happening to them as are their physicians, who are unable to find an organic basis for these complaints. At first, such people receive solicitous attention from their families. Later, however, they may elicit resentment. Most of these patients do not recognize the possibility that their complaints may have emotional and psychological rather than physical explanations.

Somatization disorder. One of my patients, a college sophomore, complained of severe menstrual cramps, back and shoulder pains, sinus difficulties, intermittent diarrhea and constipation, and heart palpitations. She was seeing a chiropractor regularly for "adjustments," and in one month, had several consultations with a gynecologist, an internist (for an electrocardiogram and a gastrointestinal diagnosis), and an eye-ear-nose-and throat physician for her sinus problems. She was also attending exercise classes regularly for "body tone." Physical problems were never diagnosed. Eventually, after a year of psychotherapy, my patient complained much less about her physical problems and consulted her physicians much less frequently. To this day, however, she claims that she has "learned to live with her physical difficulties," while she continues to discount their emotional origins.

This patient is typical of a large number of people with an array of physical "problems" and complaints whose medical histories are complex, vague, and chronic, often beginning in early adulthood. The DSM-III calls this syndrome somatization disorder. Its incidence is much more frequent in women than men (about one in one hundred women fall into this category, according to the DSM-III). Many patients with somatization disorders insist that they have always been "sickly," depressed, and anxious, and that they have always relied on medical consultations for "help." Rarely can they point to specific physical problems in their histories, however.

Patients with somatization disorders tend to use sedatives, tranquilizers, and other medications dispensed by their physicians to ease their pains. Thus, an additional problem with some of these patients is that they may develop severe drug-dependency—often difficult to treat, because such patients tend to rely heavily on their "medicines."

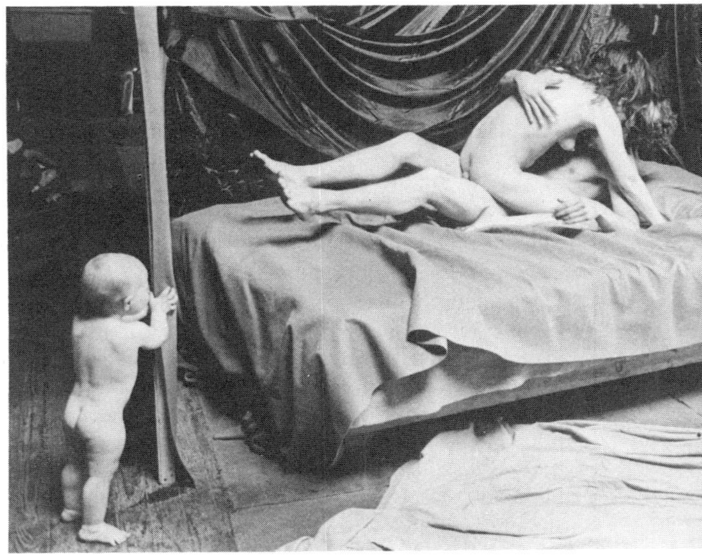

A child's accidental witnessing of the sexual activities of his or her parents was thought by some clinicians to be a shameful event that is repressed from consciousness, later to surface in a "hysteria prone" individual as a symptom. (Charles Gatewood/ Magnum)

*Conversion disorder (or hysterical neurosis, conversion type).** Conversion disorder is the label applied to a highly specific loss of function of an organ or body system, without (known) physical explanation, and presumably without conscious or voluntary control. According to the DSM-III, the gender distribution of this disorder is not known.

Conversion symptoms are extremely rare but were reported more frequently several generations ago. Today, they would tend to appear, if at all, in military settings, especially during times of war. The specific symptoms often follow the fashions of the times, differing from era to era and culture to culture. Conversion symptoms, thus, can cover a

* Conversion disorders have for decades been grouped with the psychoneuroses. For many, this traditional classification still holds. Conversion disorders are described in this chapter along with other psychophysiological disorders, rather than in Chapter 9, to conform to the newer diagnostic system of the DSM-III.

Case 8.2 Sally: Conversion Disorder

Sally is a twenty-year-old typist who is pretty, childlike, flamboyantly dramatic, and fun. She cries easily, laughs easily, has many friends, is popular with men, and rather bubbly and chatty.

One day, when Sally was about nineteen years old, she was sent from her desk to the firm's physician, then by her family to the family physician, then from an opthalmologist to a neurologist, and then back to the company physician, who recommended a visit to a psychologist for treatment. She suddenly found that she could not see. However, she did not stumble or bump into things and showed normal pupillary reflexes. Although there was no organic basis for this loss of function, Sally was convinced that her blindness was "real." She did not show much fear or anxiety about her situation.

In therapy, she gradually learned, with the aid of occasional hypnotic sessions, that when she was about five years old she had witnessed her father making love to her baby sitter. On this occasion, she had crept out of bed to go to the bathroom, and heard noises in the living room, next door to her own room. She never mentioned what she had seen to anyone. A month after this incident, her father died suddenly. Soon, she repressed all memory of what she had seen. She went through high school without incident and was relatively happy in her first real job.

These events happened just before the onset of her conversion symptom: The typist in the next cubicle confided to Sally that she was having an affair with their boss, a married man. Sally did not believe the confession, but even if true, she felt that it was not morally wrong. She did not think much about it anyway. The next week, on a Friday night, Sally returned to the office to get her sunglasses which she had (purposely?) left on her desk. She saw her friend and their boss in one of the offices in deep conversation. Nobody had seen her either enter or leave.

From the moment she sat at her desk on Monday morning, she was irrationally convinced that she would be fired. When word was relayed to her that her boss wished to see her the next morning, Sally kept the appointment, despite her fears. During the interview (the therapist learned later that she was actually being assigned a somewhat better position with a slight increase in salary), Sally complained of severe headache, dizziness, faintness, and spots before her eyes. By the time she was sent to the company physician for a check-up, she was no longer able to see.

After five twice-weekly sessions, with the occasional use of hypnotic methods and suggestion, Sally's symptoms completely disappeared. She has continued in treatment because she wants to find out more about her responses so that she can avoid future problems. She is learning about the shock, dismay, and anger she experienced when she "caught" her father with the babysitter and the subsequent guilt she experienced after his death. In fantasy his death became something she had willed in vengeance.

She also learned about the shock, dismay, and anger she experienced toward her boss, followed by a sudden upsurge of guilt—a symbolic repetition of the earlier situation. Above all, Sally learned that she wants to remain a child, and is afraid to grow up, to see, to acknowledge, to learn from, and to become part of the real, complex world around her.

A year later, Sally became supervisor of four other typists at the same company. Her friend is no longer there, for she is married, pregnant, and does not want to work. Nobody knows how the boss is getting along, because he was transferred to a subsidiary in Europe. He never did learn the reason for Sally's blindness and dramatic recovery. Only she and her therapist knew for sure.

wide range: blindness, deafness, paralysis of limbs, aphonia (loss of speech), inability to walk or stand, and various kinds of anesthesias (loss of sensation) in different parts of the body. In each instance, the "impaired" organ or body part is actually quite normal and intact. Conversion symptoms generally involve only one disturbance, unlike the multiplicity of complaints in the somatization disorders described above.

Symptoms may appear suddenly after an

acutely stressful event, such as the death of a close relative or after an emotionally traumatic event, as in battle. Some clinicians claim that there may also be some predisposing personality patterns. Thus, presymptomatic people may be dependent, suggestible, and in need of sympathy. They are often described as dramatic, "histrionic"—in need of attention. Sometimes, but not always, they may display a neutral, bland, non-worrying attitude (called *la belle indifférence*).

Most Freudians insist that such symptoms reflect repressed, taboo wishes that date back to early childhood. A contrasting view is that brain disorders such as head injury may play some role in conversion symptoms (Whitlock, 1967). In any event, "true" conversion disorders are so infrequent that it is difficult to assess the specific causes that may be involved.

Conversion symptoms are fairly easy to distinguish from "real" symptoms. Patients with conversion blindness avoid objects and situations that might injure them. In examination, their pupils react to light. Also, certain kinds of anesthesias ("glove" or "stocking" anesthesias) follow the naive person's conception of anatomy rather than actual neurological structures. As might be expected, there are objective tests for distinguishing actual blindness or deafness from conversion symptoms (Grosz and Zimmerman, 1965; Pankratz, Fausti, and Peed, 1975).

Conversion symptoms can often be dramatically relieved by suggestion, hypnosis, drugs, and placebos. The so-called miracle cures reported to take place at various spiritual centers or revival meetings are more likely responses to suggestion than anything else.

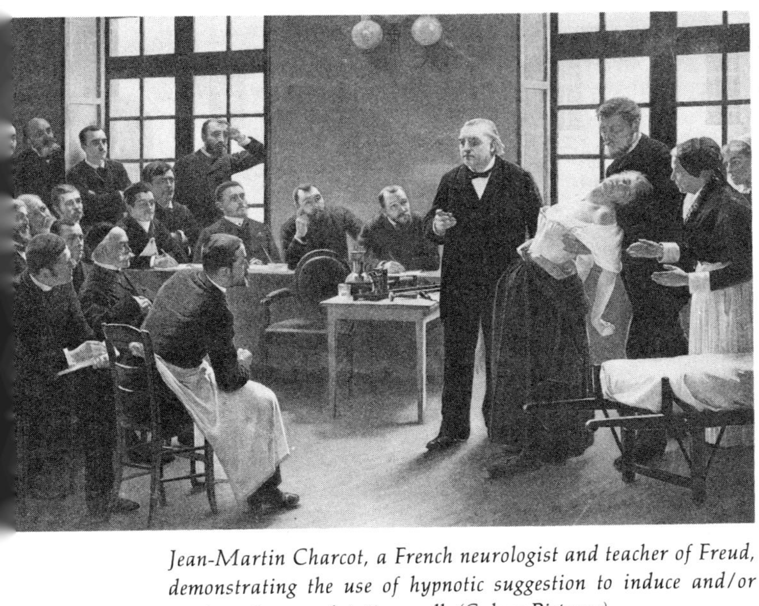

Jean-Martin Charcot, a French neurologist and teacher of Freud, demonstrating the use of hypnotic suggestion to induce and/or treat a seizure or fainting spell. (Culver Pictures)

Psychogenic pain disorder. A large group of patients complain of severe, chronic pain, but physical and neurological examinations do not indicate any physical basis for their complaints. Even if there is some associated physical problem, the pain is described as grossly excessive or protracted in the light of its actual physical cause. The pain may "mimic" an actual disease (such as a back injury) but no tissue damage is detected.

"Pain patients" often have "pain careers"—life styles that consist of chronic complaints, doctor-shopping, incapacitation, and, for a good part of their lives, considerable attention-getting. Like many of the patients described in this chapter, they run the risk of excessive dependence on drugs and medications. Often, they get no help from these sought-out remedies.

Because the onset of pain, which can occur at any age, often coincides with some stressful life event, and because clinical exploration yields many psychological "reasons" for the continuation of these symptoms, such as dependence on others and avoidance of responsibilities, this group of disorders is called psychogenic. Patients diagnosed as having psychogenic pain generally describe pain symptoms as their major complaint, even though there may be some depression and anxiety associated with their pain. According to the DSM-III, psychogenic pain is more commonly diagnosed among women than men, but overall prevalence data about this syndrome are not available.

It is common knowledge that we all differ in "thresholds" (sensitivity) for pain. Even more striking is the generally observable phenomenon that under conditions of severe stress, for example in battle conditions or in an athletic contest, pain in response to an injury is often not experienced at all. Here are other pain "facts": sensitivity to pain decreases with age; men are less sensitive to pain than women; and the side of the body opposite to the dominant hemisphere of the brain is least sensitive (Schmeck, 1979).

Many of these individual thresholds to pain may be learned. But recent findings indicate that brain biochemistry may play a more important role than was thought to be the case in how the body defends against or deals with pain. In the past several years, a group of chemicals called endorphins have been isolated. (Chemicals discovered earlier called enkephalins have the same function.) It seems that the body produces these brain chemicals in response to hormonal discharges during stress (fighting or fleeing responses). Electrical stimulation of parts of the brain also produces higher levels of endorphin in the brain. And endorphins are produced when there are pain signals in the brain produced by *other* chemicals. Apparently, the brain's biochemistry "fends" against pain when necessary to do so.

In some people, the biochemical defense against pain may be limited, increasing the subjective experience of pain or may be in ready or excessive supply, perhaps explaining why some people experience little or no pain, even under ordinarily painful stimulation. It could be that the brain's way of handling pain in trances, highly suggestible states, or during some religious rites is also related to these biochemicals. The level of natural "opiates" in the brain may also bear some relationship to heroin addiction, but it is not entirely clear how, as yet.

Many pain patients have already been successfully helped with hypnosis, suggestion, placebo, and biofeedback (see Spotlight 21.2, pp. 645–46). Intriguing possibilities for treating pain patients also lie in the biochemistry of the brain—possibly when the endorphins are more clearly understood. Perhaps drugs will one day be manufactured that trigger the body's own natural substances to "take over" in its defenses against pain. It is too early to tell. These researches offer exciting possibilities in helping pain-sufferers. In addition, they suggest that "psychogenic pain" may, at least in part, have some biochemical origins.

Hypochondriasis (or hypochondriacal disorder). You may be familiar with some people who, on the basis of an everyday, minor ache, feel that they are coming down with an infectious disease or that they are dying from cancer. These people fall into the diagnostic category of hypochondriasis, which refers to an unrealistic interpretation of ordinary aches and pains as symptoms of a major disease. According to the DSM-III, hypochondriasis is fairly common and occurs in equal frequency in men and women.

Although people with this diagnosis may not have specific complaints and dysfunctions (as in somatization or conversion disorders), they seem preoccupied with their bodily activities and functions. According to the DSM-III, such patients can be differentiated from some of those described earlier in this chapter in that they do not have a long, complicated medical history. Instead, it is more likely that these fears of ill health develop later in life. They become preoccupied with their bodies despite little physical or organic evidence that there is an actual body problem and despite any professional reassurances that they receive. These hypochondriacal preoccupations differ from the shifting reports of bizarre symptoms that some schizophrenics display (see Chapter 11).

Factitious disorders. Patients who voluntarily "fake" various symptoms with no apparent reason or goal—even going to great lengths such as inflicting injury upon themselves—are diagnosed as having factitious disorders, according to the DSM-III. These disorders, sometimes called the Munchausen syndrome (after the Baron, teller of tall tales), are known to hospital personnel all over. People with this syndrome often show bizarre behavior and

Spotlight 8.7 Factitious Disorders: Neither Rhyme nor Reason?

During times of war, some men have "faked" certain symptoms to be relieved of combat duty or to avoid the draft. Others have pretended to be physically or mentally ill to avoid conviction for a crime. These are examples of malingering, which is not regarded as a pathological symptom. Malingering involves a conscious and voluntary act and serves an adaptive purpose for the subject, whether or not you approve of the act itself or the goals that are involved.

There is another group of related behaviors which seem purposeless, without observable goals—without "rhyme or reason." According to the DSM-III, these are factitious disorders which characterize a group of unusual patients who voluntarily and consciously simulate actual physical or mental disorders so that they can achieve the attention and status associated with being sick. Factitious disorders are not common, but when they do appear, they are manifested mostly by men, according to the DSM-III.

Here are some examples. One of my patients injures himself by inflicting burns and scissor cuts all over his body. He does this periodically until he receives medical and psychological attention. Another patient, described in an earlier version of the DSM-III, "presents" to his doctor a physical symptom, hematuria (urine that contains blood). Blood tests indicate that he has probably taken anticoagulants (which he denies) to create this medical problem. Still other patients are known as "hospital hobos." At first they are not labeled as such in the hospital setting, then their medical record emerges. They have been patients in innumerable hospitals in innumerable cities. They have undergone an extraordinary number of surgical procedures. They have dislocated their own shoulders, swallowed poison to develop abdominal pains, ingested drugs or medicine (like penicillin) to which they are allergic. Such patients spend most of their time in hospitals, discharging themselves angrily if they do not receive "proper" medical attention, but soon admitting themselves to other hospitals. They make a career of voluntarily carving out for themselves one physical or mental symptom after another so that they remain hospitalized more often than not.

Are these factitious pathologies different from malingering because the individual seems to lack motivation for his bizarre acts? Is it pathology because the medical simulation seems illogical, senseless to the observer? Actually, these deviant behaviors may have some very stong motivations. It may be that some patients seek care and attention, but do not know how to get it except by demanding medical intervention. The care becomes symbolic for being looked after, watched out for, and loved. It may also be that the hospital with its medical routines and physical interventions may actually help some patients to feel alive, to feel that they are *somebodies.*

These cases do not comprise a large enough group for study nor are they recognized "early" enough to allow generalizations about successful psychological intervention. Furthermore, they do not necessarily seek help for changing or modifying their "factitious" behavior. If you were a hospital administrator would you turn down such patients? Remember, their symptoms are real—even if self-inflicted.

some of them may be schizophrenic. Spotlight 8.7 describes people with factitious disorders with physical symptoms in a little more detail. Factitious disorders with psychological symptoms (often mimicking psychosis) may involve memory loss, hallucinations, and conversion symptoms that are brought about by the ingestion of various substances.

Spotlight 8.8 Primary and Secondary Gain

Primary gains refer to the "rewards" a psychological symptom or a psychogenic illness achieve for the individual on deep psychological levels, such as anxiety-reduction or repression of conflict or shameful thoughts. Sally's conversion symptom, described earlier, is a good example of primary gain. Most symptoms also carry some *secondary* gains. These refer to the supports, attention, controls, or rewards that sick people achieve from their illnesses, whether real or imagined. You all have experienced periods of relief when a headache or a disease "took you off the hook" from an examination at school, for example, or from some possibly stressful social situation. Secondary gains can be reasonably good rewards for illness.

Two patients, an older man and a younger woman, aptly illustrate this point. Both patients had been repeatedly diagnosed, over a period of years, as having multiple sclerosis, and indeed, many of the appropriate symptoms were present in each case, such as tremors, occasional remission of pain, nystagmus (a shifting oscillation of the eyeballs), and ataxia (poor coordination of the voluntary muscles as in walking or reaching for objects). Both had had a long history of hospitalization, medications, and medical consultations. Both had been suffering in a kind of cheerful, sweet, "martyrdom." When finally, each, under different circumstances, had been told that the disease had been misdiagnosed, one patient—the younger—developed symptoms of intense panic, phobias, and excruciating headaches. She continues to be the center of attention in her family, including her bewildered husband. The older patient left his wife, went into a severe depression, and is currently functioning on a marginal basis, although "well," physically.

OVERVIEW

By now you should be aware of the fact that no matter what the etiology of a disease is, psychological variables play a crucial role in determining its course. The loss of a close person, for example, and the sense of hopelessness or helplessness the survivor experiences (see Engel, 1968; Schmale, 1958) can not only exacerbate illness, but also can even cause death. One report indicates that there were ten times a higher death rate among a group of widowed spouses within one year after bereavement than among a group of peers controlled for age and sex (Brody, 1979a).

In general, one's attitude towards one's self, sense of despair, hopelessness, or feeling of powerlessness, and conversely, control and power over one's fate, are very much related to the outcome or course of an illness. Most health practitioners are becoming more aware that their patients' emotional attitudes toward recovery, toward getting better, can make the difference between speedy recovery and a long protracted illness. The intricate embroidery—the interwoven fabric—of mind, body, emotions, feelings, and thoughts may be difficult to unravel, but is dramatically palpable, nevertheless, in illness or in health.

The ubiquity of emotions in health or disease is one of the reasons that in recent years many psychopathologists have been loath to label certain diseases "psychosomatic." The implication would be that *other* diseases are not. Further, calling a disease (for example, asthma) "psychosomatic" implies that we know the precise emotional and psychological mechanisms that precipitate the physical condition; but this is far from the case.

Yet the compelling evidence seems to justify the use of *some* way of indicating the powerful role that psychological factors may play in a particular disease. It is for this reason that some are continuing to use the expressions psychophysiological and psychosomatic. Even the DSM-III, which had abandoned the label psychosomatic, is suggesting that the physical conditions and diseases listed on Axis III be rated according to the extent to which psychological factors play a role in their etiology and maintenance.

We look to the future of this exciting area. Perhaps we will one day be in a position to isolate and weigh the exact contributions of our emotions and of individual responses to stressors to our physical condition.

SUMMARY

Part II introduced the clinical syndromes with a brief summary of some of the major treatment approaches to aid in understanding the subsequent text discussion. This chapter focused on the body's response to emotional conflict and stress. Accordingly, it considered the role of stressors and life events in the development of psychopathology and various body disorders. The chapter then reviewed Selye's general adaptation syndrome, including the signs that might be indicators of a maladaptive stress response and went on to discuss and illustrate psychophysiological (or psychosomatic) disorders, with special attention allocated to peptic ulcers, cardiovascular disorders, asthma, and migraine headaches. Sleep, dreams, and several eating disorders—obesity, anorexia nervosa, and bulimia—were also given special consideration. Finally, the chapter described relevant DSM-III diagnostic categories (somatoform disorders). These include somatization disorder, conversion disorder (or hysterical neurosis, conversion type), psychogenic pain disorder, hypochondriasis (or hypochondriacal disorder), and factitious disorders.

Highlights

1. Life events research explores the possibility that a series of important life changes (for example, the death of a close family member) may predispose an individual to physical or psychological pathology. Recently, this research thrust indicates that number of *undesirable* events and especially how these are perceived are more significant than the *number* of events, independent of their desirability, in determining onset of pathology. The empirical evidence also suggests that there is a pre-existing susceptibility or resistance to the impact of life changes which include such variables as personal competence and the presence of social support systems.
2. Selye's hypothesis about the stress response, the body's way of dealing with stressful demands made upon it, is used as a backdrop in considering symptoms with probable or prominent emotional origins—that is, psychophysiological or psychosomatic disorders.
3. A review of hypotheses about the etiology of psychophysiological disorders indicates that "psychodynamic" explanations, special "body type" hypotheses, and the "organ vulnerability" approach have generally not received empirical support. Instead, more favorably viewed approaches are those that acknowledge individual differences in the nature and intensity of the body's response to stressful stimuli in interaction with learned factors.
4. Ulcers, which tend to run in families, are probably not as closely linked to personality type and emotional conflict as they were once thought to be. Although biochemical predisposition may be involved, not all people with the appropriate "chemistry" develop ulcers. Obviously, a more refined examination of the personal and environmental variables that contribute to the onset of this psychophysiological disorder, including the individual's appraisal of stressful situations, is required.

5. Cardiovascular problems, such as essential hypertension and coronary heart disease, may have strong emotional components. Certain personality types ("Type As") apparently show increased risk to coronary heart disease.
6. Although the etiology of disorders such as asthma and migraine headache is not entirely clear, these and many other psychophysiological disorders may reflect an interaction of personality factors and the individual's way of responding to stressful situations in physiologically prone individuals.
7. Sleep, which is not the passive opposite of wakefulness, is an active state that involves a regular, orderly sequence of events. There are four stages of sleep, each characterized by its own type of EEG pattern. Sleep researchers also differentiate between REM sleep and NREM sleep, which are also characterized by many physiological differences.
8. Sleep disorders such as insomnia, sleepwalking, sleep terrors, and narcolepsy were described. The study of sleep cycles, sleep disorders, and the function and origins of dreams offers many possibilities for understanding more about the brain and brain pathology.
9. Hypotheses in connection with the development of obesity include various psychodynamic explanations, Schachter's "externality hypothesis," and Nisbett's "fat cells" approach. It was concluded on the basis of the relevant literature that no one explanation for obesity accounts for all the facts.
10. Anorexia nervosa was described and illustrated. The evidence suggests that some organic or endocrinological dysfunction interacts with personal, familial and cultural variables to produce this condition.
11. Conversion symptoms, which are relatively easy to distinguish from "real" physical symptoms, are now extremely rare although they were once quite common. They seem to be easily treated by suggestion, hypnosis, and placebo, possibly explaining the "miracle cures" reported to have taken place in spiritual centers all over the world.
12. Although individual responses and sensitivity to pain may have a large learning component, there is evidence suggesting that brain biochemistry may play an important role in how the body defends against pain.

ISSUES AND QUESTIONS

1. You have seen that many physical disorders do not appear to have any organic basis. There is even evidence for "mass psychogenic illness." For example, a large number of women factory workers suddenly complained of such severe headache, dizziness, and weakness, that the plant had to be closed down (Peterson, 1979). No physical explanation, such as pollutants, poison, or other environmental stimuli were found.

   Such incidents of "contagious" psychogenic response are apparently more frequent than is generally thought to be the case. They tend to occur in highly structured, "assembly-line" social systems such as schools, prisons, and factories.

   It may be that employers could screen those at risk for such responses through "psychological profiles" based on test scores and interview ratings. Of course, many potential employees would be eliminated who might never display these symptoms, for such screening methods are not entirely accurate. What is your opinion about using psychological tools in this way? Whose rights should be protected, the potential employee or the employer?
2. Some critics of psychology claim that psychophysiological symptoms should be treated primarily through medical and physical remedies. These critics suggest that emotional and psychological factors be given, at best, secondary consideration, since there is only moderate

agreement as to their nature. They cite the time and expense involved as well as the disagreement among the experts as some of the reasons for questioning the routine referral of asthma or pain patients, for example, for psychotherapy. Do you agree? Remember, a strong case can be made out not only for psychological etiology, at least in part, for many of the syndromes described in this chapter, but also, for the impressive significance of psychological factors in the course and prognosis of *most* illnesses.

SUGGESTIONS FOR FURTHER READING

Bruch, H. *The golden cage: The enigma of anorexia nervosa.* New York: Vintage, 1979. The author, a specialist in anorexia nervosa, has written this book for easy reading by the lay person. The title refers to the feeling, common among anorexic patients, that they are a "sparrow in a golden cage." Often, according to Dr. Bruch, anorexic patients are bright, attractive adolescent girls from well-to-do homes. Despite these apparent advantages, they feel inadequate, unable to keep up with the standards of their golden cages and so starve themselves as a way of being different, special, and in control of their lives. Although the author's portrayal of anorexia nervosa reflects her own particular theoretical views and clinical experiences, this book is well worth reading, for the picture she paints is a vivid and compelling one of the physical and emotional pain suffered by victims of this disease.

Cartwright, R. D. *A primer on sleep and dreaming.* Reading, Mass.: Addison-Wesley, 1978. Paperback. This book provides an up-to-date introduction to research related to sleep and dreaming for use by both professionals and students. A brief account of the history of dream research and reviews of diverse aspects of sleep and dreaming are presented. This book also discusses clinical issues related to sleep disorders and the relevance of sleep patterns in understanding individual differences.

Dement, W. C. *Some must watch while some must sleep: Exploring the world of sleep.* San Francisco: Freeman, 1972. Paperback available. This book is delightful to read and informative as well. The author, a pioneer in sleep research, discusses scientific research into such questions as: Do we really need sleep? What function does sleep serve? What happens when we are dreaming? What causes insomnia and how does it feel? Why is it that serious sleep disturbances often accompany mental illness? These are just some of the issues presented by Dement in a readable, anecdotal, yet scholarly manner.

Glass, D. C. *Behavior patterns, stress, and coronary disease.* Hillsdale, New Jersey: Erlbaum, 1977. In this book, Glass presents in a clear, systematic manner, a series of experiments designed to explore the relationship between Type A behavior, methods for coping with and responding to stress, and coronary heart disease. Factors that may explain why certain people develop Type A behavior patterns are also explored. This book provides an excellent review of the literature on Type A behavior, stress, and coronary heart disease.

Selye, H. *The stress of life.* New York: McGraw-Hill, 1978. Rev. ed. Paperback. This popular book is a revision of the classic, first published in 1956. The author's original explorations, dating back to 1936, demonstrated a relationship between various diseases and the body's stress response to injury, harm, threat, and invasion from an outside source (such as germs). Selye's work, perhaps more than any other single body of research, laid the groundwork for much of the current thinking about stress, life events, and "psychophysiological" disease. This book is not only of general interest but also provides an excellent annotated list of books on stress.

9

Anxiety, Dissociative, and Personality Disorders

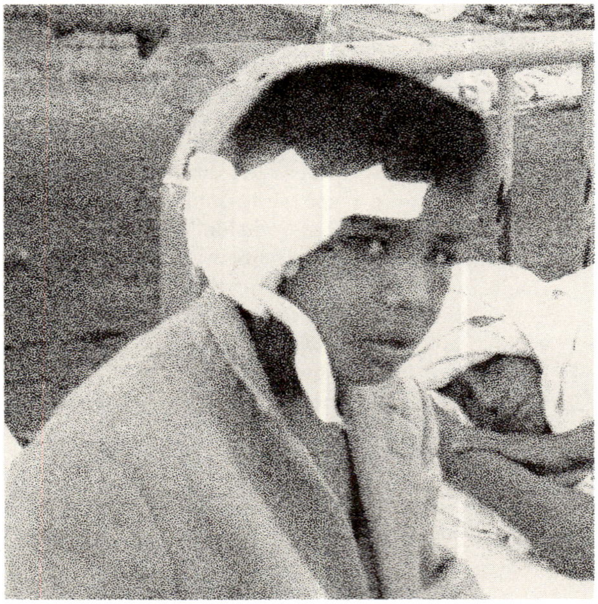

This chapter surveys most of the clinical syndromes labeled neuroses or psychoneuroses. These syndromes roughly share a common ground: the ways in which anxiety and conflict are handled. In addition, they are usually differentiated from the psychoses along several important dimensions noted in this chapter.

The neuroses usually include the conversion disorders, now classified by the DSM-III with the somatoform disorders (see Chapter 8). The neuroses have also traditionally included neurotic depressions, which will be discussed in Chapter 10.

Anxiety is a distressing emotional state characterized by high levels of autonomic arousal and strong feelings of tension, apprehension, and anticipated dread, often of an irrational nature. Because anxiety is such a central concept in this and other chapters, we will take a closer look at it later.

Section II of this chapter considers a group of syndromes referred to as personality disorders. These are usually classified neither as psychoses nor as neuroses. Yet they are associated with extremely maladaptive behavior patterns that are often quite disruptive both to those people who manifest them and to others with whom they are involved.

SECTION I
ANXIETY AND SOME OF THE NEUROTIC DISORDERS

WHAT ARE THE NEUROSES AND HOW DO THEY DIFFER FROM THE PSYCHOSES?

The psychoneuroses are mild forms of emotional disturbance, rarely requiring hospitalization and generally characterized by an underlying current of great anxiety and conflict. Clinicians usually distinguish the psychoneuroses from the psychoses, which are more severe forms of emotional disturbance. Dividing lines and boundaries in the arena of human behavior and pathology are rarely clearcut. Drawing the specific boundaries between the neuroses and psychoses therefore is no easy task. And yet such distinctions often make the difference in the choice of treatment offered the patient—for example, whether hospitalization is recommended or a major tranquilizer introduced.

1. Although there are instances in which a severe form of neurosis can be more painful or incapacitating than a milder form of psychosis, a distinguishing feature sometimes employed is severity. It is thought that the psychoses involve more personal disorganization, incapacitation, and disruption of daily living than do the neuroses.

2. Another distinguishing feature is overall adjustment. People with neuroses are thought to function better in most life areas than those with psychoses, to have a greater capacity to relate to others, and to conform to social standards. Psychotics, especially those who have been chronically disturbed, are less able than are neurotics to get along with others in social situations, probably because of personal eccentricity.

3. Still another major distinction between neurotic and psychotic disturbances is the degree of reality testing present. Reality testing generally comprises the group of behaviors and actions that people engage in as they ascertain whether something really works—is true or valid. It is the capacity to determine the boundaries, limits, and contours of the real, external world as separated from the subjective, internal world. In psychotic conditions there may be mild to extreme impairment of this ability, for example, hallucinations or delusions. There may be disorientation in time and place, and confusion about personal identity—where I am and who I am. In neurotic conditions, however (with the exception, perhaps, of certain dissociative states, see pp. 210–15), there is generally intact awareness of reality.

4. Related to reality testing skills is the degree of insight that the patient has into his or her emotions and condition. People with neurotic symptoms often have greater insight into their disturbance than do psychotics.

5. Chapter 6, when discussing defense mechanisms, noted that at one time or another all of us employ various maneuvers for reducing anxiety. However, there seems to be more extreme, per-

Listing 9.1 DSM-III Categories Described in Chapter 9

Section I*

Anxiety Disorders

- Phobic disorders (or Phobic neurosis)
  - Agoraphobia with panic attacks
  - Agoraphobia without panic attacks
  - Social phobia
  - Simple phobia
- Anxiety states (or Anxiety neuroses)
  - Panic disorder
  - Generalized anxiety disorder
  - Obsessive-compulsive disorder (obsessive-compulsive neurosis)
    - Atypical anxiety disorder
    - Posttraumatic stress disorder
      - Acute
      - Chronic or delayed

Anxiety Disorders of Childhood

- Separation anxiety disorder
- Avoidant disorder of childhood or adolescence
- Overanxious disorder

* The listings in Section I are generally classified as neuroses or psychoneuroses in the DSM-II and in traditional classification systems. The conversion disorders described in Chapter 8 are also usually classified with the neuroses, as are the dysthymic disorders or depressive neuroses described in Chapter 10.

Dissociative Disorders (Hysterical Neuroses, Dissociative Type)

- Psychogenic amnesia
- Psychogenic fugue
- Multiple personality
- Depersonalization disorder (depersonalization neurosis)

Section II

Personality Disorders

- Paranoid personality disorder
- Schizoid personality disorder (or Schizoid disorder in childhood or adolescence)
- Schizotypal personality disorder
- Histrionic personality disorder
- Narcissistic personality disorder
- Antisocial personality disorder (in children, Conduct disorders)
- Borderline personality disorder (Identity disorder in childhood or adolescence)
- Avoidant personality disorder (Avoidant disorder of childhood or adolescence)
- Dependent personality disorder
- Compulsive personality disorder
- Passive-aggressive personality disorder (Oppositional disorder in children)

sistent, and florid use of defense mechanisms in psychotic conditions than there is in most neurotic conditions. Psychotic regression, for example, is a very dramatic state. The psychotic may behave as if he or she were a child, defecating and urinating in clothing, using baby talk, or crawling on all fours. It is rare for neurotics to display such extreme behavior, although they may well use the mechanism of regression in a more moderate way to ease their subjective discomfort.

6. The emotional outbursts, swings, and behavior changes displayed by many psychotic patients are generally much more extreme, less comprehensible, and less in tune with what is happening in the real situation surrounding them than is the case for people with neurotic conditions.

7. The psychotic expresses the primary process material described in Chapter 6—the inner, private thoughts, fantasies, desires, and dreamlike material—more than does the neurotic. Neurotics tend to go to rather extreme lengths to repress this material, preventing it from surfacing to the level of subjective experience and objective expression.

8. Finally, many psychotic patients, especially those diagnosed with schizophrenia, show disordered thought processes in judgment, reasoning,

and problem-solving. Chapters 11 and 12, which describe schizophrenia, elaborate on these and other features of psychotic conditions.

Incidence

According to most authorities, the major portion of a mental-health practitioner's practice is devoted to the diagnosis and treatment of the neuroses. Many surveys indicate that 30 to 40 percent of patients who seek help at hospitals, clinics, and private offices suffer primarily from a neurotic problem (Kolb, 1973). Other estimates suggest that anywhere from one in five to one in ten people can be regarded as neurotic or as showing neurotic symptoms, and that women are characterized in this way more frequently than are men (Chesler, 1972; Kolb, 1973; Rosenthal, 1971). The high incidence figures of neurotic conditions may actually underrepresent their occurrence in the general population because many neurotic states are probably undiagnosed and unrecorded.

Among children, boys are more frequently diagnosed as showing neurosis than girls until adolescence, when this pattern is reversed (Eme, 1979). The causes of these disparities may contain a large cultural component, for example, differing expectations and diagnoses for boys and girls or for men and women.

THE CLINICAL SYNDROMES: ANXIETY DISORDERS

The anxiety disorders described in the following pages have in common either the subjective experience of anxiety or symptoms that arise from the individual's attempts to deal with intense anxiety. Spotlight 9.1 describes what anxiety feels like and some of its physiological manifestations.

Spotlight 9.1 Symptoms of Anxiety

What are the symptoms of anxiety? How can they be recognized? In most anxiety states there is typically some form of motor tension (tics, shakiness, postural "tightness"), a sense of apprehension and dread, intense autonomic arousal, and excessive watchfulness and vigilance—a kind of overalertness to the possibilities of being overwhelmed by acute panic. Also, somatization disorders (see Chapter 8) may sometimes accompany anxiety states. That is, there is an accompanying focus on aches, pains, and bodily discomforts, but these, unlike conversion and psychophysiological disorders, tend to be constantly shifting in quality, intensity, and location.

Translated into specific symptoms, the array of possible indicators of anxiety is truly impressive. In addition to subjective sense of dread, these include difficulties in falling asleep, recurrent, terrifying nightmares, facial tics, bodily tensions, tremors of the hand, jitteriness, restless movements (fidgetiness), startle responses, interruptions of the flow of speech, such as stammering, changes in blood pressure and heart rate, faintness, dizziness, diarrhea, nausea, a feeling of choking or inability to breathe, increased perspiration, pallor, and occasionally, in extreme states, confusion and disorganization with accompanying panic.

Anxiety can appear in many different forms. Anxiety levels can be low or intense; anxiety can be persistent or episodic. Sudden acute episodes of anxiety can last a few minutes to an hour or more. These episodes are called anxiety attacks and often occur at night, awakening the sleeper abruptly, catapulting him or her into a state of terror. Some anxiety states can have specific content. For example, one rare form of anxiety disorder specifically focuses on the dread and danger of an impending disease, such as cancer. Typically, however, anxiety is felt as a vague, free-floating fear, unattached to specific content or to real danger.

Case 9.1 Steven: Phobic Disorder

Steven is a thirty-five-year-old engineer for a huge corporation in the suburbs of one of the big cities. His field is computers, and he is in charge of training a large staff of engineers who sell computers. He has successfully trained many "waves" of engineers from all over the country using the facilities, conference rooms, and technical hardware at the home office. He is intelligent, charming, and poised, and is married to a social worker in the community mental-health clinic. They have a three-year-old boy.

Steven and his wife just bought a ranch house in preparation for their next child, for his wife is in her fourth month of pregnancy. Almost simultaneously, he was given a promotion and a huge raise. Sounds ideal? It may not be your idea of the good life, but it had been Steven's dream. The only problem was that, to the surprise of all concerned, Steven turned down the offer. A few weeks later, he sought help for depression, excessive drinking, and unemployment.

What happened was this: Steven had been a phobic person for years. He was an organized and meticulous person who inhibited the expression of his emotions. Ten years ago, on his way to meet the first wave of computer engineers at a sales conference twenty miles from the home office, he became panicky and could not get himself to drive over a high bridge that spanned a wide river. He telephoned his wife, who managed to get to him. She drove him over the bridge in their car while he crouched fearfully on the floor of the back seat. He arrived late for his meeting and was so shaken up that he had to leave early. Since that time, his irrational fear of bridges had generalized to driving cars. He was almost always fearful of reexperiencing the acute panic he had felt—of losing control and "going crazy" in front of others. He "solved" his problem by avoiding all such risks.

Since that time, he worked things out sufficiently well, he thought, so as to get on with his life. This took a good deal of planning, but it worked. His wife drove him to work each day. By going twenty miles upstate (and twenty miles downstate), he avoided high bridges. He had his salespeople come to him. He rarely had to travel anywhere because conferences, presentations, and sales meetings were always at the home office. He stayed at the office later than the others, giving an impression of dedicated ambition. In reality, this was the way he avoided the embarrassment of having his wife pick him up each evening. He also turned down after-hours meetings, cocktails with colleagues, and anything else that required driving.

During this period Steven was at ease, except for twinges of anxiety when he had to turn down certain business invitations. For ten years he managed to impress his supervisors, eventually earning the promotion mentioned earlier. Then his world collapsed! For with his new job went new responsibilities: the training of regional personnel in twenty states all over the country rather than in the home office. This would entail flying to the nearest city, renting a car, and meeting with salespeople in their offices; then, again in cars, the group was expected to visit potential customers so that they (the salespeople) could be observed making their presentations. No wonder he panicked!

When Steven first came for help, he and the therapist both participated in a detailed assessment procedure (see Chapter 20) followed by appropriate behavioral interventions designed to eliminate his phobias. Gradually he learned to take increasing risks toward reaching the goals of showing up at work, driving over high bridges (at first with help from his wife), and traveling to distances from home. Finally he was helped to learn to go about the business of his new job. He is still a bit shaken by his experiences and continues in psychotherapy to help him to better understand "what happened."

Phobic Disorders (Phobic Neuroses)

Phobias are avoidance responses arising from an irrational fear of social or interpersonal situations (for example, public speaking), or activities (for example, driving through tunnels), or things (for example, bugs, snakes, or pigeons). The DSM-III states that 1 to 5 percent of the general population suffers from phobic symptoms, and that these symptoms appear most often among women. Although the patient knows that his or her fear is unreasonable, for there is no real threat or harm, the phobia guards the person from experiencing fear by simply arranging circumstances so that the feared situation, activity, or thing is avoided. Phobic patients thus do not actively experience fear or anxiety as a primary symptom.

Many phobic people report that they initially experience intense anxiety or panic in connection with an essentially harmless situation or object. This, they continue, is followed by sturdy, ingrained avoidance responses. These avoidance responses soon generalize to many situations or circumstances that carry risks of exposure to the feared situation or object. For example, avoidance of elevators generalizes to windowless rooms, tunnels, and other enclosed spaces. Phobic patients state that they think that they might "go crazy," "fall apart," or be helplessly victimized by extreme panic if exposed to the feared situation.

Phobias are generally categorized into several types. The most common and the most severely incapacitating is agoraphobia, with or without panic attacks. People with agoraphobia avoid public places, crowds, streets, and unfamiliar situations. In the most severe form, the phobic person retreats entirely and is housebound. Most often, however, people with agoraphobia are able to perform daily routines, such as work, but often need to be accompanied by a close intimate or family member for psychological support.

Social phobias include some familiar ones such as fear of public speaking or of eating or of writing in front of others. A common phobia in males is of urinating in public toilets. One patient, for example, had gone from job to job until he found the perfect one in an advertising agency: he was given a key to a private men's toilet which he shared with only two other men.

Simple phobias include the avoidance of specific objects or activities, for example, furry animals, insects, rats, snakes, pigeons, knives, or windows. Simple phobias also include those for heights and enclosed spaces; the latter is called claustrophobia, fear of small enclosed spaces, such as elevators or airless rooms. Fear of flying frequently reflects claustrophobia rather than the fear of an accident.

The DSM-III describes a related disorder, common in children and adolescents, called separation anxiety disorder. This syndrome has much in common with agoraphobia and is characterized by extreme anxiety in situations that involve separation from a close figure, such as a parent. Children with separation anxiety are often excessively concerned about the parents' involvement in a major catastrophe; or they fear that the parents, out for dinner, will never return; if they are not with their parents, they fear that they will be kidnapped, hurt in an accident, or killed.

People with intense fear of heights would avoid occupations like window-washing. Their phobic responses, thus, would permit them to be free of anxiety in connection with the feared situation. (Steven M. Stone/The Picture Cube)

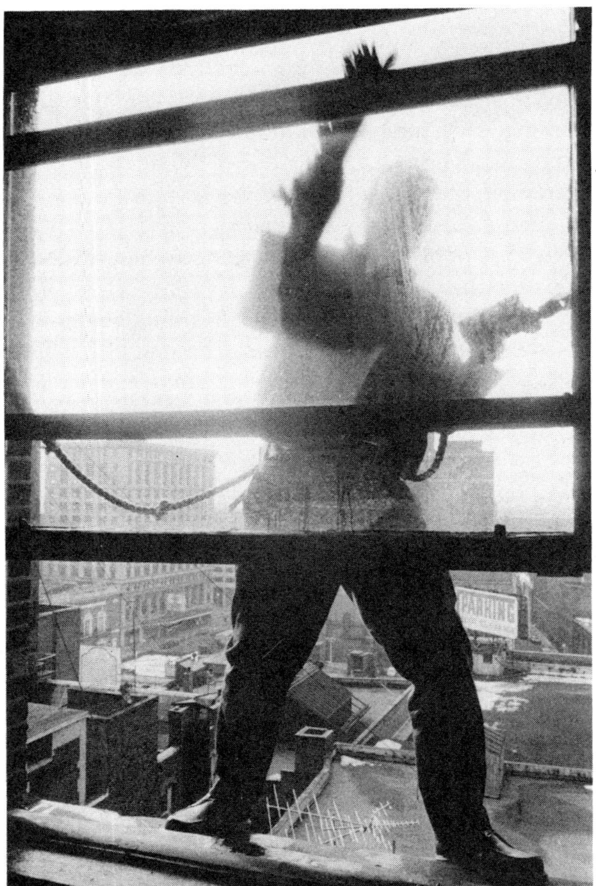

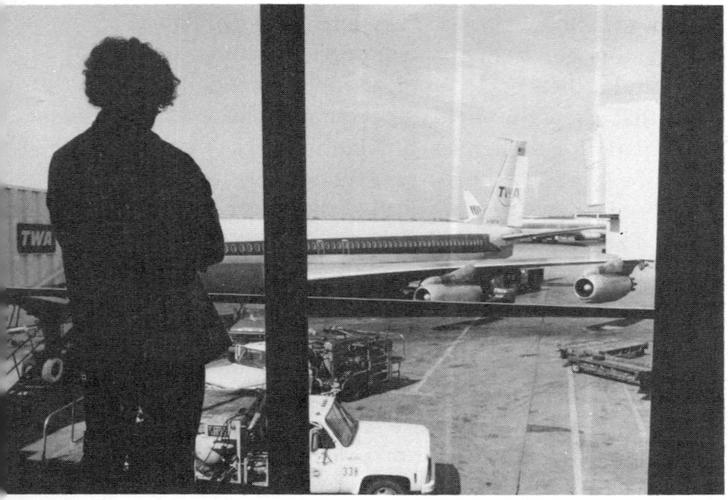

Fear of flying often reflects claustrophobia rather than the more "rational" fear of an accident. (Read D. Brugger/The Picture Cube)

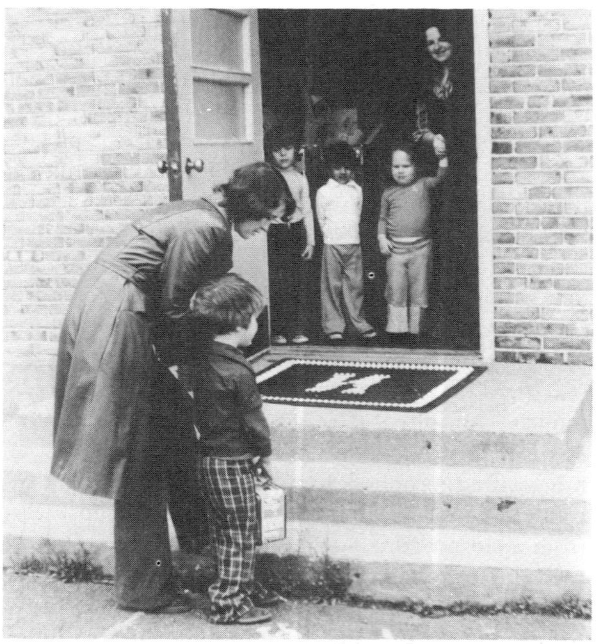

Separation anxiety disorders in children are often expressed as school phobias; but they can also be manifested by fear of being alone in bed at night. (Elizabeth Barry/The Picture Cube)

Separation anxiety disorders are often expressed as school phobias (reluctance or refusal to go to school) or as sleep problems, for example, fear of being alone in bed at nighttime. These disorders are sometimes accompanied by various physical symptoms such as headache or nausea before going to school, nightmares with separation themes, and extreme agitation (sometimes panic) in anticipation of separation from the attachment figure.

Anxiety States (Anxiety Neuroses)

Panic disorders. Some people experience sudden, heightened levels of intense autonomic activity of an acutely distressing nature called panic. Episodes of panic are characteristically accompanied by feelings that one is "going crazy," losing control, or dying. Panic is most commonly associated with an intense, overpowering urge to flee. Physiological symptoms include paresthesias (sensations such as prickling, burning, tingling of the skin), breathing problems, heart pounding, feelings of choking, lightheadedness, dizziness, feelings of unreality, fainting, sweating, trembling, and inability to talk. Panic attacks occur more frequently among women than men, according to the DSM-III.

Panic disorders are distinguished from the panic that phobic people experience when forced to confront the feared situation, for they most often occur without clearcut external stimuli, usually taking the individual by surprise. The panic that may be a consequence of a life-threatening situation (a threatened rape, assault, or near collision, for example) is not regarded as a panic disorder.

Generalized anxiety disorders. These anxiety disorders are characterized by persistent feelings of anxiety with symptoms of the sort described in Spotlight 9.1, such as restlessness, jitteriness, trembling, lightheadedness, pounding of the heart, sweating, and so on. Present also is a sense of dread, apprehension, and anticipated catastrophe accompanied by a constant vigilance (watchfulness and hyperattentiveness) as to possible danger. *But*

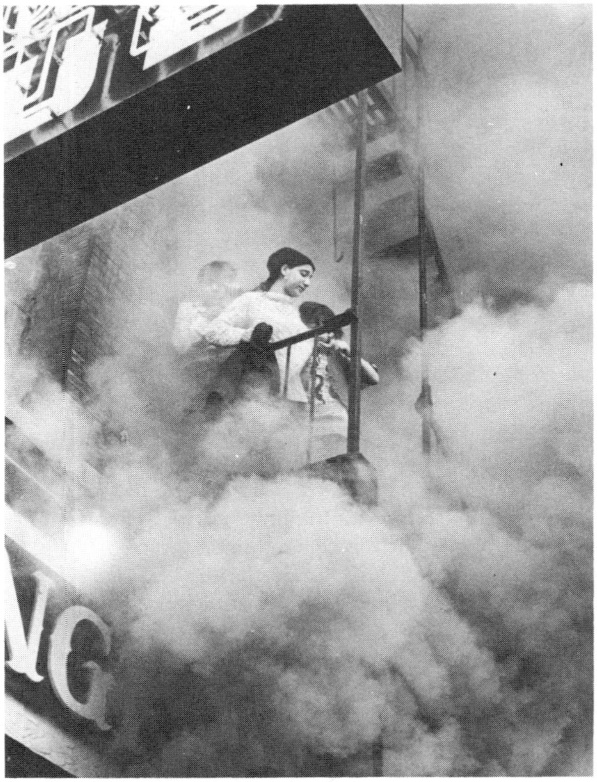

Panic that involves intensely disturbing autonomic responses might arise in a situation, such as this one, from which there is no escape. Panic disorders, however, generally involve acutely distressing episodes of panic when there is no external cause. (Jack Prelutsky/Stock, Boston)

no immediate or real danger is present. That is, the distress typically does not arise as a response to stressors or to life events such as a death in the family.

According to the DSM-III no information is currently available as to the gender distribution of adult anxiety disorders, but among children the pattern (called over-anxious disorder), occurs more often among boys than among girls, and is frequently accompanied by worry about future events, overconcern with competence, excessive need for reassurance, somatic complaints with no physical basis, self-consciousness, and susceptibility to embarrassment.

Obsessive-compulsive disorders (obsessive-compulsive neuroses). These disorders are characterized by recurrent obsessions, compulsions, or both. Obsessions are unwanted, persistent thoughts, ideas, images, or urges that enter one's mind without conscious intent. Compulsions are irresistible, involuntary recurrent acts—also without conscious intent—such as repeated hand-washing or button-touching rituals. The DSM-III notes that about 2 percent of the general population receives a diagnosis of obsessive disorder. Incidence and gender distribution of compulsive disorders are not reported.

People with these obsessive-compulsive disorders regard their obsessions or compulsions as irrational and senseless (although children may not do so). As a matter of fact, symptoms are generally regarded as ego-dystonic—unwanted, unacceptable, repugnant to the person experiencing them. Examples of behaviors that do not qualify as reflecting an obsessive-compulsive disorder because they are not ego-dystonic or ego-alien are brooding and worrying about an examination or public appearance, as unpleasant as these preoccupations (ruminations) may be. According to the DSM-III, excessive eating or gambling are sometimes erroneously called compulsive eating or gambling; but these are not true compulsions because they are not ego-alien, that is, these activities are often pleasurable, sought-after behaviors.

One form of obsessive thinking has been called, in French, *folie du doute* (roughly, "madness of doubting"). People with this pattern are characterized by an inability to make decisions and to be endlessly in doubt about their behavior. They check and recheck an act, convinced that it was never completed or even attempted. Obsessive patients may return again and again to check the burners on the stove and the electric lights in the house before going out, always doubting, never feeling secure. Even while doing so they may be aware of the irrational nature of these persistent and recurrent thoughts. Some obsessive content may reflect taboo areas, such as incestuous desires toward a member of one's family or murderous feelings toward a "loved one." The stronger the efforts to dispel such

Case 9.2 Tom: Anxiety Disorder

When Tom was eighteen years old and a senior in high school, he recalls being at the "top of the heap." He was a star athlete on the football team, popular, and a very good student. Although he sometimes worried about grades (he was much more conscientious than his teammates), he always felt happy. He said he had no physical or social complaints at that time. Before exams he occasionally had difficulty falling asleep, and on rare occasions, recalls even having had nightmares. But he was used to this infrequent pattern and did not worry about it. His parents were proud of him and he felt good about their approval.

Two years later he tried out for the sophomore team in a big Eastern university. He not only failed to make the team but also was severely criticized by the coach for some misplay in the tryout period. Soon after, his grades fell and he began to stammer and to develop facial tics. At nighttime, instead of occasional difficulty in falling asleep, a new pattern emerged: a few hours of sleep were interrupted by an "anxiety attack" forcing him to suddenly sit up in bed gasping for breath. At these times he felt his heart beating so rapidly that he thought he was going to die. He reported feeling terrified. After several weeks of suffering in this way, he refused to lie down in bed for he was extremely fearful of falling asleep and then being overcome by intense, overwhelming anxiety. He dropped out of college and returned home.

Tom's parents finally convinced him to seek treatment, which he did by first consulting their family physician for an appropriate referral. After a year of twice-weekly psychotherapy, he returned to college.

Tom's acute picture of anxiety was treated through medication and some "traditional" talking therapy during which time he came to understand his symptoms and their connection to his conflicts about achievement. With reassurance and continued therapy, he learned that he was not dying and that his physical complaints were triggered by emotional events. He learned also that criticism or failure to meet some standard did not mean that love and friendship would be taken away from him. He learned that his strong need to please authorities arose from his desire to please his parents, a method of dealing with anxiety that he learned early in life. He discovered in therapy that when he was quite young, he anticipated all possible criticisms—structuring his life so that a minimum of criticism (and supervision) would be directed to him.

Tom also began to realize that he had had little experience dealing with anxiety, and was totally unprepared for it when he felt its full impact. When he accepted his low tolerance for anxiety, and saw that he could live through such experiences without dying, his dread of its possible appearance began to lessen. Thus, with the aid of some specific therapeutic techniques, he gradually developed more adequate ways of dealing with his world.

Today, Tom occasionally experiences tension, nightmares, and fleeting anxiety. But most of his symptoms have subsided. He no longer experiences acute anxiety attacks, is currently doing well at college, feels physically fit, and plans to go to graduate school.

obsessions, the more persistent these obsessions seem to become. It is extremely rare for such taboo thoughts to be actually carried out, however.

One patient, for example, an eminent pediatrician, was plagued by the recurrent rumination that she wished to choke the babies she was treating. With support in the therapeutic situation, she forced herself to continue her medical practice, knowing that her intense subjective distress and fear were symptoms—traced to earlier wishes and guilt—that would not be enacted. And indeed, they were not enacted. She experienced less and less anxiety with successive years of practice, although her fears and obsessions never subsided completely.

Many people experience senseless repeated ideas. Examples include a tune that keeps running through one's mind or words that repeatedly pop into one's consciousness. Some people may experience urges to laugh out loud or to shout obscenities in a public place such as in church or at a lecture—desires that may be repugnant to them. Obsessional thoughts, however, are often not as innocuous as these examples. For obsessional thoughts are generally extremely distressing and guilt-and anxiety-producing to the people who experience them.

A common compulsion reflects a preoccupation with cleanliness and neatness. Often a patient exhibits an excessive fear of becoming diseased or contaminated by contact with something others have touched. People who suffer from this type of compulsive disorder are trapped by their symptoms. For they must compulsively wash their hands after touching a doorknob or railing, are often "forced" to wear gloves even in stifling weather, or feel themselves compelled to wash anything before touching it. Many patients are helpless prey to a continuous dread that they have failed to wash themselves properly. Often they perform elaborate rituals, such as complicated prayers and incantations or placing objects of furniture in a certain design. Simpler compulsive rituals such as touching, counting, skipping certain cracks or lines on sidewalks, and other "magical" rites appear most often among children, and tend to disappear with age.

Many patients report that attempts to resist the urge to act out a compulsion are met with a rising sense of tension and anxiety—until they "give in." Yet they feel that they can "almost" control their behavior but would feel extremely distressed and anxious were they to do so. Recently developed therapeutic methods offer many such patients strategies for employing self-control techniques to help them deal with this dilemma.

Posttraumatic Stress Disorders

The person has been back from Vietnam for about one and a half years. He has done ostensibly well, has been able to get a job and to marry. He feels somewhat estranged from his peers at work and does not discuss combat experiences with them. Recently he has begun to have difficulty sleeping, has intrusive daytime images and some nightmares of combat scenes although not necessarily one repetitive "story." These commonly involve atrocities whether or not he was involved in committing them himself.

During the daytime he is often suspicious and, when frustrated or in fear-arousing situations, feels that he is in great danger of losing control over his hostile and aggressive impulses. With growing hostility and suspicion he may conceal firearms to protect himself. There is also fear of going crazy and guilt over his own pleasurable responses to his intrusive ideas of committing severe physical violence to others. There may be startle reactions, psychosomatic syndromes, anxiety attacks, loss of motivation and depression.

The person often turns to drugs such as heroin or sedatives because they temporarily relieve the depressive, anxious, fearful and hostile mood states. Interpersonal difficulties may supervene because of the patient's continued and uncontrollable suspicions, moodiness, surly behavior or excessive dependency. Threats by the person are frequent and will also alienate interested friends and family members. The person wants to ward off any reminders that may create intrusive and repetitive experiences and will tend to be defensive in any inquiry by others as to his past experience. . . .

Horowitz and Solomon, 1978, p. 272

The foregoing is a "composite" based on real veterans of the war in Vietnam.

Returning war veterans have been extensively studied through interviews and observations (Figley, 1978; Grinker and Spiegel, 1945; Haley, 1978; Kardiner, 1943; Neff, 1975; and Shatan, 1978). Many veterans display behaviors after returning home that resemble the anxiety symptoms described in Spotlight 9.1. However, in addition to these symptoms, for example, startle responses to sudden stimuli (new or similar to original combat stimuli), also found are explosive aggressive reactions, suspiciousness, restlessness, guilt, and a sense of interpersonal alienation and detachment. These reactions can be immediate or delayed and have been variously called battle fatigue, traumatic war neurosis, or combat neurosis.

Although observations such as the foregoing have been reported since World War I, only recently have clinicians concluded that some people respond in similar fashion to other types of ca-

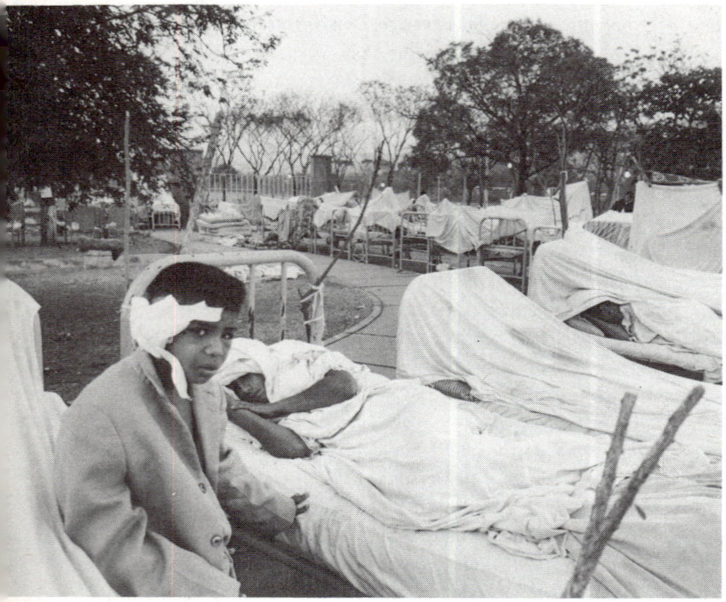

Psychological symptoms can emerge immediately or months after a natural catastrophe, such as an earthquake, and can be acute or chronic. (© Sepp Seitz 1980/Woodfin Camp)

tastrophic events, and that these responses form a more or less predictable pattern or syndrome. In the light of increasing clinical experience with victims and survivors of various traumatic stressors that are generally outside of the range of ordinary experience, the DSM-III now includes appropriate diagnostic categories of a more formal nature than did the earlier DSM editions. These are the posttraumatic stress disorders, classified as either acute, in which symptoms appear within six months of the trauma, or chronic or delayed, in which symptoms last for over six months and/or appear many months, even years, after the severe stressor.

The severe stressors that can provoke these disorders cover a wide range and include not only the experiences of combat but also such traumas as rape or attempted rape. Natural disasters, such as floods and earthquakes, and socially induced traumatic experiences, for example, concentration camp or prisoner-of-war internment, large fires, airplane crashes, and victimization as a hostage are also capable of eliciting emotional difficulties of intense, extremely maladaptive proportions.

Typically the patient may experience a brief stress response immediately after the stressor that includes painful resurgence into consciousness of the trauma and nightmares that recapture the anguish of the event. There may, in some instances, be a "psychic numbing," in which the individual feels dazed, distanced, strange, and detached from the world around him or her. Acute symptoms of terror and autonomic arousal might follow soon afterward, or onset of symptoms can be delayed up to fifteen years after the catastrophic event and can persist for decades (Klonoff et al., 1976). For example, a study of a marine explosion resulting from a collision at sea in which ten men were killed disclosed that most of the survivors reported some symptoms, such as sleep disturbances and "nervousness," immediately after the disaster. However, symptoms tended to *increase,* rather than decrease, over a four-year period (Leopold and Dillon, 1963).

Acute or delayed symptoms include some or many of the following (these may be intensified in circumstances that contain elements present during the traumatic event): depression, anxiety and subjective distress, heightened autonomic responsiveness and arousal, concentration and memory difficulties, headache and dizziness, suspiciousness, irritability, impulsivity, explosive aggressiveness, nightmares, and various types of sleep disturbances.

DISSOCIATIVE DISORDERS

Dissociation refers to a group of dramatic behaviors with a common thread.* This thread is a loss, modification, or dramatic change in consciousness (awareness), identity, or motor behavior. It is as if

* Despite the usual assumption of the psychogenic nature of all such disorders, follow-up studies of some instances of dissociative disorders tend to implicate organic etiology, such as head injury with concussion, in a number of these cases (Martin, 1971).

certain aspects of an individual's functions become detached or "dissociated" from other aspects: the individual no longer functions as a whole. These behaviors include psychogenic amnesia, psychogenic fugue, multiple personality, and depersonalization disorder (depersonalization neurosis).

Psychogenic amnesia. This disorder, in which the etiology does not lie in some physical disturbance, such as a blow on the head or a brain tumor, is characterized by a sudden inability to retrieve personal information from one's memory. The memory disturbance is more dramatic and inclusive than is ordinary forgetfulness. Often there is a severe social or interpersonal stressor (bombing in wartime, combat duty) that precipitates the amnesic period. According to the DSM-III, psychogenic amnesia rarely occurs in the elderly, appearing most often in young adult females and young males in combat. Amnesic states frequently end as suddenly as they begin, and they rarely reoccur.

There are several kinds of psychogenic amnesias. They are localized amnesia, in which the patient cannot remember anything immediately after an extremely stressful event, such as a flash flood or ravaging fire; selective amnesia, in which the patient is unable to recall only some events but has no difficulty with others; generalized amnesia (quite rare), in which the patient cannot recall any aspects of his or her life; and continuous amnesia, in which the patient cannot recall events or identity from a specific time in the past to the present.

Psychogenic fugue. This relatively rare state, which tends to occur during great disasters, wartime, or after an acutely distressing event, involves actual physical flight from the traumatic situation accompanied by an abrupt cessation of usual routine activities and an assumption of a new identity. Psychogenic fugue states are diagnosed only when they are without an organic basis. According to the DSM-III, there is no information about gender distribution of this disorder.

Typically, the individual in a fugue state is in a daze, without awareness as to how he or she entered the new pattern of behavior and "identity." He or she may travel for weeks, appearing "normal" to an unknowing stranger. Suddenly the individual "returns" to the former self and to awareness of who he or she is, confused and perplexed as to the strangeness of the new surroundings. Generally, there is complete amnesia for the circumstances preceding the onset of the fugue state.

Multiple personality. The most dramatic of the dissociative states is multiple personality, sometimes called "dual personality." This state does not refer to "split personality," a phrase sometimes inappropriately applied to schizophrenia. In states of multiple personality, two or more dramatically different personalities can coexist in the same person for a short period of time to several years. This rare disorder is most common in young adult females. Onset is sudden, and shifts from one personality to another generally appear after a severe stressor.

Frequently, the prime or "dominant" personality has no awareness of the other personalities. The alternate personality (or personalities) is often somewhat aware of the prime personality, however. Often the prime personality is shy, inhibited, and

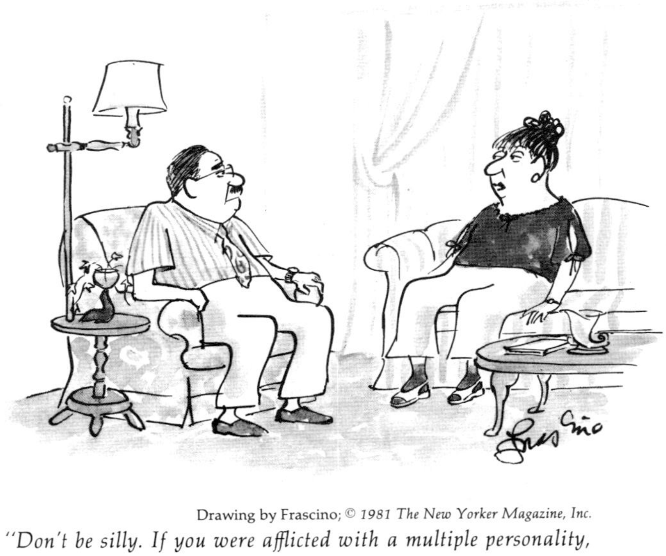

Drawing by Frascino; © 1981 *The New Yorker Magazine, Inc.*

"Don't be silly. If you were afflicted with a multiple personality, I'd have noticed something."

conventional whereas the other personality is aggressive, seductive, sexually flamboyant, and harsh.

Instances of multiple personality are extremely rare, but are so absorbingly dramatic that they tend to be described in great detail in the clinical literature. Their stories also appear in movies, TV, and the popular press. Spotlight 9.2 presents a case study of Eve, who suffered from multiple personality. A movie and several publications were based on Eve's story.

Clinical data from Eve (and from Evelyn, another case of multiple personality who was thirty-one years old when referred for treatment and diagnosis, see Jeans, 1976) were analyzed in a "blind" procedure in which psychologists interpreted test responses from the different personalities without knowing which of the personalities they came from (Osgood and Luria, 1954; Osgood, Luria, and Smith, 1976). The test was the Semantic Differential Test (Osgood, Suci, and Tannenbaum, 1957),

Spotlight 9.2 A Case of Multiple Personality: The Three Faces of Eve

Although many nineteenth-century physicians described cases of dual and multiple personalities, many clinicians readily admit that they have rarely, if ever, encountered as dramatic a case as Eve, who has been described in detail by Thigpen and Cleckley (1954, 1957).

Eve White was a twenty-five-year-old married woman being treated for severe headache, marital conflicts, and various emotional difficulties. There was a history of occasional blackouts after a headache, and at least one report of a trip the patient made for which she had complete amnesia. Hypnosis cleared up the amnesia immediately.

In a relatively early interview, Eve appeared agitated, distressed, and reported hearing voices. During this interview Eve White suddenly became a totally different person. She referred to Eve White as "she" or "her" and in manner, style, language, gesture, eye motions, use of language, quality of voice, and general expression, she differed dramatically from Eve White, who was a controlled, demure, self-contained, and conventional person. The new personality called herself Eve Black. The amazed therapist was in a state of wonderment and awe as Eve Black emerged during the course of therapy as a distinct, strong, and colorful personality, distinguished from her counterpart in thousands of different ways:

Eve White	Eve Black
Demure, retiring, in some respects almost saintly	Obviously a party girl. Shrewd, childishly vain, and egocentric
Face suggests a quiet sweetness; the expression in repose is predominately one of contained sadness	Face is pixie-like; eyes dance with mischief as if Puck peered through the pupils
Clothes: simple and conservative, neat and inconspicuously attractive	Expression rapidly shifts in a light cascade of fun-loving willfulness. The eyes are as inconstant as the wind. This face has not and will never know sadness. Often it reflects a misleading and only half-true naiveté
Posture: tendency to a barely discernible stoop or slump. Movements careful and dignified	
Reads poetry and likes to compose verse herself	Voice a little coarsened, "discultured," with echoes or implications of mirth and teasing. Speech richly vernacular and liberally seasoned with spontaneous gusts of rowdy wit
Almost all who know her express admiration and affection for her. She does not provoke envy. Her	

Eve White	Eve Black
strength of character is more passive than active. Steadfast on defense but lacking initiative and boldness to formulate strategy of attack	A devotee of pranks. Her repeated irresponsibilities have cruel results on others. More heedless and unthinking, however, than deeply malicious. Enjoys taunting and mocking the Siamese alternate
Consistently uncritical of others. Tries not to blame husband for marital troubles. Nothing suggests pretense or hypocrisy in this charitable attitude	All attitudes and passions whimlike and momentary. Quick and vivid flares of many light feelings, all ephemeral
Though not stiffly prudish and never self-righteous, she is seldom lively or playful or inclined to tease or tell a joke. Seldom animated	Immediately likable and attractive. A touch of sexiness seasons every word and gesture. Ready for any little, irresponsible adventure
Her presence resonates unexpressed devotion to her child. Every act, every gesture, the demonstrated sacrifice of personal aims to work hard for her little girl, is consistent with this love	Dress is becoming and a little provocative. Posture and gait suggest lightheartedness, play, a challenge to some sort of frolic
Cornered by bitter circumstances, threatened with tragedy, her endeavors to sustain herself, to defend her child, are impressive	Never comtemplative; to be serious is for her to be tedious or absurd
This role in one essentially so meek and fragile embodies an unspoken pathos. One feels somehow she is doomed to be overcome in her present situation	

Source: C. H. Thigpen and H. M. Cleckley, A case of multiple personality, *Journal of Abnormal and Social Psychology, 49,* 141–42.

After many sessions, Eve Black's personality came to be better understood. In contrast to Eve White, who knew nothing at all about Eve Black (learning about her only in the course of therapy), Eve Black knew all about Eve White. She knew all about her failure in marriage, love for her child, and difficulties and problems. She thought much of this was "silly." As she went on her buying sprees, bar-hopping binges, and flirtatious jaunts, she was sardonic and derogatory about Eve White. "When I go out and get drunk," she says, "*she* wakes up with the hangover. She wonders what in the hell's made her so sick" (1954, p. 141).

Later, a new personality emerged:

> . . . [*with*] *Eve White's maladjustment still growing worse generally, a very early recollection was being discussed with her . . . a painful injury she had sustained when scalded by water from a wash pot. As she spoke her eyes shut sleepily. Her words soon ceased. Her head dropped back on the chair. After remaining in this sleep or trance perhaps two minutes her eyes opened. Blankly she stared about the room, looking at the furniture and the pictures as if trying to orient herself. . . . Slowly, with an unknown husky voice and with immeasurable poise, she spoke. "Who are you?" (Thigpen and Cleckley, 1954, p. 144).*

Jane was different from the two Eves in innumerable ways, in maturity, a sense of fulfillment, and in initiative, without the faults and inadequacies of either. She was more colorful and vivid than the sweet and bland Eve White, and favorably impressed the therapists working with her. It later emerged that Jane was actually a role being played by Eve Black in an attempt to "win the competition with Eve White" over her therapist (Osgood et al., 1976, p. 256).

At the end of treatment, the three personalities presumably evolved into a unified whole, Evelyn, who has remarried and who is living a relatively more adjusted life than her predecessors (Lancaster and Poling, 1958).

and the goal was to explore whether or not the patient's different personalities could be differentiated through objective procedures that yielded data that were analyzed apart from the patient. Results for both Eve and Evelyn's personalities were fairly impressive, agreeing quite well with clinical observations regarding the distinctive aspects of each of the personalities.

Depersonalization disorder (depersonalization neurosis). Did you ever experience a sense of unreality in which you feel that you are existing outside of yourself, watching yourself (generally from above) as a stranger? Most young adults experience such feelings from time to time and these sensations are momentary and fleeting. As a matter of fact, many people are familiar with related feelings of *déjà vu* (a sense of having experienced an entire scene or situation before without actually having done so) and *jamais vu* (failure to recognize a familiar situation). These common, fleeting experiences are not disorders.

When such feelings of unreality persist over a period of time, at least a half-hour, recur frequently, and interfere with social or occupational functioning, the DSM-III refers to this state as depersonalization disorder, another of the dissociative disorders. Depersonalization is diagnosed most often in young females, and generally appears suddenly after a severely stressful event such as an airplane crash, accident, or acute pain. In such recurrent episodes of depersonalization, the patient experiences persistent feelings of being separated from his or her self, body, or surroundings. The sense of unreality, as if in a dream, sets him or her at a distance from the real world. People report even being able to observe themselves from this distance.

Other dissociative disorders resemble the self-induced trancelike states practiced by some follow-

Spotlight 9.3 Existential Neurosis

Many patients do not neatly fit into the DSM-III categories. For example, some do not complain of specific symptoms, but of persistent feelings of uselessness and hopelessness in their lives. They are not going anywhere, have few goals, and feel alienated from the world. They sense despair and futility—but not necessarily depression—a kind of aimless meaninglessness in their existence. They are unhappy with their jobs, marriages, college goals, and friends. They are bored. Sometimes they seek various sexual, religious, or drug experiences to relieve their boredom, or they may think that changing jobs, spouses, colleges, or friends is the answer. They find, often, that any such move is not the answer. "Who am I? What do I want? What am I doing here? Why am I so busy doing these meaningless things?" These are the kinds of questions such people ask of themselves and of their therapists, even though they do not seek help for an anxiety attack in the middle of the night or for a specific phobic symptom.

Some people call these general states of hopelessness and lack of purposeful identification "existential neurosis" (Maddi, 1967), but most clinicians, familiar with these states, need no diagnostic category when they are confronted with this all-too-familiar syndrome: an unhappy person, who is possibly even "successful" from society's viewpoint, who feels detached and alienated from the world of people and events.

Everyone has at some time asked questions like, "Is this what I really want?" As a matter of fact, one of the normal stages that adolescents in our society are expected to go through is the establishing of one's ego identity (see Spotlight 6.4 describing Erikson's thoughts in this area).

ers of certain Eastern religions, or instances of religious ecstasy achieved by some people at revival meetings. There are, in addition, certain types of "twilight" states in which the individual's attention seems focused, yet is far away while he or she remains unresponsive to ordinary stimulation and the surrounding social and interpersonal environment. If a pencil is placed in the hands of such a person, he or she may engage in automatic writing, without (seeming) awareness of what is being written.

ANXIETY: A CLOSER LOOK

In the preceding pages as well as in the pages ahead, anxiety emerges as a central concept. People do many things to handle their anxieties, from the defense mechanisms described in Chapter 6, such as rationalization or sublimation, and avoidance in the form of phobias, to irrational actions as in compulsions. This section takes a closer look at anxiety. How does it arise? Are some people more anxiety-prone than others?

Anxiety-Engendering Situations

All of us are often exposed to situations that engender anxiety; this section describes some of these circumstances.

1. Anxiety appears when there is a *threat to survival*—a sinking ship, a separation from a nurturant mother or caretaker, an inescapable collision with a car coming from the opposite direction. The aftermath of near-death experiences in great disasters, accidents, drastic (for example, open heart) surgery, or combat can produce heightened states of anxiety. Near-miss exposures to death thus are sources of anxiety.

2. Anxiety can arise when one feels *a loss of touch with reality* or *a disorientation* in time, place, or identity. This is especially so when one *feels* one thing to be the case and *knows* another thing to be the case. Thus anxiety can be experienced by people who are becoming senile or who are suffering from some type of brain dysfunction that can cause this kind of incongruity. Anxiety can also be experienced when people realize that they are misperceiving reality, as in hallucinatory experiences, or when there is some unexplainable distortion of an expected sensation or perception. A sudden rise of ambiguity or loss of structure or meaning of a situation can also yield anxiety, as in certain drug states. For example, "bad trips" during LSD use may sometimes result from generally heightened levels of anxiety and panic due to the uncertainty that the individual feels when there is no longer an ordinarily stable, predictable world with expected types of sensory input.

3. *Overarousal* by excessive internal or external stimulation, or states of heightened awareness and sensitivity, have sometimes been associated with feelings of anxiety. Such heightened states may diminish very slowly in some individuals, even after the source of the original arousal is no longer present.

4. *Stranger anxiety* in infants (see Ainsworth et al., 1978) represents still another source of anxiety. An infant can experience anxiety at very young ages, even only several months old in situations that engender unfamiliarity and uncertainty.

5. A *primary loss of support*, a feeling of sudden dislocation as in falling, also engenders anxiety, especially when these sensations are not expected. When anticipated, as for example in parachute jumping, anxiety levels are drastically reduced, although in some instances they are not entirely eliminated.

6. High levels of anxiety are experienced by some people under conditions of *sensory deprivation* (see Solomon et al., 1961) which can be best characterized by imagining oneself cooped up in endless dark in a space ship on an extended trip in a noiseless room, or in a situation in which any other kind of sensory input in the visual, auditory, or tactile areas is at a minimum or so diffuse and vague that nothing is perceived. Similar effects are produced by monotonous or repetitive stimulation with little change over time. In experimental sensory depri-

vation situations subjects also report changes in judgment, memory, and time perception, as well as hallucinatory experiences and various bizarre body sensations.

7. Still another source of anxiety is sometimes called *existential anxiety,* a sense of powerlessness, helplessness, and having no options in the face of a threat to survival. Existential anxiety is present not only in the face of immediate danger, for it also reflects the fear of ultimate death—of having no self and of being nonexistent—that some people experience.

8. *Helplessness* and the feeling of no options is often a question of how an individual perceives the situation he or she is in. States of autonomic arousal can give rise to feelings of anxiety if an individual sees himself or herself in a no-options, no-way-out situation, that is, as having no choices for problem solving (Mandler, 1972; Seligman, 1975; see Chapter 10, pp. 248–50). Such states of helplessness thus are not entirely dependent on the situation but on how individuals view the situations they are in and how effective they estimate their coping skills to be. The blocking of a planned sequence of behavior toward a goal when no alternative actions are possible can create feelings of helplessness and anxiety, whereas an organized plan of behavior (even if not completely relevant) serves to reduce the helplessness associated with anxiety. Mandler (1972) feels that chronic anxiety is related to feelings of self-esteem in that people with low self-esteem do not regard themselves as likely to find alternate plans in the face of disorganization. That is, persons who think poorly of themselves will more likely experience interruptions in planned behavior as overwhelming and final, and thus will be more prone to chronic helplessness, hopelessness, and anxiety than those people who think highly of themselves.

9. *Failure to live up to cultural expectations and standards,* or acting out or fantasizing about taboo themes in one's culture (for example, extreme aggressive or sexual fantasies about members of one's family) leads in many instances to guilt and/or to anxiety. Although there are many clinical indications that guilt and anxiety are not synonymous, nor necessarily experienced as similar feelings, for purposes of the current discussion, guilt-provoking situations are included in this list of sources of anxiety.

10. Spotlight 6.5 in Chapter 6 described some of the work of Harlow and his associates regarding the *relationship of infant and mother* or mother-surrogate (in monkeys) in engendering feelings of well-being or anxiety in the individuals studied. In humans, also, the mother or the mother-surrogate is essential for the survival of the infant in regard to feeding, toileting, and warmth, as well as in providing opportunities for the clinging, touching, cuddling, and physical attachments that seem an integral necessity for normal growth. Little or no opportunity for this kind of attachment may result in anxiety and depression in the developing individual, who in turn may display poor mothering skills regarding her own offspring. Deprivations of this sort may leave their durable imprints, even though primary needs for food, sleep, and other forms of nurturance are gratified.

11. Competing drives or responses under conditions of high motivation can also lead to anxiety states. For example, under a threat to survival, the drive to escape from either one of two situations (for example, from either a wild animal or an incontrollable fire) would lead to excruciatingly high levels of anxiety (and panic). These have been called *avoidance-avoidance conflicts.*

Experimental psychologists have for years produced conflict in animals that are sometimes referred to as experimental neurosis. It is not entirely clear how much relevance experimental neurosis and experimental conflict in animals bears to the psychopathology of humans. However, surprisingly interesting parallels can be drawn from this work to conceptualizations on the human level that point to the high levels of autonomic arousal and/or depression resulting from unpredictable situations (Mineka and Kihlstrom, 1978; Seligman, 1975; Thomas and Dewald, 1977). Another parallel on the human level is the double bind where choices between two contradictory options cannot be made (see Chapters 6 and 12.

Spotlight 9.4 Experimental Neurosis

There is a long history of inducing conflict in animals (for example, rats, cats, dogs, sheep, goats, and pigs) through experimental procedures. Various methods have been used, such as punishing errors an animal makes when solving problems not capable of being solved, introducing excessive numbers of uncontrollable or predictable shocks in training procedures, consistently punishing consummatory responses such as eating, or attempting to train subjects to distinguish between stimuli that are extremely difficult to discriminate (see Mineka and Kihlstrom, 1978, for a review of some of these studies).

Responses of animals under such experimental conflict conditions can be illustrated by Pavlov's descriptions (1927) of work in his laboratory on classical salivary conditioning with a dog. In a discrimination procedure, meat powder followed the presentation of a circle but was not offered when an ellipse was shown, in an attempt to demonstrate salivary conditioning to the circle (conditioned stimulus—see Chapter 6) but not to the ellipse. The animal learned the discrimination rapidly (salivating with the presentation of the circle but not the ellipse). The animal was then required to make increasingly finer discriminations during which the ellipse was modified during successive presentations to resemble the circle more and more, until the axes of the ellipse became 9:8, thus:

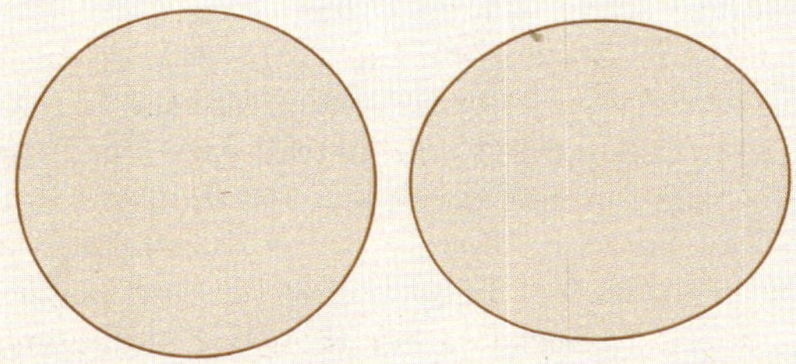

Perfect circle   9:8 ellipse

Then this happened.

After three weeks of work on this differentiation not only did the discrimination fail to improve, but it became considerably worse, and finally disappeared altogether. At the same time the whole behavior of the animal underwent an abrupt change. The hitherto quiet dog began to squeal in its stand, kept wriggling about, tore off with its teeth the apparatus for mechanical stimulation of the skin, and bit through the tubes connecting the animal's room with the observer, a behavior which had never happened before. On being taken into the experimental room the dog now barked violently, which was also contrary to its usual custom; in short it presented all the symptoms of a condition of acute neurosis. On testing the cruder differentiations they were also found to be destroyed. . . . A fresh development of the latter differentiation up to its previous exactness progressed twice as slowly as at first, but during the re-establishment of this crude differentiation the animal gradually became quieter, returning finally to its normal state. . . . The 9:8 ellipse at its first application was completely discriminated from the circle, but from the second application onwards no trace of a discrimination was obtained, and the animal again entered a state of extreme general excitation with the same results as before (Pavlov, 1927, p. 291).

Do you see a possible connection between the foregoing and some forms of human psychopathology?

Anxiety Traits and Anxiety States

The research literature on anxiety is voluminous. Between 1950 and 1966, there were 3,500 publications on this subject (Mandler, 1972), much of it contradictory and confusing. One attempt to bring some order into this chaotic area was to employ a distinction between state and trait anxiety (Spielberger, 1972). Trait anxiety is the propensity that an individual has to experience anxiety in various situations. It can be inferred from the frequency and intensity of anxiety responses over time. State anxiety is the actual anxiety engendered and experienced by an individual in specific anxiety-producing situations. State anxiety thus is more directly observable and measurable whereas trait anxiety is generally inferred. The difference between trait and state anxiety can be illustrated by self-report statements such as "I feel on edge, upset" (state anxiety) or "I tend to worry about unimportant things" (trait anxiety).

There is some evidence (see Kendall, 1978; Mellstrom, Zuckerman, and Cicala, 1978) to suggest that trait anxiety may not be an entirely stable feature in an individual but will instead vary from situation to situation. For example, even though some people may be more anxiety-prone than others, a few high-trait-anxiety people may become particularly anxious in social rather than test situations, whereas others may become particularly anxious in test rather than social situations.

Even so, we now know that most high-trait-anxiety people do not develop specific anxiety disorders. Fortunately, most do not. Why do some people develop severe neurotic problems, such as irrational fears or compulsions, and others do not? The next section addresses itself to this question in some specific ways.

SOME APPROACHES TO UNDERSTANDING ANXIETY DISORDERS

Chapters 6 and 7 reviewed some of the major approaches to understanding the development of psychopathology, such as the Freudian, learning, cognitive, and strictly biological models. Some of the major theories presented in Chapter 6, especially those of Freud and the neo-Freudians, were devised primarily as attempts to understand the neuroses, especially the anxiety, conversion, and dissociative disorders, and the various maladaptive symptoms that arise from the individual's attempt to deal with guilt, anxiety, and conflict. These general views are now supplemented by some additional specific considerations about anxiety and anxiety disorders.

Eysenck's Approach

Hans Eysenck, a prodigious writer and researcher, has some very specific views about abnormal behavior (Esyenck, 1947, 1960, 1976; Eysenck and Beech, 1971; Eysenck and Rachman, 1965). A central feature of these views is that abnormal symptoms can be conceptualized as maladaptive behaviors that arise from either faulty conditioning or a lack of conditioning. Because people have differing constitutional makeups, some will condition (make associations, learn; see Chapter 6) more or less easily than others.

Because so much of the conditioning in human culture is social conditioning designed to inhibit impulsive actions, people who condition more easily will tend to be more socialized and consequently will be more inhibited in their activity, think more than act, and tend to be shy and subdued. Eysenck has labelled this type of person introverted. People who condition less easily will be more impulsive, outgoing, and active. Eysenck calls this type of person extraverted. The Introversion-Extraversion dimension occupies an important place in Eysenck's views.

Eysenck developed much of his position from empirical work with personality inventory scores of thousands and thousands of subjects. Intercorrelations of these scores (how various scores vary with each other, their degree of association; see Chapter 3) were then examined further through a technique called factor analysis, to see whether or not common dimensions or factors emerged. Not only was the Introversion-Extraversion (IE) factor found, but also the Neuroticism (N) and the Psychoticism (P) factors as well. Eysenck claims that most of the differences among people can be expressed by their scores on these three dimensions or factors.

The Psychoticism factor, which is a score that reflects an individual's awareness of and contact with reality, does not concern us for our current purposes. Eysenck explains neuroses on the basis of the first two factors, Introversion-Extraversion and Neuroticism. The Neuroticism factor can be understood by considering the fact that some people respond with greater autonomic arousal and emotion to stressful situations and events than do others. These people are less adaptable and will tend to experience disruptive emotions more frequently and intensely than others, causing them to be less "stable." Such people score high on Neuroticism, which is a measure of emotionality and stability. High-N people are thus more emotional, less stable, less able to cope with stressful situations than low-N people.

According to Eysenck, people with different combinations of Introversion-Extraversion and Neuroticism factors show or develop different types of neurotic behaviors. For example, high-N and high-I people will be highly emotional and will condition easily. Thus they will experience aversive (punishing, negative) stimuli quite strongly, learning quite readily to avoid such stimuli. This results in anxious, phobic, or extremely shy neurotic behaviors. Eysenck calls these dysthymic disorders. Low-N and high-E people, on the other hand, tend to be resistant to such disorders (Eysenck and Rachman, 1965). High-N and high-E people are highly emotional and unstable but do not condition easily. They show a deficit in learned social behaviors and tend to be impulsive, a characteristic of psychopaths or sociopaths (people with strongly ingrained patterns of antisocial behaviors; see Chapter 18). Eysenck notes that criminals do not "improve" with punishment (condition less easily than do people with high-I scores) and cites this observation as empirical confirmation of his views. However, there is some disagreement with Eysenck's views about people who show antisocial behaviors ("criminal types"). Many psychologists, for example, do not go along with designating them as high in Neuroticism, although the "lack of conditionability" description tends to elicit less controversy.

Other specific disorders of the kind described in this and other chapters have also been conceptualized on Eysenck's axes. For example, hysterical (conversion and dissociative) disorders are viewed as high in Neuroticism and high in Extraversion (like the sociopath), whereas obsessive-compulsive disorders are conceptualized as high in Neuroticism and high in Introversion. In fact, a moderate number of studies reviewed do indeed support the notion that the hysterical and the obsessive types fall within the Neurotic dimension but at opposite ends of the Extraversion-Introversion dimension, but these findings are not completely consistent (Pollack, 1979).

Eysenck's views are less popular in this country than they are abroad, possibly because of their basic commitment to a constitutional and physiological basis for maladaptive behaviors. In addition, many critics claim that these views are too mechanical and simplistic in the light of the complexities of neurotic behaviors.

Phobic Disorders: A Closer Look

Researchers and clinicians have been especially interested in phobic disorders, and in particular agoraphobia, because of the widespread incidence of these disorders and because of the relative success of some of the behavioral and cognitive methods in treating them (Barlow and Wolfe, 1981; Coleman, 1981; Hollon, 1981).

At one time, psychodynamic formulations seemed to "make sense" in that often, in therapy, the origins of a phobic reaction could be traced to earlier taboo wishes and forbidden fantasies. These wishes become associated with the later-to-be-avoided object or situation. For example, a patient with murderous wishes and fantasies toward his child became phobic about kitchen implements such as knives, garbage disposal sink units, and household chemical agents such as ammonia and rat poison. The initial panic developed from an urge to employ one of these everyday items for a terrifying purpose. Similarly, suicidal or murderous impulses, in another patient, eventually produced excessive fear of heights. One patient refused to cook for anyone but herself, and was phobic about entertaining guests at home. Later, in therapy, her phobia was traced to guilt over the horrifying rumination that she would poison her guests, especially other, older women.

This type of understanding, however, as well as

insight into other "dynamic" aspects of agoraphobics—for example, their dependency, or the role that family members have in sustaining symptoms—has not been especially helpful in alleviating their extremely distressing problems. As a matter of fact, psychotherapy and psychoanalysis generally have failed to ameliorate the special problems of anxiety disorders, in particular, phobic responses.

Another way of looking at these clinical problems is to view them as responses that can be understood in the context of conditioning and learning approaches. For example, one aspect of such disorders is that the anxiety generalizes quite rapidly to similar aversive contexts and is easily conditioned to stimuli present at the time of the acute response. Anxiety responses show a durability generally lacking in the array of responses that humans are capable of making. In addition, responses that a subject learns to avoid anxiety or other aversive stimuli are also extremely persistent and durable (Martin, 1971).

In other words, strong anxiety responses can be conditioned easily to many situations and tend to persist over time. Phobic patients quickly learn ways to reduce or avoid anxiety. These soon become strongly ingrained avoidance responses associated to situations in which the individual has experienced acute anxiety or panic. Imagery and cognitive responses play an important role in the development of phobic responses. For at the prospect of thinking about or in conjuring up an encounter with the phobic situation, the individual experiences a rising sense of anxiety that elicits the avoidance behavior (Beck, Laude, and Bohnert, 1974). The immediate reduction of anxiety thus reinforces the phobic response.

This conceptualization helps us to understand a so-called paradox: if the individual simply avoids all anxiety-producing situations by anticipating them, there is no anxiety and therefore no anxiety-reduction. If this is the case, the phobic response should extinguish, because there is no reinforcement, that is, no anxiety reduction. According to one view, the persistence of avoidance responses despite the absence of reinforcement is explained in part by the principles of "partial irreversibility" (Solomon and Wynne, 1954). This principle states that extreme fear and anxiety responses evoked by certain stimuli tend to persist, that is, they can be described as a permanent fear reaction. To some observers, this "principle" only restates the empirical observation and is, in fact, no explanation.

A more acceptable approach to understanding this paradox is to introduce cognitive variables: the failure of the avoidant response to extinguish readily can be explained by cognitive and imaginal responses that include images, thoughts, fantasies, and ideas about the future and about feared responses. That is, the individual imagines himself or herself in the feared situation as falling apart, being flooded by anxiety, "going crazy." Avoidance is reinforced when the individual feels safe and no longer has to anticipate (that is, to see himself or herself in) the dreaded situation.

Clinicians experienced in work with agoraphobics (see Chambless and Goldstein, 1980; Coleman, 1981; and Goldstein and Chambless, 1978) have drawn a distinction between agoraphobics and other phobic patients. Whereas phobic patients avoid objects or situations because of expected anxieties associated with them, it is felt that agoraphobics, although at first experiencing panic attacks, avoid the feared situation because of their *fear of experiencing anxiety*—of losing control, or being overwhelmed with extreme feelings that they will "go crazy." This fear of fear is a special characteristic of agoraphobics that arises from a set of irrational beliefs about the dreaded consequences of anxiety and panic as a result of strong dependency, feelings of inadequacy, and a self-image that involves poor skills to cope with external threat.

Some Differences Between Anxiety Patients and Control Subjects

The human organism's normal capacity to experience anxiety is based on a sudden autonomic and endocrinological surge that is apparently designed to cope with a threatening event: fleeing, fighting, fending in some way for survival. An intriguing strategy that might be able to aid us to understand why some people develop anxiety symptoms and others do not do so is to look for differences between patients with anxiety symptoms and control subjects without such symptoms.

The evidence indicates that high- and low-anxiety people differ significantly on various tests of perception, learning, and personality (Eysenck, 1957). Are there more direct comparisons of high- and low-anxiety individuals? Perhaps such evidence can shed additional light on how anxiety symptoms develop. Typical of this research are efforts to measure various autonomic and hormonal indices of groups of patients and controls (a) before experimentally induced stress, (b) at various times during experimentally induced stress, and (c) after the stress is removed. An example of experimentally induced stress is to require the subjects to perform some speed task under conditions deceptively designed to suggest "failure," such as severe censure. Physiological indices include such measures as heart rate, volume of blood flow, blood pressure, muscle tension, skin resistance, and level of adrenocortical hormone in blood plasma and urine.

Chapter 7 describes the sympathetic and parasympathetic aspects of the autonomic nervous system (see Figure 7.6). The sympathetic system, when strongly aroused, produces increased heart rate and respiratory responses, and a lowered salivation response, resulting in dryness of the mouth, sweating on the palms and feet, and shivering and shaking. On the other hand, when the parasympathetic system is activated, the individual experiences diarrhea, frequent urination, fainting, a drop in blood pressure, and other related consequences of a decrease of blood supply to the brain. Chapter 8 discussed the body's stress response—a generalized response to strong stress that involves the powerful release of hormones from the pituitary-adrenocortical system, activated by the release of ACTH (adrenocorticotropic hormone) into the blood stream.

These responses occur in acute situations of fear and panic for all humans. Are people who develop anxiety disorders different in some way in these patterns of autonomic and hormonal response? More and more research evidence suggests an answer of *yes* to this question.

Adrenocortical and autonomic arousal levels. Anxiety patients show higher adrenocortical and autonomic arousal levels before the experimental stress is introduced, and higher arousal levels during stress, than do control subjects (Davis, Malmo, and Shagass, 1954; Kelly and Walter, 1968; Lader and Wing, 1964; Malmo and Shagass, 1952; and Persky et al., 1959).

Groups of subjects were injected with drugs such as epinephrine or lactic acid. Whereas normal subjects responded only with limited or moderate responses (shakiness, for example), anxiety patients tended to respond with full-fledged anxiety attacks that lasted for long periods of time. Whether or not this is due to arousal because of cognitive responses (that is, anxiety patients may have responded to moderate physiological changes with apprehension, bringing on the full-fledged attack), there is no doubt that anxiety patients are more highly aroused than are normal controls.

Figure 9.1 shows the higher blood pressure scores (which continue to rise) during a mirror drawing test (Malmo and Shagass, 1952). The subjects were psychoneurotic patients (with the majority being high-anxiety patients), controls, and chronic schizophrenic patients whose task involved tracing the outline of a circle while watching their hands in a mirror. This involved reversing the usual procedure and presumably induced some stress in the subjects.

In another study (Kelly and Walter, 1968), blood flow to the forearm was indicated by blood volume in the forearm measured at one-minute intervals while blood circulation was temporarily stopped. The amount of dilation of the blood vessels—a sympathetic response—was used to indicate the response to stressful stimulation (that is, subtracting numbers under timed conditions while being continually criticized by the experimenter). Chronic anxiety subjects are at the top of the list in regard to both prestress and stress periods. One ex-

Figure 9.1 Mean blood pressure during mirror drawing test. The blood pressure of the psychoneurotic—mostly high-anxiety—patients was not only higher than that of the other subjects but also continued to rise during the test situation. (Reprinted by permission of the publisher from Studies of blood pressure in psychiatric patients under stress, *Psychosomatic Medicine, 14,* 90. Copyright 1952 by The American Psychosomatic Society, Inc.)

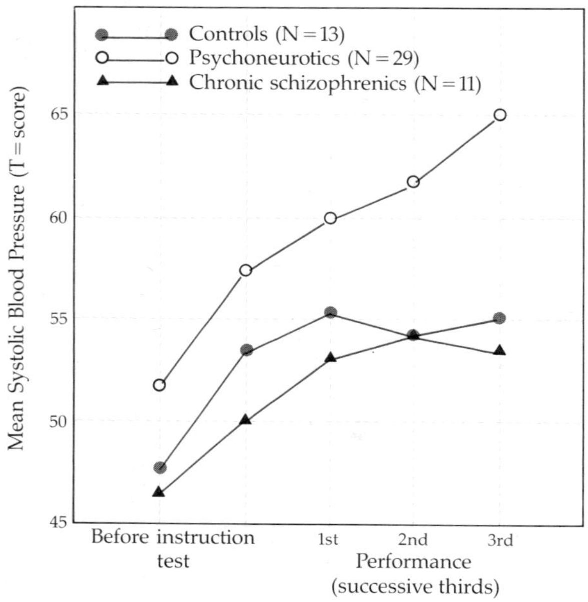

planation for the high autonomic levels of anxiety subjects in the prestress period, of course, is that the *anticipation* of the experimental procedures was itself viewed as stress by these subjects, thus preventing a "pure" picture of basal level from being obtained.

Most of the findings indicate higher basal levels before stress for anxiety subjects than for the other groups of patients and controls. Such patients, according to some researchers, are physiologically "different" from others. One explanation is that there is a constitutional predisposition in some people for prolonged exposure to stress to produce a chronic condition of higher autonomic levels, much in the way that a needle that indicates (and controls) room temperature might not return to normal levels after a prolonged period of heightened positions. Malmo (1975) calls this an archaic feature of our brains that "seems to involve a set-point that remains elevated after it should have returned to a normal level" (p. 20)—a so-called "sticky" set-point that is biologically maladaptive for some people. The precise mechanisms that underlie the differences among individuals in "sticky set-points" are not yet clear, but even if they were clear they are not within the scope of this book.

Habituation. Under ordinary circumstances, various autonomic responses adapt or habituate; generally, such responses return to lower levels or to baseline levels after continued exposure to a series of stimuli. Anxiety patients tend to adapt, or habituate, less well than do other groups of patients.

A typical method for assessing habituation or adaptation is to present subjects with a series of arousing stimuli and measuring responses before and during the period of stimulation. This was the procedure used in a study of the GSR (galvanic skin response) under stimulus conditions consisting of first a rest period of ten minutes followed by twenty auditory stimuli of 100-decibel intensity of one-second duration each at intervals randomly varying between forty-five and eighty seconds (Lader and Wing, 1964). Figure 9.2 presents the findings of this study.

This figure shows not only that the anxiety subjects had higher GSRs during the rest period than had the controls, and maintained this higher level throughout the stimulus situation, but additionally that their GSRs *rose* in contrast to the control subjects, whose GSRs habituated, as expected, with successive stimulus presentations. Anxiety subjects also showed more spontaneous GSR fluctuations unrelated to stimuli than did the control subjects. Observations of the patient group also showed significant correlations between anxiety level and habituation rate: the more anxious subjects showed slower rates of habituation.

Similar findings have been reported with other

Figure 9.2 Skin conductance effects of twenty auditory stimuli. Anxiety patients had a significantly slower rate of habituation than did the normal controls. (From M. H. Lader and L. Wing, Habituation of the psychogalvanic reflex in patients with anxiety states and in normal subjects, *Journal of Neurology, Neurosurgery and Psychiatry*, 1964, *27*, 212. Reprinted by permission of the authors and the *British Medical Journal*.)

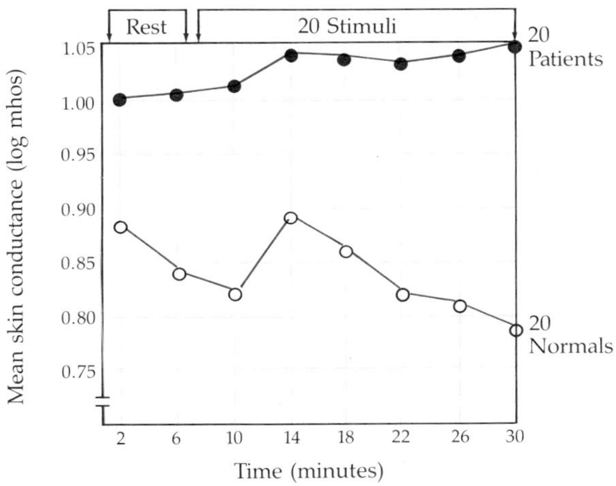

groups of anxiety patients and normal controls in which this general procedure produced the same pattern of habituation and fluctuation rates. Among various groups of neurotic patients, for example, habituation rates were slowest in those with anxiety with depression, and progressively increased in the various groups up to normal controls (Lader, 1967). In addition, spontaneous fluctuation rates of the GSR were *highest* in group 1 (see below), progressively decreasing to group 6. The groups were:

1. anxiety with depression
2. anxiety states
3. agoraphobia
4. social phobia
5. specific phobias
6. normal controls

In general, habituation findings employing other measures such as muscle tension or blood pressure confirm the slower habituation rates of anxiety patients compared to controls (Davis, Malmo, and Shagass, 1954; Malmo, Shagass, and Heslam, 1951).

Recovery responses. Normal physiological responses to sudden arousal involve a return to normal levels within a matter of seconds. These recovery responses—for example, homeostatic returns after a startle response to a sudden loud noise—can be measured through such indicators as muscle tension. Experimental findings indicate that anxiety patients, even though showing the same increase (compared to normal subjects) in muscle tension after a sudden noise do not return quickly to normal levels. Normal subjects do so within a fraction of a second. Instead, anxiety patients return slowly to a level higher than the relaxed level, and remain that way (for example, during a period of auditory stimulation [Malmo, Shagass, and Davis, 1950]).

Hereditary and Constitutional Factors

There is moderate evidence, based on twin studies, that there may be some constitutional predisposition to responding to stressful circumstances with high levels of anxiety. In one study of identical and fraternal twins, 41 percent of the identical twins, whereas only 4 percent of the fraternal twins, shared the diagnosis of "anxiety reaction" (Slater and Shields, 1969). This comes as no particular surprise, for there are strikingly high correlations for such autonomic measures as heart rate or skin resistance for MZ (identical) as compared to DZ (fraternal) twins. For example, at the end of an experimental session during which auditory stimuli were presented to the subjects, the correlation coefficient for heart rate for identical twins was .78, and for fraternal twins, —.38 (Lader and Wing, 1966).

Introversion-extraversion. Anxiety patients, as contrasted to other neurotic patients, presumably differ along the introversion-extraversion dimension, according to Eysenck. Is there some evidence that this tendency is inherited? That is, are there predispositions as to sociability or social fear and shyness? Here again some evidence indicates (see Martin, 1971) a moderate, even fairly high degree of correlation between MZ (reared apart or together) twins and little or no relationship between DZ twins on scores on self-report questionnaires, such as the MMPI. In one study, as a matter of fact (Shields, 1962), MZ twins actually showed *higher* correlations on an introversion-extraversion scale when reared apart than when reared together, whereas the DZ twins showed little or no correlation. Raising MZ twins together apparently created environmental and social pressures for greater dissimilarity between the twins, presumably because in such relationships one of each pair becomes dominant and the other more submissive.

Overall, reviews of some of this material (see Martin, 1971; Rosenthal, 1971) show moderate support for predisposition but do indeed point to the important role of environmental and familial factors in sustaining neurotic involvements. Even findings that show that diagnosed neurotic individuals come from families in which more parents also show neurotic symptomatology (see Shields and Slater, 1961) must be interpreted very carefully, for social, environmental, and familial conflict may well have produced the neurotic symptoms in the offspring.

The foregoing material suggests that anxiety patients do indeed differ from normal subjects in their tendency to experience higher levels of autonomic arousal and in maintaining these levels over more prolonged periods before returning, if at all, to basal levels. Prolonged experiences of these heightened levels may produce a chronic anxiety condition, and some evidence exists that there may be constitutional elements in this predisposition to remain at heightened levels. Beyond this, however, the evidence no longer is incontrovertible. For even though some people have built-in capacities to experience greater subjective distress in fight-flight situations, there is strong support for the importance of learned strategies for coping, situational components, as well as cognitive elements—questions of interpretation and meaning.

TREATMENT OF ANXIETY AND DISSOCIATIVE DISORDERS

The attempt to treat the anguish of neurotic symptoms was central to the development of psychoanalysis and its various offshoots (see Chapter 19). In addition, many of the other methods discussed at the end of this book were developed in conjunction with treating the disorders described in the current chapter, as well as Chapter 8 (for example, the conversion disorders), and Chapter 10 (the neurotic depressions). These methods include psychotherapy, hypnosis, biofeedback, direct suggestion, placebo, and various techniques to induce relaxation. Behavioral methods, in particular (see Chapter 20), and methods that employ various cognitive strategies have been rather successful in treating phobias, anxiety, panic disorders*, and obsessional symptoms. Hypnotic methods have been especially useful in treating the conversion and pain disorders as well as dissociative disorders, for example, multiple personality. Finally, some of the pharmacological interventions described in Chapter 21 have been particularly aimed, with some success, at reducing the distress of anxiety.

SECTION II
PERSONALITY STYLES AND PERSONALITY DISORDERS

TWO FAMILIAR PERSONALITY STYLES

Certain personality types are not characterized by symptoms and are not regarded as disorders. Rather, they refer to the general "flavor" of the personality, how it adjusts to life, other people, and

* Treatment approaches to panic disorders must first rule out physical causes (hyperthyroid condition, for example) that may produce similar symptoms.

daily living. We acknowledge this when we talk about someone's "personality." Sometimes the personality is so clearcut in its general approach to the world that there are both consistency and predictability associated with it. These consistent qualities can be abrasive, attention-getting, "difficult," or troublesome. Troublesome or not, these qualities add up to the common, long-term thread which appears to determine how the person perceives his or her personal world and how he or she thinks about this world. It seems that people with these ingrained, pervasive personalities experience their worlds in ways that sharply differentiate them from others.

Described in this section are two such personality styles.

The Obsessive-Compulsive Personality Style

The obsessive-compulsive personality is familiar to us all and is described in great detail in the clinical literature (see Pollack, 1979; Shapiro, 1965). Freud referred to this personality style as the "anal character" and even suggested some constitutional vulnerability: some people may have more intense sensitivity (are more highly "eroticized") in the anal area. As babies, they were more predisposed to pleasurable stimulation in this body area—during toilet training, for example—than in other areas. Regardless of etiology, this distinctive style can be sharply differentiated from other styles by evidencing the following traits: perseverence, thriftiness, self-control, and orderliness. Attentional skills are sharp and focused, and there is concern with details to the extent that the whole picture may be missed. A great focus on "should" is found, with reliance on rules and regulations. The personality seems rigid and "tight." These people are often constricted and lack spontaneity in emotional expression; they tend also to lack playfulness. Some people suggest that far from being "negative," these qualities are highly rewarded in our culture (the "Protestant ethic"), providing for the people who display these traits feelings of self-worth and confidence (Paykel and Prusoff, 1973).

This particular personal style elicits considerable agreement as to its objective qualities, according to an extensive review of the literature, but there is little evidence as to the purported relationship between the anal character and actual toilet-training methods (Pollack, 1979). It is of considerable interest that there seems to be little overlap between this general style and the obsessive-compulsive neurosis described earlier (Pollack, 1979).

The Hysterical Personality Style

The hysterical personality is also a familiar, frequently described style (see Shapiro, 1965). This style is evidenced by emotional, impressionistic, histrionic people who tend to repress their conflicts, ignore what they do not want to see, and focus on "global" impressions that help them to ignore or avoid details of situations, unlike the obsessive-compulsive personality. They tend to be nonanalytic, forming quick, intuitive impressions of others. They may even seem shallow, but they are dramatic, have a flair in terms of personal expression, and tend to be romantically inclined. Although they are temperamentally changeable, they are generally mild-mannered and easygoing, despite transciency in emotional expression.

PERSONALITY DISORDERS

Personality disorders are not so much neuroses with their specific symptoms, such as obsessions, phobias, or high anxiety levels, as they are long-term maladaptive personal and distinctive styles. They differ from the styles described above in that they are extremely troublesome, distressing, and dysfunctional ways of dealing with people, society, work, and indeed life in general, whereas the foregoing personality styles are not this disruptive.

These personality disorders were at one time called character neuroses, character disorders, neurotic personalities, or neurotic character disorders. Such rigid, ingrained, "difficult" personal styles are not easily modified, in or out of treatment, nor do the people with such disorders usually seek help for their difficulties. It may be that some of these so-called disorders reflect social and cultural judgments as to how people should behave, and not actual pathology. Certainly serious questions can be raised as to whether many of the categories delineated by the DSM-III as "personality disorders" are indeed pathological.

Clinical Description

A brief description of childhood and adult personality disorders as presented in the DSM-III, coded on Axis II, follows. These disorders can be regarded as enduring, inflexible personality traits that are maladaptive for the individual, causing impairment in occupational and social functioning, and often creating great subjective distress. It is important to remember, that these "disorders" are without specific symptoms, generally characterize an individual's long-term functioning (rather than emerge as a flare-up of responses as in a disease), do not fit appropriately into other categories (such as schizophrenia), and tend to create great interpersonal and social difficulties.

Several childhood disorders have equivalents, as will be discussed, on the adult level of personality disorders. If these persist into adulthood, the DSM-III suggests that their diagnosis should be changed to the appropriate adult category. Otherwise, most of the disorders listed here can also characterize children.

1. *Paranoid personality disorder.* This disorder, more frequently diagnosed in men, is characterized by suspiciousness and mistrust of others, tendency to take offense quickly, guardedness and vigilance (watchfulness), expectation of trickery and the possibility of threat, overconcern with the hidden motives of others, readiness to counterattack to perceived threat, a generally cold and aloof temperament with a poor sense of humor, and frequently, pathological jealousy.

2. *Schizoid personality disorder.* (This disorder in children is called *schizoid disorder of childhood or adolescence.*) According to the DSM-III, the gender distribution of this disorder is not known. Its characteristics include few close friends, inability to form interpersonal relationships, insensitivity to the feelings of others, lack of social skills, great reserve and seclusiveness, solitary interests and employment preferences (night clerk, for example), bland affect, that is, an inability to express emotion, but no disorder of thinking. According to the DSM-III, such people deliberately choose isolation and are not interested in social participation or peer contact.

3. *Schizotypal personality disorder.* Although some qualities of the personal style in this disorder may resemble those found in schizophrenia (see Chapter 11), these are not severe enough to warrant the diagnosis of schizophrenia. The gender distribution of this disorder is not known. Characteristics of schizotypal personalities include oddness and peculiarities in language, communications, and thinking (for example, magical thinking and superstitions); tangential, vague, or overelaborate speech; social isolation, suspiciousness, paranoid thinking (feelings of persecution), and ideas of reference (events and conversations interpreted egocentrically—"they meant that for my ears"); illusions about or sense of hidden forces; aloofness, coldness, and interpersonal distance; and hypersensitivity to real or imagined criticism.

4. *Histrionic personality disorder.* (This is similar to some qualities of the hysterical style already described.) This disorder, more commonly diagnosed among women than men, is characterized by self-dramatization, self-centeredness and vanity, shallowness, egocentricity, and a need to draw attention to oneself. People with these disorders seem affectionate but insincere, are emotionally excitable, impulsive, and occasionally irrationally angry, displaying outbursts or tantrums. They are often dependent, helpless, and constantly seeking reassurance. Occasionally they make suicidal gestures.

5. Narcissistic personality disorder. This disorder is characterized by grandiosity, self-importance, preoccupation with fantasies of success and power, exhibitionism, constant need for admiration, response to criticisms with indifference or rage, lack of empathy (compassion, being able to understand how others feel), expectation of special favors without assuming reciprocity, exploitiveness, and disregard for the integrity of others. The DSM-III does not indicate the gender distribution of this disorder.

6. Antisocial personality disorder. In adults this disorder is characterized by chronic antisocial behavior in which the rights of others are violated. Several of the following are present in this diagnostic category: poor performance as a responsible parent; frequent unlawful behavior, for example, illegal occupations, several arrests; several divorces, separations, or desertions of a spouse; assaultiveness; a limited sense of financial responsibility; impulsivity; repeated lying and "conning"; and recklessness. In children the diagnosis, which the DSM-III labels conduct disorders, is based on characteristics that include truancy, expulsion from school, running away from home, lying, stealing, bullying, assaultiveness, vandalism, theft, resisting authority, and later in adolescence, by aggressive sexual behavior and substance (for example, alcohol) abuse. The DSM-III indicates that with children as well as adults, this disorder is more common in males than in females. These disorders will be described more fully in Chapter 18.

7. Borderline personality disorder. According to the DSM-III, this disorder is more frequently diagnosed in women than in men. Characteristics of this disorder include: impulsivity or unpredictability in at least two areas such as excessive spending, sexual activity, or substance abuse; unstable, intense relationships with others that contain marked shifts as well as manipulation for one's own ends; inappropriate displays of anger; identity problems (Who am I?); mood shifts from normal levels to depression or anxiety that usually last only for a few hours; inability to be alone; and self-damaging behavior, for example, suicidal gestures, self-mutilation, accidents, and fights. In children and adolescents a corresponding diagnosis is called identity disorder, according to the DSM-III. Some, but not all of these features can be found in existential neurosis, described in Spotlight 9.3.

8. Avoidant personality disorder. According to the DSM-III, this is a common disorder characterized by extreme hypersensitivity to rejection, avoidance of relationships, low self-esteem, and strong desire for affection. In children it is called avoidant disorder of childhood or adolescence, is also quite common, and is similarly characterized by an extreme avoidance of strangers, including peers. There are generally good relationships with family members and caretakers, however. Avoidant disorder in children should not be confused with schizoid disorders of childhood, the DSM-III states, in that the former children are interested in social participation while the latter children are not. Once entering into relationships, children with avoidant disorders are capable of enjoying themselves and even of establishing good relationships.

9. Dependent personality disorder. This disorder, the DSM-III states, is more frequently diagnosed among women than among men. It is characterized by long-term patterns of allowing others to assume responsibility for major decisions and actions regarding one's life and an accompanying willingness to submerge self-reliance. People with this disorder often "put up" with abuse from others, because in return, dependency needs are gratified. Other characteristics include extreme intolerance for being alone, low self-esteem, and feelings of helplessness and stupidity.

10. Compulsive personality disorder. This is more commonly diagnosed among men, according to the DSM-III, and is a long-term pattern of behavior that involves limited ability to express warmth and tenderness, excessive preoccupation with details, rules, schedules, and lists so that person is unable to "grasp the whole," insistence that others submit to his or her way of doing things, extreme devotion to work so that "fun" and pleasure are minimized, and indecisiveness, postponement of planning for fear of making mistakes, and inability to plunge into work because of ruminations about priorities. It is important to note that a compulsive personality disorder does not facilitate an individual's adjustment. Rather, it is typically dysfunctional. Compulsive "styles," on the other hand, are often helpful and useful for the individual. Obsessive-compulsive neuroses are differentiated both from disorders and styles because of the presence of specific symptoms. Obsessive, ego-alien thoughts, or compulsive actions and rituals over which the individual seems to have little control, are present in obsessive-compulsive neuroses, but not in the disorders or styles.

11. Passive-aggressive personality disorder. According to the DSM-III, this disorder describes people who are unable openly to express intense feelings of hostility and anger. Rather, they resort to hidden, covert ways to do so, leading to ineffective functioning in interpersonal and occupational areas. The DSM-III states that a related disorder in children is called oppositional disorder. In adults there is a pattern of procrastination, dawdling, stubbornness, intentional inefficiency, and "forgetfulness," whereas in children, in addition to these qualities there is a pervasive oppositional pattern toward parents, school, and authority figures; argumentativeness and stubbornness; learning problems despite ability; and general belligerence. Gender distribution of this disorder is not known among adults, but among children oppositional disorder appears more frequently in boys than among girls, according to the DSM-III, which notes that a diagnosis of oppositional disorder is not made if there is violation of rights of others or if societal "rules" are violated, in which case diagnosis of conduct disorder is made.

Personality disorders, many clinicians believe, are difficult to treat. In actuality, most psychologists do not have a wide array of practical or research experience with the personality disorders, primarily because such people tend not to seek help or to volunteer for research. It is further held by some, as already noted, that these so-called disorders should not be regarded as "abnormal" and should not, therefore, be included in the DSM-III's list.

For example, the DSM-III lists identity disorders arising in childhood or adolescence that should be diagnosed as such if there is

1. Severe subjective distress regarding uncertainty about a variety of issues relating to identity including three or more of the following:
   long-term goals
   career choice
   friendship patterns
   sexual orientation and behavior
   religious identification
   moral value systems
   group loyalties
2. Impairment in social or occupational (including academic) functioning as a result of the symptoms in 1
3. Duration of the disturbance of at least three months
4. A disturbance not due to another mental disorder
5. If 18 or older, does not meet the criteria for borderline personality disorder

There is considerable controversy regarding this category, because the conflicts described may arise from healthy, normal adolescent concern with identity and with assuming the responsibilities of adulthood. Should identity disorder be included, then, in a list of abnormal behaviors? Should we raise a similar question about some of the other personality disorders, for example, dependent or avoidant personality disorders?

SUMMARY

Chapter 9 focused on clinical syndromes traditionally labeled neuroses or psychoneuroses, disorders that share a common denominator—the ways in which anxiety and conflict are handled. Following a presentation of the major differences between the neuroses and the psychoses, the chapter described and illustrated the different anxiety and dissociative disorders. These clinical entities include among others, the anxiety disorders (phobic disorders, anxiety states, and posttraumatic stress disorders) and the dissociative disorders (psychogenic amnesia, psychogenic fugue, multiple personality, and depersonalization disorder). Anxiety is a central concept that underlies many of the foregoing conditions. Accordingly, the chapter examined in close detail situations conducive to its development and reviewed some hypotheses in connection with why some people develop anxiety disorders. The chapter then explored the differences between anxiety and nonanxiety patients, especially those having to do with autonomic and hormonal indices. Section II of this chapter briefly presented the DSM-III's classification of personality disorders.

Highlights

1. Distinguishing between the neuroses and psychoses is often extremely important for both research and applied considerations—for example, for choosing among different treatment strategies. Some distinguishing criteria are the severity of the disorder, the degree of adjustment to many interpersonal and social demands, the quality of reality-testing skills, the level of insight, the floridity of symptoms, and the presence or absence of thought disorders.
2. In the case of anxiety disorders, anxiety is often acutely experienced either without external cues or when the defenses of the individual are dropped (for example, when phobic avoidance is not possible). In the case of dissociative disorders, anxiety, as such, is rarely experienced. In these disorders, there is a loss or change in awareness or consciousness, as if some mental functions become detached or "dissociated" from other functions.
3. Although instances of multiple personality are extremely rare, they are dramatic illustrations of dissociative states. In these disorders, two or more distinctively different personalities coexist in the same person. Often the dominant personality has little or no conscious awareness of the others.
4. There are many anxiety-engendering situations, including threats to survival, instances of disorientation in time or space, states of physiological overarousal, stranger anxiety in infants, and states of helplessness in perceived no-options situations. It is often possible to distinguish these and other anxiety states from anxiety traits. Not all individuals who experience high levels of anxiety or even those who show high trait anxiety develop anxiety disorders. Hypotheses about the development of these disorders, ranging from those of Freud to those of Eysenck, have attempted to deal with this question.
5. Eysenck's views are in sharp contrast to those of Freud (see Chapter 6). Many of Eysenck's notions derive from the observation that people differ in the degree to which they become conditioned to stimuli. People high in "conditionability" who receive high N (Neuroticism) scores and high I (Introversion) scores on a specially developed personality inventory will experience aversive stimulation strongly and will tend to develop anxious, phobic, or shy neurotic behaviors. On the other hand, high N scorers who also receive high E (Extraversion) scores will tend to develop conversion and dissociative (hysterical) disorders. Eysenck's views have not been popularly received by many psychologists because of their basic commitment to constitutional factors as underlying the etiology of the neuroses and other types of disturbed behavior.
6. Psychologists have focused special attention on the origins of phobias, which by their nature can be understood more easily than can many other types of symptoms in the context of conditioning and learning approaches. Of particular interest, however, is a so-called paradox

about the "sturdiness" of such responses. If avoidance of a feared situation reduces anxiety, then anxiety reduction serves as the reinforcing agent that maintains the phobic response. But if the individual *avoids* the anxiety producing situation at all costs, there is no anxiety and therefore no anxiety reduction. Therefore, the phobic response should extinguish over a period of time. How is it, then, that phobias persist quite stubbornly and with great resistance to change? The answer is still not entirely clear to researchers, but cognitive variables may play a significant role in explaining the paradox.

7. Major differences between anxiety and non-anxiety patients have been demonstrated. A review of this material indicates that anxiety patients tend to differ from other subjects and especially from normal subjects in their tendency to experience higher levels of autonomic arousal and in maintaining these levels over more prolonged periods of time before returning, if at all, to basal levels. There may be constitutional elements in this predisposition, but the importance of environmental and cognitive factors in the development of anxiety disorders was stressed.
8. Personality disorders—for example, passive-aggressive or antisocial personality disorders—are difficult to treat and there is not a wide body of practical and research experience with them. Many people question the inclusion of some of these disorders, for example, identity disorders, in the DSM-III's list of diagnostic categories.

ISSUES AND QUESTIONS

1. Do you think that you are an anxious person? Are you generally anxious? Or do you tend to have specific anxieties that arise in predictable circumstances? Or perhaps you have episodes of anxiety unrelated to circumstances you can specify or of whose origins you are not conscious.

   This chapter makes reference to some of the causes of anxiety. Trace some of the sources, circumstances, events, and contexts—interpersonal or in fantasy—of your anxiety. What about a near-death accident or a sudden separation from your parents when you were very young? Were you ever suddenly disoriented in time or space? Did the anxiety that was experienced under these circumstances subside or persist? Did you experience any generalization of anxiety—spread of effect—to other situations? Or are you unable to trace its course?
2. If you have a phobia—and many people do—can you trace its origins, the history of generalization, and describe the intensity of the avoidance response? In Chapter 20 illustrations of how phobias are treated through principles of learning will be presented. Perhaps you can use some of these principles to modify your own phobic response.
3. This chapter described experimental procedures that increase anxiety levels in various groups of subjects. What is your opinion about the ethics of such procedures? Do you approve of such studies if volunteers are used and if subjects are informed about the purpose of the experiment? If you needed to have a group of high-anxiety patients but had to depend only on volunteers, would you not be screening out some of the subjects you most wanted to include in your work? How would you solve this dilemma?

SUGGESTIONS FOR FURTHER READING

Fenichel, O. *The psychoanalytic theory of neurosis.* New York: Norton, 1945. In this classic work, Fenichel presents a Freudian examination of all of the neuroses. Essential reading for anyone desiring to fully understand the psychoanalytic viewpoint, it is filled with case illustrations, traditional Freudian insights, and references to the psychoanalytic literature. This encyclopedic work also covers schizophrenia, depression, mania, and character disorders. But the reader is forewarned that the going is rough and the psychoanalytic interpretations, heavy.

Figley, C. R. *Stress disorders among Vietnam veterans: Theory, research and treatment.* New York: Brunner/Mazel, 1978. This collection of papers provides a picture of stress disorders, particularly as experienced by men who fought in Vietnam. Clinical material sheds light on the etiology, onset, and prolonged effects of combat stress reactions as well as on various aspects of the veterans' postcombat adjustment. Therapeutic issues are also discussed.

Schreiber, F. R. *Sybil.* New York: Warner, 1973. Paperback. This book is a fictionalized account of the life and treatment of Sybil, a woman who suffered from multiple personality disorder. It presents Sybil's subjective experience of "waking up" after having lived as one or another of her sixteen selves, of her eleven-year psychoanalytic treatment and exploration of those selves, and of the childhood experiences that, according to Sybils' psychoanalyst, were the causes of her illness. Written on a popular level, this is an interesting and readable case illustration.

Shapiro, D. *Neurotic styles.* New York: Basic Books, 1965. Paperback. This chapter has already described Shapiro's obsessive-compulsive and hysterical styles. If you wish to read more about neurotic styles, read this book. Shapiro paints an interesting picture of the ways in which obsessive- compulsive, hysterical, paranoid, and impulsive people experience themselves and their worlds, and how they appear to others. In addition, Shapiro provides a psychoanalytic explanation as to why their symptoms take the forms that they take.

Wheelis, A. *The quest for identity.* New York: Norton, 1958. This essay was written by a psychoanalyst concerned with the difficulties he believes all contemporary people experience in finding their identities in a rapidly changing culture. According to this author, the individual in today's society must carve his or her identity out of the confusing complexity of a modern world in which knowledge is rapidly expanding and constantly changing. At the same time, traditional truths, once the bedrock of society, are no longer accepted unequivocally. This interesting and thought-provoking comment, although written about twenty-five years ago, seems relevant today, especially in the light of some of the identity problems described in this chapter.

10

Depression, Affective (Mood) Disorders, and Suicide

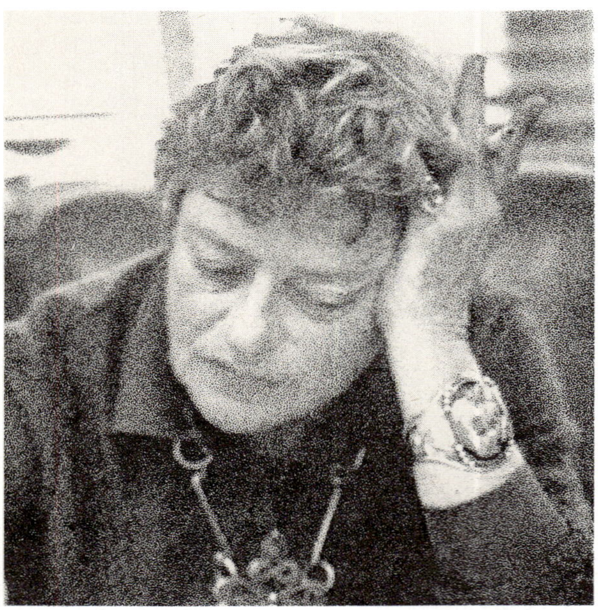

DEPRESSION: GENERAL BACKGROUND

Depression and disorders of affect (emotions, mood, and feelings) are among the most prevalent of mental disorders, with estimates ranging from 4.5 to 15 million depressed persons in the United States (Berger, 1978; Fischer, 1979; Kline, 1974). Each year, about 125,000 Americans are hospitalized for depression, and it is projected that about 15 percent of American and European adults will have a depressive episode at least once in their lives (Berger, 1978; DSM-III; Lehmann, 1971).

It is well known that these estimates drastically underestimate the prevalence of depression, for official records depend on clinic attendance or hospital admission and most instances of depression are probably untreated. Actually, only one person in five suffering from depression is treated professionally, and only one in fifty goes to a hospital (Lehmann, 1971). If, in addition, one considers that many instances of alcoholism or drug addiction may represent "masked depression" (Lesse, 1974), the resulting total figures of depression reach staggering proportions.

Definition and Symptoms of Depression

As this chapter unfolds, you will see that there are many different types of depression and that we are just beginning to understand how to distinguish among them. But before considering problems in diagnoses, etiology, and theory, we will first look at the common ground that the depressive spectrum occupies.

Depression is best defined as an inability to experience pleasure or to obtain reinforcement through pleasurable activities. The predominant mood is one of great sadness, hopelessness, or despair. These feelings are generally accompanied by low self-esteem, feelings of guilt and worthlessness, low energy and motivation, and poor concentration. Depressed people are self-absorbed, show little interest in others, and may cry easily, with little or no provocation. Some severely depressed people have dried-out feelings, an inability to feel any emotion or even to cry. These people complain that they feel like a piece of cardboard—flat, empty, and two-dimensional.

Although some depressed people are retarded in motor activity—sluggish or virtually immobilized—others may be extremely agitated, pacing the floors restlessly, like caged animals. Some, but not all, depressed people have suicidal thoughts, may make suicidal attempts, or may even become "successful" at suicide. There may be additional symptoms, such as somatization (the conversion of mental states into physical symptoms) or delusional thinking. Not all symptoms, however, are present in all instances of diagnosed depression.

Affect and mood can assume a variety of intensities and colorations. One's feelings can range from mild "blues" to great depths of despair. These feelings can also be judged as to their appropriateness or inappropriateness. Judgments of this nature are not always valid, however, for there may be cultural and social styles that determine these responses, as noted in Chapter 2. Even so, within familiar cultural settings, most people can probably make such judgments with a fair amount of reliability and validity. Hilarity in a situation calling for seriousness is an example of inappropriate affect. Flatness of affect, on the other hand, refers to the inability to respond with any emotion at all—pleasure, displeasure, anger—in a situation in which some emotional response is appropriate and called for. Depressive states are frequently characterized by flat affect; schizophrenic states, by inappropriate affect. These distinctions do not always apply, however, because schizophrenic patients may also show flat affect and some depressive patients may show inappropriate affect.

Spotlight 10.1 lists some of the symptoms of depression.

Sociocultural Aspects of Depression

Chapter 2 drew a broad relationship between culture and psychopathology. Is there a more specific relationship of depressive symptomatology to various cultural and social factors? Just how depression is expressed seems very much associated with one's culture (King, 1978). For example, depression in African cultures is more likely to be manifested by somatic complaints, motor retardation, and depressed mood but by *less* guilt, suicidal ideation, and anxiety than depression in European cultures (Binitie, 1975; Mendels, 1970).

Spotlight 10.1 Depression: Characteristic Symptoms

Mood: sadness, unhappiness, a feeling of being blue, frequent crying; feelings of hopelessness and despair; pessimism about self, one's future, and world events; inability to experience pleasure (anhedonia)

Self-image: poor self-confidence; feels that he or she has nothing to offer or is unable to meet the standards of others; feels guilty, unworthy, unattractive, unable to sustain anyone's interest and incapable of being loved; a deep sense of one's helplessness and inability to cope with or to solve problems

Interpersonal relations: withdrawn, ingoing, isolated; occasional irritability or impatience with others

Motivation, energy, and interests: lowered motivation and energy levels, inability to pull self together to act or to make decisions and plans; lowered activity level (psychomotor retardation) but sometimes an increase in activity level; loss of interest in usual activities; difficulty in maintaining a conversation or sustaining verbal flow; difficulty in concentrating and in sustaining attention to external events

Appearance: slouched posture, limp body tone; sometimes, inability to look at other person or make eye contact; neglect of cleanliness and personal appearance

Somatization: may have somatic and bodily complaints, aches, and pains; appetite loss; dryness of skin and clouding of eyes; poor sleep pattern, such as great desire for sleep or insomnia; frequent constipation; waning sex interests or difficulties in sexual performance; weight loss (but in some instances, weight gain); chronic fatigue and weakness

Several additional symptoms may be present:

Delusional thinking

Flat and/or inappropriate affect

Suicidal thoughts, threats, attempts

Anxiety, extreme agitation

Impaired thinking, judgment, and reality orientation

About 15 percent of the population will have a depressive episode at least once in their lifetimes. (Left: Arthur Tress. Right: Joel Gordon)

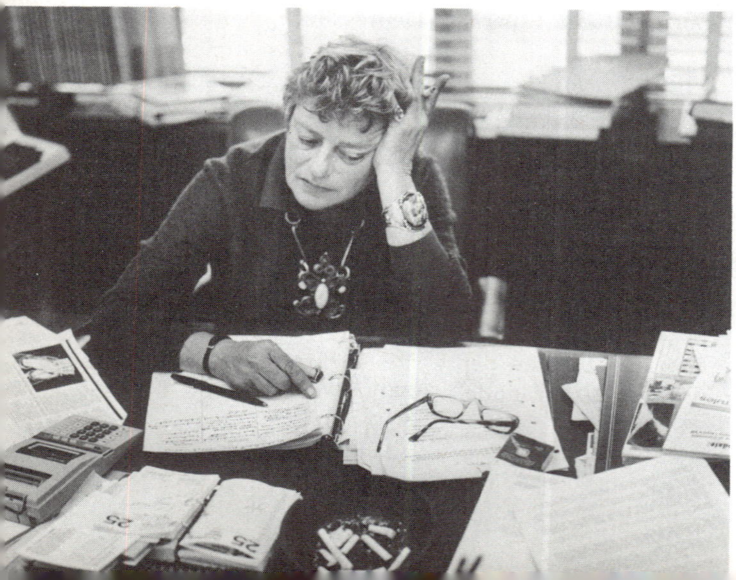

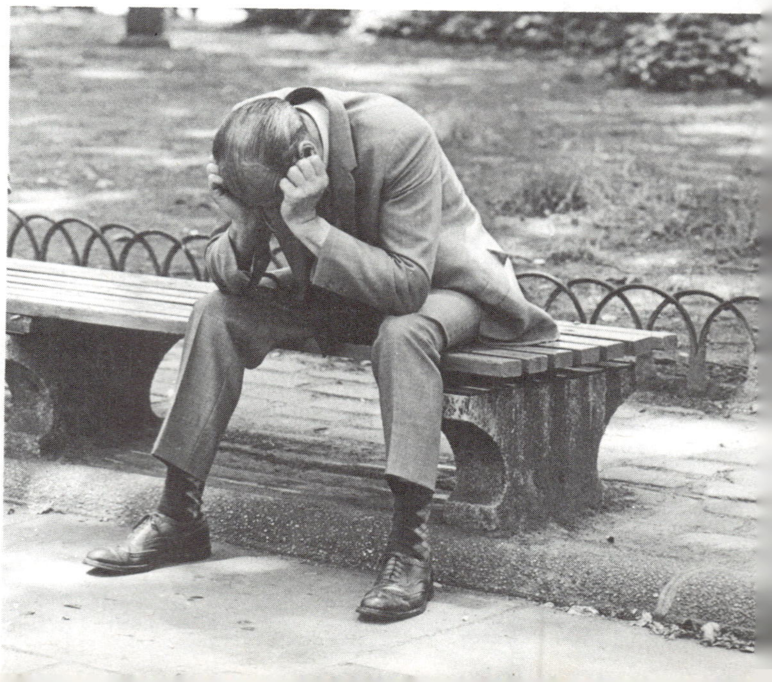

SES. Later, under the topic of manic-depressive illness,* we shall see that social class variations do not play an important role in incidence of that condition. However, there is some agreement that almost all other kinds of depression and depressive symptoms do tend to vary along social-class lines, with lower socioeconomic status (SES) associated with greater incidence (Hollingshead and Redlich, 1958; Srole et al., 1962).

Race. As for racial variations in incidence, the data are difficult to interpret. For it seems likely that blacks in our society are less readily diagnosed as depressed than whites, yielding a distorted picture of less depression among blacks than whites. When this diagnostic bias is removed, however, incidence of diagnosed depression among blacks increases (Zubin et al., 1975).

Racial incidence figures also appear to be dependent on sociocultural variables such as urban versus rural residence, northern versus southern location, attitudes of blacks toward whites and each other, and changing social patterns. For example, a 1959 U.S. Department of Statistics report states that depression and suicide are much less frequent among southern blacks than among southern whites, northern blacks, or northern whites (Mendels, 1970). Possible explanations for these data are that aspirations and therefore frustrations were lower among southern blacks than southern whites in the 1950s, or that extended families and religious beliefs offered positive emotional supports to blacks. It is also possible that hospital admission and suicide data for southern blacks may not have reflected "true" incidence at that time (Prange and Vitols, 1962).

Gender. There is virtually no disagreement about the relationship between gender and depression: the incidence of depression is greater among women than men (Amenson and Lewinsohn, 1981; Angst, 1974; Lehmann, 1971; Rosenthal, 1971; Silverman, 1968; Weissman and Klerman, 1979; Weissman and Paykel, 1974). Further, more women attempt, but do not complete, suicide than men. Within this culture as well as throughout the world, even though more women than men are diagnosed as depressives (according to the DSM-III, twice as many females than males), this is particularly so for "neurotic" depressions, that is, those presumably without biological, biochemical, or genetic bases (Weissman and Klerman, 1979).

What are the possible reasons for such consistent findings? Social and cultural factors affecting women's ability to feel adequate and to cope, such as dependent role, induced feelings of helplessness, exposure to more stressors than males, cultural permissiveness about expressing symptoms (males tend to be judged more harshly when expressing symptoms) may explain some of these differences (Hammen and Peters, 1977; Radloff and Rae, 1979). Other explanations may lie in the hormonal and physiological differences between men and women. However, these factors are not consistently associated with particular syndromes, and they have been questioned as determinants of the striking differences in incidence figures. Still another explanation lies in the attachment bonding hypothesis (Weissman and Klerman, 1979), which proposes that through a combination of biological and learned factors, women are more responsive to disruption of attachments (divorce, separation, reduction of family ties) than are men, showing their reactions through depressive symptomatology.

Whatever the true reason for the incidence figures, most explanations are strongly biased in favor of sociocultural variables. As a matter of fact, the DSM-III no longer employs a special diagnostic category that was once called involutional melancholia, a severe depression generally thought to be brought on by menopausal or postmenopausal changes in physiological and psychological status. Today, most clinicians and researchers find no evidence that this diagnostic category is associated with the endocrinological changes of menopause. The lack of invariant relationship between physiological factors and this kind of depression is fur-

* Now generally called bipolar affective disorder.

ther confirmed by the finding that replacement (hormone) therapy does not necessarily improve depression in some menopausal women. Severe depression in this age group may actually reflect feelings of being unneeded and worthless as well as the marginal social roles associated with becoming older in our culture among both men and women, rather than the physiological changes that may be taking place at this time.

THE CLINICAL SYNDROMES

Thus far, we have been hinting that depression is not a unitary illness, not a single disease. What are the different kinds of depression? Although there continues to be considerable debate as to subtypes, it will help you if you distinguish between the *primary* and *neurotic* types. The primary group consists of the major affective disorders, which probably

Case 10.1 Janice: Neurotic Depression

Two months before her thirtieth birthday, Janice's boyfriend left her for someone else. She was angry, hurt, and humiliated. Just as these emotions were beginning to subside, Janice's mother, with whom she had been living, died suddenly. There was a week of busy activity (during which Janice felt numb) as she prepared for the funeral, sorted out her mother's things, and greeted a stream of well-wishers and sympathizers.

When there was no longer any company, Janice spent a sleepless, restless, anxious night. The next day, many symptoms appeared. Not only did these persist for many months but also they seemed to increase in intensity before she sought help. She showed poor concentration and had crying spells, insomnia, and weight loss. When she was not crying, she mulled over her hurt feelings and petty grievances against others. Although she continued working (she was an elementary-school teacher), she gradually gave up all social activities. Janice's friends, in turn, began to forsake her, for she was unable to respond to their reassurance or interest in any way. On weekends she stayed home, showing little interest in anything but her television set. She would sit in front of the screen, feeling anxious and preoccupied with her sense of worthlessness. Although she shopped and cooked for herself, she felt no interest or excitement in life.

A few sessions after therapy began, Janice's therapist diagnosed her condition as neurotic depression. There was no history of previous episodes of depression, no family history of depression, and no distortion of reality. In therapy, Janice learned that she always wanted to be a model child. She ran for approval—in appearance, grades, achievements—to her mother (her father had left her mother when Janice was a baby). In recent years, she interpreted her mother's insistence that she get married as a lack of confidence in Janice's ability to fend for herself. Janice's increasing sense of failure was compounded by guilt, also engendered in many subtle ways by her mother's Victorian attitudes toward sex, for Janice had been sleeping regularly with her boyfriend. When her boyfriend left her, Janice's mother said, "I always knew he was no good. All he wanted was your body."

Just before she became "ill," Janice suppressed a rising sense of anger toward her boyfriend and her mother. But she felt guilty about the anger. She did not deserve anyone's affection or love. Even her father had abandoned her. She was useless: unloved and unlovable. Everybody had left her, so there was no point in life. She was getting old, unattractive. Soon, she would be over the hill. The death of Janice's mother, occurring at the peak of Janice's guilt, self-doubt, and suppressed anger, had pushed her into the severe depression just described.

In therapy, Janice was helped to understand the origins of her irrational beliefs about herself. She began to reevaluate herself and her future options and learned to trust herself and her feelings, even anger, without being overwhelmed by them. She especially learned that she could exert some control over her own destiny. Today, Janice is married to one of her colleagues at school, and feels alive, worthwhile, and eager to live her life.

arise from internal (endogenous) biochemical factors, in contrast to neurotic depressions (Akiskal et al., 1979). Although the DSM-III does not directly refer to neurotic depression,* many clinicians and researchers do indeed find that the distinction between neurotic depressions and the major affective disorders is a useful one, especially in regard to response to treatment.

Neurotic Depression

All of us get depressed from time to time. We feel cheerless, dejected, and unhappy. Often, this is in response to an event: a rejection, a failure in school or at work, a plan that went awry. What distinguishes such temporary normal states from pathological depression is the intensity and duration of the depressed episode, the extent to which our daily lives are disrupted, and the ease with which we can "snap out" of the depression, given time and a diminution or disappearance of the causal circumstance.

A good example has to do with the normal mourning that follows the death of a close relative: a husband, wife, mother, father, sister. Time, emotional support from friends, and a gradual restoration of one's daily routine help the mourner to get over the depression. It may be a question of weeks, months, or even a year. But when the depression is intense and prolonged and characterized by agitation, excessive guilt, extreme preoccupation with the dead person, and some of the other symptoms listed in Spotlight 10.1, we talk of a grief reaction, rather than of normal mourning.

We are beginning to learn as already noted that there are several distinct types of depressions that can be distinguished from the normal fluctuations of mood that make us unhappy from time to time. Because these distinctions are still being explored in the experimental laboratory and in the clinic, you may find it somewhat confusing if all of the debate concerning the fine points of classification is presented. For this reason, I will simplify some of the discussion, without overlooking the main points of its thrust.

For clarification and ease of understanding, therefore, the so-called neurotic depressions will be described first. These are neither the everyday fluctuations of mood or states of happiness or unhappiness nor the deep, intense, protracted depressions that may require hospitalization. Neurotic depressions have been called, from time to time, reactive, situational, or nonendogenous depressions, but the terms matter less than your understanding that these states are distinguishable from the primary affective states described in the next section by several important features.

Neurotic depressions comprise a significant portion of the clinician's practice. Although they may sometimes present the same depressive picture as the primary or major disorders, they are not generally treated by similar methods. For this reason,

We all get depressed from time to time. Clinical depression, however, lasts longer, is deeper, and is more disruptive to daily living. (Jim Pozarik/Liaison)

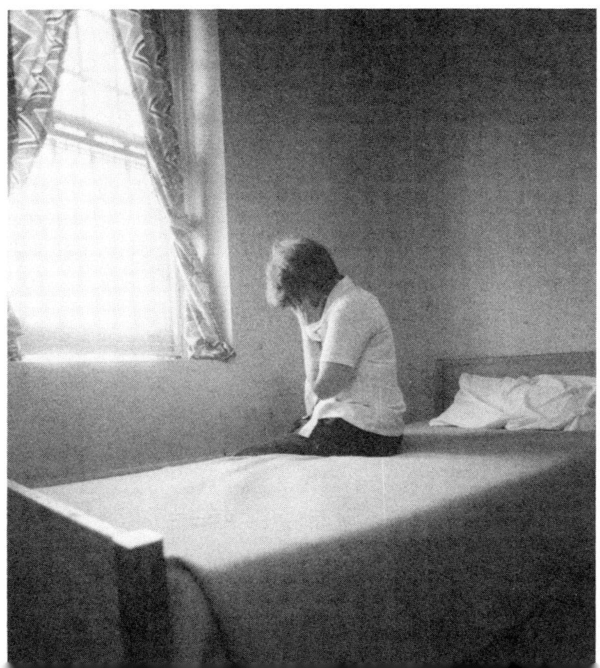

* Actually, the DSM-III category, dysthymic disorder, is the depressive neurosis of the DSM-II.

the debate as to the distinguishing features of this group of depressions is not an entirely academic one, for it has many practical consequences such as choice of most effective therapy.

From a burgeoning literature,* we can learn about the features that characterize neurotic depressions. Many of these features distinguish such depressions from the primary ones.

1. People with neurotic depression comprise a more heterogeneous group of people than those with primary or major depressions, for they tend to coexist with (are "superimposed on") many of the anxiety disorders described in Chapter 9, such as the obsessive-compulsive syndromes.
2. Neurotic depressions sometimes arise from stressful events. Often, however, there is no social stressor, but rather a more subjectively defined conflict, feeling of helplessness or inability to cope. Primary disorders do not seem to arise from such stressors.
3. Neurotic depressions are differentiated from primary ones in that in the former, there is not necessarily a history of depression or a family history of major affective disorders.
4. Neurotic depressions are not characterized by psychotic features such as delusions, hallucinations, impaired judgment, and lack of insight. More often than not, even though the depressive symptoms can be quite severe, the patient is able to meet most of the demands of job, school, and family.
5. Neurotic depressions are not generally accompanied by the physiological correlates of the major affective disorders such as biological retardation (psychomotor sluggishness and slowness) and certain kinds of sleep patterns, for example, early morning awakening. Neurotic depressives sometimes perceive pain and fatigue differently from the primary depressives: the latter group can withstand greater heat or work before reporting pain or withdrawing, and may often even fail to report pain (Miller, 1975).
6. Neurotic depressions are often quite responsive to verbal, behavioral, and cognitive therapies (see Chapters 19–21), whereas primary affective disorders often are not responsive to these treatments. Additionally, neurotic depressions are often only moderately responsive—if at all—to the pharmacological interventions that have been so helpful in remediating the symptoms of the major affective disorders.

The important thing to bear in mind is that even though there is not complete agreement as to what to call these depressions, or even a consensus as to their distinguishing characteristics as a group, these heterogeneous neurotic depressive disorders do not seem to possess the qualities of deep despair, sometimes leading to suicide, that characterize the major affective disorders.

Bipolar Affective Disorders

For many generations, even centuries, observers of human behavior noticed that some people periodically displayed high, euphoric, excited (manic) states or were plummeted into episodes of deep despair. These extreme affective (mood) states are opposite poles of the manic-depressive illness or disease, first labeled by Kraepelin in 1896 (see Kraepelin, 1921). Until then, even though one person displayed these swings, the polarities were thought to be two separate diseases. Kraepelin was the first to recognize these swings as poles of the same disease. It took many generations of researchers after Kraepelin to suggest that some people may have only recurrent manic episodes, and others only recurrent depressive episodes, but that both types of patient may be suffering, nevertheless, from a disorder very much related to Kraepelin's manic-depressive illness. These disorders represent an affective dysfunction that many people label endogenous. The term endogenous captures the etio-

* Akiskal and McKinney, 1973, 1975; Akiskal et al., 1979; Depue and Monroe, 1978a,b; Fowles and Gersh, 1979; Gersh and Fowles, 1979; Lader, 1975; Miller, 1975; and Thomson and Hendrie, 1972.

logical nature of this illness in that it seems to arise in response to "inside" rather than external factors (e.g., psychosocial stressors) and bears some relationship to biochemical and genetic variables.

The DSM-III no longer labels manic-depressive illness and related syndromes as such, but lists only the various subtypes under the general category of major affective disorders. However, in its classic form this condition is characterized by sudden episodes of a charged, euphoric, elevated mood that suddenly subsides as quickly as it erupted (for example, after a few weeks or months), soon plunging the patient into a severe, retarded depression that also can last for several months. These swings or cycles from manic to depressed phases can occur several times in the lifetime of the patient. In this classic form, we speak of a bipolar affective disorder.

Case 10.2 Frances: Major Affective Disorder, Bipolar type

Frances, now twenty-eight years old, has been picked up on three separate occasions by the local police, who claim that she was soliciting, or "hustling." Frances was indeed looking for men in the various bars she would go to, but not for income or for sex. She was looking for good times, fun, and action. She got plenty. She was restless, excited, euphoric. She could not stay home.

Frances, a social worker, was an A student at school. She was popular, a leader, and radiantly warm and outgoing. She attracted people as honey attracts bees. She was always talkative, eager, tireless in energy, and the initiator of projects, trips, parties, and action wherever she was. In her senior year at college she suddenly fell into a deep depression. She dropped out of college, returned home, and secluded herself for three months. She saw a therapist once a week, but for the most part she sat silently during the interviews.

As suddenly as the depression occurred, it subsided. Frances felt chipper, expansive, even elated. She returned to college, finished her courses with honors, and applied to and completed social-work school, all within two years. She was offered many jobs and accepted the best paying one as assistant to the director of a residential center for delinquent girls. Her performance on the job was outstanding. She assumed many special projects, gradually becoming indispensable to the institution and its administrative staff. Some people, however, were beginning to feel irritated by her pushy good will, activity, and social expansiveness. They were beginning to resent her taking over in social situations, her constant self-centered talk, and her unceasing need to be "on."

During the second year on the job, Frances had to quit. She had become deeply depressed, isolated, and unable to work, or even talk. She had frequent suicidal thoughts. She went home for several months on sick leave, suddenly "got better," and returned to her job when she felt that old drive, push, and elation. She worked for another year. This time, the elation became more frantic, pressured, excited, and exuberant. She began to prowl the neighborhood for action—and mostly ended up in one-night stands with anyone who would have her. She drank excessively and the next morning did not remember her sexual and drinking bouts. She was just about to be fired when she became depressed. She left suddenly for home, finding a bewildered, resentful family.

When she "got better," she was no longer employable. She had switched over into a period of manic excitement that was no longer controllable at home. She vaguely knew she was ill, but her parents were sure—finally recognizing this fact. Frances was admitted to a hospital and remained in a closely supervised ward for two months. After a period of therapy and medication, she was sent home.

Frances is still under supervised medication. She no longer is picked up by the police. Although she becomes moderately depressed each year, the depressions are not as deep as formerly. She feels good after each depression, but does not enter a phase of manic excitement. Frances now works in a community mental-health program a few miles from home, is soon to be married, and understands her illness well enough to consider genetic counseling to help her face the question of whether or not to have children. Frances has her blood chemistry checked every few weeks to make sure that everything is satisfactory. Both her mother and maternal grandmother, she discovered, had periodic episodes of deep depression. Frances' two sisters, incidentally, one aged twenty-two, and the other aged thirty-five years, have experienced neither extreme depression nor manic excitement.

Frances is happy now that she knows she can control her extreme emotional fluctuations. She had lost confidence in herself and had felt guilty about her behavior. The fact that she was a burden to her family had been very troubling to her. She now feels more confident about her job, her "sanity," and her effect on others. In the past few years, psychotherapy proved to be essential in helping her overcome her fears about her future, her identity, and her need for medication.

The DSM-III estimates that about 1 percent of the population suffers from bipolar affective disorder, the incidence of which is equally distributed between men and women. However, other estimates are lower—about 0.3 percent, with about 600,000 identified and treated people in the United States each year (Berger, 1978). It has also been suggested that the incidence of this condition is more frequent in upper-SES levels (Silverman, 1968). This might be explained, however, by unreliability of diagnoses on lower-SES levels or by confusion with other syndromes such as schizophrenia, as well as by greater sensitivity in detecting instances of this illness on upper-SES levels.

Symptoms of mania and depression. Spotlight 10.1 described the symptoms of depression, which in the depressive pole of this illness can range in severity from mild or moderate to extremely intense. In the extreme form, there can be delusions of body deterioration, deep despair and hopelessness, suicidal threats, thoughts, and gestures, and many completed suicides.

Symptoms in the manic pole can similarly range from mild or moderate in expression to extreme, excitable, unmanageable states often requiring hospitalization. Spotlight 10.2 describes some manic symptoms; but these symptoms may never reach the extreme form. In hypomania, for example, you might find the individual to be a warm, outgoing, likable, talkative, friendly chatterbox who shows much energy and a high activity level, and who is always on the "go." Hypomanic people may be a little inattentive and a little stubborn and egocentric; they are often self-absorbed in that much of their talk, activity, and interests revolves around themselves. But they are often generally likable, although they may also be irritating from time to time.

In acute manic states the foregoing is exaggerated. The verbal flow is uninhibited. There may be "bad" punning, an excess of wit. The patient is relentlessly "on." There is flight of ideas, a rapid verbal shifting of ideas with sequences of associations based on a minimum of logic or reason. Ideas are not completed—there seems to be an inner distractibility so that the stream of thought is never brought to a goal or endpoint. For example, one patient was asked if he felt sad. He replied:

> *Yes, you have to be quiet to be sad. Everything having to do with "s" is quiet—on the q.t.—sit, sob, sigh, sin, sorrow, surcease, sought, sand, sweet mother's love, and salvation. This is my first case—I am kind of a bum lawyer or liar—too damned honest to be a lawyer, so had to be a liar (Kolb, 1973, p. 103).*

There may also be sudden swings from humor to anger accompanied by a general disregard for social customs in language, gestures, and behavior.

In the extreme manic phase, hospitalization is generally necessary. Such patients are out of contact with reality. There is rapid and incoherent speech, meaningless or bizarre gestures, and frequently, hallucinations and delusions. Sometimes these patients display uncontrollable bursts of anger or violence or sudden senseless actions that can be harmful to themselves or to others.

Spotlight 10.2 Manic States: Characteristic Symptoms

The following symptoms and behaviors characterize manic stages of bipolar affective disorders (see Spotlight 10.1 for a list of depressive symptoms). Behaviors of the sort described here are not all present when a diagnosis is made. Many patients show more moderate forms of manic expression, from mild (hypomanic) levels to more euphoric, active, heightened states, stabilizing at these levels without going into the frankly psychotic state that is accompanied by delusions and extreme impairment of judgment that may require hospitalization.

Researchers are coming to believe that the disease has a wide spectrum of manifestation so that predisposition for it may in some people never develop into a full-blown episode. For example, many people are changeable and moody, fluctuating from the blues to elation or euphoria for no apparent reason, a state called lability. Labile people are not necessarily suffering from a bipolar disorder, although some researchers suggest that such lability may reflect the presence of a disposition or tendency toward this type of pathology.

Mood: Euphoria, elation, excitement; sometimes irritability, fleeting anger; there can also be contagious hilarity

Self-image: high, uncritical, unrealistic self-esteem; there can be grandiosity or delusions of affiliation with powerful persons or with a celebrity, in extreme cases, with God

Interpersonal behavior: sociable, outgoing, likable; in more extreme forms, expansive, intrusive (telephoning people at all hours), promiscuous; fluid, transitory relationships; involvement with many people and their projects, schemes, and business endeavors without being qualified to do so

Motivation and energy: high, energetic activity level; pressure to keep talking, with many puns and quips; physical restlessness; flight of attention and ideas ("racing thoughts"); and quick changes of attention; highly distractible

Sleep: decreased need for sleep, with early rising and little fatigue; can go for days, in extreme instances, without sleep

Judgment and attention: in extreme form, impairment of judgment and illogical, incoherent presentation of ideas; buying sprees, grandiose unrealistic schemes; may give away financial holdings or life savings in moments of expansiveness

Delusional thinking: can be frankly psychotic; in extreme forms, mistaken notions about one's identity and achievements

The DSM-III Classification

The affective disorders cover a wide spectrum of symptoms and intensity of expression. As noted, we are only now beginning to distinguish, even if crudely, among their different manifestations. There is by no means uniformity or consensus among the experts as to these distinctions. The DSM-III listings of affective disorders are presented in Listing 10.1. As can be seen from this list, the affective disorders are classified into the major affective disorders (consisting of the bipolar disorders and major depression), other specific affective disorders (including cyclothymic disorder and dysthymic disorder—the latter is the depressive neurosis already described), and atypical affective disorders.

Older, more traditional classifications generally distinguished between neurotic and psychotic depressions, or *endogenous* (not arising from outside factors such as stress; and *reactive* (presumably touched off by severe stressors) depressions. Specifically the DSM-II distinguished in its category of major affective disorders, involutional melancholia and various subcategories of manic-depressive ill-

Listing 10.1 The DSM-III Categories for Affective Disorders

- Major affective disorders
  - Bipolar disorder
    - mixed
    - manic
    - depressed
  - Major depression
    - single episode
    - recurrent
- Other specific affective disorders
  - Cyclothymic disorder
  - Dysthymic disorder (or depressive neurosis—DSM-II)
- Atypical affective disorders
  - Atypical bipolar disorder
  - Atypical depression

The major depressive episodes are coded: in remission; with psychotic features; psychotic features as mood-congruent or mood-incongruent (see text); with or without melancholia (see text).

Manic episodes are coded: in remission; with or without psychotic features; psychotic features as mood-congruent or mood-incongruent (see text).

ness. In addition, there were separate categories for psychotic depressive reaction and for depressive neurosis. We have already noted that the category for involutional melancholia is no longer in use; instead, a major depression is used when applicable.

The bipolar designation was illustrated in Case 10.2, which described Frances's episodic bouts with manic and depressive episodes. A major depression is illustrated in Case 10.3, which describes Christopher and the single, anguished psychotic depression he experienced.

The cyclothymic disorders, according to the DSM-III, describe a mood disturbance with periods of depression and hypomania that are not as severe as those included in the major affective categories. There are periods of depression including feelings of inadequacy, low self-esteem, excessive need for sleep, and problems in attention and concentration alternating with periods of heightened self-esteem, outgoingness, and focused productivity. These less extreme mood disturbances are not characterized by psychotic features such as delusions, hallucinations, or thinking disturbances. The dysthymic disorders, which can also characterize children, refer to the neurotic depressions already illustrated. These, of course, are characterized by an absence of psychotic features.

The major affective disorders, the DSM-III suggests, should be classified as with or without psychotic features. If psychotic features are present, a rating should be made as to whether or not the psychotic "content" is congruent with the mood disorder.

Mood-congruent psychotic features in depression or in a manic episode refer to the degree to which the delusions are consistent with expectation. In depression, the delusions or hallucinations are expected to have themes of great guilt, deserved persecution, and hypochondriasis. In manic episodes, mood-congruent ideation refers to delusions or hallucinations related to inflated self-worth; excessive power, skills, and talents; or identification with a powerful person, historical figure, or celebrity.

Mood-incongruent psychotic features in depression are delusions and hallucinations of being thought-controlled from without (thought insertion) or thoughts being known to others (thought broadcasting) rather than those associated with guilt, persecution, or hypochondriasis. In manic episodes, mood-incongruent psychotic features include delusions of persecution and of thought insertion and control, rather than the expected themes of grandiosity.

Case 10.3 Christopher: Major (Unipolar I?) Depression

Five years ago Chris, a 55-year-old senior partner in an old, respected Wall Street law firm, was offered the presidency, with a sizable financial reward, of a major corporation. A few days later, he became acutely depressed; within a few days he went into a full-blown psychotic depression that coincided with the announcement of his new position in the newspapers. There was no history of depression in his personal or family background.

His symptoms included excessive crying, threats of suicide, paranoid thoughts (feelings of persecution), delusions (his insides were rotting), and much verbalization of guilt. He became convinced that he was being punished because he was undeserving, worthless, and a fraud—unable to deliver the goods, to produce in any area that was expected of him. Between crying spells Chris was angry, agitated, sometimes hallucinatory, and at other times obsessed with his rotting insides. Often he sat in one position, staring into space. He lost weight, his face was pale, his eyes were clouded, and he avoided eye contact with others.

Chris was hospitalized because of his agitated suicidal threats. His wife—his third—and grown daughter could not take care of him at home because they were both working. He remained in the hospital for only a few weeks. During his stay and after he was discharged, he saw a psychotherapist daily. The therapist was available to him by telephone, also, to offer support, reassurance, and compassion. During this period, he was "maintained" on a moderate level of antidepressant medication (see Chapter 21).

In therapy, Chris learned that his "flight" into depression was a flight from success. Gradually, he was helped to put the pieces of his life together. He was the only child of an extremely successful father and was very dependent on his mother. Until he entered graduate school, he shirked responsibilities, did unevenly at school, and had many financial difficulties. He left college twice, but returned because he was not "making it" in the outside world either. Everyone was better off than he was, he thought, and he harbored great fantasies of aggression—toward males in particular. In these fantasies he would compete with men in sports, games, the classroom, sexual activities, always emerging as the winner. In graduate school he began to "act out" some of these fantasies, compulsively entering various competitions. With great effort he consistently won, as in his fantasies. Yet he felt undeserving, fraudulent, and guilty.

Later, as he began to build a successful career, he found himself in and out of three marriages, each terminating with a stormy divorce. His wives were weak, submissive women whom he bullied. Yet he felt emotionally dependent on them. Of interest is his realization that although he felt he could never win his mother's approval, he consistently discounted his wives' approval. Chris also came to realize his enormous reservoir of anger toward his (now dead) father, who he felt ruined his life.

Chris's poor self-confidence, feeling of being undeserving, basic dependency, and hidden appeal to his wives and mother (help me—I can't make it on my own) were just below the surface of his push for success. When success did come, he was sure that he could not meet the demands of his position. This irrational thought, together with the enormous surge of guilt (finally really winning out over all the others) and "grief" over his lost dependency and pattern of failure, catapulted him into severe conflict and the acute psychotic reaction. Chris now understands this and has come to terms with his poor self-confidence, guilt about being assertive, and need to bully and yet be dependent on women. He thinks he will soon remarry but remains somewhat wary of his ability to sustain a marriage.

Chris is now happier than ever before, but he looks back on his life, many wives, and current aloneness with wonderment that he survived it all. Today, he is sometimes depressed, occasionally has bouts with indecision, often gets severe headaches and backaches, and from time to time experiences great, overwhelming anger—feelings that subside as quickly as they erupt. He does not know what he is angry about. The memory (not of the circumstances but of the suffering) of the psychotic episode of five years ago, after he was informed of his great success, is only now beginning to fade.

The DSM-III recommends an additional subclassification of the major depressive episode: *with* or *without melancholia.* This is a historically early label that applies to extremely severe depression that the DSM-III characterizes as especially responsive to physical therapies. Melancholia is present when there is virtually no pleasure at all in any activity and when, in addition, at least three of the following are present: depressed mood (not grief and not response to separation or loss); depression is worse in the mornings; extremely early awakening; either severe psychomotor retardation or severe agitation; considerable weight loss; excessive guilt.

Table 10.1 Another Model: Subtypes of Bipolar and Unipolar Disorders

Type	*Definition*
	Bipolar
Bipolar 1	Personal history of both depressive and manic episodes, both usually requiring hospitalization
Unipolar mania	At least one hospitalization for mania, but no episodes of depression; family history of bipolar disorder
Bipolar 2	Hospitalizations for depressive episodes, but no manic or hypomanic symptoms leading to hospitalization; family history of bipolar disorder
Bipolar 3	At least one hospitalization for depression; no personal history of mania or hypomania, but family history of bipolar disorder
Bipolar other	Treated on an outpatient basis for depressive and hypomanic symptoms, but never hospitalized
	Unipolar
Unipolar 1	At least one hospitalization for depression; no personal or family history of mania or hypomania
Neurotic	Relation to Unipolar 1 unsettled
Unipolar other	Sought help or been treated for depressions only, but not hospitalized; no family history of bipolar disorder

Source: R.A. Depue and S.M. Monroe, Learned helplessness in the perspective of the depressive disorders: Conceptual and definitional issues, *Journal of Abnormal Psychology, 87,* p. 10. Copyright 1978 by the American Psychological Association. Reprinted by permission of the authors.

The DSM-III listings have both advantages and disadvantages. They distinguish between major and minor disorders; and within the major disorders they classify the presence of psychotic features. They permit distinctions between bipolar and unipolar disorders (see Table 10.1), and they contain suggestions for the kinds of depressions that might be responsive to medications. On the other hand, the DSM-III reflects the shifting grounds of the field in general in its lack of decisiveness and precision in defining the various types of depression. The failure of the DSM-III to classify the depressions with fine gradations reflects the limitations of our knowledge about depressions.

Researchers are continuing to provide more valid classificatory schemes, especially in the light of biochemical distinctions, family and clinical history, and differential response to medications among various groups of depressed and bipolar patients (Akiskal et al., 1979; Depue and Monroe, 1978ab; Fieve and Dunner, 1975). One such model is presented in Table 10.1. Although the fine points of this scheme are still being debated, there are already some encouraging implications as to the effectiveness of differing treatments for the different subtypes, offering some promise for the validity of this model.

Unipolar depressions are particularly troublesome to clinicians and researchers. Spotlight 10.3 looks at unipolar depressions more closely.

THEORIES AND MODELS OF DEPRESSION

The first set of theories described in this section stresses psychological factors. These theories are probably more relevant to the neurotic depressions described earlier in this chapter. The second set of theories, stressing a biological orientation, is probably more relevant to an understanding of the

Spotlight 10.3 Unipolar Depressions: A Mixed Bag

The understanding of severe unipolar depression, now regarded as a diverse category (Akiskal et al., 1979), is receiving considerable attention among clinicians and researchers, especially because its incidence is much greater than that of the bipolar disorders (Berger, 1978; DSM-III; Depue and Monroe, 1978a,b). For, according to Winokur (1979), depression outnumbers mania in the general population nine to one.

Here are three separate attempts to separate out the contents of this mixed bag, each with some biochemical, clinical, genetic, and pharmacological evidence in its favor. This is no idle taxonomic (classificatory) game, because not only treatment strategies but also further understanding of the etiology of mental disorders can be illuminated as progress in this area is made.

1. *Secondary versus primary depressions* (Akiskal and McKinney, 1975). Primary depressions have a family history of depression, do not occur in response to stressors (seem endogenous), and are generally not associated with neurotic disorders. In this scheme, people with secondary disorders never show psychotic features and respond differently to medications than do those with primary disorders.
2. *Pure depressive versus depressive spectrum disease* (Winokur, 1979). This classification is a simple one, holding that pure depressive disease is diagnosed in persons with a family history of depression but no alcoholism, whereas depression spectrum disease, a more variable, heterogeneous group, is diagnosed if a first-degree relative (father, mother, brother, sister) has alcoholism or an antisocial personality.
3. *Biologically retarded depression versus nonretarded depression* (Lader, 1975; Noble and Lader, 1972). A review of psychophysiological evidence—for example, indices of autonomic reactivity such as skin conductance, forearm blood flow, and resting salivary secretion—in a large number of patients independently assessed on a diagnostic scale suggests that the meaningful distinction among depressions is related to the presence or absence of retardation, a slowing up of physiological processes. The simple scheme suggested rests on the distinction between retarded and nonretarded depression.

   Retarded depressed patients, compared to normal, anxious, agitated, and depressed patients can be distinguished in several ways. They show reduced galvanic skin responses (GSR) and generally little autonomic reactivity, secrete less saliva, have frequent sleep disturbances such as awakening still tired, and show many endocrinological characteristics such as low epinephrine and norepinephrine excretion (Lader and Wing, 1969; Shagass and Jones, 1958).

major affective disorders just discussed. Many proponents of either "camp" however, claim the relevance of their approach to most, if not all, depressions.

Psychoanalytic Formulations

Psychoanalytic attempts to understand and treat depression rest largely on the view that depression entails inverted anger. The anger is turned against the self because of the guilt, anxiety, and fear of retaliation engendered as a result of intense hostility toward someone (such as a parent) on whom there is great dependency (Fenichel, 1945; Jacobson, 1971; Ostow, 1970). This repressed hatred, or rather self-hatred, seems to be a dynamic that exists in personalities in which there has been deprivation at the oral stage of psychosexual development, resulting in fixation at dependent levels.

Attempts to verify these formulations have proved to be largely inconclusive, primarily because such hypotheses are not empirically testable (Akiskal and McKinney, 1975). In fact there has been little experimental research on the psychoanalytic aspects of depression, although there is a plethora of case and clinical material. Further, a review of the few studies that explore the significance of early factors like parental deprivation, birth order, early childhood conflicts, and parental loss yields no consistent evidence supporting the view that these factors are of any importance in later depression (Becker, 1974; Granville-Grossman, 1968). The inconclusive status of psychoanalytic formulations is especially true for the major affective disorders.

Behavioral Formulations

The reinforcement model: Lewinsohn. Many behavioral positions have stressed inadequate or insufficient reinforcers as causing depressed behavior or the reduced frequency of social reinforcement in the maintenance of the depression (Costello, 1972; Eastman, 1976; Lazarus, 1968).

One such theoretical approach suggests that the depressed person's mood and behavior can be explained on the basis of a low rate of "response-contingent positive reinforcement." Depressed people show a "low rate of behavior" that can be explained by the low number of events in their environment that are reinforcing for them, and by the difficulties or limited skills they have in eliciting reinforcing events (Lewinsohn, 1974).

Indirect, moderately confirming evidence has accumulated regarding this hypothesis. For example, one study showed that depressed people tend to report fewer pleasant events engaged in than nondepressed people (Lewinsohn and Libet, 1972; MacPhillamy and Lewinsohn, 1974). Also, treatment programs designed to help depressed people increase those activities that produce positive reinforcement through pleasure are somewhat successful (MacPhillamy and Lewinsohn, 1974).

That depressed people receive fewer social rewards—one aspect of Lewinsohn's approach—because they do not elicit them from their environment also receives moderate confirmation. That is, a low rate of motor, verbal, and social activity results in reduced reinforcement in the individual's environment. For example, in one study, subjects were asked to converse over the telephone with depressed or nondepressed people. After the conversation, subjects who had conversed with depressed people reported more depression, anxiety, hostility, and negative feelings toward these people than did subjects who conversed with nondepressed individuals (Coyne, 1976).

Still another study attempted to test the prediction that "depression is a response to a low rate of reinforcement" (Wener and Rehm, 1975). The authors presented 200 female high-school and nursing students with a one-hundred-word list to which they were asked to respond with what they thought to be the most commonly or frequently associated word (for example, black–white, up–down). Positive reinforcement as to correctness of response was given at a high rate (four out of every five trials) to one group of subjects. Another group was positively reinforced at a low rate (one out of every five trials). Subjects were told that the correct association was not necessarily the one they themselves would make but what they think most other people would make. Speed and self-confidence of responses were measured as the subjects proceeded in the experimental presentation of the words. A measure of depressive affect was administered at the end of the experimental procedure. The findings were consistent with the authors' prediction in that depressive affect, self-confidence ratings, and latency (speed) of response were all related in the predicted direction to rates of reinforcement. Infrequent reinforcement, as expected, was associated with higher depressive affect scores, slower responses, and lower self-confidence ratings.

An extensive review of studies designed to explore this model yield only mild support regarding low rates of response-contingent reinforcement as a cause of depression, because most studies were of a correlational nature (Blaney, 1977). However, a low rate of social reinforcement might sustain, or result from, depressed behavior, rather than cause it.

Overall, because many findings in this area were based on normal or moderately depressed volunteer subjects, this model tells us very little about clinical depression.

The cognitive model: Beck. The many studies that attempt to relate lack of positive or insufficient reinforcement to the origins of depression stress the environment, overlooking internal variables. But even when depressed subjects were induced to participate in pleasurable activities, their depressed mood did not change (Hammen and Glass, 1975). These and similar studies suggest the strong possibility that feelings about, and perception and evaluation of the meaning of, the so-called reinforcing events are of extreme importance in characterizing depressed people. According to Beck (1967; Beck et al., 1961, 1974), depressed people are prepared to view events around them negatively. They have a cognitive set of helplessness and hopelessness. Depression results from perceiving environmental events in one's experience, or world, as negative; of anticipating one's future as negative; and of viewing one's self in a negative light.

Moderate empirical evidence supports this view (see Blaney, 1977 for a review). Correlational studies, for example, indicate that depressives recall negative material with greater facility than positive material (Lloyd and Lishman, 1975). Clinical evidence also supports the cognitive approach in that depressives do indeed, as Beck suggests, tend to have gloomy views of interpersonal events, incorrectly label happenings as negative, and draw arbitrary negative inferences from data, all designed to enhance their pessimism and negative self-view.

Even if cognitions do not directly cause some of the deep, severe, intense depressive states described in this chapter, they may certainly play an indirect role in sustaining or continuing them. And if, in the course of helping depressed people, we can modify their beliefs about themselves that may be distortions, illogical inferences, or overgeneralizations that "justify" and "confirm" their feelings of worthlessness, self-blame, and guilt, then indeed Beck's views offer some promise. As we shall see in Chapters 19, 20, and 21, which deal with various approaches to modifying behavior, this cognitive thread plays an extremely important role in the success of some treatment methods.

The self-regulation model. Depressed people, even if performing on the same level as nondepressed people, reward themselves less than do their controls. These experimental findings find support not only in a college population but also in clinical populations.

This approach is consistent with Bandura's (see Chapter 6), which emphasizes the role of an individual's selective responses to environmental events by a personal evaluation of his or her own failures and successes and by devising his or her own goals and rewards. People themselves play an important self-determined role in the nature of their own experiences. In other words, the consequences of a person's acts are "processed" in different ways by different people; the "environment" is not the same for all people; and equal behaviors do not have equal consequences.

There is some empirical evidence for this view. For example, depressed patients were less likely to reward themselves, or rewarded themselves consistently lower, than nondepressed patients following their responses in simple tasks (for example, word associations or word recognitions), despite equal levels of performance between the two groups (Lobitz and Post, 1979; Rehm, 1977; Rozensky, Rehm, Pry, and Roth, 1977). These low levels of self-reward were also accompanied by low levels of self-expectation and self-evaluation. But these negative views applied only to themselves, for when rewarding, evaluating, or setting levels of performance for others, depressed patients were considerably more generous than they were for themselves (Lobitz and Post, 1979). Depressed people thus are not universally negative. They perceive themselves as less deserving, less competent, and with a more pessimistic outlook than they perceive others.

Overall, these empirical findings cannot be viewed as suggesting causal factors in depression.

Spotlight 10.4 Beck's Inventories

In the course of their work, Beck and his colleagues found it essential to develop objective and reliable methods for assessing the views that subjects have about themselves, their worlds, or their futures. They did indeed develop instruments that have served highly useful research purposes, especially since they have been found to show good reliability and validity (for example, appropriate variations in scores were obtained by patients judged to vary in depth of depression).

One of these instruments is the Beck Depression Inventory (Beck, 1967; Beck, et al., 1961), which requires subjects to rate themselves not only regarding the presence of symptoms such as those described in Spotlight 10.1, for example, somatic preoccupation, guilt, fatigability, or social withdrawal, but also regarding their cognitive views. Here are two examples of ratings from this inventory:*

	Sense of failure
0	*I do not feel like a failure*
1	*I feel I have failed more than the average person*
2	*As I look a back on my life, all I can see is a lot of failures*
3	*I feel I am a complete failure as a person*

	Body image change
0	*I don't feel I look any worse than I used to*
1	*I am worried that I am looking old or unattractive*
2	*I feel that there are permanent changes in my appearance that make me look unattractive*
3	*I believe that I look ugly*

An area of interest to Beck, as noted, is the subject's view of the future, specifically, his or her sense of hopelessness. Here are some true-false items from the Beck Hopelessness Scale (Beck, Weissman, Lester, and Trexler, 1974):*

I just don't get the breaks, and there's no reason to believe I will in the future. (T)

The future seems vague and uncertain to me. (T)

I happen to be particularly lucky, and I expect to get more of the good things in life than the average person. (F)

These, and instruments and inventories like them, have been particularly useful in assessing level of depression or sense of hopelessness before or after some experimental manipulation.

* Items excerpted from the Beck Depression Inventory and Beck Hopelessness Scale, copyright © 1978 by Aaron T. Beck, M. D. Further information about these scales and/or permission for their use may be obtained from: CENTER FOR COGNITIVE THERAPY, Room 602, 133 South 36th Street, Philadelphia, PA 19104.

They do suggest that depressed people view themselves differently from the way they view others, perceptions that may result from, rather than cause, the depression. Once again, if modification of depressive behaviors based on these empirical findings helps to change expectations, self-evaluations, and self-rewards, then these findings might have some therapeutic implications, but only if empirical findings demonstrate equivalent changes in mood and depressive affect, which after all, is what depression is all about.

The learned helplessness model: Seligman. The term *learned helplessness* was first suggested by Seligman as a model for depression in humans, as a result of experiments with dogs (Seligman and Maier, 1967).

This model proposes that belief in one's own helplessness emerges as a result of having learned that one's own actions have little or no relationship to events or outcomes (Miller and Seligman, 1973; Seligman, 1972, 1973, 1974, 1975; Seligman, Klein, and Miller, 1976). This viewpoint suggests that helplessness, a sense of not being able to exert control over one's environment, is the primary cause of nonendogenous depression. At times, learned helplessness is equated with—is employed as a definition of—depression.

The original work, later demonstrated with other animals and humans, specifically demonstrated that dogs exposed to repeated, inescapable, uncontrollable, or unpredictable aversive stimulation, such as shock, subsequently in escapable or controllable situations did not attempt to avoid this stimulation. The subjects remained passive (depressed) despite options to solve the problems before them. On the other hand, if the subjects in the preexperimental period had not been exposed to inescapable, uncontrollable stimulation, they actively attempted to escape the subsequent aversive situation.

The learned helplessness paradigm applied to humans suggests that when people learn that they cannot affect their environments—that they are powerless to control what happens to them—they become passive, immobilized, and restricted in coping ability. They have learned that whatever they do will have little effect on what happens to them. Depression thus can be characterized as consisting of low levels of problem-solving behaviors in the face of aversive stimulation, even when it is possible to do something about what is happening. The learned helplessness model implies that depressed individuals have had a long history of training in helplessness and have learned to respond with great passivity in situations requiring active behavior. This state of affairs is accompanied by self-perceptions of not having any control over one's fate.

Much of the experimental evidence for the applicability of this model to humans was derived from experiments that placed college subjects into situations that paralleled the no-escape, escape, and control situations of the animal experiments. In one study, for example (Miller and Seligman, 1975), it was demonstrated that nondepressed college students, as a result of learned helplessness training in an aversive no-escape noise situation, subsequently performed like clinically depressed subjects on anagram tasks. Depressed subjects presumably employed a learned helplessness strategy in the perception of new learning situations—a strategy that can be trained in nondepressed subjects by prior exposure to certain kinds of situations in which no matter what is done, avoidance of a negative stimulus cannot be achieved.

It is claimed that some of Seligman's findings have specific treatment implications. In an early study, for example, when dogs, trained for helplessness by pretreatment exposures to inescapable shock, were later forced to escape from the aversive stimulation by being dragged across the electrified area of the experimental box to the nonelectrified (safe) area, they eventually learned to escape the aversive stimulation. This has implications for the treatment of depressed people: directive treatment that forces depressed, passive people to obtain reinforcement through their own actions may be effective in reducing depression. That is, by creating and sustaining situations in which people can learn that events and outcomes are controllable, learned helplessness (and depression) can be reversed.

These intriguing studies have been carefully evaluated by many researchers and clinicians, especially because their findings seem provocatively relevant to the understanding and treatment of depression. Some of the reported experimental findings have not always been duplicated (replicated) (Blaney, 1977). For example, the expected transfer of learned helplessness effects across situations among pretreated subjects was not found, nor was depressive affect always induced by helplessness training (Cole and Coyne, 1977).

By and large, the most compelling arguments are that the model from animals is not relevant to clinical depression. Further, the experimental evidence based on college students whose level of depression is assessed by checklists and inventories such as the Beck Depression Inventory (1967) simply does not apply to the full range and complexities of what is known about clinical depression (DePue and Monroe, 1978a; Eastman, 1976; Costello, 1978; Buchwald, Coyne, and Cole, 1978; Huesman, 1978). For example, the subtypes of depression previously described, especially the endogenous type, which apparently has a large nonlearned etiological component, are not effectively dealt with by Seligman's approach. Although some efforts have been made to redeem the utility of this approach by suggesting that it applies specifically to "reactive depressions" (Klein and Seligman, 1976), most researchers claim that even this large group of depressions is heterogeneous, requiring a more complex etiological model than that offered by the learned helplessness paradigm.

Separation and Anaclitic Depression

In Chapter 6, when Harlow's work was discussed, mothering, cuddling, and physical closeness to a peer or mother surrogate in young infancy were described as some of the consequences of deprivation in these areas. This discussion focused mainly on research with monkeys. More recent research with adult monkeys has continued this general thrust: the removal of social supports, social systems, and social interactions can engender depressive behavior. In one study, Suomi et al. (1975) demonstrated that separation of adult monkeys from their families resulted in depressed behavior unless the separated monkeys were housed with other monkeys. Depressed monkeys groomed themselves less, showed self-clasping behavior (hugging or holding some part of their bodies for a length of time), or rolled themselves into balls, their physical appearance deteriorated, and they showed stereotyped movements.

Spitz (1945, 1946) had made similar observations much earlier in work with human infants. He used the term *anaclitic depression* to describe the striking impairment of development in cognitive, motor, and speech areas when there had been a sudden separation from the mother. Spitz's clinical observations were that infants separated from their mothers between the ages of six and twelve months first went through an early phase of great anger and protest. This phase was followed by anaclitic depression—a period of withdrawal and a plateau, developmentally speaking. If the baby and the mother were returned to each other within three to five months, the baby recovered. Continued separation from the mother resulted in "hospitalism" (a pattern of extreme apathy, loss of body tone, and nonresponsiveness), with a strong possibility that there would be mental and physical deterioration. So frequently have such clinical cases been reported that the DSM-III now recognizes this syndrome by referring to it as reactive attachment disorder of infancy, applicable to children below the age of thirty-six months who have had disruption of caretaking and affectional bonds, with a subsequent display of apathy and nonresponsiveness.

These observations have been generally confirmed by Bowlby (1969, 1973), who described a similar sequence of protest and despair in older (two-to-three-year-old) hospitalized children separated from their mothers. Bowlby suggested that the inability to tolerate such separations with its ensuing grief and despair was basic depressive affect. Even though these authors regard separation and loss as primary precursors of a depressive reaction, it is not clear whether or not substitutes for mothering in the form of peer or mother-surrogate interactions are sufficient to ward off depressive behaviors in humans, as some of Harlow's work would suggest (Spiro, 1974).

Although some of the foregoing discussion suggests that depression and separation or loss of a loved object are always associated, a review of investigations of the relationship of such events as loss and separation in adults to onset of depression disclosed that only a portion of clinical depressions can be so accounted for (Paykel, 1973). Loss and separation do not occur in all depressions, nor do all individuals who suffer loss or separation become depressed (Klerman, 1974; Scott and Senay, 1973). Further, parental death does not predispose a child to adult depression, according to a review of controlled studies (Crook and Eliot, 1980).

Biological Approaches to the Primary Affective Disorders

Although many of the foregoing theoretical models seem relevant to understanding depression, and even offer some possibilities for treating depression, the thrust of recent conceptualizations about the primary affective disorders has recently taken a somewhat different direction, focusing mainly on the body and its biochemistry. These conceptualizations are particularly interesting in the light of findings that many depressive disorders do not arise as a result of external stressors or life events (Akiskal and McKinney, 1975). These are not new notions, for they go back to the ancient Greeks, who thought that physical factors, the body humors, controlled the emotions. The word melancholia, in fact, means "black bile," the substance causing depression, according to their theory.

The evidence that has been accumulating slowly but steadily comes from genetics, biochemistry, neurobiology, and from the relatively new advances in psychopharmacology. Although such material is considerably beyond the scope of this book, the next several pages will briefly touch on some of the major implications of this work. Important to bear in mind is that in the decades to come you will undoubtedly see some remarkable advances in knowledge about how the brain and its biochemistry fits into the overall scheme of behavior, both normal and abnormal, especially in the areas of mood, alcoholism, depression, suicide, and schizophrenia.

Genetic and familial factors. About 10 percent of first-degree relatives (parents, siblings, and offspring) of manic-depressive bipolar patients also develop this illness. When both parents were diagnosed as having manic-depressive disease, the risk for their children developing this illness falls between 20 and 40 percent (Schulz, 1940). These and similar data that disclose a high familial incidence among members of a family in which there is some type of affective disorder have led many researchers to conclude that there are strong genetic components in the transmission of this condition (Dunner, 1975; Kety, 1979; Winokur et al., 1969).

Can these findings be due to similar environment? Twin and adoptee studies can shed light on this issue. Identical (MZ) twins (same genetic information) show 50 percent concordance, while fraternal (DZ) twins show 10 percent concordance, as do siblings, for this disease. When adopted, ill children's adoptive and biological families are compared, the illness most often runs in their biological families, whereas the incidence in their adoptive families runs at about the same rate as in the general population (Kety, 1979).

There is not a one-to-one relationship between inherited genetic structures and the expression of this disease, however, even though earlier work tended to stress absolute genetic determinism in its incidence (for example, Kallmann, 1952). But there is some agreement that genetic transmission plays an important, if not invariant, role in this illness, leaving room for the influence of other variables. There are many investigations of considerable relevance to the current discussion (see, for example, Cadoret and Winokur, 1975; DeFries and Plomin, 1978; Dunner, Gershon, and Goodwin, 1976; Trzebiatowska-Trzeciak, 1977; Winokur, 1971; Winokur et al., 1969, 1975) that provide some of the following findings. Family incidence for people with either bipolar or unipolar illness is considerably greater than that for the general population. Moreover, bipolar and unipolar depressions probably represent different subtypes, because their familial incidence differs: incidence among families of bipolar patients is much larger than among unipolar patients. There may even be some genetic subtype within the bipolar and unipolar categories. However, the exact nature of genetic transmission continues to remain unknown.

Biochemical factors With the development of sophisticated methods for studying the neurochemistry of the brain, it is becoming possible to explore the relationship of behaviors, especially pathological behaviors, to brain chemistry. These explorations, unfortunately, yield speculative and indirect rather than direct evidence, because it is not possible to study the brain neurochemicals of a living person directly. Nevertheless, technology now includes the study of biochemicals in the urine, blood stream, cerebrospinal fluid, and postmortem examination of brain tissue of depressed people or suicides through highly developed methods.

Through these methods, as well as through the examination of the responses of different groups of depressed patients to medications (for example, becoming more agitated, manic, improving, not responding), it has become increasingly clear that there are (a) significant biochemical underpinnings to the major depressive states and (b) differences among clinically distinguishable depressive subtypes.

The earliest conceptualizations in this area suggested that clinical depression is correlated with the actions of certain neurotransmitters, specifically, the biogenic amines (Bunney, 1971; Schildkraut, 1965; Schildkraut and Kety, 1967). These are the catecholamines (dopamine and norepinephrine) and the indoleamines (serotonin and tryptamine). In the early version of this biochemical model, it was thought that depressions were associated with a deficiency of the catecholamines (especially norepinephrine) at some receptor sites, whereas the switch to manic excitement was associated with an excess of these brain chemicals.

Initially there was encouraging support for this and related views. For example, many of the drugs that lift mood and reverse depression (see Chapter 21) tend to raise the level of these biogenic amines in the brain (Akiskal and McKinney, 1975).

Since the early catecholamine hypotheses, it has become clear that the proposed relationships are not that simple and that interactions of several of the biogenic amines are probably involved in producing different kinds of mood states (Schildkraut et al., 1977). For example, low levels of serotonin (an indoleamine) were found in the cerebrospinal fluid of some, but not other, equally depressed patients. (Is there a serotonin subtype in primary affective disorder (Åsberg, Thorén, and Träskman, 1975)?

Still other biochemicals, such as sodium or potassium—especially their distribution on either side of neuronal membranes—have great influence on the activities of the neurons in the brain. These chemicals, called electrolytes, are ions or electrically charged atoms that are of great significance in the processes of neural transmission. Although their complex influences on neural transmission are not fully understood, evidence has begun to accumulate that electrolyte imbalances are associated with some states of depression and manic excitement (Coppen, 1967; Tosteson, 1981). The effectiveness of lithium carbonate in remediating some affective disorders may reflect this electrolytic imbalance.

Evaluation of biological approaches to depression. What is the status of these relatively new developments? Various neurotransmitters and neurochemicals and their interactions are very much implicated in determining the onset and course of the major affective disorders. It is probably through these chemicals that genetic structures work their influence. However, it is now clear that no single neurotransmitter or neurochemical is responsible for moods, depression, or depressive subtypes. But the functional relationships and interactions among neurotransmitters, hormones, and electrolytes in determining these states are not yet understood and are very much open to further study (Ghose and Coppen, 1977; Sourkes, 1977; Van Praag, 1977).

Largely as a result of differential response to medications as well as of some indirect genetic evidence, the biochemical model supports the notion that there are distinct subtypes among the major affective disorders, especially between the bipolar and unipolar types (Akiskal and McKinney, 1975; Depue and Monroe, 1978a; Schildkraut et al., 1977, 1978). There is thus considerable promise for alleviating many types of depressive disorders through gaining more complete knowledge about the effectiveness of specific pharmacological interventions with different groups of patients. In the meanwhile, we are still far from being able to control the levels of deficiencies or excesses of brain chemicals because there is not enough information about their interactions. Also, it may be that depression precedes or is a precursor to some of the chemical states found, rather than the other way around. Further, as has already been noted, although we are discussing brain processes, our actual methods for assaying the biochemistry of the brain yield only indirect speculation, not "facts." And finally, although the role of stressors and cognitive variables in controlling the levels of various neurochemicals in the brain are not completely understood, they may play an important part in this complex arena (Akiskal and McKinney, 1973, 1975).

A Theoretical Integration of Some of These Models

The compelling nature of many of the foregoing models has led to an attempt to integrate several of them into a "unified" theory (Akiskal and McKinney, 1973; 1975). In this model, depression is the final "common pathway," the end product, of reversible deficits or dysfunctions in certain neural centers that provide reinforcement to the organism. That is, depression comes about if the reward system in the central nervous system (CNS) is not working properly.

Thus, although depression is conceived as a failure to respond to reinforcement in the usual, expected ways, these researchers suggest that many different types of events and circumstances can contribute to this final common end stage. This includes genetic predispositions, physiological stressors (such as hypothyroidism or viral infection), psychosocial stressors and predispositions (such as separation and loss), and psychological predisposition (such as learned helplessness). Each of the foregoing can contribute to or cause brain dysfunctions in levels of biogenic amines, neurotransmitters, and other biochemicals that alter the functions of the reward centers, thus leading to depression.

Figure 10.1 graphically illustrates the interlocking contributions of the various components

Figure 10.1 Schematic representation of melancholia as a final common pathway that can originate from many sources. (H. S. Akiskal and W. T. McKinney, Jr., Overview of recent research in depression: Integration of ten conceptual models into a comprehensive clinical frame, *Archives of General Psychiatry,* 1975, 32, 300. Copyright 1975, American Medical Association.)

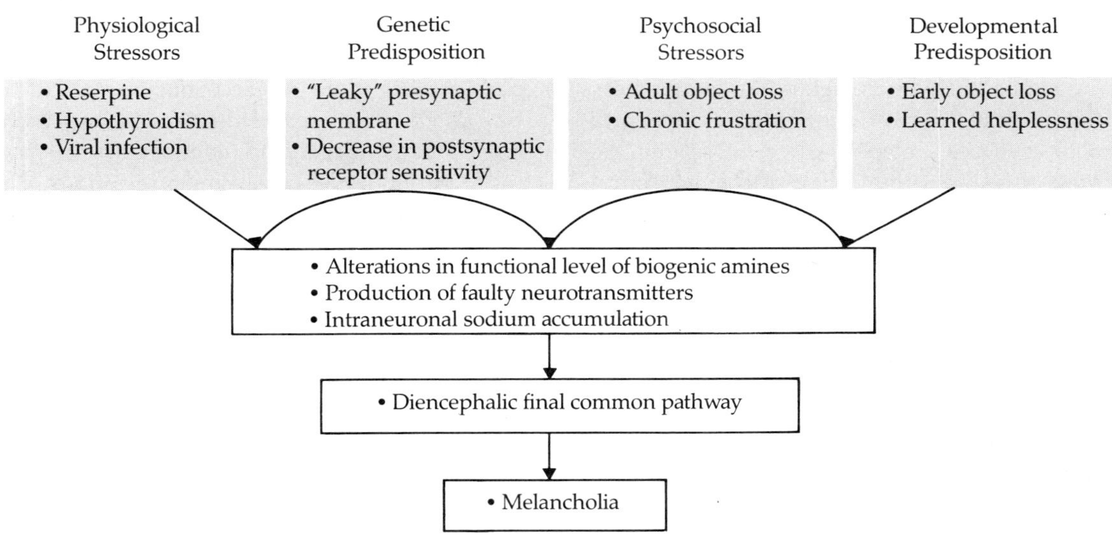

that can contribute to the end state of depression, unifying many of the separate models previously discussed. In sum, this model suggests that biochemical interactions can be secondary to, rather than always a primary cause of, depression.

TREATMENT AND ASSESSMENT OF DEPRESSION

The treatment of depression varies with the position that one adopts as to its etiology. Therapeutic interventions thus range from psychoanalytic approaches and various cognitive strategies (for example, those of Beck) to pharmacological methods. The final "common pathway" approach (see p. 253) not only implies that depressive states are reversible, but also suggests to some people that intervention at any level (for example, biochemical, psychosocial, psychological) would be appropriate in reversing depressive affect.*

Chapters 19–21 discuss these and various other interventions. It should be noted, however, that whatever the specific method, the significance of support, reassurance, and compassion in the treatment of depression should be underscored. Most therapists are familiar with the desperately depressed patient who has experienced inappropriate therapy: for example, a silent therapist, or an active, interpretative one who is "heavy" with psychoanalytic insights but who is lacking in compassion. Friendly and empathic listening, reassurance, and availability—even a telephone conversation—are sometimes more important than one's theoretical orientation.

If any of the interventive methods is to work on an optimal level, the correct assessment of the patient is required. Neurotic depressions are not "lifted" (if at all) by the same medications as are some of the endogenous types. And even among the latter, inappropriate medications may switch a depressive into a manic phase, speed up "cycling" between manic and depressed phases, or have no beneficial effects at all (for example, lithium carbonate for many subtypes of depression). Similarly, cognitive psychotherapeutic or behavioral interventions are probably more effective in modifying neurotic depressions across many situations than are the pharmacological ones.

In attempts to assess the patient, are psychological methods of the sort described in this book helpful? Projective instruments have not fared too well in this regard except in generally reflecting the lack of productivity and responsiveness of the patient. Various inventories especially developed for depression such as the Beck Depression Inventory or the Zung Depression Status Inventory (Zung, 1972), are more effective instruments, judging by their reliability and validity. They can be quite useful, thus, in selecting depressed subjects or in assessing level of depression before or after an experimental manipulation. These inventories, however, do not substitute for the rich, multifaceted impressions a good clinician can derive from a face-to-face situation, during which the nature and intensity of symptoms, family history, previous response to medication, recurrence of episodes, nature of sleep disturbance, history of suicidal attempts, or presence of delusional material can be assessed. Nonetheless, the pinpointing of appropriate treatment, even with this information, awaits considerably more research not only as to the nature of the subtypes of depression and their etiologies but also regarding the most effective methods for modifying their clinical manifestations.

SUICIDE

There are at least 26,000 reported suicides annually in the United States (Berger, 1978). Suicide is among the ten leading causes of death in this country (Beck, Kovaks, and Weissman, 1979). In the 20-to-40-year-old age group, suicide is the third lead-

* It should be noted, however, that Akiskal and McKinney (1973, 1975) do not specifically imply that interventions other than biochemical would be effective.

ing cause of death (Schuyler, 1974). In the younger group, estimates of suicide vary from the fourth most common cause of death (Jacobs, 1971; Mendels, 1970) to second only to accidents (Nemy, 1973).

These figures vastly underestimate the "true" number of suicides, for many are unrecorded. "Accidental" deaths in automobiles, for example, or death as a result of overdose of sleeping pills, may actually be suicides. Thus, some estimates run as high as 50,000 to 75,000 suicides annually (Schuyler, 1974). It is further thought that there are about 250,000 to 1,000,000 unsuccessful suicide attempts, possibly even more, each year (Jacobs, 1971), with a high proportion of these among youth (Dublin, 1963; Jacobziner, 1960).

The many unanswered questions about suicide pose a challenge to the mystifying nature of suicide. The next section touches on some aspects of this challenge.

Not all suicides can be prevented, but many can be. (Nancy Hays/Monkmeyer Press Photo Service)

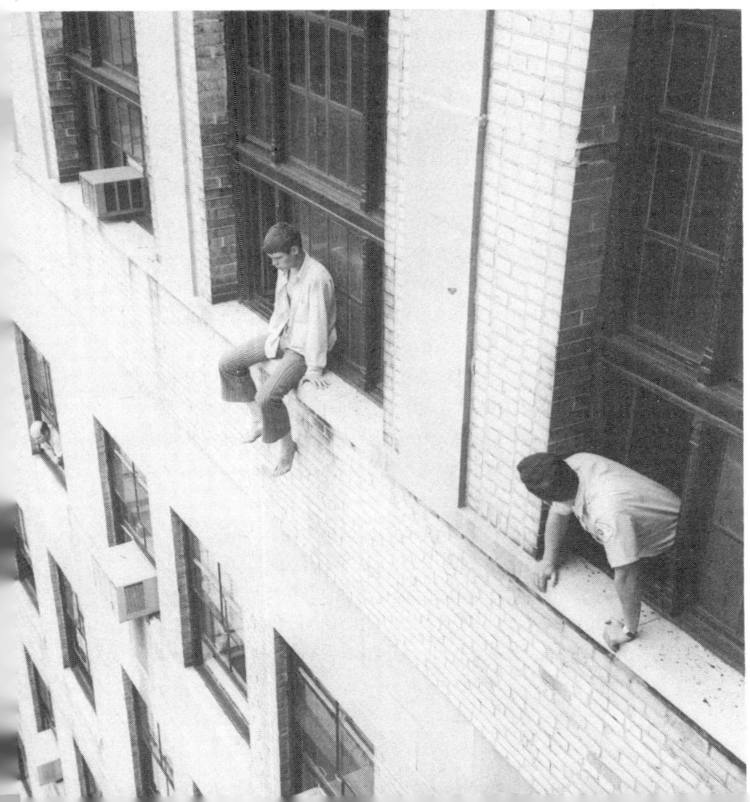

Suicide and Society

How would one explain some of the following facts about suicide? Suicide rates tend to decrease in wartime, and to increase during periods of economic depression. In New York City, young black adult men have twice as high a suicide rate as young white adult men (Hendin, 1969). On the other hand, suicide rates in racially segregated southern communities in the 1950s show blacks to have *lower* suicide rates than whites. And suicide rates in various immigrant populations in the United States are higher than those found in their countries of origin.

One unifying classic hypothesis might account for some of these data about suicide. Durkheim (1897), a French sociologist, proposed that the less integrated or looser the social organization of a group, the greater will be its incidence of suicide. Thus, the cohesiveness of a wartime society might explain the drop in suicide rates during war years. Whether or not one subscribes to Durkheim's conceptualizations, the epidemiology of suicide tends to confirm the more general view that sociocultural factors are of extreme significance in efforts to understand suicide.

The wide variation in suicide rates from nation to nation is a well-known fact. Table 10.2 presents such figures per 100,000 in population. Why does Hungary have the highest rate and Italy the lowest? Why are the disparities between male and female rates so different in various nations? For example, in Israel, Japan, and England—each with strikingly different religious systems and cultural mores—the frequency with which women commit suicide is two-thirds of that for men, an extremely high rate when compared to most of the other nations.

Even methods of suicide vary from culture to culture and through the ages. Thus the usual methods, through guns, knives, poison, hanging, jumping from heights, slashing the wrists, or breathing noxious gases, follow the fashion in the same way that symptoms do (Monk, 1975; Rosen, 1975). Men have always tended to use more violent (more lethal) methods than women (guns, for example,

Table 10.2 Suicide Completion Rates per 100,000 in Selected Countries

Country	Both Sexes	Male	Female
Australia	19.2	27.0	12.2
Austria	28.3	42.0	16.9
Canada	11.1	17.3	4.9
Czechoslovakia	28.2	40.9	16.5
Denmark	24.2	32.4	16.2
England	15.1	18.3	12.2
Finland	29.0	47.7	12.3
France	20.7	32.3	10.0
Germany	24.1	33.3	16.2
Hungary	33.9	48.9	20.3
Israel	10.1	11.9	8.2
Italy	7.1	10.2	4.2
Japan	24.7	29.0	20.6
Netherlands	9.1	11.5	6.8
New Zealand	13.0	18.0	8.0
Norway	10.0	15.7	4.5
Poland	12.8	21.9	4.7
Scotland	11.4	15.2	8.1
Sweden	21.7	32.0	11.6
Switzerland	23.3	33.9	13.2
United States	15.6	24.0	7.7

Source: Modified from Public Health Paper No. 35, "Prevention of Suicide." Geneva: World Health Organization, 1968. From Schuyler, 1974, p. 83. Reprinted with permission.

rather than barbiturates), explaining their greater success in completing the suicide attempt.

Social attitudes toward suicide have also varied through the ages (Rosen, 1975). During the early Greek and Roman classical periods, for example, suicide for personal reasons (for example, to maintain one's honor) was acceptable. In the Middle Ages, on the other hand, suicidal acts were harshly rejected, and great shame and guilt were cast upon the families of the suicide. Social censure was so extreme that the corpses of suicides were degraded and their properties confiscated; further, they could not be buried on consecrated ground. Vestiges of this harshness remain today, for suicidal acts still elicit repulsion and other strong feelings such as shame and guilt.

Causes and Risks of Suicide

Suicide occurs most frequently in the spring, with its highest incidence among white Protestant males (Farberow and Shneidman, 1961). The reasons why some individuals take their lives, and others in the same set of circumstances do not, continue to baffle even the experts in the field. The major obstacle to research, of course, is that the subject is dead. Inferences from relatives and other surrounding circumstances such as suicide notes can only approximate the motivation of the person who has successfully completed the suicide.

Is there a satisfactory theory of suicide? Durkheim's model is too broad to account for individual cases; at best, it can explain only some of the data, and that only on a general sociocultural level. Freudian explanations are equally general and cover too many possibilities, for example, intense hostility turned inward (anger against the self) or a death instinct. Neither approach accounts for the individual attempt or act. As a matter of fact, there are few explanations that can satisfactorily predict or "explain" this violent act against the self. Reasons that seem to work for some suicides do not work for others, and there is no general common denominator that cuts across the diverse people who comprise the population of suicides or attempted suicides. For many people often feel helpless, trapped by their circumstances, and hopelessly depressed, yet they do not commit suicide. It is thus easier to present some epidemiological and incidence data and to describe possible suicide risks than to talk as if we have definitive answers.

Suicide occurs in diverse SES groups, age levels, and psychopathological categories: agitated depressives; the very young and the elderly; the terminally ill; people with intractable diseases or various entrapping neurotic or psychotic symptoms; the alcoholic; the grief-stricken; and the lonely. Most researchers agree that a wide range of motives and causes seem to account for individual suicides, especially because the diversity of people who take their own lives is a striking feature of the suicide data. Neither the individual traits alone nor the environmental, psychosocial stressor can predict suicide (Braucht, 1979).

Spotlight 10.5 Suicide Notes

From a seventeen-year-old boy:

To my family and friends:

I'm sorry it has to be this way. For some reason, I have set unattainable goals for myself. It hurts to live and life is full of so many disappointments and troubles. What I would really like to say is that I can't face up to problems the way I should. Society is always judging you and telling you what to do. My problem I think is that I have always thought only of Bill [himself]. Everything I have done hasn't satisfied me. Why this is I cannot tell you. It is a very funny feeling that I get inside when I sit down to do something. Maybe like what I write or do won't be accepted by society. Competition is another thing I hate. Maybe I expected too much out of life. Please don't cry or feel badly. I know what I am doing and why I am doing it. I guess I never really found out what love or responsibility was.

Bill

I might also add that I had had in recent years no great desire to continue living. Saying goodbye to all of you who I was close to would only make things harder for me. Believe me I tried to cope with my problems but I couldn't.

(from Jacobs, 1971, p. 88).

From a widow with grown children:

Dear D——— and D———:

I didn't know how you felt. I am sorry for anything I caused. I have always enjoyed card games with you and D———, when you and he liked to play. But I guess I expected too much. I have always been afraid to be alone in the Eve's, that's my only fear, loneliness. Each day I looked forward to you and D——— coming home in the Eve. I am sorry believe me. This way will be better for you & D———. I don't want to stand in your way.

The house will be yours and D———'s equally to live in as long as you 2 wish I'm no good by myself & don't want to stop you and D——— from having fun. So this is the only thing I can think of.

I never realized before how much I was in the way. God bless and keep you both safe. All my love.

Mother

(from Tuckman, Kleiner, and Lavell, 1960, p. 1105).

And from a husband to his wife:

Dear Mary. You have been the best wife a man could want and I still love you after fifteen years.

Don't think to badly of me for taking this way out but I can't take much more pain and sickness also I may get too much pain or so weak that I can't go this easy way. With all my love forever—

Bill

(from Shneidman and Farberow, 1957, p. 203)

Do suicide notes shed light on the causes of suicide? It is known that a little over one-third of the suicides leave notes (Farberow and Schneidman, 1961). These notes ascribe a variety of reasons for suicide, including depression, a deep sense of failure and an inability to cope, loneliness, marital difficulties, bereavement, financial difficulties, intractable pain, and terminal illness. Some notes stress the no-way-out-no-other-options theme. Others ask for forgiveness and understanding. Still others are accusatory, angry.

But what of the other two-thirds who left no notes? Are these individuals different in some way from the note writers?

Although depression is a frequent cause of suicide, it is by no means the only cause, and a one-to-one relationship between depression and suicide has not been established (Mendels, 1970). On the other hand, it is estimated that half of all suicides are associated with endogenous depressive disorder. Even more moderate positions also tend to implicate primary affective or endogenous depression in many suicides (Robins et al., 1959), with estimates ranging from 3 to 14 percent of suicide among people with manic-depressive illness (Rosenthal, 1971), still a staggering proportion. Severely depressed patients who are retarded, withdrawn, silent, and virtually immobilized, however, rarely commit suicide (Mendels, 1970). Interestingly, when the depression "lifts," these patients are at a higher risk, presumably because there is more motivation, energy, and directed effort in executing a suicide plan. Alcoholics are also a fairly high suicide risk, as well as drug abusers in instances when there is a mixture of drug and alcohol ingestion.

Suicide is not always a response to a crisis or an emergency act executed under the pressure of intense emotion and sudden impulse. The model that portrays a trapped individual under severe stress who becomes agitated enough to commit suicide simply does not account for the many instances of deliberate acts of self-destruction preceded by a calm, planned meeting of obligations, putting one's papers in order, and the like.

Although rates for women are lower than those for men, they are increasing (Sainsbury, 1968), possibly a reflection of the less "protected" status of women in recent times. About three times as many women than men attempt suicide, but, as noted, men are more often successful in completing the act. The peak suicide risk in women is in the 40-to-60-year-old group. This might result from the separation, loneliness, or bereavement many women of this age experience in the context of the dependent role women have traditionally filled.

Who, then, are the high-risk people? Suicidal risks are high for over-40 males living alone with a history of previous suicide attempts, endogenous depression, schizophrenia, or alcoholism. Elderly depressives are among the highest suicide risks. Married males are the lowest risk. All risks increase with age in both sexes, but young widowed males are also a rather high risk (Monk, 1975; Sainsbury, 1968; Schuyler, 1974).

A clinician facing a patient who is isolated or lonely with several of these characteristics, especially when there is endogenous depression and a history of alcoholism and drug abuse, agitation, intense guilt, feelings of extreme inadequacy, unrelieved insomnia, and worry about real or fantasied disease should immediately consider the possibility of a serious suicidal attempt (Sainsbury, 1968). In actuality, however, the prediction for the individual case cannot be made with a high degree of accuracy, for the vast majority of people with some or even all the foregoing characteristics do not commit suicide.

Classification of Suicides

Is it possible to distinguish among types of suicides so that homogeneous groups can be studied? According to Resnick and Hathorne (1973), who have described one such classification system, the answer is yes.

1. An accurate classification scheme would most certainly employ a distinction between *suicide attempters* and *successful completers*. Attempters and completers come from demographically different populations. Most suicide attempters are female and tend to be younger than the completers. Successful suicides tend to be among older, socially isolated, urban, unemployed, retired, separated, or widowed males (Schuyler, 1974).

2. Still another distinction resides in *intent*—differentiating between an act that is planned with deliberate intent to die and a vague, almost accidental act that cannot be characterized in this way. For example, an "accidental" death resulting from driving when drunk may have been planned only on an unconscious level, while a death achieved after the purchase of a gun and patient waiting until the fam-

ily is away must be construed as an intentional, conscious wish to die.

3. *Lethality of method* chosen for the suicide should also be assessed. A mild drug overdose can be sharply contrasted with a bullet through one's head or a leap from the top of a skyscraper. Men, as noted, tend to choose more lethal methods than women. Lethality of method and seriousness of intent do not bear a one-to-one relationship. An individual might be seriously determined to die, yet survive an attempt because of the low lethality of the method chosen to do so.

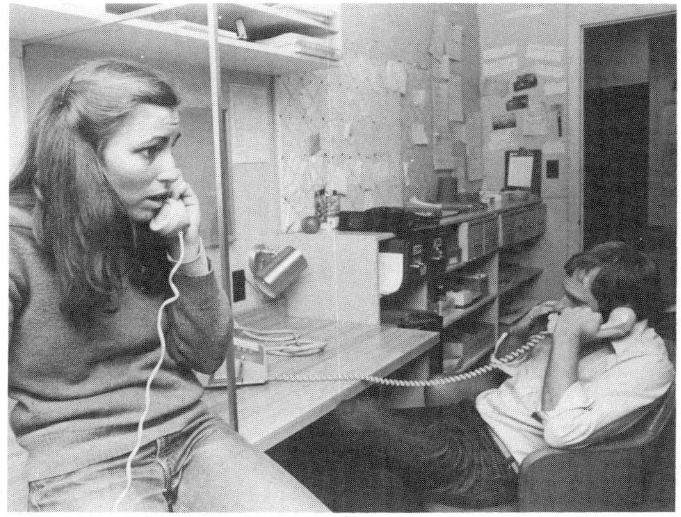

Suicide hotlines in operation. (© 1982 Paul Fortin/Stock, Boston)

Suicide Prevention

One of the first strategies in suicide prevention is to dispel some popular myths that tend to perpetuate the notion that suicides are difficult, if not impossible, to prevent. For example, the myth that people who threaten or talk about suicide are not "doers" is clearly not substantiated. Another is that once a person makes up his or her mind to commit suicide, the act cannot be prevented. Such people, it is claimed, do not want to be stopped. They want others to go away, to turn their backs. Still another myth—this one frequently subscribed to by suicidal persons themselves—is that "no one is there to turn to." People do in fact respond to the pleas for help proffered by a suicidal person. Spotlight 10.6 describes one such set of responses.

Possible clues to prevention of a suicide lie not only in the belief that suicidal people actually are crying out for help, but also in the fact that socially isolated people with a lack of social supports and few interpersonal relationships are greater risks that those who have some ties and life-lines to family and community (Jacobs, 1971). Thus prevention, in the case of an individual who is threatening suicide, is to make available immediate, interpersonal emergency aid, through listening and supportive actions to anyone reaching out for help. Suicidologists like Shneidman, Farberow, and their associates (see Farberow, 1977, for example), have had a long, dedicated involvement with research into suicide and activities in conjunction with suicide prevention. Their activities at the Suicide Prevention Center in Los Angeles have served as a model for many suicide crisis centers throughout the nation. A primary purpose of these centers is to provide immediate help, in the form of telephone support and counseling, to anyone who avails himself or herself of this service.

The anonymous availability of sympathetic listening to a suicidal person is not as easy as it sounds. In one training manual, for example (see Farberow, Heilig, and Litman, 1968), the importance of first airing the feelings of the telephone volunteers themselves toward life, death, suicide, and suicidal people was stressed. Volunteers can be easily "thrown," made to feel anxious and threatened, by a desperate suicide call. Unless the volunteers' own personal responses are clearly understood and dealt with, an emergency call can easily be fumbled.

The training manual for volunteers noted above also gives the following guidelines:

1. A telephone relationship should be established

Spotlight 10.6 M 21 STUDT GIVES SELF 3 WKS BEFORE POPPING PILLS FOR SUICIDE. IF YOU KNOW GOOD REASONS WHY I SHOULDN'T PLEASE WRITE BOX D-673

This was an ad placed by a Harvard student in a Boston newspaper. It ran for two weeks. The student had no plans for suicide. His ad was partially stunt, partially bravado—he had been showing off with friends over beer. But also, he was genuinely curious about the kinds of responses he would receive. To his amazement, he was inundated with responses. He was especially struck with the fact that people did seem to care, did reach out to help others, and were willing to dig into their own emotions—especially if they had been there before, at the brink of death.

The student's name is Leland Moss. His analysis of the 169 letters he received appears in a book edited by Shneidman (1972), which also contains several other brief essays on death and suicide written by Harvard students. Moss's informal analysis of these letters disclosed that there were more female responses than male. Of the 169 respondents, 102 offered more direct contact by providing a name, phone number, or address.

Moss analyzed the responses according to their content.

1. The largest category of respondents made some reference to themselves. Many of these wrote of their own misery. Some had attempted suicide themselves. One person wrote: "I've contemplated it. Eventually I did it—committed suicide—here in Cambridge. It was a matter of killing certain sensitivities, burning them out. . . . I'm *still* committing suicide. Everyday I do it so that I may live." Some referred to the sense of "well-being" that replying gave them. One woman wrote, ". . . thanks (sic) for making me feel happy inside tonight because you made me feel for you." Still others wrote out of a sense of personal, moral responsibility: "I felt a moral obligation to write to you."

2. The second largest category of responses made references to "Nature" as providing a reason to live. According to Moss, these "ran the full gamut of suggestions I go to the beach and look at all the beauty there to sending me a packet of morning glory seeds with instructions on how to plant them and watch them grow."

3. Many people read the suicide ad as an "other-oriented action," a plea for love in a lonely world. More than forty respondents used the phrase "I care" or "We care" in their letters. One wrote, "it might be pointed out that a world in which people try to respond to (you) . . . might indeed be a world in which life could well be worth living." Some went even further and said that in order to help him they needed to know him better, encouraging him to call or write to them.

4. Others urged the author to "fight" or called him a "coward." If you don't hold some firm beliefs or have some high-reaching goals to attain in life, then life really isn't worth living, so take your damn pills!" Moss found such notes "offensive."

Because "many writers were so upset by my plea that at one point in their letters they broke down and simply pleaded back "Don't" or "You just can't," Moss decided that he owed these concerned individuals the message that he "didn't." To communicate that message, he placed another ad in the newspaper that had run the original ad. This one read, "'Tis spring and I'm still alive, thanks to all of you. Box D-673."

and maintained so that contact is not lost. While this is done, information is gradually obtained.

2. The volunteer should attempt to clarify the significant and crucial problems that are at the core of the suicidal plan.
3. Throughout the call, the volunteer should attempt to assess the risk for suicide of the caller: Is there depression? agitation? Does the caller sound psychotic?
4. The next step is to survey the "assets" and "significant others" of the caller. These re-

sources include family, friends, clergy, police, and available hospital facilities.

5. These steps are followed by actual mobilization of such resources.
6. Finally, a therapy plan, some action in behalf of the patient, should be adopted.

Clearly, not all suicides can be prevented by such intervention. But some can be prevented by the simple expedient of being there, of offering some form of contact, even if just through listening, reassurance, and support. Special police units all over the country know this principle: the handling of the immediate crisis in person or on the telephone through compassionate presence such as a nod, some talk, some distraction, and providing an atmosphere of personal interest, may make all the difference between life and death.

The inability to cope, a feeling of utter helplessness—of being trapped with no options (as in a terminal disease, real or fantasied)—and a deep sense of despair because of these conditions may lead some people to choose an ultimate way out, a final answer, through suicide. Even in this context, however, the suicide gesture more often than not is a desperate call for attention, a cry for help (Farberow and Shneidman, 1961). If viewed thus as an interpersonal affair that calls for the involvement of others, many experts believe that a fair number of suicides can be prevented.

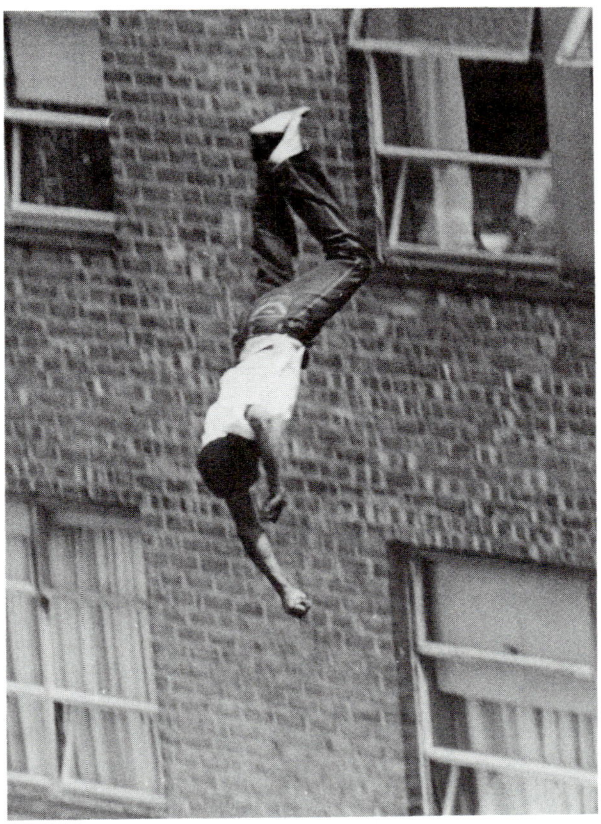

This suicide attempt was thwarted; the police were below with a net. Such attempts may be repeated—sometimes with grim results—unless social supports and counseling are available. (David Handschuh/Wide World Photos)

SUMMARY

Chapter 10 surveyed depression, affective disorders, and suicide, by outlining the characteristics and signs of depression; presenting various sociocultural considerations, for example, the extent of depressive disorders and its relationship to such variables as SES and gender; and describing the clinical syndromes with case illustrations. Diagnostic problems, and especially the differentiating characteristics of various types of depression, are still not entirely clear. But generally it appears helpful to distinguish the neurotic depressions from the major affective disorders. Some of the numerous theories of depression include various behavioral formulations and biological approaches. The last pages of this chapter explored the phenomenon of suicide from several viewpoints that include incidence, possible causes, risks, and classification schemes.

Highlights

1. In our society, depression is one of the most prevalent of all mental disorders. Empirical data suggest that there is more depressive

symptomatology among women and low-SES groups than among other groups.

2. Although depression probably reflects diverse diagnostic categories about which there is not complete agreement, many clinicians differentiate between neurotic depressions and the nonneurotic, or primary, depressions. Some of the differences between these types of depression are that in neurotic depressions there may be accompanying anxiety disorders; stressful events may precipitate onset; and there is no family history of major depression, psychotic features, or special physiological signs such as psychomotor retardation and certain types of sleep patterns.
3. Psychoanalytic hypotheses about the etiology of depressions have not received convincing empirical confirmation. Faring somewhat better are behavioral formulations, for example, those of Lewinsohn (the reinforcement model), Beck (the cognitive model), and Seligman (the learned-helplessness model). Moderate support has been found for various biochemical hypotheses as to the underpinnings of some types of depression—the major affective disorders in particular. Even so, it is clear that no single neurochemical or group of neurochemicals is responsible for mood, depression, or subtypes of depression. Further, definitive knowledge in this area is still forthcoming.
4. Suicide, among the ten leading causes of death in this country, continues to present a major challenge to mental-health professionals in regard to causes and prevention. There are many sociocultural variations, not only in incidence of attempted and completed suicides, but also in methods used, and attitudes toward victims and their families. Suicides occur among diverse groups, ages, and diagnostic categories, not only among depressed people. These and other unexplained data about suicide make it difficult for a unified theory of suicide to emerge.
5. Objective studies of suicide would be aided by a reliable classification system. One such scheme classifies subjects into groups comprised of failed versus completed suicides, level of intent, and lethality of method chosen.
6. Empirical studies show that high risks for suicide can be found among the following groups: over-40 males living alone with a history of previous suicide attempts; endogenous depressives; schizophrenics; alcoholics; and elderly depressives. Prediction for individual cases cannot be made with great accuracy, however.

ISSUES AND QUESTIONS

1. Surveys suggest that the frequency of reports of mild to severe depression on campuses is so large that 75 percent of a group of respondents in a major American university reported various symptoms of depression (Bosse et al., 1975). Academic pressures were described as the most frequent cause, but boyfriend and girlfriend problems, adjustment to college life, concern about identity, the future, and various interpersonal problems were also cited. Conduct your own survey. Are there additional causes that contribute to depression around you?
2. Most of us have a strong will to live, to remain alive forever. We may fantasize being cloned, or being frozen at death for future "thawing." Ernest Becker (1973), a Pulitzer Prize winner, has suggested that our lives comprise attempts to solve the one universal, ever present problem—how to avoid death. To deny death, to ward it off, to pretend there is life forever—these are universal responses that produce terror because they force us to acknowledge that our lives must end. Thus, Becker would have us understand much of what we have covered in this book in the light of this one key motivational thread. Can you think of personal examples that illustrate this theme?
3. The cultural taboos about facing death and discussing it openly are beginning to wither away.

The relatively new discipline, thanatology, the study of death, is beginning to focus on the problems of the terminally ill, the bereavement and grief of the living, and the interpersonal dynamics between the dying person and the survivors (see Kastenbaum and Costa, 1977, for a review).

As an aid for the families of the dying person as well as to help the dying person himself or herself, the stages that many people go through as they face death have been classified. One such classification is that of Kubler-Ross (1969): At first there is *denial* ("It's not true"). Then there is *anger*, indiscriminate rage against the world, followed by a *bargaining* stage, an attempt to "make a deal" ("I'll ask God nicely and if I'm good, He'll postpone death"). The final stages are *depression* then *acceptance*, the giving up of the fight. There has been some criticism that these stages are not entirely valid. Have you had any opportunity to judge for yourself as to the validity of these stages by observing the death of a close relative?

4. *Do you think a person has the moral right to end his or her life when this person is suffering great pain and has no hope of improvement?*
Do you think a person has the moral right to end his or her life when this person has a disease that is incurable?
Do you think a person has the moral right to end his or her life when this person is an extremely heavy burden on his or her family?

(© 1975 by the New York Times Company. Reprinted by permission.)

These questions were used in a Gallup Survey of 1,535 adults in 300 different locations (Most in poll. . ., 1975). The results indicated that the majority of Americans believe that it is morally wrong to commit suicide, even when in great pain (51 percent), or with an incurable disease (53 percent), or when the subject is a heavy burden to his or her family (72 percent). Men and women did not differ in their opinions, but age was a significant factor in that a reversal of findings was found for the eighteen-to-twenty-nine-year-old age group. The majority of respondents in this age group (with or without college education) said that they believed that a person does have the moral right to end his or her own life if suffering great pain and terminal illness.

What is your opinion? Should people be left to determine their own fates, that is, should they alone be ultimately responsible for their own actions? Are you concerned about the legacy left for the survivors of the suicide: guilt? confusion? angry bewilderment?

One interesting aspect of this issue has been elucidated by Farberow (1977), who states

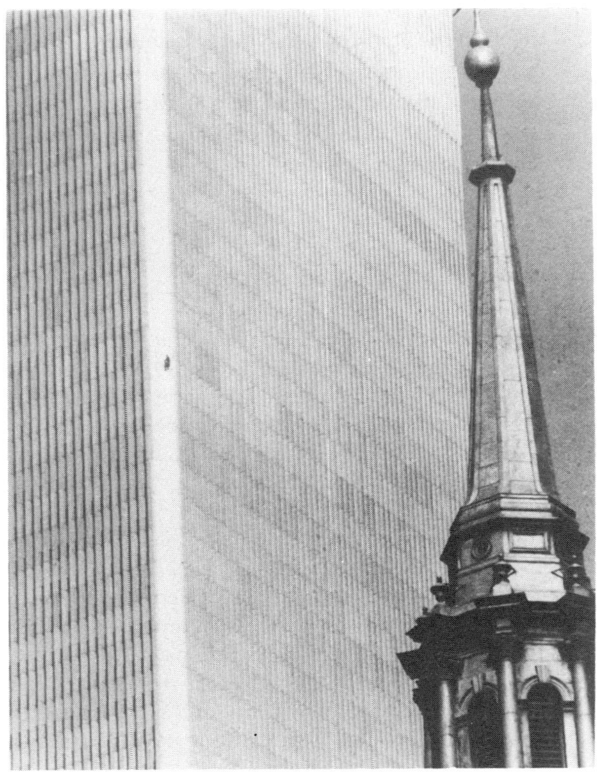

George Willig at the half-way mark in his successful scaling of the 110-story World Trade Center in 1977. The steeple of St. Paul's Church is in the foreground. Society tolerates—and sometimes even glorifies—some high-risk stunts that court death, but it generally takes a strong negative moral stance on suicide. (United Press International Photo)

that society hypocritically frowns on the overt suicide, claiming a moral right to intervene with its execution. Yet, society looks the other way, even encourages and glorifies, indirect suicides in the form of many risk- and excitement-seeking activities. To choose a few examples: death-defying motorcycle and automobile stunts, high-wire performances, and even skyscraper climbing. Are there mitigating circumstances in some suicides? Are some more socially acceptable than others?

5. Spotlight 10.6 contains an ad from the classified section of a Boston paper asking for reasons why the writer should not kill himself. Write your own response to this ad. Compare the dominant theme in your response to those in the responses of others in your class. What are the different themes? appeals to family? responsibility? moral and religious beliefs? life and its values?

SUGGESTIONS FOR FURTHER READING

Beck, A. T. *Depression: Causes and treatment.* Philadelphia: University of Pennsylvania Press, 1972. Paperback available. This classic book describes not only the psychological literature on depression, but also presents the author's stimulating views about cognitive aspects of depression, based on the careful study of more than 1,000 depressed patients. Chapter 10 has already presented some of these views: The depressed person's experience is shaped by his or her negative beliefs. Treatment of depression, then, should attempt to assist the patient in understanding and altering self-defeating cognitions.

Bowlby, J. *Attachment and loss. Vol. I: Attachment.* New York: Basic Books, 1969. *Attachment and loss. Vol. II: Separation.* New York: Basic Books, 1973. Paperback available. These classics grew out of the author's intense concern with the responses of children who had been separated from their mothers or caretakers early in life and the apparent relationship of that separation to later psychopathology. The first volume looks at the nature of the original attachment of a child to his or her mother; the second examines the effects of disturbance of that attachment upon the child's later emotional development.

Fieve, R. R. *Moodswing: The third revolution in psychiatry.* New York: Morrow, 1975. "Moodswing" refers to manic-depressive illness and the "third revolution" refers to recent advances in the pharmacological treatment of that illness with lithium. This book consists primarily of the author's account of his treatment of manic-depressive patients, initially as a psychoanalyst and later as a psychopharmacologist. In addition to vivid pictures of the lives of these patients, Fieve describes the dramatic changes that took place as a result of lithium treatment. He also presents captivating accounts of the role that moodswings seem to have played in the lives of many famous or historical figures, for example, Balzac, Lincoln, and Theodore Roosevelt. This is a popular-level book that is quite frankly a biased presentation of the effectiveness of medication in treating this disease.

Seligman, M. E. P. *Helplessness: On depression, development, and death.* San Francisco: Freeman, 1975. Paperback available. This book is recommended for those who are interested in more details about Seligman's learned helplessness theory and research than were given in this chapter, for it is the culmination of more than ten years of work. Seligman presents his research, theory, and therapeutic suggestions in a very readable manner and includes many provocative ideas related to learned helplessness, for example, how helplessness may develop in early childhood, the effects of poverty on helplessness, and how to remediate learned helplessness in the classroom.

Shneidman, E. S. (Ed.) *Suicidology: Contemporary developments.* New York: Grune & Stratton, 1976. This book of essays, collected by a renowned suicidologist, covers a wide range of issues, including the epidemiology of suicide, the development of scales for the estimation of suicide risk, the thought patterns of the suicidal person, student suicide, and suicide prevention. In addition, there is a set of essays that deals with the "philosophic and legal aspects of suicide." Readers will find this collection thought-provoking and emotionally compelling.

Weissman, M. M., and Paykel, E. S. *The depressed woman: A study of social relationships.* Chicago: University of Chicago Press, 1974. Paperback available. This book reports a study of the social adjustment of forty women during an acute depressive episode and afterwards. The depressed subjects, who were in treatment, were compared to forty normal controls on rating scales of social adjustment, self-reports of mood, and, on the basis of self-reports, social relationships at work and with family and friends. In addition, the results of various types of therapy (all were treated with drugs, while half received psychotherapy as well) were evaluated. This book provides an interesting view into the daily life of the depressed woman and contributes significant data to the understanding of depression.

11

Schizophrenia and Paranoid Disorders

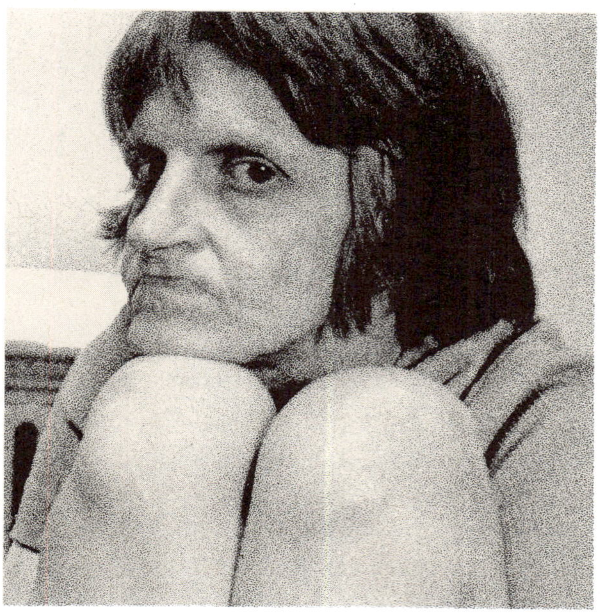

SCHIZOPHRENIA

The mind must have a filter that functions without our conscious thought, sorting stimuli and allowing only those which are relevant to the situation in hand to disturb consciousness. And this filter must be working at maximum efficiency at all times, particularly when we require a high degree of concentration. What had happened to me in Toronto was a breakdown in the filter, and a hodge-podge of unrelated stimuli were distracting me from things which should have had my undivided attention. . . . My brain, after a short time, became sore with a real physical soreness, as if it had been rubbed with sandpaper until it was raw. It felt like a bleeding sponge. . . . I had very little ability to sort the relevant from the irrelevant. The filter had broken down. Completely unrelated events became intricately connected in my mind. (MacDonald, 1960, pp. 218–19; originally published in Canadian Medical Association Journal. *Vol. 82, January 23, 1960)*

The foregoing is an account of what it was like for one person during a schizophrenic episode. The terror and confusion, the chaotic feelings and thoughts that characterize the subjective tortures of "madness" are also described by a great writer, Franz Kafka:

When it was becoming unbearable—once towards evening in November—and I ran along the narrow strip of carpet in my room as on a race track, shrank from the sight of the lit-up street, then turning to the interior of the room found a new goal in the depths of the looking glass and screamed aloud, to hear only my own scream which met no answer nor anything that could draw its force away, so that it rose up without check and could not stop even when it ceased being audible, the door in the wall opened towards me, how swiftly, because swiftness was needed and even the cart horses down below on the paving stones were rising in the air like horses driven wild in a battle, their throats bare to the enemy. (Kafka, 1913)

Most patients and ex-patients suffer their agonies privately, with neither the skill nor artistry to describe their inner feelings. Even so, almost all subjective accounts of a schizophrenic episode portray a bewildering array of bizarre and terrifying sensations and thoughts.

Schizophrenia—thought to be one of the most serious health problems in Western civilization—comprises a group of psychoses that has baffled clinicians for generations because of its widespread incidence, relative resistance to treatment, and bizarre, outlandish symptoms. It is likely that more research attention has been devoted to schizophrenia than to any other clinical entity. But still there continues to be widespread disagreement as to its definition, diagnosis, measurement, and etiology. Schizophrenia is frequently listed among the *functional* disorders (no known physical etiology) in contrast to *organic* disorders (pathologies that arise from physical causes, as in certain kinds of brain damage). As we shall see later, especially in Chapter 12, many researchers no longer regard schizophrenia as having a purely psychological etiology.

No two schizophrenias are really alike. Although many of the behaviors described in this chapter characterize schizophrenia, they do not always apply to all schizophrenic patients. In fact, some patients show only one or two of the behaviors I will be describing and otherwise may appear to behave quite normally. To make matters worse, some of these symptoms also appear in other pathologies, for example, some central nervous system (CNS) dysfunctions (see Chapter 13).

Generally, the odd, bizarre, and peculiar (idiosyncratic) behavior of many schizophrenic patients can be roughly described as follows. One of the most important distinguishing characteristics of schizophrenia is some impairment in cognition and thinking. Broadly, this area includes such mental processes as reasoning, judgment, and logicality of associations. Frequently there are language and communication difficulties, with content of communications "off," peculiar, and odd. There generally are attentional difficulties with uneven, scattered focus and an inability to maintain task completion. Most often there are delusions and hallucinations and various kinds of bizarre sensory and perceptual experiences, sometimes accompanied by a distorted sense of self, such as being without boundaries, alone, floating, or not belonging to oneself.

Disturbances of affect are usually present, in-

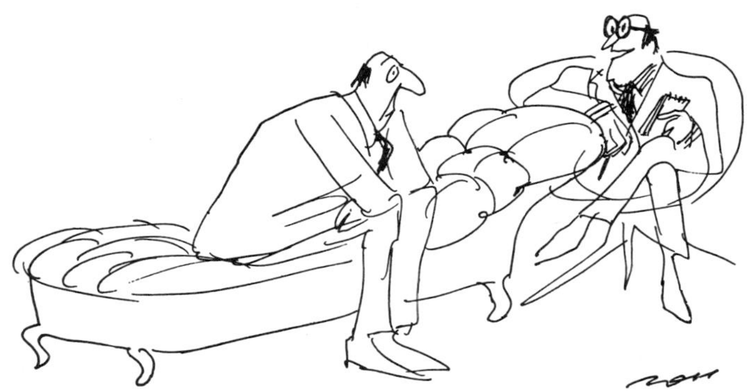

"First the good news. You have a strong, healthy ego. Now the bad news. It has no basis in reality."

cluding inappropriate affect (for example, a patient describes being tortured while smiling broadly); blunted affect, in which the intensity of emotional expression is reduced; anhedonia, involving an inability or reduction of capacity to experience pleasure; and flatness of affect, a constricted, narrow, even entirely absent repertoire of emotional behavior. There may be rapid shifts of affective expression—from mirth and hilarity to angry outbursts. There may also be a great loss of motivation in the schizophrenic process, with apathy and a withdrawal into a subjective world of fantasy, self-concern, and egocentric expression of ideas unrelated to the external world.

There are many additional symptoms and groups of symptoms including disturbances in posture and motor behavior (for example, repeated stereotyped movements or assumptions of bizarre, prolonged postures) that will be described in the pages ahead when case illustrations are presented. Spotlight 11.1 presents a list of some of the symptoms associated with schizophrenia.

Spotlight 11.1 A Partial List of Schizophrenic Symptoms and Behaviors

Not all—as a matter of fact, very few—of the symptoms and behaviors associated with schizophrenia are found in each person diagnosed with schizophrenia. Many of these behaviors are present only to a mild degree whereas others are very marked, especially in chronic, deteriorated cases. Some types of symptoms, for example those associated with thinking disorders, are more consistently associated with the schizophrenic process than with other pathological processes; while others, for example, body preoccupations, are not exclusive to schizophrenia.

affective difficulties flatness, poverty (paucity, emptiness), blunting, or shallowness of affect; inappropriate affect; lack of consistency or congruence between mood and thought

anhedonia little or no ability to experience pleasure

attentional difficulties scattered, uneven attention; inability to focus attention; unusually distractible

autism excessive daydreaming and fantasy behavior; interpretation of reality is based primarily on personal and subjective needs

catatonic stupor, catatonia lacking the will or ability to talk, move; patient may sit, lie, or stand in one position for hours or days, often in awkward, strained, peculiar postures

delusions grotesque, bizarre, grandiose, or persecutory beliefs unfounded in reality and often containing sexual or bodily content; early in the disease process, these may bear some similarity to the excessive obsessional ideation already described in some psychoneurotic states; see also ideational symptoms

depersonalization feeling of not existing, of watching one's self from without, of having no identity, no sense of self

"derailment" loosening of the flow of ideas so that they seem to go off onto another track that may be only minimally related to the main idea

hallucinations perceptual experiences that can occur in any sensory area without external stimulation; most frequent in the auditory area and less often in visual, tactile, olfactory, and taste modalities; auditory hallucinations often consist of hearing one's thoughts aloud, voices arguing or talking about patient, voices telling patient what to do or think, or voices that accuse patient of some "evil" characteristic

ideational symptoms poverty (paucity) of ideas; ideas of influence (thought control), that is, ideas are controlled by outside influences such as electricity or someone's "remote control" apparatus; patient is sometimes overwhelmed by obsessive, anxiety-provoking ideas; ideas of reference—remarks and events are interpreted as directly related to patient; thought broadcasting—others are aware of one's inner thoughts; see also, delusions

insight, lack of lack of awareness into or understanding of own motives or feelings, or of understanding that one's perceptions and thought may be abnormal, or that one is "ill"

mannerisms stereotyped movements, postures, and facial expressions are repeated, purposeless, and peculiar

mutism voluntary or involuntary speechlessness

negativism in some patients, contrariness, stubbornness, or resistance to or refusal to comply with requests or expectations of others without apparent reason

neologism a coined, manufactured word, often complex, to express one's ideas or conflicts, for example, love-spinachhead

paranoid ideation ideas of persecution or of grandiosity

perceptual, sensory, attentional dysfunctions impaired sense of time; variability or slowness of reaction time to simple tasks; heightened, sluggish, or distorted perceptual responses

persecutory ideas ideas of reference—people, groups, gangs, organized syndicates are "out to get me"

ruminations, body bizarre, irrational, obsessional thoughts about the body: "it is being drowned from within, gradually filled with poisonous fluids"; "it is falling apart, disintegrating"; "my blood is turning to water"; "my body is being gradually mutilated"; "I am dying of cancer caused by emitted rays from another planet"

ruminations, moral, philosophical, religious bizarre, irrational, obsessional thoughts about the meaning of life, God, philosophy, creation, the symbolic structure of the universe, evil versus good

ruminations, sexual bizarre, irrational, obsessional thoughts about sexual orientation, performance, prowess, and anatomy: "my penis is withering away unless I masturbate every morning at 10 A.M."; "everyone wants me because my genitals are visible"; "I am a homosexual but no one knows it; I will be killed when this is found out"

speech and communication difficulties overelaborate speech; incoherent speech; subjective, bizarre references in speech; stilted, overabstract, or pedantic speech, stereotyped or set, mannered phrases

stereotyped movements see mannerisms

suspiciousness ideas of reference, attribution of malevolent motivation to neutral acts on the part of others; distrustfulness without objective evidence

thought disorders cognitive impairment in judgment or in logical or causal thinking; difficulties in abstracting, forming categories and groups; loose associations and fragmented thinking (ideas do not seem logically connected to each other); primary process thinking; over-abstract thoughts and generalizations with inappropriate reference or relevance to what is going on

waxy flexibility in catatonic states (see catatonic stupor, catatonia), patient maintains whatever posture he or she is placed in by someone else for an unusually long time, despite discomfort or awkwardness

History of the Concept of Schizophrenia

Schizophrenic-like behavior has been described throughout the centuries in the writings of historians and poets. Even the Bible alludes to "madness," which was probably schizophrenia. In the nineteenth century, a fourteen-year-old boy who suddenly developed disorganization in behavior, aggression, and "stupidity," but yet who had had a history of outstanding intellectual functioning, was labeled as evidencing *dementia praecox* ("precocious madness"). The phrase was obviously based on the observed early onset of the pathological process in this and similar cases. At about the same time, labels for specific symptoms began to appear. For example, the term *catatonia* (literally, tension insanity) was used in the nineteenth century to describe patients who sat motionless for days on end, staring into space, unresponsive to stimuli. We still use this term today to describe the same set of behaviors.

Emil Kraepelin, in 1896, suggested that many seemingly unrelated symptoms such as those listed in Spotlight 11.1 were actually aspects of a single illness, dementia praecox. According to Kraepelin, this disease was characterized by early onset (generally during adolescence) in individuals for whom there was no history of mental illness. Progressive deterioration and chronicity (long duration of illness) was inevitable, he thought. In 1911, Eugen Bleuler introduced the term *schizophrenia* (splitting of the mind, "split personality"—not to be confused with multiple personality, described in Chapter 9). Bleuler thought that this phrase was descriptive of the lack of congruence between thought and emotion that characterized this group of patients.

Both Bleuler and Kraepelin perceived schizophrenia as a reflection of some kind of disturbance of the brain. Later, Adolph Meyer, an American psychiatrist of Swiss descent, popularized the view that schizophrenia is a maladaptive reaction to a series of negative and traumatic events in the life history of the individual.

Incidence and Prevalence of Schizophrenia

It is expected that about 2 percent of the population will have episodes of schizophrenia at some point in their lifetimes, this figure increasing to about 6 percent in the urban slums (Schizophrenia: Is there an answer?, 1974). Some estimates, however, are a little lower, hovering around the 1-percent level (Berger, 1978). There is considerable agreement among epidemiologists that these figures have remained fairly stable over the generations, despite the advent of medications to treat schizophrenia and the general trend to "deinstitutionalize," that is, to discharge people from hospitals as rapidly as possible and to choose other ways than hospitalization to deal with patients (see Chapter 21 for a discussion of these circumstances).

In recent years, at any point in time, about 1 million people in this country can be regarded as diagnosed schizophrenics (a little under 200,000 inside, and the rest outside of, hospital settings). The hospital population of schizophrenics, thus, even though declining in the past two decades, continues to be substantial: about 25 percent of available beds in general hospitals are occupied by diagnosed schizophrenics, whereas about 50 percent of available beds in mental facilities are occupied by diagnosed schizophrenics (Berger, 1978; Gunderson et al., 1974).

Crosscultural considerations. Even with declining hospital rates, incidence remains fairly stable. Is this true for all cultures? Is schizophrenia universal? All cultures in all areas of the world where there are records report cases of schizophrenia, even though the descriptions of its manifestations (symptoms) vary. Some experts go so far as to suggest that the incidence of schizophrenia across various cultures is so stable that variations in prevalence figures reflect unreliability of diagnoses, not "true" incidence (Dunham, 1966).

Table 11.1 shows considerable variations in prevalence rates across various nations. Some incidence rates are consistently higher than others. For example, an extremely high stable rate (3 percent of the population) is reported in an isolated area of northern Sweden (Rosenthal, 1971). Why is this so? Can it be related to inbreeding, or perhaps to the social isolation in this region.

Not all researchers agree as to the universality of schizophrenia, suggesting that the stability of rates across cultures may be true only for *process* types of schizophrenia (chronic, deteriorating states, see later) in societies exposed to Western culture (Torrey, 1973). According to another view, however, even rates for process schizophrenics will vary according to the prevailing social attitudes as to the causes of insanity (Murphy, 1968). In those

Table 11.1 Some Prevalence Rates for Schizophrenia

			Cases	
Date	*Place*	*Population*	*Number*	*Rate per 1,000*
1929	Thuringia, Germany	37,546	71	1.9
1930–31	Bavaria, Germany	8,628	22	2.5
1935	Bornholm, Denmark	45,930	150	3.3
1936	Finland	418,472	1,798	4.2
1939–44	Northern Norway	1,325	6	4.5
1944	Western Sweden	8,736	40	4.6
1946–49	Northern Sweden	8,931	85	9.6
1947	Denmark	5,500	50	9.0
1947	Rural Sweden	2,550	17	6.6
1948	Rural Scotland	56,000	235	4.2
1940	Hachizo, Japan	8,330	32	3.8
1941	Tokyo, Japan	2,712	6	2.2
1941	Komoro, Japan	5,207	11	2.1
1946–48	Formosa, China	19,931	43	2.1
1933	Baltimore, U. S.	56,044	127	2.3
1936	Baltimore, U. S.	57,002	158	2.9
1938–40	Rural Tennessee, U. S.	24,804	47	1.9
1950	New Haven, U. S.	236,940	845	3.6
1951	Hutterites, U. S.	8,542	9	1.0

Source: J. M. Murphy, Psychiatric labeling in cross-cultural perspective, *Science 191* (March 1976), 1019–28 (Table 12); based on Dunham, 1965, pp. 18–19. Copyright 1976 by the American Association for the Advancement of Science.

Note: These data are based on different epidemiological investigations by various researchers employing a variety of diagnostic methods and data-collection procedures. Not all cases reported are hospitalized cases.

societies in which schizophrenia is attributed to external causation such as poisoning or witchcraft, this hypothesis predicts that there would be fewer chronic manifestations of the disease than in those societies that attribute schizophrenia to internal characteristics such as genetic endowment or an individual's personal strength.

In any event, the facts remain: Almost all cultures report some form of schizophrenia, despite variations in incidence figures. The variations themselves, it should be noted, are not totally explained by diagnostic differences or poor reliability of diagnostic judgments. Nor are there other satisfactory explanations for them. For example, the fact that relatively more Norwegians in Minnesota than in Norway have schizophrenia might be explained by social selection or drift in that the "unfit" may have migrated to the United States from the homeland (Dunham, 1966). An equally plausible explanation implicates the stresses and strains experienced by the displaced immigrant trying to survive in a foreign culture, rather than the drift of the "unfit."

Some Sociocultural Relationships

Social class. Although the incidence of schizophrenia cuts across all socioeconomic status (SES) groups, a consistent, clearcut inverse relationship exists between rates of schizophrenia and social class: the lower the social class, the higher the rate of schizophrenia (Dohrenwend and Dohrenwend, 1969, 1974; Garmezy and Streitman, 1974; Kohn, 1976; Strauss, 1979; and Torrey, 1973). This finding applies to "true" prevalence, that is, to treated as well as nontreated cases (Dohrenwend and Dohrenwend, 1974).

Chapter 2 has already described some of the classic studies that have yielded a relationship between social class and psychopathology. More recent explorations, based on SES indices, occupational levels, or residence, have consistently confirmed this association. These dramatic correlations appear to exist mostly for urban populations, especially the larger cities, however, according to Kohn (1976).

Hollingshead and Redlich (1954, 1958), like so many other investigators, interpreted their New Haven findings of higher incidence of schizophrenia in lower-class groups to be a result of the social stresses, strains, frustrations, family disorganization, and harshness of the poverty that characterizes the experiences of lower-SES groups. This is a social causation view supported by many investigators.

An opposing view emerged from the classic work of Faris and Dunham (1939), who found extremely wide variations of rates of schizophrenia in various sections of Chicago. The highest rates—1 in 100—were found in Chicago's inner city of single-room occupancy, transiency, and social disorder. Rates decreased as one moved away from the inner city, with rates shrinking to 1 in 1,000 in peripheral sections. These findings were explained by the notion of drift or social selection mentioned earlier. Ill or about-to-become-ill people, finding it increasingly difficult to cope with life, gradually drift to inner-city areas because there are fewer pressures there. Downward mobility, the drifting toward lower SES levels, is thus held as an explanation for the greater incidence of psychopathology in general and of schizophrenia in particular in dense city areas, where there is the greatest concentration of low-SES people.

Unfortunately, neither the downward mobility nor the social factors explanations account for all the accumulated data (Dohrenwend and Dohrenwend, 1974; Kohn, 1976). As we shall see in Chapter 12, a combination of several causative factors best describes the empirical data.

Gender. Some investigators suggest that because of the problems and frustrations attendant to being a woman in Western civilization, there is a trend for more women than men to become mentally ill (Gove and Tudor, 1973). This speculation does not seem to hold for schizophrenia, however. Most of the data suggest that sex differences in incidence of schizophrenia do not exist (Samuels, 1978, 1979; Schumer, 1979). This generalization is a little tenuous, however, because "true" prevalence data (that include untreated or unrecorded cases) are difficult to obtain, and research that seeks to identify male-female differences in incidence in schizophrenia is quite meager (Wahl, 1977) and sometimes difficult to interpret (Lewine, 1979).

Reviews of the literature suggests that being male or female and attitudes toward maleness and femaleness do affect the expression of the illness and its course to hospitalization or recovery, but not incidence rates (Lewine, 1979, 1980; Schumer, 1979). Females have more difficulty remaining in the community, after hospital discharge, than do males, or their families are less able to function when they are schizophrenic and their husbands healthy than when their husbands are disturbed and they are healthy. Further, there are differences between males and females in severity of symptoms, age of onset, and premorbid (before onset of disease) competence. Overall, being male or female shapes many of the events attendant to the history of the patient and his or her schizophrenic episode, despite equal male-female incidence figures.

Ethnic and racial considerations. There may be special cultural subgroups characterized by heightened

Listing 11.1 DSM-III Categories Described in Chapter 11

Schizophrenic Disorders
- Disorganized (formerly Hebephrenic)
- Catatonic
- Paranoid
- Undifferentiated
- Residual (no blatant psychosis, but patient still shows sign of illness such as eccentric behavior, inappropriate affect, social withdrawal)

Paranoid Disorders
- Paranoia
- Shared paranoid disorder (folie à deux—see text)
- Acute paranoid disorder
- Atypical paranoid disorder

Psychotic Disorders Not Classified Elsewhere
- Schizophreniform disorder
- Brief reactive psychosis
- Schizoaffective disorder
- Atypical psychosis

stresses, strains, frustrations, and social conflicts in which higher rates of schizophrenia are found. In New York City, for example, with SES variables matched, persons of Puerto Rican origin have a higher rate of schizophrenia than those not of Puerto Rican origin (Rendon, 1974). This finding can be explained by language problems, unrealistic goals, and the clash of cultural, familial, sexual, and interpersonal values, especially among young Puerto Ricans, whose rates were especially high. By and large, however, racial and ethnic factors are not directly related to incidence of schizophrenia, except when low SES is also involved.

THE CLINICAL SYNDROMES—THE SCHIZOPHRENIAS

The early Kraepelinian distinctions among the different types of schizophrenic disorders still hold sway today, with minor elaborations and variations. Diagnostic differentiation among the subcategories of schizophrenia continues to be troublesome.

The disorders described here generally have an onset during adolescence and early adulthood. They are characterized by many different types of symptoms, often involving marked deterioration from previous levels of functioning. Usually there is a prodromal phase (early indications of an illness before the actual onset itself), during which changes in the personality and the emergence of certain types of symptoms become apparent. These include social withdrawal, peculiar behavior, changes in grooming and personal hygiene, lowering of performance at school or work, flat or inappropriate affect, odd thinking, and changes in cognitive and perceptual responses. Sometimes these changes occur rapidly and dramatically: the patient appears to be catapulted into an active psychotic state; such onset is called acute. At other times the changes follow a slow insidious course, taking place over a period of years. The slow, gradual prodromal process is generally associated with poor prognosis, whereas the rapid downhill plunge is associated with a better prognosis, frequently with a return to premorbid levels.

Diagnoses of schizophrenia are typically made if there is a continuous picture over a period of at least six months of active symptoms that are characterized by one or more of the following: bizarre delusions such as of being controlled, thought broadcasting, thought insertion, or thought withdrawal*; grandiose or religious delusions without persecutory content; delusions of persecution if also

* These terms refer to feelings that one's thoughts are controlled from without, by some force or person, so that one's thoughts are known to others, inserted by others, or removed by others.

accompanied by hallucinations; various kinds of auditory hallucinations; thought disorder if accompanied by flat or inappropriate affect; delusions or hallucinations; and catatonic or disorganized behavior.

The Disorganized (Hebephrenic) Subtype

The hebephrenic subtype of schizophrenia is characterized by incoherence of speech; blunted, inappropriate affect that is sometimes incongruous or silly, for example, giggling and laughing for no apparent reason; and many grimaces and facial mannerisms. There are peculiarities in behavior, social withdrawal, and sometimes bodily complaints. Delusions and hallucinations are not systematized or organized but are fragmentary and isolated from one another, in contrast to the delusional or hallucinatory systems of the paranoid subtype to be discussed later.

Generally, this subtype has a slow, early onset. There is a poor premorbid adjustment (isolated, lonely, "peculiar" person with few inner resources),

Case 11.1 P.R.: Schizophrenia, Hebephrenic Type

P. R., a girl, twenty years old, who had been employed as a nurse, was admitted in a restless, agitated state, but a few minutes later was smiling and happy. These phases rapidly alternated, even in the course of a few minutes. . . .

"Do you hear voices?" "No—yes—very seldom. I seem to be sort of dead." Later she admitted that she did hear voices, and that they terrified her dreadfully. . . .

She behaved in a disturbed, excitable way, and made such a noise that she had to be removed to a room by herself. . . . She refused food, so that for a time it was necessary to tube-feed her. Still later she deliberately poked her fingers into her eye and caused conjunctival hemorrhage.

During her residence in the hospital she continued to be hallucinated, and talked freely about her experiences. She said that voices told her things had been done to her during the night. During the day also she hallucinated, and often sat gazing at the ceiling in an ecstatic way.

Here is a sample of her speech:

Losh, I don't know what it is. You see—she says—I don't know, I'm sure. There's Cinderella. There is a much better play than that. I don't know, I said. He is an awful idiot. O dear God, I'm so stupid. That's putting two and two together—saying I really don't know—saying Cathie, and so I observe and—flowers. An orange, and shoe laces. A gaberdine skirt. Pettigrew's and the jazz band, with cream cakes. She says no. They like my hair bobbed, but I'm so stupid. Contrary Mary. Statues at Copland and Lye's. Oh, I said, yes, yes, yes. I'd go off to sleep immediately afterwards, I said, I know quite well. Nothing, I said. I forget all that I saw next. The next thing was—eh? The poor man's mad. They'll be chopping off our heads next, and—calendars tied with blue ribbons. Oh, dear God. Contrary Mary again. What period—that's right. I don't like acting the goat at all. A cream-sponge sandwich. My memory is so slow, that all I'm sure. It was caramels then and fruit cakes. Well, well, I said, I can't help it—I don't want to help it, and well, I don't care. Contrary Mary again, and says—Nurse Grant—dogs barking. What's the matter with me anyway? I'm so terribly stupid. I'm fed up with this place—that's all. Sago pudding. She looks pale and tired often, but not—I know that. (Sings) Take me over there, drop me anywhere, Manchester, Birmingham, Leeds, Well I don't care. I should like to see my best girl—Mrs. Patrick, she says—though 'tis time for parting, that's it, Jean and my tears are starting. I've got the Kruschen feeling. —Blue belts and medals—three eggs for tea. No, that won't do. Oh, dear God, I'm so stupid. I won't see my way—white rabbits. Back home in Tennessee—that the way it's spelt. Oh, I don't know what I am going to do now. It's all wrong. Dear God, I'm so silly. It's killing, isn't it? Cream cakes, French cakes, and meringues. Flies, fleas, butterflies, and so on.

Source: Henderson and Gillespie's *Textbook of Psychiatry,* (pp. 775–76), revised by I.R.C. Batchelor,

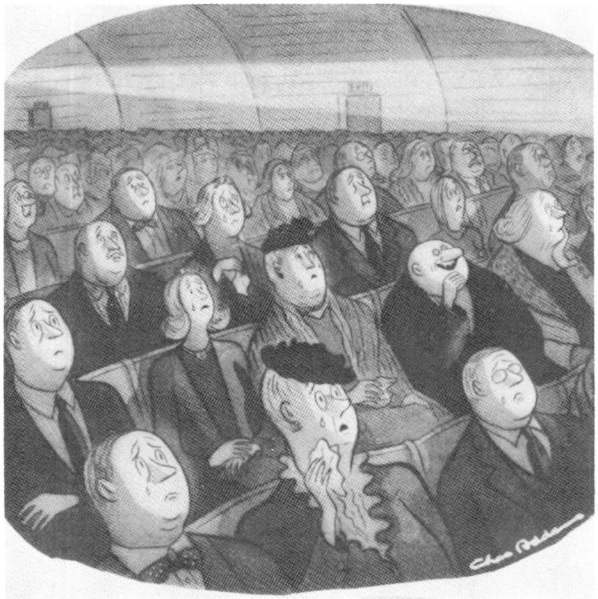

Drawing by Chas. Addams; © 1946, 1974 The New Yorker Magazine, Inc.

and most often, a chronic course. In advanced, deteriorated chronic cases there is soiling and wetting, incoherent speech, neologisms, and pronounced posturing and mannerisms.

The Catatonic Subtype

The catatonic subtype has become relatively rare in Europe and North America, where it was once quite common. This subtype is characterized by disturbances in psychomotor responses that can take several forms. One form is stupor or mutism in which there is little or no responsiveness to the environment. There can be rigidity of posture, in which a "tight" posture is maintained against all attempts to stimulate a change. There might be catatonic posturing, in which the patient assumes an inappropriate or bizarre posture for a length of time, or there can be an excited phase of seemingly purposeless motor activity. There may be shifting from one of these forms to another without predictability. Negativism and mutism, which are particularly common, and waxy flexibility (see Spotlight 11.1) may also be present.

In the excited state, there is marked agitation and motor activity. The patient may shout and be destructive and violent, with uncontrolled outbursts unrelated to environmental events. These may be dangerous to the patient as well as to others. Catatonic patients often require physical restraint lest they do themselves or others harm. They may break windows, attack a bystander, or rip and destroy their own clothing. Such patients—probably more than any of the others described in this book—typify the popular version of "crazy," violent, ward behavior; in catatonic excitement there is unpredictable behavior that includes mystical, ecstatic, or terrifying experiences and transitory hallucinatory and delusional behavior.

The withdrawn type is characterized by a dramatic reduction of all activity. Catatonic stupor, in which the patient lies for days in one position without seeming to respond to environmental stimulation, may abruptly end in a violent phase of the sort already described. The patient may close or avert the eyes downward, and stare blankly with fixed expression. He or she may stand in an extremely uncomfortable position without change for unusually long periods, leaning partially against the wall or semicrouching in midair with one arm raised. These positions may be accompanied by

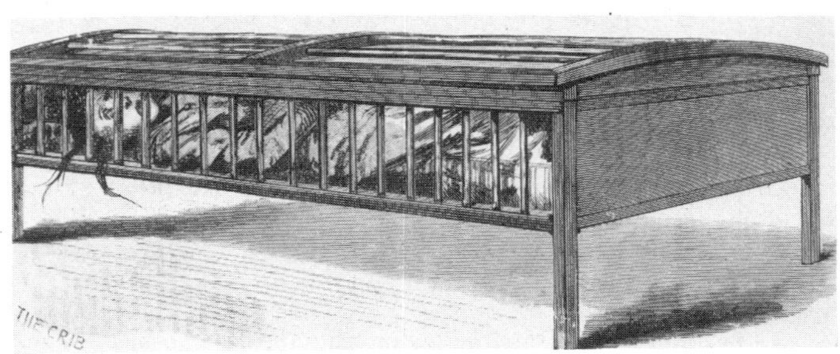

Treatment of mental disease in the Victorian Age: the crib—a device to restrain unmanageable cases, probably excited catatonic schizophrenics, in a New York institution. Woodcut, 1882. (The Bettman Archive)

refusal of food and care. The patient may be defecating and urinating into his or her own clothing. In this state, there may be little responsiveness to stimulation—some movement before the patient's eyes, pinpricks, or sudden pain. When the patient recovers, however, he or she can sometimes render a detailed list of all of these environmental events, despite apparent lack of responsiveness to, or perception of, them at the time they took place.

Patients may gradually or suddenly return to normal even after months of the most dramatic catatonic withdrawal. Prognosis (course of the disease) is often quite good with this subtype, especially if an acute phase has preceded the catatonic phase, which is often the case. Remission (freedom from or reduction of symptoms) is often as rapid and sudden as onset.

The Paranoid Subtype

Onset of paranoid types of schizophrenia tends to be at a later age than onset of the other types. This form of schizophrenia is characterized by marked delusional beliefs centering around ideas of persecution, reference (see Spotlight 11.1), jealousy, or grandiosity, accompanied by guardedness, suspiciousness of others, hostility, and aggressiveness. Generally, in paranoid schizophrenia, there is greater cohesion of cognitive and intellective processes and less dramatic disintegration of personality than in the other types described. Many researchers are beginning to believe that paranoid and nonparanoid schizophrenia represent two rather different disease entities; a later section of this chapter will explore this possibility.

Case 11.2 Male, Schizophrenia, Catatonic Type

[Patient] had been an average scholar but introspective and solitary at school, with no liking for games and no hobbies. He became a mill-worker at the age of 15 and was "more a boy for home, never keen on girls." He served in the Army during the Second World War and had some sort of transient mental breakdown, of which no records are available. After demobilization he was idle for six months: he appeared depressed and mixed up, seemed to take no interest in things around him and did not even respond to questioning. Then he had a job for six months, but was dismissed and again hung around the house, making no attempt to seek further employment. Thereafter he became even more dull and apathetic, looked vacant and faraway, refused to get out of bed or take food. He declared that people were trying to take a rise out of him, that some unknown individual was "making him think about things," and that he himself was a "riddle of bones." In the year following his demobilization from the Army he was admitted to a mental hospital, aged 23 years.

In hospital at first he lay in bed with an occasional vacant smile, and refused food. He was correctly orientated and could give his history with reasonable accuracy, but he had little insight, saying that he had been sent to the hospital on account of fits of bad temper. He was both auditorily and visually hallucinated: he complained of hearing buzzing noises, sounds like someone squealing and voices which he could sometimes understand but whose messages he could not remember, and he described flashes of light and shadows in the middle of the room. He expressed the belief that the doctors and nurses could manipulate their shadows, and that there was another person in his bed. Later he complained of tasting soap in his mouth and of receiving poison from the post beside his bed. Often he could not be engaged in conversation, sat vacantly by the hour and had both to be taken to his meals and pressed to eat. At times he was incontinent, chewed the end of his tie and hoarded rubbish. For weeks on end he would be in a state of stupor or near to it, showing catalepsy and flexibilitas cerea *[waxy flexibility]. Then a period of excitement would intervene, when for days or weeks on end he would be hyperactive and talk a great deal in a disjointed and usually incoherent way. At these times he would strike out impulsively at the nursing staff. On occasion he clowned in a crude way and would walk on his hands.*

Source: Henderson and Gillespie's *Textbook of Psychiatry* (pp. 278–79), revised by I.R.C. Batchelor, © Oxford University Press 1969. Reprinted by permission of Oxford University Press.

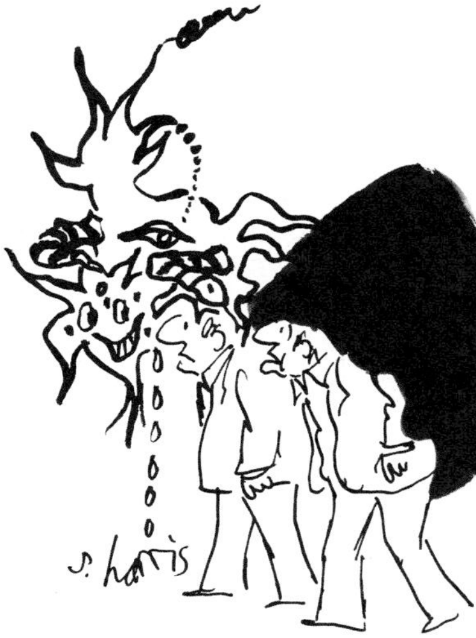

"BUT YOU MUST ADMIT HALLUCINATIONS ARE MORE INTERESTING THAN DEPRESSION."

Sidney Harris

In premorbid and early phases of paranoid schizophrenia, there is rigidity and humorlessness, extreme guardedness, sensitivity, grudge-holding, and suspiciousness. Later, delusions, bizarre ideas of persecution, ideas of reference, and hallucinations with either persecutory or grandiose content become apparent. With the continued course of the disease, the delusions shift and become more unsystematic. There may be neologisms, pronounced incoherence, and a general disintegration of the personality.

Often there is great preoccupation with body processes and fear of body disintegration. There may be concern with abstract ideas, for example, evil versus good, or powerful electronic devices that can manipulate and control one's mind. Numbers, religious systems, and world schemes often preoccupy the paranoid schizophrenic. There may be grandiosity, or there might be identification with great historical figures such as Napoleon or Joan of Arc.

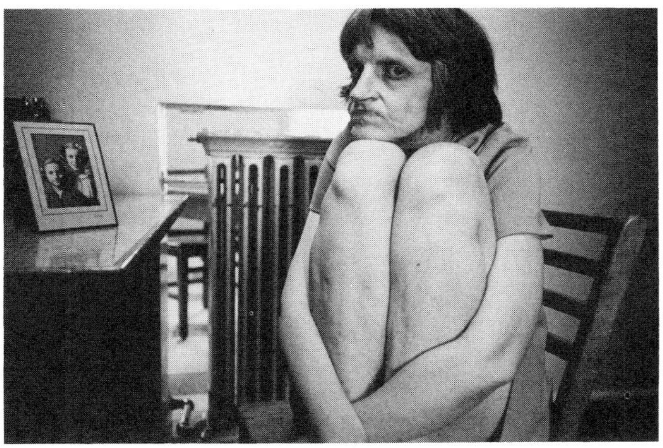

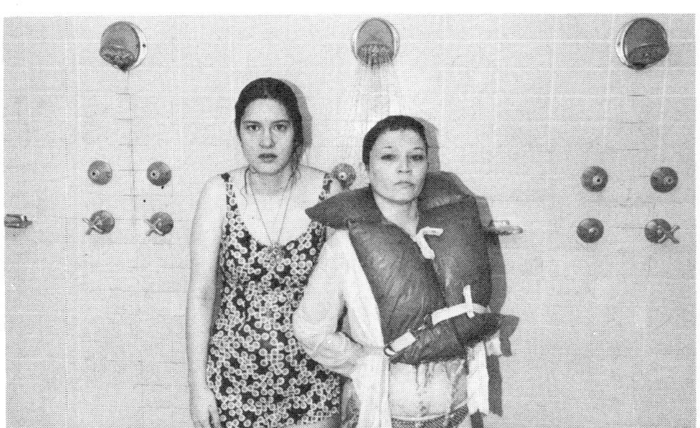

Photographic portraits of schizophrenic patients. (Mary Ellen Mark)

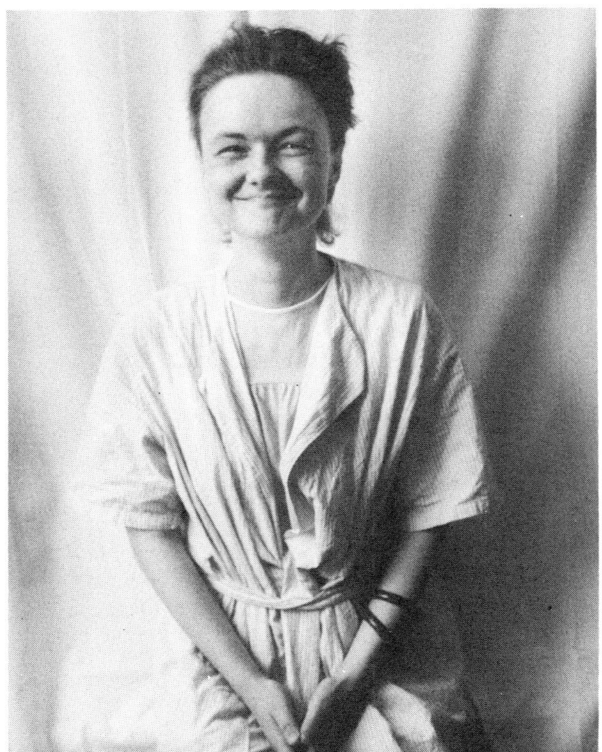

Case 11.3 C.R.: Schizophrenia, Paranoid Type

The year C. R. became fifty years old he left the assembly line in the automotive factory, grabbed some heavy equipment in an adjoining tool shop, and brutally assaulted his foreman, who after weeks of hospitalization with some crushed limbs and a broken nose, finally recovered. He's been after my wife for years, C. R. said. And the radio waves that go back and forth between them are so strong that I saw them on Gunsmoke last night. All the neighbors are complaining about the interference with their TV sets. Last year he tried to get to me by thinning my blood with the remote control machine he has in his garage. But I smashed it. And he never knew who did it.

Three months before this first acute episode, he had expressed scattered delusional fears of persecution, was agitated, and described intermittent auditory hallucinations. He was extremely frightened by these symptoms, but he felt that the persecution was real, as were the hallucinations. He was preoccupied with a stream of thoughts (ruminations) that centered chiefly on his wife's supposed infidelities, "making it with everybody."

After a legal hearing that was attended by the company psychiatrist and a court-appointed psychiatrist, the judge had C. R. committed to a state hospital. During the hearing and the first week of hospitalization, C. R. was dazed, confused, disoriented, and mute. At the end of two months, during which C. R. was on medication and had daily visits with a medical resident, weekly meetings with a psychologist, and biweekly group sessions with other patients (to which he made little or no contribution), he was discharged into the care of his wife. In the year after discharge he visited a day clinic two times a week for group sessions. At these meetings, continued use of medication was encouraged by the counselor.

Soon C. R. was back at the job and seemed to be getting along all right—for about two years— until he had a recurrence of acute symptoms. Once again, he was hospitalized with acute panic and hallucinations, after displaying assaultive behavior toward his wife. He became well quickly, at least up to the level of his moderately adequate premorbid adjustment, and once more was released into the care of his wife.

Now, five years later, he is on continuous medication and attends group meetings once weekly at the local mental hygiene clinic, where he is becoming more open and articulate about his problems. He knows that he is not "well," and although he grumbles bitterly about having to do so, he takes his medication regularly. With his average intelligence, secure job, and compassionate (but complaining and harried) wife and family, he is no threat to the community, himself, or others, and can probably live out the rest of his life marginally well.

The Undifferentiated and Residual Subtypes

The DSM-III lists an undifferentiated subtype that does not fit any of the foregoing categories but that nevertheless meets the general criteria for making a diagnosis of schizophrenia, such as delusions, hallucinations, thought disorders, and peculiar, odd behavior. The residual category is used when there has been a previous psychotic episode, no current flagrant or prominent symptom, and yet continued indications of illness such as blunted or inappropriate affect, social withdrawal, eccentric behavior, illogical thinking, or loosening of associations.

The Simple Type

For years most diagnosticians and the DSM-II recognized the category *schizophrenia, simple type.* The DSM-III no longer uses this category. It is unclear whether or not the following clinical description and case illustration should be classified among the schizophrenias at all, and there is no evidence to suggest a genetic link or overlap between this and the other types of schizophrenia. Yet for many years the diagnosis was sufficiently accepted as a valid subtype of schizophrenia as to warrant hospitalization, as in the case of A. R., Case 11.4. At the end of this chapter the issue is raised as to whether or not people like A. R. should be hospitalized against their wills. As you read the case description, bear this question in mind.

This disorder presumably starts in puberty with a gradual loss of interest and drive accompanied by increased apathy and withdrawal. The youngster stays away from social contacts, becomes reclusive, and does extremely poorly in school. Although generally there is apathy, there might be occasional violent rages. The personality picture worsens through the years and may end in marked deterioration. Delusions and hallucinations are usually not present. This kind of personality shows shallowness of affect and inability to form attachments or relationships. Many of the bums, drifters, vagrants, hoboes, and tramps that aimlessly float through life may be schizophrenics of this type.

Simple schizophrenics show a meagerness—an impoverishment—of emotions that gradually becomes more and more pronounced. Diffidence, lack of concern, and a minimal level of interest, motivation, drive, or energy level—but without depression—characterize these states. Such people find it difficult to meet responsibilities and they are not responsive to environmental pulls, demands, pressures, and exhortations. They are shallow, flat, emotionally "withered," and two-dimensional.

THE PARANOID DISORDERS

The paranoid disorders refer to those conditions that are primarily characterized by persistent persecutory or grandiose delusional systems, or sys-

Case 11.4 A.R.: Schizophrenia, Simple Type

A. R. was committed to the hospital when twenty-one years of age following his arrest for window-peeping. In describing his childhood characteristics, the patient's family stated that he "was always a little hard to understand," but was a quiet boy who never entered into rough games. His school record was excellent and he always stood high in his class. At age seventeen, when in the fourth year of high scoool, he was obliged, because of a long illness of his father, to leave school and secure gainful employment. He secured work with a large manufacturing company where he soon came to be considered the second best operative on a certain type of machine. For two years he worked steadily, seemed ambitious, and appeared to have a normal and wholesome but not marked, interest in girls. At age nineteen he gave up his position, showed no interest in securing another, and when asked if he worked replied, "What do I want to work for? I have a father and sister working and they are enough." He appeared quite self-satisfied and felt that he should have a position of importance.

At about this time he was first arrested for peeping into women's bedrooms. Through the influence of his father, the charge was dropped. He became careless of his personal appearance and remained unoccupied except for occasional periods, when he set up pins in a bowling alley. A year later he was again arrested but again was released on the intercession of his father. He came to say little unless addressed and grew antagonistic toward his father and sister. He would remain out until midnight and then come home, eat a large meal, read until 2 A.M., and sleep until noon. Finally, after his third arrest for peeping, he was committed to a hospital for mental disorders.

On arrival at the institution, the patient was found to be of asthenic physique and slightly effeminate in appearance. His emotional responses were shallow and inadequate. He showed no concern over his situation, laughed about it in a silly manner, and referred to his offense as "just a foolish idea." His hospital residence was characterized by apathy, preoccupation, and inactivity. During the summer he would at times take part in the patient's baseball games, but in winter he refused ground privileges. He never expressed any delusions and denied hallucinations. At times he would be seen, apparently much preoccupied, walking alone about the hospital reservation, laughing to himself.

Source: L. C. Kolb, *Modern clinical psychiatry,* 8th ed. (Philadelphia: Saunders, 1973), p. 331.

tems of jealousy, that are not accounted for by the other diagnostic categories. They include paranoia, shared paranoid disorder, and acute paranoid disorder. These disorders cannot be diagnosed as reflections of schizophrenic or affective disorders because the generalized thought disorders of the former (incoherent ideas, illogical thought processes) and the mood dysfunctions of the latter are not present. These paranoid disorders are characterized by delusional systems that are persistent and single-minded without affecting other areas of functioning. The individual appears to be intact, especially with regard to thinking processes. Yet there appear to be disturbances in interpersonal relationships as well as eccentric behaviors that include suspiciousness and frequent litigious activities—suit-bringing and various legal involvements. Great anger may also be displayed. People with paranoid disorders rarely seek treatment, for they have little insight into the quality of their thinking. According to the DSM-III, the gender distribution of paranoid disorders is not known.

It may be difficult to distinguish paranoia from some of the other syndromes just described such as paranoid personality disorders (Chapter 9) and paranoid schizophrenia. Those suffering from paranoid personality disorders or styles (Shapiro, 1965) are not characterized by the delusions, hallucinations, and the bizarre behavior of the paranoid schizphrenic, or by the single grand scheme of the paranoic. People with paranoid personality disorders are suspicious, unspontaneous, rigid, and narrowly focused people who are always searching for clues to confirm their suspicions. They often feel tense, because they live in constant anticipation of their worst fears coming true and they may be furtive or arrogant and aggressive, but they do not have the delusions about mind control, electricity, or gamma rays "rotting away their insides," for example, of the paranoid schizophrenic or the grandiose master plan of the paranoic.

The person with classic paranoia, on the other hand, with his or her grand overall scheme, is completely enmeshed in a logical, tightly woven system without showing any of the bizarreness and fragmented delusions of the schizophrenic or the "normal range" behavior of the individual with the personality disorder.

Paranoia. "True" paranoia is so rare that many clinicians have never come into face-to-face contact with it. Paranoic people do not show up in clinics or seek help, for they possess little insight into themselves; nor do they become deteriorated or helpless, thus requiring care. In paranoia, intellectual function, life style, employment pattern, marital status, and general personality may remain stable and intact, with no bizarre or inappropriate functioning and apparently with no incursion of the disease process. With the exception of a logical, internally consistent, unshakable, and single-minded delusional system—which may be elaborate and incredibly grandiose— the individual suffering with paranoia may show little evidence of his or her disease.

Case 11.5 F.R.: "True Paranoia:"

F. R. is a twenty-eight-year-old successful stockbroker in a prestigious firm. He thinks he will be made a full partner one day. He has many important accounts and is highly respected by the senior people—especially for his mathematical acumen and his knowledge of economic trends in world markets. He gets along well with his colleagues. But nobody really knows him. He eats lunch alone, does not drink or smoke, loves to listen to classical music, and is an excellent chess player. He is married. He and his wife, who works for one of the big computer corporations, have decided not to have children. They live quietly and with considerable reserve in a quiet and considerably reserved neighborhood that matches their personalities. They have few friends. They love to read, go to bed early, and rise early. They claim they have good sexual relations and are "simpatico" with each other.

F. R. sought consultation because of occasional, terrifying panic attacks accompanied by acute headaches that awoke him from time to time from a nightmare. He claimed, actually, that these were not nightmares and that his panic attacks resulted from real terror that he would be kidnapped by a syndicate representing one of the Near Eastern nations. He knows too much, he said. At which point, he proceeded to present his detailed, elaborate "story."

They were out to kill him, he said, and would do so at any moment. His life is in peril, but he cannot do anything about it, because if he did, the "big shot" in Washington whom he was protecting would be killed. He named names.

F. R. then presented a lengthy, complicated story beginning on the day of his twenty-first birthday, when he was kidnapped. And for an hour the patient told a bizarre tale of harrowing escapes, murders, spy and espionage activities, mind control, surgical procedures, and international intrigues that have lasted for years, all revolving around the fact that he was privy to certain information about the "big shot" in Washington. The story made sense: the parts fitted together and seemed to have a logical intactness as to sequence and organization of ideas. The patient otherwise showed no symptoms. He was intelligent, did not hallucinate, worked productively and creatively for his firm, and enjoyed a pleasant relationship with his wife.

F. R. claims that he plans to clean up this mess, starting next year, and he has a five-year-plan to do so. Whether he plans to go into politics, initiate public action, write an expose, or start a social-political national organization is not clear. He has intelligence, foresight, and organizational ability; he is also well-spoken and articulate. Who knows? Perhaps his "story" is real, after all! And perhaps he will do something of great social significance. Stranger events and circumstance have been made public.

In any event, he did not seek psychotherapy. He was even shocked at the suggestion. He wanted an evaluation of his headaches and, more important, an opportunity to present the names and details and dates in his "story" to someone in strict confidence before they "got to him."

His wife later disclosed that there were several periods of hospitalization for "nervous breakdown." There was also one acute period of depression and anxiety. She also said that apart from the complex delusional superstructure he has built, there are no other symptoms that she can think of, and certainly no bizarre, unusual, or peculiar characteristics in his behavior, language, or thinking. She was with him on the day of his twenty-first birthday, the day of his presumed kidnapping. They were counselors in a summer camp, and he never missed a day's work. He was the music counselor and ran the chess program, doing a brilliant job in both capacities. The campers, however, never liked him. His wife accepts his delusional system, knowing that she can do nothing about it.

Some paranoic people feel themselves to be endowed with unusually superior abilities. As a matter of fact, many great movements, social revolutions, and ideological upheavals have been sponsored by people who may have been suffering from paranoia. Celebrated "deliverers"—the Joans of Arc—with grand delusional belief systems and no other thinking disorder—may have contributed immeasurably to the world's progress. Case 11.5 describes a man whose ultimate life contribution is still undetermined but who seems to meet some of the criteria for a true paranoic.

Shared paranoid disorder (folie à deux). A variation of paranoia arises in the form of two (or more rarely, more) closely interrelated people, such as husband and wife or adult identical twins, sharing a common delusional system. The French term *folie à deux* (madness for two) reflects this rare pathology. Such an enmeshment (symbiosis) of two people—with its spilling over of delusional systems to which both people are committed—creates a fascinating clinical picture. For example, if the wife of the "primary" patient described in Case 11.5 had cooperated with him in his delusional system, we would have a picture of *folie à deux.* The DSM-III notes that if one member of the symbiotic system can be separated, the delusional beliefs of the secondary patient will diminish or disappear.

Acute paranoid disorder. This disorder is diagnosed, according to the DSM-III, when there is a paranoid disorder of six months' duration or less. The symptoms are the same as those found in other paranoid disorders, for example, persecutory delusions, but no prominent hallucinations, and no bizarre delusions or associations. Onset, which is sudden, is sometimes found when there is a sudden relocation of an individual, as in time of war, deportation, military induction, immigration, and similar abrupt changes in the social environment. This disorder rarely becomes chronic, according to the DSM-III.

Atypical paranoid disorder. This is a residual diagnostic category that fits into the general classification of paranoid disorders but yet cannot be classified in any of the foregoing categories.

Spotlight 11.2 Border Disputes: To Label or not to Label?

Ever since Bleuler in 1911 described latent schizophrenia (1950) there has been an ongoing debate about whether or not there is a borderline diagnostic group that, although not psychotic, shares many of the behavioral and symptomatic manifestations of schizophrenia (see Grinker, 1979; Gunderson, 1979; Gunderson & Singer, 1975; Kernberg, 1979; Liebowitz, 1979; Rieder, 1979; Siever & Gunderson, 1979; and Spitzer & Endicott, 1979). The diagnostic befuddlement over this issue still continues, and a few years ago almost an entire issue of the *Schizophrenia Bulletin* (5, 1979, no. 1), a scholarly quarterly journal, became a forum for the pros and cons of this debate.

Most clinicians are familiar with some of the features of the so-called borderline syndrome and with many of the labels that have been employed to reflect this fuzzy category, for example, schizophrenic character, pseudoneurotic schizophrenia, borderline, ambulatory, or latent schizophrenia (Gunderson, 1979; Gunderson & Singer, 1975). To make matters worse, in Chapter 9, when the personality disorders of the DSM-III were listed (see page 202), additional classifications were introduced that are relevant to the current discussion: schizotypal personality disorder and borderline personality disorder. This spotlight highlights some of the problems and issues that clinicians face when, even if not working entirely in the dark, they are groping for more light. No answers are offered here, only a sharper presentation of some of the problems in this area.

What are so-called borderline patients like? Not all clinicians would agree as to borderline traits. Many, however, would go along with the following description: Although borderline people are not psychotic, do not distort, modify, or perceive the real world totally subjectively, or have delusions and hallucinations, they get by in their worlds rather poorly. They show disturbed interpersonal relationships, such as great dependency or inability to have any but superficial, transitory relationships. They may show intense hostility, impulsive behavior, anxiety, depression, and disorganization in ambivalent or unstructured situations. They may even have psychotic episodes. There may be a history of drug abuse and irresponsible, shifting patterns in regard to marriage, children, family, jobs, and finances. "Borderlines" may also show oddness in language and thinking, some suspiciousness, and extreme sensitivity to criticism. In fact, their condition appears to be a combination of the DSM-III's schizotypal and borderline personality disorders (see pp. 226–27).

Why do people want to clarify this issue? One important reason is that these individuals are difficult to treat by the usual methods. If we knew more about them and could feel certain that we were talking about a diagnostic entity that contains a common ground, perhaps we could be of more help to them by carving out effective therapeutic approaches or by devising workable preventive methods. A second reason has to do with the general quest of scientists for rigor of observation and definitions, beginning first with a valid classificatory scheme. Still another reason concerns the mountain to climb—the baffling problem of schizophrenia and its related disorders.

What are some of the issues that have to be solved regarding the so-called borderline classification? (a) Is the borderline diagnosis a milder form of schizophrenia? Is there a schizophrenic spectrum of which the borderline diagnosis is one part? (b) Is the borderline classification, instead, some aspect of an affective disorder, a wavelength on the affective spectrum? (Yes, according to Liebowitz, 1979). (c) Does the distinction between schizotypal and borderline categories make sense, as suggested by Spitzer and Endicott (1979)? (d) If the borderline classification bears some relationship to either schizophrenic or affective disorders, or both, is there genetic evidence that it runs in families in which these disorders have a high preponderance? (e) Is there emerging some common denominator regarding successful treatment of people diagnosed as borderline? Or are different borderline subtypes responsive to different types of treatment? Is there a higher risk of schizophrenic episodes for borderline patients than for other diagnostic groups?

PSYCHOTIC DISORDERS NOT CLASSIFIED ELSEWHERE

The DSM-III includes several other diagnoses that are classified as psychotic because they describe conditions that include delusions, hallucinations, incoherence, repeated derailment (see pp. 268–69), marked poverty of content of thought, strikingly illogical thinking, and behavior that is grossly disorganized or catatonic. Yet these conditions do not meet the criteria of the other disorders. They include schizophreniform disorder, brief reactive psychosis, and schizoaffective disorder. The category *atypical psychosis* is a residual category for instances of psychosis in which a diagnosis fitting any of these or the other categories already described cannot be made.

Schizophreniform disorder. This diagnosis applies to psychotic conditions that are of brief duration (more than two weeks and up to six months), have sudden onset with acute symptoms such as turmoil and confusion, and are characterized by good prospect for restoration of premorbid levels of adjustment. The symptoms of schizophreniform disorders are similar to those of the various schizophrenic conditions, including delusions, hallucinations, incoherence, and grossly disorganized behavior, but this diagnosis is made when the psychotic episode is of brief duration. In this designation, the incidence of schizophrenia in the patient's family is not greater than in the general population, a criterion that presumably differentiates this disorder from the other schizophrenias (see Chapter 12).

Brief reactive psychosis. This diagnosis indicates a psychotic episode lasting from a few hours up to two weeks, following an event of major proportions that would be extremely stressful to most people. Usually the psychotic symptoms disappear in a few days. According to the DSM-III, symptoms include emotional turmoil and at least one of the following: incoherence or loosening of associations; delusions; hallucinations; and behavior that is grossly disorganized or catatonic.

Schizoaffective disorder. This is a category for which the DSM-III presents no diagnostic criteria, noting only that the diagnosis has been a confusing one for many clinicians. The DSM-III suggests using this category when there is uncertainty about whether or not the "correct" diagnosis is affective disorder, schizophreniform disorder, or schizophrenia. The World Health Organization in 1977 defined schizoaffective psychoses as "mental disorders in which manic or depressive syndromes are mixed with schizophrenic syndromes simultaneously or successively during the course of illness." According to Angst et al., (1980), this diagnosis should be made when a diagnosis of neither an affective disorder or schizophrenia can be made; this clinician also indicated that although patients with schizoaffective disorders have a high rate of relapse, there is excellent functioning between episodes.

Atypical psychosis. According to the DSM-III, this is the appropriate diagnosis when psychotic symptoms such as delusions, hallucinations, incoherence, loosening of associations, illogical thinking, or disorganized or catonic behavior are markedly present, but when the overall pattern does not fit any of the foregoing categories.

PROBLEMS IN THE DIAGNOSIS OF SCHIZOPHRENIA

A good diagnostic system, in addition to reliability and validity, should be able to predict outcome and should implicitly convey some directions for best type of treatment. Further, it should be capable of consistent interpretation and application. The "traditional" system just described does not satisfy these and several other criteria for a workable diagnostic scheme. For not only do clinicians differ in the narrowness or breadth of what they assume is schizophrenia, but also there are differences among them as to just what schizophrenia is.

There are, for example, cultural variations in the application of the traditional scheme. British clinicians tend to apply affective diagnoses (as long as there is some mood disorder) more frequently than American clinicians, who tend to designate the patient as schizophrenic as long as there is *some* thinking disorder. American clinicians employ a diagnosis of schizophrenia in a much wider variety of clinical conditions (Professional Staff of the United States-United Kingdom Cross-National Project, 1974). In general, the broadness or narrowness of the scope contained within the diagnosis of schizophrenia and the confusions in diagnosing schizophrenic, affective, and schizoaffective disorders add to what is an already confusing picture (Kuriansky, Deming, and Gurland, 1974; Taylor, Gaztanaga, and Abrams, 1974).

An interesting demonstration of culturally based diagnostic confusions and differences was provided by Zubin and his staff (see Gurland et al., 1972), who worked with video tapes of diagnostic interviews. Spotlight 11.3 describes some of this work. One strategy for tackling some of these diagnostic problems is to systematize and objectify observations about symptoms and then to see whether certain symptoms or clusters of symptoms actually add up to the same diagnosis in repeated trials. Spotlight 11.4 describes some of this work.

Reactive-Process Classification: A Valid Subtyping of Schizophrenia?

There is poor agreement as to what constitutes the subtypes of schizophrenia even among experienced clinicians (Blashfield, 1973; Hohman, 1964; Zigler and Phillips, 1961; Zubin, 1967). Concern with solving these problems has led some investigators to consider breaking away entirely from the traditional subtypes.

One major break from tradition is to classify schizophrenic patients on the basis of prognosis—prediction of the outcome of their disease. Some patients get progressively worse, ending up in a deteriorated, vegetative state, whereas other patients recover fairly rapidly and go about the business of living with little impairment in functioning. A diagnosis that contains within it some implication for outcome may make better sense, it is thought, than

Spotlight 11.3 Crosscultural Biases in Diagnostic Practices

In a cross-national study of differences in diagnostic practices (see Professional Staff of the United States-United Kingdom Cross-National Project, 1974), Zubin and his staff presented videotaped interviews to psychiatrists in New York, London, throughout the United States, and parts of Canada and the British Isles, for diagnoses. Americans generally tended to diagnose schizophrenia more frequently than the British, who used the manic-depressive diagnosis more frequently. Canadian clinicians seemed to use diagnostic practices in between the British and American extremes. American psychiatrists also tended to rate the interviews as showing greater pathology. Figure 11.1 shows the diagnoses made by groups of American and British psychiatrists watching eight videotaped interviews.

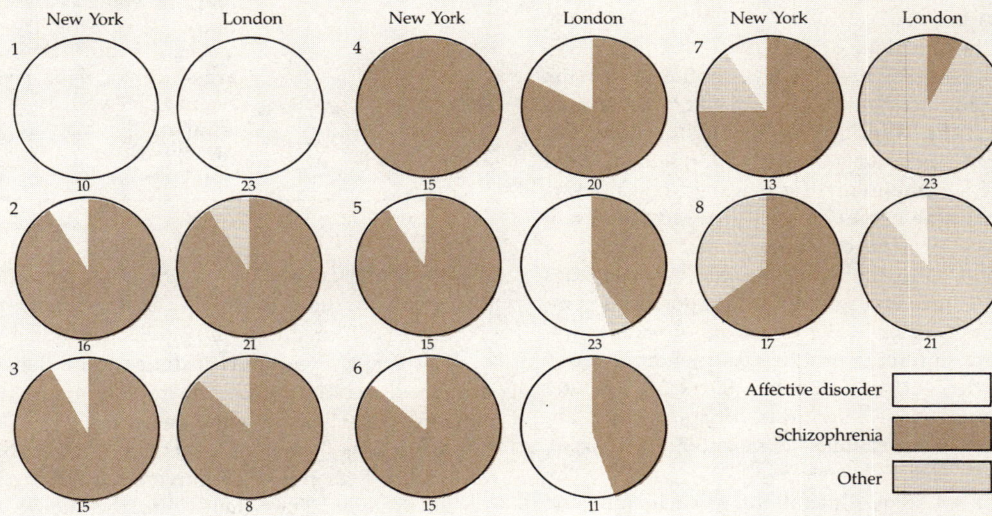

Figure 11.1 Eight different videotaped interviews diagnosed by clinicians in the New York State Psychiatric Institute or the Maudsley Hospital in London. The smaller numbers represent the number of clinicians who rated each interview. (From *Schizophrenia Bulletin,* 1974, No. 11, p. 87)

a diagnosis that is unrelated to what happens to the patient.

A classification system that considers outcome need not contain any bias in favor of one etiological position over another. Nor would such a system necessarily incur the disfavor of those who believe that schizophrenia is a disease process that subsumes many etiologies. For example, a diagnosis of measles A might be made for patients with speedy recoveries and no residual physical difficulties after

Spotlight 11.4 Objectifying the Diagnosis of Schizophrenia: A Symptom Approach?

Have the traditional psychological tests been useful in the diagnosis of schizophrenia? Projective methods have failed to provide the objective, reliable means to diagnose schizophrenia with predictive validity as to outcome (Schumer and Zubin, 1972; Zubin, Eron, and Schumer, 1965). Objective inventories have fared better, however. Other approaches to classifying patients include the computer-based diagnostic schedules developed by Spitzer and his colleagues (for example, Spitzer and Endicott, 1968) already described in Chapter 4; these offer considerable promise.

Some investigators believe in the systematic use of symptoms in making a diagnosis of schizophrenia. The World Health Organization has sponsored such an attempt (International Pilot Study of Schizophrenia) for many years, gathering data from nine countries, each markedly different in sociocultural flavor. From a vast reservoir of behavioral data, statistical analysis has yielded a system of signs and symptoms that possess a common denominator in the diagnosis of schizophrenia in the different countries (Carpenter, Strauss, and Bartko, 1974; Carpenter, Bartko, Carpenter and Strauss, 1976; Sartorius, Shapiro, and Jablensky, 1974; and Strauss, Carpenter, and Bartko, 1974).

Here are some illustrations of such signs and symptoms and their corresponding observation or question from the examination employed in the WHO study (Carpenter, Strauss, and Bartko, 1973):

Sign or Symptom	*Observation or Question*
restricted affect	blank, expressionless face; very little or no emotion shown when delusion or normal material is discussed which would usually bring out emotion
poor insight	overall rating of insight
thoughts aloud	do you feel your thoughts are being broadcast, transmitted, so that everyone knows what you are thinking? do you even seem to hear your thoughts spoken aloud? (as if someone nearby could hear them?)
nihilistic delusions	do you feel that your body is decaying, rotting? do you feel that some part of your body is missing, for example, head, brain, or arms? do you ever have the feeling that you do not exist at all, that you are dead, dissolved?

Newmark et al. (1976) compared ratings of observers as to the presence of certain symptoms according to four different systems, including their own system. Symptoms included such behaviors as loose associations, autism, flat affect, withdrawal, hallucinations, and delusions. They designated a large group of patients as schizophrenic and others as nonschizophrenic on the basis of these systems. Then they compared the accuracy of these designations with the diagnoses obtained in usual clinical procedures. They found good agreement for some systems and poor agreement for others.

One of the systems that was found to be inadequate is a fairly popular one proposed by Schneider (1959; see also Mellor, 1970). Schneider's system states that any one of eleven "first-rank" symptoms is of special significance in the diagnosis of schizophrenia. First-rank symptoms include three types of auditory hallucinations (for example, voices arguing), the presence of delusions, and several types of persistent thoughts that are experienced as bearing a relationship to or being controlled by external forces (for example, ideas are stolen out of one's mind by an outside force, or "broadcast" to others, or inserted by an external agent). The use of first-rank criteria resulted in a large number of "false positives"—that is, a large number of patients who were not schizophrenic were incorrectly labeled schizophrenic.

The general finding that no one sign or group of several signs or symptoms successfully categorizes all schizophrenics was supported in a larger study based on diagnostic data obtained from nine countries (Carpenter and Strauss, 1974). That is, the presence of one symptom or category of symptoms alone—no matter how important—does not define schizophrenia exclusively. On the other hand, fairly (but not entirely) successful differentiation of schizophrenics from nonschizophrenics was obtained on the basis of skilled observations of the presence of several symptoms, especially if weighted in empirically established ways.

recovery, whereas measles B might be assigned to patients with slower recoveries and some residual symptoms after recovery. These diagnoses need not make any assumptions about the cause of measles, such as viral contagion, genetic predisposition, or various combinations of circumstances and predispositions.

One such distinction that seems to make sense is the reactive-process distinction. In the *reactive* type, generally, there is no longstanding history of poor premorbid adjustment, onset is sudden, symptoms are acute, frequently there is remission in a relatively short period of time, and there is a favorable prognosis. In *process* schizophrenia there is a long history of poor premorbid adjustment; the onset is gradual, insidious, and earlier, and there is a chronic and progressively worsening pattern of illness usually ending in deterioration, with obviously poor prognosis.

Because of the early researches of Zigler and Phillips (Phillips, 1953; Zigler and Phillips, 1962), we are not only aware of the greater heterogeneity of premorbid levels of schizophrenics, but we are also beginning to acknowledge the relationship of premorbid competence to outcome of the disease. As a matter of fact, according to these investigators, a valid evaluation of premorbid competence is a significant clue to prognosis in *all* psychopathology, not just schizophrenia (Phillips, 1964). This makes sense, because the adaptive resources in a "good" premorbid individual may help that person cope with a psychotic episode more effectively than would be the case for a "poor" premorbid individual in whom coping resources had been eroded over a period or were never really adequate.

It thus became important to develop methods for evaluating the early social adequacy of the patient. Such scales are in fairly widespread (mostly research) use (see Kokes, Strauss, and Klorman, [1977] for a review and presentation of the most important of these). One widely used scale is the Phillips Rating Scale of Premorbid Adjustment (Phillips, 1953) which assesses a patient's social and sexual premorbid "competence" on the basis of his or her case record (see Spotlight 11.5).

Do process schizophrenics really differ from reactive schizophrenics? According to a review of relevant studies (Rolf and Harig, 1974), the answer is yes: it may be that chronic (process) and short-term (reactive) illnesses reflect different clinical entities. For example, in one long-term longitudinal study, schizophrenic adolescent patients with a chronic course tended to have parents who were more frequently disturbed, more relatives with chronic schizophrenia, lower IQs, and earlier onset than a group of adolescent schizophrenics with more favorable adult adjustment (Roff, 1974).

It has also been proposed that each group of

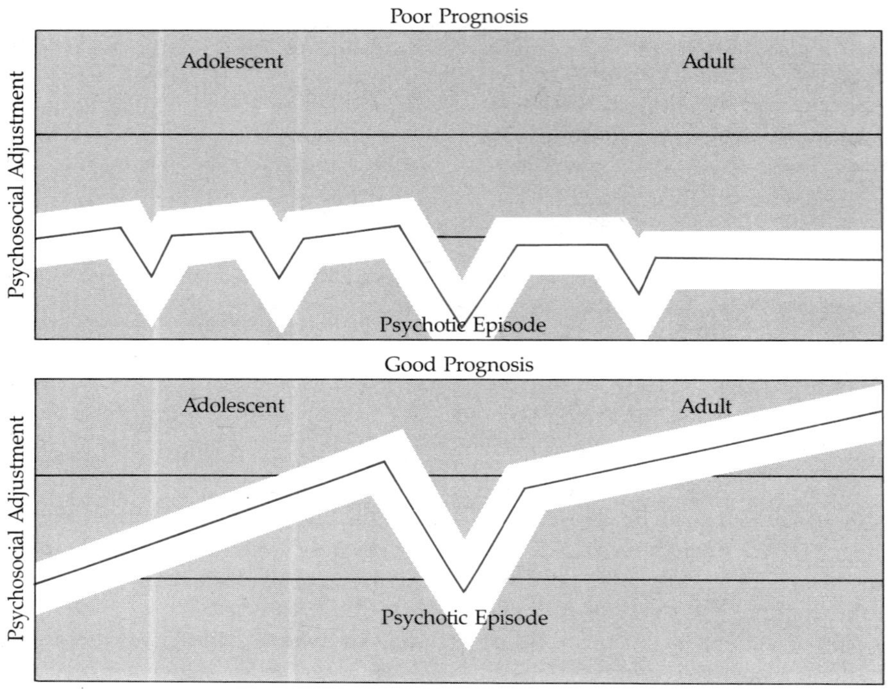

Figure 11.2 "Good" and "poor" schizophrenic histories. Premorbid competence is related to prognosis and outcome in schizophrenia. (From *Schizophrenia Bulletin*, 1977, *3*, No. 2, pp. 180–81)

patients perceives or "handles" threatening stimuli differently. Reactive patients are said to be more responsive to threatening, external stimuli (lower thresholds to threat) whereas process schizophrenics, because they are more retreated and withdrawn, are thought to be less responsive to stressful stimuli (DeWolfe, 1974; Sappington, 1975). The greater responsiveness to "dangerous" external stimuli would thus explain the disorientation and disorganization in the acute schizophrenic episode.

Because of developmental and social difficulties, process schizophrenics are thought to have more idiosyncratic (odd, peculiar, personal) thought processes, greater lack of involvement in the demands and requirements of the tasks presented to them, and lower responsiveness to relevant information in the situation they are asked to handle, than do reactive schizophrenics, who have not had an equivalent history of social retreat. Conversely, reactive schizophrenics, in an acute episode or under stress of admission to a hospital, will show greater responsiveness to irrelevant, external stimuli, displaying fragmentation in thinking processes (lack of connectedness and logical flow of ideas). As a result, there will be greater reduction of performance under stress among reactive schizophrenics than among process schizophrenics, despite more improvement among the former group of patients later on.

The literature is filled with demonstrations of differences between process and reactive schizophrenics in many cognitive areas, including the way in which they utilize information, how they form concepts and perceive events, the manner in which

Spotlight 11.5 An Abbreviated Form of the Phillips Rating Scale: Predicting Outcome?

Harris (1975) described an abbreviated version of the much widely used Phillips Scale (1953) as an economical, reliable, reasonably valid brief method of assessing case history material. Such assessment is often required not only for research purposes, but also for planning of treatment and making prognostic decisions. The Phillips Scale weights inadequate premorbid adjustment so that the higher the score, the poorer the adjustment. Poor premorbid adjustment is presumably correlated with later process schizophrenia.

In the abbreviated and longer versions, high weights are assigned for homosexual orientation and preference as well as single status. Although sexual and marital variables might have had predictive validity at one time, one wonders whether these variables continue to be predictive, in the light of changing attitudes in these areas. On the other hand, the scale for premorbid social and personal adjustment (see the abbreviated version following) seems to contain content that might well assess the social competence of the subject with a fair degree of reliability and validity.

Abbreviated Scale of Premorbid Social-Personal Adjustment

	Score
(A) A leader or officer in formally designated groups, clubs, organizations, or athletic teams in senior high school, vocational school, college, or in young adulthood.	0
(B) An active and interested participant, but did not play a leading role in groups of friends, clubs, organizations, or athletic teams in senior high school, vocational school, college, or in young adulthood.	1
(C) A nominal member, but had no involvement in, or commitment to, groups of friends, clubs, organizations, or athletic teams in senior high school, vocational school, college, or in young adulthood.	2
(D) From adolescence through early adulthood, had only a few casual or close friends.	3
(E) From adolescence through early adulthood, had no real friends, only a few superficial relationships or attachments to others.	4
(F) From adolescence through early adulthood (i.e., after childhood) quiet, seclusive, preferred to be by self; minimal efforts to maintain any contact at all with others.	5
(G) No desire to be with playmates, peers, or others, from early childhood. Either asocial or antisocial.	6

Source: Harris, 1975, p. 13.

they learn, and the coherence and integration of their delusions (Heilbrun and Heilbrun, 1977). Consistent differences are not found in all empirical studies, however.

Because of the failure of the process-reactive distinction to account for all cases in the schizophrenic spectrum, some authorities (for example, Mosher, Gunderson, and Buchsbaum, 1973) have concluded that although extreme cases can be differentiated on the basis of premorbid histories, the majority of patients cannot be neatly categorized into either process or reactive categories.

Paranoid versus Nonparanoid Schizophrenia

Related in some ways to the process-reactive distinction is the paranoid-nonparanoid dichotomy. Evidence is beginning to accumulate that patients showing paranoid symptomatology differ from the nonparanoid group along several dimensions. For example, there is some (not entirely consistent) evidence that premorbid social competence and adjustment (and level of maturity—developmental level) are related to this distinction, with more adequate premorbid status being associated with later paranoid, rather than nonparanoid, status (Goldstein, Held, and Cromwell, 1968; Strauss, 1973; Zigler and Levine, 1973; Zigler, Levine and Zigler, 1976).

Paranoids have later age of onset and less frequent familial schizophrenia than nonparanoids (Tsuang and Winokur, 1974). In autonomic responses, paranoids habituate to stressful stimuli more quickly than nonparanoids. That is, compared to nonparanoids, stressful stimuli become less disturbing over a period of trials for paranoids, who resemble normal subjects in this respect (Payne and Shean, 1975). Paranoid schizophrenics were also shown to be more sensitive to threatening stimuli than nonparanoid schizophrenics (Heilbrun and Norbert, 1971); less "regressed" than nonparanoid schizophrenics (that is, less likely to produce word associations similar to those of children, Youkilis and DeWolfe, 1975); and less perceptually but more cognitively oriented than nonparanoid schizophrenics (McDowell, Reynolds, and Magaro, 1975).

Deficits in the thought processes of schizophrenics, such as overinclusive thinking—difficulty in focusing on relevant variables—are thought to be especially characteristic of paranoid schizophrenia. That is, delusional processes in such patients might stem from overgeneralizations based on thought processes that contain irrelevant details (Payne, 1961), an interpretation that has some empirical basis.

What might one infer from these and similar findings? Paranoid schizophrenics do indeed seem to differ from nonparanoid schizophrenics. They seem more intellectually and cognitively oriented, more mature in terms of word associations, more intact, and more aware of threatening simuli. They also evidence more adequate premorbid histories.

The mysteries of etiology, prognosis, and treatment for schizophrenic patients will not be uncovered and placed into coherent patterns unless some coherent way of "explaining" these differences emerges. Are these two types of patients genetically, biochemically, and cognitively different from each other? Are they extensions of the schizophrenic spectrum as a result of processes we still do not understand? Or does learning alone account for the development of paranoid symptoms—a point of view put forth by Ullmann and Krasner (1969), who stated that learned selective attention is responsible for the persecutory delusions of the paranoid.

Whether the reactive-process and paranoid-nonparanoid distinctions make sense will be determined by the different paths that prevention, treatment, and outcome take for these classifications. If, for example, as some people believe, the etiology of the process type is organic and the etiology of the reactive type is psychological (that is, if life circumstances play a siginificant role in the development of the reactive type), then prevention, treatment, and outcome variables will differ accordingly for these types in predictable ways. These open up fascinating research possibilities.

TREATMENT

Schizophrenia is difficult to treat.* Evaluations of effectiveness of different methods yield a generally gloomy picture, with the exception of approaches that employ medication. Unfortunately, however, defining effectiveness of treatment is extremely tricky. For people who are not in hospitals, perhaps

* Most of the methods touched on in this section are described in detail in Chapters 19–21.

length of stay outside of a hospital is a good criterion. For chronic patients within hospitals, improved behavior on the ward as judged by aides and nurses might be the criterion. For acute patients, length of stay *within* the hospital might be the best criterion. The final chapters of this book deal with some of the problems in measuring the effectiveness of different treatment approaches. This section briefly describes and evaluates some of the major methods in treating schizophrenia. Mental hospitals are considered at some length in Chapter 21.

Individual psychotherapy. A review of studies of effectiveness of various individual psychotherapy methods has yielded a picture that is not very optimistic: generally, psychotherapy with medication seems to be more effective than psychotherapy alone (Feinsilver and Gunderson, 1972; May et al., 1976).

Psychoactive medication. In general, the phenothiazines and related drugs (see Chapter 21) are the most effective controls for schizophrenia in or out of hospital settings. Further, there is some agreement that whether combined with individual, group, or socially oriented therapies or alone, medication is superior to any of the other therapies used alone (Feinsilver and Gunderson, 1972; Lehmann, 1975). However, it is often difficult to get schizophrenics in nonhospital settings to take medication (Van Putten, 1974).

Group therapy. Group treatment of schizophrenic patients after hospitalization and discharge into the community has been popularly endorsed by many practitioners, although its effectiveness alone (as a substitute for individual therapy and medication) has not been adequately demonstrated. By and large, however, patients treated in group situations have been encouraged to continue medication and to become more interpersonally active (O'Brien, 1975). Further, group methods are appropriate in various professional settings and can be easily coordinated with a variety of other treatment approaches, such as medication, family methods, and various clinic programs.

Family methods. Treating the schizophrenic's family is viewed with favor by those who regard family processes as significant in the development of schizophrenia (see Chapter 12). Although studies that evaluate family treatment methods in schizophrenia are sparse, there are some indications that such methods are effective in helping the family to maintain its equilibrium in the light of the crisis it is facing. Unfortunately, subjective opinions of the therapists or the self-reports of the patients themselves rather than more objective measures have often been used as measures of improvement (Massie and Beels, 1972), making it difficult to assess the effectiveness of family treatment of schizophrenia.

Community support systems. After discharge from the hospital, many routes can be chosen for the patient, who can go home or to a "self-help" apartment, live with a foster family or in a boarding home, or attend a daycare center or night hospital. Regardless of the posthospitalization route, fewer and fewer patients are expected to stay in hospitals for great lengths of time as a result of the general policy of deinstitutionalization and the widespread use of psychoactive drugs, which make it possible for large numbers of patients to be discharged into the community.

Community support systems are networks of community facilities designed to help expatients, even severly disabled ones, to remain in the community by providing as much aid in as many areas as possible (Turner and TenHoor, 1978). This network includes crisis and emergency facilities such as hospitalization, training and rehabilitation services, appropriate living arrangements, opportunities to develop social skills, medical and mental health care, and community advocacy to protect the patient's rights.

About half of discharged patients return to their families, but the other half cannot yet live independently in the community. Halfway houses and other types of special residences are non-

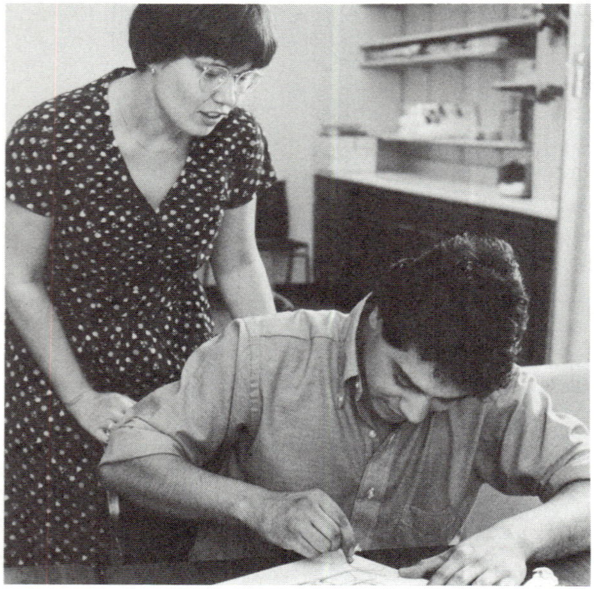

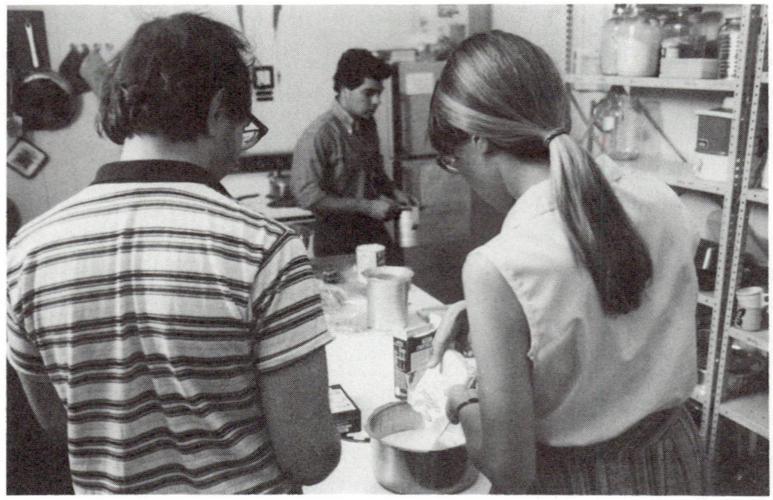

Nonhospitalized schizophrenic patients in a day-treatment center in an art-therapy session and helping to prepare lunch. (© Susan Lapides 1982; all rights reserved)

medical, supervised residences in the community that are transitional facilities for discharged mental patients who have no home to return to. Presumably, these residences are a stepping-stone to the community by offering social and vocational skills and opportunities to increase self-confidence for independent functioning. Foster homes can also provide the same services. Actually, not too much is known about these residences, which apparently differ from one another in many respects (Carpenter, 1978). Patients prefer such settings to hospitals, however. They are less expensive and they can provide excellent preparation for living independently in the community.

Overall, community care programs that involve well-controlled, supervised programs in social-service, medical, and psychological areas can be quite effective in helping patients to remain out of the hospital (Davis, Dinitz, and Pasamanick, 1974; Pasamanick et al., 1967).

Behavioral interventions. Behavioral methods, in or out of hospital settings, have been successfully employed to modify inappropriate behaviors of schizophrenics. For example, many facilities make use of the token economy, in which various types of responses are reinforced with tokens later to be turned in for a reward or privilege of some sort. Grooming, relating to others, speaking in more coherent fashion, and performing various tasks are reinforced, gradually preparing patients for independent community adjustment. Chapter 20 describes these methods in greater detail.

OUTCOME RESEARCH

Social planners, mental-health professionals, hospital administrators, drug manufacturers, and relatives of patients tend to ask the same questions: What is the course of this disease for this particular patient? What can we expect in the patient's future?

Outcome research typically explores the capacity of single variables alone and in various combinations (such as premorbid status, employment patterns, age of onset, social class, urban versus rural residence, ethnic membership) to predict some outcome variable such as length of hospital stay, degree of symptom-free status in the recovery phase, or number of future hospitalizations (readmissions). In such research (Bromet, Alto, Harrow, and Kasl, 1974; Depue and Dubicki, 1974; Heffner, Strauss, and Grisell, 1975; Klorman, Strauss, and Kokes, 1977; Larson and Nyman, 1974; and Strauss and Carpenter, 1974ab), the following variables were the best predictors of future outcome: employment patterns; social and interpersonal relationships (friends, sexual experiences, and marriage); age of onset (the earlier, the poorer the prognosis); intelligence; and current status of the patient (is this an "established" chronic patient?).

Where does all this lead? If a patient has a generally good premorbid history in social relationships, is intelligent, has had some sexual involvement, is married, has not been labeled a chronic case, has developed his or her disease later in life, and is not from a low-SES level, he or she can expect shorter-term hospitalization, fewer readmissions, and a more symptom-free recovery status. It would seem that an individual's capacity to meet stress and to obtain social, external, and emotional supports from his or her community or spouse are related to the course of the disease. The fragile and tenuous opportunities to deal with the constant bombardment of stressful situations in the slums, on low-SES levels, or when socially isolated may thus well be related to the question of outcome.

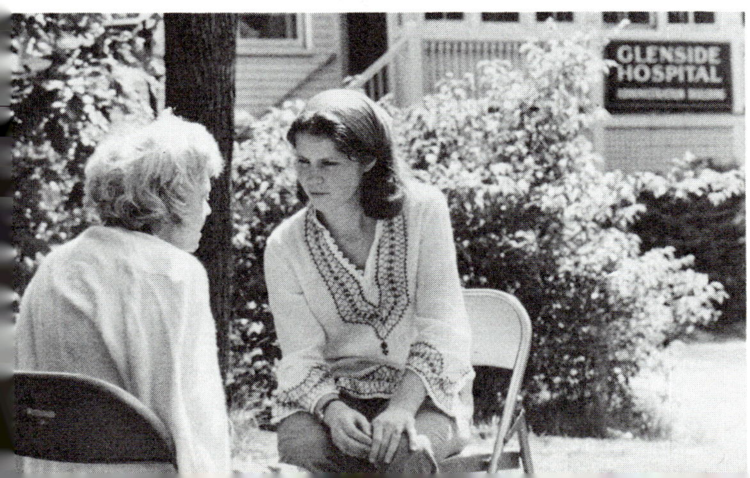

Recovery from a schizophrenic episode can take many paths, depending, in part, on the social supports available to the about-to-be-released patient. (Julie O'Neil/Stock, Boston)

SUMMARY

This chapter surveyed the incidence and prevalence of schizophrenic and paranoid disorders and their relationships to social class, gender, and ethnicity, and discussed the kinds of behaviors and cognitions generally associated with a diagnosis of schizophrenia such as thought disorders, delusions, and hallucinations. Different clinical subtypes, presented with case illustrations, include the disorganized (hebephrenic), catatonic, paranoid, and simple types. Paranoid disorders were described, as were several problems in connection with diagnosing schizophrenia. Possible simplification and objectification of diagnostic procedures include using a reactive versus process distinction, which rests heavily on premorbid criteria, or a paranoid versus nonparanoid distinction. The chapter concluded with a brief presentation of typical treatment strategies and touched on the nature of schizophrenia outcome research.

Highlights

1. Schizophrenia, one of the most baffling of the mental disorders, is a group of clinical syndromes that is manifested by bizarre and unpredictable symptoms in a wide number of areas: peculiar, idiosyncratic behavior; thinking disorders of various types; language and communication difficulties; delusions; hallucinations; and disturbances of affect and motivation. Onset is often in adolescence or early adulthood and can be sudden or slow and insidious. There may be many periods of remission in the course of the illness.
2. The incidence of schizophrenia appears to be stable across many cultures. In our own society, rates of schizophrenia range from about 1 percent to about 6 percent in urban slums. Schizophrenia is found in all SES groups but rates increase as one goes down the SES scale. Racial and ethnic variables as well as gender are apparently not related to the incidence of schizophrenia.

3. Many clinical subtypes of schizophrenia can be roughly distinguished. The disorganized (hebephrenic) type is generally characterized by slow, early onset, poor premorbid adjustment, unsystematized delusions and hallucinations, and blunted, inappropriate affect, with silliness and incongruousness in overall behavior.
4. The catatonic subtype, now relatively rare, appears in two different forms: a withdrawn type, frequently characterized by mutism, negativism, and waxy flexibility; and an excited form, frequently characterized by agitation, violent outbursts, and dangerousness.
5. Onset of the paranoid subtype is generally later than the other types. In this subtype of schizophrenia there is less disintegration of cognitive skills than in the other subtypes; the personality is dominated by delusional beliefs having to do with ideas of persecution, reference, and grandiosity.
6. Simple schizophrenia, a condition that worsens over the years, is a category no longer retained by the DSM-III. It is characterized by slow onset in puberty with a gradual loss of interests, drive, and motivation, general apathy, and shallowness of affect; there are no delusions or hallucinations.
7. Paranoid disorders, which include paranoia, shared paranoid disorder, and acute paranoid disorder, are marked chiefly by persistent persecutory or grandiose delusional systems with general unimpairment of cognitive functions and thinking processes outside of the system. People with paranoid disorders are often litigious and may show great anger from time to time. They rarely seek treatment and have little insight into their disturbance.
8. The relationship of the so-called borderline classification to schizophrenia is still not clear, and individuals with borderline characteristics continue to present many diagnostic and treatment difficulties to most clinicians.
9. There are many crosscultural differences in criteria used to diagnose schizophrenia. This fact and other problems of reliability of diagnosis have motivated researchers to seek more reliable diagnostic procedures. Among procedures proposed is the reactive versus process dichotomy, which rests heavily on the prognosis of the patient and a related criterion, premorbid competence. In process schizophrenia, for example, there is a long history of poor premorbid adjustment and a poor prognosis involving a chronic, deteriorating picture. There is some evidence that this classification "holds" up for various clinical populations.
10. The paranoid-nonparanoid distinction is another simple classificatory system. Paranoids, in contrast to nonparanoids, have a later age onset, more adequate premorbid status, fewer instances of schizophrenia in the family history, and various types of autonomic, perceptual, and cognitive (differentiating) characteristics, for example, overinclusive thinking.
11. A brief review of treatment strategies indicates that psychotherapy alone is not particularly effective. The psychoactive medications, either alone or combined with individual or group therapies, seem to be most effective in controlling and modifying symptoms of schizophrenia. Behavioral methods for modifying many of the inappropriate behaviors of schizophrenics have also shown some success.
12. Results of outcome research indicate that shorter-term hospitalizations, fewer readmissions, and a more satisfactory recovery course can be predicted for schizophrenics who have had good premorbid histories and who developed schizophrenia later in life; also, for those who are bright, married, and have higher social-class status.

ISSUES AND QUESTIONS

1. Case 11.4 describes A. R., a simple schizophrenic. Can you morally justify incarcerating A. R. in a mental institution? Does society have other alternatives? According to Thomas Szasz, this man should have been held responsible for his illegal acts and punished by the legal codes,

rather than incarcerated in a mental institution—eventually becoming a helpless, ineffectual, and noncontributing member of society. Do you agree? If familial, community, vocational, or other types of social support had been available, would this man's life have unfolded differently?

Consider the case of C. R., the paranoid schizophrenic described in Case 11.3. This patient got into trouble and might do so again. Some people say he is mentally "unfit" and dangerous and should be hospitalized for life. Thomas Szasz would like *legal* redress, holding the man legally responsible for the harm to his foreman, rather than the peremptory incarceration that befell him. Do you agree?

2. Rosenblatt (1974) made a strong but unpopular plea for making custodial care available to mentally disturbed people who do not have emotional and personal supports in the community—especially if they are impoverished, homeless, or aged. His approach challenges the proposition that everyone can be "cured" and that "sick" people do better on the "outside." Custodial care need not imply societal failure, Rosenblatt thinks, for some patients simply cannot be "cured." Custodial residents who choose this life would be free to leave if they wish. Society is obligated to offer this option, Rosenblatt states, as a refuge and haven for the misfits and the incompetents with no place to go. Because little treatment is offered to custodial residents, Rosenblatt continues, research and therapy efforts can be directed elsewhere, to those who want help and who can profit by it. The "dependence without punishment" aspect and the pessimistic undercurrents of this approach, Rosenblatt admits, are not popular themes in our mental-health orientation. But he is firmly convinced that custodial care alone is neither old fashioned nor unnecessary. What is your opinion?

SUGGESTIONS FOR FURTHER READING

Bernheim, K. F., and Lewine, R. R. J. *Schizophrenia: Symptoms, causes, treatments.* New York: Norton, 1979. Paperback available. This concise book covers the basics of schizophrenia from diagnosis to treatment in a straightforward and readable manner. Written for the nonpsychologist—for families of schizophrenics, the general public, and schizophrenics themselves—it provides a limited but accurate overview of this very complex syndrome.

Bettelheim, B. *Love is not enough: The treatment of emotionally disturbed children.* New York: Free Press, 1950. Paperback available. This book is an account of a psychoanalytically oriented residential treatment center for emotionally disturbed children. The focus of the school was on providing a safe, structured environment that would be conducive to ego development and the development of life skills. (For an alternative approach, see Lovaas and Bucher [1974], described at the end of Chapter 20).

Cancro, R., Fox, N., and Shapiro, L. E. (Eds.) *Strategic intervention in schizophrenia: Current developments in treatment.* New York: Behavior Publications, 1974. The treatment of schizophrenia has taken many directions—some more successful than others. This book covers many of these treatment directions, including pharmacological, behavioral, family, and individual approaches. Also described are hospital, posthospital, and various aftercare procedures. For those interested in the question of what is being done about schizophrenia, this book provides an excellent, straightforward overview of an extremely complex field.

Kaplan, B. (Ed.) *The inner world of mental illness: A series of first-person accounts of what it was like.* New York: Harper, 1964. Paperback. This fine collection of reports, essays, and autobiographical accounts (not all on schizophrenia and some written from the clinician's viewpoint) provides a touching bird's-eye view of the tormented and terrifying perplexities of emotional disorder. But be warned that these are literate, edited, articulate communications that are not representative products of the spectrum of people who suffer from mental illness.

12

Schizophrenia: Etiological Theories and Research Strategies

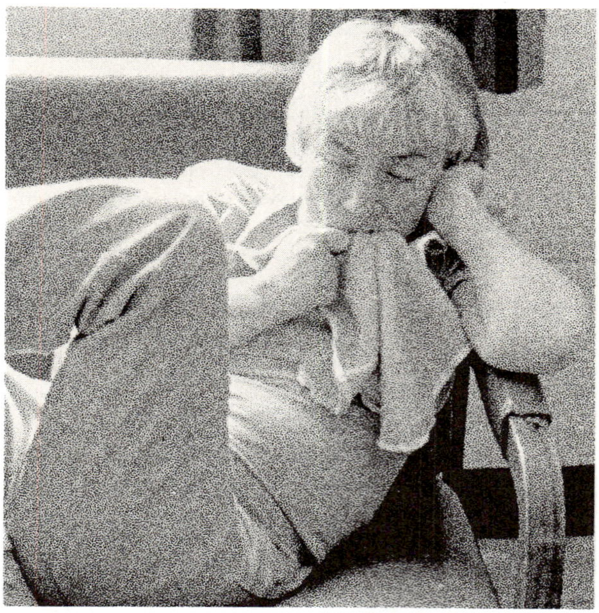

Chapter 11 introduced you to the major clinical manifestations of schizophrenia and its subtypes and to some of the problems clinicians face in diagnosing its many manifestations. Now you are ready to explore the puzzle of schizophrenia more deeply. Why do some people, living out the harshest of lives, emerge relatively unscathed, while others, experiencing the same deprivations, fall back again and again into the so-called "schizophrenic solution"? Why does a disorganized "sick" family produce one schizophrenic child among several healthy ones? Why do many schizophrenic people get well and remain so for many years only to get "sick" again? These are only a few of the many unanswered questions surrounding the enigma of schizophrenia.

Section I of this chapter surveys some of the prominent theories and hypotheses about the etiology of schizophrenia. Section II will describe some correlates and research strategies that help us to understand the performance of schizophrenic people or to identify those who are at risk for becoming schizophrenic.

SECTION I
THEORIES AND MODELS: WHAT CAUSES SCHIZOPHRENIA?

Our survey of etiological models is presented in three parts: a section that describes psychological approaches, one that describes physical approaches, and a third that describes some hypotheses that attempt to integrate findings from both viewpoints.

PSYCHOLOGICAL APPROACHES

Psychoanalytic Formulations

Regression in schizophrenia

. . . reaches back to much earlier times than does any regression in neuroses, specifically, to the time when the ego first came into being. . . . The infant starts out in a state of "primary narcissism," in which the systems of the mental apparatus are not yet differentiated from each other, and in which no objects exist as yet. The differentiation of the ego coincides with the discovery of objects. An ego exists in so far as it is differentiated from objects that are not ego. Therefore, the following formulae mean one and the same thing, only varying in point of view: the schizophrenic has regressed to narcissism; the schizophrenic has lost his objects; the schizophrenic has parted with reality; the schizophrenic's ego has broken down (Fenichel, 1945, p. 415).

Schizophrenia truly baffled Freud and his followers. Yet it did not take much ingenuity to come up with a view of schizophrenia that could be easily embedded within the master plan. Stated simply, this view—and there are variations on the general theme—is that schizophrenia is a defensive maneuver against overwhelming anxiety that primarily employs regression to an early, primitive, infantile level of development. The regression is more extreme, more profound than in the neuroses, with instinctual drives—id impulses and forces—becoming liberated, unrestrained by ego and superego. One result is the defective interpersonal ("object") relationships of the schizophrenic.

In schizophrenia the individual's attempts to deal with anxiety have failed and a total breakdown of defenses has occurred. It should be noted that the anxiety that precedes this schizophrenic "break" is thought to be generated mainly by internal psychological factors rather than by external stressors (Arieti, 1974).

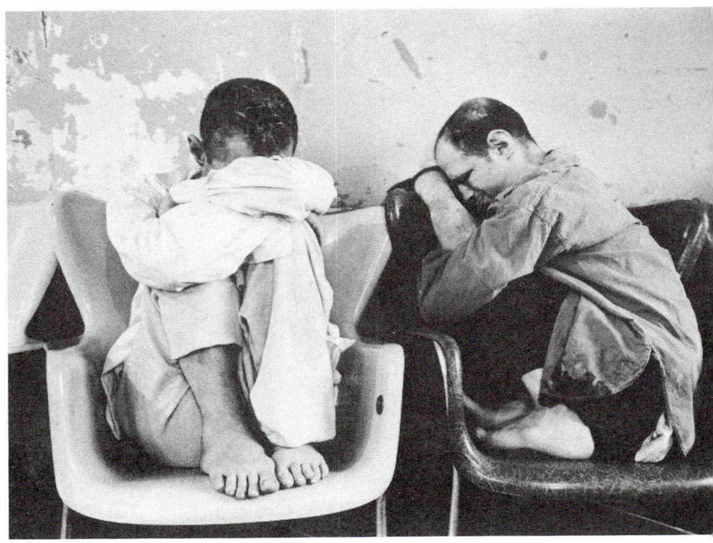

Schizophrenic regression? (Bill Stanton/Magnum)

In psychoanalytically oriented explorations of regressive behavior, much has been made of the so-called similarity between schizophrenic thinking and the thinking of normal children. Some investigators go so far as to suggest that children who later become schizophrenic never give up their normal behaviors and thinking processes (Betz, 1973). But the fact that they never progress beyond primitive levels of cognitive development eventually distinguishes them from their peers.

Primitive levels of thinking include prelogical, magical attribution of causes, reliance on fantasy interpretation of events, fluid associations of ideas, the tolerance of mutually exclusive ideas, and the primary process thinking that has already been described. Such mental processes, from a psychoanalytic perspective, stem directly from drive-directed and instinct-directed inner cores without the tempering and curtailing provided by the ego and superego, which are in tune with reality and society.

Unfortunately the claims made for schizophrenia as a return to childhood modes have failed to acquire a body of confirming experimental evidence. Nor are many of these claims stated in ways that allow empirical validation. Psychoanalytic formulations have thus incurred the disfavor of many researchers who feel that the "regression" approach is merely descriptive or illustrative of schizophrenic behavior, not explanatory (Chapman & Chapman, 1973). Because of the minimum acknowledgement of genetic and biochemical variables by most psychoanalytically oriented interpreters of schizophrenic behavior (see later sections of this chapter), dissatisfaction is found even among those prone to viewing Freudian hypotheses sympathetically, for example, Arieti (1974).*

* Harry Stack Sullivan, an analytically oriented American theoretician, was especially interested in schizophrenia (1962). He acknowledged the organic components in schizophrenia by suggesting the existence of two distinct types. One is the chronic, organically determined disease, while the other is a disorder of living—an episode in an individual's career that abruptly begins after a period of panic and terror in response to extreme conflict when the security defenses and systems of the "about-to-be-schizophrenic" have failed.

Life Events, Stress, and Environmental Variables

Broad views that early childhood events, such as birth complications, separations from parents, bizarre interactions between parent and child, experiencing parental conflict, and various types of harsh occurrences during development are causally related to schizophrenia are no longer held by most researchers. Nor are the brutal realities of poverty and lower-class status held responsible as etiological factors.

Are stressful life events in *adulthood,* such as separation from a spouse through disease or death, associated with schizophrenia? Although there are many problems in defining "stressful event" (what may be stressful for one person may not be equally stressful for another), the consensus is that stressors and life events play only a minimal role in the etiology of schizophrenia (Spring, 1981). It is possible, however, that when a person has a predisposition to

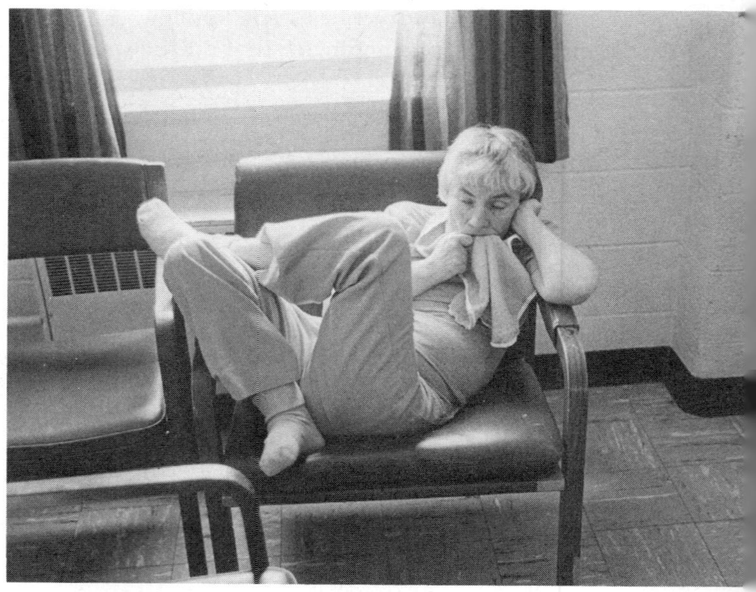

Older psychoanalytic formulations viewed schizophrenia as a defense against overwhelming anxiety, with regression to an early infantile level of development as the principal strategy. (© T. Simon 1979/Liaison)

schizophrenia, certain triggering events (such as an argument with a neighbor) may be crucial in precipitating a schizophrenic episode (Zubin, 1981). However, the role of stressors as generally defined may be less crucial than commonly believed (Rabkin, 1980); but even here, there does not seem to be a consensus among the experts (Dohrenwend and Egri, 1981).

Schizophrenia and Learning Models

1. *Are the symptoms of schizophrenia learned?* Learning models of schizophrenia generally hold that the poor coping skills and the inadequate personality of the schizophrenic, as well as such symptoms as "disattention," delusional beliefs, poor judgment, and inadequate communication and language patterns, can be explained by one or another of several learning paradigms (see Chapter 6). For example, schizophrenic behavior may be accounted for by imitation of disturbed parental behavior or inadequate reinforcement or training for competency. Furthermore, modifiability of some aspects of schizophrenic behavior is held to be a strong point in favor of learning approaches.

2. *Mednick's heightened autonomic arousal* approach makes use of the concept of *drive*, a strong inner, and sometimes outer, stimulus that seems to energize behavior, causing the organism to take action to reduce its intensity. In this model, anxiety is regarded as a compelling drive. Preschizophrenics can be distinguished from other groups because they operate under an extremely high drive state. Mednick and his colleagues (Mednick, 1958; Mednick and Schulsinger, 1968) derived these hypotheses from studies of responses of high-risk children (see Spotlight 12.4), a fair percentage of whom later became schizophrenic. Some of their findings indicated faster conditioning, greater stimulus generalization, slower learning in more complex situations, and speedier recovery from autonomic arousal in GSR (galvanic skin response) situations among high-risk subjects compared to controls.

Spotlight 12.1 Pregnancy and Birth Complications in the Etiology of Schizophrenia

It has been noted that a greater number of birth and pregnancy complications occurred among the offspring of schizophrenic mothers who later become schizophrenic than among comparable controls who did not become schizophrenic (Mednick, et al., 1971). Complications include such conditions as anoxia (oxygen deprivation), prolonged labor, umbilical cord problems, prematurity and low birthweight, and illness during pregnancy such as excessive bleeding. It has also been noted that a greater frequency of fetal and neonatal deaths occur among the offspring of schizophrenic mothers than in the general population (Rieder, et al., 1975). When monozygotic (identical; coming from the same genetic material) twins discordant for schizophrenia are examined, the twin who became schizophrenic was more likely than the other twin to have had a perinatal (present at birth) complication (Pollin & Stabenau, 1968; see Spotlight 12.3). Are such babies truly at greater risk for becoming schizophrenic than their healthier counterparts?

Can we suppose, then, that extreme stresses at birth could be one of the intensely damaging environmental events implicated in the etiology of schizophrenia? Unfortunately subsequent explorations have not fully confirmed these findings, and the general conclusion seems to be that they are not of major etiological significance in the production of schizophrenia (Hanson, Gottesman, and Heston, 1976; Sameroff and Zax, 1973; Zax, Sameroff, and Babigian, 1977), despite the fact that such complications may well reduce the person's capacity to cope, to learn, and to deal with the stressors of life effectively. Moreover, it appears that schizophrenic mothers do not necessarily have more birth complications or neonatal deaths than mothers from other diagnostic groups and that chronicity and severity of illness, rather than diagnostic category, is related to greater frequency of perinatal complications (Zax, Sameroff, and Babigian, 1977). As we shall see, however, if early stresses and subsequently impaired competence occur with predisposing genetic factors, they may bear a relationship to the later clinical expression of schizophrenia.

Mednick regarded such states of high arousal as anxiety. The schizophrenic learns to avoid these uncomfortable states by fragmented, bizarre, loose associations and by withdrawal, with a consequent drop in anxiety level. This theory states quite simply that the schizophrenic *learns* his or her symptoms to escape the consequences of heightened levels of arousal and anxiety.

3. *Broen and Storms' approach* (1966) also employs the concept of high drive levels, along with certain experimental findings about the conditions under which stimuli and responses are connected. Responses are habits evoked as a result of habit strength, with potential responses to a given stimulus falling into a hierarchy of strength so that the response on the top of the hierarchy is the one that is evoked. High drive generally increases or facilitates the evocation of the dominant response. Among schizophrenics, however, rather than increasing the probability that the dominant response will be evoked, high drive states actually increase the probability that nondominant responses will be evoked. In other words, among schizophrenics, one cannot count on the expected because the usual response hierarchies are disrupted. Competing responses, even though not dominant, have a high chance of becoming evoked under conditions of high arousal or drive. According to Broen and Storms, this would explain the unusual, "remote," bizarre, and farfetched responses of schizophrenics.

4. Another approach characterizes schizophrenic behavior as evidencing *extinction of attentional responses to social stimuli* (Ullmann and Krasner, 1969), which explains the finding that chronic, hospitalized schizophrenics cannot be "shaped" as easily as other subjects by positive social reinforcers such as praise or approval. On the other hand, in studies that involve the shaping of continuous speech, as well as in other verbal conditioning demonstrations, many positive verbal reinforcers were successfully employed in modifying the behavior of schizophrenic patients (Caulfield and Martin, 1976; Salzinger, Portnoy, and Feldman, 1964a).

These and other attempts to examine the conditions under which schizophrenic performance has been learned and the conditions under which schizophrenic behavior can be modified are well within the experimental fold; the hypotheses under consideration are open to verification and replication. Further, such approaches have a positive view of schizophrenia: Schizophrenic behavior is modifiable and changeable by means of learning techniques.

Family Forces

The possibility that some types of family interactions and family systems might induce or sustain psychopathology was raised in Chapter 6. Now we return to a more detailed consideration of family forces as they bear on the etiology of schizophrenia. Many researchers believe that schizophrenic patients have been reared in families in which the communication systems and interaction patterns are disturbed and that these patterns can be differentiated from those of families that do not produce a schizophrenic patient. The former families are called schizophrenogenic. Elucidation of the processes by which such a family generates and sustains schizophrenia in one of its members can generally be said to be the purpose of family studies of schizophrenia. These studies focus not only on learning more about the etiology of schizophrenia but also on developing treatment strategies.

How can disturbed family processes produce pathology? Some early investigators of family interactions sensed hidden, covert processes within families they referred to as "homeostasis"—the maintenance of a steady state—which entails processes by which the family maintains its "intactness." These processes

. . . serve to keep it from falling apart, and which in certain circumstances may also serve to produce disturbances or illness in one member of the family in order to preserve the health or the intactness of the inclusive family (Spiegel, 1958, p. 24).

A family might assign certain fixed roles to family members in order to maintain its integrity

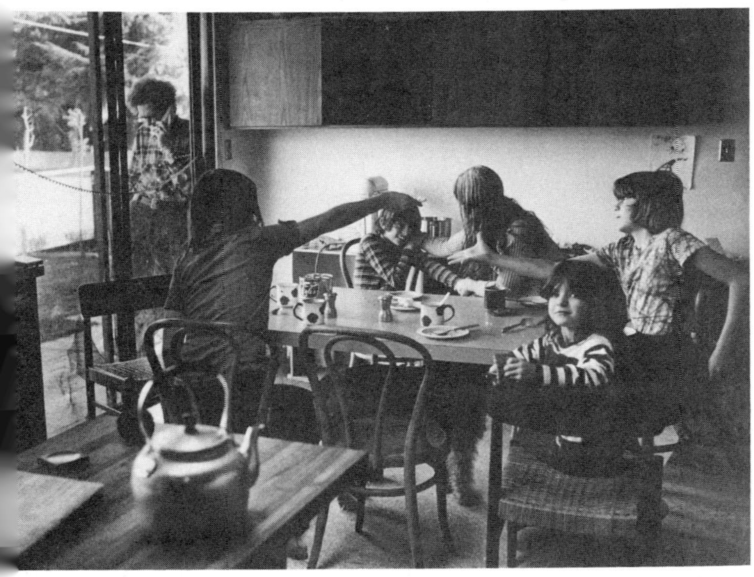

A disorganized family "climate" may contribute to the pathology of a family member, according to one view. (© Hella Hammid 1975/Rapho-Photo Researchers)

and its continuity. For example, a child who is relentlessly scapegoated within the family system or regarded by family members as emotionally disturbed is selected and inducted into that role. Although the end result may be harmful to the child, the process, it is felt, is nevertheless essential for the family's maintenance of its solidarity. Another example would be the induction of the wife-mother into the role of a helpless, hysterical, incompetent, and much-abused person. Thus some families could be called "sick" if the processes within it produce, indeed *require,* pathology in any individual member (Kluckhohn and Spiegel, 1954; Spiegel, 1957).

A dominant theme in studies of schizophrenogenic families concerns the disturbed reality-testing, faulty thinking, distorted handling of affect, and disorganized and scattered communication processes that presumably characterize them. Generally, it is thought that communication patterns, "communication deviance," and communication *forms* rather than content characterize the schizophrenogenic family (Morris and Wynne, 1965; Wynne and Singer, 1964). If the family is viewed as a subculture (a system that generates rules for behavior, thinking, and communicating), then it is hypothesized that these rules, as well as family myths and legends, stresses and strains, and unwritten codes, can produce and indeed enforce and sustain pathology in an individual member. An example is the "double bind" form of communication (Bateson, Jackson, Haley, and Weakland, 1956, 1963) in which messages transmitted by a family member contain overt and covert mutually exclusive and contradictory meanings (see Chapter 6, p. 124).

According to some researchers, many of the familial environments of schizophrenic patients can be characterized by a variety of problems at the time of onset of the pathologic process. These include incestuous fantasies or fluid, vague boundaries between the generations (in assigning discipline or assuming authority, for example); poor role differentiation (such as small children becoming the caretakers of alcoholic parents); incompetence of parents in filling parental roles; and lack of parental coalition (no parental alliance or "togetherness"). Many of these familial qualities result in or reflect family schism or skew (Lidz, 1958; Lidz, 1973; Lidz and Lidz, 1949).

In schismatic families, the parents are at odds with each other and attempt to impose contradictory or opposing (generally distorted) values on their children, who internalize conflicting, unresolved views and perceptions of the world around them. According to Lidz and his colleagues, the patient in such families is usually female. In skewed families, the generally distorted value-orientation, viewpoints, and role assignments revolve around one of the parents only, usually the mother, with the rest of the family passively and unquestioningly accepting such distortion; the patient in such families is generally male. Throughout this family approach is a common thread: The thinking disorders, irrationalities, and distortions in schizophrenic patients arise as a response to the family environments that surround them.

In addition to distortions of perception, thinking, and communication, pseudomutuality in schizophrenogenic families is also described (Wynne, Ryckoff, Day, and Hirsch, 1958). Pseudomutuality is a surface stability and equilibrium to which each member of a family contributes in order to "not make waves." The result is an illusory peace, an atmosphere in which serenity and harmony seem to prevail. Although everyone meshes with everyone else, this "mesh" is achieved by a thoroughgoing, pervasive family culture of myths, legends, and beliefs to which all family members subscribe.

Measuring and observing nonverbal aspects of family systems require a focus that differs from that required for measuring variables such as aggressiveness, passivity, or seclusiveness. How do researchers measure and quantify the verbal interchanges within an experimental or control family, the number of discussions, the pathways (who talks to whom), the number of contradictory messages, the disruptions, the arguments, the coalitions and alliances (who takes sides with whom and against whom), the interferences and interruptions, the amount of noise (background disruption preventing clarity of communication), the order in which members of families talk to each other, or the rules with which communications are expressed?

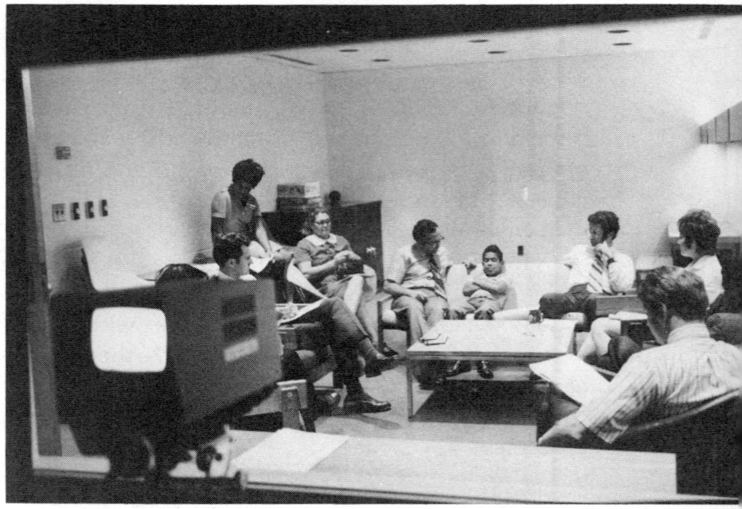

Family research often involves technically sophisticated methods of data collection. (Constantine Manos/Magnum)

The methods used to objectify such variables do not usually employ conventional individual psychological tests, interviews, and similar one-to-one interactions. Instead, these methods tend to rely on the use of videotapes, group observation through one-way screens, and observations in actual rather than laboratory settings so that natural interactions can occur.

Through either traditional or more technologically sophisticated methods, what has been learned thus far? In a review of fifty-seven direct-observation studies that compared the family behavior of disturbed and normal families (Jacob, 1975), little consistency was found except in the area of family communications. One distinctly positive, consistent finding was that normal families communicated with greater clarity than schizophrenic families (families containing at least one person diagnosed as schizophrenic). Clarity of communication denotes such variables as attention, explicitness of information presented, and acknowledgement of others' responses. In addition, normal families tended to display more frequent interruptions, while schizophrenic families tended to show more disagreement among their members.

On the whole, despite some positive findings, there is little definitive evidence that directly confirms the transmission of schizophrenia via family interaction patterns (Hirsch and Leff, 1975). Several crucial issues remain unresolved. Even if communication difficulties and reality-distortion problems characterize schizophrenic families, such qualities may arise from the expression of genetic predisposition in some family members. A contrasting interpretation is that disturbed family patterns result from or are in response to a schizophrenic member; that is, they emerge as an adaptation to the deviant behavior of a disturbed family member, rather than being a cause of that member's disturbance. Also, if family interactions are disturbed in these pathological families, why does only one member, rather than several members, develop schizophrenia? These remain essentially unanswered questions.

Yet, most clinicians are very much aware of the "special" quality or flavor of interactions in some families in which pathology seems to permeate its climate so relentlessly as to leave significant emotional scars on some family members. We will continue to explore the quality of these interactions in the sections that follow.

R. D. Laing

We are discussing Laing's views, noted in Chapter 6, in more detail here not only because of his eloquent statements about schizophrenia, but also because many of his formulations are based on his therapeutic observations of familial interaction and communication patterns. Within his framework, the wishes and hidden messages of family powerholders force some members to become unwitting victims if they are to "play the game."

Laing does not acknowledge schizophrenia as a biological or psychological "fact" (1960; Laing and Esterson, 1964). He does, however, acknowledge a set of behaviors that society labels "schizophrenia." According to Laing, this occurs for "political" reasons—to isolate and control the people who display such behavior. Laing insists, however, that from the patient's point of view, such "sick" behaviors are sensible and rational; he or she employs them to deal with or confuse the people who have confused *them*, the patients. If understood from the perspective of the sick patient, bizarre behavior is *not* bizarre or irrational.

It is especially the family of the patient that has made the patient respond in the way that he or she does: The double bind—the contradictory, impossible-to-meet demands, rules, and regulations that the family imposes—so confuses and baffles the patient that he or she adopts ways of baffling and confusing the family in turn. The world created by such patients is complex but logical as a response to an impossible family situation. The patient retreats into a subjective, tortuous world of perceptions and interpersonal vagueness, distrust, and distortions that spell safety. This inner world is perhaps illustrated by Laing's own poetry published in a collection called *Knots* (1970). Here is a knot:

Jack does not see something.
Jill thinks Jack does see it.
Jack thinks Jack does see it and Jill does not.
Jill does not see herself what
    she thinks Jack does see.

Jack tells Jill
        what Jack thinks Jill does not see.
Jill realizes
    that,
        if Jack thinks
            Jill does not see that,
            which Jill thinks she does,
        Jack does not see
            what Jill thought
                Jack saw.

(From R. D. Laing, Knots *(London: Tavistock, 1970), p. 65)*

The retreat into mystification is illustrated by still another Laingian description:

One of the greatest barriers against getting to know a schizophrenic is his sheer incomprehensibility: the oddity, bizarreness, obscurity in all that we can perceive of him. There are many reasons why this is so. Even when the patient is striving to tell us, in as clear and straightforward a way as he knows how, the nature of his anxieties and his experiences, structured as they are in a radically different way from ours, the speech content is necessarily difficult to follow. Moreover, the formal elements of speech are in themselves ordered in unusual ways, and these formal peculiarities seem, at least to some extent, to be the reflection in language of the alternative ordering of his experience, with splits in it where we take coherence for granted, and the running together (confusion) of elements that we keep apart.

Yet these irreducible difficulties are practically certain to be much increased, at least in one's first encounters with the patient, by his or her deliberate use of obscurity and complexity as a smoke-screen to hide behind. This creates the ironical situation that the schizophrenic is often playing at being psychotic, or pretending to be so. In fact, as we have said, pretence and equivocation are greatly used by schizophrenics. The reasons for doing this are, in any single case, likely to serve more than one purpose at a time. The most obvious one is that it preserves the secrecy, the privacy, of the self against intrusion (engulfment, implosion). The self, as one patient put it, feels crushed and mangled even at the exchanges in an ordinary conversation. Despite his longing to be loved for his 'real self' the schizophrenic is terrified of love. Any form of understanding threatens *his whole defensive system. His outward behavior is a defensive system analogous to innumerable openings to underground passages which one might imagine would take one to the inner citadel, but they lead nowhere or elsewhere. The schizophrenic is not going to reveal himself for casual inspection and examination to any philandering passer-by. If the self is not known it is safe. It is safe from penetrating remarks; it is safe from being smothered or engulfed by love, as much as from destruction from hatred. If the schizophrenic is incognito, his body can be handled and manipulated, petted, caressed, beaten, given injections or what have you, but 'he', an onlooker, is inviolable.*

(From The divided self *by R. D. Laing, published by Tavistock Publications, Ltd. (1960), pp. 163–64)*

Schizophrenia and Parent-Child Interactions

Whereas the preceding material implicated global family systems and processes in the etiology and maintenance of schizophrenia in one of its members, the current section considers more specific, one-to-one interactions and behaviors of parents and children (predominantly *mothers* and children) as might be expected in the light of traditional, culturally engendered paradigms.

Aversively controlling mothers. An intriguing and once-popular hypothesis (Heilbrun, 1973) is that the offspring of mothers who are aversively controlling—that is, who exercise strict control over their children and who at the same time tend to be critical and rejecting of them—will be less independent, more sensitive to criticism, and more withdrawn than the offspring of mothers who are nurturant, accepting, and not aversively controlling. Presumably this pattern of passivity and hypersensitivity to criticism may lead to severe disturbance in functioning, even to schizophrenia in extreme cases.

Heilbrun explored this hypothesis in a series of related researches that focused on how the mother is *perceived* by the subject rather than on her actual behavior. In one study, for example, he compared the perceptions of twenty-six hospitalized schizophrenic women with those of twenty-six control subjects of their mothers' childrearing attitudes, as measured by an objective inventory (Parent Attitude Research Instrument). The schizophrenic women perceived their mothers as being significantly more controlling than did the normal women. In other studies, typical findings were that male subjects who reported mothers as being highly controlling with low nurturance scored higher on the schizophrenic and social introversion scales of the Minnesota Multiphasic Inventory (MMPI; see Chapter 5) than the males who reported their mothers as showing low control and high nurturance.

Still other findings indicated that schizophrenics with high-control, low-nurturance mothers responded to censure on a cognitive task with larger decrements (decreases in performance) than did other types of schizophrenics. These results are consistent with hypotheses about the disruptive influence of censure on schizophrenic performance (Rodnick and Garmezy, 1957).

Is it possible, then, to conclude that aversively controlling, nonnurturant mothers can be implicated in the induction of schizophrenia in some of their children? Not exactly. For the opposite could be an equally plausible hypothesis. That is, mothers may become controlling and rejecting in response to schizophrenic children. Or, it could be that subjects who become or are schizophrenic tend to perceive their mothers in this way. The issue is not resolved because perhaps the way in which a mother is *perceived* is important in the etiology of schizophrenia. In any event, there seems to be little evidence that overcontrolling mothers, per se, produce schizophrenic children. (Hirsch and Leff, 1975).

Bizarre parent-child interactions. A child raised by a schizophrenic parent will not necessarily become schizophrenic (Bleuler, 1974). As a matter of fact, in one nine-year longitudinal study in Denmark (see: No worse, 1976), it was found that children raised by schizophrenic mothers are no different and in some ways better off than those raised in orphanages and foster homes. Bleuler hypothesized that the necessity to cope with irrational behavior forced the pathologically reared children to contend with their psychotic mothers by discounting or ignoring their behavior. He also suggested that the basic mothering skills of the schizophrenic mother may have been intact during her child's infancy.

And yet, the bizarre or at least highly unusual interactions between the schizophrenic mother (or father) and a child (often even an adult child) who later becomes schizophrenic, perhaps "borderline" schizophrenic, is well known (see Spotlight 12.2). Some of these accounts are of explicit sexual interactions. Such sexual episodes between parent and child frequently occur when the child is too young to handle the erotic excitement that is induced, and becomes overwhelmed with guilt and anger.

Spotlight 12.2 Bizarre Family Interactions: Remembrance of Things Past

The experiences of children growing up with schizophrenic parents have only recently received systematic attention. According to one long-time researcher (Bleuler, 1978), many such children suffer their agonies in silence and later, when able to talk, prefer to bury the horrors of their past lives because they feel ashamed and guilty. Offspring raised in deeply disturbed family settings in which one or both parents are schizophrenic experience great fear, which is always near the surface in very young children. Later, communication disorders develop, along with extreme shyness and periods of fantasy, daydreaming, withdrawal, or aggression. Sometimes, *"folie à deux"* develops, in which a child shares the distortions of a sick parent (see Chapter 11, p. 281). What are some of these experiences and interactions like?

A mother worries obsessively about her young son's penis. Is it developing in a normal way? Ritually, she takes her son to a physician each week for examination and reassurance. A father has a daily morning bathroom visit with his young son in which he, the father, is completely nude for about a half-hour, has a bowel movement, looks for blood in his stool, and examines his mouth in the mirror for sores. The son has witnessed this ritual each morning for years—since the age of two. A mother, until her son is 19 years old, sits on the edge of the bathtub each morning as the son urinates, defecates, and showers. Later, when he enters the army, he is picked up as a voyeur. Wolberg (1968), in a paper characterizing the family interactions of borderline patients, describes these and other bizarre, implicitly or explicitly sexual interactions between parent and child.

The recollections of other children who have had schizophrenic parents or who have been schizophrenic themselves are described by clinicians everywhere. Some of these memories may be colored by the bizarre distortions and perceptions of the patients themselves, but others have been confirmed as accurate. These lurid recollections include such events as a daily early-morning ritual in which the feces of all members are examined and then disposed of; nightly sexual encounters between a father and a child; and forcing children to witness sexual encounters between adults. Other memories are of physical abuse—of one or more children being brutally assaulted, scarred, burned, disfigured, or mutilated by their parents. The abusive action may take many forms—for example, enforced prostitution, participation in criminal behavior (rape, burglary, arson), or being locked out of the house on a cold, rainy night without food.

Yet, an amazing phenomenon persists: The most unfavorable familial, environmental, and even biological circumstances (see the next section) do not necessarily produce schizophrenia. As a matter of fact,

. . . only a minority of the children of schizophrenics are in any way abnormal or socially incompetent. The majority of them are healthy and socially competent, even though many of them have lived through miserable childhoods. . . . Keeping an eye on the favorable development of the majority of these children is just as important as observing the sick minority. . . . In studying a number of the family histories, one is even left with the impression that pain and suffering has a steeling—a hardening—effect on the personalities of some children, making them capable of mastering their lives with all its obstacles, in defiance of all their disadvantages (Bleuler, 1974, p. 409).

How is this possible? Who are these invulnerables? This is a perplexing yet optimistic question, yet to be explored.

Some thread of agreement among diverse investigators, clinicians, and researchers does suggest an unusually close, interdependent, mutually intimate relationship between mother and child (schizophrenia is said to emerge as a result of a "disturbed symbiotic relationship" between mother and child, according to some views). This view portrays their relationship as a suffocating, enmeshed one in which the child never develops a sense of self, and never feels that he or she can be independently responsible for solving problems, coping, and learning. Empirical demonstration of the validity of this hypothesis is still an open question, despite ample clinical illustrations.

Thus we see that hypotheses implicating family factors in the etiology of schizophrenia, though intriguing, have not led to conclusive findings. However, we can assume that disturbed family interactions will be present whenever schizophrenia occurs in any of the family's members.

The approaches just discussed all have some limitations. Why do schizophrenics frequently experience remission (get better)? Why does schizophrenia generally develop in adolescence or later rather than following periods of early stress? How do the strict environmentalists account for the importance of genetic and biochemical variables (see the following sections)? Why is it that the cruelest deprivations or the most bizarre upbringings by schizophrenic parents do not necessarily produce schizophrenia in the offspring (Bleuler, 1974)? We will now turn to other models that may better "fit" the data.

PHYSICAL APPROACHES

Genetic Predisposition

The genetic model of schizophrenia generally states that there is a genetic vulnerability or predisposition (genotype) to schizophrenia which may or may not be expressed (phenotype) as clinical schizophrenia depending on as-yet-unspecified sociocultural and environmental circumstances. What evidence has accumulated for this model?

Exploration of the genetic model generally involves a search for identical twins, one (or both) of whom is schizophrenic, or for children of schizophrenic parents who have been "adopted away." Naturally, the number of subjects involved is very small, because schizophrenia occurs very infrequently in the general population—at the rate of about 1 percent. Luckily, many of the Scandinavian countries have national registers of births, adoptions, and medical and hospital histories, which provide a rich opportunity for family, twin, and adoption studies, some of which will be described in the following discussion.

Adoption strategies. One of the earliest adoption studies demonstrated that the incidence of schizophrenia (actual hospital cases) in children born to hospitalized, chronic schizophrenic mothers, separated from them within the first few days of life, and adopted or raised elsewhere, was about 20 percent (Heston, 1966). If the definition of schizophrenia were broadened to include "spectrum," "soft-core" (not flagrant or fullblown) symptoms without hospitalizations, the percentage would be even higher. No psychopathology was found in a matched group of children born of nonschizophrenic mothers and raised in similar adoptive or foster-home environments.

In subsequent Danish studies (Kety, et al., 1975; Rosenthal, 1975a; Rosenthal, et al., 1971; Rosenthal and Kety, 1968; Wender, et al., 1974), adoption study methods were improved over the original work, but conclusions drawn were generally the same. Through use of the national registers noted earlier, the size and comprehensive quality of the samples were greatly increased by locating all adoptees in Copenhagen over two decades. Knowledge of the diagnosis of the subject, mother, or relative was withheld from the experimenters, and direct methods for assessing the status of the subjects and their relatives through interviewing were employed (in contrast, for example, to data obtained from hospital records and "old" case material).

Table 12.1 presents a summary of some of these Danish studies. In this table, it can be seen that 18.8 percent of "adopted-away" children of schizophrenic parents are schizophrenic.

Other studies yield more or less the same findings. Combining data from several studies, it was found that 15.5 percent of children of schizophrenic parents raised in adoptive or foster homes become schizophrenic. However, children of *normal* parents raised by schizophrenic parents have been found to

Table 12.1 Summaries of Prevalence Data from Some of the Danish Adoption Studies*

	Number of Subjects	*Percentage of Schizophrenia***
Adopted-away children of schizophrenics	69	18.8
Adopted-away children of normals	79	10.1
Biological parents of schizophrenic adoptees	66	12.1
Biological parents of control adoptees	65	6.2
Adoptive parents of schizophrenic adoptees	63	1.6
Adoptive parents of control adoptees	68	4.4
Biological half-siblings of schizophrenic adoptees	104	19.2
All adoptive siblings plus full and half-siblings of control adoptees	143	6.3

Source: Adapted from I. I. Gottesman and J. Shields, A critical review of recent adoption, twin, and family studies of schizophrenia: Behavioral genetics perspectives, *Schizophrenia Bulletin*, 1976, *2*, No. 3, p. 365.

*Kety, et al., 1975; Rosenthal, 1975a; Wender, et al., 1974.

**The percentages given include definite plus doubtful cases but do not include "soft spectrum" cases, according to the authors.

Table 12.2 Concordance Rates in Several English, American, Norwegian, Danish, and Finnish Twin Studies*

	Kringlen (1967)	*Fischer (1973)*	*Gottesman & Shields (1972)*	*Tienari (1971)*	*Pollin et al. (1969)*
MZ (identical)					
Number of pairs	55	21	22	17	95
Concordance	45%	56%	58%	35%	43%
DZ (fraternal)					
Number of pairs	90	41	33	20	125
Concordance	15%	26%	12%	13%	9%

Source: Adapted from I. I. Gottesman and J. Shields, A critical review of recent adoption, twin and family studies of schizophrenia: Behavioral genetics perspectives, *Schizophrenia Bulletin,* 1976, *2,* No. 3., p. 373.

*If one twin has schizophrenia, percentage of other twin diagnosed with schizophrenia—data are not age-corrected.

be at no higher risk than children in the general population (Hanson, Gottesman, and Meehl, 1977; Heston, 1966; and Wender, et al., 1974).

In sum, large-scale, elegant adoption studies have generally confirmed Heston's earlier conclusions that biological children of schizophrenics who are adopted away show more schizophrenia and related disorders than carefully selected control adoptees of normal parents.

Twin studies. Twin-study strategies are among the most incisive methods for exploring a genetic hypothesis of schizophrenia. Even the earliest studies tended to suggest a genetic hypothesis of schizophrenia in finding greater concordance (percentage similarity) for MZ (monozygotic—identical) twins who share the same genetic material than for DZ (dizygotic—fraternal) twins who share roughly 50 percent of the genetic material (Kallmann, 1946; Slater and Shields, 1953).

Comparisons of DZ and MZ twins reared in the same family assume the constancy of the familial environment while varying the degree of resemblance of genetic variables. By and large, most of these studies arrive at the same general conclusion: a high concordance rate for MZ twins (about 46 percent) and a considerably lower one (about 14 percent) for DZ twins, similar to rates for siblings in general (Gottesman and Shields, 1972; Kety, 1979).

Family studies. Another strategy for exploring the viability of the genetic model is to study the incidence of schizophrenia for different degrees of blood relationship. First-degree relatives include siblings, parents, and children. The first-degree relatives of schizophrenics should show the highest incidence of schizophrenia, and the relatives of normals, the least. As distance of relationship to schizophrenic patients increases, the percentage of schizophrenia found among the relatives should decrease. Offspring of dual matings, in which both parents are schizophrenic, should show an even higher incidence of schizophrenia than when only one parent is schizophrenic. This should hold true even for adopted-away offspring of two schizophrenic parents. All of the foregoing relationships are in fact found (DeFries & Plomin, 1978; Gottesman & Shields, 1972; Gottesman & Shields, 1976; Gottesman, Shields, and Hanson 1982; Kety, et al., 1975). Table 12.3 summarizes some of these data.

Some interesting data emerge from Table 12.3. The risk for children with one schizophrenic parent is about 13 percent, while that for offspring of *two* schizophrenic parents is about 46 percent. (A Soviet

Spotlight 12.3 Monozygotic Twins Discordant For Schizophrenia: Another Perspective

The study of the concordance of schizophrenia in monozygotic twins (percentage of expression of the disease in both twins) has yielded support for the importance of genetic factors. But an interesting question arises from the empirical finding that there is a rather large percentage of *discordance* in monozygotic twins. (The designation of discordance may, however, be inaccurate, because a twin not showing schizophrenia at the time of a study may do so at a later date.)

What are the differences in life experiences, parental handling, birth weight, and other circumstances that might account for the fact that one monozygotic twin develops schizophrenia while the other does not? This research path may shed light on the "benevolent" variables in the life course of a vulnerable child. Perhaps we can learn to construct our interventive programs by studying pairs of discordant twins more closely.

Here are some of the major findings in a review of relevant studies (Wahl, 1976):

1. Discordance is relatively rare in chronic, deteriorated schizophrenics. That is, discordance is more likely to occur in twin pairs in which the schizophrenic partner has a milder degree of impairment. Also, discordant twins have fewer family members with schizophrenia. Such evidence suggests the occurrence of two types of schizophrenia—one a genetically determined type, the other an environmentally determined type (Rosenthal, 1959). More recent evidence has led most investigators to lean toward the genetically determined type, with some of them acknowledging that environmental factors may interact in significant ways with genetic factors.

2. Schizophrenic discordance in monozygotic twins seems to be a result of environmental disparities between them; lower social class, more environmental stress, and greater social isolation from others are posited as possible circumstances of the sick member. The environments of concordant twins seem to be less disparate. Additional environmental factors may also be relevant to discordance: discordant twins may have been separated from each other; or one of the pair may have received preferential parental treatment, had more social contacts, or come from an upperwardly mobile socioeconomic class (Kringlen, 1967).

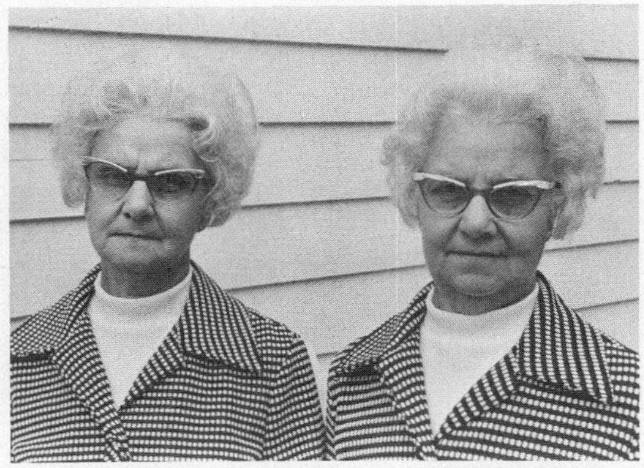

Many MZ (identical) twins show discordance for schizophrenia. Why one of a pair of MZ twins—reared in similar circumstances—develops schizophrenia and the other does not is of great current interest to scientists. (Copyright © Harvey Stein, 1980)

3. Female discordance rates are lower than those for males (that is, if one twin of a female pair has schizophrenia, the other is more likely to develop the disorder, compared to pairs of male twins)—a finding that requires some explanation in the light of another finding that females do not seem to be more genetically vulnerable than males (Rosenthal, 1970). One explanation is that female twins lead a more consistently similar life, with more homogeneous environments (Slater, 1968). The fact that this situation is changing suggests that in the future, discordant rates among female twins will increase. Another explanation is that female monozygotic twins identify more with each other and therefore have more homogeneous psychological environments (Rosenthal and Kety, 1968). Still another explanation is that these differ-

ences are really sampling artifacts—errors in obtaining the sample—and that true differences between male and female discordance rates do not exist (Samuels, 1979).

4. What are the positive factors in the upbringing of twins operating to prevent one of them from developing schizophrenia? The limited amount of data indicate that the unaffected twin was less submissive, had a less difficult birth, was physically healthier, submitted less to the co-twin, was more often the "spokesperson" of the pair, did better in school, and showed a better employment adjustment (Slater and Shields, 1953; Tienari, 1968).

Overall, the following factors seem to be of some significance regarding which twin develops schizophrenia: birthweight, neonatal medical complications, eating and sleeping problems; perception by family members as weaker and more vulnerable; some minor neurological signs; and personality differences in that the twin who becomes schizophrenic is more submissive, depressed, fearful, and less socially skilled (Pollin and Stabenau, 1968).

study of dual matings in which both parents are schizophrenic yielded even higher risk figures for their offspring—57 percent, and up to about 80 percent when flexible, "soft" criteria were used [Moskalenko, 1972]). Also, although second- and third-degree relatives—for example, first cousins, nephews, and nieces of schizophrenics—have relatively low risk, siblings of a schizophrenic, whether or not a parent is schizophrenic, are at considerably higher risk.

Overall, there is little agreement about the genetic processes involved in the transmission of schizophrenia. Many unanswered questions remain regarding the precise nature of the genetic mechanisms that may be involved. For example, the issue of whether there is a specific gene for schizophrenia or whether several genes are involved (polygenic hypothesis) has not been resolved. The inability of geneticists to interpret many of the relevant behavioral findings on the basis of the specific mechanisms of heredity is not our concern for current purposes. These important areas are still under exploration (Gottesman and Shields, 1976; Hanson, Gottesman, and Meehl, 1977; Rosenthal, 1977). However, "It should be noted as a source of hope that the overwhelming majority of all relatives of schizophrenics are *not* themselves schizophrenic" (Gottesman, Shields, and Hanson, 1982, p. 84).

The Biochemistry of Schizophrenia

An impressive array of evidence points to at least some biochemical bases for the schizophrenic process. Despite intriguing research findings, however, no one major biochemical factor has been thoroughly confirmed (different pathways may lead to the same phenotype), and for most of the major hypotheses, studies yield contradictory findings (Bowers, 1980; Matthysse, 1976; Meltzer, 1979ab; Wyatt, Termini, and Davis, 1971).

Why does this area generate excitement among many researchers? If the biochemical underpinnings of schizophrenia are more clearly understood, they can point the way to the possible control, even remediation, of the pathological process through biochemical or psychopharmacological intervention. Further, exciting possibilities would then open up for understanding many of the perplexing problems of schizophrenia, such as why some people become schizophrenic and others, either from the same genetic background or under the same stressful circumstances, do not. Perhaps also, we could shed light on another mystery: why "sick" people, even with acute disturbance (hallucinations, delusions, bizarreness in behavior) become better without intervention.

You are already familiar with some of the prob-

Table 12.3 Risks of Schizophrenia for Relatives of Schizophrenics

Relationship	*Number of studies*	*Number of relatives*	*Number of schizophrenics**	*Percentage schizophrenic**
First degree				
Parents	14	8020	447	5.6
Siblings—all	13	9921	1002	10.1
Siblings—no parent schizophrenic	9	7264	698	9.6
Siblings—one parent schizophrenic	5	624	104	16.7
Children	7	1577	202	12.8
Children of two schizophrenics	5	134	62	46.3
Second degree				
Half siblings	5	500	21	4.2
Uncles/aunts	3	2421	57	2.4
Nephews/nieces	6	3966	120	3.0
Grandchildren	5	740	27	3.7
Third degree				
First cousins	3	1601	39	2.4
Spouses	4	399	9	2.3

Source: Adapted from I. I. Gottesman, J. Shields, and D. R. Hanson, *Schizophrenia: The epigenetic puzzle* (New York: Cambridge University Press, 1982), p. 85.
*Includes schizophrenic and *probable* schizophrenic patients.

lems in drawing inferences about differences in biochemical makeup among groups of patients and controls (for example, see pp. 251–53 on the biochemistry of depression). One type of inferential evidence, however, remains impressive: the differences in the effects of medication on the behavior of patients and nonpatients. Is the psychotic behavior reduced? In some instances does pathological behavior increase? Is it possible to establish models that could account for the internal biochemical events responsible for the increases or decreases in the behavioral pathology? As we shall see, proponents of some of the major biochemical theories rely heavily on this type of evidence.

Differences in performance between schizophrenics and nonschizophrenics in response to some intervention, such as medication, may be due to the long-term status of schizophrenic subjects as a result of diet, hospitalization, previous medication, and the related consequences of having been a patient. Under such circumstances, it would be premature to conclude that the intervention bears a direct relationship to the etiology of schizophrenia. What is required is a control group composed of young, unmedicated, nonhospitalized schizophrenic subjects, so that the effects of intervention would not be confounded by either preexisting conditions, or by other interventions and effects of long-term patient status. It is also difficult to obtain reliably established, homogeneous groups of schizophrenic subtypes.

Despite such difficulties, many promising models are being explored, with some provocative possibilities for understanding schizophrenia. The following list describes some of these hypotheses.

1. *The dopamine hypothesis* has for many years been the most reputable of the biochemical hypotheses about schizophrenia (Langer, Brown, and

Docherty, 1981). This hypothesis proposes that dopamine (one of the catecholamines; see Chapter 7), a neurotransmitter, is implicated in producing schizophrenia. More specifically, it proposes that an excess of dopaminergic activity or dopaminergic transmission occurs in some of the special brain cells that release and are dependent on dopamine. That increased dopamine levels or "supersensitivity" of dopamine receptors in certain sections of the brain might underlie, activate, or create the schizophrenic process has been chiefly based on the two lines of inferential evidence mentioned above: (a) the antipsychotic or antischizophrenic medications (phenothiazines) that reduce the bizarre, delusional, or hallucinated behavior of active schizophrenia, reduce, block, or "antagonize" dopaminergic transmission; and (b) conversely, drugs that *increase* such activity, that is, activate the dopaminergic system, such as the amphetamines, can produce psychotic-like states or dramatically increase schizophrenic symptoms in "partially remitted" or actively ill schizophrenics (Barchas et al., 1978; Langer, Brown, and Docherty, 1981; Meltzer, 1979ab).

Increased dopaminergic activity does not necessarily mean that such abnormalities bear an easily detectable one-to-one relationship to schizophrenia. Such enhanced activation might be due to a decrease in release of other neurochemicals such as norepinephrine or serotonin (Meltzer and Stahl, 1976; Meltzer, 1979ab). It may be that such increased levels may be activated by the body's response to stress or to early experiences in some but not all individuals (Barchas, et al., 1978; Meltzer and Stahl, 1976). Further, levels of dopamine activity in the brain are apparently not related to *all* schizophrenic dysfunctions, because some of the medications that block dopaminergic activities do not reduce bizarre behavior in all schizophrenic individuals. Are some schizophrenic conditions simply not due to dopaminergic physiology? For example, elevated norepinephrine levels in the cerebrospinal fluid were found in a group of paranoid schizophrenics (Lake et al., 1980). Or is dopamine excess a secondary response to *other* biochemical imbalances (Meltzer, 1979ab; Meltzer and Stahl, 1976) or is it related to a general psychotic, rather than to a specifically schizophrenic pattern (Alpert and Friedhoff, 1980)?

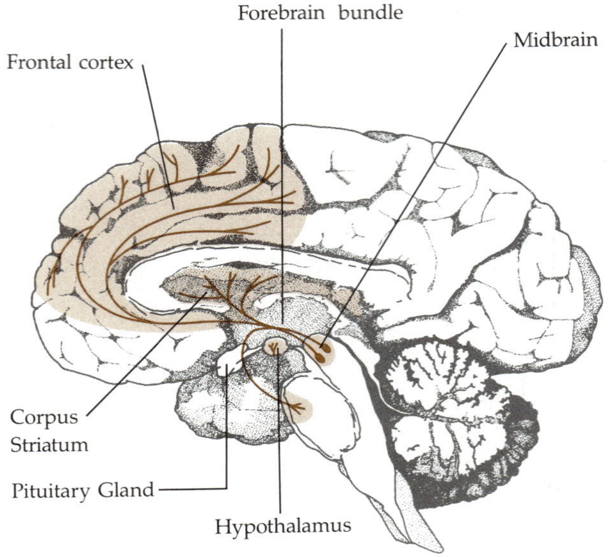

Figure 12.1 Major dopamine pathways in the human brain, shown schematically. The neurons that contain dopamine have their cell bodies clustered in two small regions of the midbrain. These neurons send out widely branching fibers that terminate in the corpus striatum, which regulates motor activity, and in the limbic forebrain, which is involved in emotion. A small group of dopamine neurons in the hypothalamus also regulates the secretion of hormones from the pituitary. (From The chemistry of the brain by Leslie L. Iversen. Copyright © 1979 by Scientific American, Inc. All rights reserved.)

Overall, the popular dopaminergic hypothesis has not received consistent empirical support and, in some cases, may even be contraindicated by some of the empirical evidence (Lake et al., 1980).

2. *The transmethylation hypothesis* (Osmond and Smythies, 1952) is derived from the fact that the body produces certain neurochemicals similar to mescaline, a derivative of the peyote plant that produces psychotic-like symptoms. It was thought that these naturally produced chemicals (endogenous hallucinogens) might play a role in creating certain

psychotic states in some types of circumstances. Empirical evidence in support of this hypothesis in relation to the etiology of schizophrenia has not been impressive. It is possible, however, that during a psychotic episode, the brain makes use of these naturally occurring chemicals in ways that differ from normal use. Thus, these natural hallucinogens could well be associated with the *symptoms* of schizophrenia (as a rash is associated with measles), rather than with its *cause* (Barchas et al., 1978; Rosengarten and Friedhoff, 1976).

3. *Monoamine oxidase* (MAO) is an enzyme (a protein that acts on other chemicals to produce change) found in many different forms of human tissue, including the blood and brain. This enzyme helps to metabolize some of the biogenic amines we have been discussing, such as dopamine and serotonin. It has been reasoned that if these MAO functions are reduced or blocked, an excess of the biogenic amines might be responsible for the bizarre symptomatology of schizophrenia. This was the line of inquiry followed in a frequently cited study demonstrating reduced MAO activity in the blood platelets (grayish bodies important for clotting) of acute and chronic schizophrenics (Murphy and Wyatt, 1972).

If reduced MAO activity is found in the tissues of schizophrenics, this would be further support for biogenic theories of schizophrenia. Unfortunately findings have not been consistent (Barchas et al., 1978; Meltzer, 1979ab; Wyatt and Murphy, 1976). Some evidence does suggest, however, that patients with acute schizophrenia without auditory hallucinations show normal platelet MAO activity, whereas patients with auditory or visual hallucinations or paranoid reactions show reduced activity (Adler et al., 1980; Wyatt et al., 1980).

Although MAO activity is sometimes viewed as being under genetic control (Meltzer, 1979ab), diet, medication, and hormonal status of the individual can also be influential controlling factors. Overall, the MAO-activity hypothesis of schizophrenia is an intriguing one, especially since, as noted, it is relevant to the promising biogenic amine models.

4. The *endorphin hypothesis* of schizophrenia is derived from recent discoveries of a group of "new" neurotransmitters called the endorphins, which have been shown to produce analgesic effects similar to those of some of the opiates (see Chapter 7, p. 148). It has been proposed on the basis of research with rats that one member of this group of naturally occurring morphine-like opiates—beta-endorphin—might be responsible for some schizophrenia-like motor behavior. Injections of beta-endorphin into the brains of rats resulted in catatonic states in which rigid, unnatural postures were maintained by the rats over a period of time. These effects could be immediately reversed by injections of naloxone, a morphine antagonist used in humans experiencing a morphine overdose. Additionally, it has been reported that the auditory hallucinations of schizophrenics can be inhibited by naloxone.

These and other bits of evidence, such as the excessive concentration of beta-endorphin in the dialysis wash (hemodialysis—blood cleansing) of chronic schizophrenics without kidney disease (Wagemaker and Cade, 1977), have suggested that one of these endorphins might be involved in producing schizophrenic symptoms. This may be a result of their interactions with and modulation of dopaminergic neuronal activities (Bloom et al., 1976; Volavka, Davis, and Ehrlich, 1979). However, because little evidence exists for directly linking the endorphin and dopamine biochemical systems within the brain, and since support for this general hypothesis is based on a limited number of schizophrenic subjects with findings that have even been contradicted (Ross, Berger, and Goldstein, 1979; Watson and Akil, 1979), most scientists reject this approach to schizophrenia, especially the portions relating to dialysis treatment (Sobel, 1981). Nevertheless, since work with the endorphins is still in its infancy, scientists are optimistically exploring the possibilities these neurochemicals offer for understanding the biochemical underpinnings of schizophrenia.

A relatively recent approach to understanding the relationship of these biochemicals to psychopathology underscores the complex interactions of these substances and stresses the fact that these chemicals are not necessarily or inherently "abnormal" but are perhaps activated and *used* in abnormal ways in the biological processes of mentally ill people at the time of their illness. It is also possible that stress and learned factors may actually alter the ways in which biochemical mechanisms function (Barchas et al., 1978). For example, events at critical stages may "lock in" certain kinds of biochemical interactions in susceptible people, thus leading to disordered behavior, much in the way that frost can stunt the growth of some, but not all fruit trees because of genetically determined structures that cause each of the plants to respond differently to severe environmental stress. In any event, we are a long way from understanding the complex interactions of neuronal transmission systems, how and when they are "locked into" producing abnormal behavior, and how and when their functions are modified, either externally, through medications, or through "normal" processes that may account for remissions.

SOME INTEGRATING HYPOTHESES

Diathesis-Stress

The diathesis-stress theory of schizophrenia (diathesis: constitution, heredity) is the general prototype of several views holding that regardless of the biological and genetic structures predisposing an individual to schizophrenia, severe stress and psychological deprivation are necessary for the disease to actually manifest itself. This interactional view makes good sense in the light of the relevant literature on schizophrenia.

The concept of schizotaxia, genetic endowment of schizophrenia that may or may not be expressed, observed, or manifested in the lifetime of the individual (that is, phenotypically), is relevant to this approach (Meehl, 1962). The interaction between endowment and environment is assumed: some stress or severe event in the lifetime of the schizotaxic individual can precipitate (trigger, cause a dormant possibility to take place) schizophrenia if there is a predisposition for it. Stressor agents can include drugs, near-miss accidents, harsh and cruel parental figures, excruciating pain and other kinds of severe anxiety-producing situations (acute or persistent), pregnancy and birth complications, severe economic deprivation, unpredictable familial environments, and events perceived as overwhelming with which the genetically predisposed individual cannot cope.

The diathesis-stress approach, appealing as it is, brings with it some important, familiar questions yet to be answered. Given vulnerable children with morbid genetic ingredients and the most stressful of possible precipitants, why do some manifest schizophrenia while others do not? And even when schizophrenia is manifested, why are there remissions? And why do some schizophrenics, but not others, get better? When unfavorable environmental circumstances are removed, why doesn't the clinical picture improve?

Vulnerability Model

A model that attempts to deal with some of these questions was proposed by Zubin (1978). The vulnerability model suggests that the common denominator among schizophrenics is vulnerability, rather than the disease. This model also stresses the self-limiting nature of the schizophrenic episode and a return to premorbid levels of competence after the episode has subsided, both well-known "facts" about schizophrenia:

> *The schizophrenic is drawn from the entire range of human variation with regard to intelligence, competence, coping ability, achievement, and all other aspects of the human condition. He may be a top executive, a gifted artist, an outstanding scientist, a blue-collar worker, or an unskilled ne'er-do-well bowery bum. No stratum of mankind is spared from this blight. The one feature that all schizophrenics have in common is not the ever-presence of their illness, but rather the ever-presence of their vulnerability. Some of them are highly vulnerable and have repeated episodes.*

Others are relatively invulnerable and have but one brief episode or none at all. When episodes develop they are not lifelong. They terminate sooner or later with or without therapeutic intervention. The majority of schizophrenics today spend the major part of their lives in the community, self-supporting and indistinguishable from the rest of the population except in the eyes of those who have labeled them. To the best of our knowledge, half the patients recover fully, another 40% have relapses but still manage to spend most of their lives in the community, and only 10% appear to remain chronically ill. . . . At the onset of an episode, the patient's competence and ability to cope adequately with life's exigencies appear to go underground. At the end of the episode, these attributes tend to reappear at their premorbid levels and the patient can resume his former place in society (Zubin and Spring, 1977, pp. 122–123).

Zubin's views are very much related to the diathesis-stress approach, suggesting that some underlying vulnerability and the presence of severe stressors may impinge on the individual's life and in some cases produce an episode (1980). His views also imply that for any vulnerable individual, provided that vulnerability can be determined, events at various life points could help to modify the so-called inevitable path to a schizophrenic breakdown. For example, increasing the competence of the individual to handle a stressor, such as a death or separation, or modifying the influence of internal biochemical events through medication might forestall an episode. This challenge to the inevitability of schizophrenia would of course require some indicator of vulnerability and signs of the imminence of an impending episode (for example, biochemical evidence), as well as an assessment of the resources of an individual to cope with the crisis he or she is facing.

If any conclusion can be drawn from the preceding material, it is that even if strong genetic and biochemical underpinnings for schizophrenia are present, the expression of pathology does not follow inevitably for any particular individual. Vulnerable people may carry their vulnerability through a lifetime, without expressing the phenotype of schizophrenia. Further, genetic predisposition may actually produce many kinds of phenotypical subgroups, with or without pathology (Cancro, 1979).

Schizophrenia in any given individual does not develop as a result of an acute life crisis alone, nor as a result of being born to schizophrenic parents alone, or as a result of being raised in a schizophrenogenic environment alone. There is apparently great environmental diversity in the pathways leading to schizophrenia, and it may be that stressors themselves may play a more important role than was thought to be the case in inducing a set of biochemical events—as a result of predisposition—that lead to repeated episodes of psychopathology. It could also be that environmental events, such as learning or medication might alter and block the pathways that lead to schizophrenia.

SECTION II
MAPPING THE TERRAIN OF SCHIZOPHRENIA: SOME CORRELATES AND RESEARCH STRATEGIES

Although theories about the etiology of schizophrenia help us to know a great deal about this disease, another research approach to understanding schizophrenia is concerned with its characteristics. How do schizophrenics think? How do they process information (handle the sensory input impinging on them)? How do they learn? What are some physiological correlates of schizophrenia?

Investigations motivated by questions such as these are less concerned with theories of etiology than with ascertaining the nature of schizophrenia as it manifests itself in various situations. The more complete our knowledge of these areas becomes, the easier it will be to find solutions to questions of causality.

For example, if we find consistent dysfunctions in cognitive or sensory processes in schizophrenics that do not appear in normals or people with other kinds of emotional disorders, perhaps closer attention to the brain will aid our attempts to understand the origins of schizophrenia. Here (as with other investigations) too great a reliance on any one area must be tempered with caution. Faulty cognitive and perceptual functions may eventually prove to be a result, rather than a cause, of the schizophrenic process.

In subsequent sections, some general areas are singled out for further scrutiny. These comprise some well-explored areas and, as popular paradigms, are representative of some of the strategies schizophrenia researchers employ.

Physiological Correlates

In several of the preceding chapters we described studies that attempted to link some of the disorders under consideration to dysfunctions in autonomic processes. For example, anxiety patients were shown to differ in several important ways from control patients in autonomic responsiveness (see pp. 220–23).

In studies of schizophrenia, a variety of physiological measures have been used, including heart rate, galvanic skin responses, EEG, pupillary size, and other measures that directly assess internal states under different kinds of stimulation. Overall, these studies demonstrate that schizophrenics do indeed respond differently from normals and other groups on various physiological measures: they tend to show distinctive patterns in levels of arousal (Buchsbaum, 1977). Why this is so, and the specific mechanisms involved (such as inborn differences, change in responses as a result of being ill, or learned responses) are still not clear. It is possible that these findings are not entirely explainable by genetic factors and that learning as well as various psychological states could account for many of these findings (Zahn, 1977). If respiration, heart rates, and pupillary responses are much more variable in schizophrenic than in normal subjects, as the findings do indeed indicate, attentional problems or the way information is processed (see next sections), rather than inborn physical differences in responsiveness, could be responsible (Lader, 1975).

Skin conductance (GSR). Generally, high amplitudes of responses, short latency (quick responses), and fast recovery are found in the offspring of schizophrenics, with fast recovery being an especially striking characteristic of schizophrenic subjects (Venables, 1977). Some evidence also indicates that schizophrenic subjects include both high responders *and* low responders (Venables, 1977), although the amplitudes of schizophrenic subjects are generally larger than those of control subjects, using various auditory and visual stimuli (Venables, 1960).

Spotlight 12.4 Pioneering Studies in Denmark

As mentioned previously, the national-register data in the Scandinavian countries make it possible to study large samples of subjects over many years. One classic, pioneering series of studies that served as a general model for many others all over the world was conducted in Denmark (Mednick, 1970; Mednick and McNeil, 1968; Mednick and Schulsinger, 1968). These studies called attention to the possibility that some very important differences in autonomic functioning might exist between high-risk children, some of whom become schizophrenic, and children not at high risk.

In 1962, Mednick and his associates studied the offspring of 207 chronic schizophrenic mothers, using various measures, and compared their findings with those of a matched group of 104 control subjects—the offspring of normal mothers with relatives who showed no major psychopathology. The offspring of the schizophrenic mothers were regarded as high-risk subjects, and indeed, five years later, 20 of the high-risk group were found to be schizophrenic. These were designated the "sick" group; those comprising the balance of the high risk-group were referred to as the "well" group. None of the controls became schizophrenic. Comparisons led to many interesting findings, including some in the autonomic area.

To begin with, high-risk subjects, whether or not they later become schizophrenic, differed from the control subjects in that they showed higher levels of autonomic arousal (as measured through skin resistance), higher amplitude of galvanic skin responses, shorter latencies (responded more quickly), and returned to basal levels more quickly (had quicker recovery times). When "sick" and "well" subjects—all of whom were at risk for becoming schizophrenic—were compared, findings demonstrated differences between them that tended to be confirmed in other studies, also. High-risk children who later became schizophrenic showed even more vigorous autonomic responses than the high-risk children who did not. The "sick" group tended not to habituate in various test situations, continuing to show high autonomic arousal, while short latencies and adaptation to the repeated stimuli characterized the control group, and to a lesser extent, the "well" group.

A related exploration confirms the possibility of psychophysiological distinctions between high-risk and low-risk subjects. High-risk subjects selected from the 9,006 children born in Copenhagen between 1959 and 1961 differed from their controls both in EEG recordings and auditory evoked potentials (averaged, computerized recordings of minute electrical activity in the brain in response to stimulation), showing many similarities in neurophysiological patterns to actively disturbed children and adult chronic schizophrenics (Itil, Hsu, Saletu, and Mednick, 1974).

Although these findings show striking differences among the groups of children studied, they do not indicate whether the origin of such differences is genetic or environmental. Mednick and his associates did feel, however, that possible pregnancy and birth complications, such as anoxia (oxygen deprivation), could have contributed to these physiological differences. Even more significantly, they felt that later schizophrenia, as we have already noted, developed as a dramatic avoidance of high drive (arousal and anxiety) states that were extremely discomforting to the subjects experiencing them.

EEG recordings (see Chapter 7, page 146). Reviews of studies conducted over the last fifty years confirm early findings of EEG abnormalities in the records of schizophrenics compared to control subjects (Itil, 1977; Itil, Saletu, and Davis, 1972; Lader, 1975). Abnormalities include differences in types of waves and greater variability and "choppiness" of waves. These findings are true even for untreated cases, which is important because treated cases may reflect the effects of medication and diet. Further, studies with autistic and schizophrenic children indicate a range of 30 to 80 percent of EEG abnormalities. Such findings are generally valid for a large spectrum of subjects, including children of schizophrenic parents, schizophrenic children, and schizophrenic adults (Itil, 1977).

Language and Communication

Most clinicians agree that the communication styles, content, "flavor," and language of schizophrenics differ from those of normals. These impressions are fully supported by empirical, objective observations and analyses of actual samples of schizophrenic speech, yielding a consistent picture

Spotlight 12.5 Smooth-Pursuit Eye Movements (SPEM)

Try to follow a moving object with your eyes—for example, a tennis ball that has just been hit or an airplane you have just become aware of overhead. You must first focus on the object so that it is centered on the fovea (the point of sharpest vision on the retina). You do so through rapid eye movements, called saccadic movements. In pursuing the moving object, the eyes move much more slowly; these pursuit movements serve to smoothly retain the image of the moving object directly on target, on the fovea, by maintaining a coordinated relationship with the moving object. These movements are all aspects of the eyes' pursuit system.

Early in the 1900s, through a rather crude method of photographing reflections of light from the eyes as they followed the movement of a pendulum, Diefendorf and Dodge (1908) discovered that the smooth-pursuit eye movements of a group of chronic schizophrenic patients were rather different from those of other types of patients (Holzman and Levy, 1977). Since that time, the methods for tracking and recording smooth-pursuit eye movements have become very sophisticated—for example, through use of infrared reflection techniques and electronic recording devices (Lindsey et al., 1978). Nonetheless, the general thrust of the findings are the same; a few of these findings follow (Holzman and Levy, 1977; Lindsey et al., 1978):

Between 65 to 80 percent of schizophrenics but only about 6 percent of normal subjects show deviant pursuit patterns. In addition, first-degree relatives (mothers, fathers, siblings) of schizophrenic patients also show deviant eye tracking movements. More specifically, about 45 percent of the nonschizophrenic relatives of schizophrenic patients, compared to only 10 percent of the nonschizophrenic relatives of nonschizophrenic patients, show deviant smooth-pursuit eye movements. Further, even in MZ twins discordant for schizophrenia, there is high concordance for deviant eye tracking patterns.

Is there some CNS defect in the processing of sensory data that could account for such findings? Is some defect in nonvoluntary attention present? The neurophysiological substrates of these findings are still not entirely clear, and, in addition, these results are complicated by the fact that deviant patterns are also associated with other psychotic states and some CNS disorders (Holzman and Levy, 1977).

of differences in the verbal skills of schizophrenics compared to nonschizophrenics (Grand, et al., 1975; Salzinger, 1973; Tucker and Rosenberg, 1975).

In what ways has it been empirically determined that schizophrenics communicate differently from nonschizophrenics? One early method that objectively explored communicability of schizophrenic speech employed the "cloze" procedure (Taylor, 1953). This method typically involves the deleting of every fifth word in speech samples of subjects and requiring another group of subjects to guess the missing words. Difficulties in understanding the speech of schizophrenics can thus be systematically measured. In one study in which a large number of speech samples from schizophrenic and physically ill subjects matched for age, sex, education, and ethnic background were compared through cloze methods (the guessers were college students), the schizophrenic subjects were consistently less understandable than the nonschizophrenic subjects (Salzinger, Portnoy, and Feldman, 1964b).

In word-association tasks, schizophrenic subjects tend to produce more idiosyncratic (unique to the individual in contrast to usual or frequent responses of a group) associations than do normals.

Examples of usual associations are: up-down; night-day; table-chair. Examples of idiosyncratic associations are: table-slimy; night-blood; up-higher universe. Schizophrenics also show more variability in their associations from day to day (Storms, Broen, and Levin, 1967).

Objective evidence indicates differences between schizophrenic and normal speech in a variety of other areas also. For example, schizophrenics use relatively more verbs, respond with greater variability to interruptions, and are more variable in verbal responses (periods of silence, hesitations, activity) than normals (Salzinger, 1973).

Do these well-established characteristics of schizophrenic speech and communication indicate a basic language defect? Studies exploring this issue do not tend to implicate central language defects in explaining these impairments. For example, schizophrenics have been shown to perceive the organization of normal speech and to respond to its syntactic structure much in the manner of normals (Carpenter, 1976; McGhie and Chapman, 1961; Rochester, Harris, and Seeman, 1973). Word-association response processes of schizophrenics and normals are probably not as different as they were once thought to be (Cohen and Camhi, 1967), and some investigators have demonstrated that schizophrenics accentuate normal associations rather than deviate from them (Miller and Chapman, 1968; see section that follows). Thus, although objective studies have yielded definite differences, they have not provided definitive explanations for these findings.

Thinking Disorder

You will recall that many of the symptoms of schizophrenia are characterized by a "peculiarity," or differentness in thinking, judgment, and related cognitive processes. Most people believe that these very characteristics—unusual, strange, bizarre, or idiosyncratic ways of thinking about and viewing the world—define, or at least are essential to, the schizophrenic process. Both Kraepelin and Bleuler characterized schizophrenia as a thinking disorder, and generations of later investigators tended to concur. The nature of these disorders, however, continues to elicit much theorizing and controversy (Chapman and Chapman, 1973).

One early group of researchers explored the performance of schizophrenic and brain-injured patients in a variety of sorting tasks that employed blocks of various shapes and colors, differently colored threads, and various objects (Goldstein, 1944; Kasanin & Hanfmann, 1938). Schizophrenics based their groupings and categories on irrelevant or subjective criteria. For example, blocks would be grouped in a row (without regard to color or size) representing a train going to "my mother's house," or into seemingly random groupings representing "school friends I dream about all the time." The free-associational, fluid, subjective quality of this sorting behavior was labeled as "impairment in the abstract attitude." In normals, the abstract attitude would have allowed sorting or categorizing on the basis of some category or concept such as color, size, shape, function, or of a complex category employing more than one criterion simultaneously (such as sorting blocks into tall rectangular ones, short rectangular ones, tall round ones, and short round ones).

Describing schizophrenic thinking as comprised primarily of an impairment in the abstract attitude has been the subject of much research and considerable criticism. For example, some theorists have held that the thinking of schizophrenics results from overinclusion, a way of dealing with stimuli that embraces or includes more of the stimulus field than is necessary for completing the task, rather than from impairment in the abstract attitude (Cameron, 1939). Although experimental investigations such as those by Payne and his associates (see Payne and Friedlander, 1962), who had their subjects sort various objects under controlled conditions, tended to confirm the hypothesis of overinclusion, recent work suggests that this concept needs more refinement (Davis and Blaney, 1976; Harrow, et al., 1972; Tucker, et al., 1969). It is highly likely that the various subtypes of schizophrenia must be considered in interpreting the concept of overinclusion. For example, paranoid patients tend more than nonparanoid patients to interpret erroneously or connect causally a wide variety of unrelated and disconnected circumstances and events (Payne, Caird, and Laverty, 1964).

A search for a unifying model to account for some of the above findings has led many researchers to speculate whether attentional processes and the ways in which stimuli are processed could serve this need.

Spotlight 12.6 A Popular Paradigm For Exploring Attention in Schizophrenia: Reaction Time

Since our receptors are bombarded continuously by a wide spectrum of both internal and external stimuli, we must have some way of separating the relevant stimuli and those that we cannot ignore—those on which our adaptive adjustment depends in a given situation—from the irrelevant, those which we can ignore with safety and continue undisturbed with the ongoing activity. This is selective attention. *Once the sector of the environment has been selected, attention is directed toward it until we attain our goal or become satiated or bored with it. . . . Since we cannot remain glued to the same sector forever, a switching mechanism must be available which directs our attention to some other sector (Zubin, 1975, p. 141).*

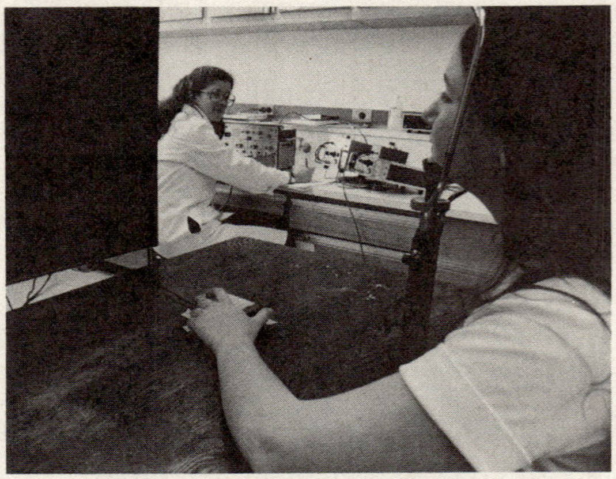

Reaction-time studies represent a popular paradigm in the ongoing experimental exploration of schizophrenia. (© Lynn McLaren 1977/Photo Researchers)

Though not presenting all of the issues, these aspects of attention have been objectively studied in various kinds of reaction-time studies, a research strategy popular because of the reliability and simplicity of the experimental methods involved. But why reaction time? The answer is that many researchers believed that one approach to studying attention and set was to measure the subject's ability to maintain a preparatory orientation to a signal that requires the immediate execution of a task (for example, pressing a lever for a red, but not for a blue, light).

One of the earliest attempts to study attention and set by means of reaction time was described by Shakow and his colleagues. Typically, in such studies (Rodnick and Shakow, 1940), reaction time to auditory or visual signals is measured in samples of schizophrenic and control subjects, with findings invariably showing that schizophrenic subjects have slower reaction times than normal subjects. In a series of subsequent studies, Shakow (1963) explored the possibility that problems in maintaining attention and set could explain many of the characteristics of schizophrenic responses, not only on reaction time tasks but also in a variety of other tasks, and that inability to maintain a major set over a short period of time is a central defect of schizophrenia.

Shakow differentiates between major, or generalized, set and segmental set:

Generalized or major *sets are called such because the minor or irrelevant individual aspects of the stimulus-response process, the ones that come to the fore in all situations, have been partialed out to leave only the principal aspects, those relevant to adaptation, in central focus. . . .*

Segmental set, *on the contrary, is disclosed by an inconsistency* within *an aspect of the response. . . .[it]involves a preparatory adjustment that is particularly directed to portions, to partial or minor aspects of the total stimulus-response situation, or in the extreme case, even to aspects entirely outside the stimulus situation.*

(Shakow, 1977, p. 131).

The difficulty in maintaining major sets could account for the fragmented, peculiar, often irrelevant responses in thinking, language, and verbal associations, as well as the reaction-time performance of schizophrenic subjects. Presumably, this difficulty is a reflection of the buffeting and distractions by segmental sets.

Not only do schizophrenic subjects respond more slowly than normal subjects, but they also do more poorly on tasks requiring them to execute a simple response after a preparatory interval of a few seconds. Typically, in this experimental model, a warning signal (such as a tone or light) precedes the actual stimulus to which the subject must respond. Variations in length of preparatory interval, as well as in stimulus complexity, affect schizophrenics' reaction-time performance.

Schizophrenic performance in crossmodal reaction-time tasks has also been shown to be slower than those of control subjects. "Crossmodal" in this context refers to the introduction of more than one sensory modality in reaction-time situations in which the signal could be in the same (ipsimodal) or a different sensory modality—for example, an auditory signal preceding a visual one. Compared to their ipsimodal performance, the reaction times of schizophrenics were found to be more impaired when there was a modality shift than were those of control subjects (Sutton et al., 1961).

In schizophrenic performance, the buffeting by minor sets and the attention to irrelevant details might be due to anxiety avoidance, fear of the new, or to other motivational factors. These behaviors could also be due to certain neural and physiological substrates that cause deficits in reaction-time performance. It is not yet clear just what these neural events are, however. One hypothesis that is reasonably consistent with most of the findings, according to a major review of reaction-time studies (Nuechterlein, 1977) is Zubin's "neuronal trace" model (1975), which holds that neural traces facilitate performance for similar future tasks and interfere with or inhibit performance for dissimilar tasks to a greater extent for schizophrenic subjects than for normal subjects. Even so, these experimental reaction-time models may be only the "tip of the iceberg" in understanding the neurophysiology of schizophrenia. In the long run, the gradual accumulation and elimination of countless findings and hypotheses in this and other areas described in this chapter should provide a clearer picture of the enigma of schizophrenia.

Attention and Stimulus Processing

A repeated element in the self-descriptions of the schizophrenic experience is the flooding of stimulation from within and without so that the patient is unable to distinguish the relevant from the irrelevant. The looseness of associations, failure to maintain a set, fluidity of ideas, and senseless notice of detail after detail (distractability) without follow-through or focus described in such self-reports are all aspects of what has come to be called attention (see Chapter 7, Spotlight 7.2).

Attention can be defined as the selective responding to portions or aspects of the wide stimulation impinging on an organism (stimulus array), with an accompanying disattention or ignoring of other aspects of the stimulus array. It is not possible for the brain to attend to more than a certain selected number of stimuli or patterns of stimulation at the same time; the rest is discarded or unattended to (Broadbent, 1958). Normal responses are those that filter out irrelevant stimulation while focusing on the relevant. The brain has a filtering mechanism that performs this function. It is thought that one of the chief characteristics of schizophrenia is some kind of breakdown in this mechanism—a failure to sort out or filter the relevant from the irrelevant in the stimulus array ("information") impinging on the subject. In schizophrenia, the implications of this faulty mechanism are far-reaching, possibly accounting for disorganization in language, thinking, attending, concentrating, and perceiving shown by such patients (Garmezy, 1977; Lang and Buss, 1965; McGhie and Chapman, 1961; Silverman, 1964; Zubin, 1975; Venables, 1964).

Although there is general agreement on this score, this is where the uniformity ends. To define attention is not easy. It is a complex construct that has been studied in a variety of different ways. And various "tests" of attention show only a low correlation with each other (Kopfstein and Neale, 1972; Neale and Cromwell, 1970). In addition, some of the fascinating experimental findings in this area are contradictory or difficult to interpret. It does seem, however, that some generalizations emerge: The performance of schizophrenics does indeed differ from those of normals in almost all experimental tasks; differences occur in performance between schizophrenic subtypes in many areas (specifically paranoid versus nonparanoid and chronic versus acute); and breakdown in the filtering mechanism or in attentional responses can account for many of these differences.

Attention and subtypes of schizophrenia. Attentional dysfunctions may account for differences among schizophrenic subgroups (Silverman, 1964), although such interpretations are regarded by some as too simple (Strauss, Carpenter, and Bartko, 1974). According to one general view, chronic (process) nonparanoid patients suffer from a restricted range of attention or reduced responsiveness to stimuli (Broen, 1968; Broen and Nakamura, 1972; Venables, 1964). The hypothesis is that they curtail excessive inputs from the environment, probably as a defensive maneuver. Acute, reactive, paranoid patients, on the other hand, suffer from "stimulus flooding"—deficiencies in ability to restrict the range of incoming stimuli (Dykes and McGhie, 1976; Silverman, 1964). These patients are overstimulated, manifesting difficulty in ignoring or disattending to irrelevant stimuli. They thus "explain" or find reasons for a wider range of events in order to make sense of their worlds.

The processing of stimulation. In many of the studies just discussed, the processing of stimulation has been implicated. The stimulus approach to understanding schizophrenic behavior, and especially to the understanding of attention, has taken several routes. Descriptions of a few of these routes follow.

1. *Stimulus overselectivity.* Schizophrenics behave in unusual or bizarre ways because they respond to a much smaller section of the stimulus array than do normals. Information is "processed" very slowly by schizophrenics, so that much of the "outside world" is lost (Yates, 1966). Some experimental confirmation of this view has been reported for simple as well as complex visual and auditory tasks (Davidson and Neale, 1974; Wishner and Wahl, 1974). A related view about the performance of autistic children refers to their "stimulus overselectivity"; such children respond to only a limited number of cues in the surrounding environment (Lovaas, Koegel, and Schreibman, 1979).

2. *Immediacy hypothesis.* Immediate but not remote stimuli are more "compelling" or controlling to the schizophrenic than to the normal subject (Salzinger, 1971ab; 1972). That is, "immediate" stimuli, in a temporal or spatial sense, are more significant in determining the behavior of the schizophrenic than are symbolic and socially learned stimuli. The short attention span of many schizophrenics, their many peculiarities and eccentricities, as well as several other perceptual and cognitive characteristics, such as concreteness, are thus ex-

Table 12.4 Frequent and Remote (Idiosyncratic) Word Associations for Normal and Schizophrenic Male Subjects

Normal Male College Subject	A Schizophrenic Male College Subject
Black ....white	black...........slime, time
table ....chair	table ....Mabel, maybe, I don't know
up ....down	up ....neighbor's cryings
night...........day	night...........day
happy ....sad	happy ....beer and suds
light ....dark	light ....fighting and who cares
cup..............saucer	cup..............up, who cares again?

Note: Test some of your friends. Do they come up with the usual associations?

plained by their tendency to respond to stimuli that are immediate rather than remote.

3. *Disattention hypothesis.* One view about responses of schizophrenics suggests that they reflect an inability to "disattend" from a preceding stimulus with the same ease and rapidity found in normal responses (Cromwell & Dokecki, 1968). This results in a "stickiness" in schizophrenic responses that prevents rapid shifts in attention to and anticipation of a new stimulus. The responses of a schizophrenic thus, appear irrelevant and frequently unrelated to the central, relevant stimulus. In this view, in contrast to Salzinger's, the schizophrenic, is responding to remote rather than to immediate stimuli.

Response Models

Response hierarchies. The work of Broen and Storms was briefly alluded to when a few learning hypotheses of schizophrenia were discussed in this chapter (p. 300). In this approach, weaker and stronger response habits of a schizophrenic compete with each other, so that the schizophrenic's responses are not the usual, dominant ones. These authors do not suggest that the sequence of hierarchies of habit strength in schizophrenic subjects differs from that in normals, but only the probability that certain remote or unusual responses will be evoked.

Response biases. Another way of characterizing schizophrenic performance is by the special way in which stimuli are processed: schizophrenics respond more easily according to "normal biases" than do normals (Chapman and Chapman, 1973). That is, although normals have a tendency to respond to stimuli according to certain biases, they are able to modify those tendencies when necessary, whereas schizophrenics are not as able to resist the pull of their biases.

For example, in one study, schizophrenics tended, more often than normals, to respond to the strong, or usual meaning of a word—the normal bias—despite the fact that the context implied a weaker meaning. Thus, schizophrenics tended to respond to the strong (or "preferred") rather than the weak meaning of the word in the following multiple-choice situation:

When the farmer bought a herd of cattle, he needed a new pen. This means:

He needed a new writing implement. (strong meaning)

He needed a new fenced enclosure. (weak meaning)

He needed a new pick-up truck. (irrelevant statement)

(Chapman, Chapman, and Miller, 1964, p. 60)

Strong meanings come readily to mind for both normals and schizophrenics. The normal subject will screen or filter this response tendency if it is inappropriate. The schizophrenic, however, is defective in this process: the dominant information becomes overweighted.*

According to this theory, the tendency to "yield to normal biases" is thought to underlie a wide variety of the cognitive symptoms of schizophrenia. It predicts that schizophrenics will tend to be overly concrete when abstraction is difficult and that their concreteness will reflect the qualities of the stimulus that by normal standards would be considered "prominent." Similarly, schizophrenics will tend to "overinclude," that is, bring too much of the stimulus field into the task when the stimuli in the field coincide with what might "normally" be included, but which, given the situation, are in fact inappropriate.

Children At Risk For Schizophrenia

A research strategy that cuts across all etiological theories emerges from several key questions. Who are the (vulnerable) people who later develop schizophrenia? Do they always have schizophrenic parents? Were they victims of unusual stress? Were they biochemically, behaviorally, and physiologically normal during infancy? Were their familial environments bizarre? If we could identify the candidates for schizophrenia early enough, perhaps we might be able to seek ways to prevent its occurrence.

One way of approaching these questions would be to study as many children from the population-at-large as possible, on the assumption that some will become schizophrenic and others will not. Many years later, when a small percentage (about 1 percent) of this sample will have become schizophrenic, their histories, characteristics, and early behaviors could then be traced. Because an extremely large sample must be carefully observed over many years, with a yield of very few schizophenic subjects, such efforts are not feasible.

It may be more practical to use already available familial data to find a greater number of potential schizophrenics. For example, a method that locates the offspring of one or two schizophrenic parents on the assumption that they are more vulnerable than a matched group of control subjects with no schizophrenic parents allows researchers to observe, test, and follow up on a population for which the risks for schizophrenia are increased. It would then be possible to isolate the early characteristics of those who became schizophrenic in comparison to those who did not.

It should be noted that even though the children of schizophrenic parents for high-risk research are selected for study, the vast majority of these offspring do not become schizophrenic (see Spotlight 12.7): 10 to 16 percent of the offspring of one schizophrenic parent actually develop schizophrenia; but the percentage rises to 35 to 44 percent, if both parents are schizophrenic (Rosenthal, 1966).

We have already touched on the Danish pioneering studies of Mednick (Mednick and Schulsinger, 1968) and his associates (see pp. 299–300 and Spotlight 12.4) that found a number of important differences, especially in psychophysiological functioning (such as heightened autonomic levels in high-risk children), between high-risk and control subjects. Since these early studies, well over 20 other high-risk projects have been initiated (Hanson, Gottesman, and Meehl, 1977). Are there additional "markers"—indicators of later pathology—that emerge from these studies? What variables are associated with high risk for schizophrenia? Some of these include: birth complications; abnormal neurological responses in infancy; unusual or deviant stimulus responsiveness; marked sociocultural deprivation, especially economic deprivation that tends to be associated with nutritional difficulties; severe physical or intellectual limitations; unsocialized aggression in boys; excessive conformity, inhibition, and withdrawal in girls; and in adolescence, peer difficulties and few, if any,

* Recent empirical evidence suggests that manic patients, as well as schizophrenic patients, differ from normal subjects in yielding to "preferred" meanings of words, even when these meanings are inappropriate (Naficy and Willerman, 1980). In other words, excessive yielding to normal biases may not be uniquely characteristic of schizophrenic pathology.

Spotlight 12.7 Inevitability of Schizophrenia? The Cheerier Side

Manfred Bleuler, who devoted his life to working with schizophrenics, has written a detailed description of follow-up investigations of their children (1974, 1978). Here are some of his findings:

Of the 208 Swiss schizophrenic subjects followed over a 20-year period, only half got married, producing 169 children. An additional group of 15 children were born out of wedlock. Schizophrenic women had more children than schizophrenic men; they married earlier and became ill later than the men. According to Bleuler, this is perhaps the reason that schizophrenics are more likely to have had a schizophrenic mother than a schizophrenic father—a simple result of fertility, pregnancy, and marriage.

Of the 184 children of schizophrenics, 10 became schizophrenic. Bleuler indicates that this figure coincides with other estimates, which range from 7 to 16.9 percent. He notes that children of schizophrenics are almost ten times more likely to develop schizophrenia than are children of nonschizophrenics. However, the percentage of children of schizophrenic parents who actually become schizophrenic themselves is small; and even smaller is the percentage of children with schizophrenic grandparents who become ill.

Bleuler concurs that 8 to 10 percent of the children of schizophrenics are doomed to schizophrenia but does not find support for the assertion that half to two-thirds of the other children of schizophrenics will be abnormal (even when not schizophrenic). The majority, 84 percent of married children, have sustained successful marriages. As many as 75 percent of these children are mentally sound. And of the rest, no clear-cut relationship to the disorder of their parents can be proved.

What about the familial environments that schizophrenic parents provide? Only 85 children lived with a schizophrenic parent for some substantial length of time. These limited data, however, suggest that living with a schizophrenic parent does not necessarily induce schizophrenia. Bleuler does state, however, that if there is a strong predisposition, such unfavorable circumstances might contribute to later pathology.

friendships (see Mosher, Gunderson, and Buchsbaum, 1973; Rolf and Harig, 1974; Watt, et al., 1970).

High-Risk Research and Preventive Programs

If it were possible to isolate those children we think show strong potential for becoming schizophrenic, how would we go about preventing the occurrence of later episodes? This general orientation underlies the goals of several projects designed to locate high-risk children at a sufficiently early age to thwart the emergence of the disease. The Vermont Vulnerable Child Development Project (Rolf and Harig, 1974) is an example of such intervention. These programs select high-risk children on the basis of various criteria, such as familial pathology, abnormal autonomic responses, abnormal EEG recordings, deviant behavior, and sociocultural deprivation, and then attempt, through intensive, enriched daycare and therapeutic settings to forestall illness by training these children for competence. Training for competence stresses such variables as independence, leadership, more focused attention, skills in coping with stress, skills in dealing with the irrationality of parents, playfulness and social responsiveness, communication skills, increased cognitive skills, and control of aggression (see Anthony, 1974; Garmezy, 1975; Rolf and Harrig, 1974). A warm, permissive social climate—thought to be conducive to the learning of educational and social

Spotlight 12.8 Torque and Schizophrenia: A Physical Marker?

Most people draw circles in a counterclockwise direction. Drawing circles in the opposite, or clockwise direction, is referred to as *torque,* more frequently evidenced by left-handed than by right-handed children. Torque seems to be a developmental phenomenon. It is frequently found among four-year-old children, for example, but occurs in only about 30 percent of the 16-year-olds sampled. It has also been found that aberrant behavior is more common among children who demonstrate torque than among children who do not (Blau, 1977).

These observations led to the hypothesis that the persistence of torque beyond the age of four is an indication that the brain is not developing normally. It was further hypothesized that brain abnormality indicated by the presence of torque might be related to psychopathology in general and to vulnerability to schizophrenia in particular.

To test this hypothesis, 106 children (54 no-torque and 52 torque) with an average age of nine years who had been seen for various problems during the 1960s at a psychological clinic were tracked down ten years later. Parents and/or guardians of these children were asked detailed questions about the adjustment of their child in the ten intervening years. On the basis of these interviews, each child was rated as to level of adjustment on a 9-point scale ranging from "good" to "bad." In addition, parents and guardians were asked if they had sought or obtained professional help for their child since their original contact with the clinic ten years before and, if so, what diagnosis was made.

Of the 52 children who had demonstrated torque when tested in the 1960s, 11 had since that time been diagnosed as schizophrenic. Only one of the 54 no-torque children had been so diagnosed. In addition, the torque children comprised 36 percent of the group that were given good-to-fair adjustment ratings and 77 percent of the group given poor-to-bad ratings. Thus the hypothesis that torque bears some relationship to schizophrenia, and to maladaptive behavior in general, was supported by these findings.

Blau's explanation of these findings suggests that some deviant brain organization is responsible for torque, and that its relationship to left-handedness and certain kinds of learning problems might well implicate dysfunctions in the corpus collosum, the bundle of fibers that connects the two hemispheres of the brain. Structural and functional impairments in the corpus collosum might result from various developmental problems from infancy on and could be responsible for difficulties in cognition, language skills, and other behaviors necessary for life adjustment, perhaps leaving the person more vulnerable to developing schizophrenia.

skills—is generally provided in such educational-therapeutic settings.

Whether such programs prove to be successful in preventing, or reducing the severity of, schizophrenia remains to be seen. Evaluation of the effectiveness of the specific interventive measure employed in these projects and their interactions with the temperaments and motivation of the teachers and therapists involved is a tricky business. In addition, have we selected the "right" preventive and interventive measures? We are limited by the paucity of basic knowledge about the causes of schizophrenia: how can we prevent or intervene in a process if we are not completely sure what caused it?

SUMMARY

Section I of this chapter surveyed the proliferation of hypotheses and theories that have been developed in an attempt to answer the puzzling question of the causes of schizophrenia. The material covered psychoanalytic formulations, life events and stressors as causative variables, learning models, approaches implicating familial patterns, Laingian views, and models based on parent-child interactions. This section also described physical explanations for schizophrenia—specifically, considerations having to do with genetic and biochemical variables—and presented views that attempt to integrate some of those models. Section II discussed some typical research strategies designed to unravel the mysteries of schizophrenia. These strategies deal with physiological correlates, language and communication processes, thinking, attention and stimulus processing, and various response models. Finally, the section described research focusing on identifying children at high risk for schizophrenia and on developing techniques for preventing it.

Highlights

1. The psychoanalytic formulation of schizophrenia as a defensive maneuver against overwhelming anxiety that results in regression to early infantile levels has not received strong empirical confirmation.
2. Stressors and life events, including pregnancy and birth complications, probably play only a minimal role in the etiology of schizophrenia.
3. Various learning models of schizophrenia, such as those of Mednick and of Broen and Storms, have received moderate confirmation and are of interest in the context of possible modifiability of schizophrenic behavior through learning techniques.
4. Although research and theories about whether or not schizophrenogenic families exist are methodologically innovative and interesting, on the whole, despite some positive findings, there is little definitive confirmation of the family transmission of schizophrenia.
5. Research studies have failed to demonstrate that aversively controlling mothers and harsh, depriving, even bizarre, parent-child interactions play a causative role in schizophrenia.
6. There is moderate evidence, through various adoption and twin strategies, that suggests that there is some genetic predisposition for schizophrenia. On the other hand, there is a large percentage of discordance for schizophrenia in MZ twins. The study of why one twin develops schizophrenia while the other does not may shed a great deal of light on why pathology develops in any given individual.
7. Impressive evidence suggests that there are some biochemical underpinnings of schizophrenia. Although several promising hypotheses exist concerning the neurochemical processes involved, we are far from understanding how complex neuronal systems interact with one another and how they set the stage for the expression of abnormal behavior.
8. The diathesis-stress hypothesis suggests that genetic predisposition for schizophrenia requires severe psychosocial or environmental stress and deprivation to trigger a schizophrenic episode. That is, it is the interaction between environment and endowment that is the crucial causal variable rather than either one alone. Unfortunately, numerous facts about schizophrenia—for example, that many genetically vulnerable children, even under the harshest of environmental circumstances do not develop schizophrenia—do not support this hypothesis. Zubin's vulnerability model fits the empirical data more adequately by suggesting that the common denominator among schizophrenics is vulnerability, rather than the disease itself.
9. Investigations show that schizophrenics and nonschizophrenics can be distinguished by many physical and physiological indices, such

as autonomic and electroencephalographic measures. In addition, different kinds of language, thinking, and attentional patterns have been shown not only to distinguish schizophrenics from nonschizophrenics, but also, in some instances, to distinguish among various subtypes of schizophrenics.

10. Additional research strategies that attempt to explore the enigma of schizophrenia stress a stimulus approach (for example, by demonstrating that immediate, rather than remote, stimuli are more compelling for schizophrenics) or a response approach (for example, by demonstrating that there are typical biases and patterns of responses to verbal stimuli among schizophrenic subjects). Although these models tell us much about schizophrenic performance and even offer possible avenues for modifying behavior, they do not shed direct light on the etiology of schizophrenia.
11. An entirely different approach to the study of schizophrenia emerges from the question: what are the characteristics of children who later become schizophrenic? Children-at-risk research requires longitudinal observations to determine the special characteristics, if any, of young subjects who later become schizophrenic compared to the characteristics of those who do not, even when they are at risk to do so. Both groups can be compared to low-risk subjects who never become ill. Findings from high-risk research make it possible to select and place vulnerable children in prevention programs designed to intervene in or offset the unfolding of what was once thought to be an inevitable process. Most high-risk children, however, do not become schizophrenic, even when "the dice are loaded" against them in terms of genetic predisposition and poor environmental circumstances.

ISSUES AND QUESTIONS

1. Because most of the children labeled "high risk" do not develop schizophrenia, even under the most unfavorable circumstances, such as extreme economic deprivation or parental abuse, on what basis do we intervene in their lives? Will the label adversely affect the child? How do we avoid the stigma of labeling and the inference that "tainted" genes are involved in an inevitable unfolding of a pathological process?
2. Is it possible to establish a controlled research setting in which we "treat" some high-risk children in ways that we hope will be advantageous in forestalling future pathology but do not "treat" an equivalent group of others? Is our deliberate failure to provide care for some high-risk children unethical?
3. Although one day it may be possible to control schizophrenia, our current interventive methods are not definitely validated. In this light, then, at what age should we require consent from the subjects themselves? How should we obtain the consent of parents of high-risk children we wish to include in an intervention program? If they are not themselves competent to judge the value of what we offer, should we decide ourselves?
4. What are the ethical and legal issues involved in preventing schizophrenics from marrying and having children? (Many states have such laws.) Civil rights advocates favor the individual's right to marry, have children, and conduct their lives in their own ways, even if they are regarded as mentally ill. Do you agree? If not, why?
5. Some advocates of intervention strategies avoid these issues entirely by suggesting that the rights of society far outweigh the rights of the individual in matters such as these, and that access to records, application of labels, and intervention without consent offer more to society and to individuals in the long run than does the elaborate process of obtaining consent from, say, nonconsenting parents. These activists say that there is an ethical obligation to intervene, rather than to stand by and wait, and that minimizing possible noxious influences that may

eventually be associated with schizophrenia (even when our confidence is low) is a must.

There are no easy answers to these issues. Our opinions about them are inevitably intertwined with our social and religious beliefs and with our political philosophies. Where do you stand?

SUGGESTIONS FOR FURTHER READING

Bleuler, M. *The schizophrenic disorders: Long-term patient and family studies.* New Haven: Yale University Press, 1978. This book represents the culmination of over 20 years of detailed study of 208 schizophrenic patients. The book describes the vicissitudes of the patients' lives and illness over those years and their relationships with members of their immediate families. It describes their histories in rich clinical detail and presents quantitative analyses of developmental and familial factors, hypothesized to play a significant role in the development of schizophrenia. Finally, the author presents his theories regarding the nature of schizophrenia. This outstanding scientific and clinical book is highly recommended.

Friedenberg, E. Z. *R. D. Laing.* New York: Viking, 1974. This little volume explains Laing's position in psychiatry and philosophy, with special stress on Laing's views on schizophrenia and the "game" that "sick" people play in attempts to do battle with their adversaries. Underscored is Laing's view that any attempts to understand such individuals must be based on the world as seen by *them,* not by us.

Salzinger, K. *Schizophrenia: Behavioral aspects.* New York: Wiley, 1973. Paperback. This is a relatively brief overview of theories of schizophrenia with a heavy emphasis on behavioral, learning, and stimulus models. The author's research orientation permeates this book, providing provocative ideas for further explorations that would be especially interesting for students planning to pursue careers in experimental psychopathology.

13

Organic Mental Disorders

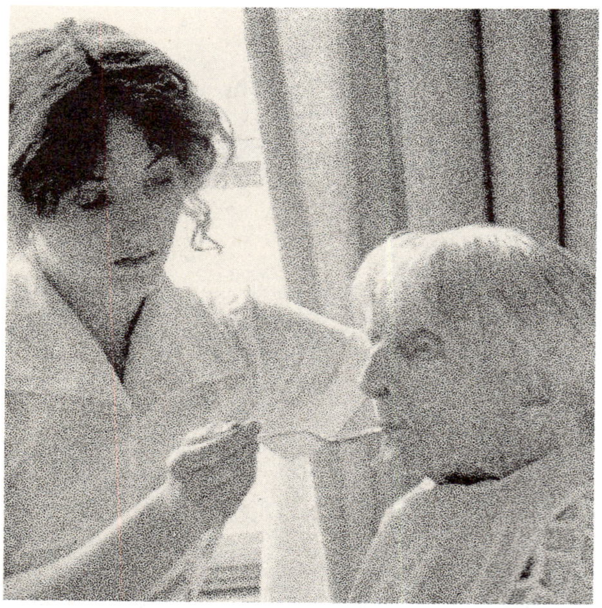

A sixty-year-old man, his wife, and one of their good friends were playing chouette, a backgammon game for three or more people. The man was the best player of the group, but that night he lost consistently. Many times during the evening he would disregard the backgammon pieces—his own and his opponents—at the extreme right of the board, missing opportunities, taking impulsive chances, and claiming victories when there were none. In the weeks to follow, his wife saw him become increasingly irritable, dependent, forgetful, and occasionally disoriented in time and space. He bumped into furniture several times, and sometimes complained of excruciatingly painful headaches. She was determined to get him "into" psychotherapy. Four months after the losing evening at the backgammon table this man died of a large, inoperable brain tumor that was undiagnosed for the first two months after the earliest symptoms appeared.

GENERAL BACKGROUND

This chapter is concerned with behavioral and emotional disorders that arise from or are associated with known physical dysfunctions of the body, especially of the central nervous system (CNS). These disorders can become evident at any time from birth to old age. It is true that some of the disorders already described may result from biochemical imbalances—certain kinds of depression, for example. But up to now, specific physical or organic impairment has been implicated only in a general way as the direct cause of the emotional disorder. The current chapter is addressed to those mental disorders for which there are specific and demonstrable physical causes such as brain tumors, toxic substances, repeated blows on the head, or cerebrovascular (having to do with blood supply to tissues of the brain) dysfunctions. Spotlight 13.1 lists some of these causes.

Spotlight 13.1 Causes of Organic Mental Disorders

The pages ahead contain descriptions of some of the clinical syndromes associated with or arising from various types of brain pathology. Many of these syndromes result from not one but several causal variables. Others have as yet unknown etiology. We cannot always pinpoint the causes of many organic mental disorders. Even when we can do so, we have much to learn about prevention and treatment. Some of these causes are clearly environmental, for example, gunshot wounds or bacterial infections, but many organic disorders are not so easily classified. The following are broad causal categories that are neither mutually exclusive nor clearly environmental or constitutional.

1. The most frequent cause of organic mental disorders is some *deficiency in the blood supply to the brain.* The brain requires one-fifth of the blood and oxygen supply of the rest of the body (Kety, 1979). These vascular dysfunctions eventually cause tissue damage and if widespread, may lead to death. Blood supply or nutriments to the brain can be curtailed by atherosclerosis, an accumulation of deposits on the walls of cerebral blood vessels that causes narrowing of the passages through which blood to that particular area of the brain can flow; cerebrovascular accidents (CVAs or "strokes") or cerebral hemorrhage resulting from a rupture of the wall of a blood vessel; high blood pressure which can interfere with the normal structures of the brain and its blood vessels; physical damage to brain tissue through tumors, blows, and wounds; cerebral thrombosis (blood clot); or cerebral embolism (any foreign matter such as an air bubble) in a blood vessel.

2. *Bacterial, viral, and other infectious conditions* contribute to a significant portion of neurological (CNS) disorders, many of which can now be treated with impressive results.

3. *Toxic states* refer to the behavioral, mental, or physiological symptoms that result from the ingestion of noxious drugs or fluids (for example, alcohol, lead vapor, or manganese) that have either a temporary or a permanent deleterious effect on the CNS.

4. *Biochemical and neurophysiological dysfunctions* account for a wide array of brain disorders. These dysfunctions include endocrinological and metabolic disturbances (such as thyroid dysfunctions) and nutritional and vitamin deficiencies (examples include pellagra, a deficiency of niacin, or beriberi, a deficiency of thiamin). We are learning a good deal more about nutritional deficiencies through studies of malnourished, low-birthweight children in developing nations (Pincus and Tucker, 1978).

It may be that many of the mental disorders described in this chapter, if fully understood, result from some "misinformation" or miscommunication among brain cells through excesses or insufficiencies in neurotransmitters and other mediator substances, for example, hormones (see Rubenstein, 1980). Some evidence already suggests that this biochemical approach, focusing on impaired communications among cells, is a valid explanation for diseases of hitherto unknown etiology such as Parkinson's or Huntington's disease (see later sections) (Mann et al., 1980).

Psychologists and organic mental disorders. The role of the psychologist in the diagnosis of brain disorder has diminished somewhat in the past decade because of remarkable technological advances—for example, in radiological (X-ray) and computer methods that do the job with greater precision (see Spotlight 13.4). Yet, psychologists can tell us a great deal about brain-behavior relationships by measuring the effects of brain damage on the patient's skills, general behavior, emotions, and mental status. They not only offer us techniques for assessing the patient's performance, but also they are equipped to develop special methods for the restoration of skills that are lost as a result of brain injury.

Sociocultural Considerations. Social conditions may predispose an individual for "diminished integrity of the brain," a point that has been made many times earlier in this book. Diminished integrity may range from lowered learning ability to severe brain impairment and mental retardation (see next chapter). In other words, children born into extreme poverty are much more likely to be positioned at the high-risk end of a life-health-disease-death spectrum than are other children. Why this is so is not difficult to understand. The conditions that are associated with brain disorders include many obvious ones such as birth complications, poor maternal health or alcoholism during pregnancy, drug addiction, disease, increased possibility of gunshot wounds, and similar circumstances that have a "differential social distribution"—that is, that are more likely to be present in low-SES groups than in other social groups. Added to these hazardous conditions of poverty are the nutritional insufficiencies that may also contribute to brain dysfunction (Wurtman and Wurtman, 1977). Yet, many of the organic syndromes described in this chapter—pathological aging, for example—do not bear a direct relationship to SES and cultural variables. As a matter of fact, the precise etiology of many of the organic mental syndromes described in this chapter is still not entirely clear.

THE CLINICAL SYNDROMES: MAJOR ORGANIC MENTAL DISORDERS

Senile and Presenile Dementias

Most experts agree that the fourth or fifth leading cause of death in the United States is senile dementia, preceded only by such killers as cancer or heart disease. Estimates range from one to four or so million people afflicted with senility, roughly 15 to 25 percent of the over-sixty-five population. About 30 percent of the over-eighty population suffers with this disease (Pincus and Tucker, 1978). As the life span increases, however, these figures are expected to rise.

What are the symptoms and what is the course of this syndrome? Senile dementia is a chronic, progressive (worsening) condition, in which a steady, relentless deterioration of cognitive, physical, and bodily functions takes place. Early symptoms include memory lapses, mild personality changes,

Spotlight 13.2 Organic Mental Disorders Described in Chapter 13 and the DSM-III Categories

Syndromes Described in Chapter 13

1. The senile and presenile dementias
2. Other degenerative diseases
3. Syndromes associated with metabolic and endocrinological dysfunctions
4. Syndromes associated with infectious diseases
5. Toxic syndromes
6. Syndromes associated with brain tumors (neoplasms)
7. Syndromes associated with trauma to the head and brain
8. Organic personality syndrome
9. Convulsive (seizure) disorders
10. The aphasias

DSM-III Organic Mental Disorders—the Dementias Arising in the Senium and Presenium

Primary Degenerative Dementia
- Senile onset (after age sixty-five)
- Presenile onset (age sixty-five and below)
- Multi-infarct dementia
  - Subtypes of categories of dementia:
    - with delirium
    - with delusions
    - with depression
    - uncomplicated

DSM-III Organic Brain Syndromes

These syndromes refer to behavioral states that are substance induced* or associated with various physical conditions such as diabetes, thyroid imbalances, gunshot wounds, brain tumors, extensive brain surgery, and infectious diseases. They are classified by their major behavioral (symptomatic) characteristics as follows:

1. *Delirium* is an acute condition with generally rapid onset, usually of brief duration of about one week; if the underlying condition is corrected or self-limited, recovery can be complete. A primary criterion for delirium is a clouding of consciousness (reduced clarity of awareness of the environment) with lowered attentional skills; additional characteristics are perceptual disturbances, illusions, hallucinations, incoherent speech, insomnia or daytime drowsiness, increased or decreased motor activity, disorientation, and memory impairment.

2. *Dementia* is, essentially, a loss of intellectual abilities of sufficient severity as to interfere with social or occupational functioning; primary characteristics include memory impairment, disturbances in abstract thinking, judgment, and various other disturbances in higher cortical functions; there may be personality changes that reflect an accentuation of premorbid traits. Although dementia is primarily associated with irreversible changes in the CNS leading to death, in many instances of treatable dementia, for example, hypothyroidism, the condition can be arrested or reversed.

3. *Amnestic syndrome* is characterized by short- and long-term memory impairment with difficulty in learning new material and retaining it; sometimes memory for the remote past is much better than for the immediate past. Disorientation and confabulation (the relating of fictitious events to fill in memory gaps) often accompany lack of insight into the severe memory loss. The amnestic syndrome (formerly called Korsakoff's disease) is most frequently associated with chronic alcohol use and thiamine deficiency.

4. *The delusional syndrome* is characterized by the presence of delusions in a state of wakefulness

* Conditions that are specifically ascribed to excessive ingestion of substances such as alcohol, the amphetamines, LSD, heroin, and PCP are described in Chapters 16 and 17.

or alertness; these delusions can be crude or highly organized and may be associated with mild cognitive impairment. Hallucinations are not prominent in the clinical picture.

5. *Hallucinosis* is a condition of persistent, recurrent, "wakeful" hallucinations, often auditory but occurring in any sensory modality depending on the cause. Certain drugs typically cause visual hallucinations (LSD, for example), whereas others typically cause auditory ones (alcohol, for example).

6. *The affective syndrome* refers to disturbances in mood that are similar to the depressive or manic states described in Chapter 10 but having a specific organic etiology such as a toxic condition or a hormonal dysfunction, for example, excessive steroids or hypothyroidism.

7. *The organic personality syndrome* refers to personality changes that possess distinctive patterns reflecting specific organic pathology, usually structural damage to the brain due to tumors or head trauma; most often, this category refers to frontal-lobe involvements (see p. 343) but other causes can also be involved. Typically, characteristics of this syndrome include emotional lability (explosive temper outbursts, for example), difficulties in impulse control, poor social judgment, sexual indiscretions, apathy and indifference, and suspiciousness or paranoid ideation.

8. *Intoxication* is a condition arising from recent or currently ingested noxious substances (for example, an amphetamine) that have abnormal effects on the CNS; this toxic state is transient, generally reversible, and disappears entirely when the substance is metabolized. Intoxication is not diagnosed in the case of social or recreational use of drugs such as alcohol if there is no maladaptive behavior. Disturbances include those of perception, wakefulness, attention, thinking, judgment, emotional control (e.g., aggression, picking fights), and motor behavior.

9. *Withdrawal* refers to various behavioral and physical conditions associated with the reduction or termination of the ingestion of certain toxic substances such as alcohol or heroin after prolonged use. Symptoms, which are often specific to the substance, include anxiety, restlessness, irritability, insomnia, and impaired attention; they can be rather extreme, as after prolonged alcohol or heroin use.

and apathy. Soon the patient suffers extensive memory loss, especially for recent events; disorientation of time, place, and person; loss of interest in surrounding situations; and nonrecognition of the familiar. Depression, paranoid symptoms, and anxiety may also appear at this time. Later stages include inability to care for oneself, incontinence, hallucinations, and delusions. At the end, the by-now-bedridden senile patient is in a vegetative state, dying in a mental hospital or nursing home.

At the age of seventy-five years, the brain generally weighs only about 55 percent of the weight of the brain of a young adult (Kolb, 1973). The young adult's brain contains about 12 billion neurons. With age, the brain shrinks because of the death of about 100,000 neurons daily. These cells are never replaced. This is a normal process and the large majority of elderly people are not senile, although they certainly may be depressed and lonely.

What causes the normal aging process to become disrupted, yielding the pathological picture just described, is not entirely known, nor is it known why more women than men, independently of the greater life span of women, become senile (Altman, 1977). Today, scientists are beginning to obtain a clearer picture of possible explanations.

In the living brain, through methods such as the CAT scan (see Spotlight 13.4) which provides a computerized X-ray glimpse of the brain, or through autopsic examination, for example with the use of the electron microscope, significant differences between the neuronal structures in the brains of senile and nonsenile subjects have been found, including a loss of neurons, and atrophy and other kinds of cellular changes (Heston, 1976). Current data also suggest that in the normal brain there are

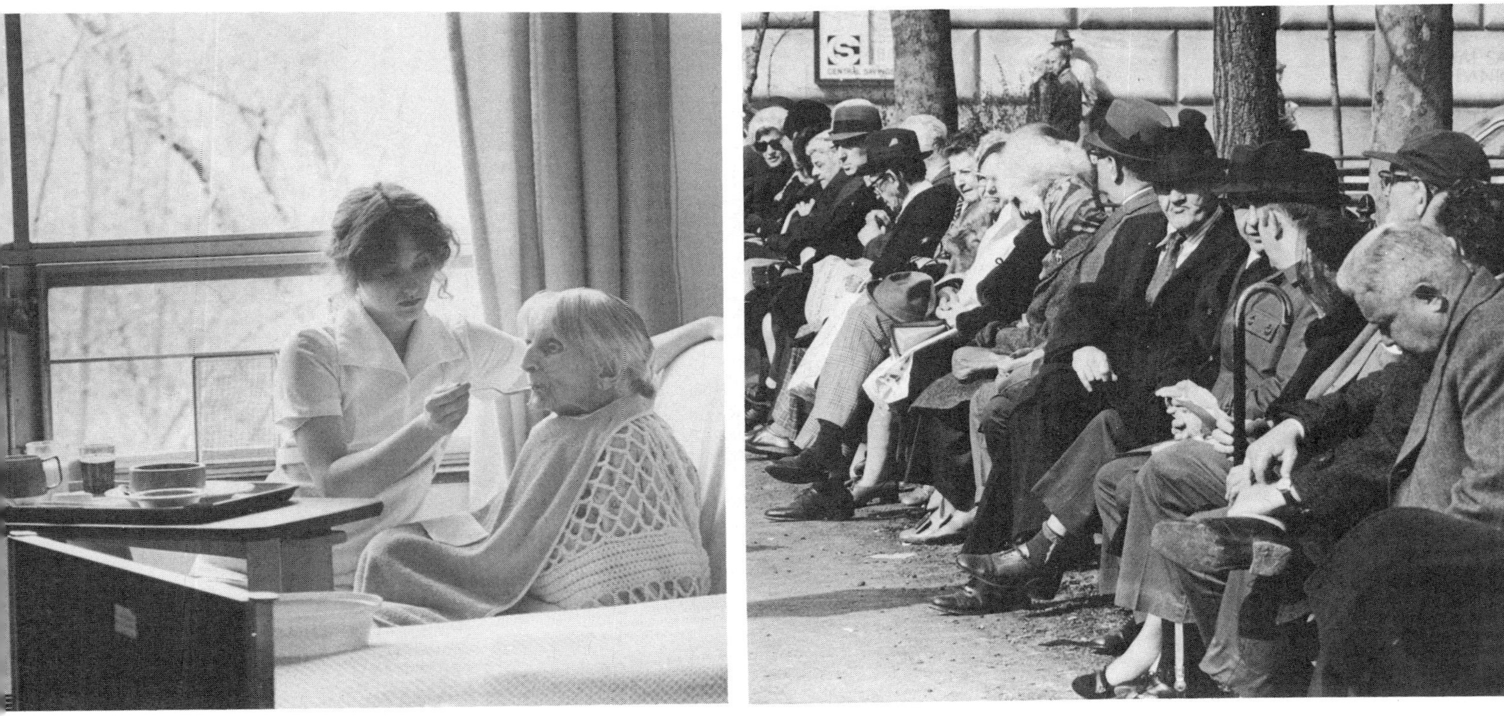

Not all elderly people are senile, but many are depressed and lonely. (Left: Jim Harrison/Stock, Boston. Right: A. Keler/Sygma)

two types of neuron, one with dying or shrinking dendritic "trees" and another with growing dendritic "trees" (see Figure 7.1) (Buell and Coleman, 1979). With age there is an increasing preponderance of the dying group. But in the senile population, the rate at which the dying group becomes preponderant is speeded up.

Why these differences occur is still being explored. One hypothesis implicates a slow-acting virus that may take years to incubate, that is, the virus is dormant for decades before symptoms appear (Kety, 1979). Other models suggest that genetic predisposition (Heston, 1976), infectious disease, or chronic toxicity as a result of excessive alcohol ingestion may be involved (Katzman, Terry, and Bick, 1978). Gaining favor are hypotheses that stress biochemical abnormalities that affect the production of essential neurotransmitters in the brain (Katzman, Terry, and Bick, 1978; Kolata, 1981). If any one of these hypotheses proves to be accurate, then one day it may be possible to find the effective prevention or control, for example through a combination of neurochemicals that can replace or manufacture the needed deficiencies within the body. In the meanwhile there is little we can do about the devastating effects of the dementias.

Presenile and other dementias. Presenile dementias are distinguished from the senile forms primarily in terms of age of onset, with the age of sixty-five years being the approximate cut-off point. Alzheimer's disease, named after Alois Alzheimer, who described this syndrome in 1907, is indistinguishable from the senile type in symptoms and brain changes, but is diagnosed when onset is younger than sixty-five years of age. Onset can occur as

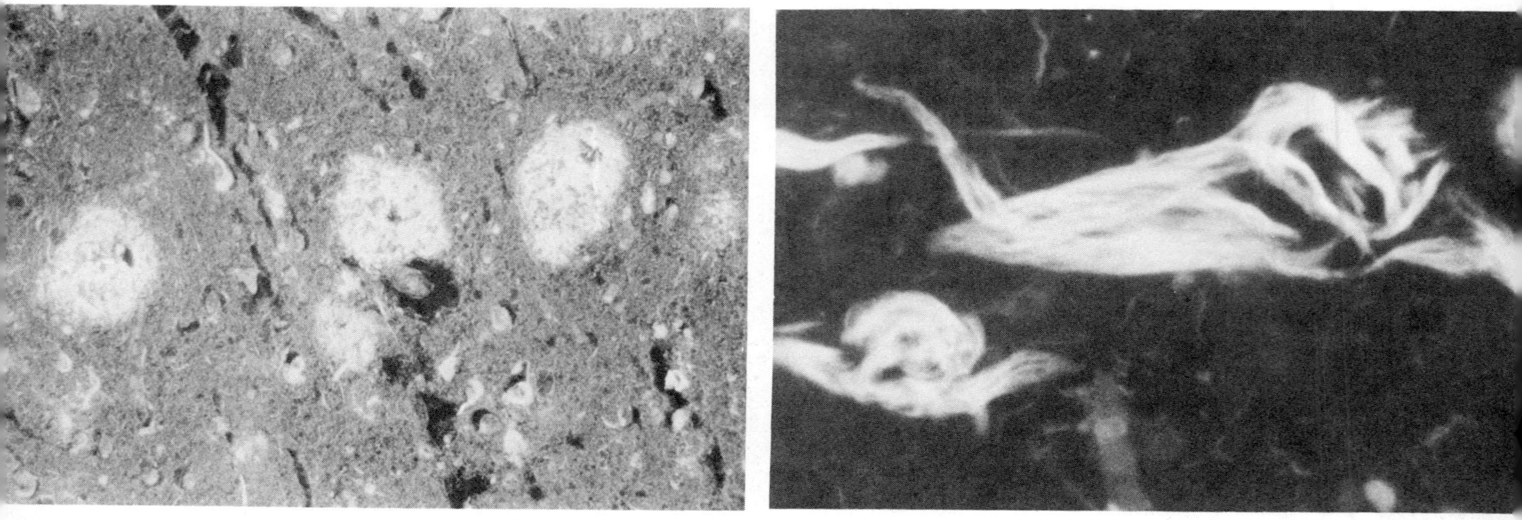

Photomicrographs of plaques (left) and tangles (right) in the brains of Alzheimer patients. (Dr. Robert Terry, Professor and Chairman, Department of Pathology, Albert Einstein College of Medicine)

young as the forties or fifties. Pick's disease, first described in 1892, resembles the course of the senile and presenile dementias in many ways but differs from the usual dementias in anatomical aspects of brain pathology.

Multi-infarct dementias. The DSM-III distinguishes this rare form of dementia from the senile and presenile forms already noted. These dementias are thought to have an earlier onset than the dementias just described; they result chiefly from a series of cardiovascular accidents that have a cumulative effect on brain tissue.

Other Degenerative Diseases

Huntington's disease (Huntington's chorea). A rare, inherited disorder (about 5 per 100,000 in the general population), this condition is found throughout the world. It wreaks progressive, irreversible damage to the CNS, eventually resulting in dementia, helplessness, and death in about fifteen years after onset. Symptoms first appear when the "carrier" (the person who transmits the disease) is an adult, between the ages of thirty to fifty years, and there is currently no known prevention or treatment for their degenerative course. The genetic transmission leads inevitably to atrophy and degeneration of neuronal brain structures, including those in the frontal cortex. In addition to marked personality changes that include severe emotional problems, depression, and suicidal ideation and acts (Pincus and Tucker, 1978), there are ceaseless choreic movements—jerky or writhing motions of the face and extremities.

There is no known method that can identify the carrier. As a result, the dominant trait is unwittingly transmitted to 50 percent of the patient's offspring before the disease appears. Is there some indirect method for identifying a carrier? A follow-up (retrospective) study of 60 potential victims—one parent already had the disease at the time of initial testing 15–20 years earlier—suggests that even before actual symptoms in these offspring are expressed, there may be a measurable deficit in cognitive performance (Lyle and Gottesman, 1979). In

Case 13.1 Huntington's Disease

The first distinctive description of the disease was given in 1872 by Dr. George Huntington, whose father and grandfather had practiced medicine at East Hampton, Long Island, for a period conjointly covering 78 years and had observed families among the adult members of which an incurable chores had existed for generations. . . .

The onset of Huntington's chorea is insidious and, generally speaking, occurs between the ages of 30 and 45 years. Frequently a change of character antedates or accompanies the appearance of the choreiform symptoms. The patient may be irritable, obstinate, and moody and lack initiative. In other cases the picture may be one of fatuous euphoria. Esthetic and ethical senses are blunted. Many patients become fault-finding, spiteful, irascible, and even destructive and assaultive. These emerging personality traits adversely affect their relations in marriage, their family, and their vocation. There is an increasing lack of spontaneity in activity, of concern as to the disease, and of solicitude as to obligations of conscience, affection, or ideals. Suspiciousness, jealousy, anmd paranoid trends, even to the extent of well-developed delusions of persecution, appear. Some patients experience hallucinations. With the increasing emotional deterioration, there is a coincident impairment of attention, memory, and judgment. Interest in life becomes progressively narrower. There is also a poverty of ideas and a disorderliness of thought. The dementia may become extreme.

Before the choreiform movements are clearly manifest and as muscle tone increases, with twitching, bobbing movements, and inability to remain still, accidents are frequent, owing to falls or collisions with objects. Complaints of soreness and stiffness of joints, weakness, and arthritis are common at this stage.

The choreiform movements usually appear first in the upper extremity, neck, and face. These involuntary movements are clumsy, irregular, jerky, stretching ones. In the early stages it appears as if the patient were merely inattentive or careless in his movements, which gradually increase in intensity and in coordination. The contractions of the facial muscles result in grimaces while those of the tongue, lips, and respiratory muscles lead to a hesitating, explosive, poorly articulated type of speech which, in advanced cases, is difficult to understand. The choreiform movements result in a shuffling, dancing type of gait associated with irregular movements of the trunk. The movements usually cease during sleep. As the disease progresses, there is interference with swallowing, walking becomes impossible, and the patient may become bedridden. . . . Suicide is not uncommon.

Source: L. C. Kolb, *Modern clinical psychiatry,* 8th ed. (Philadelphia: Saunders, 1973), pp. 301–302.

this study, the largest deficit, as indicated by such tests as the Bender Visual Motor Gestalt and the Wechsler Intelligence scales, appeared for those who were soon to show symptoms. The least deficit was shown by those who were still normal at the time of the follow-up testing. Whether or not this kind of indirect prediction, based on test performance, will be useful depends on future research that employs considerably larger samples, long-range follow-up, and crossvalidation to determine whether or not results hold up with new samples. There may be some promise in this approach, especially if more precise, direct physical predictors or markers are not found.

Parkinson's disease. Another progressive, degenerative, deteriorating disease of unknown origin was first described in 1817 by James Parkinson, who was himself afflicted with this disease. About 50,000 people each year in this country become afflicted with Parkinson's disease (Kety, 1979). The overwhelming disabilities of its victims, however, are now dramatically reduced because of great advances in pharmacological treatment.

Symptoms, which generally manifest themselves in midlife, first appear as involuntary rhythmic movements of the arms, especially while at rest, which later spread to the legs, neck, and jaw. There is increased muscle tone resulting in rigidity of pos-

Spotlight 13.3 The Gilles de la Tourette Syndrome: A Nondegenerative Neurological Disorder

A few years ago, the *New York Times* ("Bizarre outbursts. . . .," 1975) described two women—an elderly mother and her middle-aged daughter—who had been leisurely strolling down the street, arm-in-arm. Suddenly, the daughter stopped and exploded with a stream of obsenities. She was gesturing excitedly and seemed out of control, with arms jerking and body twisting. This woman was suffering from Gilles de la Tourette's syndrome, a rather rare disease with onset in childhood, generally between the ages of two and four years. At first there may be only facial tics. In the course of this illness, these involuntary movements cover a wider area, for example, the shoulder and arms. There is poor coordination, sometimes accompanied by grunts, barks, and unprovoked obscene utterances that are extremely embarrassing to the patient, who has no control over them.

The pattern of bizarre behavior described above for many years was thought to result from a variation of schizophrenia, especially because there were periods of remission in the course of the illness. For many years, Gilles de la Tourette's syndrome was unsuccessfully treated by psychotherapy, hypnosis, or behavior modification methods—attempts to deal with it only as a *psychological* disorder. Today, however, researchers think that biochemical (possibly dopamine?) dysfunctions in brain processes, together with inherited disposition and psychological factors such as stress, contribute to its expression (Goforth, 1974; Perera, 1975). The patient suffers no intellectual deterioration in this neurological disorder and responds dramatically to medication (haloperidol).

ture; difficulty in initiating and ending voluntary motions such as walking; often immobilized, expressionless facial features; and rigid, bent-over gait characterized by extremely small, shuffling steps. Although there are generally no symptoms such as disorientation or decreased cognitive skills, emotional problems may occur such as depression, anxiety, and helplessness.

Parkinsonism has been attributed to many causes such as encephalitis (acute inflammation of the brain) or metabolic defects. An increasingly popular etiological hypothesis suggests that a slow-acting virus is the cause (Pincus and Tucker, 1978). Eventually, whatever the cause, damage to neural tissues focuses on lower brain centers that control movement and involves destruction of the dopamine pathways to the brain. Dopamine is an important neurotransmitter, as we have already seen. Although dopamine cannot enter the brain directly, a precursor chemical, called L-DOPA, can enter the brain directly if administered orally. This chemical is then transformed into the needed dopamine, resulting in control and reduction of the dramatic symptoms of Parkinson's disease in the majority of cases. Although dosages of L-DOPA have to be extremely large, resulting in occasional side effects such as nausea, confusion, psychotic episodes, agitation, and in some instances, choreiform movements such as those described above (Pincus and Tucker, 1978), it has been of enormous significance in making ordinary living—job, marriage, daily activities—possible for countless victims of this disease.

Parkinson's disease provides a perfect example of the control of a degenerative disease through understanding some of the biochemical mechanisms involved in its expression. It is possible that Huntington's disease as well as the previously mentioned senile dementias can also one day be controlled—perhaps even prevented—through similar research efforts.

Syndromes Associated with Metabolic and Endocrinological Disorders

Some disorders can be ascribed to *specific* metabolic and endocrinological deficiencies or dysfunctions. However, many of the other disorders described in this chapter may also result from biochemical dysfunctions.

Certain vitamin deficiencies, if extreme enough, can result in dramatic clinical syndromes. One of these, Wernicke's disease, is found largely among chronic alcoholics in whom there is a thiamine and niacin deficiency. Wernicke's disease involves memory loss and confabulation, various ocular disturbances, and eventual dementia.

A fairly well-known syndrome resulting from endocrinological dysfunction is Graves' disease, a result of hyperthyroidism (an excess of thyroid hormone in the blood). Behaviors associated with Graves' disease include hypermotility, anxiety, vigilance (overalertness), and excitability. In extreme cases, excitement, manic or paranoid states, acute delirium, or systematized delusions may appear.

In these endocrinological and metabolic disorders, the pathological condition generally disappears when the deficiency is balanced. However, some cases may be too advanced to be reversible.

Syndromes Associated with Infectious Diseases

The *New York Times* (Altman, 1980) recently reported worldwide concern about an infectious disease that was devastating livestock throughout Africa and that was threatening to affect humans on an epidemic scale. On the human level, symptoms include headache, malaise, muscle ache, blindness, and in some cases, encephalitis (inflammation of the brain). This is a viral disease, researchers discovered, mostly transmitted by mosquitos. But the virus can be inhaled directly, and might even be transmitted through ticks and other insects.

The *New York Times* was describing a disease that is typical of a wide variety of other diseases that are caused by viral, bacterial, or protozoan agents. These agents are easily transmitted to humans through ticks, mosquitos, parasites, or directly through personal contact (sexual contact, for example). What concerns us currently is that a large number of these microorganisms can infect or inflame brain tissue directly (as in Rocky Mountain spotted fever or African "sleeping sickness"), resulting in a wide array of mental symptoms that can include severe headache, disorientation, loss of judgment, delirium, hallucinations, memory impairment, seizures (see pp. 343–45), aggressive outbursts, and even coma and death if they are not brought under control. Fortunately the incidence of many of these diseases has diminished dramatically as a result of early detection, advances in immunological methods, and the development of powerful drugs such as the antibiotics. Generally, the mental conditions just described clear up when the infection is treated, and there are little or no residual effects if the treatment is introduced in the early stages of the illness.

An important infectious disease that in advanced stages can result in serious CNS damage is syphilis. This infection is caused by a spirochete, *Treponema pallidum,* one of several spiral-shaped bacteria, usually transmitted through sexual contact. In the past, patients suffering from the more advanced stages of this venereal disease had accounted for 10 to 20 percent of admissions to mental facilities (Golden, Strider, et al., 1979), but with the advent of powerful antibiotic treatment methods, the number of patients at the advanced stages of this disease (neurosyphilis) has decreased sharply to about 1 percent (Kolb, 1973).

Neurosyphilis interests us once more because of the rapid increase in sexual activity and in venereal disease and the possibility that there are new bacterial strains that are resistant to ordinary treatment methods (Golden, Strider, et al., 1979). As a result, there may be a rise in frequency of the last stages of syphilis (the infection remains dormant or resting, without symptoms, for years), which, if untreated or treated too late, ends in progressive neurological degeneration, dementia, and death. How does this final stage of meningoencephalitis,* sometimes called general paresis, general paralysis of the insane, or dementia paralytica, develop?

After the initial stage, which involves a chancre or sore (usually in membranes such as those in the genitals) that disappears after several weeks, a general rash appears that also eventually disappears. In the majority of cases, invasion by the spirochete is controlled by the body's own system, so that only in a minority of cases (about 10 percent) do the powerful bacteria infect the CNS, penetrating the blood-brain barrier very slowly, over a period of many years.

The asymptomatic stage, in which the primary syphilitic condition seems under control or eliminated entirely, is actually a latent period or period of incubation that can last from ten to twenty years, and in a small number of cases, even longer. The earliest symptoms of neurosyphilis are personality-behavioral ones such as depression, neglect of attire and personal grooming, fatigue, irritability, and argumentativeness. Soon follow loss of concentration, periods of confusion, sometimes grandiosity and expansiveness, and occasionally delusions. These symptoms are succeeded by rapid deterioration in personality, memory, orientation, judgment, and other intellectual skills. There may be convulsions and stupor; eventually, coma and death bring the untreated disease to its conclusion.

If not treated (penicillin is the preferred treatment), general paresis results in death two to five years after the first symptoms of the final stage appear. If treatment comes too late, the disease leaves permanent effects such as memory impairment and various other cognitive deficits. The final stages of syphilis will undoubtedly continue to be rare but earlier, more frequently occurring stages of general paresis may be confused with other mental disturbances and thus not be properly diagnosed and treated. For this reason, most mental facilities routinely check for this infection in all new admissions.

* The first part of this word derives from meningitis, which is an inflammation of the membranes of the brain or spinal cord.

Toxic Syndromes

Lewis Carroll's character, the Mad Hatter, was probably developed around the knowledge that one of the hazards of eighteenth- and ninteenth-century hatmaking was exposure of workers to mercury derivatives, resulting in mercury poisoning. Some of the symptoms that arose were tremors of the lips, tongue, and limbs, muscle weakness, apathy, memory impairment, loss of confidence, and angry outbursts (Kety, 1979; Kolb, 1973).

There are many other toxic chemicals that, when ingested, can cause serious mental symptoms ranging from mild intoxication, confusion, suspiciousness, and disorientation to acute excitement, panic, paranoid ideation, and delirium. These symptoms may subside when the poison is metabolized, or there can be permanent symptoms as a result of repeated ingestion of the toxic substance. Some acute toxic states are difficult to differentiate from the so-called "functional" psychoses such as schizophrenia. One such example is amphetamine psychosis—a condition of heightened suspiciousness with marked delusional symptomatology, induced by excessive amphetamine use.*

Exposure to dangerous noxious chemicals can be unwitting, as in the case of workers exposed to mercury or manganese used in manufacturing processes; or accidental, as in the case of children raiding the medicine cabinet. A fairly large number of toxic reactions are self-induced—through abuse of so-called recreational drugs, excessive use of self-

* Toxic states due to excessive use or abuse of "recreational" drugs such as alcohol and the amphetamines are described more fully in Chapters 16 and 17.

medications, or ingestion of drugs in a failed suicide attempt. In addition, some toxic states can be created by a doctor's prescription of powerful medications such as cortisone or one of the psychoactive drugs.

It is possible to control or prevent exposure to many noxious chemicals. An example is lead poisoning, an occupational hazard of workers in the painting or building trades, who could become poisoned through inhalation of lead vapor used in their materials before lead was prohibited by law from being used in paint. Children who have ingested old paint peelings and chips from woods and painted surfaces in apartments that have been painted with paints containing lead can also show a chronic syndrome that researchers claim to have long-range effects. These include impairment in growth and attentional skills, learning disabilities, and general behavior difficulties. Repeated, excessive ingestion of this material can lead to irreversible brain damage, even death.

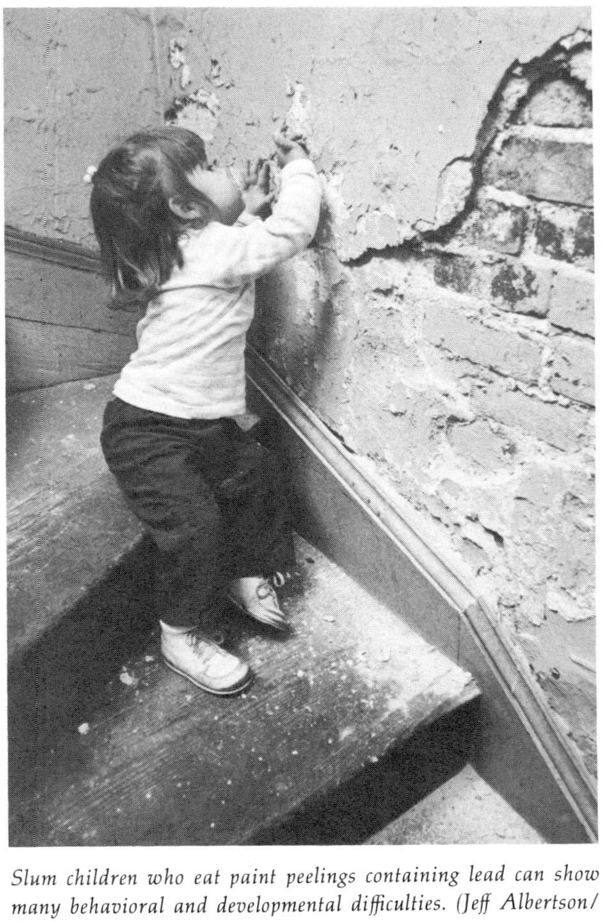

Slum children who eat paint peelings containing lead can show many behavioral and developmental difficulties. (Jeff Albertson/Stock, Boston)

Syndromes Associated with Brain Tumors

Tumors (neoplasms, or abnormal growths) of the brain can be malignant—growing and destroying healthy tissue in their wake—or benign. Even benign tumors can cause disruption in normal brain functions. Upon autopsy, 2 to 3 percent of patients in mental and other types of hospitals have been found to have abnormal growths of the brain, according to Kolb (1973), possibly accounting for at least some of their mental symptoms. Although advanced methods in diagnosis, determination of exact location, surgical treatment, and control (for example through cobalt treatment) of such tumors have reduced the disabilities and deaths attributed to them, brain tumors continue to account for a significant portion of organic mental difficulties.

Early symptoms of brain tumors vary according to their location, and can include headache, vomiting, dizziness, a number of ocular symptoms, some disorientation, motor difficulties or memory impairment, as well as specific neurological and electroencephalographic (EEG) signs (see Spotlight 13.4) that reflect damage to healthy brain tissue. Even before some of these symptoms make their presence known, some personality changes might be evidenced, for example, irritability, fear of the unknown, increased sloppiness in attire, or angry outbursts. Later, if the damage is widespread, patterns or syndromes of deficits and disabilities emerge, depending, generally, on the location of the tumor (see page 343). For example, advanced occipital lobe tumors may be accompanied by visual hallucinations such as flashes of colored lights, frontal lobe

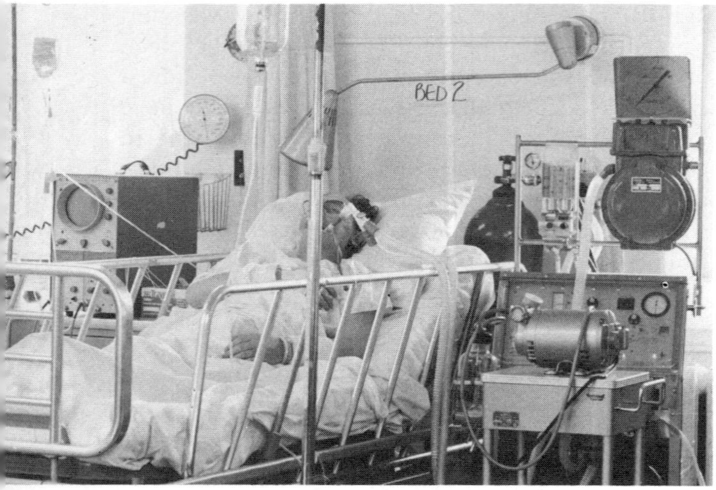

This comatose, terminally ill patient is being kept alive by various life-support systems. At what point, if at all, should the question of "pulling the plug" arise? And who is to make the decision? (Jan Lukas/Photo Researchers)

tumors by poor social judgment and poor impulse control, and tumors on the undersurfaces of the cerebral hemispheres by olfactory hallucinations.

Syndromes Associated with Trauma to the Head and Brain

Traumatic organic syndromes are behavioral states ensuing from various kinds of blows and injuries to the head through falls, automobile accidents, industrial accidents, prizefighting and other athletic events, fights, and extreme exposure to electricity. Depending on the extent of the injury and nature of tissue damage, symptoms can range from temporary confusion and disorientation to "secondary" chronic syndromes that persist over many years. An example of the latter is the "punch-drunk" ex-prizefighter who shows a chronic posttraumatic syndrome characterized by impairment in coordination, attention, and concentration, thickness of speech, silliness, and general disorientation.

After a traumatic event there may be concussion, a brief disruption of cerebral processes with a period of unconsciousness followed by complete recovery. There may be, however, a short period of confusion and disorientation and a gradual reduction of symptoms, a period that may last for several weeks. During this time there may be dizziness, concentration difficulties, memory difficulties, or lowered tolerance for loud noise and extreme light. Some traumatic events, however, result in coma, during which there is no response to stimulation—a period that may last for several hours, days, weeks, or months. Coma generally implies that there has been brain-tissue damage (tears or lacerations or capillary hemorrhages called contusions). The patient may have periods of semicomatose or stuperous responses to stimuli but then will return to a comatose state. Consciousness may clear completely after periods of stupor, delir-

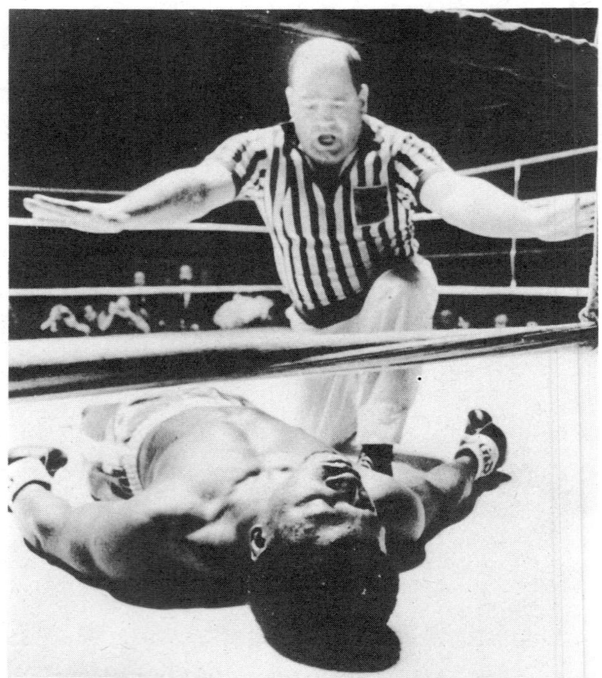

This prizefighter may be lucky. Others can show, after repeated blows to the head, a posttraumatic syndrome characterized by "punch drunk" behavior. (United Press International Photo)

ium, or amnesia as the patient emerges from coma, or the comatose state may continue, ending in a vegetative plateau or death.

An Organic Personality Syndrome?

The DSM-III lists a diagnostic category called organic personality syndrome. Is there an "organic personality"? Yes, according to many clinicians, referring to a constellation of traits called the frontal-lobe syndrome. This group of personality characteristics appears with some frequency among patients who have suffered destruction of cortical tissue of the frontal lobe through surgery, injury, or tumor (see page 350). The frontal-lobe syndrome generally consists of impairment in impulse control, poor social judgment, lack of planning ability, limited concern with the consequences of one's acts, apathy and indifference, occasional suspiciousness, temper outbursts, and often little or no cognitive impairment. Relatives of "frontal-lobe" patients speak of an unexplainable change from the premorbid personality.

In addition to the frontal-lobe syndrome, other clinicians refer to the catastrophic reaction of brain-damaged patients to their injury—a global response to awareness of limitations, disabilities, and inability to cope with all the attendant ambiguities and confusions that surround them. This total bewilderment presumably cuts across the personalities of *all* brain-injured people, according to early researchers like Goldstein (1942) and Goldstein and Scheerer (1941). There is an accompanying concrete attitude, consisting of rigidity, inflexibility, and stubborn adherence to the familiar—all aspects of the injured individual's attempt to achieve mastery over his or her world.

Today, clinicians who work with brain-injured individuals are not so willing to assume that all brain-injured people show similar patterns in personal response to their deficits. Although the frontal-lobe syndrome, the catastrophic reaction, Graves' disease (hyperthyroidism) syndrome, and the concrete attitudes of some brain-damaged persons can be clearly identified, there is no one personality syndrome that cuts across all types of brain damage. There is an extremely wide range of personal responses to brain injury, more so than was once thought to be the case. (At one point, people referred to specific syndromes associated with specific kinds of dysfunctions, for example, the "epileptic personality," which was thought to be explosive, shallow, unpredictable, and egocentric.)

It seems highly likely that the premorbid personality of the injured individual and his or her typical defenses shape the responses to the threat and stress of injury and lowered capacity to cope. Symptoms can include depression, a sense of helplessness and powerlessness, great reliance on orderliness and meticulousness, or enormous energy thrown into strategies for hiding and covering up the deficit. Anger, anxiety, paranoid vigilance, terror in new situations, and childish dependency are other possible symptoms. The clinician working with a brain-damaged patient in attempts to restore lost functions cannot ignore the personal responses to threat that each individual makes, even though in instances of severe frontal-lobe damage or specific endocrinological dysfunction, for example, some common denominators may be found.

Convulsive (Seizure) Disorders: The Epilepsies

Epilepsy is not one disease entity but is, rather, a "catch-all" name for a group of disorders that have, as a primary symptom, various types of convulsions or seizures. It is estimated that there are about two million epileptics in this nation (Sauer, 1979). Generally, we can say that epilepsy is characterized by the abnormal simultaneous rhythmic firing of a large number of neurons spread over a relatively large area of "normal" neurons (Kety, 1979). This firing triggers the seizures. The causes of such widespread neuronal activity are not actually known, but there are several reasonable hypotheses that might explain some of the different epilepsies.*

* What was once called idiopathic epilepsy is not a diagnosis or even a description but rather a general reference to seizure states with no known cause.

A small percentage of epilepsies can actually be traced to scar tissue in the brain as a result of injury such as automobile accidents, infection, prenatal or perinatal damage, and brain tumors; the scar tissue becomes the focal point of the abnormal electrical activity. But this is not the case for most epilepsies (Kety, 1979). Most of these disorders, it is now thought, are brought about by the abnormal electrical activity of certain "epileptic" cells as a result of biochemical dysfunctions. Today, it is generally agreed that *some* biochemical triggering, whether genetic or not, accounts for the seizure. One of the chemicals specifically implicated is gamma-aminobutyric acid (GABA), assumed to be an important inhibitory neurochemical in the brain, functioning as a suppressor of electrical activity. When there is a GABA deficiency, there is thus a tendency for excessive CNS neural activity.

Seizure-prone individuals—even those with identifiable EEG abnormalities such as brain tumors (8 percent of patients with brain tumors have seizures) or cortical lesions—do not always have seizures. The body apparently produces suppressor measures so that seizures do not always take place. Sometimes "triggering" can be traced in seizure-prone individuals. One list of precipitating conditions for different individuals is presented in Listing 13.1.

The traditional classification of seizure disorders that appears here was previously thought to account for most instances of these abnormal states. More refined diagnostic methods, however, have somewhat expanded this older version. A somewhat reduced version of this newer classification appears in Listing 13.2.

Grand-mal seizures. These seizures comprise convulsions, the loss of consciousness, falling to the ground, and confusion, disorientation, and depression in the immediate, postseizure period. About 50 percent of patients with such seizures report an aura, unpleasant subjective sensations preceding the seizure, such as tingling, olfactory hallucinations, or flickering lights. Grand-mal seizures can be dangerous to the subject because they can involve injuries such as tongue biting and head and

Listing 13.1 Factors That May Precipitate Seizures in Susceptible Individuals

- Hyperventilation (overbreathing, sometimes associated with anxiety or stress)
- Sleep (usually within the first 30 minutes or shortly before awakening)
- Sleep deprivation
- Sensory stimuli
  - Flashing strobe lights
  - Reading, speaking, coughing, laughing
  - Touch, pain
  - Sounds of various types
- Trauma (blow or injury to head)
- Hormonal changes
  - Menses, puberty
  - ACTH, adrenal steroids
- Fever
- Emotional stress
- Drugs
  - Phenothiazines (antipsychotic drugs—see Chapter 21)
  - Tricyclic drugs (antidepressants—see Chapter 21)
  - Antihistamines
  - Alcohol
  - Anticonvulsant drugs—overdose

Source: Adapted from *Behavioral neurology,* second edition, p. 5, by Jonathan H. Pincus and Gary J. Tucker. Copyright © 1978 by Oxford University Press, Inc. Reprinted by permission.

Listing 13.2 The International Classification of Epilepsy: Major Categories

Partial Seizures
a. focal (sensory or motor)
b. psychomotor or temporal lobe (see text for description)

Focal seizures generally involve a localized sensory or motor event in a hand, arm, leg, face; these seizures may entail a "Jacksonian march"—a progressive sequence of these sensory or motor events on the same side of the body

Primarily Generalized Seizures
a. "absences" or petit-mal seizures (see text for description)
b. tonic-clonic or grand-mal seizures (see text for description)

Source: Extracted from *Developmental disabilities: Etiologies, manifestations, diagnoses and treatments,* pp. 35–36, by Robert J. Thompson, Jr., and Aglaia O'Quinn. Copyright © 1979 by Oxford University Press, Inc. Reprinted by permission. See also Gastaut, 1970, and Merlis, 1970.

facial bruises. These violent convulsive episodes consist of alternating phases, a tonic phase (stiffening of the body through muscle contractions) and a clonic phase (jerking of the body as a result of alternating muscular flexion and extension).

Petit-mal seizures. These seizures, often referred to as psychological absences or absences because they involve a momentary lapse of consciousness lasting up to about 30 seconds, are generally characterized by twitching of the eyelids or head, loss of muscle tone, pallor, and a dreamy look on the face of the patient. Petit-mal seizures generally appear among children, with onset from about four to eight years. These seizures begin and end suddenly.

Petit-mal seizures usually disappear by the age of eighteen years, with the majority of patients manifesting grand-mal seizures in adulthood. Absences may occur quite frequently, from a few to several hundred episodes daily.

Psychomotor seizures. These seizures occur primarily with adults (Kolb, 1973) and last longer than the petit-mal seizures described above—up to a few minutes. Typically, they are accompanied by repetitious, automatic (stereotyped) movements (automatisms) such as chewing, lip-smacking, or verbalizing; feelings of depersonalization; and visual hallucinations. Sometimes the patient reports intense emotion such as rage, terror, ecstasy, or religious exaltation.

Treatment of seizure disorders varies according to causes. Medication is the most important method of control.* In a small number of cases, surgical intervention has also been used. Behavioral methods, such as relaxation training and biofeedback, have also been used with some success (see Chapters 20–21). About one-half of the patients with seizure disorders can be free of seizures entirely, the seizures of another one-third can be controlled; the remaining group does not yield to current methods of treatment (Mostofsky and Balaschak, 1977).

Important is the gradual disappearing—through public education and education of the patients themselves—of the stigma and superstition surrounding seizure states. A convulsive disorder is not equivalent to mental illness, does not necessarily indicate mental retardation or a propensity to violence or crime, and does not consign the individual to a life of restriction, celibacy, or protected social and vocational environment.

* Of the anticonvulsant medications, the usual methods, such as phenobarbital and Dilantin are now being supplemented or replaced entirely by newly developed drugs that have fewer side effects, such as drowsiness.

Spotlight 13.4 Probing Organic Brain Syndromes: Some Diagnostic Aids

Although clinical observation and psychological assessment can tell us much about the functions of the brain by pairing "known" lesions or tissue damage with loss of function, no matter how reliable the method or astute the clinician, close scrutiny of the living brain is not possible through available behavioral and clinical methods. Described here are several methods that attempt to probe the structures and events of the living brain more directly. You can probably assume that in your lifetime you will see technological advances that will permit even greater accuracy in attempts to understand the living brain than those provided by these methods.

1. Chapters 7 and 8 describe electroencephalography (EEG), and Figure 8.3 shows the EEG waves of a subject during different stages of sleep. The EEG has also been used to record the electrical activity of various parts of the brain during other states of arousal and awareness, for example, during imagery or seizures or while hallucinating or experiencing anxiety or panic.

The EEG, a technique first described by Hans Berger in 1929, measures changes in electrical potential between different parts of the brain by attaching wires to the scalp and then amplifying and recording the extremely weak voltage generated by the billions of neurons in the brain. These amplified oscillations in voltage show up as waves having amplitude, frequency, and characteristic patterns, depending on the state of arousal of the subject and his or her mental activity. Many patterns of brain waves have been identified and some of these have been specifically associated with different kinds of abnormal states. Figure 13.1, for example, shows the changes of an individual's EEG tracings from a normal state to a seizure state. The common kinds of waves found among humans are shown in Figure 13.2.

The EEG has become an important diagnostic tool because of the association of certain EEG patterns with different pathological conditions. It is important to remember, however, that diagnosing brain dysfunction on the basis of the EEG alone is

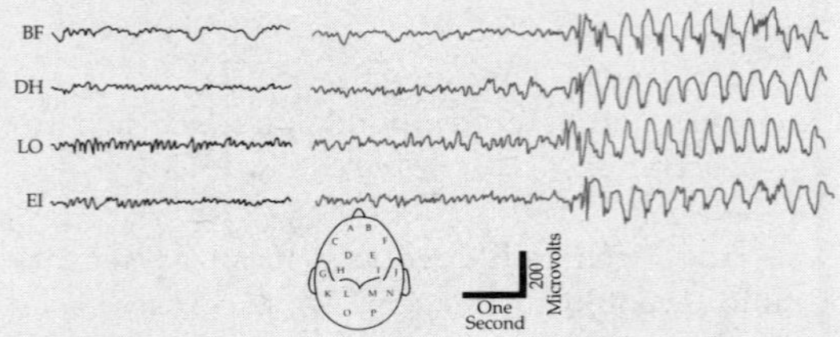

Figure 13.1 Electroencephalogram of an epileptic. Each trace records how the voltage between two areas of the head (see diagram of the head) changed over time. The black traces show the normal electrical activity in the brain of a normal person. The colored traces of an epileptic show normal activity until the onset of a seizure at about the halfway point. (From Disorders of the human brain, by Seymour S. Kety. Copyright © 1979 by Scientific American, Inc. All rights reserved.)

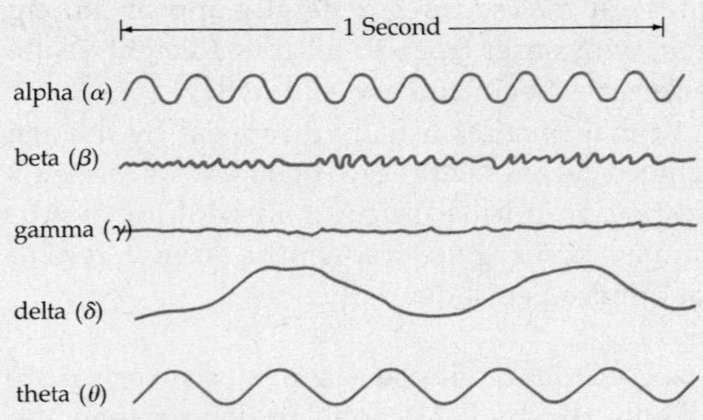

Figure 13.2 Examples of the five most common types of human brain waves. (From R. F. Thompson, *Introduction to physiological psychology* [New York; Harper & Row, 1975], p. 118. Reprinted by permission of the publisher.)

not warranted, because some abnormal wave patterns can be found in normal subjects, and normal EEGs have been associated with pathological brain tissue (Maher, 1966; Yates, 1966).

2. Conventional X-ray methods are useful in localizing obvious structural problems of the brain, such as tumors or blood vessel defects, by specialized methods such as pneumoencephalography, which forces air into the cavities (ventricles) of the brain; and cerebral angiography, which visually depicts blood vessels of the brain by injecting into them a nontoxic fluid opaque to X-rays. Conventional X-ray methods, however, are sometimes not definitive, for they are frequently not precise enough to distinguish minor structural defects.

3. The CAT scan (computed axial tomography, sometimes called computer-assisted tomography), developed in 1973, meets many of the problems unsolved by the cruder methods. Simply stated, this technique "summarizes" or "integrates" X-rays taken from many different angles to yield cross sections of the living brain that provide precise localization of hitherto undetected or unlocalized defects such as displaced ventricles, small tumors, swollen tissues, blood clots, blood masses through hemorrhages, and atrophied tissues. Despite the enormous expense of the equipment, in 1979 there were well over 2,000 CAT scanners all over the world, with hundreds being manufactured and installed each year (Di Chiro and Brooks, 1979). Computer-assisted tomography has been of such great significance in physiology and in medical diagnosis that its developers, A. M. Cormack and G. N. Hounsfield, shared a Nobel Prize in Medicine in 1979.

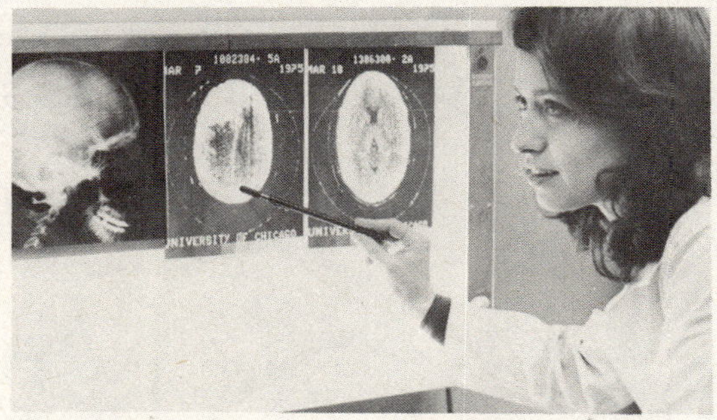

CAT scans can be extremely useful in detecting defects in living brain tissue, such as tumors, blood clots, and blood masses. (United Press International Photo)

The Aphasias

Aphasia is the general term for an impairment of one of many skills having to do with the production, understanding, reception, reproduction, and manipulation of written or spoken words and symbols. The sensory and motor mechanisms for hearing and speech are not involved; aphasics can, thus, articulate, hear, see, and form words. Aphasic conditions arise from lesions (actual physical damage) in certain sections of the cerebral cortex, generally in the dominant, usually left, hemisphere.

The first recorded observation of aphasia is attributed to a Frenchman, Paul Broca, who noted, in about the middle of the last century (through postmortem examination), that injury to a small area of the frontal lobe in the left cerebral hemisphere was consistently associated with a peculiar kind of speech disorder that had been generally referred to as aphasia. Patients with lesions of Broca's area, as this section of the brain has since been called (see Figure 13.3), have difficulty in speaking or writing grammatically. The patient's labored verbal constructions make sense, however, and Broca's aphasics can often sing with great fluidity and articulation, for there is no motor or cognitive difficulty as a result of this particular type of tissue damage.

In Broca's asphasia, both speech and writing

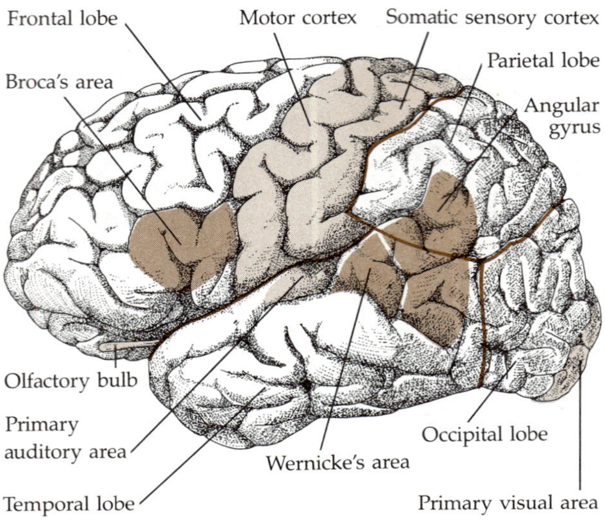

Figure 13.3 This diagram of the cortex indicates the areas whose specialized functions are known. Most of these regions involve motor, sensory, and perceptual functions. Broca's and Wernicke's areas are involved in language production and comprehension. The angular gyrus is thought to mediate between visual and auditory information.

have a "telegraphic style." For example, asked about an appointment at the dentist's, a patient hesitantly and indistinctly said (but might have written), "Yes . . . Monday . . . Dad and Dick . . . Wednesday nine o'clock . . . 10 o'clock . . . doctors . . . and teeth" (Geschwind, 1979, p. 186).

In the 1870s, a German researcher, Carl Wernicke, discovered that damage to another area, this time in the left temporal lobe, also resulted in an aphasic disorder. Wernicke's aphasia, however, unlike Broca's, is associated with grammatical, fluent speech and "correct" sentence structure, which appear to make sense but actually do not do so, except in the most roundabout way. One Wernicke's aphasic, for example, in describing a picture of two boys stealing cookies unseen by a woman said, "Mother is away here working her work to get her better, but when she's looking the two boys looking in the other part. She's working another time" (Geschwind, 1979, p. 186).

Since these early observations, it has been possible to construct a precise model of how these two areas are neurally connected and what they are reponsible for in terms of reading, writing, speech production, comprehension of speech, and ability to utilize grammar and syntax.

There are many types of aphasia. *Apraxia* is an inability to perform a previously possible, intended motor activity. There is no accompanying physical problem such as weakness or paralysis that causes this condition. In *nominal aphasia* the patient has difficulty in naming an object, even though there is understanding of its use or what it is. In *syntactical aphasia* there is difficulty in placing words into their usual sequence. *Alexia* is an inability to understand the written word, although the patient may be able to read the word correctly. He or she may write and speak a word, but will have difficulty in comprehending its meaning. *Agraphia* refers to an inability to write spoken words. *Agnosia* is the general term used to describe an impairment of recognition of objects. A patient can describe an object with all its qualities—yet that object looks unfamiliar, and he or she cannot say what it is used for. *Prosopagnosia,* a startlingly narrow type of aphasia, is an inability to recognize faces:

> *In the normal individual the ability to identify people from their faces is itself quite remarkable. At a glance one can name a person from facial features alone, even though the features may change substantially over the years or may be presented in a highly distorted form, as in a caricature. In a patient with prosopagnosia this talent for association is abolished.*
>
> *What is most remarkable about the disorder is its specificity. . . . for example, the patient can usually read and name seen objects. What he cannot do is look at a person or at a photograph of a face and name the person. He may even fail to recognize his wife or children. . . . when a familiar person speaks, the patient knows the voice and can say the name immediately. The perception of facial features is also unimpaired, since the patient can often describe a face in detail and can usually match a photograph made from the front with a profile of the same person. . . .*
>
> *(Geschwind, 1979, p. 189)*

What is fascinating about this disability is that its lesions can be specifically located, time after time, on the "underside of both occipital lobes, extending forward to the temporal lobes" (Geschwind, 1979, p. 189).

Many of these aphasias have been specifically localized in various neural systems. Is this true for other human cognitive abilities? Seeking the answer to this question has for decades fascinated scientists studying the brain.

Localization of functions in the brain. It was once thought that each small section of the brain was responsible for a specific set of behaviors or sensations. This view—localization of functions—might apply to simple movements and simple sensory processes, but the specific one-to-one correspondence of brain area and behavior, it is now thought, does not apply to higher cognitive processes. As a matter of fact, it had become popular to believe, along with Lashley (1929), that different parts of the cortex are actually equal in potential for learning, training, and thinking (brain equipotentiality) and that the functions lost by damage to one area can be assumed equally well by other areas of the brain. In this approach, the extent, rather than the localization, of damage determines the deficit after brain injury.

Actually, the truth lies somewhere in between. As you shall see, for most complex functions the one-to-one localization theory does not hold up. Most brain experts now believe that neural circuits and systems than can involve far-reaching sections of the brain are responsible for high-level abilities such as memory and verbal problem-solving. These complex functions

> *cannot be localized in narrow zones of the cortex or in isolated cell groups, but must be* organized in systems of concertedly working zones, each of which performs its role in complex functional system, *and which may be located in completely different and often far distant areas of the brain (Luria, 1973, pp. 30–31; italics are Luria's).*

It is the very lack of specificity in the brain for complex functions that provides the basis for the amazing recovery that so many victims of cerebral injury are able to make. Restoration of function and rehabilitation after injury is the subject of the final section in this chapter.

FUNCTIONS OF SOME CEREBRAL REGIONS

The study of brain-behavior relationships when there is brain injury provides us with an opportunity to learn a good deal about the structure and function of various parts of the brain.* That is, in instances when there is brain injury (for example, through tumor, hemorrhage, surgery, gunshot wounds, or cerebrovascular accidents), and when such injury can be localized, deficits in the patient's performance can tell us a great deal about the functions of the injured portion of the brain.

Parts of the brain bear a complex, functional relationship to one another, and the more complex functions such as thinking, judging, reasoning, writing, spatial orientation, and language involve the interactions of many brain areas and neuronal systems. For example, one neuronal system that is essential for higher-level functions has to do with attention and arousal (see Spotlight 7.2). According to many brain scientists, this system (the reticular activating system, RAS), involving neural structures in the core of the brain stem, maintains us in wakeful, alert, aroused states that form the backdrop for most of our behavior.

Figures 7.5 and 13.3 illustrate the division of the cerebral cortex roughly into major sections or zones. Here I describe some of the functions, in a general way, of these areas, and some of the "typical" disabilities that may result from damage to these areas. This is a limited summary, for there are many important brain areas not touched on.

---

* Chapter 7, pp. 137–44, gives a brief overview of the functions and structures of the CNS. Much of the current section is derived from Luria (1973).

The frontal and prefrontal lobes. Even extensive bilateral frontal-lobe brain damage, that is, damage to both the left and right cerebral hemispheres, does not necessarily result in sensory or motor difficulties. Even so, frontal-lobe injury has a special quality, of great importance to human behavior, that is sometimes referred to as the frontal-lobe syndrome, as was already noted.

In humans, the frontal lobes are the most specialized parts of the brain, occupying about one-fourth of the total mass. These lobes are intricately connected with all other sections of the brain and cerebral cortex, more so than is the case for any other part. The functions of the frontal lobes are of the highest intellectual order, including planning, intent, foresight, conscious activity, and the activating, alerting, and attentional responses necessary for goal-directed action. The frontal lobes are involved in thinking, defining a problem, assessing the effectiveness of its solution, and checking the results against the initial requirements. These functions are concerned with awareness of the future, the consequences of one's actions, and the ability to assess the external world in relation to goals and whether or not one's behavior is moving toward these goals.

Frontal-lobe patients may understand words and simple sentences but not complex forms of narrative speech. They show poor problem-solving skills because they cannot keep goals in mind. They are impulsive and often resort to unselective guessing. They do not check their results, show poor judgment, and cannot focus, concentrate, and employ voluntary attention in the solution of problems, especially complex ones that involve speech. However, they may be entirely capable of solving the problem, of performing the actions involved, and of remembering what the problem is.

The occipital lobes. These brain areas specialize in vision and in the processing of visual information. The primary (projection) areas of these lobes are the terminal points of excitations beginning with the nerve fibers from the retina, which send signals through the optic nerve and optic tract. The left fields of each eye terminate in the *right* hemisphere occipital lobe, while the right fields of each eye terminate in the *left* hemisphere. Lesions in these primary zones cause only partial visual disturbances, for the patient can adjust to losses of vision by making eye movements and retinal adjustments. The primary visual cortex "processes" simple visual information from the eyes, while the secondary visual cortex is responsible for visual perception that combines, organizes, and puts together visual information into more complex perceptions. Lesions in these zones do not create losses in visual acuity or of visual "information" such as color, light, dark, etc. Rather, they result in deficits in visually recognizing whole objects or in synthesizing separate parts into a meaningful whole. Patients with such lesions can deduce what an object is by logically putting together its separate visual parts. For example, although a bunch of grapes is not perceived as such, the patient may be able to figure out that a group of round, small purple stimuli may be a bunch of grapes by logically putting together bits and pieces of visual information.

The temporal lobes. Unlike excitation from the retina to the visual cortex, fibers from each of the ears go to *both* hemispheres. The predominant neural connection, however, is in the opposite hemisphere. Primary temporal zones are responsible for auditory sensitivity whereas the secondary zones are responsible for auditory perception—the combining of sounds, pitches, rhythms, and the differentiation of pitches, especially in the analysis and perception of speech sounds. Less is known about lesions in the right temporal zones than in the left, but it is known that right lesions are unconnected to speech, producing instead disturbances in hearing music or in rhythm perception.

Lesions in the left temporal regions (especially of the secondary area) can result in sensory aphasia—inability to understand speech, even though hearing is intact. In such patients, the general meaning of a verbal communication can often be understood from its context and there is no disturbance in written or visual verbal activities.

Left-hemisphere temporal activities also involve memory for words as well as the "point" of a problem, such as its possible verbal solution, and therefore lesions here affect thinking and problem-solving skills. This difficulty is eased if one presents a problem to such a patient in writing rather than verbally. Left temporal patients also have difficulties in drawing a picture of a named object, and in writing from dictation.

The parietal lobes. Among many diffuse functions, the parietal regions seem to be involved in the pulling together of complex spatial information. Parietal-lobe patients suffer impairment in visual-spatial orientation, for example, right-left orientation or location of one's bearings on a map, even if their sensory processes are intact. Lesions of various parietal zones in combination with lesions of other zones produce a variety of symptoms. For example, left temporal-occipital-parietal patients cannot read, write, or grasp the meaning of verbal communications; left temporal-parietal patients show difficulty in the naming of objects; left occipital-parietal patients cannot fit blocks together to make a pattern similar to a visually presented one, that is, they cannot deal with visual-spatial relationships, even though they know what the problem is. Interestingly, in addition to having difficulty in finding their bearings, such patients show difficulties in understanding symbolic relationships, numerical systems, and logical-grammatical structures. As a result, the reception and analysis of information are impaired.

The sensorimotor cortex. Virtually all regions of the body have corresponding regions in sections of the sensory and motor cortex (Geschwind, 1979). The motor cortex is responsible for voluntary control over the muscles, sending out impulses (efferent system) for movement. Signals from the skin, joints, and muscles, in turn, are received in the sensory cortex (afferent system). These systems regulate one another through constant feedback and corrections.

Lesions in the motor cortex result in various disabilities in which control over voluntary movement is lost (efferent motor aphasia) despite intact intent, understanding, and capacity to perform the act. Lesions in the sensory cortex produce afferent apraxia, a disability arising as a result of disturbances in receiving impulses from one's own body. Patients suffering from afferent apraxia show coarse, undifferentiated, uncorrected movements despite intact muscle strength because kinesthetic signals are not properly processed in the brain. In general, lesions in the sensorimotor cortex result in difficulties in executing skilled, smooth, coordinated movements.

The left-right cerebral hemisphere functions revisited. In Chapter 7, Spotlight 7.1 discussed right-left hemisphere differences in function (called lateralization). It was noted at that time that the left hemisphere specializes in linguistic skills whereas the right hemisphere specializes in spatial, artistic, musical, and imaginative skills. Because the right hemisphere makes little or no contribution to speech functions, it stands to reason that brain injury in either the left or the right hemisphere (depending on lateral dominance, of course—that is, whether one is normally right or left handed) makes an enormous difference in any behavioral disabilities resulting from such an injury.

In general, left-hemisphere patients, although they lose various linguistic skills, retain the perception of melodies and visual patterns. Right-hemisphere patients, on the other hand, show certain types of perceptual difficulties while retaining basic linguistic skills. For example, they show disturbances in perception of information arising from their own bodies. They can show little or no perception of a left-sided paralysis stemming from their right-hemisphere tissue damage. It is almost as if they have no knowledge of the left side of their bodies. Right-hemisphere patients show lack of concern about, and inappropriate emotional responses to, their own injuries, in contrast to left-hemisphere patients, who experience a deep sense of loss, even depression, in response to their disabilities (Geschwind, 1979).

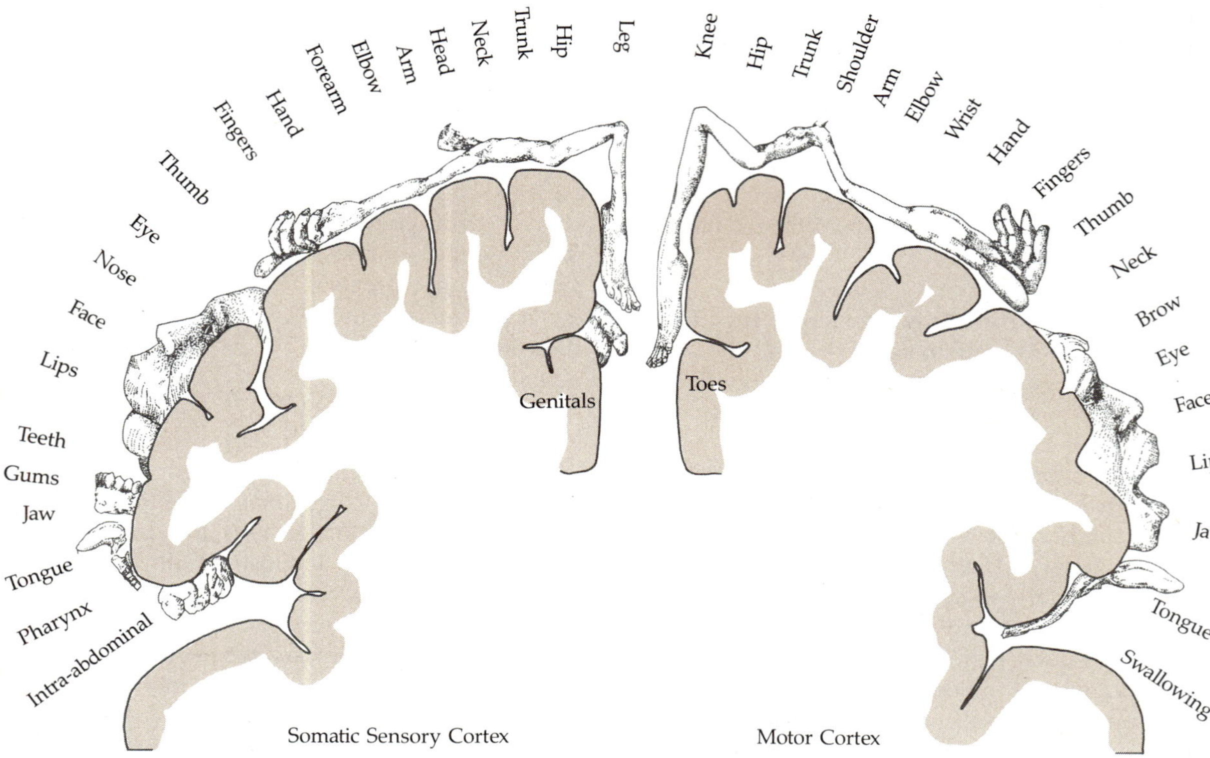

Figure 13.4 Sensorimotor regions of the cortex. The cerebral cortex is highly specialized; each area controls a specific part of the body, and the greater the precision required, the larger the area of the brain devoted to it. (From *Specializations of the human brain* by Norman Geschwind. Copyright © 1979 by Scientific American, Inc. All rights reserved.)

In day-to-day behavior, this strict lateralization of function is much less obvious. Both hemispheres are in communication with each other, interacting and communicating through complex neuronal circuits. The right hemisphere even has some rudimentary linguistic ability. Only when the connections between the hemispheres are severed, or when there is brain damage, are the resulting symptoms striking reminders to us of the general lateralization of functions in the human brain (Geschwind, 1979).

ASSESSMENT AND RECOVERY OF FUNCTIONS AFTER BRAIN DAMAGE

Although the role of the psychologist in diagnosing brain damage is diminishing in the light of such methods as the CAT scan that in many instances do the job better, there are ever expanding areas of activity for the psychologist. These include (a) the clarification of brain-behavior relationships; (b) the assessment of disabilities and deficits that result from brain damage; and (c) the development of methods to help in the restoration of lost functions. The first of these areas has already been discussed. The following section examines the other two areas.

Assessment

Early indications of brain involvement can sometimes be detected even before there are dramatic deficits in abilities. In these as yet "undiagnosed" instances, an astute clinician will be sensitive to changes in personality and behavior—organic personality changes—of the kind already described in this chapter, such as an increase in irritability, sloppiness, or concreteness. In addition to personality changes, other deficits appear, such as disorientation, memory impairment, or faulty perception in the different modalities. Traditionally, to arrive at a clinical picture that taps these areas, in addition to observations the clinician has relied on many of the instruments described in Chapter 5, such as the Rorschach test and the Thematic Apperception Test (TAT). These and other special clinical instruments are used in a battery, often for differential diagnosis (deciding among diagnostic possibilities). Findings tended to be used qualitatively, to suggest the possibility of brain damage rather than to survey systematically the nature and extent of performance difficulties.

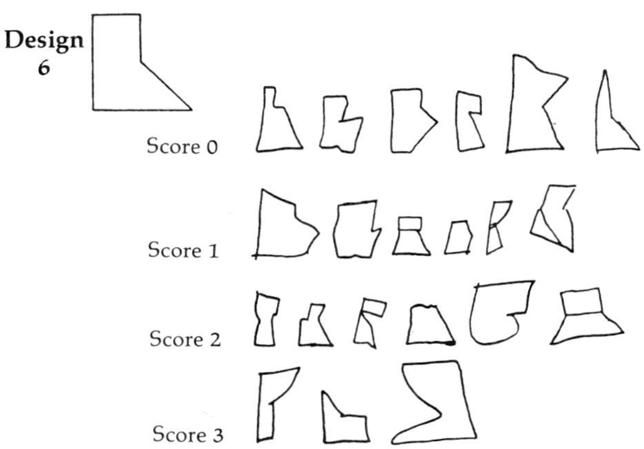

Figure 13.5 One of the Graham-Kendall designs, followed by attempts to reproduce it from memory by different subjects. Higher scores are assigned to the poorer reproductions, produced by people with various types of motor and perceptual difficulties. (From F. K. Graham and B. S. Kendall, Memory-For-Designs Test: Revised general manual, *Perceptual and Motor Skills Monograph Supplement*, 1960, *11*, 147–88.

Thus it is possible to conclude from test findings and clinical observations that a patient is not schizophrenic, for example, but suffering from brain damage. Using this approach, the clinician might find impaired "recent" memory, a large discrepancy between verbal and performance IQs with the latter being quite low, good vocabulary but poor skills in making abstractions, poor memory for briefly presented designs, distorted and childish figure drawings, and poor visual-motor coordination.* The clinician might correctly suspect some type of brain involvement.

However, such tests are not diagnostically precise. And they are only minimally useful in systematically surveying the *specific* disabilities and deficits that different brain-damaged patients show. Because of their lack of specificity as well as narrowness in failing to tap a broad range of cognitive, perceptual, linguistic, and motor abilities, neuropsychologists have developed other more systematic, standardized, and reliable test batteries.

One such instrument is the Halstead-Reitan Neuropsychological Test Battery (Reitan and Davison, 1974), which is administered with several other tests that specifically "screen" for aphasia and other types of sensory and perceptual defects in the different modalities, as well as assess IQ and personality (a Wechsler scale and the MMPI, respectively). Because this battery requires six to eight hours to administer, it is not routinely administered to all

* These findings can typically be gained from the Bender Visual Motor Gestalt Test (Bender, 1938), Benton Visual Retention Test (Benton, 1955), Graham-Kendall Memory-For-Designs Test (1960), Wechsler Memory Scale (Wechsler, 1945), the Wechsler Intelligence Scales, and many other special clinical tests too numerous to cite.

patients who seek help or who are in a mental facility. The formal Halstead-Reitan battery is comprised of several subtests that include a categories test for abstracting ability, a tactile performance test performed blindfolded with blocks; a rhythm test that assesses discrimination of various rhythms; a speech-sounds perception test requiring discrimination between similar-sounding consonants, and a finger-tapping speed test.

Another test, the Luria-Nebraska Neuropsychological Battery, is claimed to be more detailed in surveying defects due to brain injury than are the Halstead-Reitan tests. This battery is based on the kinds of qualitative observations the Russian neuropsychologist A. R. Luria has described in his careful work with brain-damaged patients (Golden, Hammeke, and Purisch, 1978, 1980). One advantage that this battery has over the Halstead-Reitan one is that it requires less than two and one-half hours to administer and yet attempts to survey as many sensory modalities (for example, tactile, auditory, visual) as well as different cognitive and verbal functions as possible within this limited time.

The Luria-Nebraska Neuropsychological Battery, which consists of 269 separate measurements or observations, seems to be a very promising in-

Table 13.1 Mean Summary Scores of 50 Brain-Injured and 50 Schizophrenic Subjects for the 14 Indices of the Luria-Nebraska Battery

	Mean of Summary Scores		
Index	*Brain-injured*	*Schizophrenic*	*Is Difference Significant?*
Motor	44.36	34.20	Yes
Rhythm	12.21	12.26	No
Tactile	19.32	13.62	Yes
Visual	16.14	12.82	Yes
Impressive speech	23.67	19.48	No
Expressive speech	33.34	24.86	Yes
Reading and writing	24.67	17.51	Yes
Arithmetic	16.15	10.07	Yes
Memory	16.25	15.84	No
Intellectual	38.32	33.24	No
Pathognomic*	34.46	22.20	Yes
Left hemisphere*	18.82	13.24	Yes
Right hemisphere*	18.00	12.44	Yes
Total	27.06	15.51	Yes

Source: A. D. Purisch, C. J. Golden, and T. A. Hammeke, Discrimination of schizophrenic and brain-injured patients by a standardized version of Luria's neuropsychological tests, *Journal of Consulting and Clinical Psychology*, 1978, *46*, 1266–73. Copyright 1978 by the American Psychological Association. Adapted by permission of the publisher and author. Roughly 50 percent of the brain-injured subjects were diagnosed with either cerebral trauma or cerebral vascular disorder, with the remaining subjects diagnosed as having neoplasms, infectious diseases, degenerative diseases, epilepsy, metabolic and toxic disorders, and congenital disorders. Of the schizophrenic subjects, roughly 40 percent were of the paranoid type and another 40 percent undifferentiated; the rest fell into the catatonic, hebephrenic, paranoid, simple, and schizoaffective categories.

*The *pathognomic* index was based on the sum of the 34 most "effective indicators" of brain damage. Left- and right-hemisphere indices were based on all measures requiring either left-hand or right-hand performance, respectively.

strument. It discriminates quite well among control, schizophrenic, and neurological patients, and between left- or right-hemisphere patients. Also, within each hemisphere, findings with this battery produce patterns of test responses that discriminate moderately well among frontal, temporal, sensorimotor, and parietal-occipital patients (Golden, Hammeke, and Purisch, 1978; Lewis et al., 1979; Purisch, Golden, and Hammeke, 1978). Table 13.1 for example, shows many significant differences between brain-damaged and schizophrenic subjects in scores derived from the Luria-Nebraska battery. Spotlight 13.5 illustrates typical items from this battery.

Spotlight 13.5 Mapping the Assets and Deficits of Brain-Injured Patients: Sample Items from the Luria-Nebraska Battery

The 269 separate observations or items that comprise the Luria-Nebraska Neuropsychological Battery (Golden, Hammeke, and Purisch, 1978, 1980) involve systematic observations in a broad spectrum of skills and abilities that help not only to specify the symptom and possibly localize the injury, but also to carve out the significant areas for the recovery of lost functions. The following are samples from this large pool of items.

Motor functions. Tasks include producing simple movements with hands, mouth, and tongue following a model or verbal instructions; tasks also assess coordination, visual perception, and drawing ability.

11. Do as I do. (Place right hand under chin with fingers bent.)
25. Without lifting your pencil from the paper, I want you to draw the best square you can.

Rhythm (acoustico-motor) functions. Tasks include discriminating between sounds of different pitches and rhythms as same or different.

62. You will now hear a rhythm on the tape. When I tell you that the rhythm is over, I want you to tap with your hand the rhythm you heard on the tape.

Tactile (cutaneous and kinesthetic) functions. Tasks reflect various body and touch sensations and perceptions of one's own body as well as of external objects.

80. (subject is blindfolded) Now I will put your left arm in a certain position; try to put the other arm in the same position.

Visual functions. Items include visual-spatial perception and orientation, identification of objects and pictures, constructing geometric patterns with blocks, and telling time from clocks with no numbers.

97. This drawing shows a stack of blocks in three dimensions. Tell me how many blocks are in the stack.

Impressive speech. Items include those that measure discrimination of English sounds, reproducing these orally or in writing; naming objects from pictures; and responding to the examiner in ways which indicate understanding of complex grammatical constructions.

100. You will hear some sounds on the tape. What I want you to do is first repeat exactly the sound you hear and then write down the letter of the alphabet that goes along with the sound.
125. Which boy is shorter if John is taller than Peter?

Expressive speech. These tasks require the production of simple speech sounds, familiar and unfamiliar words and phrases or sentences, naming and classifying objects, and producing narrative descriptions.

133. Repeat after me: a (as in late); I (as in light); m (as in milk); b (as in baby); and sh (as in shine).
164. Tell me what's happening in this picture.

Reading and writing.

178. Copy these in your own handwriting.

192. What sound is made by the letters g-r-o? p-l-y?

Arithmetic skills.

219. What is the missing number?
12 - ? = 8

Mnestic (memory) processes. Tasks include level of skills for remembering and recalling visual, acoustic, and kinesthetic material, both verbal and nonverbal, under various conditions of no interference and interference with direct memory.

231. I want you to remember some words that I am going to say: house-tree-cat. Now, look at this picture—what do you see? (After 15 seconds): What were the words?

Intellectual processes. Items require the subject to interpret themes of pictures, define words, form concepts, classify objects, understand analogies, perform arithmetic computations, and demonstrate reasoning skills.

249. In what way are table and sofa alike? In what way are an ax and saw alike?

Source: C.J. Golden, T.A. Hammeke, and A.D. Purisch, *The Luria-Nebraska Neuropsychological Battery Manual.* Reprinted by permission of Western Psychological Services, 12031 Wilshire Blvd., Los Angeles, CA 90025. Copyright © 1980 Western Psychological Services.

Recovery

The restoration of a mind after brain injury is often a slow, agonizing process. Spotlight 13.6 describes in his own words the struggle of a psychologist to recover his role in life after such injury.

Not all patients are as knowledgeable as the psychologist in this Spotlight, but most can profit from the attention and skills of an expert. A frequent first step is the thorough assessment of the deficits and assets of the patient in as many performance areas as possible. This step is often crucial, because the establishment of immediate recovery paths may make the difference between the restoration of lost skills or the relative failure to do so. The next steps depend on the introduction of the appropriate strategies that best fit the needs of the patient. I will not describe the vast reservoir of techniques that has been developed for the restoration of lost functions in visual, tactile, or auditory perception, speech and writing, attention, body perception, spatial orientation, and visual-motor coordination. In general, the specific strategies also make use of the same principles that are involved in most learning situations, for example, reinforcing the correct response, using short training periods, eliciting the attention and cooperation of the subject, and being concerned with transfer to real-life situations.

The important thing to remember is that most specialists in this area have an optimistic view about recovery. For the brain has a certain amount of plasticity and neuronal systems for higher functions are not irrevocably fixed or localized. As a result, many functions that are lost can be assumed by healthy, intact brain tissue (Geschwind, 1979; Luria, 1973; Pincus and Tucker, 1978).

Not very much is known about what actually takes place in the recovery process. There are several possibilities. For example, lost linguistic functions as a result of left-hemisphere damage might be recovered through the use of dormant, "underused" *right* hemisphere neuronal circuits that have been "silently learning" all along. Or tissues near to the damaged tissue might take over (Geschwind, 1979). Of course, the more widespread the damage—that is, the greater the number of disrupted neuronal systems—the greater the deficit in performance, because there is less healthy tissue available to take over recovery functions. For these reasons, certain patients do better than others, for example, patients with less extensive damage or damage to only one hemisphere. Because of the plasticity of the developing brain, children younger than eight years do very well in the recovery process. Left-handed people (or those with left-handed relatives) in the case of left-hemisphere damage often show excellent recovery, presumably because their *right* hemispheres are "experienced" in performing executive functions in intellective areas.

Still, there are many mysteries. There is often spontaneous recovery in the first month after injury (Pincus and Tucker, 1978). But why does spontaneous recovery take place, with some patients, three to six months after the injury was sustained? Perhaps the biggest mystery of all is the remarkable role that human motivation—the will to get better—plays in the recovery process.

Spotlight 13.6 Recovery from Brain Injury: One Man's Struggle

The excerpts below are taken from an article written by C. Scott Moss (1980). It appeared in a professional journal with a few spelling errors that are apparently the author's and that are left intact. The carotid arteries are the large arteries on each side of the neck.

The loss of an arm, the impairment of mobility, the reduction of sight or hearing are all grievous problems of adjustment to anyone, but one of the most cataclysmic of all, especially for a psychologist, is brain injury. In 1967, at the age of 43, while employed as a professor at the University of Illinois, I suffered a permanent blockage of the left internal carotid artery. In a single moment I was transformed from a very much alive, energetic, enthusiastic husband and father, teacher and professional person to one who was profoundly brain injured. The area of affected (dead) cortical tissue extends about the size of my palm implanted over the parital area of the left side of the brain, including the speech center. The motor area, fortunately, was relatively untouched.

When I regained consciousness the next morning in the hospital I was completely unable to talk, read or write. Also, I was unable to handle any abstractions, my way of thinking had become totally concrete. My memory for past events literally was wiped away and even the future was meaningless; so I existed only in the "here and now." I was unable to converse with anyone about anything; I could not decipher the meaning of headlines in the newspaper and I could make only "henmarks" in writing. I could not even silently summon up words for my nonexistant speech. I had lost the ability to dream. So for approximately two months, I lived in a complete vacuum of conventional symbols (words). During the daytime I had no words to express what was happening either internally to myself or externally to others, and at night I had no dreams. Amazingly, this experience did not bother me because I really had somehow become resigned to approaching death. . . .

*In a twelve-day period the hospital performed its medical-diagnostic function and then simply threw us back into our home, totally on our own resources—*sans *advice,* sans *medication,* sans *knowledge of whatever community resources were available for rehabilitation. The next three years were spent on a strictly trial and error basis, constantly trying to devise ways to break through the "brain and speech paralysis." Since I had no memory to speak of for preceding events, my wife constantly sought to stimulate my mind with names, places, and associations. I began to put together a huge box of family photographs that eventually filled twelve albums. Painstakingly my wife and I began to work on the first of five papers that I had obligated myself to write prior to the stroke. We lived a daring life throughout, traversing a very thin line between what I thought I could do and that which I could not. In terms of formal therapy, I had to take the initiative for seeking out hypnotherapy, speech therapy and behavior modification—anything that was available. . . .*

Three years after the stroke, out of sheer frustration with my inability to carry on a life any longer as a professor, I left the University of Illinois. . . . I finally settled on a much less threatening position as the Mental Health

Coordinator at a large federal prison on the West Coast . . . no one in the new surroundings knew that I had had a stroke. Bette and I have always disagreed about whether I should represent myself as a handicapped person. Her thinking was that I should not try to hide the fact that I had major language and thought disturbances since no one would expect me to function at my former level of performance. Saving me from instant anxiety was not the point, however. Instead, my whole strategy was not to give in to the concept that I was an "ill" or "sick" or a "handicapped" person who would trade upon his disease for solace or sympathy. After earlier transitory attempts at "normal" role-playing in the university setting, in the prison setting it became a deadly serious act. I had learned full well that society's tendency to label people whom it supposedly wanted to help can produce more of the very deviant behavior which it hopes to extinguish. Fortunately, life was still full of surprises and as I continued to improve I was once again caught up very actively in the daily problems of both personal and professional life. Today I feel that I can let down at times because after twelve years I have recovered 85–90 percent of my former capacity and an error here or there does not bother me.

I still possess a dozen residuals of my stroke but to my mind I do a grand job in glossing over and covering them up. For instance, I still cannot engage in cursive writing (I print or type or make use of a recording device); I still do not know what is left and which is right (I try not to direct anyone to anything and my wife touches my shoulder to direct me when she is back-seat driving); and I still get five hours sleep per night arising at 4–5 A.M. to prepare for the day's forthcoming events. The result is that I must battle against constant fatigue. . . . In time I came to realize that every single interaction of mine had two implications; it was partly altruistic (as a father, husband, teacher and clinician I was still busy doing things for other people), but underlying it was the factor of self-service, that is, every encounter was also therapy or rehabilitation for me. . . .

Source: C.S. Moss, Recovery from Brain Injury, *Clinical Psychologist,* 1980, *33,* No. 2, 5–6. Reprinted by permission of the publisher and author.

SUMMARY

This chapter focused on mental disorders arising from ascertainable organic conditions, especially of the central nervous system (CNS). Following a description of the sociocultural correlates and general causes of these organic disorders, the chapter discussed presenile and senile dementias, degenerative conditions such as Huntington's and Parkinson's diseases and various mental conditions associated with metabolic, endocrinological, and infectious diseases and disorders, toxic reactions, brain tumors, and trauma to the brain and head. It also described convulsive disorders and the aphasias, presented the general functions of various cerebral regions (for example, the frontal and prefrontal lobes or the temporal lobes), and raised the question of whether or not there is localization of brain function. The chapter concluded with a discussion of assessment methods and problems in connection with restoration of functions after brain damage.

Highlights

1. Although some mental conditions resulting from organic involvements are more likely to occur under conditions of poverty—for example, conditions that arise from poor maternal health or disease, drug addiction, or alcoholism during pregnancy—many of the other states described in this chapter, for example, pathological aging, do not bear a direct relationship to SES.
2. Although the precise etiology of many organic mental conditions is not clear and may reflect

the interactions of several causal variables, several broad categories seem to be implicated. These include deficiency in the blood supply to the brain caused by such conditions as atherosclerosis, cerebrovascular accidents, actual physical damage to the brain, embolisms, and blood clots; bacterial, viral, and other infectious conditions; toxic states as a result of the presence of noxious substances in brain tissues; and various biochemical and neurophysiological dysfunctions that may arise from several sources.

3. Senile dementia, the fourth or fifth leading cause of death in our country (it affects more women than men, independently of the longer life span of women), may arise from biochemical abnormalities in the brain. However, there are many other hypotheses about the causes of senile dementia, including a slow-acting virus. Examples of other degenerative diseases include Huntington's disease, a rare, inherited disorder; and Parkinson's disease, probably caused by nongenetic, biochemical dysfunctions that can in most instances be pharmacologically controlled.
4. Although some clinicians believe that there may be special personality syndromes associated with certain types of brain involvement—for example, the frontal-lobe syndrome, manifested by poor impulse control and social judgment, difficulties in evaluating future consequences of acts, and apathy—most researchers agree that there is no one personality cluster that cuts across all types of brain disability. The premorbid personality and typical defenses of the injured individual may play an important role in determining that person's emotional responses to injury.
5. Epilepsy is a "catch-all" label for many types of seizure disorders that are characterized by abnormal firing (probably triggered by biochemical factors) of large numbers of special neurons. Seizures and various types of seizure-related conditions can arise from a variety of causes and are roughly classified into grand mal, petit mal, and psychomotor types. The causes of these abnormal conditions determine treatment and control whenever possible, but medication such as Dilantin is probably the most important treatment approach. In a small number of cases surgical intervention has been successful, as well as various types of behavioral methods.
6. The aphasias—a general term for impairment in specific types of skills in reading, writing, speaking, and understanding words and symbols—arise from lesions in specific areas of the dominant (usually left) hemisphere of the cerebral cortex. Much is known about specific aphasic disabilities as a result of injury sustained in Broca's and Wernicke's areas and there is considerable clinical experience also with other types of asphasia, for example, apraxia, alexia, and agraphia. Yet clincians now believe that the specific localization of functions suggested by work with aphasics does not apply to most cognitive processes. The lack of specificity in the brain for many complex functions is responsible for the fact that patients with cerebral injuries can often recover a variety of lost functions.
7. Broadly defined cerebral areas are associated with general functions with distinctive qualities, so that extensive injury in these areas produces "typical" types of impairment. The frontal lobes, for example—the most specialized parts of the brain—are responsible for planning, foresight, problem solving, evaluation of solutions, goal orientation, and awareness of the consequences of one's actions. Frontal-lobe patients can be easily identified by their impulsivity, poor concentration, lack of foresight, and poor judgment in problem-solving activities. Similarly, injury sustained in the occipital, temporal, and parietal lobes and the sensorimotor cortex produces identifiable, distinctive kinds of impairment.
8. Psychologists work with brain-damaged patients not only for diagnostic purposes but

also to clarify brain-behavior relationships, aid in the assessment of deficits arising as a result of injury, and develop techniques to help restore lost functions. Assessment methods for reliably surveying an array of specific disabilities in cognitive, perceptual, linguistic, and motor areas include the Halstead-Reitan Battery and the Luria-Nebraska Neuropsychological Battery. Such instruments have many advantages over the broader clinical tests because they can specifically pinpoint areas of disability, for example, in the perception of rhythm or in certain types of recall, that require retraining.

9. Recovery of lost functions after brain injury is often a slow process requiring high levels of motivation in the patient. Immediate assessment of deficits to establish recovery routines is desirable. Although little is known about what specifically takes place in the brain in the recovery process, one hypothesis suggests that undamaged portions of the brain (for example, the right hemisphere in the case of linguistic abilities), which have been "silently learning" all along, take over some functions. Another hypothesis is that tissue near to the damaged tissue now take over for new learning. There are individual differences in recovery patterns. Younger, more motivated patients, and those with less extensive damage, do better than others. Still, there are many unanswered questions about the recovery process, for example, why in some instances spontaneous recovery takes place three to six months after injury.

ISSUE

In 1976 California was the first state to permit the "living will," protecting the rights of patients to die, should they wish to do so, by suspending life-support methods used to extend their lives if they are terminally ill (Natural Death Act). Since that time, many other states have adopted similar laws.

The use of artificial methods to delay death when "brain death" has occurred is opposed by many people. Yet how is "brain death" defined? There are many, not very clearly delineated, criteria for judging the precise moment of death. Further, who makes the decision to "pull the plug"? The courts? In California, only a mentally competent person can make such a will, which expires five years after such a will is witnessed and signed. Who is to decide or judge the mental competence of the will-maker?

The issue becomes even more complicated when there is no "living will." Think about some of the degenerative diseases described in this chapter that can result in a vegetative state before death occurs naturally. Who decides to "pull the plug," if indeed this position is legally acceptable? The closest relatives? The courts? A team of doctors? These questions can invoke strong feelings. What is your reaction?

SUGGESTIONS FOR FURTHER READING:

Gardner, H. *The shattered mind: The person after brain damage.* New York: Knopf, 1975. Paperback available. This book presents descriptions of various organic syndromes in nontechnical, readable fashion. Disorders of language, memory, recognition, visual perception, and musical and artistic ability as a result of brain damage are not only discussed but placed in the context of the underlying brain functions of the injured area. The author explains the functions of the normal brain in the light of what is learned about the injured brain. This book is highly recommended for students interested in brain damage syndromes and in neuropsychology.

Golden, C. J. *Diagnosis and rehabilitation in clinical neuropsychology.* Springfield, Ill.: Thomas, 1978. As a basic introduction to clinical neuropsychology, this book is excellent. It begins with a brief review of brain physiology and theories of brain function.

This is followed by a discussion of various neuropsychological assessment techniques for adults and children, with particular emphasis on how different tests can help to identify which part of the brain is dysfunctional or damaged. Case examples illustrate conditions and rehabilitation techniques. As a readable and fairly thorough overview of the field, this book is highly recommended to the interested student.

Luria, A. R. *The man with a shattered world: A history of a brain wound.* New York: Basic Books, 1972. Paperback. This is the account of a man's courageous, tenacious struggle to overcome the disabilities incurred as a result of a bullet wound in the temporal-parietal area. Initially unable to recognize his own name, Zasetsky, the wounded man, gradually recovered some speech, some ability to read, and eventually, some ability to write. Luria, the renowned Russian neuropsychologist who worked with and studied this man over a period of twenty-five years, presents verbatim excerpts from the patient's autobiographical notes, reports his own observations of him, and presents brief and simple lessons—"digressions"—on brain anatomy, verbal memory, and the psychology of grammar. This book is short, fascinating, informative, and incredibly moving.

14

Mental Retardation and Developmental Disabilities

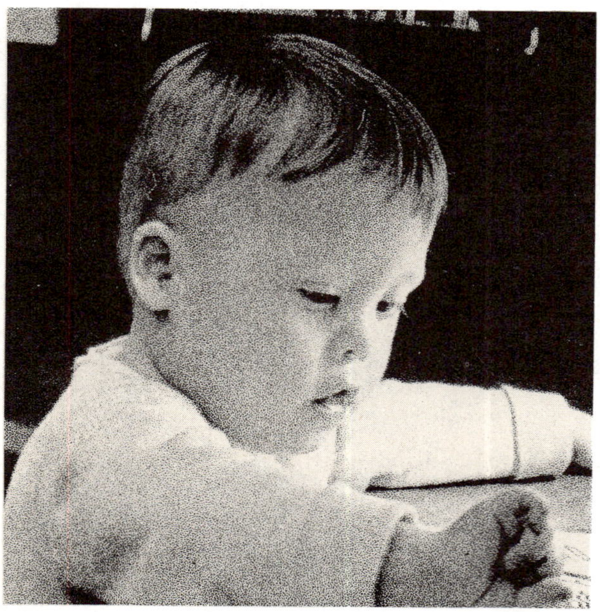

SECTION I
MENTAL RETARDATION

GENERAL BACKGROUND

Case 14.1

When Richard was eight months old, he was diagnosed as having cerebral palsy (see p. 396).

His mother had suspected that something was wrong for some time before that because he was so inactive and wouldn't reach for anything. His physical development was very slow. He did not sit up until he was more than a year old, and he never learned to walk at all. When he was 14 months old, he had a series of . . . seizures. The doctor put Richard on anticonvulsant medication and the seizures ceased. As he grew older, he became an increasing problem to his family. He began to say a few words when he was three, but his control over his articulators was so poor that no one could understand him except his immediate family. . . . at five [he] was still not toilet trained, was confined to a wheel chair, and drooled almost continually. . . . [at age ten], Richard still could not take care of his most basic needs, and his parents began to look for a . . . permanent placement for him. He was finally admitted to a state institution for the retarded. His psychological evaluation on admission determined that Richard was functioning at the level of the average three year old mentally. Immediately after he was admitted, he began having violent seizures again, which subsided only gradually as the doctors experimented with various medications. At the institution, the staff eventually taught him to signal his toileting needs so that he could be brought to the bathroom, and a speech therapist devoted considerable time to improving his language, but with little success. He is still unable to walk or dress himself, and there is little hope that he will improve very much or ever be released except to some other total care facility.

Source: Mental retardation: The changing outlook, pp. 13–14, by R. P. Ingalls,

Case 14.2

Roy was the second of two boys born in New York City's Harlem. His father disappeared when he was two years old. Roy's family

moved three times before Roy started school, once because the building they lived in was being torn down, once when they were evicted because of nonpayment of rent, and once when they moved voluntarily because the landlord refused to provide enough heat during a cold winter. There was nothing unusual about Roy's early physical development. His mother was a hostile and authoritarian woman who was continually yelling at her children and who would beat them with a hairbrush at the slightest provocation. As a result, Roy spent as little time as possible at home, even when he was very young.

In the first grade, Roy did not like his teacher, and

she did not like him. She complained that she couldn't understand much of what he said because he slurred his words and that he was frequently dirty and smelled of urine. Roy spent most of his schooltime trying to avoid work. . . . He had a great deal of difficulty sitting still for any length of time. . . . When he was promoted to second grade, he was placed in a special section for slow learners. . . . With special remediation he was able to learn all of his letters and could read a few simple words, in spite of the fact that he really had no interest in schoolwork. . . . In the third grade, he was suspended for three days for fighting. He started to skip school with increasing regularity and hang around with his older brother and his friends. A year later he was arrested for shoplifting, but was released with a warning. After his third suspension from school in the fifth grade, he was given a thorough examination by the school psychologist, who administered a standard intelligence test to him and determined that Roy's IQ was 63. As a result, he was placed in a special class. Here there were fewer students and the teacher could give him more individual attention. . . . and by the end of the year (Roy) was reading at the second-grade level.

By this time, however, his older friends were getting into bigger trouble. The next year, he was arrested for stealing money from a cash register and again released with only a warning. A short time later . . . he and his brother were arrested again for stealing a car and taking it on a joy ride, and this time he was referred to a private residential school for delinquent boys upstate. There he received intensive counseling and some special tutoring. A year later, he was returned to his mother. After that, Roy managed to stay out of trouble for awhile and even attended school regularly because he liked to work in the machine shop in the high school. However, he still could not read very well. . . . When he was 16, he quit school. He could not find a job, and a few months later, he was arrested for the armed robbery of a liquor store. He was sent to prison for six months and then was let out on parole. The parole board found him a job in a gas station. His boss taught him a good deal about fixing cars, and Roy became a fair mechanic. He got married a year later and settled down. Most of his former friends were in prison. . . . it was easy for him to stay out of trouble if there was no one to encourage him to transgress. He is still working at the gas station and spends most of his spare time fixing cars, watching television, or drinking beer at the local bar.

Source: Mental retardation: The changing outlook, pp. 8–9, by R. P. Ingalls,

Both Roy and Richard had been diagnosed as mentally retarded, but they are as dissimilar as two people can be. As you can see, the label *mental retardation* applies to a diverse group of people with less in common among themselves than one might expect.

Definitions and Classification

The American Association on Mental Deficiency (AAMD, Grossman, 1973) and the DSM-III define mental retardation in similar ways: mental retardation is diagnosed when there is significantly subaverage general intellectual functioning associated with or resulting in deficits or impairments in adaptive behavior, and with onset before age eighteen.

The DSM-III and the AAMD determine intellectual functioning on the basis of individually administered, standardized intelligence tests that yield IQ scores, and although they both set 70 or below as an arbitrary boundary, they caution us to regard this boundary flexibly (say 65 to 75). They also caution us that if there is no problem in adaptive behavior, we should not make a diagnosis of mental retardation, even if the IQ is lower than 70.

The AAMD and the DSM-III both define adaptive behavior as the effectiveness or degree with which the individual meets the standards of personal independence and social responsibility expected of his or her age and cultural group. During infancy and early childhood, these criteria include the development of sensorimotor skills, communication skills (speech and language), self-help

Listing 14.1 Syndromes Described in Chapter 14

Mental Retardation
Attention Deficit Disorder with Hyperactivity
Pervasive Developmental Disorders
  Infantile autism
  Childhood-onset pervasive developmental disorder
Cerebral Palsy
Specific Developmental Disorders
"Idiot Savants"

skills, and social skills such as learning to interact with others, getting along with others, and later, participating in group activities. In addition, adaptive behavior includes the use of adequate reasoning and judgment in achieving mastery over one's environment. Later, during adolescence and adulthood, the adequacy of adaptive behavior would be judged on the basis of the individual's ability to meet certain standards of vocational and social performance so that independent functioning can be expected.

The standard four-part classification of mentally retarded individuals is mild, moderate, severe, and profound. Spotlight 14.1 describes these levels in greater detail. The first level, mild mental retardation, applies to about 80 percent of the mentally retarded; mildly retarded people are educable and eventually self-supporting, a fact that many of us are likely to forget.

The "new look": some changing perspectives. The older view was that *mental deficiency* (an alternate label that is no longer popular) is an incurable, inherited condition that produces a socially incompetent, mentally subnormal individual who reaches a fixed "ceiling" (upper limit) of development that is much lower than is the case for the rest of us (Doll, 1941). This view has undergone some remarkable changes.

1. Mental retardation is no longer diagnosed on the basis of the so-called fixed IQ determined at birth. The newer view acknowledges the importance of the individual's capacity to get by in the real world outside the tester's office or the schoolroom. Especially at upper levels of IQ (near 70), adaptive ability can be sufficiently adequate so that the label of retardation would not apply.

2. Clinicians now recognize that there are many causes of retardation. Organic, physical, or biological variables may operate alone, or psychosocial causes or an interaction of several causes may produce retardation. In the vast majority of mentally retarded people, however, there is no known physical cause.

Not all neurologically impaired individuals, such as this child, are mentally retarded, despite appearances. (© David E. Kennedy)

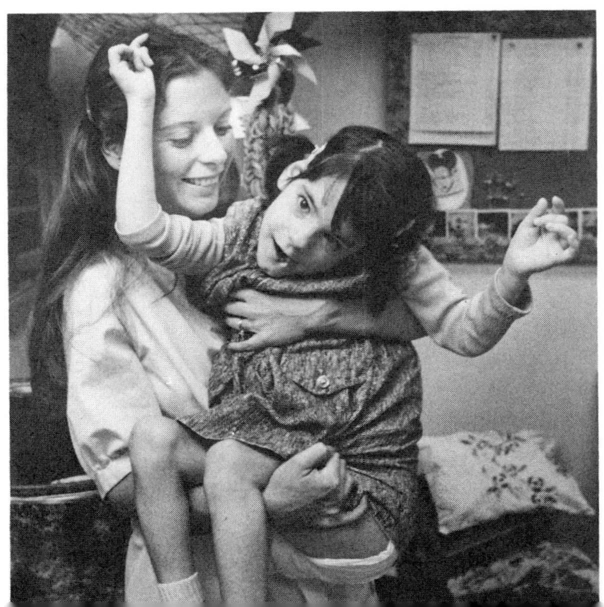

Spotlight 14.1 Classification and Description of Levels of Mental Retardation According to the DSM-III

Category	Rough IQ Range	Percentage of Retarded	Description
Mild ("educable")	50 to 70	About 80%	Individuals with this level of mental retardation can develop social and communication skills during the preschool period (ages 0–5), have minimal impairment in sensorimotor areas, and often are not distinguishable from normal children until a later age. By their late teens they can learn academic skills up to approximately the sixth-grade level; and during the adult years, they can usually achieve social and vocational skills adequate for minimum self-support, but may need guidance and assistance when under unusual social or economic stress.
Moderate ("trainable")	35 to 49	About 12%	Those with this level of mental retardation during the preschool period can talk or learn to communicate, but they have only poor awareness of social conventions. They may profit from vocational training and can take care of themselves with moderate supervision. During the school-age period, they can profit from training in social and occupational skills, but are unlikely to progress beyond the second-grade level in academic subjects. They may learn to travel alone in familiar places. During their adult years they may be able to contribute to their own support by performing unskilled or semiskilled work under close supervision in sheltered workshops. They need supervision and guidance when under mild social or economic stress.
Severe ("moderately trainable")	20 to 34	About 7%	During the preschool period there is evidence of poor motor development and minimal speech, and they develop little or no communicative speech. During the school-age period, they may learn to talk and can be trained in elementary hygiene skills. They are generally unable to profit from vocational training. During their adult years they may be able to perform simple work tasks under close supervision.
Profound ("limited training")	Below 20	Less than 1%	During the preschool period these children display minimal capacity for sensorimotor functioning. A highly structured environment, with constant aid and supervision, is required. During the school-age period, some further motor development may occur and the children may respond to minimal or limited training in self-care. Some speech and further motor development may take place during the adult years, and very limited self-care may be possible, in a highly structured environment with constant aid and supervision.

Spotlight 14.2 Some Worn-Out Myths About Mental Retardation

The past two decades have seen a dispelling of many myths about mental retardation such as those listed here, that offers millions of stigmatized and labeled people and their families a new lease on life.

1. Most mentally retarded people are unemployable and a drain on society. They should be put away ("warehoused") for life, because their condition is unchangable, incurable.
2. Because the IQ is fixed at birth, an individual with subnormal intelligence can never change, learn, or fit into society.
3. Most mental retardation is genetically determined, inborn, and therefore not preventable.
4. The principles that underlie teaching and training of "normal" individuals do not apply to the mentally retarded.
5. The mentally retarded should be treated like children, even when they are adults. They are incompetent, unable to care for themselves, and will forever remain dependent on others.
6. The mentally retarded should not be allowed to marry and have children, because they will produce other mentally retarded children.
7. Like the poor, the mentally retarded will always be with us.
8. The more severely or profoundly retarded the mental retardation, the less preventable it is.
9. The mentally retarded are mentally ill.
10. The mentally retarded are to be pitied and should be sheltered and coddled.
11. The mentally retarded are crazed, aggressive, sexually uncontrolled (for example, Lenny, in Steinbeck's *Of Mice and Men*).
12. The mentally retarded are pure "innocents," "good" people from whom we can learn spiritual values.
13. The mentally retarded are subhuman and animal-like and are justifiably objects of ridicule (for example, town fools or village idiots).
14. The mentally retarded should be "hidden" by their families.
15. The mentally retarded are not responsible and should have no legal rights.

Source: From Begab and Richardson, 1975; Crissey, 1975; Ingalls, 1978; Kurtz, 1977; and Wolfensberger, 1969.

3. The newer view does not assume the incurability and the inevitability of many forms of retardation. Most mentally retarded people are educable or trainable. Further, some of the more severe types of retardation are probably preventable, if not now, in the forseeable future.

4. Finally, it is acknowledged that mentally retarded people have feelings, emotions, desires, and egos, just like the rest of us.

Prevalence and Sociocultural Variables

Mental retardation is regarded as the fifth leading disability in the United States (preceded by mental illness, cardiac disease, arthritis, and cancer) and probably the primary disabling condition affecting children. According to the DSM-III, at any one point in time, approximately 1 percent of the population meets the criteria for mental retardation. Some estimates are as high as 3 percent, however (Ingalls, 1978; Kurtz, 1977). This means that in this country, even using the lowest of these estimates, there are well over two million individuals, ranging from the mildly to the profoundly impaired, who can be regarded as mentally retarded. Most of these people fall into the mildly retarded category.

The figures remain staggeringly large even if only the numbers of individuals with IQs below 50 are considered. According to one estimate, these number from three to five per thousand in the general population (Abramowicz and Richardson,

1975), suggesting that up to about one million people in this country may require some kind of special supervision and training, with a small percentage of these requiring institutional settings.

SES and racial-ethnic distribution. Most experts agree that of the mildly impaired group—where there is no known organic etiology—almost all fall into low-SES groups (Ingalls, 1978; Kurtz, 1977; Thompson and O'Quinn, 1979). Generally speaking, there is a familial pattern to this distribution in that family members of mildly impaired individuals also tend to show mild retardation. Retardation due to organic factors cuts across all SES groups, however, and there is no familial pattern except, of course, in instances of genetically transmitted retardation such as phenylketonuria (PKU) or Tay-Sachs' disease (see later sections of this chapter).

There is a consistent, empirically established relationship between mental retardation and ethnicity or racial, minority-group membership. This is so because minority status, especially being black or Mexican-American, is associated in our society with poverty and its accompanying high-risk variables such as drug abuse, alcoholism, malnutrition, poor medical supervision, exposure to noxious substances, and infectious diseases (Heber, 1970; Ingalls, 1978; Kurtz, 1977; Mercer, 1973).

In one prevalence study in Riverside, California, Mercer (1973) looked at SES and racial variables as they related to mental retardation. There were large SES differences of the sort already described, but racial differences were even larger with many more Mexican-Americans and blacks than "Anglos" among the mentally retarded population than expected on the basis of the actual distribution of these groups in the community. For example, although almost one-third of the mentally retarded sample was of Mexican-American descent, only 10 percent of the people in the community were of this ethnic background.

Sex distribution. Studies tend to agree that there is a higher rate of all levels of mental retardation among males than among females and especially so in the mildly impaired group (Farber, 1968; Ingalls, 1978; Kurtz, 1977). Estimates run as high as two to one. Are males more susceptible to prematurity, brain damage, or physical dangers in the environment after birth, factors that are related to mental retardation? Yes, according to many experts (Ingalls, 1978, for example). But these factors can account for only some male-female differences in incidence, because most differences are found in the mildly impaired group for which there are generally no known physical causes. It may be that being classified or labeled as mentally retarded is more likely for boys than for girls because of sociocultural reasons:

> *Parents treat boys and girls quite differently, and these differences in treatment might well contribute to differences in mental functioning. For example, parents are frequently more tolerant of aggressive and acting out behavior among boys than among girls, and this means that boys are less likely to apply themselves to schoolwork and other intellectual pursuits. Some families encourage their sons to be independent while they encourage their daughters to be dependent, and this means that boys have a greater opportunity for social failure . . . boys who are doing poorly are more likely to be diagnosed as retarded than are girls. Boys who are not doing well in school tend to become behavior problems to a much greater extent than do girls. They tend to call attention to themselves and make themselves obvious, while a girl who is having academic difficulties is more likely to sit quietly in the back of the class and not cause any problems. Many teachers tend to prefer quiet children to disruptive children, even if they are not as bright. As a result, boys are much more likely to be referred to the school psychologist for testing or the principal for disciplining than are girls. Thus, they are more likely to be diagnosed as retarded.*

(From *Mental retardation: The changing outlook,* p. 73, by R. P. Ingalls, Copyright © 1978 by John Wiley & Sons. Reprinted by permission of John Wiley and Sons, Inc.)

Some confirmation of this interpretation is suggested by a finding in the Mercer (1973) study that did indeed show many more boys than girls listed as mentally retarded by community social agencies, schools, and clinics. However, in the same community, when an adaptation measure and an IQ test were used on a representative sample of this community, thereby eliminating bias attributable to referral patterns, these differences were not observed.

TYPES OF MENTAL RETARDATION: CAUSES AND CLINICAL EXAMPLES

There are no known organic causes for most instances of mental retardation. The much smaller group of organically caused instances of retardation are comprised of a diverse group of etiologies, many of which, it appears, are or one day will be preventable (Hansen, Belmont, and Stein, 1980), contrary to popular opinion.

Infections and Intoxications

Infections and intoxications can cause mental retardation by adverse affects on the fetus (prenatal), newborn (perinatal), or developing child (postnatal). A well-known example of infection as a cause of mental retardation is *rubella,* or German measles. This viral disease can seriously affect the developing fetus if the mother contracts it during the first one-third of the pregnancy. As a result of a rubella epidemic in 1964–65 in this country, 30,000 children were affected with a variety of symptoms that included mental retardation (almost half the sample), hearing and visual defects, and cardiac problems (Holmes et al., 1972). Immunization prior to pregnancy has made striking inroads into the incidence of this infectious disease, however, with a consequent reduction in its potency as a cause of mental retardation.

Other congenital infections are the herpes, encephalitic, meningeal, and syphilitic infections (see Chapter 13), which have adverse effects on the developing fetus and which may result in mental retardation. Congenital syphilitic infections have more than doubled recently (Thompson and O'Quinn, 1979) and are of special significance if the mother develops syphilis after the sixteenth week of pregnancy. A child might appear to be normal at birth but can be actively affected later in life at ages ten to fifteen years because of the slow-developing virus involved in these conditions. Administration of antibiotics to the newborn is the recommended treatment.

Prenatal and postnatal intoxication. These conditions are important causal factors in mental retardation. Adverse effects of radiation on the developing fetus can also result in infant death, birth defects, or mental retardation. The increase of birth defects in children born to women who were exposed to nuclear blasts is by now well known. Less well known, but receiving increasing public attention, are the severe effects on the developing fetus of drugs such as heroin and prescribed medications.

Listing 14.2 The American Association on Mental Deficiency's List of Major Causes of Mental Retardation

1. Infections and intoxications
2. Trauma or physical agents (for example, child abuse, falls)
3. Disorders of metabolism or nutrition
4. Gross brain disease (postnatal)
5. Conditions due to unknown prenatal influence
6. Chromosomal abnormality
7. Gestational disorders (having to do with pregnancy)
8. Following psychiatric disorders
9. Environmental influences

Note: For purposes of clarity and simplicity, the section in the current chapter on causes of mental retardation is organized somewhat differently.

Source: Grossman, 1973.

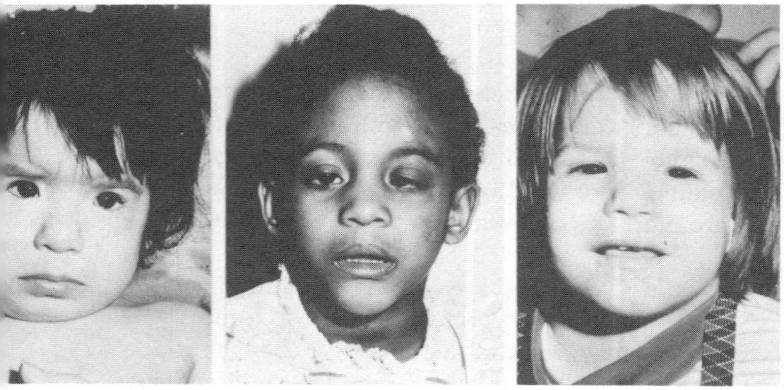

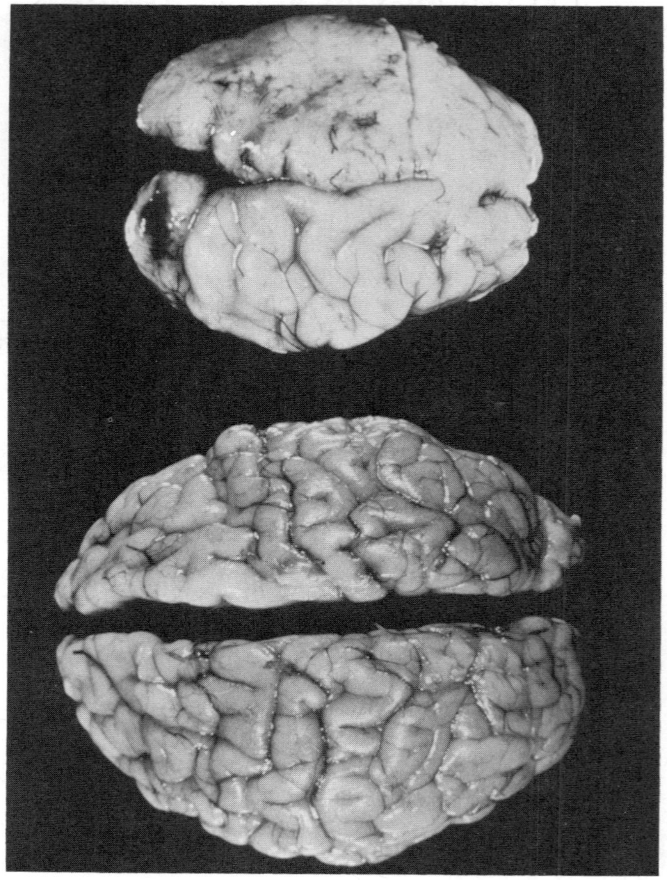

Figure 14.1 Right: The brain at top was taken from an infant with FAS who died five days after birth; note the small size, abnormal shape, and primitive development. The other brain is that of a normal infant. Above: These children, from three racial backgrounds—American Indian, black, and white—all have FAS, and all are mentally retarded. (From P. Streissguth et al., Teratogenic effects of alcohol in humans and laboratory animals, *Science, 209,* 1980, 353–61.)

The past decade has witnessed increased concern with an unsuspected teratogen (an agent that causes birth defects), alcohol. The fetal alcohol syndrome (FAS) has been identified in one to two per 1,000 births, and occurs among children born to alcoholics (Abel, 1980; *British Medical Journal,* 1976; Kirman, 1978). The FAS comprises an array of symptoms in the newborn, such as poor growth; physical deformities in the limbs and cranium—for example, microcephaly, a small, peculiarly shaped skull with a receding forehead and a furrowed scalp; cardiovascular dysfunctions; and later, behavioral and learning difficulties and mental retardation.

Neurological examinations of two-to-three-day-old infants at Boston City Hospital, for example, disclosed that 65 percent of the babies born to nondrinking or moderate drinkers were normal, whereas only 29 percent of the babies of heavy drinkers were normal (Ouellette and Rosett, 1976; Ouellette et al., 1977). The FAS infants were smaller, more jittery, and showed poor muscle tone; a few were microcephalic. It is entirely possible that some of their behavioral and physical defects can be due to related variables, such as the diseases or malnutrition of the chronic alcoholic mother, rather than to the alcohol itself, but there is some evidence that even moderate drinking may also affect the newborn (Abel, 1980; Kirman, 1978).

High risk for the FAS occurs when the mother takes about six alcoholic drinks or more daily, but what the safe *lower* limits are have not been clearly established (Abel, 1980).

Medicines prescribed for pregnant women. Medicines, especially those traditionally regarded as safe if given at the end of pregnancy, have also been very much implicated in some of the behavioral defects newborns have shown (Kolata, 1978a). These "officially" permitted procedures and medications include anaesthesia during birth, tranquilizers of various types (for example, Librium), and some of the sedatives prescribed to help the pregnant woman feel more comfortable.

One large longitudinal study* of 3,500 healthy babies born to healthy mothers (to rule out the possibility that birth or pregnancy complications can account for the results) found that the amount of obstetric medication given to the mothers affected the behavior of their children at least up to the age of seven years, confirming dozens of similar studies conducted with smaller samples ((Kolata, 1978b). Children born to heavily medicated mothers showed developmental lags in motor behaviors such as sitting and standing, difficulties in "inhibiting" abilities (for example, in adapting to repeated stimuli or to stop crying when comforted), and later, slower language and cognitive development.

Tens of thousands of babies, prenatally exposed to heroin or methadone because they were born to women addicted to narcotics (see Chapter 17) show abnormal behaviors from birth (the withdrawal syndrome) in addition to being very small for their age (Kolata, 1978b; Thompson and O'Quinn, 1979). Behavioral symptoms include irritability and excitability, high-pitched crying, sucking problems, tremors, and diarrhea. Prenatally exposed babies may later show disturbed speech, hyperactivity, and learning problems. Perhaps some of these children are also mentally retarded.

Many of these children (often born to unmarried women) are "difficult to live with." As a result, they are shifted from home to home because foster parents are unwilling to keep them. Thus, it is suspected that such children are also exposed to a variety of unstable environmental circumstances as well as to narcotics—all possible causes in producing low levels of intelligence. It may be too early, thus, to jump to conclusions about the specific effects of the behavioral teratogens and their contribution to mental retardation, for other factors may be involved. A good case can be made, however, for continued efforts to explore these relationships.

* This was part of a study of more than 50,000 babies in a project supervised by the National Institutes of Health. The data in connection with this report were analyzed by Yvonne Brackbill and Sarah Broman.

Trauma and External Physical Causes

Next to brain infections, physical injuries—accidental or otherwise—are the most frequent causes of postnatally acquired mental retardation (Ingalls, 1978). Interestingly, nature's remarkable insulation of the fetus during pregnancy protects it from physical injury. It is during the birth process and in the early childhood years that most physical trauma occurs. During birth (the perinatal period), the newborn's vulnerability to physical injuries can arise from difficult labor, mechanical injuries through use of instruments, and oxygen deprivation (anoxia) because of the premature separation of the fetus from the placenta during birth (that is, a period during which the child cannot breathe on his or her own). In the postnatal period, children can fall or have accidental blows on the head as well as other traumas, especially in unpredictable environments of the ghetto street or in emotionally disturbed, alcoholic, or "schizophrenogenic" family settings.

Child abuse—the battered child. Wilful physical blows to the infant and developing child can produce skull fractures, internal bleeding that causes intracranial pressure, or unconsciousness that can have serious effects on behavior, including learning difficulties or retardation depending on the seriousness of the brain injury. Understandably, incidence of such wilful injury is greatly underestimated, for parents cover up, make excuses ("it was an accidental fall," or "there was this violent fight between the two boys") to the attending physician in the emergency room—if indeed, the child is brought to a hospital at all.

The most serious effects of injury on development occur during the early childhood years while the brain is still developing. This makes all the more dramatic the finding that about two-thirds of the victims of child abuse are under three years of age, and one-third, under six months of age. Of about 300,000 identified instances of child abuse per year, there are 2,000 deaths and 60,000 instances of serious injury, of which about 6,000 involve permanent brain damage with mental retardation (Elmer and Gregg, 1967; Kempe, 1976; Kempe et al., 1962; Martin et al., 1974).

Only recently has this hidden violence within the family come to light. Such explosiveness occurs within many types of families and across all social and economic levels, contrary to the stereotype of the lower-class home and the Saturday-night drinking bouts. We are also beginning to learn more about how to help control these behaviors, for example, by first encouraging parents to acknowledge their violence and by offering "hotlines" and counseling services to them if they wish to but cannot control their violent behavior. Chapter 18, which presents material about violence and antisocial behavior, discusses in more detail some of the causes for such destructive behavior within the family.

Endocrine Disorders

Certain dysfunctions of the hormonal system (endocrinological disorders) are associated with mental retardation. The most frequent of these is an insufficiency of the thyroid hormone (hypothyroidism). Its extreme form is called congenital hypothyroidism or cretinism, a rare condition that appears at birth, and that may result from several causes including drugs, radiation during pregnancy, iodine insufficiency, even genetic factors (Ingalls, 1978). If undetected and untreated congenital hypothyroidism can lead to physical and mental retardation. But if appropriate thyroid therapy is introduced by four months of age, its dramatic effects can be controlled and there is no retardation (Ingalls, 1978; Rosman, 1976). Untreated instances of hypothyroidism have relatively set characteristics that include, in addition to moderate or severe retardation, coarse hair, dry coarse skin, short stature, large tongue, poor motor coordination and awkwardness, language difficulties, sluggishness, anemia, and chronic constipation (Clarke and Clarke, 1974; Ingalls, 1978; Thompson and O'Quinn, 1979).

Malnutrition

Severe malnutrition in the early years may affect the biochemical and functional development of the brain. The strength of this relationship, if it exists at all, is not entirely clear (Pincus and Tucker, 1978), however, because severe malnutrition tends to occur in low-SES groups that can be characterized by many other variables that can cause mental retardation. There is little doubt, however, that if extreme enough, malnutrition can produce mental retardation. For example, *Kwashiorkor*, a disease of infancy and early childhood due to extreme deficiency of protein, is related to mental retardation in India. Such starvation is rare in developed nations, however (Ingalls, 1978; Pincus and Tucker, 1978).

The effects of malnourishment of the mother on the developing fetus are not clear. Here again, the mother's malnutrition as a cause of mental retardation cannot be definitely implicated unless the effects of poverty in causing mental retardation are also clearly understood.

Mental Retardation and Congenital Physical Deformities

Many mentally retarded individuals have accompanying physical defects. Physical defects do not necessarily mean mental retardation, however. Some of these conditions are congenital (present at birth but not inherited) malformations with unknown causes, although it is generally acknowledged that in these and related conditions, infections, physical trauma, radiation, and drugs can be responsible. Many of these congenital defects involve cranial anomalies such as microcephaly (an abnormally small skull), and hydrocephalus, a condition in which an excess of cerebrospinal fluid in the head exerts pressure on the brain, resulting in an abnormally large skull. Prognosis for these conditions is "mixed" (Ingalls, 1978), but in some of these conditions surgery immediately after birth can arrest the condition so that there is no intellectual deficit.

Inherited and Inborn "Errors": Chromosomal and Genetic Syndromes

A small percentage of the mentally retarded population (under 10 percent) became so because of inborn factors that result from chromosomal abnormalties or genetic transmission.* Below are a few of the more well-known syndromes. According to the National Genetics Foundation, there are over 2,000 genetic diseases, most of which are unrelated to mental retardation. You are reminded that scientists have made amazing discoveries as to the prevention or control of some of these disorders.

Down's syndrome ("mongolism"): A chromosomal abnormality. As described in Chapter 7, there are 23 pairs of chromosomes in the human cell. Children born with Down's syndrome have three instead of the usual pair of chromosome 21.* Down's children are almost invariably retarded, but many only mildly. Contrary to popular belief, the range of retardation is extremely broad with many Down's children leading useful, contented lives for decades.

Down's children are recognizable at birth by certain physical characteristics that include a large, protruding tongue with deep fissures at the back, slanting eyes, a small round head, transverse (simian) crease on the palms, eyes that are set close together, no Moro reflex (the "startle" reflex in normal infants: the extension of the extremities in response to a sudden loud stimulus), small stature, dry skin, short stubby fingers that curve inward, inflammation of the eyelids, and at least a dozen other abnormal physical characteristics (Thompson and O'Quinn, 1979; Trunca, 1980). In addition to these distinctive physical features, many children born with Down's syndrome have heart and respiratory defects or acute leukemia. For this reason, in the past such children rarely survived into middle or old age, for they were subject to many infections and illnesses that resulted in early death. Recently, this picture has changed somewhat.

About one in every 700 births produces a Down's child. Each year there are about 5,000 new cases of Down's syndrome in the United States (Omenn, 1978). Risk for giving birth to a Down's syndrome infant increases with age (see Table 14.1), so that if a mother is older than forty-five years, the probability is 1 in 65 that her offspring will have this syndrome, compared to 1 in 1,500 for women under thirty years of age. Relatively new evidence has implicated older *fathers* in producing Down's children, but the mechanisms involved are not clear (Thompson and O'Quinn, 1979).

The advent of new medications has permitted a longer life span for many of these children, so that even if 20 to 30 percent die in the first few years,

---

* Only the most frequent syndromes will be described, but there are many other CNS hereditary disorders that are frequently associated with mental retardation. One type that shows up after birth are the neurocutaneous dysplasias, of which one is neurofibromatosis, transmitted through a dominant gene and found in about one in 3,000 live births. This condition involves multiple growths in the peripheral and central nervous systems as well as fairly large "café au lait" spots on the surface of the skin. About 10 to 25 percent of children born with this disease are mentally retarded, mostly in the mild range (Thompson and O'Quinn, 1979). Another inherited brain disease that is transmitted by a dominant gene is tuberous sclerosis which results in the development of many nodules on the cerebral cortex. Most victims of this disease become increasingly retarded with age, generally accompanied by seizures (Ingalls, 1978).

* The chromosomal abnormality (trisomy 21) was discovered only a few decades ago by a French scientist named Lejeune (Lejeune, Gautier, and Turpin, 1959).

Table 14.1 Risk of Having a Down's Syndrome Child as a Function of Mother's Age

Age of Mother	*Risk*
Under 30 years	One in 1,500 births
30–34	One in 750 births
35–39	One in 280 births
40–44	One in 130 births
Over 45	One in 65 births

Source: U.S. Department of Health, Education and Welfare.

the majority live at least to the middle years or older (Robinson and Robinson, 1976; Kirman, 1978). This greater longevity produced a challenge for society, with a surprising result: that despite speech, motor, and other developmental delays in learning, Down's children can be taught many skills. Moreover, work is possible for a good number of such individuals. Interestingly, empirical evidence indicates that those who live at home or in the community learn more, survive longer, and develop more skills than those who are institutionalized, a trend that is true for other types of mentally retarded individuals as well (Thompson and O'Quinn, 1979; Kirman, 1978).

Although there is no known cure for Down's disease, it is now possible to detect the chromosomal abnormality that produces the defect in the fetus during the mother's pregnancy. The technique by which this is done is called amniocentesis, a painless, rather simple method of removing cells from the amniotic fluid surrounding the fetus. If the fetus indeed shows chromosomal or other genetic abnormalities, the mother can choose to terminate the pregnancy. Spotlight 14.3 describes this and related procedures in more detail.

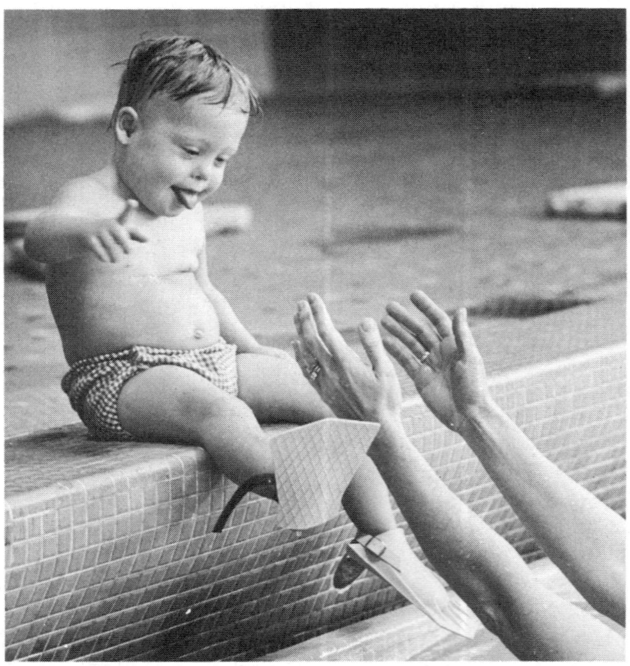

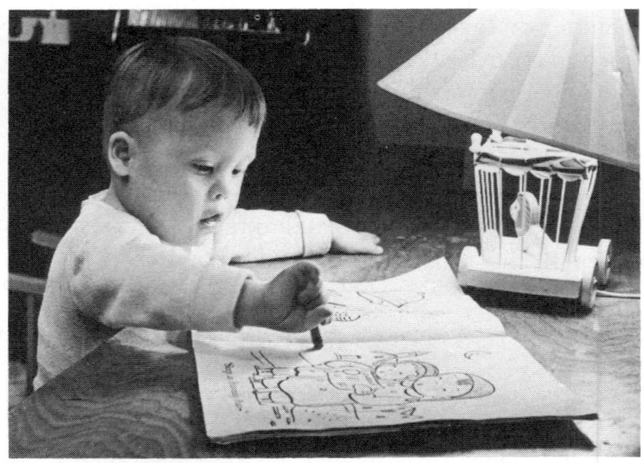

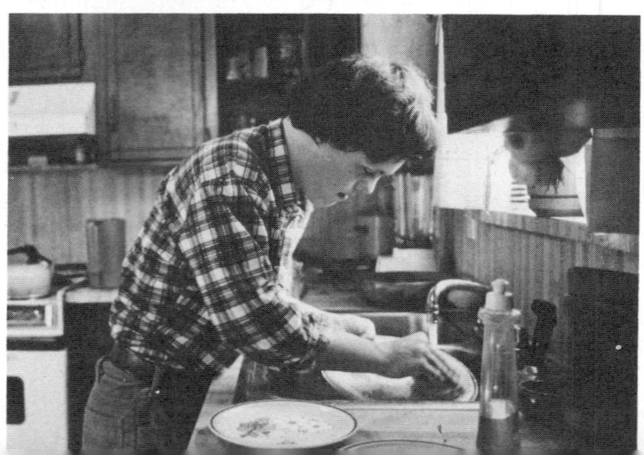

This Down's syndrome child, photographed at different ages, has been successfully taught many skills. (© Bruce Roberts)

Spotlight 14.3 Genetic Counseling and Assessment of Risk in the Newborn

Genetic counseling attempts to aid prospective parents (especially those in high-risk groups) by informing them of the risks they face in giving birth to physically defective, mentally retarded, or otherwise abnormal children. A counselor, for example, might tell the parents about the rates of a particular defect in the general population (say, 1 in 1,000), what their own personal rates are (say, 1 in 65), the availability of screening methods after the baby is born (for PKU, for example, see p. 378), and what their options are, such as amniocentesis and abortion, if the fetus is defective.

The decision to do something about such risks rests with the potential parents, not the counselor. For example, parents who have had several Tay-Sachs' babies (see p. 378) may decide to have no more children after they have been informed that as Tay-Sachs' carriers, there is a one in four chance their offspring will have this fatal disease. Other parents may wish to go ahead with the pregnancy, but in any event, the decisions of both sets of parents are based on knowledge. Some people might feel that they would even be within their rights to sue the obstetrical staff if they were not forewarned about such risks.

How can one know about a birth defect before the offspring is born? There are several methods that can be used. The genetic counselor not only discusses the availability of these techniques but also what the risks to the fetus and mother are as well as errors in connection with their use.

Amniocentesis. This is a procedure wherein a small sample of amniotic fluid is taken from a women 15 to 17 weeks into pregnancy. The sample is obtained with a needle that is carefully guided by ultrasound to aid in determining the position of the fetus. The pregnancy is allowed to progress this far before the amniocentesis because there is not enough amniotic fluid, which surrounds the fetus, until this time. Amniotic fluid consists primarily of cells from the urine, skin, and respiratory tract of the fetus. The rather complicated analysis of these cells to detect defects and chromosomal "errors" takes about three weeks to complete. Although this method is used chiefly for Down's syndrome, there are about seventy-five other hereditary, biochemical disorders that can also be detected by this method, for example, neural tube closure defects in which infants are born with no brain. There is almost 100 percent accuracy in the diagnoses that are made but there is a small risk to the fetus: miscarriage in about 1 or 2 percent of the cases (Fuchs, 1980). Amniocentesis is recommended for pregnant women in their late thirties and for those who have had other children with genetic disorders or when there is a family history of such disorders.

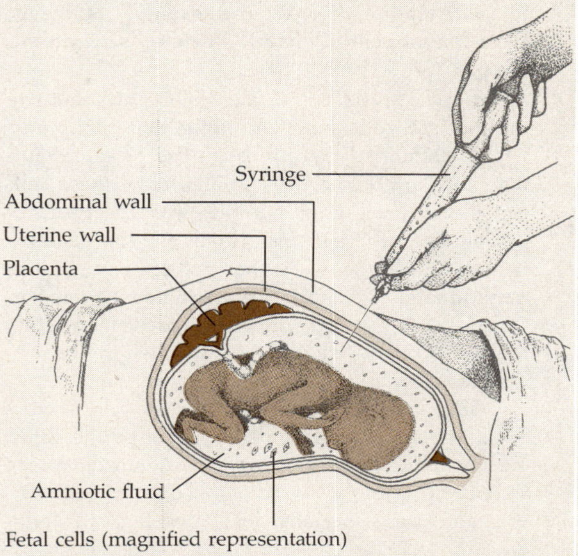

Figure 14.2 Amniocentesis. Withdrawing a sample of amniotic fluid from the fetal sac is the first step in checking for possible genetic defects in the unborn child.

Issues in connection with amniocentesis are (Omen, 1978): Given the small risk of miscarriage, should *all* women over the age of thirty-five years be tested for Down's syndrome? If other disorders are found, should the parents be informed so that an appropriate decision can be made? If there is a family history of certain sex-linked disorders, should amniocentesis automatically be recommended to determine the sex of the fetus in order to rule out the disorder (for example, a female fetus cannot possibly have Klinefelter's syndrome; see p. 377)?

Analysis of fetal cells in maternal blood. About two million fetal cells are found in the maternal blood, having circulated there through the placenta (Altman, 1979a; Omenn, 1978). Samples of these cells can directly tell us about the presence of chromosomal and other abnormalities, for example neural tube defects. Further refinements of this method might result in its replacing amniocentesis, especially as a routine measure for women under the age of thirty-five years, for the risk in this procedure is lower than that in amniocentesis.

Other new developments in fetal medicine. Fetoscopy is a method that allows parts of the fetus, such as fingers, limbs, genitals, and hair details, to be viewed directly, by bringing light into the uterus and using specially developed lenses (Mahoney and Hobbins, 1979). In this way, in the early months of pregnancy, missing limbs, trunk abnormalities, neural tube defects, and other gross malformations can be directly observed. Along with this method is the relatively new technique of obtaining samples of fetal skin for biopsy (the removal of tissue for diagnostic study). In addition, samples of fetal blood can be obtained directly from the placenta. When perfected, these methods will eventually allow the prenatal diagnosis of many inherited diseases not detectable through amniocentesis. Currently, such procedures involve some risk to the fetus, for they are invasive. But technology will one day undoubtedly make these methods safer, permitting further progress in the fight against diseases that cause retardation (Mahoney and Hobbins, 1979). For example, fetal therapy, actual treatment of defects in the fetus, is in the foreseeable future, as in treating a defect with appropriate chemicals or in withdrawing excessive cerebrospinal fluid from a fetal head (Schmeck, 1981).

Case 14.3 Karen: Down's Syndrome

Families that produce a Down's syndrome child must make many decisions about the education, training, and future of their retarded child. This is illustrated in the case of Karen.

Both her parents were college graduates, and they lived in a middle-class suburb. . . . She was diagnosed at birth as having Down's syndrome. . . . Her parents were horrified when the physician told them that their child would be retarded, but they accepted the fact and tried to raise her as they would any other child. . . . Karen's development was quite slow. She didn't sit up until she was a year old, and didn't walk until she was nearly two years old. Her mother, after a good deal of effort, had her completely toilet trained by the time she was five, but the local school system had no facilities for a child as severely retarded as Karen, and so she was excluded. She stayed at home with her mother for another year and a half, and her mother conscientiously taught her . . . self-help skills such as dressing. . . . Karen was able to talk in short sentences, although she was hard to understand. . . .

A year later, the school system initiated a classroom for trainable level children, and Karen was a charter member. In school, she continued to learn social and self-help skills, and an attempt was made to teach her to read, write, and count. She attended school until she was 17. . . . At this time, she was able to count, although she had little idea of what numbers meant. She could write her name, but she had no functional reading skills. A psychologist determined that she was functioning at the level of the average six year old, and she told Karen's parents that her IQ was 40.

After Karen left school, her parents became increasingly concerned about her future. She would always need some sort of supervision, but they were totally opposed to institutionalizing her. They had visited the state training school and were horrified by what they saw. They could not afford to place her in a private facility, and so she just stayed at home with them. . . . She had no friends, and the only socializing that she did was attending a dance once a week sponsored by the community association for the retarded. . . . After several years . . . they [the parents] were finally able to enroll Karen in a sheltered workshop where she was given jobs of assembling simple parts for a local factory and stuffing envelopes. . . . Karen is still at the workshop. Her father recently had a heart attack, and her parents are now more concerned than ever about Karen's future since they know that they will be too old to care for her much longer. . . .

Source: Mental retardation: The changing outlook, by R. P. Ingalls, pp. 12–13, Copyright © 1978 by John Wiley & Sons. Reprinted by permission of John Wiley & Sons, Inc.

Klinefelter's syndrome. This chromosomal disorder is a sex-linked dysfunction in which the male offspring is born with 47 chromosomes instead of the usual 46. There is an extra X chromosome attached to the XY (male) pair. The XXY syndrome occurs in about one in every 1,000 male live births. Its features, which become especially apparent at puberty, include development of the breasts, slim body build, a high voice, and sparse hair growth. These males also show infertility and underdeveloped penis and testes. Usually, mild or moderate retardation is present, but in many instances there is no retardation at all (Ingalls, 1978; Sarason and Doris, 1969). These and other sex-related (chromosomal) disorders make up about 1 percent of the institutional population (Clarke and Clarke, 1974).

Phenylketonuria (PKU). Some types of mental retardation are associated with recessive inheritance, for example PKU, which is determined by a single recessive autosomal gene. This defect results in an enzyme deficiency that produces dysfunctions in

Case 14.4 S. B. F.: An Untreated PKU Child

S. B. F. was referred for evaluation of developmental delay at 4 years 8 months of age. . . . The initial PKU screening test (in infancy) revealed a phenylalanine level of 8.8 mg% after one day of milk feedings. For unknown reasons, a followup of this elevated level (normal up to 3.6 mg%) was not done.

Motor milestones (rolling, sitting, pulling to stand) were achieved appropriately during the first year. However, S. B. F. did not walk until 18 months of age. He began to follow simple commands at 24 months of age, and to speak in a few 2 or 3 word combinations by 2 years 6 months. Now, at 4 years of age, he is unable to dress himself, is messy in feeding himself, and his coordination has been slow to develop. His behavior has been difficult to manage because of frequent temper tantrums and screaming.

On developmental testing . . . at 3 years 11 months of age, he was found on the Stanford-Binet to have a mental age of 2 years 4 months and an IQ of 50. At that time his language was echolalic and perseverative. The family did not follow through with further developmental evaluation and therapy. . . .

When he was seen for the first time . . . he presented as an attractive blond, blue-eyed youngster who looked bright and smiled readily. He seemed to be in terror of the physical examination, however. . . . Phenylalanine level was grossly elevated. . . . A repeat of the Stanford-Binet yielded a mental age of 2 years 3 months and an IQ of 35. . . . Speech and language skills receptively were at the 2-year 4-month level and expressively at the 24-month level. Fine motor skills were at the 20–24-month level, and gross motor at the 24–28-month level.

Dietary modification will be undertaken so as to substantially decrease the intake of phenylalanine. Whether this will be tolerated at this time or whether it will produce any amelioration of the retardation or behavior remains to be seen.

Source: Thompson and O'Quinn, 1979, pp. 35–36.

the metabolism of protein. As a consequence, there is moderate to severe retardation accompanied by seizures, poor motor coordination, and perceptual difficulties. Recessive, inherited disorders like PKU can be carried by normal individuals with a 25 percent chance that PKU will occur in their offspring.

The past decades have witnessed remarkable advances in controlling and preventing retardation due to PKU, which occurs in about 1 in 10,000 to 20,000 live births. National screening for PKU babies has become possible as a result of the discovery that babies with PKU can be diagnosed in early infancy (at one time, through an examination of their urine, but now through blood tests). If PKU is found, the dangerous buildup of the toxic substance that causes the brain damage—phenylalanine—can be controlled through diet. If dietary control is introduced immediately, retardation can be prevented. But if untreated, mental retardation inevitably follows and is irreversible.

PKU and related inborn metabolic disorders (for example, galactosemia, a failure to metabolize properly a carbohydrate called galactose) are examples of the fact that environmental interventions can prevent certain inherited disorders. This is a challenge to the traditional view that genetic disorders are neither preventable nor treatable.

Tay-Sachs' disease. This genetically transmitted disease—its infantile form is the one we most often hear about—is also caused by a single recessive autosomal gene. As with PKU, even if both parents are healthy but carry the recessive gene for this defect, there is a one in four chance that their baby will have the disease.

Tay-Sachs' is a degenerative neurological disorder resulting essentially from inborn metabolic errors that create "fatty" deposits in the nervous tissue. There is no known cure for Tay-Sachs' disease, and severe degeneration of the infant beginning at about three to four months inevitably occurs. There is progressive muscular weakness, blindness, loss of previously developed skills, extreme sensitivity to sound, loss of body tone, and frequently, convulsions. Death usually occurs by the age of two to four years.

Tay-Sachs' disease occurs largely in Jewish populations with origins in a small area of Eastern Europe and is carried by three or four in 100 people of this particular population. Incidence was about one in 3,600 live births until fairly recently. Although Tay-Sachs' disease was always extremely rare in other populations, its expression has been virtually eliminated in the target population as a result of technical advances that permit its detection in utero (see Spotlight 14.3).

Gestational Disorders: Prematurity

Empirical research clearly establishes a relationship between prematurity* and mental retardation, both through retrospective studies (examining birth records of mentally retarded individuals) and longitudinal studies (observing and testing low-birthweight babies as they develop), according to Ingalls (1978). Below-weight babies have ten times greater risk for mental retardation than normal-weight babies (Hurley, 1969). Moderately low birthweight is associated with mild impairment, and extremely low birthweight with more severe impairment. Prematurity may not *cause* mental retardation but may result from the same factors that cause mental retardation—for example, alcoholism or drug abuse of the mother.

Prematurity is more frequent among nonwhites, but this is undoubtedly related to lowered socioeconomic, nutritional, and medical care among the racial minorities. Further, the striking relationship between prematurity and mental retardation occurs primarily among low-SES groups (Birch and Gussow, 1970). Many studies indicate that premature babies in higher SES groups show only small differences in intelligence compared to control full-term babies in the same SES level, while premature babies in *low*-SES groups show signifi-

* Prematurity, a gestation period of less than 37 weeks, is usually indicated by birthweight rather than by length of pregnancy, for time of conception is usually difficult to ascertain with exact accuracy.

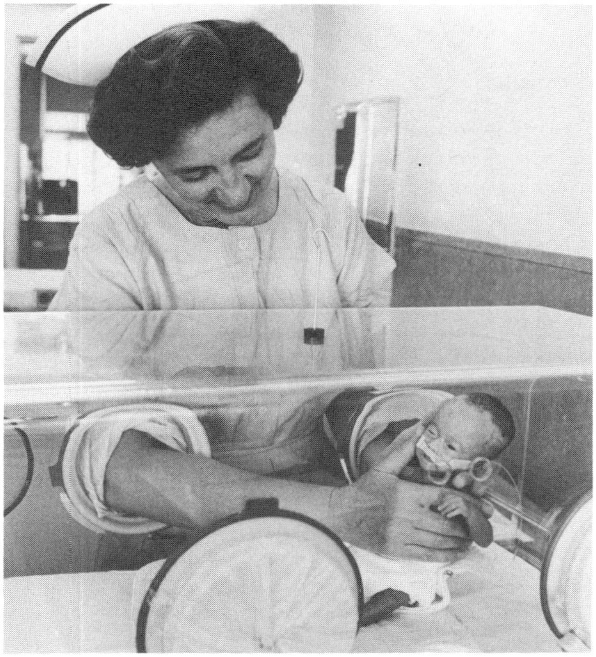

Premature babies are at higher risk for mental retardation than full-term babies. (Werner Wolff/Black Star)

cantly lower intelligence than their controls. Such babies apparently begin with a disadvantage that is never made up (Ingalls, 1978).

Psychosocial Retardation

About 75 to 80 percent of the mentally retarded (mild impairment, primarily) come from low-SES groups with no apparent organic (inherited, congenital, infectious) etiology. More often than not, this type of retardation is not diagnosed until the child's performance becomes obviously discrepant with some norm, some expectation for performance at school. When the individual leaves school and blends into society, the label tends to dissolve.

What lies behind the poor learning ability, dullness, inability to keep up at school found in the schoolrooms of the poor all over the world? Apparently the impoverished conditions in the slums of the cities and of the shacks of the rural poor are the breeding grounds for this kind of retardation. The child enters school with no motivation to learn, poor language preparation, inability to understand classroom rules like daily attendance, listening, or not speaking out of turn. The inconsistent and disorganized communication rules within the family, its lack of stress on language, and the empty psychosocial backdrop of the poor everywhere offer little opportunity for curiosity, intellectual growth, and preparation for school. These conditions have been implicated in the development of various disorders frequently in this book.

Psychosocial retardation thus makes its insidious presence during the early years—deficits that increase as the child of poverty gets older. It may be that this type of deficit is not true retardation, only a different language style, a deevaluation of learning and of abstract, conceptual thinking that we tend to measure in our schoolrooms and intelligence tests. Are we unfairly labeling the children of our poor by our biased testing methods?

Many slum children have educational deficits that reflect psychosocial deprivation rather than "true" mental retardation. (Copyright © Harvey Stein 1977)

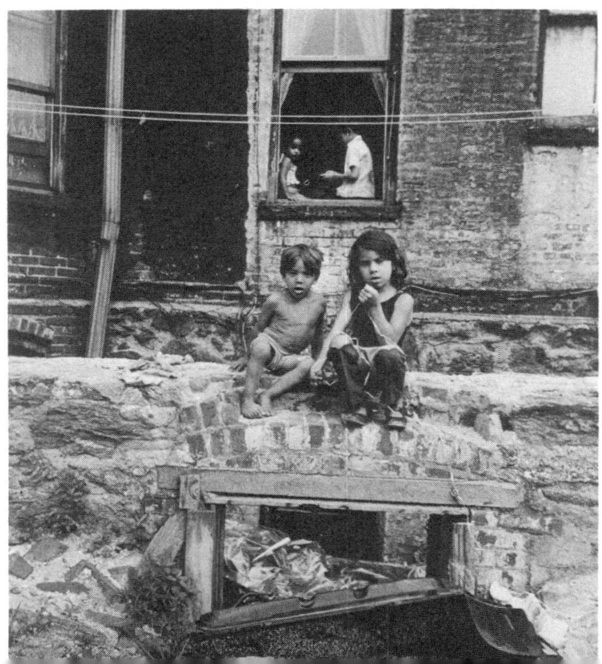

Spotlight 14.4 "Idiot Savants"—Are They Mentally Retarded?

We have all heard about the amazing mental feats performed by "mentally retarded" children, the so-called idiot savants. Such children may not be able to carry on a normal conversation, read, or keep up with their peers at school. If tested, their IQs would fall into the retarded range. But they may be able to hear a musical work for the first time and sing sections of it the next day. Or they can perform "calendar calculations": when asked, they can rapidly state the months and years in the next century in which the twelfth day of the month, for example, falls on a Thursday. Or they can identify the manufacturer of any automobile that they see. Despite difficulty in understanding ordinary language, they may have exceptional skills in writing or spelling in a foreign language, or they may be able to work with complex electronic equipment.

These extraordinary children, it is estimated, appear in about one of ten autistic children, one in 2,000 mentally retarded children, and about one in three million in the general population (Rimland, 1978). It would seem that they are neither retarded, judging by the usual standards, nor are they like the typical autistic child. We are just beginning to learn more about these children, especially through interest generated by Bernard Rimland, Director of the Institute for Child Behavior Research in San Diego.

Why do these children have such overdeveloped abilities in narrow, highly specialized areas while at the same time they are so deficient in other areas? Early theories held that the savants' skills are genetically determined, "built-in" quirks (Rife and Snyder, 1931). Later researchers believed that the special abilities of savants are actually skills that were developed to compensate for other handicaps, just as blind persons may develop extra skills to compensate for their blindness (Lindsley, 1965).

One theory that seems to be at least descriptively accurate suggests that the savants' abilities are due to their extraordinary skill in focusing—attending and concentrating—on the task at hand. Rimland (1978) refers to this as "high fidelity attention." He holds that savants are able to focus on a very narrow range of stimuli, but are unable to "pull back" to integrate larger aspects of their environment. In addition, they are not easily distracted by other stimuli, even when it would be to their adaptational advantage to be so.

The prodigious feats of many savants with numbers, music, and spatial relations have led to the belief that their right-hemisphere functions are overdeveloped, used in out-of-proportion balance to the left hemisphere, which is stifled, in some way, from proper growth. If this imbalance is further associated with the extreme attentional deficit that permits only narrow intense focus, then perhaps the unusual behavior of such people can begin to make sense.

Of interest is the study of identical twin savants, George and Charles, first reported in *Life* magazine who performed amazingly complex mental calculations with impressive speed and accuracy. The twins were later studied by psychologists who were interested in determining the "system" they used and the processes underlying this system. The researchers asked a psychology graduate student to learn the system they thought the twins used for such calculations. After much study the student learned the system, but he was slower in his calculations than the twins were. Then he "suddenly" developed the ability to calculate with speed that matched theirs. This led the investigators to hypothesize that the calculating rules worked by the left hemisphere had somehow "migrated" to the right hemisphere, "which grasps patterns of information all at once" (Rimland, 1978).

In any event, these fascinating savants offer a rich opportunity for furthering our knowledge about the remarkable capacities of the human brain. Perhaps some of the answers will lie in discovering the neuroanatomical, neurochemical, and neurophysiological underpinnings of the brains of these people, who, after all, are probably not metally retarded, just neurologically "different."

ASSESSMENT

There is considerable dissatisfaction with the IQ test as a measure of adaptive ability and educational potential. Especially criticized is the notion of the inherited, fixed IQ. A single score can label and stigmatize a child through his or her school career, obscuring underlying assets the child may have.*

Children of poverty may have IQs in the 60s, but they may also show lively ability to get by in their worlds. They get around their communities, can deal with other people, and can function fairly independently. They can "survive." When IQ alone was used to determine who the mentally retarded in a community were, the rates were very high (Mercer, 1973). But when adaptative ability was included in this determination, the rates declined among blacks from 44.9 per 1,000 to 4.1 per 1,000, and among Mexican-Americans from 149.0 per 1,000 to 60.0 per 1,000. The rates remained the same for the "Anglos" (4.4). It would seem that particularly among minorities and the disadvantaged, an assessment of adaptative ability may negate the label, mental retardation.

The SOMPA and Estimated Learning Potential.

The SOMPA (System of Multicultural Pluralistic Assessment) is a set of evaluative procedures that acknowledges the fact that a child may do poorly at school for a variety of reasons, including the possibility that his or her cultural background and language may differ radically from that of the school (Mercer, 1979). The SOMPA was standardized in California on 700 black, 700 Hispanic, and 700 white children, ages 5 to 7 years.

The assessment methods that are employed in this procedure survey a variety of social, physical, medical, adaptive, and intellectual areas as well as determine the sociocultural level, SES status, stability, cohesiveness, and acculturation of the subject's family into the mainstream culture of the school. This is accomplished by individual testing of the child in physical areas as well as by the administration of the Revised Wechsler Intelligence Scale for Children (WISC-R, see Chapter 5). There is also a detailed parent interview that helps in assessing the health and developmental history of the child.

This pluralistic assessment provides several layers of information. Is the subject at risk in medical and physical areas? Is the child's conventional IQ markedly divergent from the average range as determined by the traditional standards? How does the child's intelligence test performance compare to the average performance of his or her own ethnic group? Most important, the SOMPA introduces a method for determining the estimated learning potential (ELP) of the child.

The ELP is an adjusted IQ based on an evaluation of the child's sociocultural level within his or her ethnic milieu. It is designed to further differentiate among low-scoring children as to their ability to profit from school. To illustrate: Two Hispanic, extremely low-SES children received identical, extremely low adjusted IQs even when compared to appropriate ethnic norms. One child, however, comes from a disorganized, marginally adjusted family with very poor role models, whereas the other's family provides the opposite: both parents are active in church and an already working older brother spends much time in sports and other activities with his "kid" brother. The sociocultural index and ELP score for the second child is higher than that for the first; family counseling and special educational help are necessary for the first child to improve his chances for getting by in life.

Competence and Adaptive Behavior

Instead of intelligence, many experts are now talking about competence (Garmezy et al., 1977; McClelland, 1973; Zigler and Balla, 1977; Zigler and

* A landmark decision that challenged the traditional intelligence test's use in labeling minority group children as retarded (with consequent placement in special classes) was the 1971 California decision regarding *Diana* vs. *the Board of Education* in which several Mexican-American families challenged the classification of Mexican-American children on the basis of an IQ test presented in English.

Trickett, 1977). It is true that not all experts agree on just what competence is, but there are some common themes in various definitions that refer to social ability and mastery over one's social environment so that the use of one's resources to cope, achieve, and get along in one's world is possible. That is, competence is a general ability to use one's abilities and aptitudes to get along in real life. Although intelligence, as we generally think about it, and competence are probably not entirely unrelated, one advantage of employing the notion of competence is that it gets us away from the fixed IQ score and the strict labeling of intellectual ability that follows from it that classifies people as mentally retarded or not.

Psychologists have employed several methods to measure people's ability to get along in life, function independently, and generally take care of themselves. One early, widely used inventory of this type is the Vineland Social Maturity Scale (Doll, 1953, 1964). It consists of a checklist of 117 items that survey the social and adaptive behaviors performed by average children at various ages as well as by adults. For example, average two-to-three-year-olds can get a drink without help or eat with a fork; or average six-year-olds can bathe themselves or go to bed without help. Retardation may be present if most of the social behaviors performed by the chronological peers of a subject cannot be performed by the subject.

The Adaptive Behavior Scale, published by the American Association on Mental Deficiency (AAMD) was especially developed to provide profiles of mentally retarded individuals (children to adults). Standardized on a mentally retarded population, it provides useful comparisons of the subject on four levels of adaptive behavior, from mild and moderate to severe or profound. The 110 items in this scale are divided into two parts that assess adaptive functional behavior and maladaptive behavior.* The Adaptive Behavior Scale is especially useful in evaluating the progress of a mentally retarded person in supervised training programs. Is he or she, for example, ready to move into a less closely supervised role in the community?

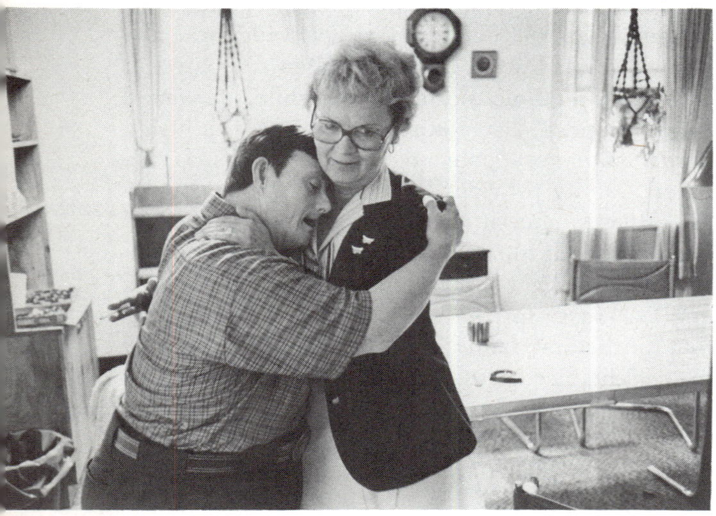

Mentally retarded people can have strong affectional ties with, and sometimes appear to cling to, familiar people on whom they have become dependent. (Alan Carey)

THE MENTALLY RETARDED AS PEOPLE

Some Characteristics of the Retarded

Many mentally retarded individuals show distinctive patterns of behavior that may tend to set them apart from their peers. They appear to cling to the familiar and to the routine and to have low self-esteem and confidence. They may mimic the behavior of others or show unvarying dependency on the initiative of people around them, sometimes displaying extreme suggestibility, even when it is not

* Part I contains 10 behavioral "domains" intended to reflect basic survival skills such as language development, numbers and time, domestic activity, and vocational activity. Part II contains 14 "domains" focusing primarily on negative affect such as violent and destructive behavior, untrustworthy behavior, withdrawal, stereotyped behavior and odd mannerisms, self-abusive behavior, hyperactive tendencies, sexually aberrant behavior, and psychological disturbances.

in their own best interests (Zigler [1973] calls this pattern "other-directedness"). They frequently show poor social skills; for example, they may retreat entirely or show excessive shyness and inability to express their wishes. As a result, they are often isolated by their peers. As a matter of fact, in social settings in which there are primarily nonretarded people, they are generally unable to form friendships.

It is not difficult to understand the origins of some of these personal and interpersonal behaviors. Most retarded people anticipate failure and do not trust their own judgment or initiative in solving problems, especially in new and unfamiliar situations. Their past experiences reinforce this self-image; they have learned that familiar, routine events are less threatening to them.

In addition, many retarded individuals suffer from the labels applied to them. Most people tend to have a set of attitudes that accompany the label of retardation and as a consequence behave differently toward a mentally retarded person than they would to "ordinary" unlabeled people. This special treatment may contribute to the isolation that many retarded people feel. The point is that the social environments of many retarded individuals may discourage the development of adequate social behavior.

The Retarded and Learning Skills

Do mentally retarded people learn on the basis of a special set of principles? Some experts say yes, suggesting that a mentally retarded adult with the mental age of ten years uses problem-solving strategies that differ from those used by an average child of ten years: they are more concrete, for example, less able to deal with abstract concepts. Other experts, however, believe that the principles are the same, although the learning process may be slower and eventually limited by a lower ceiling (Zigler, 1969).

It may appear that retarded individuals learn by a special set of rules because of their special motivational patterns and expectations about their performance that they bring to various tasks. A mentally retarded child may attend to irrelevant aspects of a task, requiring many trials to solve an easy problem. This may be a consequence of trying to please the experimenter and of wishing to remain within the social situation as long as possible. These and related hypotheses were experimentally tested and confirmed by Zigler and his associates (Zigler, 1966, 1969; Zigler and DeLabry, 1962; Zigler, Hodgden, and Stevenson, 1958).

In well-controlled experiments, for example, it was found that retarded subjects tended to spend more time performing an easy, "boring" task such as placing pegs into a pegboard than did their controls, who were matched in mental age. Zigler and his associates also found that socially-deprived (prior to institutionalization) institutionalized retarded children spent more time on such tasks than a control group of institutionalized children who had not been "starved" for social interactions. Apparently, the former group of subjects had greater need to please the adult experimenters and to conform to the social requirements of the experimental situation than did the control subjects.

These researchers hypothesized that mentally retarded children showed a pattern called negative reaction tendency which reflects their wariness of strange adults. This tendency conflicts with the positive reaction tendency just described, the desire to please adults. This model received some empirical confirmation in that mentally retarded subjects were found to spend more time on the second than on the first of two boring tasks, once having got over the initial fear of the experimenter (Zigler et al., 1958).

Sex and Marriage

Even staff members who work closely with the retarded share the popular stereotype: sexual activity between mentally retarded people is wrong and should not be allowed. In one study that employed a questionnaire administered to staff members at three residential facilities for the mentally retarded, findings indicated that almost one-third of the staff "felt that no sexual behavior, not even simple physical contact, was acceptable for retarded persons" (Mitchell, Doctor, and Butler, 1978).

And yet there is general agreement that sexual development in most mentally retarded people is similar to that of normal people. Sexual strivings, satisfaction of the need for intimacy and affection that sexual relations provide, as well as the stages of excitation and climax of sexual encounters are similar for both groups. Although homosexuality was once found to be more prevalent among the retarded than among normal people, this was probably due to segregation of the sexes in institutions for the retarded (Gebhard, 1973).

Adequate sex education and training is a "must" for mentally retarded individuals, especially in the light of the United Nations Bill of Rights for retarded individuals, passed in 1970, which stipulated that such individuals should have the right to cohabit and marry. Mentally retarded persons are often keenly aware of the responsibilities entailed in sexual activity and are quite receptive to sex education and guidance (Edgerton, 1973).

When the mentally retarded have children, can they care for them adequately?* Many mentally retarded persons living on their own, whether they are married or single, tend to need assistance from social agencies. This is true for mentally retarded persons with children as well. One study of thirty-two mentally retarded couples found that only six of the forty children of these couples had to be removed from their parents' care, however, and in most cases this was due to the retardation of the child. Most couples with children were able to provide adequately for them (Mattinson, 1973).

Do marriages between retarded persons work? The same study found that not only do they work, but also that most couples reported that the affectionate relationships with their spouses greatly enriched their lives. Indeed, many couples, by "pooling" their skills, functioned better than they would have if each had been on his or her own.

The Advances of the 1960s: The "Rights" of the Retarded and the New Outlook

Because President John F. Kennedy was particularly interested in mentally retarded people, he instituted a President's Panel on Mental Retardation whose report in 1962 had far-reaching consequences. The spirit of this report, together with the growing concern about the civil rights of many different types of minority groups, spurred a succession of court battles and eventually resulted in the enactment of many public laws that generated a new outlook for the retarded.

One cornerstone of this new outlook, which has been tested in the courts, challenged the traditional policy of institutionalizing mentally retarded or mentally ill people against their wills without adequate treatment. Additional legal mandates held that the treatment or education of such patients be provided in the least restrictive setting, that is, a setting that least restricts the freedom of the patient. These court decisions and laws resulted in the release of hundreds of thousands of people who had been "warehoused" in large institutions all over the nation. At the same time, stress was placed on how best to educate and treat these ex-inmates in "normal" community facilities. Thus, the deinstitutionalization" of the mentally retarded yielded the principles of normalization and mainstreaming regarding their place in the community.

Normalization holds that mentally retarded people should be encouraged to live their lives as closely to the social norm as possible. This concept applies to jobs, living arrangements, mobility within the community, sex, marriage, and other life events. Normalization also applies to the quality of life within institutions. Residents were formerly forced to have standard haircuts, for example—close-cropped for males and a pageboy for females.

* The mentally retarded tend to have fewer numbers of children than normal people, with about half having no children at all (Reed and Anderson, 1973; Mattinson, 1973).

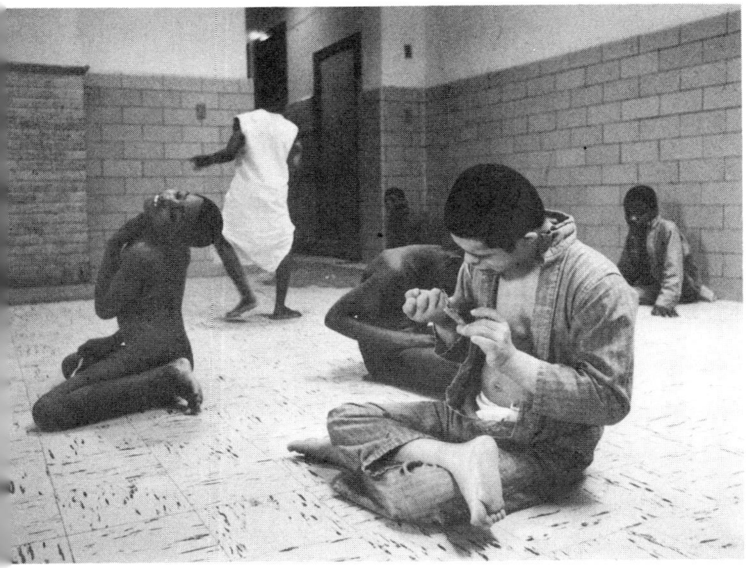

Warehousing mentally retarded people in large institutions throughout the nation is becoming a less frequent practice, as a consequence of "least restrictive" mandates. (Steve David/Sullivan Assoc.)

Today, residents can choose whatever cut they wish. Normalization also has yielded a policy that favors small cottages over large wards, which, like prisons, housed hundreds of inmates.

It is outside of institutions, however, that normalization has faced its greatest challenge. Where can mentally retarded people live? Should they be supervised? How will they support themselves? This chapter returns to these questions in later sections.

Mainstreaming, another guiding principle, refers to the teaching of as many mentally retarded children as possible in regular classrooms so as not to promote the stigma of "differentness" that is associated with special treatment in special classes. Opponents of mainstreaming insist that such children are likely to be isolated and stigmatized by their peers in regular classes and that they would experience less failure in special classes than in regular ones. Further, it is argued that their presence in regular classrooms would slow the progress of normal children. Although the issue is still being debated, the principle of mainstreaming seems to be winning out in many communities all over the nation.

Living Arrangements

The "least restrictive" alternative to institutional residence is to live alone in one's own home, be self-supporting, and to have only occasional supervision by a social worker or family member. This ideal arrangement represents the outcome for a good many of the mildly retarded group, most of whom marry, function independently, and blend into society without identifying labels.

For many retarded individuals, however, other alternatives are necessary because of some emotional impairment or physical disability that might prevent a completely independent living arrangement. These alternatives include living in a foster home or with one's own family. Group homes and residences (supervised, permanent "hostels" for a few dozen people) have also become a viable alternative to institutions for many retarded people. These community-supported facilities are especially appropriate for mildly or moderately retarded people who are educable and can support themselves, but who may require supervision in the management of their financial or medical affairs as well as in daily social activities.

Such living arrangements are not without their problems. For example, some foster homes may simply provide a room to the resident and little else. Group homes can become small "warehouses" for the retarded, still forgotten and wasted. The quality of these facilities and the follow-up of the individuals who reside in them, thus, must be the constant concern of an administrative network that sets standards and provides supervisory and follow-up resources.

Another problem in these alternative living arrangements is the alarm created in many communities regarding having mentally retarded people in their midst. Group homes, it is thought, threaten the well-being of neighbors and reduce values of community properties. For these reasons, some communities have brought legal action against such residences, invoking community zoning ordinances that had been designed to restrict multiple dwellings and rooming houses. Advocates of the rights of the retarded, however, have challenged zoning ordinances that bar group residences, stating that such restrictions defy the normalization principle and restrict the civil rights of the retarded. They argue that most residences do not degrade the architectural quality of the neighborhood, nor are they even labeled as halfway houses or hostels. Further, their residents are rarely harmful or destructive to their neighbors or communities. These battles and issues—won and lost, challenged and argued—are not yet resolved. Do you see a solution?

THE TRAINING AND EDUCATION OF THE RETARDED

Legislation has mandated that all mentally retarded people must be given the maximum training possible. Furthermore, this training must be provided within the community, when possible.* Accordingly, community training centers have appeared all over the nation. These centers focus mainly on two concerns:

1. *The training of retarded individuals for independent living and social skills,* for example, money management, traveling, social behaviors, getting along with others, care and purchase of clothing, shopping for food, and preparation of meals.

2. *The training of the retarded individual for economic self-support.* Training in independence and social skills is clearly necessary if a retarded individual is to get and hold a job. If specific training for specific jobs is adequately met, there is a wide variety of jobs that mentally retarded people can hold. You would be surprised to learn that most retarded individuals are able to keep their jobs. Even people who are moderately retarded can do some work in sheltered workshops that provide close supervision and training for simple jobs, such as stuffing envelopes. Table 14.2 lists some of the jobs in which mentally retarded individuals were placed after a training program (Becker, 1976).

Unfortunately, there are some individuals who are so severely retarded that they are not even able to hold a job in a sheltered workshop. Activity centers have been established to offer various recreational opportunities and simple training programs to these people, who might otherwise stay at home watching TV day after day.

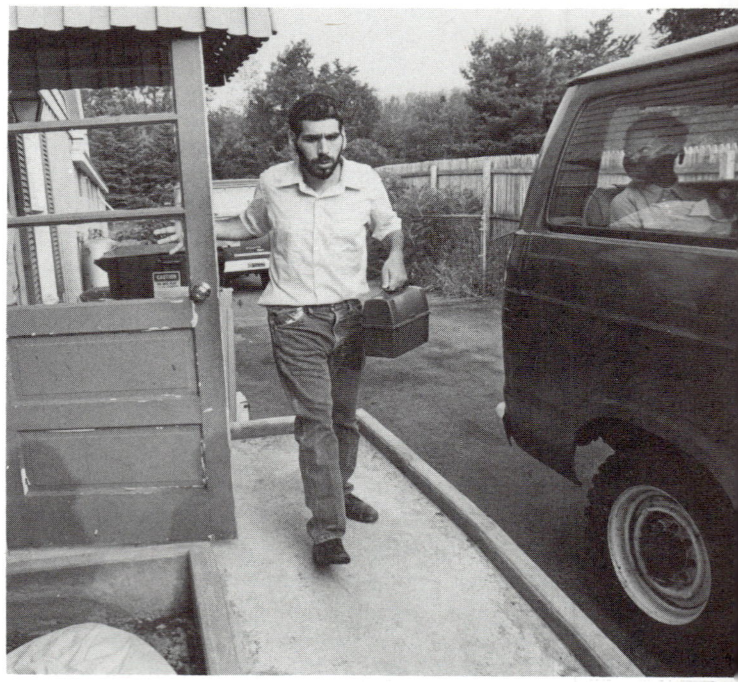

A retarded resident of a group home heads toward a van that will take him to work in a sheltered workshop. (Alan Carey)

* The sweeping mandates of Public Law 94-142 and the extension of the Vocational Rehabilitation Act to cover handicapped as well as mentally retarded individuals have guaranteed the education and training of all retarded individuals regardless of level of impairment. This includes severely and profoundly impaired as well as mildly and moderately impaired individuals.

Table 14.2 Job Assignments for 1,438 Mentally Retarded People in a Training Program

Job	Number of Trainees
Janitor	156
Dishwasher	92
Bus boy/girl	80
Kitchen helper	59
Stock boy/girl	59
School cafeteria helper	52
Automobile washer	41
Motel maid	38
Waitress	37
Nurse's aide	34
Construction worker	25
Nursemaid	25
Dietary aide	24
Assembler	23
Short-order cook	19
Bagger (grocery store)	19
Service station attendant	19
Pantry girl/man	18
Office boy/girl	18
Groundskeeper	17
Child day-care center worker	17
Cement mason helper	15
File clerk	15
Orderly (medical facility)	15
Materials handler	15

Source: Adapted from *Mental retardation: The changing outlook,* p. 411, by R. P. Ingalls, Copyright © 1978 by John Wiley & Sons. Reprinted by permission of John Wiley & Sons, Inc. After Becker, 1976.

Training Methods

Most retarded individuals are educated in regular public school classes. There they learn basic academic skills such as reading and arithmetic. However, the more severely retarded individuals offer a great and different challenge to their teachers. For this group of retarded people, who are deficient in hundreds of important skills, traditional methods have generally failed (Dunn, 1973). Fortunately, operant learning techniques have provided a successful alternative to the traditional teaching methods (see Mori and Masters, 1980).

Many skills and behaviors can be taught by operant conditioning, as the following list of a few of the available programs attests.

- brushing one's teeth
- toileting
- dressing
- making a bed
- putting on shoes
- answering simple questions
- playing a simple game
- identifying oneself
- walking or running
- eating without help
- eating without drooling
- paying attention
- listening to music
- drinking from a cup unaided
- asking for directions
- selecting clothes to wear
- washing one's face
- serving oneself in a cafeteria

Each program isolates or breaks down the component parts of a particular behavior, such as the various steps taken in making a bed. The component parts are "trained" through reinforcements (usually tangible rewards such as food) and gradually combined into longer sequences so that eventually the full behavior can be easily performed. At each step of the way, the subject experiences success—built-in rewards—before the next step in the sequence is introduced.* Thus, the usual frustrations that retarded individuals experience when traditional teaching methods are used are reduced. Furthermore, these methods have the virtue of being systematic, individualized, and objective, so that a trainee's progress can be easily charted.

* Actually, most programs use a method called "backward chaining," which is more complex, and which begins with the completed task, working back to the beginning step.

Most of these programs are applicable in a variety of settings—large institutions, group residences, foster homes, sheltered workshops, activity centers, nursing homes, or at home—and can be used by teachers, nurses, supervisors, students, employers, and family members. As a matter of fact, there are distinct advantages to involving parents in the training of their retarded child: The child is becoming more capable while at the same time the parents are becoming deeply involved in changing what they might have seen as a hopeless situation.

In ward or other sheltered settings, many work-related behaviors and skills can be trained (for example, work output in a sheltered workshop) through the distribution of tokens that can be exchanged for material things such as money or food. This is called token reinforcement and the social setting is called a token economy. Chapter 20 describes these methods in great detail.

Retarded people can be successfully and productively employed in a variety of jobs. (Will McIntyre/Photo Researchers)

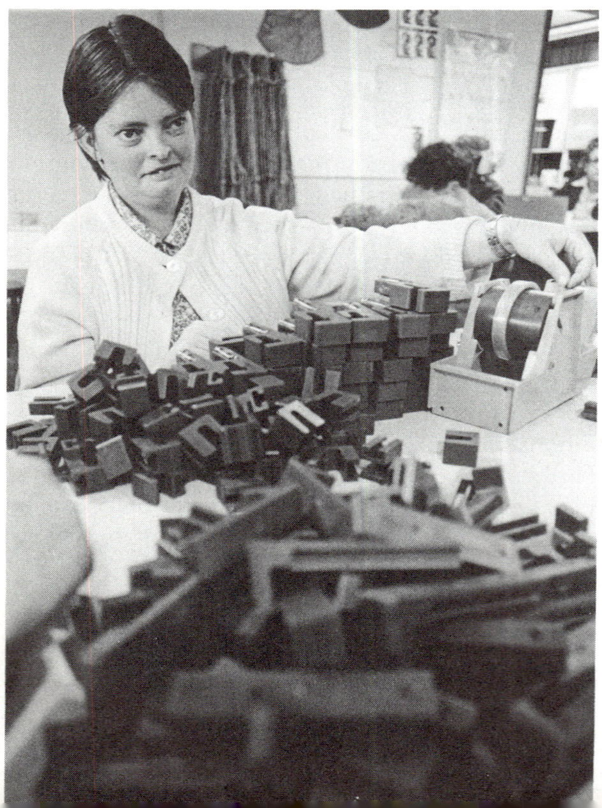

INTERVENTION AND PREVENTION

Many of the most severe forms of mental retardation are now, or will soon be, entirely preventable. These organic and physically caused inherited or congenital diseases can be either reduced or avoided entirely through genetic counseling and massive prenatal and early-infancy screening programs (see Spotlight 14.3). Thus, not only can the incidence of Down's syndrome, PKU, and Tay-Sachs' disease be reduced, but many other kinds of chromosomal defects, congenital malformations, and genetic errors associated with retardation can also be reduced or eliminated entirely (Hansen, Belmont, and Stein, 1980). In addition, improved medical care during pregnancy, at birth, and during the early childhood years can eliminate or reduce retardation caused by infectious diseases, trauma, and reduced oxygen supply in the perinatal periods, and meningitis and encephalitis during childhood.

It is with the mildly impaired group that the greatest challenge is found. For these retarded people cannot be "cured" by medical or physical means. Can we intervene with or prevent mild levels of retardation?

Early Compensatory Education: Head Start

In the 1960s as an aspect of the nation's War on Poverty, preschool programs—Project Head Start—were instituted, targeted at children from low-income homes to compensate for the more enriched family backgrounds of their middle-class peers. It was thought that these preschool programs could raise the level of the children's limited preparation in cognitive, language, motor, social, and interpersonal areas by the time they were of school age. Presumably, children who were receiving adequate stimulation at home were better prepared for school and for coping with life. The underlying hope was to intervene with and prevent the developmental and educational delays and/or retardation associated with lower-class status.

Various evaluations indicated that these pre-

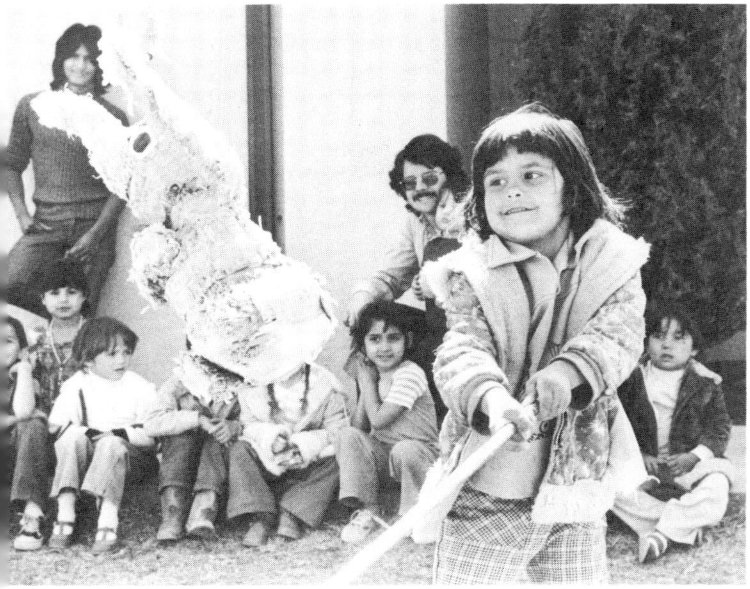

Head Start programs with high teacher-to-children ratios are more effective than those with lower ratios. (Michael D. Sullivan)

school programs did not fulfil the promise of the original expectations. Although there were some immediate gains in various areas, within a fairly short period of time Head Start children were performing no differently from those children (controls) who did not participate in the preschool enrichment programs (Westinghouse Learning Corporation, 1969). It had become obvious, however, that these preschool enrichment programs were extremely varied in goals, methods, and activities, and that an examination of some of the more successful programs might yield some lessons. This kind of review did yield some lessons: the most successful programs were those that were well supervised, highly organized, stressed language goals, and had a high ratio of adults to children (Spicker, 1971).

Most follow-up studies of children who had participated in Head Start programs compared to those who did not have indeed indicated that early IQ differences disappeared after several years. For example, in one impressively ambitious follow-up of children who had participated in eleven different urban and rural preschool enrichment programs in the 1960s in three different parts of the nation, these general findings were confirmed: IQ differences disappeared after several years of schooling (Darlington et al., 1980).* However, of special interest is the chief finding of this extensive investigation: Children who participated in preschool enrichment programs were less likely to be judged mentally retarded and less frequently assigned to special classes in their schools as a result than those children who did not participate in such programs. Extensive statistical exploration also indicated that these results were not due to differences between the enriched group and control group before preschool intervention was introduced, that is, to the possibility that the preschool-enriched group had higher initial ability, or SES status, or differed from the control group on any other background variable.

Intervention with Infants: Richard Heber and the Milwaukee Project

Preschool enrichment programs are generally introduced after the child has experienced the impoverished cultural and low-level stimulation of his or her family milieu. Intervention programs with children who are at risk for developmental delays and mental retardation might pay off if the intervention begins in infancy. The assumption here is that the earliest experiences and interactions of the child are of essential significance in shaping later competence, cognitive skills, and emotional health. The goal of primary prevention is to work with high-risk populations early enough to avert the insidious process of reduced competence and lagging development that soon appears to take its inevitable toll.

* Of 2,700 subjects in the original projects, 1,599 were followed up. These children (94 percent of whom were black), were from low-SES families and ranged in age from nine to nineteen years.

Based on this preventive assumption, as well as that of challenging the notion of a fixed IQ about which nothing can be done, a spectacularly successful program called the Milwaukee Project was initiated in 1965 by Heber and his associates (Heber, 1971; Heber and Garber, 1975). These researchers worked with high-risk infants beginning at three months of age in an intensive, seven-day-a-week home and educational center stimulation program, designed to forestall their inevitable decline into low-level intelligence.

How was risk defined? Infants born to retarded mothers (IQ of 75 or below) living in a Milwaukee low-SES neighborhood were selected as being at risk. Black families were used because these families tended to have lower mobility than other low-SES families, and the researchers did not want their subjects and families to drop out of the research program. Twenty subjects were selected on the basis of these criteria and carefully matched to a group of twenty other subjects with the same backgrounds to serve as controls for whom no enrichment was provided. None of the children had any CNS dysfunction.

The overall idea was to improve and enrich the cultural and familial environment of the experimental children in as many ways as possible but with special stress on language and cognitive skills. The intensive work, therefore, was with both children and their mothers, with whom educational and vocational training was attempted. Up to 15 months of age, the ratio of teacher to child was one to one. Later, the ratio never exceeded one to four.

The progress of control and experimental subjects was carefully evaluated at extremely frequent intervals. Variables evaluated fell into a variety of areas—medical, cognitive, and interpersonal. At one year of age there were no significant differences in medical and physical criteria, but by the age of six years, the enriched group had a mean Stanford-Binet IQ of over 30 points higher than the controls and scored higher than they did on many other tests of language development and problem-solving skills. By nine years of age, the experimental group was still 20 IQ points ahead of their controls and were showing truly impressive capacity to learn as well as to guide and assume leadership regarding interactions with their low-IQ mothers. Thus, it may be entirely possible, given the dedication of these researchers and a rather heavy financial investment, to forestall and to prevent the low-level intellectual functioning of many children of our nation.

SECTION II DEVELOPMENTAL DISABILITIES

ATTENTION DEFICIT DISORDER WITH HYPERACTIVITY*

Most of you are familiar with children who are noisy, distractible, "motorized," "always on the run," unable to concentrate. "He's driving me up the wall—driving me crazy," are common reactions to such children at home and at school.

The hyperactive syndrome is generally thought to emerge at about school age. Actually, its onset occurs earlier, at about the age of three years, but the classroom, with its confinement and its requirements to sit still, attend, and conform to its rules suddenly makes such children "stand out in the crowd" because of their difficulties in meeting these standards. Generally, there are no intellectual or cognitive difficulties with children showing this syndrome, but there may be learning problems because of attention and concentration difficulties. In most instances, symptoms diminish or entirely dis-

* The DSM-III also lists a related syndrome, attention deficit disorder without hyperactivity, which contains the same features except that its symptoms are generally milder and there is no hyperactivity. Other names for these syndromes: hyperkinetic reaction of childhood, hyperkinetic syndrome, hyperactive child syndrome, minimal brain dysfunction, minimal cerebral dysfunction.

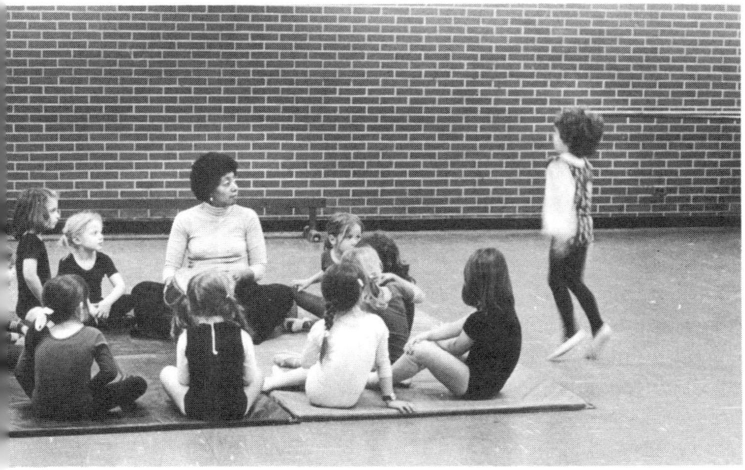

Hyperactive children can show attention difficulties and be extremely disruptive in a classroom. (Michael Weisbrot)

appear around puberty, but sometimes concentration difficulties or impulsivity may persist into adulthood.

The DSM-III Criteria

The DSM-III lists the following categories for this diagnosis. In each category the presence of two or three criteria is sufficient for making a diagnosis of attention deficit disorder.

Inattention: (a) often fails to finish tasks that are started; (b) often does not seem to listen; (c) is easily distracted; (d) has difficulty concentrating on schoolwork or other tasks requiring sustained attention; and (e) has difficulty sticking to a play activity.

Impulsivity: (a) often acts before thinking; (b) shifts excessively from one activity to another; (c) has difficulty organizing work (not due to intellectual difficulties); (d) frequently calls out in class; and (e) has difficulty awaiting turn in games or group situations.

Hyperactivity: (a) runs about or climbs on things excessively; (b) has difficulty sitting still or fidgets excessively; (c) has difficulty staying seated; (d) moves about excessively during sleep; and (e) is always "on the go" as if "driven by a motor."

According to the DSM-III, this syndrome occurs in about three out of 100 prepubertal children, with up to ten times greater frequency among boys than girls, for some unknown reason. Estimates of this ratio vary and are actually somewhat lower—5:1 to 9:1—but all experts agree that the syndrome occurs with strikingly greater frequency among boys than girls (Weiss and Hechtman, 1979). Sometimes there is a familial pattern, that is, the syndrome is more common among family members than among the general population.

Causes and Correlates

It had been thought in the past that the learning and attention difficulties, poor coordination, right-left confusion, perceptual difficulties, or EEG abnormalities shown by some hyperkinetic children meant that they were suffering from some type of brain dysfunction. The fact of the matter is that nobody can detect specific brain difficulty and that only about 5 percent of these children have a diagnosable neurological disorder (Weiss and Hechtman, 1979).

There is a strong possibility, on the other hand, that the hyperkinetic syndrome emerges as the "final common pathway" from many diverse etiological factors, especially because up to now the search for a single common cause has been fruitless. For example, some children may "act out," are not able to concentrate because their life styles are not in tune with the classroom as a result of their chaotic and disorganized environments. Some hyperactive children may be suffering from sensory defects or may have emotional problems; they may fear authority or need attention from the teacher on a one-to-one basis. Still other children may have congenital heart malformation that can cut off blood supply to the brain, a prediabetic condition, or insufficient calcium in the diet—all of which can produce behavioral difficulties.

One controversial, not entirely confirmed, view implicates additives such as synthetic colors and flavors. There are claims of 50 percent improvement among hyperactive children who followed the special Feingold diet (he is an allergist) that excludes all foods containing such presumed toxins. Controlled studies have since refuted these broad claims (Kolata, 1978c). But moderate empirical evidence does suggest an increase in "aversive" behaviors in a small sample of 22 young children who were placed on the Feingold diet and then fed ("challenged") with a blend of seven artificial colors (Weiss et al., 1980).

Overall, most experts agree that there is no genetic etiology in these behaviors. Instead it is thought that the syndrome emerges, as already suggested, from diverse etiologies (Deutsch and Schumer, 1970; Dubey, 1976; Kolata, 1978b; Lambert et al., 1976; Weiss and Hechtman, 1979). It may be that some diffuse biochemical dysfunction underlies these behaviors, brought about by congenital or perinatal factors such as anoxic conditions at birth, nutritional deprivations or excesses (for example, excessive sucrose consumption [Prinz et al., 1980], excessive smoking or alcohol ingestion during the mother's pregnancy, lead poisoning in early childhood, or other toxic conditions unknown to physicians or parents who took care of the child. We simply do not know enough to point to definitive answers.

Control and Treatment

Stimulant drugs, specifically Ritalin (methylphenidate), became the major method of "controlling" hyperactive children in the past decade. The widely touted "impressive" results these drugs effected in curtailing motoric behavior, controlling impulsivity, and raising levels of attention among these children created a climate in which entire classrooms of unsuspecting children were administered medications, often without parental consent. The wholesale use of such drugs is by now an event of the past, owing to challenges by parents and the community.

But are stimulant drugs the recommended treatment for individual hyperactive children when there is informed parental consent? An immediate challenge to what had almost become a routinely recommended procedure was that its use overlooked the specific causes that can account for a particular child's behavioral problem. Use of such drugs have also been questioned because of their many side effects, including fatigue, irritability, modified growth, and increase in heart rate and blood pressure (Schrag and Divoky, 1975; Weithorn and Ross, 1976).

Another challenge is leveled at the claim that medication is said to improve symptoms in 70 percent of hyperactive children. Follow-up studies actually indicate that despite immediate short-term results (perhaps giving everyone a "breather") there are few if any long-term benefits. This conclusion is based on follow-up of hyperactive children when drugs were used compared to control subjects who received no medication (Kolata, 1978b; Weiss and Hechtman, 1979). Specifically, there seem to be no differences among these groups in subsequent measures of emotional adjustment, delinquency, IQ, visual-motor coordination, and academic performance.*

Today, most clinicians stress the importance of diagnosing the child on the basis of his or her individual history. Once this is done, counseling, curriculum and school changes, behavior modification methods, even placebo should be considered before controversial drugs are introduced.

PERVASIVE DEVELOPMENTAL DISORDERS

There are certain disturbances of childhood that intrude on so many areas of development in such pervasive ways that the DSM-III chooses to refer to

* It had once been thought that the paradoxical effect of controlling and calming a child by administering a stimulant was evidenced only among hyperactive children. It is now known that stimulant drugs have a similar effect on normal children as well; they increase cognitive skills and reduce motor activity (Rapoport et al., 1978).

them as pervasive developmental disorders. The DSM-III divides this general category into infantile autism and childhood-onset pervasive developmental disorder. The latter has sometimes been referred to as childhood schizophrenia, but this may suggest a link to adult schizophrenia, which has not been established.

The distinctions between infantile autism and childhood-onset pervasive developmental disorder are not at all clear, nor are their etiologies definitively established. Some people prefer to place all these severe childhood disorders into one category, childhood psychosis. However, a good case can be made for distinguishing between infantile autism and childhood-onset pervasive developmental disorder (Rutter, 1978). Generally, infantile autism is regarded as reflecting pathology from the very beginning of life or at least very early in life, while childhood-onset pervasive developmental disorder presupposes normal or adequate functioning prior to the onset of pathology (Margolies, 1977).

Infantile Autism

Seth, at the age of two and one-half years, not only did not talk, but also seemed not to respond to others when they attempted to get his attention. Occasionally, however, there was echolalia (seemingly senseless repetition of words spoken by others). There was prolonged staring, frequently at shiny illuminated objects or lights, exaggerated responses or none at all to various stimuli, and an absence of any kind of responsiveness to social or personal stimuli. He failed to establish any emotional relationship to his older brother. Seth behaved as if he were looking right through the people around him, yet would listen intently to music for hours. He would spend sustained period of time manipulating toys and objects with senselessly repeated ritualistic mannerisms and behaviors. Order, sameness, and familiarity were essential to this child, who went into violent, screaming rages, sometimes hurting himself by head-banging, when the location of his toys was changed in any way.

Seth's parents were told that he was suffering

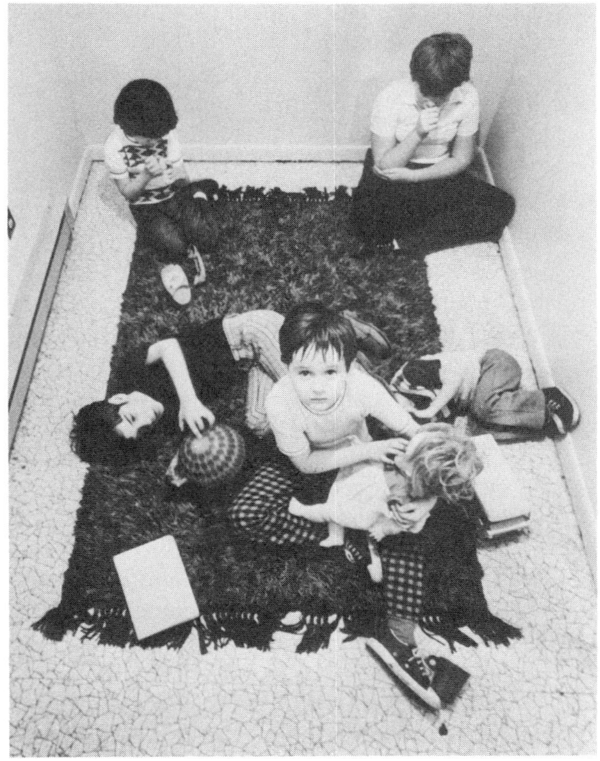

A group of autistic children at "play." (Steve Potter/Stock, Boston)

from infantile autism and that they were to "blame" because of their rigidity in dealing with him, their preference for another sibling, and the rejecting characteristics of his mother. They were to get into psychotherapy immediately, if they wished to "save" him.

Infantile autism is actually quite rare, occurring in about four in 10,000 individuals. It is diagnosed about two to four times more frequently in males than in females (Margolies, 1977; Rutter, 1977, 1978). Some researchers point out that autistic children are "overrepresented" in upper-SES groups. There is apparently no relationship to adult schizophrenia, whose incidence is not greater for autistic children. The DSM-III notes that the prevalence of this syndrome is *50 times greater* among the siblings of autistic children than in the general population, a fact that can be explained equally well by environmental as by nonenvironmental factors.

Diagnostic criteria for infantile autism vary. One of the earliest systematic descriptions of infantile autism was made by Kanner (1943), who designated some of the following criteria for its diagnosis:

1. The autistic child shows a separation, an aloneness and aloofness from the world, as if in a shell—shutting out social stimuli.
2. The autistic child seems "different" in posture, attitudes, and general behavior, from the very beginning (in contrast to the childhood schizophrenic).
3. Even in infancy, there is no preparatory "reaching out" response (usual at about four months of age) when parents attempt to pick up the baby.
4. The child does not use language and speech for purposes of communication, although he or she may have excellent rote memory for verses as well as echolalia.
5. There is often an early refusal of or struggle connected with ingesting food.
6. The child exhibits an extraordinary, obsessive need for sameness and order together with a generally excellent memory for previous arrangements of toys and objects.
7. The child engages in repetitive activity with objects; mannerisms and rhythmic motions.
8. Autistic children avoid eye contact with people, looking right through them: they do not show normal social responsiveness to words, gestures, or being picked up.
9. Autistic children look intelligent and in many ways indicate that they possess good intelligence especially in the light of excellent rote memory for complex material.
10. Fine motor coordination (such as finger dexterity) seems good but frequently there is gross clumsiness and awkward gait.

Many of the above criteria appear with other childhood disorders. However, certain invariant qualities tend to be present when infantile autism is diagnosed. These include failure to establish attachment behavior or to establish relationships with others, for example, in the form of play with other children; an obsessive need for order and sameness and for repetition of stereotyped behaviors (especially with objects); and the failure to use speech, language, and gestures to communicate (DeMyer, Churchill, Pontius, and Gilkey, 1971; DSM-III; Eisenberg and Kanner, 1956).

Seth's parents would have been surprised to learn that today there is little agreement as to the etiology of this disorder. But it is no longer believed that "psychodynamic" explanations, for example, an ungiving, cold, punitive mother, can account for this dramatic childhood syndrome.

Is there some genetic predisposition for the expression of this disorder? On the basis of a thoroughgoing review of the literature, Hanson and Gottesman (1976) concluded that infantile autism probably does not require genetic predisposition for its expression. Instead, various biological and environmental circumstances may be associated with producing the symptons of autism, especially the way in which stimuli are processed. These contributing circumstances include pregnancy and birth complications, epilepsy, viral infections, and anatomical and CNS abnormalities and dysfunctions not due to genetic factors.

What becomes of autistic children? According to the DSM-III, most autistic children, roughly two-thirds, develop into limited adults unable to lead fully independent lives. The rest, however, do moderately well as adults, working and living independently with only a minimum residual of earlier symptoms (for example, some social awkwardness).

Childhood-Onset Pervasive Developmental Disorder

If onset of some of the above behaviors occurs after two and a half or three years but before twelve years of age, the DSM-III suggests the diagnosis of childhood-onset pervasive developmental disorder. Whatever the label, this syndrome, like infantile autism, is a rare condition that occurs two to four times more frequently in boys than in girls (Rutter, 1977, 1978).* Behaviors associated with this childhood syndrome are bizarre and extremely inappropriate. Unlike adult schizophrenia (as already noted, sometimes this disorder has been called childhood schizophrenia), there are no hallucinations or delusions.

Such children may have high, but unevenly displayed intelligence. They tend to have rigid, peculiar, obsessional behavior patterns. Generally, there are poor social skills, inappropriate emotional responses, clinging behavior, social isolation and withdrawal, poor peer relationships, and rigidity and lack of empathy with people.

According to the DSM-III (see also Goldfarb, 1974, p. 7), symptoms of childhood-onset pervasive developmental disorder include:

1. Sudden excessive and seemingly illogical anxiety manifested by such symptoms as free-floating anxiety, catastrophic reactions to everyday occurrences, an inability to be consoled when upset, unexplained panics
2. Constructed or inappropriate affect, including lack of appropriate fear reactions, unexplained rage reactions, and extreme mood liability
3. Resistance to change in the environment (for example, upset if dinner time is changed) or insistence on doing things in the same manner every time (for example, putting on clothes always in the same order)
4. Oddities of motor movement, such as peculiar posturing, peculiar hand or finger movements, or walking on tiptoe
5. Abnormalities of speech, such as questionlike melody, monotonous voice
6. Hyper- or hyposensitivity to sensory stimuli, for example, hyperacusis
7. Self-mutilation—for example, biting or hitting self, head banging.

Although clinicians may come to a uniform diagnosis of childhood-onset pervasive developmental disorder based on case history material and observations, there is little consensus as to etiology of this condition (Goldfarb, 1974; Gunderson, Autry, Mosher and Buchsbaum, 1974). Some approaches suggest the possibility that such children lack adequate CNS integration or neurological integrity. Many researchers stress attentional dysfunctions: for example, the overselectivity in attention that characterizes such children can explain their peculiarities in responses, especially as displayed in interpersonal situations.

In any event, these childhood states are a "mixed bag"—probably a combination of neurological, genetic, and psychological difficulties. As with autistic children, the more simple view that disturbed parental behavior causes these difficulties is now being replaced with a more sophisticated view that acknowledges the possibility that some parents may have baffled, defensive, confused responses to children who display bizarre, nonresponsive, peculiar behavior (Schopler and Reichler, 1972).

Treatment of autistic children and those diagnosed as manifesting childhood-onset developmental disease have yielded surprisingly positive findings. Important among these general approaches is the therapeutic community—a residential treatment center that offers schooling, training, and individual therapy (Bettelheim, 1950; Goldfarb, 1970, 1974) while at the same time providing an accepting, yet organized, orderly, structured daily routine that is essential for working with such children. Although traditional psychotherapy has not been very successful, behavioral methods, often using parents as models and trainers (Margolies, 1977), as well as various psychopharmacological approaches have been shown to be quite effective in increasing focused attention, reducing irrelevant and inappropriate motor behaviors, improving

* An interesting explanation for the preponderance of males in these disorders was suggested by Eme (1979), who noted that these childhood pathologies may be associated with differing traits for boys compared to girls. Girls show patterns of inhibition, reclusiveness, and sensitivity, while boys show patterns of flagrant, unsocialized aggression. The boys' "off" behavior is more salient and detectable, and thus they may be counted more readily among the ill or potentially ill.

communicational skills, and modifying social and interpersonal behavior (see Chapters 20–21).*

CEREBRAL PALSY AND OTHER DEVELOPMENTAL DISORDERS

There are millions of handicapped children in this country (estimated to be about 12 percent or almost 8 million) who, although not retarded or "mentally ill," have also been institutionalized despite their educability and/or trainability. Today, federal law requires that such children be mainstreamed—not segregated in special schools or institutions but educated along with "normal" children to the maximum extent possible.** The law explicitly states that all such children be given maximum educational opportunities and advantages, be encouraged to follow and to train for vocational careers of their choice, and be placed in the most appropriate setting so as to avert emotional and mental damage as a result of segregation due to their disabilities. Of this group of "handicapped" individuals, this section will touch only on cerebral palsy and specific developmental disorders.

Cerebral Palsy

Because of various injuries sustained at or about the time of birth such as difficult labor associated with oxygen deprivation, some children may show abnormal development of the CNS. These children are diagnosed as having cerebral palsy, which is characterized, among other difficulties, by defects in the motor area, for example, in reaching, walking, talking, and maintaining posture. These difficulties become more pronounced as the child develops. There may also be perceptual and ocular-visual problems.

The motor difficulties of cerebral-palsied individuals have been classified into two general categories: spastic (rigidity, tension, paralysis of certain affected areas) and athetoid (characterized by involuntary, slow, worm-like movements of fingers, toes, hands, and feet). People with spastic defects, it is claimed, show more disability in visual systems than those with athetosis (Breakey, Wilson, and Wilson, 1974).

Most cerebral-palsied individuals show little cognitive impairment, despite overt symptoms, and are able to attend regular schools, eventually falling into normal employment patterns. In a few instances, there may be associated features such as epilepsy or mental retardation. By and large, the majority of people with cerebral palsy can lead normal lives without severe emotional problems.

Specific Developmental Disorders

The DSM-III lists several "disorders" that many psychologists feel should not be included in a list of mental disorders. These are the developmental delays (in a generally "normal" child) in reading, arithmetic, language, and articulation that are sometimes referred to as learning disabilities. Such disabilities are generally diagnosed and treated in an educational, rather than a psychological, setting. They reflect discrepancies between expected level of skill and actual performance in the light of the child's grade, chronological age, and intellectual capacity. The level of skill and of intellectual capacity is determined by standardized, individually administered tests. According to the DSM-III, with the exception of the developmental arithmetic disorder, these developmental disorders appear twice as frequently among males than among females.

Developmental disorders are not diagnosed as such if there is brain damage, vision or hearing impairment, mental retardation, cultural deprivation

* Treatment centers for disturbed children are no longer isolated, self-contained centers that offer psychoanalytically oriented psychotherapy to young patients "removed" from their parents. They are more likely to stress family approaches that employ parents as "change agents" and to use various innovative behavioral methods (Davids, 1975; Goldsmith, 1976).

** The label *handicapped* is broad: the law includes drug addicts and alcoholics as well as the mentally retarded, the mentally disturbed, the hard-of-hearing, the deaf, the speech-impaired, the visually handicapped, the orthopedically impaired, and those with learning disabilities not due to sociocultural factors.

due to low-SES membership, autism, or other mental disorders. What causes such difficulties? No one is really sure, but neurological dysfunction is sometimes implicated (Ingalls, 1978).

Developmental reading disorders—sometimes called dyslexia—afflict about 5 percent of the school population. Children with such reading disorders manifest enormous difficulty in reading even simple words long after their peers are reading complex material. Despite repeated help, for example, they continue to make such errors as reversing *b* and *d*, or failing to recognize simple words, or "seeing" only the first few letters of words, or only the first and last letters.

Some of these children grow up to become adults who cannot read at all. These people get along by relying on careful listening, absorbing, and retaining as much as possible by using other cognitive methods. They often hide their disabilities, although sometimes not too successfully, by using amazingly ingenious tactics, as in the case of the successful businessman whose secretary handled all his correspondence by reading to him or into a tape machine everything that came across his desk.

The etiology of reading disability is not clear, but one widely held hypothesis was proposed by Orton (1937), who suggested that dyslexia is caused by a "functional asymmetry" of the brain—that is, it occurs in instances of asymmetrical dominance of the cerebral hemispheres. Specifically, dyslexia would arise when there is impaired left cerebral (linguistic) functioning. This hypothesis has not been clearly substantiated, however, according to a review by Witelson (1977), who in her own researches hypothesized and confirmed a somewhat different (but related) approach. Witelson's hypothesis proposes that dyslexic children do not have the expected specialization of spatial and wholistic functions in the right hemisphere and linguistic functions in the left. Instead, *both* hemispheres have highly developed spatial and wholistic functions. This cerebral organization of "bilateral neural involvement" interferes with the development and specialization of the usual left-hemisphere functions, with consequent disabilities in spelling, speech, and reading.

As we learn more about the functions of the brain and how differences in neural organization affect sensory processes and behavior, we will no doubt learn more about the detection and control of many of the disabilities described in this section, such as dyslexia. Those of us who have worked with children with such difficulties will attest to the perplexity and anguish they (the children) feel, when, even after trying as hard as possible, these children cannot seem to get the grasp of "doing what comes naturally." Perhaps the next generation of children will profit from the continued efforts of people in the many disciplines relevant to this challenging area.

SUMMARY

Chapter 14 discussed mental retardation and developmental disabilities, presented definitions of retardation and the standard classification scheme, and described incidence and relationship to sociocultural variables. It then presented the causes for mental retardation and different types of retardation, with case illustrations. These include infections and intoxications, trauma and physical injury, endocrine disorders, malnutrition, genetic "errors" such as Down's syndrome and Tay-Sachs' disease, and prematurity. A special section discussed psychosocial retardation, the category that contains the largest number of so-called retarded individuals. The chapter next considered the assessment of retardation, especially in the light of the fact that competence or adaptive behavior and IQ as determined by traditional tests are not the same constructs. After a survey of the psychological characteristics and problems of the retarded, viewed as people, including a description of their social rights, this chapter described not only the training and education of the retarded but also prevention and intervention approaches. The chapter concluded with a presentation of attention deficit disorders with hyperactivity and pervasive developmental disorders, including infantile autism.

Highlights

1. Mental retardation is diagnosed when an individual displays subaverage intellectual functioning and impairment in adaptive behavior, defined in terms of personal independence, social responsibility, and capacity to achieve mastery over one's environment. The class of mild retardation applies to about 80 percent of the retarded. The other categories are moderate retardation (about 12 percent), severe retardation (about 7 percent), and profound retardation (less than 1 percent). Mildly retarded people are educable, and moderately and severely retarded people, trainable. Only the profoundly retarded are regarded as possessing limited potential for training.
2. In recent years, an entirely new look has dominated the field of mental retardation. Chiefly, changes in perspective revolve around the challenge to the notion that retardation reflects incurable, inherited, low-level IQs. The more contemporary approach is that there are many causes of retardation, most types can be prevented or modified, and that most retarded individuals are not only educable but also have feelings, emotions, and social and individual rights.
3. Most of the mildly impaired group, in which there is no known organic etiology, fall into low-SES groups. Although more males than females are diagnosed as mentally retarded (this is especially so in the mildly impaired group), it is likely that some of this disparity can be attributed to certain aspects of the labeling process.
4. For most instances of mental retardation, there are no known physical causes. The smaller group of retarded individuals for which there are known or assumed physical causes comprise a more severely retarded population. Causes include infections such as rubella, if contracted by the mother during the first third of pregnancy, or syphilitic infections; pre- and postnatal intoxications (the fetal alcohol syndrome, for example); trauma and other physical causes (child abuse is a significant contributor to this cause of retardation); endocrine disorders (for example, congenital hypothyroidism, which is modifiable up to about four months of age); and malnutrition.
5. Less than 10 percent of the mentally retarded became so because of chromosomal abnormalities or genetic transmission. A relatively frequently occurring example of this type of retardation is called Down's syndrome, which reflects a chromosomal abnormality that consist of three, rather than the usual pair, of chromosomes 21. Although Down's children are usually retarded, many are only mildly retarded and educable. Amniocentesis is a procedure used to examine cells from the amniotic fluid that can determine the presence of this chromosomal abnormality in the fetus.
6. Examples of genetically transmitted diseases are phenylketonuria (PKU) and Tay-Sachs' disease, both of which are transmitted by a single recessive autosomal gene. PKU babies can be diagnosed in early infancy and retardation can be prevented by dietary control. If untreated, mental retardation is inevitable and irreversible. In the case of Tay-Sachs' disease, there is a degenerative course ending in death at about three to four years of age for which there is no known cure. But detection of this disease in utero through the use of amniocentesis is possible.
7. Most mentally retarded individuals are only mildly impaired with no apparent organic cause. These people, classified in the psychosocial category, tend to come from low-SES groups. There are frequently labeled because they seem to be unable to keep up with their peers at school. Later, when they are older, they blend into society. Children of poverty may sometimes be misdiagnosed as retarded because the skills they do possess—competence to get by in their own worlds—are not tapped by the schoolroom requirements or the traditional intelligence test. Many psychologists are concerned with the development and use of procedures that assess adaptive and coping skills, rather than the verbal-abstract culturally biased

content frequently found in the usual intelligence test.

8. Principles of normalization and mainstreaming and that the education and training of the retarded be in the "least restrictive setting" have created issues that are still being debated. Yet many would argue that the civil, emotional, and individual rights of the retarded individual far outweigh any practical difficulties created by attempts to implement these principles.
9. Training for independent living, social skills, and economic self-support are the prime goals in educational programs for the retarded. Even when education and training for these goals are not possible—as in the case of severely retarded individuals—operant learning techniques have been successfully applied in the training of many skills, such as putting on shoes or drinking from a cup unaided.
10. Most of the severest forms of mental retardation are or will be preventable. The greatest challenge concerns the mildly impaired group. Intervention attempts with children who are at high risk for psychosocial retardation show considerable promise.
11. The hyperkinetic syndrome apparently emerges as the "final common pathway" from diverse etiological factors. There is probably no genetic etiology for this troublesome, perplexing childhood behavior pattern. A great deal of controversy surrounds the use of stimulant drugs for the control of hyperactive behavior, not only because of their many side effects, but also because of their questionable long-range value and effects.
12. Infantile autism, which many believe reflects dysfunctions from the very beginnings of life, occurs in about four in 10,000 individuals and is diagnosed two to four times more frequently in males than in females. Some of the chief characteristics of infantile autism are failure to establish attachment behavior, an obsessive need for orderliness and regularity, the presence of stereotyped, repetitive behavior and severe problems in speech and communication.
13. The onset of childhood-onset pervasive developmental disorder (sometimes referred to as childhood schizophrenia), which presupposes normal functioning prior to the pathology, is any time after two or three years up to about twelve years of age; this condition also occurs more frequently in males than in females. Symptoms are characterized by bizarre and inappropriate behavior, frequently high but uneven intelligence, and poor interpersonal skills, for example, social isolation. There are generally no delusions or hallucinations.
14. Early hypotheses about the causes of the foregoing childhood syndromes that assume disturbed parental or mother-child relationships exclusively are no longer proposed by many clinicians, who are beginning to acknowledge the importance of various CNS dysfunctions (not necessarily genetically acquired) in accounting for some of the symptoms of these puzzling childhood disturbances.
15. Cerebral palsy refers to injuries sustained at or about the time of birth that may produce some abnormal development of the CNS, resulting in motor difficulties and/or perceptual and ocular-visual problems. Most cerebral-palsied people show little cognitive impairment and can lead normal lives without severe emotional problems.

ISSUES AND QUESTIONS

1. "One bright October day, fourteen years ago, there came to the Training School at Vineland, a little eight-year-old girl. She had been born in an almshouse." This was Goddard's introduction to his fascinating little book (1912) about the Kallikaks.

   Deborah, the little girl, came from a long line of Kallikaks, whom Goddard traced genealogically. His charts showed a strikingly large number of "feebleminded" and "bad stock" people in Deborah's family: prostitutes, criminals, alcoholics, vagrants, and paupers. Goddard traced all of them to the earliest known

Kallikak, Martin Kallikak Sr., whose illegitimate son spawned the 480 descendants with "bad blood." But Martin Kallikak Sr. was married to a woman of "good stock." The descendants of this union, according to Goddard, contained no defective people and the vast majority of them were prominent, educated, landowning, and prosperous members of the community. Goddard concluded that heredity is directly responsible for "feeblemindedness" and for the undesirable, criminal, socially marginal elements of society. His conclusions inevitably followed: The solution lies in "segregation through colonizaton" of people with "bad blood"—a "leper colony" of tainted people.

Following this line of reasoning, most of the states of our nation wrote "eugenics" laws into their books requiring compulsory sterilization of the "unfit"—motivated, perhaps, by humane and compassionate social considerations that would permit mentally retarded people to live productive lives without burdening them or society with the "inevitability" of bringing more retarded children into this world. Between 1924 and 1972, for example, the state of Virginia sterilized, without permission, 8,000 mentally retarded people (Reinhold, 1980) on the assumption that if "bad blood" were prevented from being inherited, mental retardation could be curtailed.

Today, most states are repealing such laws, for compulsory sterilization of the "unfit" is considered both unethical and inconsistent with scientific knowledge about mental retardation.

a. Can you think of instances in which involuntary sterilization of a mentally retarded child might be appropriate, provided that there is parental consent and very good reason for this step? What would constitute "very good reason"?
b. Experts on ethical issues in the sciences are concerned with "sunset" provisions in lawmaking that would establish a set of procedures for cancellation or at least modification of legislation that had emerged from the lawmakers' well-intentioned but inaccurate interpretation of the sciences. Sunset procedures would require a review of a law in the light of changing scientific, popular, and ethical attitudes concerning its merit, with an appropriate adjustment of that law if necessary. Can you think of examples of legislation (other than "eugenics" laws) that have become archaic and that would profit from a sunset provision?

2. In 1980, a couple refused cardiac surgery on their 13-year-old Down's syndrome child that could have extended his life to a normal old age. The state of California had been legally pressing to perform such surgery in the light of medical findings that this institutionalized child, with an IQ of 30 to 50, would die in about 20 years. The parents' legal action claimed that if the child outlived them, he would end his days simply being "warehoused" and forgotten with other old, mentally retarded people. On the basis of this appeal (*Bothman* v. *Warren B.*), the parents won their battle in the highest court of the land.

   What do you think about the state's view that this child had a "right to life" despite the parents' concerns? Do you see the parents' point of view?

3. The use of stimulant drugs to control the behavior of hyperactive children was already discussed. Are there some circumstances in which you think their use would be appropriate? For example, a teacher claims that she can teach more to a class of thirty children if one of them was on medication for hyperactivity. Does the majority have "rights" in this connection? Should the parents of the others be concerned about the poor quality of education for their children because of the one disruptive, unruly child in the classroom?

   A child who is "motoric," constantly interrupting, "bad" in the classroom. is beginning to be disliked and avoided by his peers. He is also picked on by the teacher. He is building up a negative self-image as he sees himself becoming more and more troublesome to the others and increasingly behind them in achievement. And yet he cannot help himself. Would we not be contributing to his welfare by permitting a recommendation of medication to the parents (accompanied of course by a full description of the pros and cons involved)? Should we not approve of an agent that might enhance the child's self-image, social skills, and cognitive focus?

4. This book has already described the stigmatizing effects of labeling certain kinds of people. Discussed also have been disadvantages inherent in the labeling process, for example, the negative self-image that is generated as a result. Can you think of any advantages in classifying mentally retarded individuals? For example, can a valid classification aid in securing special help and training in social skills, or in reading and speaking?
5. What is your personal view of buying a house that is next door to a residential center for mentally retarded people? Does your personal view conflict with your more abstract approval of the "normalization" principle?

SUGGESTIONS FOR FURTHER READING

Ingalls, R. P. *Mental retardation: The changing outlook.* New York: Wiley, 1978. This is an excellent, college-level textbook about mental retardation that is written in clear, simple language, and that covers a wide variety of topics. It includes many case illustrations of the different levels and types of retardation, a discussion of etiology and problems in assessment, and a detailed summary of how to educate, train, and modify the behavior of the different types of retarded individuals. In addition, there is descriptive, as well as research, material on the emotions, personality, and families of the retarded.

Itard, J. M. G. *The wild boy of Aveyron.* New York: Appleton-Century-Crofts, 1962. Paperback. This is a classic book, written in the early 1800s, by a physician who took on the formidable task of educating a feral (living in a wild state) boy of about twelve years of age who was found in a forest near Aveyron, France. Itard applied some of the methods he developed while treating the deaf (such as sensory training) in intensively working with this animal-like boy. He assumed that Victor could be "socialized," amd that eventually he would behave, speak, and think like people reared within human societies. After several years, Itard gave up in defeat. Victor, the Wild Boy, died at about the age of forty without acquiring language, without becoming "civilized." Was Victor retarded? Was he neurologically defective? Was Victor a fascinating picture of what humans would be like without culture, without the contact of other humans that the rest of us take for granted in our own lives? Could Victor have learned to communicate if other teaching methods had been used? If you are interested, you might look at another book that addresses itself to questions regarding Victor's inability to "catch up": Lane, H. *The wild boy of Aveyron.* Cambridge, Mass.: Harvard University Press, 1976.

Meyers, R. *Like normal people.* New York: McGraw-Hill, 1978. Roger and Virginia Meyers, both retarded, were married on June 18, 1977. This book, written by Roger's brother, Robert, is the story of their lives. Originally published as a series of articles for the *Washington Post,* it presents the life histories of Roger and Virginia from birth through 1978. The struggles that Roger's parents went through—first to arrive at an understanding of what was wrong with Roger, and later to combat the prevalent advice of the times to institutionalize him—are sensitively portrayed. No less impressive are the accounts of the efforts of Roger and Virginia to live on their own "like normal people." This book also presents a history of the attitudes and policies toward the mentally retarded in America.

Rutter, M., and Schopler, E. *Autism: A reappraisal of concepts and treatment.* New York: Plenum, 1978. The papers presented in this book cover a wide range of issues related to childhood autism, including definition and diagnosis, the language of the autistic child, neurophysiological and biological studies, family characteristics, and education and treatment. Although it is not easy reading, this collection will provide the student who is seriously interested in the problem of autism with an overview of research in this area.

15

Sexual Behaviors: Variations and Dysfunctions

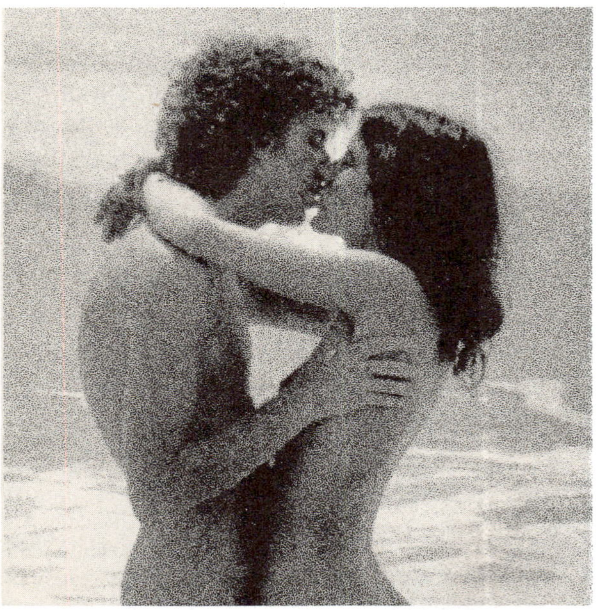

THE COMPLEX SEXUAL ARENA

In the pages ahead, a variety of sexual behaviors are described. You will consider some of these to be "normal" and some "abnormal." What yardstick are you employing in making this determination?

Are you judging by your own preferences and standards? Is there some universal criterion that defines "normality"?

In no other arena of human behavior are there such difficulties in distinguishing pathological from nonpathological. The shifting sexual practices, mores, and standards within and across cultures and through the ages do not permit such clearcut boundaries. It is safe to say that almost every conceivable kind of sexual practice and interaction has been tolerated or accepted at one point or another in the history of humanity.

Spotlight 15.1 Some Myths about Sexual Behaviors and Responses

Am I normal? Does everyone masturbate? Do most women require clitoral stimulation to reach orgasm? How big is my penis compared to other men's? What do other people *do?*

Most societies provide strict taboos, codes, "scripts," and legal and social pressures about sexual behaviors, interlaced with myths and misconceptions about sexual practices. Although today people discuss sexual practices openly, many myths about these practices continue to prevail. Here are some of them. Can you add to this list?

1. Sex is a monopoly of the very young—diminishing with age and virtually disappearing by the time people are in their sixties or seventies.
2. Homosexuality is a disease, not "normal."
3. Frequent masturbation is unhealthy.
4. Women rarely masturbate.
5. There are two types of orgasm in women: vaginal and clitoral.
6. Vaginal orgasms are emotionally mature, whereas clitoral orgasms are not mature.
7. Homosexual pairs—whether male or female—are comprised of one masculine and one feminine type.
8. Most women are frigid—incapable of being aroused or of having orgasms.
9. Male homosexuals like to get dressed up in *drag* (female makeup and clothes).
10. Unless a woman is always orgasmic, she is "neurotic."
11. During sex, women rarely have fantasies, whereas men often fantasize.
12. Transvestites (people who become sexually aroused or excited through cross-dressing—getting dressed in the clothing of the opposite sex) are homosexuals.
13. Rapists are sexually starved people with little or no sexual outlets.
14. Homosexuality is a result of glandular or endocrinological dysfunctions.
15. Most females unconsciously want to be males ("penis envy").
16. Mental-health experts tend to regard only one or two (at the most three) coital positions (positions during intercourse) as "normal."
17. There is more promiscuity on college campuses than ever before.
18. Too much sex is unhealthy.
19. Sex without love is unhealthy.
20. Female prostitutes are really lesbians.
21. In most instances of rape, the victim provokes the assault.
22. Sexually aggressive women are not normal.
23. Women are less erotic, less easily aroused, than men.
24. Black male rapists tend to assault white women.
25. The size of a man's penis determines the sex-

ual enjoyment and gratification he can offer to a woman and is an indication of his virility.

26. Women do not enjoy intercourse during menstruation.
27. It is emotionally more mature for sexual partners to have simultaneous orgasms than otherwise.
28. Most men are turned off by women who are sexually aggressive in bed.
29. Most men enjoy sex for its own sake and are not concerned with giving and receiving affection or with the sexual satisfaction of their partners.
30. Sexual variations (for example, oral sex) that depart from the usual male-female vaginal penetration are, if not abnormal, deviant and unhealthy.

Chapter 2 described fads and fashions in symptoms from era to era and from culture to culture. Such cultural variations appear in the sexual area also. For example, in ancient times, being "turned on" by statues (not only for arousal, but to climax) was fairly common (Scobie and Taylor, 1975). Today we would question the "sanity" of a bum in the park who regularly had his sex in front of General Sherman's statue. Another example: In India, a belief that cuts across all SES levels (but that is more frequent in lower than higher levels) is that semen is more than a procreative substance. As the "elixir of life," it endows an individual with great health and mystical power. No wonder, then, that in India

Listing 15.1 DSM-III Categories of Psychosexual Disorders

The organization and content of Chapter 15 differ considerably from those of the DSM-III list. However, most, if not all of these topics are touched on in the pages ahead.

- Gender Identity Disorders
  - Transsexualism
    - With sexual history of: asexual, homosexual, heterosexual, unspecified
  - Gender identity disorder of childhood
  - Atypical gender identity disorder
  - Paraphilias
    - Fetishism
    - Transvestism
    - Zoophilia
    - Pedophilia
    - Exhibitionism
    - Voyeurism
    - Sexual masochism
    - Sexual sadism
    - Atypical paraphilia
- Psychosexual Dysfunctions
  - Inhibited sexual desire
  - Inhibited sexual excitement
  - Inhibited female orgasm
  - Inhibited male orgasm
  - Premature ejaculation
  - Functional dyspareunia
  - Functional vaginismus
  - Atypical psychosexual dynsfunctions
- Other Psychosexual Disorders
  - Ego-dystonic homosexuality
  - Psychological disorder not elsewhere classified

some emotionally unstable people manifest the *Dhat* syndrome—an obsessive bodily preoccupation, with anxiety bordering on panic, that focuses on the possible loss of semen through nocturnal emissions (Mathotra and Wig, 1975).

The point is that sexual "symptoms" or hang-ups vary from culture to culture and that the expert has great difficulty in deciding what is normal and what is not normal.

The sexual scene within our own culture. Today, sex is out in the open. The proliferation of sex shops, sex magazines, picture books and manuals, X-rated movies, "sexploitation" films for whatever-your-sexual-tastes-are, massage parlors, topless and bottomless dancers, nudity on stage and screen, and sexual slang in the media attest to this fact. There is rising permissiveness toward different kinds of sexual expression and preference. We are told that everyone—at least of reasonable age—should enjoy sex. And in case enjoyment lags or is absent, clinics and counseling centers are ready to meet the challenge.

Some of the changes. There is an increase in the numbers of unmarried people living together, the figures more than doubling in the past decade (Ferrell, 1979). This increase is largely accounted for by people under the age of twenty-five years. "Living in sin" is still a minority variation in homemaking, however, for although there are over one million unmarried households, there are almost fifty million married households.

New sexual styles and living arrangements are emerging (see Murstein, 1978). "Open marriages" that involve a more flexible view toward extramarital sex, bisexual arrangements that permit heterosexual as well as homosexual simultaneous relationships, three-way households (for example, two females and one male), "wife-swapping," and group sexual activities, if still not the ways of the majority, are at least acknowledged by the majority as alternatives practiced by a minority.

Attitudes toward sexual variations and toward premarital sex are also changing. Today's teenagers

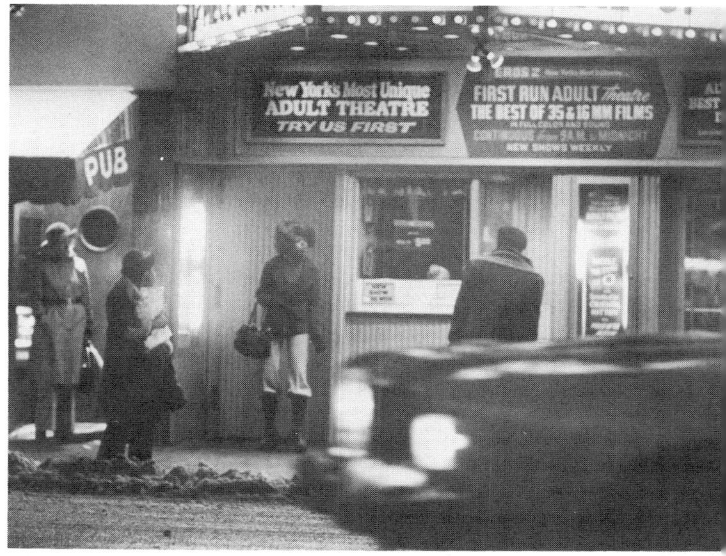

"Sexploitation" films have become part of the American scene. (James H. Karales/Peter Arnold)

tend to have attitudes toward sexual matters that differ from those expressed by their parents. One study of middle-class subjects (Chess, Thomas, and Cameron, 1976) disclosed that today's generation shows more freedom in discussing sexual matters. They evince less guilt, conflict, and concern about masturbation, venereal disease, and issues such as birth control or unwanted pregnancies. There is greater acceptance of sexual "deviations"—alternative sexual practices—and less stress among the teenage females on pushing toward marriage. Yet, interestingly, among the youngsters studied there were few ongoing sexual activities of a casual nature—that is, little promiscuity.*

* Has the "sexual revolution"—the liberation of attitudes toward sex, the availability of contraceptive methods and of abortions, and the pressure to be free and open about sex—increased promiscuity on campus? No, according to most observers of the scene, and this holds for both men and women. Even though students may be more sexually active than their parents were at this age, "relationships" or living together, rather than casual affairs and "one-night stands," are highly valued (Finger, 1975; Oswalt, 1974).

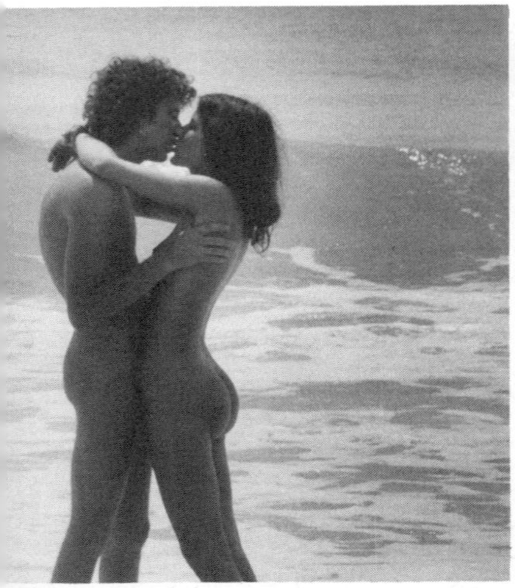

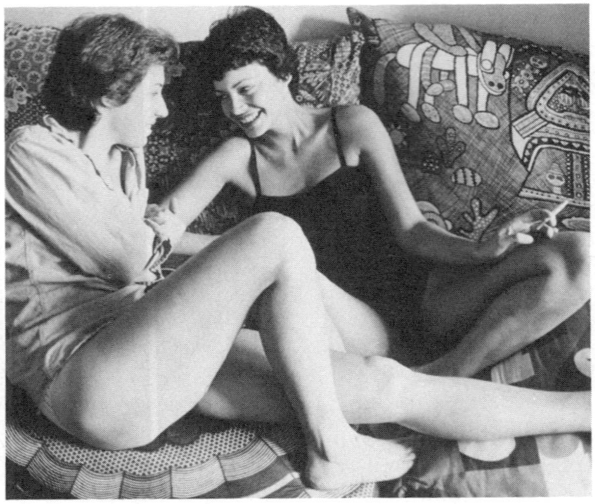

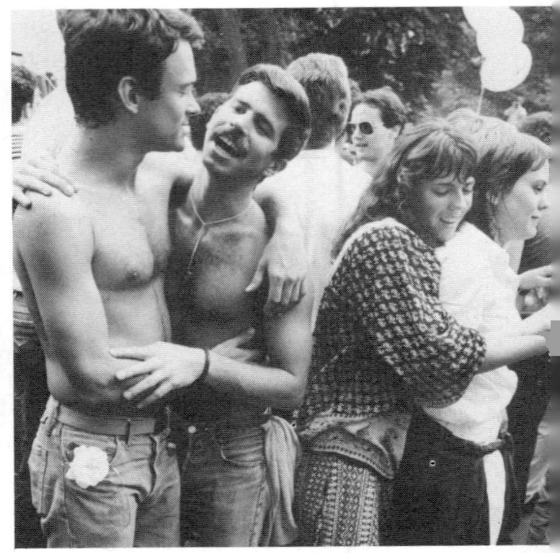

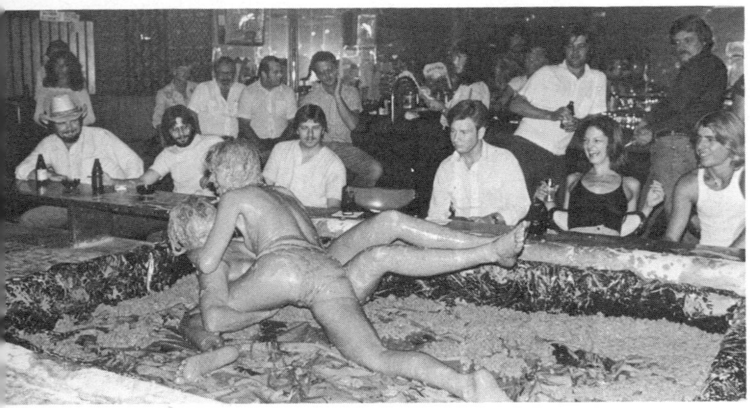

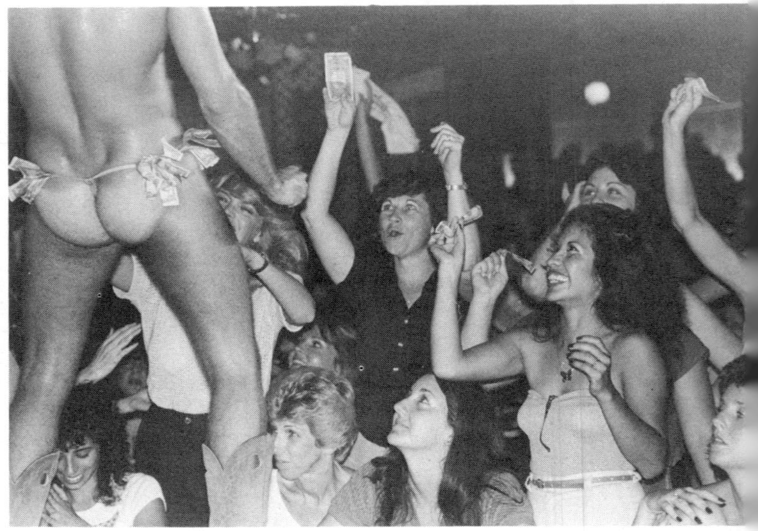

Sexual "turn ons," inclinations, and attractions can take many different forms. (Clockwise, from upper left: Peter Simon/Black Star, Joel Gordon, Jim Anderson/Woodfin Camp, David Hurn/Magnum, David Hurn/Magnum)

Some of the problems. The divorce rate is rising, more than doubling in recent years. In 1960, for every 1,000 married persons, there were 35 divorces, whereas in 1975, out of 1,000 married persons, 75 were later divorced (Ferrell and Adams, 1977).

About one-third of all girls between the ages of fifteen and twenty years have had at least one unwanted pregnancy. Many of these pregnancies are terminated through abortions. Is lack of sex education and sex information implicated in accounting for these pregnancies? No, according to one study (Kane and Lachenbruch, 1973), which indicated that teenage pregnancies did not occur more frequently among the noninformed than among the informed.

The sexual scene has generated some other negatives—over one million cases of sexually transmitted diseases (STD) were reported in 1975. The Center for Disease Control estimates, however, that

Table 15.1 Changing Attitudes Toward Premarital Sex?

	At age 18		*At age 25, 7 years later*	
N	Males 393	Females 397	Males 206	Females 143
"Sexual intercourse before marriage is all right for men but not for girls."				
Agree	23%	42%	6%	11%
Don't know	21	14	2	7
Disagree	56	44	91	82
"Most men want to marry a virgin."				
Agree	66%	69%	61%	59%
Don't know	19	19	9	9
Disagree	15	12	30	33

Source: Adapted from Schofield, 1973, p. 194.

Note: This British study of sexual attitudes and behavior of young adults was based on data obtained from 1,873 interviews of a representative group of male and female teenagers. There were 790 male and female eighteen-year-olds at the time of the first interview, and about half of these subjects were interviewed again seven years later. Although answers to the first question indicate a shift in permissiveness toward premarital intercourse, conjectures about how "most men" feel about marrying virgins remain surprisingly stable.

there are *three times* as many actual cases of STD, for most go unreported for obvious reasons (Kolata, 1976). The highest incidence is in the twenty-twenty-four year age group, and 20 percent of the reported cases are repeaters—a core group of reinfected and reinfecting sexually active people.

Why treat? If sexual behaviors are so varied, and if legal and social codes regarding them are so changeable, then whom are we treating and why? There are several reasons why many professionals treat, counsel, and otherwise try to help people with sexual problems, even though a good many of these problems would not be considered to be indications of abnormality.

Complaints about sexual difficulties tend to fall into three general groups. The first represents a large group of people who feel that they are not getting full satisfaction from their sexual lives. Problems in this area have a broad range, but they generally pertain to difficulties in maintaining levels of sexual arousal or in experiencing orgasm; these are the sexual dysfunctions. Although complaints of sexual dysfunctions are frequent, these conditions are not equally distressing to the people who experience them. Many women who do not experience orgasm, for example, may seek no help at all. Both heterosexual and homosexual people may complain about sexual dysfunctions.

A second, smaller group of people seek help because they are distressed or burdened by their privately enacted sexual practices that deviate from the practices of the majority. These sexual behaviors include various forms of "kinky" sex. The DSM-III calls these the paraphilias, but they have also been called sexual deviations, sexual variations, or sexual minorities. Many people think that as long as these practices are with adult consenting partners, they should not be considered "disorders."

A third group of paraphilias involves such behaviors as sadistic acts with nonconsenting partners or sexually abusive acts (for example, molestation of children). In addition, there are violent, assaultive acts such as rape. These behaviors reflect deep pathology and also pose a very real threat to victims, ranging from psychological and physical harm to mutilation or death. They are criminal offenses, and society possesses the legal codes to convict and incarcerate the people who commit them. At the same time, many practitioners feel that society has an obligation to seek ways to intervene into these deviant behaviors and to offer help to those offenders who wish to change.

HUMAN SEXUAL RESPONSES

To understand disordered sexual behavior or sexual dysfunctions, it is helpful first to look at male and female sexual responses as they actually occur. Perhaps only then will it be possible to determine the extent to which a particular sexual act is in some way "unusual." The surprising aspect of research into sexual behavior is that only in the past few decades has it been possible to systematically examine and observe a wide range of sexual responses. We are able to do so because of the generally less restricted attitudes toward doing research involving observing humans in sexual performance.

The Kinsey Research

Investigation of human sexual behaviors was pioneered in the late 1940s by Kinsey (1948, 1953), a biologist, who through intensive, confidential interviews with thousands of subjects, sought to uncover the sexual practices, beliefs, attitudes, and past experiences of a large sample of men and women from various educational, occupational, age, and SES levels. Kinsey and his staff were interested in the frequency and age at which sexual practices such as heterosexual and homosexual play, petting, masturbation, premarital intercourse, intercourse, involvement with prostitutes, and sex with animals occurred. The subjects' responses were then analyzed according to age and various social factors such as level of education, religious preference, and rural versus urban residence.

Kinsey's methods have elicited some criticism. For example, in both the male and the female studies, white subjects only were interviewed. Further, notoriously unreliable retrospective self-reports were used. Also, attitudes and emotions were not surveyed. An additional criticism is that although diverse educational and social groups were approached, a random sample was not obtained; and the responses of those who did not volunteer remain an unknown quantity.

Yet the Kinsey researches represented a significant advance in the study of human sexuality. They not only showed that it was possible to explore sexual responses objectively and systematically, but that people were willing to "open up" in taboo areas in surprisingly candid ways. As a result, we learned that the extent and diversity of sexual outlets in the American population were never properly estimated. Listed here are a few interesting findings from the Kinsey researches. The incidence figures are probably underestimates, making their import at that time even more striking.

1. One unexpected finding was the relationship of sexual practices to social class and educational level. Lower-SES males, for example, more rigidly adhere to behaviors that reflect a narrow view of sexual responses; penetration and ejaculation are the "point" of sexual activity. More educated, higher-SES males, however, more frequently engage in sexual foreplay of various types (manual or oral-genital stimulation, for example) and are more responsive to erotic visual stimulation and literature than are lower-class males. Although some reseachers believe that these social-class distinctions have now become blurred because of the equalizing influences of television and other media and the general upward mobility of lower-SES people, recent data suggest that social class continues to be influential in the development of sexual practices and attitudes (Weinberg and Williams, 1980).

2. The extent of sexual activity in the American population is greater than was thought to be the case, judging by the incidence of premarital and extramarital sex as well as by the sexual interest and activity among older people.

3. The extent of homosexual experiences, especially among males on all social and educational levels, is relatively large. For example, more than one-third of the males interviewed had experienced orgasm as a result of a homosexual experience after adolescence.

4. Masturbation (autoeroticism resulting in orgasm) is an extremely frequent first source of orgasm for both males and females and an active sexual outlet at all age levels. For example, among males, 60 percent of first ejaculation and 40 percent of first orgasm for females occurred during masturbation.

As a result of Kinsey's researches, masturbation is now acknowledged to be a normal sexual outlet. Yet, guilt and anxiety over masturbatory activity still plague many people, especially those with available sexual partners, and aspects of the myths about masturbation described in Spotlight 15.2 continue to prevail, even if in more moderate form (Gagnon, Simon, and Berger, 1970).

5. American males are fairly active users of prostitutes. Their patronage decreases as educational level rises.

6. Kinsey's data also disclosed that there is a relatively high frequency of sexual intercourse with animals. Although many people were aware of the open practice of "bestiality" in the last days of the Roman Empire (Lorand and Schneer, 1967) few experts were prepared for the extent of this sexual practice today. It is practiced almost entirely among males in rural areas.

Spotlight 15.2 Masturbation: A Normal Sexual Outlet

Almost everyone in your parents' or grandparents' generation has heard something about the evils of masturbation. There were many popular myths about the consequences of masturbation (for example, penises rotting away, hair growing on the palms of one's hands, or malformation of the genitalia). But also, more "respectable" warnings have been disseminated by the church and by physicians even as late as this century. Masturbation is sinful, immoral, and can cause serious diseases, blindness, tuberculosis, even epilepsy. As a matter of fact, a diagnosis of "masturbatory insanity" was once fairly common in mental hospitals not too many decades ago. One harsh Victorian method of controlling offending females was to perform a clitorectomy—surgical removal of the clitoris. Nonetheless, although some of these misconceptions about masturbation may still persist, most people know that masturbation is a normal sexual outlet.

Kinsey found that between 92 and 97 percent of all males engaged in masturbatory activity at some time in their lives. Masturbation was more prevalent, and engaged in more frequently, among upper-class, college-educated males than among lower-class males. This seemed to reflect the lower-class males' greater access to other modes of sexual outlet, including premarital intercourse and prostitution, as well as the greater tendency of lower-class males to view masturbation as an immoral, "abnormal" activity or as a sign of sexual inadequacy.

In general, Kinsey's data showed that masturbation was most prevalent among adolescent males, with incidence declining with increasing age (see Table 15.2).

Kinsey also found that although masturbation was practiced by females, fewer females than males masturbated and those that did so masturbated less often than their male counterparts. Females tended to discover masturbation through self-exploration, whereas males tended to learn about masturbation through erotic literature and social communication. Whereas 89 percent of all males had erotic fantasies while they masturbated (72 percent almost always fantasized during masturbation), only 64 percent of Kinsey's female subjects reported ever having fantasized during masturbation, and only 50 percent reported fantasizing on a regular basis.

A 1967 study found that the incidence of masturbation among males and females had not changed to any great extent since Kinsey's original research (Gagnon, Simon, and Berger, 1970). But it is likely that masturbation among females has become more prevalent over the past decade as a result of the rapidly changing sexual attitudes and practices among females in our society.

Table 15.2 Masturbation: Mean Frequency per Week for Single and Married Females and Males of Different Age Levels

	Females				Males			
	Single		Married		Single		Married	
Age (years)	*Mean freq. per week*	*% total* outlet*	*Mean freq. per week*	*% total outlet*	*Mean freq. per week*	*% total outlet*	*Mean freq. per week*	*% total outlet*
0–15	.3	85	—	—	2.02	71	—	—
16–20	.3	60	.17	9	1.46	51	.17	4
21–25	.3	46	.2	6	1.10	42	.21	6
26–30	.4	41	.2	7	.94	36	.20	6
31–35	.4	42	.2	8	.73	31	.16	6
36–40	.5	37	.2	10	.76	38	.13	5
41–45	.5	45	.2	11	.61	35	.11	5
46–50	.4	52	.2	11	.62	33	.09	5
51–55	.4	70	.1	13	—	—	.10	6
56–60	.3	78	.1	13	—	—	.04	4

Sources: (Adapted from Kinsey et al., 1948, Table 51, pp. 240–41; and Kinsey et al., 1953, Table 23, p. 178.

*Total outlet refers to the percentage of total sexual outlet provided by masturbation activity.

Spotlight 15.3 Prostitution: Commercial Sex

Prostution, the sale of sexual favors, is the world's oldest profession. Most prostitutes are young, female, and in "the life" because of money. Many of them, however, earn very little money ("trap") because they give most of it to their "pimps." They are likely to be poor, uneducated, abused runaways of ethnic minority status, pushed into drug use so that they must turn to prostitution to support their habit. This is not the whole picture, however. For some prostitutes, in business for themselves, do very well financially. Many "call girls," for example, amass a nest egg and then get out of "the life" at a relatively early age, sometimes even marrying one of their customers ("johns").

There are over 2,000 streetwalkers in New York City alone, who in one working "day" turn over thousands upon thousands of "tricks." Who knows how many other "hookers" there are who are not working the streets, and who may spend an entire evening with their "johns." One estimate is that there are about one-quarter of a million prostitutes in this country (Sheehy, 1974).

The streetwalker and the call girl are not the only kind of prostitute. There are also male prostitutes (some of them very young boys) who work for a homosexual clientele. Interestingly, society tends to downgrade the female prostitute while protecting her "johns," who may be of higher SES status. In homosexual circles, it is the *client* of the prostitute who is downgraded. According to Gagnon (1977) many male "hookers" disappear into the crowd as they get older, often leading a normal life as homosexuals.

Are prostitutes "sick"? Who enters "the life"? Most studies of female prostitutes are based on ex-

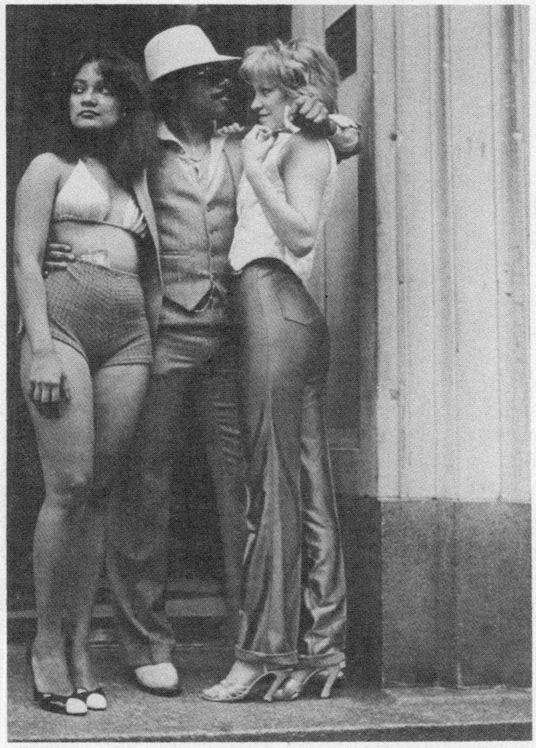

Prostitutes and their pimp. (© *Joel Gordon 1981)*

tremely limited samples. Conclusions, however, have a familiar ring: personality studies disclose a pattern of anger as well as fear and dependency toward men, sexual victimization and abuse as a child (rape, incest), weak parents, and an extremely poor self-image (James and Meyerding, 1977; Sheehy, 1974).

What are the clients like? Through the ages, most users of prostitutes have been men. At the end of the nineteeth century, patrons were mostly single, working-class males who went to prostitutes regularly and often. Since World War II, however, there has been a general decline in prostitute use, possibly because of changing mores that have increased the availability of "free" sex.

In the United States, according to Kinsey's researches, most contacts with prostitutes are made by males of low social and educational levels. For example, 74 percent of males who never went beyond grade school had used prostitutes, while only 28 percent of males with at least some college education had used the services of a prostitute. Married males, especially college-educated males, rarely use prostitutes. The use of prostitutes by single men increases sharply with age, if they remain single.

Most men, however, do not use prostitutes. Those who do so seek a prostitute's service for many reasons, according to Gagnon (1977): (a) the desire to have the kind of "kinky" sex not available through ordinary channels, for example, with more than one person or involving sadomasochistic rituals or anal sex; (b) sex without negotiation or seduction: it is paid for, does not involve persuasive tactics or dinner out; (c) sex without emotional involvement may be necessary for some men to reach orgasm; (d) combining sex with sociability, as in going out with a call girl for the evening; (e) sex away from home (at a convention, for example); (f) sex for the deformed, ugly, and disabled who may be spurned or fearful in ordinary interactions; and (g) sex for older men who are no longer "turned on" by their wives or who have waning sexual interest.

Are prostitutes "sicker" than their "johns"? You decide.

The Studies of Masters and Johnson

William Masters and Virginia Johnson (1966, 1970) led the way, by their precise and objective observations and measurements, to a vastly increased understanding of what happens during the human sexual cycle from arousal to orgasm. From their observations—over 14,000 acts in about every conceivable condition and position were observed—one thing became increasingly clear. The physiological

Table 15.3 Phases of the Sexual Response Cycle of Men and Women

Phase	*Women*	*Men*
Excitement—initial stage of arousal: in both men and women there is heavy breathing; heart rate and blood pressure begin to increase	Vascular engorgement of vaginal tissue, vaginal lubrication, clitoris may become erect, uterus changes position, breasts begin to swell, erection of nipples, vagina begins to enlarge	Erection of penis, elevation of testes, thickening of scrotum
Plateau—advanced stage of arousal just before orgasm: in both men and women genitalia are engorged with blood	Skin mottling, discoloration, and swelling of genitalia; uterus is elevated and clitoris changes its position	Testicles are in an elevated position and are greatly increased in size
Orgasm—in both men and women an acutely pleasureable response	Several .8-per-second rhythmic contractions of the vaginal walls (regardless of sexual method, clitoral stimulation is essential to trigger female orgasm); no refractory phase—within a few seconds orgasm can be reached again	Ejaculation of seminal fluid in several .8-per-second spurts following contractions of internal organs; this is immediately followed by a refractory period during which erection and ejaculation are not possible
Resolution—in both men and women, physiological responses of first three phases return to normal levels	Clitoris and uterus return to normal position, swelling, discoloration, blood pressure, and heart rate return to normal	Detumescence of penis, testicles return to normal position, blood pressure and heart rate return to normal; in older men, erection and ejaculation may not be possible again for several hours

Source: These phases were reliably measured by Masters and Johnson (1966, 1970) during a variety of sexual acts—beginning with erotic feelings and ending with orgasm—that included masturbation and homosexual and heterosexual stimulation (manually, orally, or through penile penetration).

cycle of both men and women, through arousal, continued excitement, and orgasm, is amazingly similar, whether through masturbation, homosexual or heterosexual encounters, or fantasy. Table 15.3 briefly summarizes these phases.

Some clinicians believe that the physiological observations of Masters and Johnson overlook the subjective and emotional components in the sexual experience of most men and women. Fantasy, feelings of love, standards of physical attractiveness, subjective sensations of pleasure and gratification—these are not necessarily mapped by physiological indicators and observations. Perhaps it is just this elusiveness that has continued to allow human sexuality to embrace love, romance, intense feelings, emotional commitment, mystery, and other very deep, enduring aspects of human relationships.

Some myths revisited. The work of Kinsey, Masters and Johnson, and their colleagues and students have cast doubt on, even shattered, some widely held assumptions—for example, about masturbation or the use of prostitutes. One commonly held belief (noted in Spotlight 15.1), underscored in sex manuals and propounded by Freud and his followers, is that there are two kinds of female orgasms, one clitoral and the other vaginal—the latter made possible only through the insertion of the penis into the vagina. Clitoral orgasms (through oral sex or masturbation, for example) are infantile, whereas vaginal orgasms are healthy, sexually and emotionally mature, experienced by truly "fulfilled" women. Scores of women, even as recently as a decade or so ago, sought help because they were made to feel "neurotic," or at the very least immature, because they were not experiencing "vaginal" orgasms. There is in fact only one kind of orgasm, subjectively experienced in the vaginal area, and clitoral stimulation is always essential for it, whether as a result of stimulation of the clitoris by the penis or by other ways.

Another now-exploded myth is that the capacity to be aroused and have orgasm markedly diminishes with age. Actually many people well into their seventies and eighties continue to enjoy good sexual relations with their partners. Elderly people may have fewer available partners, however (there are many more widows than widowers so that there is a smaller percentage of elderly women than men who are sexually active), or illness may intervene.

Still another unfounded belief is that homosexuality is abnormal—a sexual deviation that should be treated as a disease. The next section describes homosexuality in greater detail and also addresses the "normality" of this sexual variation.

HOMOSEXUALITY: A NORMAL SEXUAL VARIATION

Homosexuality can be defined as a sexual pattern in which the primary sexual interest is toward a partner of the same sex.*

One of the most provocative (at that time, surprising) findings of the Kinsey researches was the high incidence of homosexuality in our society among both males and females. Kinsey's survey estimated that 4 percent of white males are exclusively homosexual and that about 10 percent are more or less exclusively homosexual for at least three years between the ages of sixteen and sixty-five years. More than one-third of white males have had at least one homosexual experience by the age of forty-five years and 50 percent, some homosexual response by this age.

The incidence figures for homosexuality among females are lower than those for males, possibly about half or a third as much. Whereas 28 percent of Kinsey's female respondents reported erotic arousal to other females, 17 percent actually had had homosexual contacts, and 13 percent reported at least one homosexual experience to orgasm by the age of forty-five years. In Kinsey's survey, some respondents reported experiencing erotic feelings toward other females as early as the ages of three or four years. The incidence of homosexual erotic arousal apparently increases up to about the age of thirty years.

Some Conceptions and Misconceptions About Homosexuals

Conspicuousness. Contrary to popular belief, the vast majority of male homosexuals are not effeminate in behavior, dress, and interests, and conversely, the vast majority of female homosexuals are not masculine in behavior, dress, and interests. Homosexuals cannot necessarily be detected or identified in a roomful of people. Some male "gays" may be effeminate (may "camp") or may be in "fe-

* There are people with sexual orientations that are neither exclusively homosexual or heterosexual—that is, they have "mixed" sexual histories. Kinsey recognized this by introducing ratings of 1–6, reflecting varying degrees of exclusively heterosexual to exclusively homosexual activity. These people are variously called bisexual or ambisexual. Estimates of incidence are about 15 percent for men and 10 percent for women (Gagnon, 1977). Bisexual people (Joan Baez, the singer, for example is bisexual), according to Masters and Johnson, actually tend to show homosexual preferences, while ambisexual people are equally aroused by and comfortable with sexual partners of either sex. Bisexual and ambisexual people may be more fortunate than most people because of the increased availability of sexual partners to them, but society does not tend to make "room" for people who do not fit the usual social role and who do not tend to have couple relationships. We still have a great deal to learn about people with bisexual and ambisexual orientations, but as yet very few objective research explorations that can shed light on the origins of these sexual variations have been carried out.

male" occupations such as hairdressing or costume design; and some lesbians might be automobile mechanics. But most homosexuals are employed in the same occupations as heterosexuals: teachers, doctors, police officers, politicians, TV repair workers, and so on.

Communities. It is true that many communities have a flourishing gay subculture that may include resorts, beaches, bars, and other recreational contexts that provide homosexuals with opportunities for social contacts as well as an atmosphere that permits contacts for sexual purposes, just as there are "singles" bars and "singles weekends" at resorts for heterosexuals. Many homosexuals point out that the gay subculture arose in response to the "straight" world's tendency to stigmatize and isolate overt homosexuals, especially if they are observed in flirtatious activity or if they are openly displaying erotic interest toward someone of the same sex. The need for exclusivity thus was in response to creating a social environment that reduces the self-conscious self-awareness imposed upon them by straights.

Promiscuousness. Some male homosexuals may be promiscuous, actively looking for different sexual partners as often as they can. But many male homosexuals seek a stable one-to-one emotional and sexual relationship that can last for years, perhaps with occasional infidelities, as may be the case for many couples in the heterosexual world.

Lesbians tend to be less promiscuous than male homosexuals, often establishing a durable couple relationship that provides emotional and psychological mutual support in addition to stability in the sexual partnerhsip. Many experts are inclined to explain this difference by pointing to the general "male" value in our culture that stresses sexual activities or "conquests" with many different partners. Although the heterosexual male often cannot "act out" upon this value, usually because of the bonds of marriage, many homosexual males are more free to do so, especially if they are not restricted by the emotional ties of a couple relationship.

The aging homosexual. Contrary to popular belief, the aging homosexual is not necessarily doomed to a life of misery and loneliness unless—as is also true for his or her aging heterosexual counterpart—vanity, stress on youth, striving for sexual conquests, and unwillingness to bend with the years have contributed to making growing old an intolerable experience.

Sexual patterns of homosexuals. There are no physiological differences between homosexuals and heterosexuals in the stages of arousal and excitement to orgasm (see Table 15.3). Yet there are probably some differences in patterns of sexual interactions between homosexual and heterosexual partners (Gagnon, 1977; Marmor, 1980; Masters and Johnson, 1979; Tripp, 1975). Homosexual interactions do not necessarily involve a masculine or a feminine role: homosexuals are not mimicking heterosexual encounters or relationships. Misconceptions about polarized "roles" may have arisen from stereotyped notions that heterosexuals project onto homosexual interactions because heterosexuals are unfamiliar with or do not care to know about the interpersonal responses of homosexual encounters.

Homosexuals are amazingly varied in their sexual methods and, compared to heterosexual couples, appear to be more caring and more concerned about the sexual desires of their partners, according to Masters and Johnson (1979), who observed hundreds of homosexual and heterosexual couplings. Homosexuals who were involved with each other in a couple relationship, as a matter of fact, tended to spend more time in the sexual act and showed more sensitivity to their partners' erotic likes and dislikes than did equally committed heterosexual couples, according to these authors. Homosexual couples, for example, generally showed greater concern for foreplay, diverse erotic activities, and communication of likes and dislikes to each other than did "straight" couples. Of course, it may be that homosexual couples seeking help from Masters and Johnson may have had a deeper, more intense commitment to each other than did the heterosexual couples who sought help, thus providing a biased impression.

Finally, it is probably true that many more male homosexuals actively seek "kinky" sexual interactions, such as fetishistic, sadistic, or masochistic practices (see page 434), than do heterosexual males or females or lesbians. It is well known, for example, that homosexual prostitutes expect "kinky" demands and do not charge extra for such services, as is common among female prostitutes. One explanation is that males in general, gay or straight, are more interested in and aroused by such practices than are gay or straight females. Once again, gay males are less constricted by marriage or by expectations of female heterosexual partners, and thus may be freer to actively seek and engage in these sexual variations than are straight males.

Causes of Homosexuality

Most experts acknowledge the great significance of cultural and social influences on the extent to which homosexuality flourishes or is repressed at any given time, and there is some agreement that homosexuality has been found in almost all societies and at all historical times (see Ford and Beach, 1951). If the potential for homosexual expression is culturally determined, what determines its variation in incidence at different times and in different cultures? The experts will be addressing themselves to this question in generations to come. One hypothesis that accounts for variations in incidence is that cultures that encourage early heterosexual attachments, that are not "macho," and that do not stress heroic, "male-oriented" values such as great bravery and courage tend to have a low incidence of homosexuality, whereas cultures that stress "epic," mythic, larger-than-life, "masculine" ideals of great strength, aggression, and courage have a higher incidence—for example, the ancient Greeks and Romans or the modern Arab nations (Tripp, 1975).

Homosexuality as a learned pattern. Why does homosexuality arise in any given individual? The search for a single cause for homosexuality has proved to be fruitless. Many experts are beginning to believe that diverse pathways can lead to the same common end, and that these pathways can be traced from stages of development early in the life history of the individual. Sexual preferences and the beginning of eroticized feelings, fantasies, and idealized notions about how bodies should look (idealizing the male body, for example), begin early in life and are learned much in the way that other inclinations, aesthetic values, tastes, and standards for attractiveness are learned (Gagnon, 1977; Marmor, 1980). In effect, what we are saying is that the potential for homosexual or heterosexual preferences is present early in life and can be traced through the reinforcements in the life history of the individual. Some experts feel that sexual preferences not only begin at a young age, but also that most people tend to sustain or "return" to the preferences that were established in these early years.

The Freudian view. Freud thought that in infancy we are all inherently bisexual—capable of being erotically aroused by many diverse kinds of stimuli, "masculine" or "feminine." Homosexuality, as a matter of fact, is an expression of the "polymorphously perverse" nature of infantile sexuality—the infant is erotically attached to both parents. Freud also believed, however, that in normal development girls learn to express passivity and receptivity whereas boys learn to express power and aggression. Both boys and girls eventually develop opposite-sex preference. As the child develops, any deviation from opposite-sex preference becomes "perversion" (a "libidinal fixation at infantile sexual levels"). Perversions include homosexuality as well as any sexual preference or practice that departs from genital, heterosexual interactions.

How do deviations from normal development arise? One Freudian view holds that distortions of the "normal" family model may produce a male homosexual. One such distortion, for example, may result from a dominating, strong, overprotective mother who is closely involved with her son, in an alliance so to speak against a weak, detached, or even absent father. Another family distortion, also involving a strong oedipal attachment to the mother, may produce intense fear of retaliation from a punitive, harsh, and aggressive father. The "castration anxiety" (see p. 115) thus engendered may cast women, because they are truly "castrated," into the role of dreaded, phobic objects. Male alliances are sought because they have "reassuring" penises. Still another view stresses the extreme narcissism of male homosexuals, who seek same-sex love objects as reflections of their vain, self-loving personalities.

Freudians have had much less to say about the development of lesbianism, possibly because lesbians are less overtly conspicuous in their sexual orientation than are male homosexuals, or possibly because generations of male professionals were more mystified, made more anxious, by male than by female homosexuals. The Freudian view nevertheless proposes that some family distortion prevents a little girl from "renouncing" the preoedipal tie with her mother, that is, the female child fails to reject her mother as a love object, fails to follow the "normal" pattern of attempting to win the father over romantically and "sexually." Such girls are at risk for lesbianism, for, because they continue to identify with their fathers in their romantic attachment to their mothers, in adolescence they seek women as love objects.

Freudians also invoke the possibility that some girls may experience deep anxiety over the absence of a penis, resulting in undue preoccupation with the clitoris as an active phallus ("clitoral penis") and a denial of the vagina as a purely passive receptacle. Because normal heterosexual women have learned to accept their vaginas as passive receivers, girls who do not do so are at risk for lesbianism.*

The problem with many of these explanations is that the same family dynamics, distortions, and interactions also produce heterosexual men and women. Although there is moderate confirmation of the hypothesis that homosexual males emerge from families with strong dominating mothers and absent or weak fathers, most of these observations were based on clinical impressions and case illustrations or were derived from poorly controlled comparisons. After all, clinicians tend to see "disturbed" patients, gay or straight, who tend to come from disturbed families.

Organic factors in homosexuality. Contrary to once popular belief, there is little evidence to suggest that genetic, chromosomal, organic, and other physical variables play any role in the development of the sexual preference for the overwhelmingly vast majority of homosexuals. Male homosexuals simply are not "female" in hormonal makeup, and lesbians are simply not "male" in hormonal makeup (Masters and Johnson, 1979; Tourney, Petrilli, and Hatfield, 1975).

Some lesbians may produce higher levels of androgens (male hormones) and male homosexuals, lower levels of testosterone, than their heterosexual counterparts (Starká, Sipová, and Hynie, 1975); or some people may be born with "androgenic sensitization of hypothalamic brain centers" during fetal development (Marmor, 1980). But most experts concur that biological factors cannot "explain" the development of same-sex erotic arousal in the vast majority of homosexual individuals. And if indeed some hormonal variations are found when straights and gays are compared, which came first? Did homosexual practices change the level of sex hormones, or is it the other way around (Gould, 1974)?

We have a great deal to learn about how homosexuality develops in any given individual, but we do know, as already suggested, that learning plays a significant role in this development, and that the pathways toward homosexuality are indeed diverse.

The Homosexual as a Person

Is there a homosexual personality? Most experts agree that there is no single homosexual personality, just as there is no unifying heterosexual personality. Homosexuals differ considerably among themselves in life style, promiscuity, work stability, and in-

* Most clinicians, Freudian or otherwise, agree that tomboyish behavior in girls bears little relationship to future development of homosexuality.

volvement in the homosexual subculture of bars or exclusively gay communities.

As a matter of fact, one criticism of Kinsey's research (for example, Gagnon, 1977) is that Kinsey classified homosexuality on the basis of frequency of sexual contact, using a six-point scale (incidental experience to exclusive homosexuality). These ratings of frequency ignored such questions as how homosexuals view themselves, what feelings they have about their sexual preferences, and the meaning or centrality of their homosexual orientation in their lives.

One investigation, for example, studied about 1,000 homosexual men and women in the San Francisco area (Bell and Weinberg, 1978). Results of intensive interviews led the researchers to classify their sample into the following five categories.

1. *Closed couples.* These homosexuals live in marriage-type relationships, are faithful, and show sexual satisfactions, general self-acceptance, and contentment. They report feeling a strong emotional commitment to their partners and an acceptance of an enduring relationship between them. These homosexuals tend to receive higher scores on measures of "happiness" than does a sample of heterosexuals.
2. *Open couples.* Homosexuals classified as open couples live with a partner but also "cruise"—look for a moderate amount of "extramarital" sexual activity. These people feel less committed to and less dependent on their partners for emotional fulfillment.
3. *Functionals.* These are the sexually active and "free-wheeling" unattached homosexuals who report feelings of exuberance and happiness with their homosexuality and their active sexual lives and "swinging" life style.
4. *Dysfunctionals.* These sexually active unattached homosexuals express regret over their homosexuality and report having various sexual problems. They tend to have a poor self-image and to lack self-confidence.
5. *Asexuals.* These are more covert homosexuals than the others described above, but they are not particularly active or interested sexually. They are less exclusively homosexual, express more regret about being homosexual, and tend to have a poorer self-image than any of the other groups.

Overall, these authors concluded that whereas groups (4) and (5), representing somewhat less than 30 percent of their sample, were lonelier, less accepting of their sexual orientation, and had more sexual problems than the heterosexuals who were interviewed, homosexuals who had no regrets about their homosexuality, and who had reasonably adjusted social and sexual lives, were no less happy or content than the sample of heterosexuals studied in this research.

Are homosexuals "sick"? Is homosexuality a disorder? Although Freud thought that homosexual orientation was "perverse," he did not feel that homosexuals were sick or should be treated because of their homosexuality—unlike some of his followers, who not only viewed homosexuality as "sick" but also recommended early detection and even obligatory treatment.* Today, however, there is growing agreement that homosexuality is a normal sexual orientation. Even the DSM-III, after years of stormy inner-circle controversy among the membership of the American Psychiatric Association, no longer lists homosexuality among its disorders.**

The shift away from the pathological aura attached to homosexuality was aided in large part by the early investigations of Evelyn Hooker (1957, 1959). Hooker's major conclusions—that psycholog-

* The once-popular view among many clinicians that homosexuality is a disorder is based not only on prevailing social attitudes, but on the artifact that most clinicians derived their impressions from homosexual patients who were disturbed about their sexual orientation or who had other emotional problems for which they sought help, rather than on the large number of homosexuals who did not seek help because they were content with their sexual preferences.

** In the 1950s, the DSM-I listed homosexuality as *pathological sexuality,* a subclassification under *psychopathic personality.* In the 1968 DMS-II, homosexuality was classified as *sociopathic personality disturbance.*

ically, homosexuals cannot be differentiated from heterosexuals—were based on comparisons of Rorschach and other projective responses of male homosexuals and matched controls of male heterosexuals. In one study (1957), judges could not correctly differentiate the homosexual and heterosexual records. Judges' ratings of adjustment also did not differentiate the groups. Hooker concluded from this and other researches that homosexuality as a "clinical entity" does not exist and that it is a "deviation in sexual pattern" that falls within the "normal range, psychologically." Homosexuality can subsume a wide variety of personality variations, she continued, and it is not a distinct personality syndrome. Homosexuals can be as healthy, psychologically, as heterosexuals. If some homosexuals are disturbed, anxious, or distressed, it is because they have been made to become that way in response to society's harsh, restrictive, and frequently punitive attitudes toward them.

The Changing Outlook

Thanks to the dedication of powerful activists and to the work of some of the organizations they lead, a new life is possible for many homosexuals. Much of this activity has been concerned with the struggle to guarantee—to fight for and then guard—the civil rights of homosexuals in jobs, the military, the ministry, and in housing. This struggle goes hand in hand with efforts to reduce the stigmatization, and fear, of homosexuals prevalent in our society.

The many aspects of this struggle can range from protesting stereotyped portrayals of homosexuals in movies to actively seeking changes in the law, even if it means bringing the issue up to the level of the highest court of the land.

Educational thrusts, publicity campaigns, demonstrations, publicly vocal complaints, slogans ("gay pride" or "gay is beautiful"), or open declarations of homosexuality by some powerful or prominent individual are all aspects of bombarding the media and subsequently the people with weapons to diminish "homophobia" (an irrational fear of homosexuals). These thrusts, activist homosexuals say, are also designed to lend support to the isolated, unattached, fearful homosexual who feels alienated and alone.

Progress has been slow but decidely present. Legal battles are still being won and lost. According to National Gay Task Force figures, as of 1976, 35 states still had "antisodomy" laws (sodomy is defined as anal penetration) on their books. Such archaic laws that attempt to control people's private sexual lives may not always be actively implemented, but until they are entirely removed from the states' statutes, there is always the possibility of some legal option being exercised.

Activists directly seek legal confrontation and challenges, instead of looking the other way. In California, for example, after more than a century of the state's jurisdiction over sex acts between con-

Gay activists demonstrate not only to guard the civil liberties of homosexuals but also to reduce the stigmatizing, stereotyping, and fear that the media sometimes promote regarding homosexual practices. (Jean-Marie Simon/Taurus Photos)

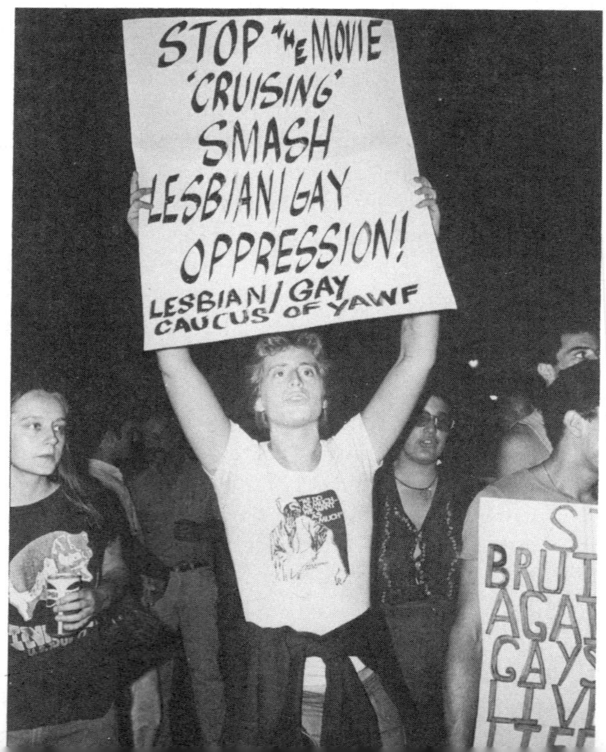

senting adults (punishment for oral sex, for example, was imprisonment up to 15 years; sodomy was punishable by life imprisonment), all sex acts between consenting adults were legalized, with penalties for adultery, oral sex, and sodomy entirely eliminated.

The changes in hiring policies of large corporations, school systems, training centers (some churches are allowing the ordainment of homosexual ministers), are not without their "backlash" reactions. In 1978, for example, the singer Anita Bryant successfully waged a campaign against homosexual rights in Dade County, Florida. Her "Save Our Children" crusade resulted in the voters' overwhelming decision to eliminate a homosexual rights' ordinance in that county. Such repeals of hard-won advances in civil rights for homosexuals have occurred in several places throughout the na-

Spotlight 15.4 Homosexuals: To Treat or Not to Treat

An extremely distressed young man has found his way into a clinician's office. He has suicidal thoughts, he claims, and wishes immediate help. He tells the clinician that he has had several pleasurable homosexual experiences (all followed by acute anxiety), frequent homosexual fantasies, and recently, heterosexual relations with one young woman whom he is planning to marry in just one month. He is contemplating suicide because he fears he is a homosexual and cannot go through with the marriage as planned. He does not wish to live his life as a homosexual, open or otherwise, and wants to become a heterosexual. The clinician is facing a dilemma, shared by many other clinicians, around which a rather spirited forum has developed: to offer or not to offer sexual "reorientation" treatment to such patients.

Clinicians who offer treatment to homosexuals do so for different reasons. An extreme position adopted by some psychoanalytically oriented therapists (see Bieber, 1976; Socarides, 1970) is to recommend reorientation treatment to *all* homosexuals: homosexuality is pathological and all homosexuals are unhappy, immature, poorly adjusted people who fear adult responsibility.

Other clinicians will extend help to homosexuals only if they manifest deep distress regarding their lives or present other cogent reasons such as a desire to have children or because they are married and wish to remain married. Masters and Johnson (1979) claimed considerable success in their attempts to help such homosexuals: among a group of 67 homosexual men and women who wished to change their homosexual orientation to a heterosexual one, they reported 65 percent long-standing success.

Still another group of clinicians offers help only to homosexuals who are dissatisfied with their sexual functioning *as homosexuals.* That is, they wish to get more satisfaction out of their sexual activities, but not as heterosexuals.

Finally, several articulate clinicians state that they will treat a homosexual client only if he or she presents a problem that has *no connection with sexual orientation.* For example, Gerald Davison, a well-known behaviorally oriented psychologist, is vehemently opposed to offering any sexual reorientation program, even if a client voluntarily requests such help (1976, 1978). Davison states that the sheer fact that psychologists offer methods for changing homosexual inclinations implies that there is something wrong with homosexuality. In this light, he wonders how "voluntary" a wish to change one's homosexual orientation really is.

Disagreeing with Davison's position are Sturgis and Adams (1978), who argue that therapists can offer reorientation programs without necessarily thinking or implying that homosexuality is abnormal.

Capsule summaries of these positions are:

Offer Programs to Voluntary Patients Who Wish to Change Sexual Orientation

If patients wish to change their orientation, we should not deny them their right to treatment. We are ethically bound to do so, even if we understand that their response may be to social pressures and that homosexuality per se is not abnormal. Distress about homosexuality or dissatisfaction with the life style attached to it may be sufficient reason for a person to wish to reorient himself or herself. Behavior methods do not necessarily imply that the behavior to be changed is abnormal, because we use such methods for many "deviances" such as excessive eating or fear of public speaking. In any event, the decision to treat, what is chosen for change, and the reasons for wishing treatment (dissatisfaction with the gay life or desire to have children) are up to the client, not the therapist.

Source: Adapted from Sturgis and Adams, 1978

Offer No Sexual Reorientation or Change Program at All

Society, not the individual, should be "treated" or changed. By accepting a patient for treatment, we are expressing our approval of his or her desire to be heterosexual rather than homosexual. If we do offer treatment to a homosexual, we should be helping him or her with problems having to do with guilt, anxiety, and depression about being a homosexual, rather than offering him or her "change programs" that, by their very existence, help to reinforce the view that homosexuality is undesirable. Homosexuals should be treated only for the problems in living that they might have without also assuming that such problems arise from their homosexuality.

Source: Adapted from Davison, 1976, 1978

What is your opinion about this extremely important issue?

tion. However, gays are not afraid of this backlash, according to some activists (see Voeller, 1980), who claim that national campaigns that include massive educational efforts, legislative battles, and confrontations with corporations, churches, and school boards, even if suffering setbacks from time to time, will ultimately change public opinion.

Ego-dystonic Homosexuality: A DMS-III Category

The DSM-III lists among its psychosexual disorders ego-dystonic* homosexuality, characterized chiefly by a "desire to acquire or increase heterosexual arousal" so that heterosexual rather than homosexual relationships (marriage or otherwise) can be maintained. The DSM-III acknowledges that societal pressure or desire to raise children within a marriage, or to have a socially sanctioned married life, may create this disturbance and that an ego-dystonic homosexual has internalized negative social values. The DSM-III, in addition, stipulates that in order to make this diagnosis, the desire to change sexual orientation be accompanied by genuine distress, anxiety, and psychological and emotional discomfort, and that the wish to "reorient" or to change homosexual orientation be present over a period of time. Temporary difficulties in adjusting to the realization that one has homosexual impulses are thus not classified in this group of psychosexual disorders, according to the DSM-III. Onset of ego-dystonic homosexuality is usually in adolescence, when the individual becomes aware of sexual arousal by people of the same sex, and feels guilty and ashamed.

The DSM-III underscores its position regarding homosexuality: it is not a disorder per se, nor are

* Ego-dystonic refers to those aspects of a person's behavior, thoughts, and attitudes, according to the American Psychiatric Association, that are viewed as repugnant or inconsistent with the total personality. Ego-syntonic, on the other hand, refers to a person's behavior, thoughts, and attitudes that are acceptable and consistent with the total personality.

occasional feelings of "life would be easier as a heterosexual" an indication of a disorder. As a matter of fact, most homosexuality is probably ego-syntonic. Lack of heterosexual arousal is not a disorder, nor is the presence of conflict, anxiety or depression in a homosexual individual a reflection of ego-dystonic homosexuality.

Many clinicians take exception to the DSM-III's new position, stating that choice of sexual partner or sexual activity is *entirely irrelevent to the diagnosis of mental illness,* and that, just as with heterosexuals, classification of a mental disorder should be made only if a disorder is present. The question of one's sexual orientation, and whether it is ego-dystonic or ego-syntonic, therefore, should not be a diagnostic consideration. This view is quite heavily represented among many psychologists, who claim that the offering of treatment services to homosexuals who wish to reorient their sexual patterns simply reinforces society's prejudices that homosexuals are "sick." This question is of special significance, for psychologists have developed many innovative methods specifically designed for and available to homosexuals who are unhappy with their sexual orientation (Adams and Sturgis, 1977). Spotlight 15.4 addresses itself to this issue.

PSYCHOSEXUAL DYSFUNCTIONS

As we have seen, there is a universality of the human sexual response—physiologically speaking—in both men and women, heterosexual, bisexual, or homosexual, in which the course of stimulation, arousal, and orgasm follows a sequential, recognizable, and measurable pattern. The essential feature of the psychosexual dysfunctions is some interference with this sexual cycle, such as an inhibition in sexual desire, disruption of the patterns of arousal, or difficulties or failures in experiencing orgasm. Homosexual as well as heterosexual people can be dysfunctional, sexually speaking.

Sexual difficulties are often a reflection of a major depression or may be accompanied by anxiety, fear of failure, or poor self-confidence. In a partnership with many interpersonal problems, sexual difficulties may reflect the strains, pulls, fears, and angers that arise when people are not getting along with each other. The sexual encounter becomes another battleground in which conflicts and tensions continue to manifest themselves.

The dysfunctions described here may result entirely or in part from organic states. Conditions such as diabetes, alcoholism, narcotic intake, multiple sclerosis, some neurological difficulties, surgical removal of some of the genital structures, various vascular problems, and certain kinds of medications that affect endocrinological and hormonal levels within the body can all impair sexual responses: arousal, erection, and/or capacity for orgasm. These states are not regarded primarily as psychosexual dysfunctions. The DSM-III lists the following conditions as psychosexual disorders.

Inhibited sexual desire. Some individuals do not feel sexually interested and are only infrequently

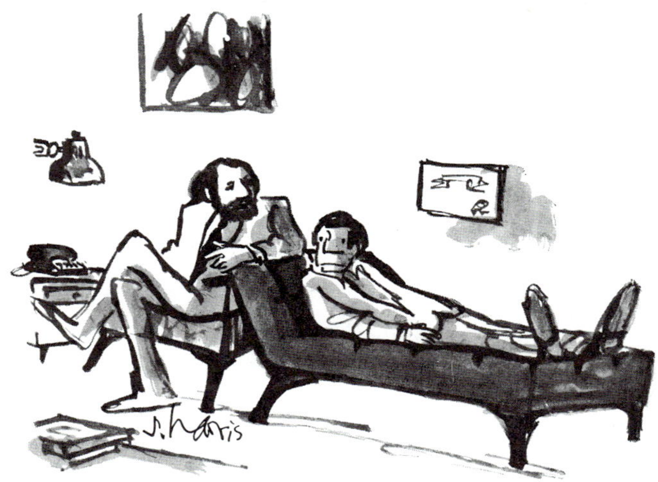

"It has been proven conclusively that as far as performance and sensation are concerned, the size of the sex organ is of absolutely no consequence. Nevertheless, if you show me yours, I'll show you mine."

aroused. This condition is not considered to be a disorder unless the individual is discomforted or distressed by it. Often, for example, a partner is not aroused by his or her husband or wife, but is "turned on" by someone else. Inhibited sexual desire does not refer to the latter, but only to those conditions that are persistent over a period of many years and are not explainable by organic or physical causes. This state is often a reflection of underlying, chronic depression.

Inhibited sexual excitement. In males, this is called impotence and in females, this has sometimes been called frigidity.* In both males and females, inhibited sexual excitement is diagnosed when there is recurrent and persistent inhibition of sexual excitement during sexual activity. The DSM-III states that in males this disorder is characterized by "partial or complete failure to attain and maintain an erection until completion of the sexual act." In females, inhibited sexual excitement refers to "partial or complete failure to attain or maintain the lubrication-swelling response . . . until the completion of the sexual act."

Inhibited female orgasm. This condition refers to a recurrent, persistent pattern in which even under conditions of adequate sexual stimulation and excitement the woman is unable to experience orgasm.

Inhibited male orgasm. This dysfunction refers to a recurrent and persistent pattern in which the male is extremely delayed in ejaculation, or unable to ejaculate after a period of adequate sexual excitement and stimulation.

* *Frigidity* has been defined in so many ways that some clinicians are no longer using this term (Sotile and Kilmann, 1977). For example, frigidity has been applied to any woman who is unable to reach orgasm during coitus, even though she can during masturbation; to women who do not experience pleasure during sexual stimulation, that is, who fail to become aroused; or to women who show little interest in sexual interactions.

Premature ejaculation. This persistent and recurrent condition (once called impotence), which is probably one of the most common of the male dysfunctions (Kaplan, 1974), refers to inadequate control of (inability to delay) the ejaculatory response. As a result, orgasm is reached quite quickly, often just prior to or soon after entry into the vagina. Frequently, males with this problem fail to arouse or to satisfy their partners and seek help for this reason.

Functional dyspareunia. In either males or females, this condition is characterized by persistent and recurrent genital pain during coitus.

Functional vaginismus. This rare psychosexual dysfunction (Kaplan, 1974) refers to involuntary spasms of the vaginal muscles so that penile penetration is not possible. Women with this condition often cannot have gynecological examinations unless they are first given an anesthetic or relaxant.

Treatment of Psychosexual Dysfunctions

One married patient, although orgasmic through other means, was still a virgin. All attempts at vaginal entry by her bewildered husband caused her great pain. She has since been helped to cope with her functional vaginismus with behavioral methods used in conjunction with hypnosis. In very broad terms the treatment of psychosexual dysfunctions, such as this vaginismus, rests on the following general considerations.

1. The very predictability and regularity of the sexual cycle (see Table 15.3) permits some of the newer sex therapies to train the body to perform various parts of the sequence through actual "tasks," including mutual caressing, fondling, and masturbation, so as to produce the required responses leading to orgasm. Such methods generally help clients to continue on a progressive course leading to orgasm through the practice of methods that allow natural, normal bodily responses to occur.

Spotlight 15.5 Sexual Concerns on Campus

There may be sexual problems that are distressing to some people, yet these do not necessarily reflect a disorder. Among these are distorted notions and expectations about sexual practices and activities of other people, as well as concerns about "maleness," "femaleness," and sexual responsiveness (Caplan and Black, 1974).

Some of the sexual concerns, fears, and hangups students presented at one college counseling facility were: misinformation; pressure to perform—to be sexually active and sexually innovative (gay liberation movement and openness on campus interpreted as pressure); couple conflicts; pain with intercourse (among females); "frigidity"; premature ejaculation and impotence; anxiety about promiscuity (mostly among females); rape (students came in with guilt and anxiety); and distress about possible homosexuality (Bauer and Stein, 1973).

Most experts agree that in addition to group and individual counseling facilities on campus, there is a need for general education about anatomy, physiology, and the sexual experiences of other people. It might be helpful to know, for example, the incidence of homosexual experiences or attractions in one's age group or the frequency of masturbation among one's peers. It might also be helpful to know certain "facts" such as: premature ejaculation is frequent in adolescent males and does not reflect deep sexual problems (Salzman, 1974), or that many males and females look for friendship, affection, and companionship as an essential aspect of their sexual interactions and do not enjoy the so-called "free-wheeling" group experiences one so often hears about.

In other words, taking advantage of any counseling facilities as well as courses in human sexuality that college offers might be of real help to many students.

2. Anxiety, which can be experienced at many junctures of the sexual encounter, as well as the tendency of some people to perform a "spectator" role ("watching" rather than "participating") can inhibit or interfere with sexual responsiveness, thus making a major contribution to male and female dysfunctions. Most sex therapists tend to curtail the "spectator" role by encouraging spontaneity and concern with one's own feelings and pleasures especially by making one's sexual desires known to the other. Psychotherapy as well as various behavioral methods are also aimed to reduce anxiety at significant junctures, for example, at just before or at the time of penile insertion.

3. Emotional and psychological factors are of enormous significance in treating sexual dysfunctions. An individual's sexual attitudes, depressive tendencies, fears and anxieties about sex, and above all, relationship to the other in the sexual partnership (for example, anger or insecurity) are probably the most significant influences in creating the dysfunction. Sex therapy must consider these variables. No amount of "mechanical" sex practice will aid the members of a marriage partnership who hate each other. Nor would sex therapy necessarily be successful with a homosexual "forced" to enter into heterosexual sex. A woman who is easily aroused and gratified by a man with whom she is in love is not "frigid," nor does she need treatment, simply because she is not easily aroused by a man with whom she is not in love.

Most sex therapies, no matter how the therapist weights the foregoing, owe a great debt to the work of Masters and Johnson (1970, 1979). These experts required that any couple seeking help stay at a motel near their clinic for about two weeks. If a single

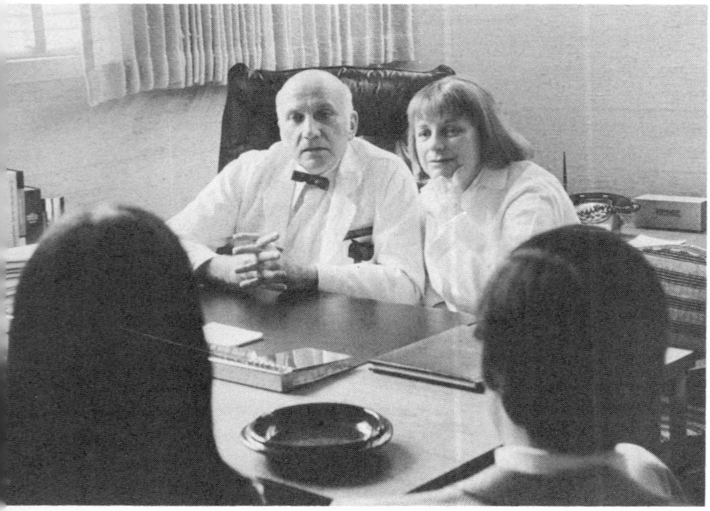

William Masters and Virginia Johnson in a sex-therapy interview session. (© 1981 Robert Levin/Black Star)

individual applied for help, a "surrogate" partner was provided. The use of surrogates—sometimes skilled prostitutes—in sexual treatment programs in clinics throughout the country has been challenged. This issue is raised again at the end of this chapter.

In the Masters and Johnson type of program, there are cotherapists, male and female, one of whom is a physician. There are individual interviews, medical examinations, and group interviews with the four participants. Then the couple is seen jointly each day, or if needed, individually, by one or the other therapist. There are many variations of this approach, especially in connection with the Masters and Johnson requirements that the couple are not at home for treatment (to remove them from the pressures of day-to-day living), that there are two therapists, that one of them is a physician, and that there is a medical examination.

In general, most programs require that the individuals at first not attempt to achieve orgasm. Instead, they are encouraged to focus on experiencing a variety of sensations. The client is given homework: tasks that have been designed to sustain sexual levels, reduce fears, and encourage "letting go"—facilitating enjoyment of the sexual response. Although the nature of the tasks, their sequence, how they are introduced, and opportunities for "reporting back" vary, most treatment approaches are oriented to increasing sexual pleasure while at the same time introducing methods to eliminate specific dysfunctions. Individuals are encouraged not to "watch" themselves. They are also encouraged to engage in fantasy to enhance the "letting go" process.

Although the general public is not aware of the many types of sex therapy programs available, the general term sex therapy refers to a wide variety of procedures, including more or less traditional individual and group psychotherapy as well as the Masters and Johnson type of program. Also used have been hypnotic methods, behavioral methods (such as systematic desensitization—see Chapter 20—in the treatment of vaginismus and other sexual dysfunctions), masturbation training, vaginal exercises, and marital counseling of couples in conjunction with any of these methods.

Moderate success has been claimed for many of these "offshoots" as well as for some of the specific exercises and methods designed to allow females to experience orgasm (Sotile and Kilmann, 1977). Masters and Johnson (1970, 1979) and Kaplan (1979) in particular report success with combining intensive psychotherapy with actual mechanical sexual practices and tasks.

To repeat, couples with disturbed interpersonal relationships—competitiveness, anger, and other reflections of marital or interpersonal discord—may seek sex therapy on an assumption that improved sexual relations can improve the interpersonal "system" between them. Marriage counseling, psychotherapy, or group therapy is often more appropriate for easing tensions in such instances. If the couple's problems are severe, direct sex therapy not only may be unsuccessful, but also may lead to an increase of the couple's difficulties (Lansky and Davenport, 1975).

Until fairly recently, most of the books and manuals in the treatment of sexual dysfunction were targeted at heterosexual couples or single individuals. Masters and Johnson (1979) recently demonstrated success in working with dysfunctional or dissatisfied homosexual male and female couples (for example, impotence in the males, inability to reach orgasm in the females) using the same methods they developed earlier with heterosexual couples. These researchers claimed 80 to 90 percent success (many were followed up after a five-year period) in helping such couples function more effectively, sexually, as homosexuals.

Many innovative, "new" methods in therapy demonstrate immediate success largely because of early "placebo" effects: strong client expectations for success (see Chs. 19–21). This may be true for some of the successful sex therapies that have flourished in the past decade. Recently, for example, therapists using the same methods of Masters and Johnson reported that they did not find the same rates of success that had been reported earlier (Adams, 1980; Zilbergeld and Evans, 1980). These disappointing results may have to do with differences in determining what constitutes success as well as the failure of Masters and Johnson to account for the dropouts or those who were disqualified for treatment when calculating percentages of improved cases. Such perennial problems in doing therapy outcome research are described in greater detail in Chapter 19.

GENDER DEVELOPMENT, GENDER IDENTITY, AND GENDER IDENTITY DISORDERS

Up to now, I have been talking about sexual acts as if they were independent of feelings, self-image, and sense of identity. In fact, an important criticism of some of the researches of Kinsey and of Masters and Johnson is that they tended to overlook these subjective variables. One aspect of this inner content concerns our feelings about being male or female. When does a child view the world from the point of view of a boy or a girl? Why do people behave as males or as females?

This section is concerned with the development of gender identity, the feeling of being male or female, and some disorders that may arise when feelings about identity and sexual structures, such as breasts, vagina, or penis, are discrepant.

Gender Differentiation

Male and female embryos, as determined by XX or XY chromosomes, are anatomically the same until about four weeks, at which time masculinizing hormones gradually change the fetus into anatomical males. By six to twelve weeks, the male sexual structures and the female sexual structures begin to be differentiated in the human embryos. If anything goes "wrong" in the masculinizing process, a complex hormonal shaping, the embryo develops into an anatomical female. That is, special hormonal "mixes" are necessary for the fetus to develop male internal and external organs, a process that is not necessary for female structures.

It is hypothesized that androgenic or estrogenic (sex) hormones also shape the development of dimorphism in the brain of the fetus: either male or female sexual orientation that helps the developing child perceive and respond to sexual stimulation as a male or female or to behave as a male or female (Green, 1980).

The strict and early polarization of male and female behaviors that is implied in the latter hypothesis has been questioned by some researchers, and it has been noted that many of these impressions have been based on extreme instances of rare biological conditions, such as unusual amounts of hormonal medications ingested by the mother during prenancy, or on the basis of animal research (Kolata, 1979c). Thus the thesis that hormonal influences in the fetus or at critical stages in the life of the organism determine gender differentiation, and that by the time a child is born or at least very early in life, he or she is "programmed" to have certain events "trigger" male or female sexual responses, is too early to confirm or disconfirm. We do know, however, that the development of feeling and knowledge that one is male or female (gender identity) and of behaviors that have to do with being identified as a male or female (gender role) are not simple questions of predetermination by the time one is born; and that the family, the culture, and the dominant and prevailing views about how males or females *should* behave play at least as important a role as does biology.

Spotlight 15.6 Gender Anomalies and Gender Rearing

Because of excessive production of androgens by her adrenals during fetal life, this otherwise biologically normal woman in her 20s was born with masculinized genitals so that her clitoris was the size of a small penis. She also had a patent vagina, and so, at birth, her mother was told that although she was a hermaphrodite, "You might as well raise her as a girl." As a result, this mother was forever uncertain as to her daughter's sex. So now, as an adult, the young woman cannot feel herself to be either a male or female but has decided that she might as well live as a woman. As a result, she feels she is a freak, is chronically depressed, and considers herself doomed to a life without adequate sexual gratification or children (although she is fertile and, with minor surgical repair, biologically competent to have children). She is sexually attracted to men but feels that they would not want her (Stoller, 1976, pp. 212–13).

Anomalies such as the one just described can arise from many conditions such as chromosomal "errors" (XXY, XXX for example), abnormal hormonal "mixes" during fetal development, or the mother's ingestion of certain types of medications during pregnancy. What kinds of biological errors of this sort can arise?

Biologically true hermaphroditism is an extremely rare condition in which the anatomical structures, for example, penis and testicles, and chromosomal makeup (XX) are in exact contradiction to each other. Such babies are raised as boys, but at puberty they develop breasts and begin to menstruate.

There can also be various degrees of male and female mixtures. Some chromosomal (XY) males may have some female internal tissues, and some chromosomal (XX) females may possess some male structures and tissues. Other chromosomal males have external organs that seem to look more like female than male organs. Instances of such incomplete or unfinished genital differentiation are troubling to new parents, for it is not clear what the sex assignment—girl or boy—should be.

The list of "errors" of this nature is virtually endless. Anomalies include undescended or missing or atrophied testicles; males with a uterus or fallopian tubes; females without any, or with a misshapen, uterus; external genitals in both sexes can be misshapen, unfinished; breast development or menstruation can suddenly develop in a boy at puberty; precocious puberty can occur in boys or girls—breasts or pubic hair can develop as early as the first few years of life; or there may be failure of puberty to take place (sexual infantilism).

Many of these biological "errors" can be recognized at birth or in the early years. Other "errors," however, are not obvious until just before or during puberty. As a result, gender assignment and gender rearing may be incorrect. Often counseling is required to help parents with the "reannouncement" of their child's gender. For the older child, counseling is very much recommended regarding decisions about gender identity. Hormonal therapy and various surgical procedures (internal as well as external) are often required to permit an individual to live out a reasonably satisfying life, including marriage, in many of the foregoing instances. In cases of sterility, adoption of children is possible. In any event, each "error" must be handled in its own way (Money, 1968).

Biological "errors" or "mistakes" in sexual differentiation offer researchers an interesting opportunity to learn more about gender identity and gender role. They afford us some confirmation, for example, that gender assignment and gender rear-

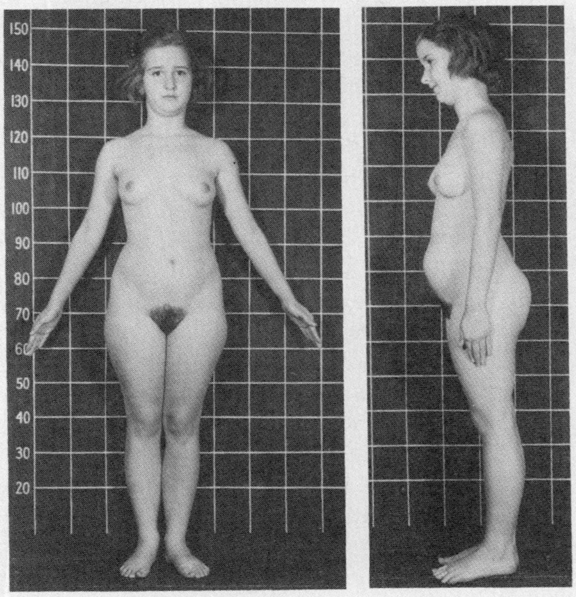

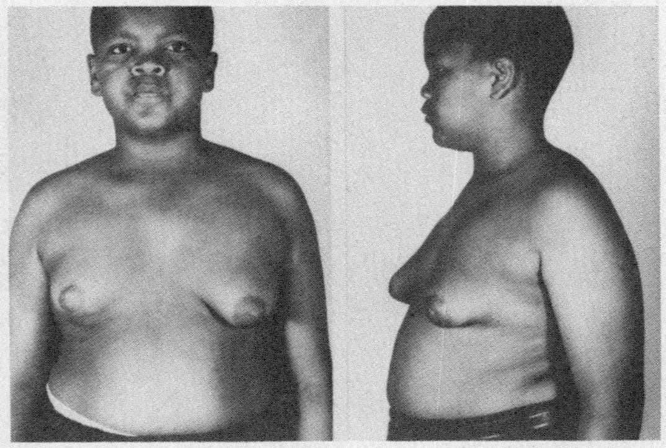

Figure 15.1 Sexual errors. The photos at left show sexual precocity in a girl nine years old, whose sexual development was first noticed at age six. The photo above shows spontaneous breast development in a boy aged thirteen, prior to corrective surgery. (From John Money, Ph.D., *Sex errors of the body* [Baltimore: Johns Hopkins Press, 1968], pp. 127, 130.)

ing, no matter what the biological "facts" or sexual structures are, are crucial determinants in gender identity: how one feels about oneself sexually and in terms of interpersonal relationships. For even when sex is misassigned, the individual feels and behaves in the misassigned role, rather than in the "true" role of the chromosomes or internal sex organs.

Gender Identity and Gender Role

As noted, the private experience of feeling male or female is called gender identity. The *public* expression—the behavior, likes, dislikes, aesthetic preferences, choices that relate to being male or female—refers to gender role. The gender dimorphism of structures that are established early in fetal development do not tell the whole story, for this is where parental influence and culture and society enter the picture.

Even those who do not stress the preprogrammed dimorphism of gender concur that gender identity and gender role behaviors become fixed or stable early in life—by the time a child is three, four, or five years old. For example, Gagnon (1977) feels that children are born more or less neutral but that they label themselves at an early age as male or female. This is a "switching" point in the life of the child, after which he or she is no longer a passive receiver of events. Instead, the child encodes all events in terms of his or her label: "I am a boy" or "I am a girl."

This label ("cognitive switch") maintains the child in a male or female role as the child develops, so that culturally assigned male role expectations or female role expectations are perceived and acted upon accordingly in different ways by girls and

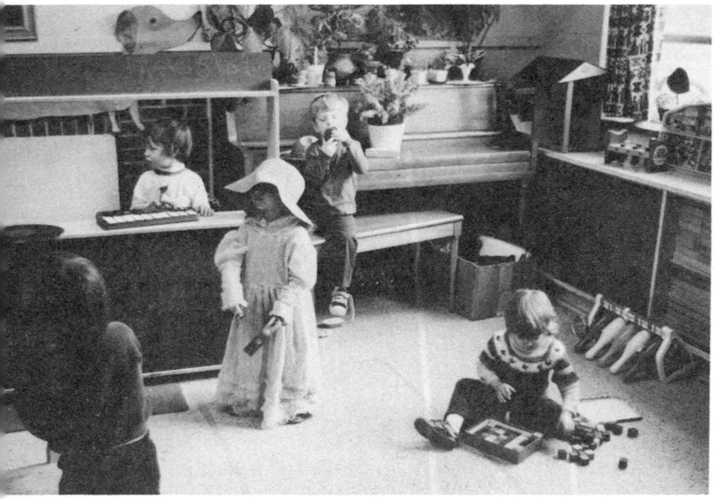

Role-stereotyped activities in the nursery schoolroom. (Copyright Michal Heron 1981/Woodfin Camp)

boys, simply because they have strong gender identities.

An examination of cultural content offers an endless array of illustrations of how the cultural shaping of gender roles takes place. The gender-differentiated influences extend to play activities, postures, aesthetic choices, habits, attitudes toward cleanliness, choices in education, career, goals, general social attitudes, and the myriads of behaviors we associate with being male or female.

At first the parents may be influential in the assignment of gender roles. Soon the school, relatives, friends, strangers, TV, and books enter in to shape the world of the individual who internalizes, picks, chooses, and codes these events in terms of the cognitive switch: the boy or girl identity. Girls and boys soon learn their roles. For example, girls are quieter, less assertive, cleaner, and pay more attention to appearances. They do not have to be "smart" but they should always be pleasant, soft spoken. Boys are strong, more aggressive, can bully. They can mess up their clothes. They can act "rough." And so on. Life provides endless opportunities for such social learning to take place.

Stereotyping of Roles and Psychological Androgyny

The rigid stereotyping of male versus female role behaviors in our culture has many negatives. For athletic or mechanically oriented girls, or girls who are more comfortable in jeans and pants, or who like to play baseball, are viewed in surprisingly disparaging ways by the stereotyping people around them. The picture *should* be, for openers, dolls, sewing, drawing, helping in the kitchen; later, lipstick, perfume, and homemaking lessons. For the girl who likes math or who is more intelligent than the rest, trouble is ahead. The boy who likes to cook or to write poetry, who is not athletically oriented, or who does not like carpentry is also in trouble. For we stereotype our expectations for gender role in ways that create anxiety or guilt in those who step over the line.

Androgyny can be defined as the possession of the physical structures of both sexes. Psychological androgyny can be defined as the freedom from viewing oneself with rigid either-or gender-role stereotypes. Many experts (see Bem, 1975) have begun to consider the possibility that psychological androgyny allows us more freedom to enjoy many aspects of life, and is emotionally "healthier" and less constricting than are the rigid roles of the "ultra feminine" or "ultra macho" male or female.

To test this and related hypotheses, the Bem Sex Role Inventory (BSRI, Bem, 1974), on which a subject can score high in masculinity, high in femininity, high in both, or in neither, was given to over 1,500 students at Stanford University. About half received scores along role expectations, about 15 percent were cross-sex-typed (they scored high on the scale of the opposite sex), and about 35 percent were androgynous, scoring high on both scales (Bem, 1975).

Summarizing experimental work of investigations of behaviors of men and women who are either highly sex-stereotyped or androgynous on the BSRI, Bem noted that feminine women were less independent than other subjects (in situations in which the response studied was conforming to incorrect judgments about whether a particular cartoon—previously rated as to its humorous value—was funny or not). Feminine women also were less assertive, or found it hard to be assertive, in telephone situations in which they were asked to conform to an unreasonable request. And masculine men were considerably less playful (with a six-week-old kitten and a six-month-old baby) than all the other subjects. Androgynous women were more playful than feminine women with the kitten, and as playful as the feminine women were with the baby.

In one situation in which a "confederate" with problems talked to the subject, masculine men were least compassionate and sympathetic, and feminine women, most compassionate and sympathetic. From these and other studies, Bem concluded that rigid sex-stereotyping was especially constricting for masculine men and somewhat constricting for feminine women. Androgynous subjects, however, behaved in all situations without constriction or limit.

In sum, Bem and others (see Spence et al., 1975) have generally found strong support for the hypothesis that psychologically androgynous people have higher self-esteem, greater flexibility, and show a richer variety of desirable traits (for example, gentleness, affection, and playfulness) than their more rigidly role-stereotyped peers.

Gender Identity Disorders: Transsexualism and Transsexual Surgery

There are some identity "mix-ups" that are particularly intriguing to researchers because of their early onset and the considerable anguish they cause to the people experiencing them. These are the gender identity disorders, characterized by an insistent, unwavering, intense belief that the anatomic sex of one's body is not one's own sex, but is in fact, some mistake, some horrible error. These disorders are called transsexual disorders, and they involve a crossgendered identity—"anatomy-identity discontinuity." In these disorders there is a persistent sense of discomfort, even revulsion about one's biologically normal genitalia and an extreme conviction that the assigned role, male or female, is inappropriate, a gross mistake. Transsexuals may dress, behave, and identify with members of the opposite sex, not for sexual arousal and excitement but as a logical expression of their identities.

Transsexuals frequently report that even when very young, they had a strong sense that their anatomy was "wrong," obscuring their real selves. Although they risked the disapproval of their parents or schoolmates, their sense of true identity propelled them to dress, behave, and play as a member of the opposite sex.

Gender identity disorders of adults and childhood are much more common in males than in females (eight to one, according to the DSM-III). Why this is so is not clear, but it has been suggested that the answer might lie in the complex hormonal differentiation between males and females that require males to "get something extra"

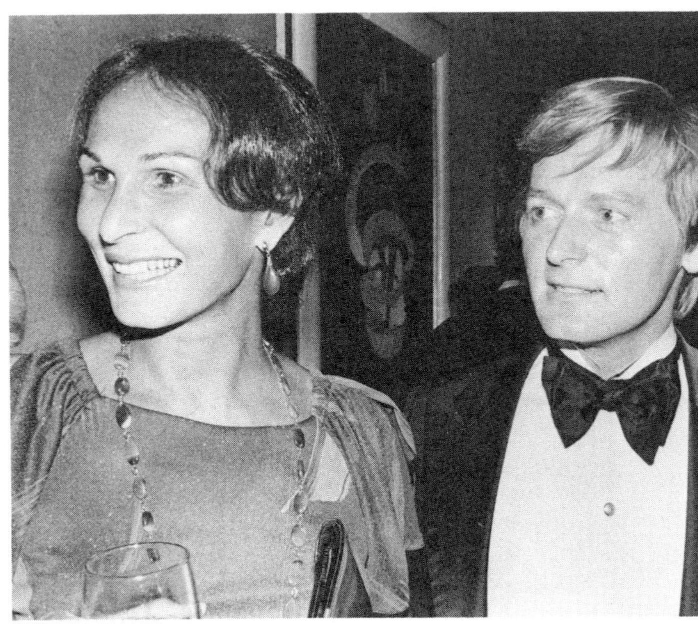

Successful transsexual surgery: Dr. Renée Richards, with a friend. (Adam Scull/Black Star)

in fetal development, possibly permitting more "errors" to occur in the process.

Many transsexuals seek to correct the discrepancy between their "true" identities and their actual physical structures through surgical and endocrinological procedures. Well over 10,000 such procedures have already been performed, at first mostly for males wishing to become females, but more recently, with an equal female-to-male ratio. In male-to-female surgery, the penis and testicles are removed but the skin of the penis is retained along with some of the skin of the scrotum to line a surgical opening that becomes the vagina. Facial hair is removed, breasts are enlarged, and female sex hormones are administered. In female-to-male surgery, clitoral tissue is surgically placed at the base of an artificial penis formed from the patient's own tissue. The penis can be made "functional" through use of artificial devices that allow penetration into the vagina. If hormonal maintenance is appropriate, erotic desire, pleasure, and capacity to achieve orgasm is retained in both males and females after transsexual surgery. Transsexuals are not homosexuals, nor do their sexual partners regard them as such, even though they were once of similar gender.

Although the research literature is contradictory as to the extent of emotional pathology in the people who seek sex reassignment (Finney et al., 1975; Roback et al., 1976), almost all clinicians working with transsurgical patients agree that the surgical and hormonal reassignment of sex is a dramatic event in the patient's life, presenting many pre- and post-surgical problems in daily living and requiring a long period of adjustment. Most programs require living in the role-to-be for many months (even a year or two) before surgery, as well as pre- and post-surgical counseling (Oles, 1977). And the experts tend to agree that severe emotional problems are not necessarily solved by sexual reassignment, and may even be exacerbated (Money and Gaskin, 1971). All agree that careful screening of applicants is required to eliminate unstable and possibly psychotic individuals.

Nevertheless, despite some of the foregoing reservations, it had been more or less thought until fairly recently that surgically reassigned transsexuals achieve a well-adjusted postsurgical life and that only in rare instances is there any severe postsurgical emotional difficulty (Van Putten and Fawzy, 1976). The initial "high" may wear off, but sexually reassigned people were thought to "blend" reasonably well into their new lives.

It is with some surprise, then, that some follow-up reports of people who have undergone these procedures yielded a less rosy picture than had once been painted, and that some of the major centers (including Johns Hopkins University, an innovator of this type of surgery) are no longer performing these procedures. Instead, some of the centers are recommending intensive psychotherapy. The Johns Hopkins staff is recommending psychotherapy in conjunction with behavioral methods to help with identity problems.

A follow-up evaluation (through interviews and objective tests) of the Johns Hopkins procedures, for example, had indicated that their transsurgical patients were faring no better than a group of controls who had been denied surgery by the staff (Meyer and Reter, 1979). As a matter of fact, some of the subjects who had been turned down by the Johns Hopkins staff went elsewhere for surgical reassignment, and these subjects showed the poorest adjustment, poorer even than those subjects who did not undergo surgery.

Follow-up evaluations are still being conducted throughout the country, however, and the picture of outcome is far from clear. Many centers (Stanford University, for example) continue to report excellent postsurgical social and personal adjustment as well as improvement in the sex lives of their sexually reassigned patients.

Transsexual surgery may not be the ultimate answer for all anguished individuals with gender-identity problems. With careful screening, pre- and post-surgical counseling, and education about risk and outcome, however, it may be the remedy for some.

SEXUAL PLURALITIES: THE PARAPHILIAS

There are certain paths to sexual excitement and gratification that do not rely on the customary homosexual or heterosexual practices. These paths have in common a persistent, unvarying reliance on certain objects, rituals, or situations that are necessary for arousal and discharge. These preferred modes for sexual expression and gratification are sometimes sought as an end in themselves. Often, orgasm is not possible through any other means.

It is not so much that many of these sexual practices deviate from the prevailing norm as that they involve an insistent, "locked-in" quality (frequently distressing to the individual) that causes some experts to regard them as "disorders." The DSM-III refers to these practices as the paraphilias (probably because the label *sexual deviations* has caused too much controversy) and includes in this group the following: fetishism, transvestism, zoophilia, pedophilia, exhibitionism, voyeurism, sexual masochism, sexual sadism, and atypical paraphilias.*

Because some of the paraphilias are quite common and harmless, privately engaged in between consenting adults or employed in fantasy by many "normal" people to enhance arousal, many theorists do not regard most of the paraphilias as "deviations" or as "disorders," especially because at some point in time or in some place each has been practiced, tolerated, even approved by the prevailing culture. However, because many of these practices can also be employed *without* consent and can range from harmless acts to the assaultive, violent use of others for sexual discharge, this discussion will separate the paraphilias into those that involve consenting partners and those that do not.

Many of the practices described in the next sections are illustrated in the writings of Stoller (1976), who worked extensively with the paraphilias. Two of the cases Stoller described are presented in Cases 15.1 and 15.2.

Some "Victimless" Sexual Practices

The practices described in this section may create distress in some individuals because these people may be unhappy about the "inconvenience" of having to repeat certain rituals or because they may be apprehensive about being caught. The distress is not intrinsic to the sexual act, however, which is not necessarily abnormal. Freud's allusion to "perverts" as "poor devils who have to pay a high price for their limited pleasure" may well apply to patients who are troubled by the rigid, inflexible nature of their symptoms or fearful about possible discovery, but not to the countless others (and who knows how many) who practice and enjoy their special sexual "thing" privately.

Today a large number of clinicians regard many of the paraphilias as trivial or harmless sexual variations that require no treatment (see Haslam, 1979). Further, if society were more tolerant, there would be less guilt and less distress about possible exposure and subsequent humiliation, probably accompanied by less of a need to seek professional help.

Fetishism. One of my patients was in the habit of stealing satin fabric samples from department stores. He would use these swatches again and again while masturbating. He is sixty years old, has never had either a heterosexual or a homosexual

---

* Pedophilia is a repeated, exclusive method of achieving sexual excitement and discharge through children. Because of its child-abuse aspects, this so-called paraphilia will be discussed in the section concerned with assaultive sexual acts. Zoophilia, according to the DSM-III, is the act or fantasy of engaging in sexual activity with animals on a repeatedly preferred or exclusive basis. Sexual contacts with animals is a frequent sexual expression, especially among the young in rural areas where there is limited availability of sexual partners. The preference for sexual contacts with animals to the exclusion of human partners, however, is an extremely rare condition, often accompanied by sadism (see later), in which sexual excitement is further enhanced by torturing or killing the animal (Stoller, 1976).

Case 15.1 Voyeurism

This single man, in his early 20s, drives to a different residential neighborhood each night and surveys homes to find rooms where he can observe women undressing, while he is safely hidden in the bushes outside the window. When he finds a room in which a young woman is undressing, he becomes excited and masturbates. Although he can exhaust himself sexually after a couple of such experiences a night, he never satisfies his desire to peep, which is an insatiable hunger.

He also goes out on dates and occasionally has intercourse without problems of potency. He enjoys this intercourse but less than the masturbating while peeping. He is not especially aroused watching a girlfriend undress. No matter how closely her nude body conforms to his ideal, looking at her under these permissive circumstances is fairly casual. . . .

Case 15.2 Sexual Sadism

This married man in his 20s requested . . . help because he feared he would soon commit murder. Since adolescence, he has been excited by fantasies and pornography depicting women bound and tortured. During courtship of his wife, he introduced mild versions of his fantasy into their sex play, and in this manner only was able to proceed on to intercourse. Now, after 8 years of marriage, they invariably have intercourse by his first binding her tightly with ropes and then, with her still bound having intercourse. She has noticed that gradually the binding has been less and less symbolic and more and more painful. . . .

It is the nature of his work to enter households of strangers to do repairs. He frequently meets housewives there, and the temptation to bind and torture them is becoming unbearable. So far, he has avoided doing so by going out to his repair truck and masturbating while looking at photographs of bound and tortured women. His fear of killing a strange woman stems not from a belief that such an act would be sexually exciting but rather that, having bound and tortured her, he would have to kill her to remove the witness.

Source: Stoller, 1976, pp. 204–205.

experience, but would like to get married. He reports homosexual fantasies during his frequent masturbation. He also recalls that when he was a child he would steal and then hide his mother's underwear, often taking it to cuddle with when he went to bed.

Fetishism is a sexual variation that entails a preferred, persistent, habitual reliance on objects or things for sexual arousal, excitement, and discharge, generally to the exclusion of other forms of sexual contact. Fetishes can be undergarments, pieces of silk or satin fabrics, shoes, boots, stockings, even soiled bras, corsets, or underwear. According to Kinsey, fetishistic behaviors are almost always practiced by males—by both homosexual and heterosexual males. The intensity with which fetishistic practices are engaged in, their domination of the individual, the objects desired for arousal, and the basic sexual orientation of the individual are as varied as the fantasies reported by patients who engage in them.

Transvestitism. This sexual variation involves the recurrent, repeated practice of crossdressing and occurs almost exclusively in males. According to Kinsey, the ratio of males to females is about 50 to 1. Transvestites dress in the clothing of the opposite sex for sexual arousal, excitement, or discharge.

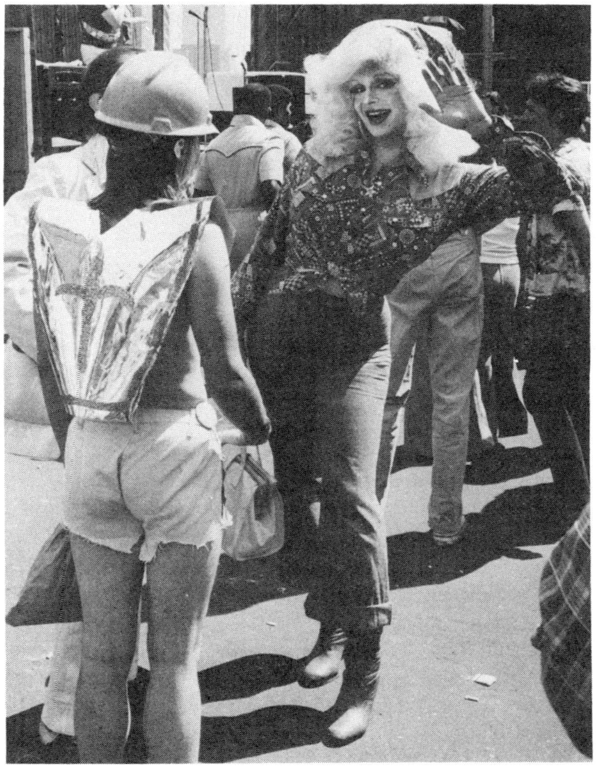

A male transvestite. (© Jan Lukas/Photo Researchers)

They are not transsexuals and they do not report problems in sexual identity such as desiring to change their genitalia to those of the opposite sex. Male transvestites feel themselves to be male. They are excited by "dressing up," but they do not feel homosexually excited. In fact, transvestites generally are heterosexuals, not homosexuals. "Drag queens" (homosexuals who dress in female clothing) are in the homosexual minority and are not necessarily attractive to most homosexuals; after all, homosexual men are attracted to other men, not to women.

No doubt a detailed history of each transvestite would disclose the earliest conditions ("imprinting") in which the touch, feel, and look of dressing up in female clothing was associated with sexual excitement and or discharge, possibly through masturbation. Some transvestites, for example, report that as children they were dressed as little girls, receiving special attention when this happened. Most experts concur that transvestite inclinations begin in childhood.

Because social attitudes in Western society toward transvestites are quite disapproving, many heterosexual transvestite men live in constant dread that they will be found out by their wives or friends. For this reason, they might seek help to modify their transvestite inclinations. If, on the other hand, a transvestite can indulge in his (or her) sexual "kicks" privately and does not feel too guilty as a consequence, there seems to be little reason to regard this sexual variation as pathological.

Other Paraphilias: Sexual Acts with Nonconsenting Victims

The first two paraphilias involve taking advantage of an unsuspecting stranger. Indeed, the "thrill" and excitement in these acts often stems from the surprise, shock, secret manipulation, and power that are involved.

Exhibitionism. This is almost entirely a male paraphilia. It involves repeated exposure of the genitals to unsuspecting strangers (mostly female children or adults) as a preferred method for sexual arousal. Most often there is no further sexual activity, although there may be masturbation during exposure. Exhibitionists ("flashers") are often picked up by the police while roaming the streets or riding the subways in secret search for the "prey" who turns them on. Surprising or shocking the observer is apparently an important component of sexual arousal for them. Exhibitionism is one of the most common of the sexual offenses, generally involves incarceration, and is often shameful to the subject. Compared to other sexual offenses, it has one of the highest rates of recidivism (repeated offenses).

Voyeurism. The chief feature of voyeurism is the repeated need to observe unsuspecting people in acts of disrobing, sexual activity, or nudity, as an exclusive, preferred method of sexual arousal and discharge (through masturbation during the voyeuristic act, or later, to fantasies generated by what was observed). Freudians describe voyeuristic needs as extensions of normal infantile curiosity (perhaps regarding sex between parents), which by now has become associated with forbidden, taboo, and sexually arousing and exciting stimulation. Although this may be true for many individuals, the question as to why this has become the preferred or exclusive sexual method is not clear.

Sexual sadism. This term refers to the need to abuse, hurt, humiliate, or debase the partner as an exclusive, preferred mode of sexual arousal and excitement. The mild or simulated playful sadistic practices that sexually tease or arouse the partner, engaged in by consenting adults are not under discussion here. Such harmless practices are relatively common in fantasy and behavior and rarely come to the attention of the clinician. As a matter of fact, according to Kinsey, 20 percent of males and 12 percent of females are aroused by fantasies of rape, bondage, chains, whips, and discipline—that is, of sadistic and masochistic themes. Even among consenting adults, however, sadistic practices (named after the Marquis de Sade, 1740–1814, a French author) can involve serious bodily harm. Sexual sadism inflicted on a "nonconsenting" partner may often accompany rape, murder, and other acts of criminal violence. Such assaultive sexual abuse is discussed in a later section.

Sexual masochism. As its chief feature, sexual masochism (named after Leopold von Sacher-Masoch, 1836–1895, an Austrian novelist) involves excitement and discharge through the experience of suffering as a result of being beaten, humiliated, whipped, bound, excreted or urinated upon. A playful, "role-enacted" variation of sexual masochism is not under discussion here as in pretending one is a servile maid during sex, nor is the use of prostitutes for mild forms of masochistic practice.

Masochistic practices are regarded as pathological and as requiring help when the voluntary submission to such acts involves severe injury or mutilation. In some instances, a life-threatening interaction that produces sexual excitement may result in death.

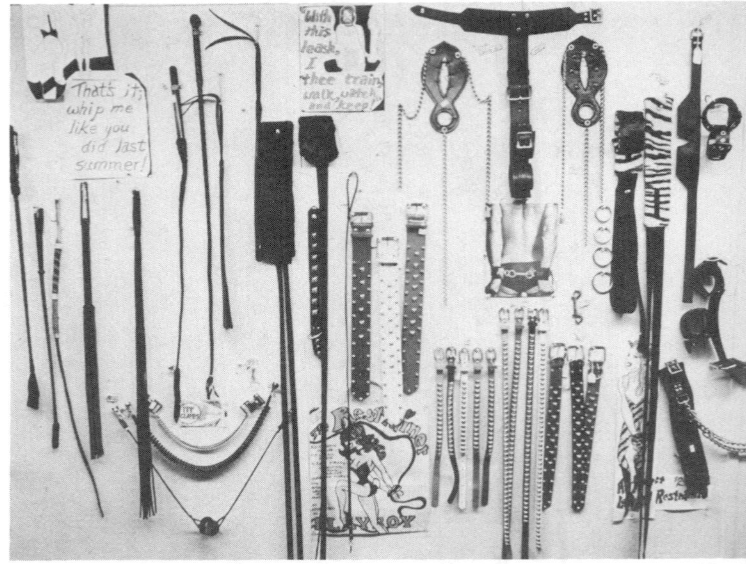

For sale: Items for sadomasochistic practices. (© Joel Gordon 1981)

Possible Causes of the Paraphilias

Most experts agree that the development of tastes, ideals of beauty, and preferences for what arouses an individual follows the general laws of learning. However, how is it that some people get "trapped" by certain paraphilias so that they become the preferred, exclusive mode for sexual release despite the individual's desire to change? The experts are further agreed that there are no biological, hormonal, organic, or genetic factors that can account for the development of the paraphilias in any individual. Freud was among the earliest clinicians to stress purely psychological factors in the etiology of what he called "perversions." However, the views of

Freud and his followers depart somewhat from the more contemporary views.

Freudian hypotheses hold that all children at the earliest and most primitive levels are "perverse"—capable of erotic attachments to and arousal by, objects and stimulation that, if development is healthy, are later modified and suppressed as genital arousal and satisfaction take their place. The normal development into genital, heterosexual modes may be disrupted by fixation or regression to infantile psychosexual levels because of some great trauma that produces overwhelming anxiety. According to Freud, "perversions" are reflections of arrested sexual development, probably as a result of guilt and anxiety arising in taboo, shameful areas.

For purposes of illustration: A forbidden sexual impulse arises when a child is watching the mother or nurse or neighbor get undressed and becomes associated with something in that context. It (the braid, article of clothing, a shoe, an undergarment) remains sexually arousing and eventually becomes essential for eliciting excitement and discharge in adult years, separated from the person because of the taboo aspects. The Freudian model also implies that there is a "return" to earlier levels in which taboo eroticized feelings arose. Thus, a child who is severely spanked by his "nanny" and who became sexually aroused at that time can later "return" to the scene of the "crime" by requiring his adult partner, dressed as a nurse, to spank him. Unfortunately, although there are ample case illustrations that presumably confirm the tie-in of such events with the later development of a paraphilia, clinical testimony of this type does not provide valid empirical confirmation of these hypotheses.

A related, more updated psychodynamic approach stresses family interactions that produce feelings of being "bad" as a consequence of sexual practices that the child is beginning to experiment with. The child then suppresses these behaviors, substituting erotic fantasies and daydreams that are more "acceptable" or at least not in overt conflict with family standards. These fantasies later become translated into the kinds of sexual requirements for arousal that are inherent in the paraphilias. In other words, the development of a paraphilia can be found in the close examination of the specific history of the child within his or her parental-familial context (Stoller, 1976).

The fact that it is possible to pair sexual arousal (as measured through penile tumescence—beginnings of erection) with previously neutral stimuli (Rachman, 1966) has been offered as bearing some relationship to the origins of fetishistic behavior. Yet largely unanswered questions remain about the development and maintenance of these paraphilias. For example, why is there such difficulty in extinguishing these behaviors in the light of the negative reinforcement usually associated with them?

Some of the experts believe that many of these behaviors are acquired and maintained through imprinting, rapidly acquired behaviors learned early in life and extremely difficult to extinguish—observed primarily in animals. In humans, an imprinting hypothesis implies that intense sexual experiences early in the life of an individual become very strongly bonded to or paired with stimuli surrounding that event. Later on, sexual arousal continues to be achieved only when stimulus elements from the early experience are present, even if appropriate partners are available.

Another unanswered question asks why the paraphilias occur almost entirely among males. It is true that males may be more aroused by visual stimuli than are females (Haslam, 1979), but this would account for the development only of paraphilias such as voyeurism. Kinsey tried to answer this question by hypothesizing that the male's sexual response is more easily paired to surrounding objects and situations than are the female's. In any event, despite many unanswered questions (for example, why are these preferred practices necessary for arousal and gratification to the exclusion of other practices?), most experts believe that the principles of learning can account for the strongly ingrained pairing or association of a specific stimulus with a specific type of sexual behavior, and that a detailed history of the individual would yield the precise circumstances of how the particular paraphilia was learned.

SEXUAL ASSAULT: RAPE AND OTHER ACTS OF VIOLENCE AND NONCONSENT

Rape is nonconsenting sexual assault, often but not always involving physical force, violence, or threat of physical injury. Because rape involves a nonconsenting victim, many experts are expanding their definition of rape to include sexual assaults on sleeping, unconscious, or mentally incompetent individuals. We are only just beginning to learn more about rape, the rapist, and the victim. Nevertheless, there is general agreement: rape is primarily an act of violence, not a sexual act, usually motivated by desire for power, control, and the expression of anger.

Some myths about rape. The many misconceptions about rape, especially those that generate guilt in the raped individual, contribute to the reluctance of victims and their families to report its occurrence. The common theme that the victim brought the whole thing on herself is exemplified by such homilies as "nice girls don't get raped" or "she was asking for it anyway." Further, victims often share their families' views: somehow the rape could have been prevented but now that it is past history, the "goods are spoiled."

Advice such as, "If you're about to be raped, relax and enjoy it" implies that rape is or can be a mutually enjoyable sexual act between partners. The myth that rape is a sexual act and that rapists are sex fiends who either need sex desperately or are sexually dysfunctional has been put to rest by empirical data that indicate that the rapist neither lacks sexual partners nor is necessarily dysfunctional with his wife or girlfriend (Amir, 1971; Groth and Birnbaum, 1979). Legalizing prostitution, therefore, will not reduce the incidence of rape. Similarly, there is very little empirical evidence that hardcore pornographic literature or films propel a potential rapist into prowling the streets for victims.

*Some facts about rape.** In 1968, there were 31,060 reported forcible rapes (statutory rape refers to sexual relations with a presumably "consenting" female younger than the age of "consent," which varies from state to state). The incidence of rape in this country is increasing, but this increase may actually reflect a greater willingness to report such assaults. All agree that the incidence of rape is considerably larger than the reported incidence, possibly four to ten times larger. Further, it is estimated that one woman in twenty-five in this country is going to be raped at some time in her life. Of rape victims, 2 to 7 percent are over 50 years of age. Rapist and victim know each other in about one-third of reported rapes; about 10 percent actually occur within the same family—stepfather and daughter, for example.

Most rapes occur in economically depressed areas and tend to be committed by single young males of low-SES levels. About half the reported rapes are committed by black men in the vicinity of their homes with black women as victims. Poverty, rather than race, seems to be related to prevalence, judging by the data in this and other countries.

Only about 15 percent of reported rapes end up in actual convictions. Jurors are reluctant to call a sexual assault rape if the rapist and the victim know each other (employer and employee, for example) or when the victim initiates the contact, as in hitchhiking. Evidence favorable to a conviction, on the other hand, include the presence of an actual weapon, witnesses, signs of penetration, indications that there was force or threat of force, evidence of lack of consent (physical injury, for example), and lack of acquaintanceship between rapist and victim. In most incidents of rape, these convincing "facts" are not easy to come up with.

Patterns of rape. The violence of a rape is usually motivated by strong feelings of anger or power that

* Sources: Abel, Barlow, Blanchard, and Guild, 1977; Amir, 1971; Freudenheim, 1978; Griffin, 1974; Groth and Birnbaum, 1979; MacDonald, 1971; Rabkin, 1979; and Walker and Brodsky, 1976.

are further ignited by the inferior status of women and the models for violence in our society (Brownmiller, 1975). In individual cases, it is thought that rape behavior is a symptom of psychological dysfunction in "weak" people who become "disorganized" under stress (Groth and Birnbaum, 1979). In their study of 500 rapists, these researchers further found that rapists tend to show little compassion or empathy with their victims, show poor judgment and lack of impulse control, and, in agreement with other studies, are not necessarily psychotic.

1. About 40 percent of the rapes in this study were classified as *anger* rapes. These rapes are usually unpremeditated, impulsive, and frequently associated with alcohol abuse. Typically, the rapist becomes "blind with rage," seeking a target upon whom to vent his explosiveness. Many rapes of elderly women are predominantly motivated by rage. The majority of such victims in this sample were brutally assaulted—beaten, kicked, knocked down.

2. More than half of the rapes (55 percent) in this sample were classified as *power* rapes in which the assailant wishes to capture, control, and conquer the victim by any means, including threat and intimidation. Physical aggression is used only if other methods fail. The power-motivated rapist tends to be a repeater, for his drive for conquest is never fully satisfied.

3. A small percentage of rapes (about 5 percent) were classified as *sadistic* rapes. These tend to be premeditated acts—for example, the victim is stalked—in which the rape takes on a ritualistic, bizarre quality. The rapist is often obsessed with repeating certain acts, such as bondage or flagellation (beating). Extreme cases may involve mutilation and murder: limbs might be severed or ritualistic disemboweling might take place. Sadistic rapists frequently have a predictable pattern that the police can recognize.

Victims of rape. Many rape victims fail to report the assault to the police because they are ashamed. Moreover, those who do so are often the butt of jokes ("the victim is a sexy lady who changed her mind") and sometimes even treated like a defendant, having to prove, for example, that the assault actually took place, that it was not provoked, and that it did involve violence.

The immediate aftermath of rape has now been objectively and systematically studied by several researchers (Feldman-Summers et al., 1979; Kilpatrick, Veronen, and Resick, 1979). Anxiety, anger, fear of unwanted pregnancy, humiliation, confusion, guilt, nightmares, and sexual problems such as lowered sexual satisfaction have all been reported.

Long-range follow-up studies indicate that many victims continue to feel guilt and continue to experience many sexual hang-ups such as lack of interest, loss of trust in the partner, or feeling that sex is "dirty." One survey reported that sexual problems such as pain, orgasmic difficulties, and lack of interest appeared in about half the victims, even up to a year after the assault (Becker, Abel, and Skinner, 1979). Many other fears were also found in a large percentage of victims, such as fear of crowds, fear of indoors, or fear of outdoors. Especially prevalent for victims as well as attempt victims were the fear of living alone and the fear of people behind them.

It is of interest that close relationships between victim and assailant are more likely associated with the victim's sexual problems than less close or stranger relationships (Becker, Abel, and Skinner, 1979). Explosive, "blitz" attacks affect the victim more seriously and with less healing than other kinds of assaults (Burgess and Holmstrom, 1979; Groth and Birnbaum, 1979). This stands to reason in that often such assaults involve physical trauma and a generally brutal assault in a life-threatening situation. In the power rape, the woman has been made to feel helpless (and sometimes even "conned"). Here she feels self-blame and guilt about not having sufficiently fought back or in some way having provoked the attack. In sadistic rape, however, the victim has many more physical and emotional scars and, if she survives, extensive psychological and medical care is required for long periods of time (Groth and Birnbaum, 1979).

SEXUAL ABUSE OF CHILDREN: RAPE, INCEST, MOLESTATION, AND COMMERCIAL EXPLOITATION

The content of this section is the sexual victimization of children. If we include in this general category the victims of parental sexual abuse, child molestation, and rape, and the sexual use of children for commercial purposes (for example, prostitution or pornographic movies), then it is estimated that at any one time, there are up to two million children who are so victimized.*

Sexual abuse within the family. An examination of the case records of a large city hospital (emergency room and pediatric gynecology clinic) disclosed many unexpected instances of sexual abuse within the family: incest, rape, and injury as a result of mutual masturbation. Rapes were sometimes committed by a mother's boyfriend with vague awareness, even compliance on the mother's part. Many of these abuses were not diagnosed properly in the initial (emergency room) contact but became evident later as a result of gynecological follow-up, at which time detailed questions were raised about symptoms that were unusual for very young children: venereal disease, sexual nightmares, certain kinds of urinary problems (Brant and Tisza, 1977).

Observations of families and children at risk for sexual abuse yield some generalizations: they tend to come from low-SES families in which children are repeatedly abused, and in which the adult abusers were themselves sexually abused as children. We are also learning that many sexually abused children come from middle- and upper-income families. We have yet to fully understand the similarities among sexual abusers of children and how they might differ among themselves regarding their capacity for violence.

Child molestation and rape. Sexual abusers of children show the full range of possible behaviors, from adult exposure of genitals, forcing the child to be photographed in the nude, hugging, kissing, oral sex, and masturbation, to rape (Groth and Birnbaum, 1979). In extreme cases, there may be mutilation and murder. Such assaults generally involve pressure—even though the child appears to be cooperating—through enticement, encouragement, threat, intimidation, or physical restraint.

Most clinical evidence points to differences between the child molester and the child rapist (DSM-III; Groth and Birnbaum, 1979). There is not enough research evidence to make this claim definitively, however, and it may be that the lines are drawn too carefully, so that potential danger of the molester may be overlooked.

Many experts (see Groth and Birnbaum, 1979) believe that rape of children is motivated by the same principles (or at least follows the same patterns) as are involved in adult rapes—anger, power, control, and sadism—and are acts of violence (often of great explosiveness), not sexual acts. The child rapist is not necessarily sexually inadequate with adults, may be homosexual, but is more likely to be heterosexual, even if the victim is a boy.

These rapes are often motivated by anger and retaliation with regard to an adult relationship in a disorganized, disturbed person who is likely to be young and from a low-SES background. Child rapists tend to "mellow out" or "burn out" as they get older.

Child molesters, according to the DSM-III, have a disorder called pedophilia, meaning love of children. No matter what the name, most clinicians and law enforcement personnel are familiar with the pattern, which is often one of repeated offenses. Pedophilia, which occurs twice as frequently among heterosexuals than homosexuals, and which is almost entirely a male pattern, is characterized by sexual attraction to and desire for a young child. The eroticization of the child in this disorder (as op-

---

* Data on about 800 female and male white college respondents indicated that about 20 percent of the females and about 10 percent of the males had been sexually abused in childhood, with considerably more reporting some incestuous experiences (28 and 23 percent, respectively), according to Finkelhor (1979)—probably an underestimate of the true population of sexually abused children.

Spotlight 15.7 Incest

Here is a "typical" profile (see Rist, 1979) of a family situation that harbors an incestuous relationship between father and daughter. The father is weak, dependent, has "deserted" his wife sexually, but longs for closeness and a long-term, nonthreatening, affectionate relationship. The mother and perhaps others in the family are aware of the sexual alliance between father and daughter but there is a "vow of silence" with the "secret" never openly expressed. The incestuous sexual relationship can last for years and often begins when the daughter is very young. The child is ashamed to talk about it, particularly because any attempt to do so tends to elicit disbelief anyway. Sometimes these children are treated as "special"—the favorite—by their fathers, who may even be jealous of the attention of others. The daughter may assume a "motherly" role in the household, taking care of the other children or handling chores. Some of these abused children report feeling "enslaved," trapped in a situation that gets "resolved" only when they run away or leave home to get married.

Incest in this country is more frequent than commonly believed (one in ten families is one estimate, although only one in twenty instances come to the attention of the authorities—Brody, 1979). Incest includes sexual relations between father and daughter (the most common form), mother and son (the least common in our culture and the most taboo), brother and sister, father and son, sister and sister, and brother and brother. Such sexual acts are among the most taboo of all cultures and ages (different cultures define incest differently—it need not be intercourse) and some cultures forbid members of the same clan (cousins, in-laws) to marry or have sexual relations. In a survey of 133 "primitive" cultures, 75 percent had some form of this taboo with regard to relatives and clan members, but all forbade sexual relations with offspring (Ford and Beach, 1951). In our culture, incest is frequently associated with alcoholism, schizophrenia, drug abuse, and low SES levels. We would be mistaken, however, to assume that incest is not found in upper-level SES families.

Follow-up data on consequences of incestuous relationships are sparse, but, as might be expected, there are many indications that there is considerable impact on the emotional, sexual, and interpersonal adjustment of abused children as they develop into adolescents and adults (Rist, 1979). Some of these children may turn to promiscuity and prostitution in the mythic search for what they thought was "special" in their lives. Others show guilt, anxiety, and many somatic complaints. In any event, we are learning more about identifying high-risk families for incest as well as other forms of sexual abuse; and one day, perhaps, we will be able to prevent their occurrence.

posed, say, to incest) involves the exclusion of adult relationships. Most child molesters are not violent, and most say that they wish for a long-term relationship that includes sexual foreplay and caressing and affection rather than violent assault as in the case of rape.

Child molesters are usually weak, heterosexual young men (most are under the age of thirty-five years) who are neither retarded nor psychotic. Most know their victims, even if only casually. They are generally unable to form attachments to other adults and tend to be sexually inadequate or impotent with them. They say that they do not feel inferior when with children (DSM-III; Groth and Birnbaum, 1979; Haslam, 1979).

Sexual abuse and commercial exploitation. Children who turn to or who are enticed into prostitution and pornography (both boys as well as girls are involved) are most often from low-SES families. They are typically runaways, unable to tolerate the physical and sexual abuse they have received at home

(Dullea, 1979). Some of these children turn to pornography or prostitution because of the money they get—no small inducement—and an illusion of "belonging" to someone or to something larger than themselves (their pimp or film producer, for example) and because they know of no other way to get by in life; they frequently do not consider returning to school or home an alternative. Counselors who attempt to rehabilitate such children with offers of job training and a clean place to stay are often disappointed, for many of these children return to their street lives. We are still casting about for effective interventions into the unhappy, disorganized lives of these children. The best approach is undoubtedly prevention, a determined attempt to identify the high-risk families and their children to forestall the inevitability of this pattern by the introduction of yet-to-be discovered methods.

TREATMENT OF OFFENDERS: RAPE AND OTHER NONCONSENTING ACTS

Child molesters and rapists have a high degree of recidivism and show poor motivation for treatment, generally not volunteering when such treatment is made available. Educational efforts directed at "accepting responsibility" for one's acts also tend to have a poor track record. For those wishing help, however, some of the behavioral methods appear promising, possibly more so than do the traditional verbal and group therapies.

A series of interventive efforts with small numbers of sexual offenders who volunteered for help was based on a "multifaceted," integrated approach that relies on many methods, most of them behavioral (Abel et al., 1977; Abel et al., 1978; Murphy, Abel, and Becker, 1980). Still in experimental stages, this general approach employs an objective, detailed assessment of the component behaviors that go into the deviant sexual arousal pattern, including inappropriate or peculiar arousal patterns and limitations in social and interpersonal skills. These and other behavioral "excesses" and "deficits" then become targets for change, using as many different techniques as possible.

It has been shown, for example, that sexual arousal in rapists, as measured by penile tumescence, occurs to inherently violent sexual stimuli (such as descriptions of a rape), but not to themes of mutually consenting, mutually enjoyable sexual activity; or that child molesters are aroused by sexual descriptions of children but not by those of adult women. Through aversive methods (see Chapter 20), a rapist's arousal to themes of sexual violence is reduced, while at the same time, sexual arousal to appropriate, nonviolent sexual activity with adult women is reinforced. The rapist might also be given help in social skills or in other interpersonal areas that may have contributed to his deviant pattern. Similarly, intervention into the child molester's pattern of arousal involve attempts to change many of his behavioral "excesses" and "deficits"—all components of the deviant arousal pattern.

Although showing some promise, limitations of these efforts lie in the dismal reality that most rapists and child molesters are undetected and unconvicted. However, the few offenders who do volunteer for such programs bring with them some potential for change by their very involvement in the program that is being offered to them.

SUMMARY

Chapter 15 described a broad range of sexual behaviors, emphasizing that in the sexual arena, designations of normal, abnormal, or pathological reflect cultural standards and practices and varying legal and social codes. Further, sexual beliefs are interlaced with myth and misinformation. The chapter then described the "normal" sexual cycle as well as a normal variation, homosexuality, in some detail. This material included a description of incidence and patterns of homosexuality as well as a discussion of possible causes. It then discussed psychosexual dysfunctions including inhibited sexual desire or excitement, inhibited orgasm, and premature ejaculation, as well as the general approach to treating such dysfunctions. The text discussed the development of gender identity and gender role and described gender identity disorders. It then, listed some sexual pluralities (paraphilias) beginning with two "victimless" practices, fetishism and transvestism, followed by other paraphilias that involve nonconsenting victims such as exhibitionism, voyeurism, and sexual sadism and masochism. The chapter concluded with a detailed section on sexually violent, aggressive, and criminal acts, including rape and sexual abuse of children.

Highlights

1. Designations of normal and abnormal sexual behavior vary from culture to culture and reflect legal and social codes. Further, there are many myths and superstitions about sexual practices, for example, that sex is a monopoly of the young, that frequent masturbation is unhealthy, or that homosexuality is a disease.
2. Sexual attitudes in our society have undergone considerable change in the past decade or two. For example, attitudes toward sexual variations and premarital sex have become permissive.
3. Despite greater permissiveness toward the so-called sexual minorities, treating some of the sexual variations, dysfunctions, and disorders may be desirable. Some people feel that they are not getting full satisfaction out of their sexual lives because of some dysfunction—for example, inability to maintain an erection to orgasm—and may seek help for this or similar reasons. Others may seek help because they are distressed by a privately enacted sexual variation, even though such a variation is not regarded as abnormal or pathological. A third group, however, involves not only deep pathology, but also poses serious threats to its victims. It comprises those offenders who commit rape, sexually abuse children, and otherwise harm their victims. These violent criminal acts are not necessarily sexual acts, even though they appear to be, and are legally punishable even as society is seeking ways to treat or to prevent their expression.
4. Kinsey's researches have taught us much about the sexual practices in our society, for example, the relationship of sexual behavior to social class and educational level, or the extent of homosexuality and prostitution in our culture. The investigations of Masters and Johnson more recently have shown us that it is possible to conduct objective observational research in the sexual area. These researchers have also confirmed the hypothesis that the physiological events leading to orgasm, through whatever means, are stable and predictable.
5. It has been estimated that about 4 percent of white males are exclusively homosexual, and that about 10 percent are more or less exclusively homosexual for at least three years in their lifetimes. The incidence of homosexuality among females is about one-third to one-half of the estimates for males. Personality makeup, sexual patterns, and life styles are more varied among homosexuals than one might expect. Homosexual behavior probably emerges from diverse pathways. Even though causes are not entirely clear, learning seems to play an influential role. Most clinicians concur that homosexuality is not a disorder and that homosexuals are not "sick." There is some controversy as to whether or not to offer treatment to homosexuals who wish to change their sexual orientation.
6. The sexual dysfunctions such as inhibited female orgasm or premature ejaculation may reflect depression, poor self-confidence, anxiety, and interpersonal and marital difficulties between sexual partners. Treatment of these dysfunctions should consider these and other psychological factors after ruling out organic causes. Sex therapies have been employed to enhance sexual enjoyment and to reduce or eliminate many sexual dysfunctions. Many of these approaches, generally based on methods

developed by Masters and Johnson, are claimed to be quite successful. However, such claims of effectiveness have recently been challenged.

7. Although biology plays an important role in shaping male and female sexual behaviors, the development of feeling that one is male or female (gender identity) is also shaped by the family, culture, and prevailing views about "femininity" and "masculinity." The public expression of behavior that relates to being male and female is called gender role. Although gender identity and gender roles are developed early in life, the chapter stresses that the culture plays a crucial part in determining the kinds of behaviors regarded as appropriate to male and female roles. Many psychologists believe that the rigid stereotyping of male and female roles in our culture creates numerous psychological "negatives."
8. Transsexual disorders—anatomy-identity discontinuities—refer to a class of behaviors arising from a deep sense of discomfort with one's assigned gender and apparent sexual structures. Transsexuals dress and behave like, and identity with, members of the opposite sex—not for sexual arousal or excitement but because they feel that such behavior is a valid expression of their true identities. Transsexual surgery, in which such discrepancies are corrected and then hormonally maintained, has proved to be successful in many instances. Recent follow-up evaluations, however, suggest that eventual outcome, judging by postsurgical emotional and interpersonal adjustment, is not as successful as had once been claimed.
9. Many of the paraphilias, such as fetishism and transvestism, are harmless practices privately engaged in without "victims." On the other hand, there are many sexual variations that involve nonconsenting partners, and some of these involve dangerous, harmful, criminal assaults. There seem to be no organic or hormonal factors that can account for the development of these behaviors in any individual, and many clinicians believe that learning plays an important role in their shaping. It is possible, according to one hypothesis, that some of these behaviors are acquired through imprinting early in the life of the individual. In any event, there are many unexplained characteristics of these sexual variations, for example, why they appear almost exclusively among males.
10. The circumstances surrounding rape are laced with myth and hearsay. We are learning a great deal about rape, however. For example, its actual incidence is probably four to ten times greater than the reported figures; most rapes occur in low-SES areas by single, young males; rape is primarily an act of violence, not of sex; rapists do not lack sexual partners; and only a small percentage of reported rapes end up in actual convictions. Rapists have been classified according to patterns of the act: most fall into anger and power categories; a smaller group can be classified by ritualistic needs to harm, mutilate, even murder their victims through bizarre, often repeated symbolic acts. The study of rape victims, which is aided by the greater willingness of subjects to come forward, has indicated that they suffer many long-range effects in a variety of emotional and sexual areas.
11. The incidence of sexual abuse of children—rape, incest, prostitution—within and outside the home can be numbered in the millions at any given time. Within the home, sexually abused children tend to come from low-SES families and the pattern is one of repeated abuse, often overlooked by other members of the family. High-risk families are only now being identified, and methods for intervention and prevention of such abuse are still only in the early stages.

ISSUES AND QUESTIONS

1. Should there be official control and censorship of literature and films that cater exclusively to minority sexual preferences and interests? What about pornographic films that employ

children? Should prostitution be legalized? In other words, what is your position on the censorship of pornography, the legalization of prostitution, and the commercialization of various sexual interests and drives? Does censorship curtail individual freedom? How can the sexual exploitation of children for commercial purposes be controlled?

2. Homosexual men and women are concerned with the many legal codes and statutes that discriminate against them, especially in connection with family issues: child adoption, child custody, divorce actions, estate problems, and so on. One current issue is the right of homosexual couples to raise children (through legal custody, adoption, or even artificial insemination). Many states permit the adoption of children by homosexual men and women; in 1976, the American Psychological Association's Council of Representatives passed a resolution which read that "The sex, gender identity or sexual orientation of natural or prospective adoptive or foster parents should not be the sole or primary variable considered in custody or placement cases." In addition, there is little evidence to suggest that homosexual couples raise children who themselves become homosexual. Do you agree that in custody battles, the issue of homosexuality is not relevant and that the relationship between parent and child and the values and attitudes of the home are more important considerations than the sexual orientation of the parent in custody and adoption cases?
3. Another issue is the licensing of marriages between homosexuals to guarantee them the same civil and legal rights, benefits, and protection (for example, estates, wills, taxes, insurance, property advantages) as are accrued by married heterosexual couples. There is some precedent for legal unions between homosexuals in a few counties in some states, but often the local courts void such marriages, and public opinion runs high against them. Test cases have generally not been won in the courts. What is your opinion of such unions? Are we denying certain rights to many individuals in our society by "archaic" marriage laws?
4. Some states specifically prohibit the use of surrogate partners (sometimes skilled prostitutes) in sex therapy programs or in other psychotherapeutic contexts, despite the claim by a few clinicians that under some circumstances with some types of sexual dysfunction, the skills of surrogate partners might be extremely important. The legal and ethical problems in the use of surrogates in sex therapy have been the subject of many professional forums. What is your opinion about this issue? Should there be guidelines for using surrogates? How should they be trained? Should prostitutes be used?
5. It has been estimated that several thousand centers and offices are offering sex treatment in this country, but that only a small percentage of them are staffed with qualified and trained professionals who use rigorously tested methods. Should centers and staff be licensed? If so, by whom and using what standards? For example, what type of educational and professional background should a sex therapist have? What sorts of views on sexual "normality" should he or she profess? How can the privacy and confidentiality of the procedure be guaranteed, and how can the rights and records of the client be protected? What concerns and problems would you watch out for if you were establishing guidelines?
6. In 1975, when he was about forty years old, Dr. Richard Raskin, opthamologist, husband, father, and a high-ranking amateur tennis player, underwent sex reassignment surgery and hormonal treatment, emerging as Dr. Renée Richards (see picture on p. 429). After these procedures, he/she successfully qualified to compete in various women's contests, over the objections of many women contestants and the Women's Tennis Association, which had wanted a sex determination test to establish "true" sex by chromosomal identification. The hope was to set a precedent for future contests in which transsexuals wished to enter.

   Do you believe that such chromosomal

tests should be routinely used in competitive matches in which strength and endurance might tip the balance in favor of one over another athlete? Should chromosomal males like Dr. Richards be permitted to enter the same contests as chromosomal females? Remember, Dr. Richards contended that she was not an imposter: she was a legal woman as well as a female in every other sense—identity, role, dress, interpersonal relationships, physical appearance, structures, and hormonal levels.

7. In some states, the law requires that sexual offenders, even if "criminally dangerous," cannot be incarcerated in mental hospitals longer than they would be if imprisoned in jail for their offense. As a result, extremely dangerous offenders, at considerable risk for recidivism, are often released into the community, not only from prisons but from hospitals. Considerations such as these have led some experts to look for ways to forcibly prevent the occurrence of such assaults in the future. Drastic methods have been suggested, to be used with recidivist rapists and child molesters, but many of these are still in experimental stages: chemotherapy, for example, or surgical incapacitation (castration). There are many legal and ethical issues involved here. Are we justified in forcing treatment on, and modifying the behavior of, unwilling subjects? Are we depriving them of their rights? But does not society have a right to protect itself? Is extending jail sentences for recidivist rapists the answer, on the assumption that they will "mellow" or "burn out" in their mid-forties?

SUGGESTIONS FOR FURTHER READING

Brown, H. J. *Familiar faces, hidden lives: The story of homosexual men in America today.* New York: Harcourt Brace Jovanovich, 1976. In 1971 the writer Merle Miller "came out," but few people were really shocked, because writers, artists, and theater people are often expected to be gay or at least unusual. When Dr. Brown, an important medical member of New York City Mayor Lindsay's staff came out—after leading a hidden, double life for many years in constant fear and near panic that he would be discovered—the step was a bold one. This book describes the experiences of many people in high political and public positions who are gay, their terror about being discovered, as well as Dr. Brown's personal anguish and road to self-acceptance. Dr. Brown, a founder of the National Gay Task Force, appeals to homosexuals to come out, to uncover their hidden identities, so that they, like the general public, can accept the notion that except for sexual orientation, gays are very much like everyone else.

Brownmiller, S. *Against our will: Men, women and rape.* New York: Simon & Schuster, 1975. Paperback available. This thorough and readable book presents myths and facts about rape, rapists, and rape victims through history and in our own time. It deals with rape during war, riots, revolutions, and in prisons. It discusses the crime statistics for rape and the treatment of rapists and their victims by our legal system. Finally, it presents the political and social efforts women are now taking to combat rape in America. It is a scholarly work and a must for any student interested in the problem of rape.

Gagnon, J. H. *Human sexualities.* Glenville, Ill.: Scott, Foresman, 1977. Paperback. This book is a beautifully written text on the spectrum of human sexuality. It deals with many of the topics that were discussed in this chapter, including gender identity, the variety of sexual responses, and the sexual minorities. The psychology of human sexuality is presented from an orientation that stresses the learned nature of sexual conduct.

Hite, S. *The Hite report: A nationwide study of female sexuality.* New York: Macmillan, 1976. Paperback available. This report, based on a survey of 3,000 women, has brought out into the open the various sexual behaviors in which women engage, and their feelings about those behaviors. Masturbation, orgasm, intercourse, clitoral stimulation, and lesbianism are some of the topics discussed. Data are given, but the bulk of the report consists of the subjects' responses to questions about feelings and sensations, for example, "Do you enjoy masturbating?" or "What do the stages of orgasm feel like?" Although this report is not based on a random sample or on a well-executed piece of research, it does provide an interesting, in-depth view into subjective aspects of female sexuality.

Kaplan, H. S. *The new sex therapy: Active treatment of sexual dysfunctions.* New York: Brunner/Mazel, 1974. In a well-written, easy-to-understand book, this author describes the many problems in sexual performance that people have. This book not only covers a wide body of knowledge about human sexuality, but also describes the various methods for treating problems—such as impotence, premature ejaculation, inability to attain orgasm—that are often unapproachable through the usual psychotherapeutic methods. Dr. Kaplan's methods, which are based on those introduced by Masters and Johnson, employ relatively simple sexual tasks that couples engage in at home (rather than in the clinic or office).

Kinsey, A. C., Pomeroy, W. B., and Martin, C. E. *Sexual behavior in the human male.* Philadelphia: Saunders, 1948. Kinsey, A. C., Pomeroy, W. B., Martin, C. E., and Gebhard, P. H. *Sexual behavior in the human female.* Philadelphia: Saunders, 1953. These scholarly, exhaustive studies of the human sexual response were truly innovative in scope and in content, for little direct knowledge had been amassed about how people from different cultural, educational, and economic groups perform sexually, or what their sexual attitudes and experiences are. These classics are a "must" for at least skimming.

Masters, W. H., and Johnson, V. E. *Human sexual response.* Boston: Little, Brown, 1966. Masters, W. H., and Johnson, V. E. *Human sexual inadequacy.* Boston: Little, Brown, 1970. From a rigorous approach that first attempted to explore and record the human sexual response (through objective, reliable procedures) of normal subjects during intercourse or masturbation, these authors, in their extensive researches, developed and empirically demonstrated methods for improving and modifying sexual performance and responses. Their assumption is that barring physical disability, everyone is capable of achieving sexual gratification through orgasm. In these two by-now-classic works, these authors describe their researches and principles.

Murstein, B. I. (Ed.) *Exploring intimate life styles.* New York: Springer, 1978. Paperback available. Open marriages, communal living, "swinging," and homosexuality are a few of the nonnormative intimate life styles explored in this collection of papers. Some of the papers are reports of research conducted in these areas; others are subjective accounts written by persons who themselves have adopted these alternative styles.

16

Alcohol Abuse

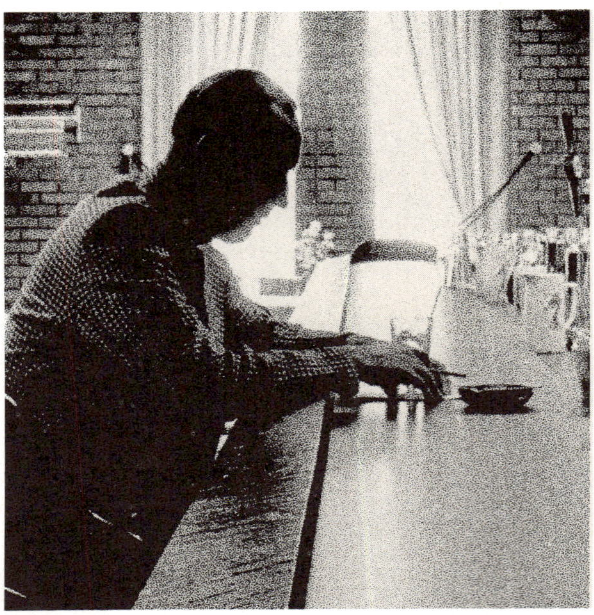

Over 100 million Americans over the age of fifteen years drink alcoholic beverages. Each year, more and more women and teenagers are joining their ranks. Although for most of these "social" and "recreational" drinkers alcohol presents no problem, it has been estimated that about ten million of them are alcohol abusers or alcoholics. What is alcoholism? Is it a disease? Why do some people throw away their lives because of alcohol? Can anything be done to help them? This chapter is addressed to these and related questions.

ALCOHOL ABUSE AND ALCOHOLISM

It has been the custom to distinguish between alcohol abuse (or problem drinking) and alcoholism. The traditional distinction implies that *alcohol abuse* is accompanied by various behavioral and interpersonal difficulties (for example, job and marital difficulties, traffic accidents) that arise as a result of heavy, uncontrolled drinking whereas *alcoholism* refers specifically to a progressive illness of addiction or physical dependence (see Spotlight 16.1).

In actuality, there is much overlap between these traditional distinctions as well as an extremely wide range of drinking behaviors and disruptive consequences for different groups of people. Because, in addition, there is some controversy as to whether alcoholism is indeed a disease, such terms as problem drinking, pathological drinking, alcohol abuse, and alcoholism will be used interchangeably to avoid becoming bogged down by problems of definition.

Pathological drinking is often characterized by some common elements and by some early signs. The problem drinker does not drink alcoholic beverages in the same way that other members of his or her social group customarily drink. The problem drinker may drink to relieve stress or anxiety, or gulp drinks, or drink too much too early in the evening, or be unduly interested in planning the next drinking occasion or in discussing the merits of various bars in town. Although this type of drinker is preoccupied with drinking—getting drunk or remaining drunk—there may be a parallel preoccupation with changing drinking patterns and drinks: no drinks until noon for the next month; no solitary drinking; white wine only during the week but vodka is all right for weekends, and so on. As heavy drinking and preoccupation with drinking continue, individual drinking patterns emerge. There can be continuous drinking, weekend drinking only, binge drinking with periods of abstinence, or lunchtime drinking instead of eating.

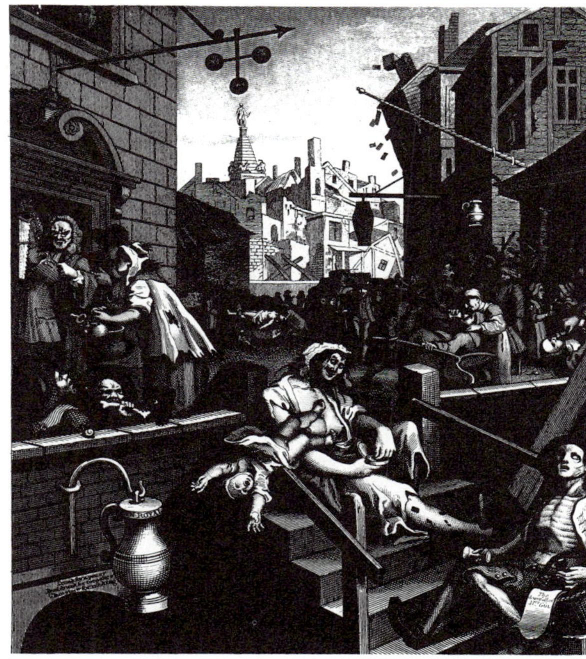

Gin Lane, *an engraving by William Hogarth, depicts the various social ills brought on by widespread addiction to alcohol, a phenomenon that occurred in England in the early eighteenth century, when alcohol became available in a cheap form as "geneva" (gin). (Culver Pictures)*

If pathological drinking or problem drinking continues unabated, there may be serious social and interpersonal consequences such as financial and marital difficulties, job problems, fights and traffic accidents, injury to self or others, and arrests. There also may be blackouts (amnesia for events during a drinking bout).

Many severe problem drinkers complain of inability to control their drinking patterns, even when warned about the deleterious effects on their health and even as they see their lives falling apart around them. They speak of "loss of control" or "craving."

Observers are familiar with a common pattern: guilt, depression, personal anguish, suicide attempts, and the repeated theme—after one sip, I just go on drinking myself into oblivion, regardless of the consequences.

It is common to describe the foregoing characteristics of chronic drinking as psychological dependence, a domination by a need to get that drink. According to the World Health Organization's International Classification of Disease, psychological dependence is "a compulsion to take alcohol on a continuous or periodic basis in order to experience its psychic effects. . . . " Most experts also characterize alcoholism as a disease of *physical* dependence, with the usual signs of (a) tolerance or (b) withdrawal (abstinence) syndrome when alcohol consumption is reduced or terminated (see Spotlight 16.1).

Spotlight 16.1 DSM-III Listings of Disorders Associated with Alcohol Abuse

In classifying types of problems associated with alcohol abuse, the DSM-III differentiates between alcohol-induced organic mental disorders, the "direct or chronic effects of alcohol on the central nervous system," and alcohol use disorders, the "maladaptive behavior associated with more or less regular use of alcohol."

Alcohol-Induced Organic Mental Disorders

Alcohol intoxication refers to "maladaptive" behaviors resulting from sufficient levels of recently ingested alcohol in the bloodstream as to produce slurred speech, impaired judgment and attention, unsteady gait, incoordination, and nystagmus (involuntary oscillation of the eyeballs). In some instances, there may be accompanying behavioral changes such as aggressiveness, irritability, and depression.

Alcohol idiosyncratic intoxication is the label applied to behaviors in the intoxicated state that are markedly unusual for a person's "typical" personality. Some highly susceptible people may show marked behavioral changes as a result of small amounts of recently ingested alcohol that are generally insufficient to cause intoxication in most people, for example, "easygoing" people who, after a few sips of an alcoholic beverage, become belligerent or assaultive. There may even be subsequent amnesia for this state.

Alcohol withdrawal (abstinence syndrome) describes conditions that can arise several days after termination or reduction of heavy alcohol consumption in a person who has drunk heavily for years. Symptoms include coarse tremors of the hands, tongue, and eyelids ("morning shakes"), and at least one of the following: nausea and vomiting; malaise and weakness; autonomic hyperactivity (for example, rapid heart beat, sweating, elevated blood pressure); anxiety, depressed mood; and orthostatic hypotension (a drop in blood pressure when the individual gets into an upright position). These symptoms tend to disappear within the course of a week or so following cessation of alcohol consumption.

Alcohol withdrawal delerium ("DTs") is a much less frequent condition than the withdrawal syndrome just described, but if it does occur, appears within the first few days after termination or reduction of heavy drinking in a person with a chronic history of drinking. Symptoms may involve autonomic hyperactivity, delusions, vivid (usually visual) hallucinations, and agitation.

Alcohol hallucinosis describes the extremely unpleasant auditory hallucinations usually of threatening voices or of hissing or buzzing sounds, that may appear a few days following cessation or reduction of alcohol ingestion in a heavy, chronic drinker. Individuals with this condition may sometimes act out on a threatening hallucination by calling the police. This state, which generally is extremely disturbing to the individual, usually subsides in a few days, but in a small number of instances, it may last for months or years. In this chronic form there is less agitation, and the clinical picture may resemble long-term schizophrenia.

Alcohol amnestic disorder (Korsakoff's disease) arises primarily as a result of the vitamin deficiencies associated with prolonged, heavy alcohol consumption and is accompanied by various neurological symptoms arising from damage to the central nervous system. Amnestic disorders may follow an acute episode of Wernicke's disease (see Chapter 13, p. 339) and may remain a chronic condition, chiefly characterized by memory impairment and confabulation (an exaggerated, glib substitute for actual facts that "covers up" the individual's sense of memory loss). A former skid row alcoholic, diagnosed with this condition, was asked, "Tell me where you worked." His reply was, "I was a test pilot for Russia but the Americans shot me down . . . and then I opened night clubs, a chain of them." He had been in a state hospital for years and it was not possible for this self-description to be valid.

Dementia associated with alcoholism applies to deteriorated states in long-term chronic alcoholics and is characterized by extreme memory impairment, loss of abstract thinking, and various other cognitive dysfunctions. According to the DSM-III, severe states of alcoholic dementia are probably not reversible. In some individuals deterioration is so marked that total care is required.

Alcohol Use Disorders

Alcohol abuse is distinguished from the organic disorders just described by its diagnostic stress on the undesirable *behaviors* resulting from excessive and more or less regular alcohol consumption, such as impairment of interpersonal relationships, family or marital disruption, occupational and financial instability, and inability to stop or control drinking patterns despite deleterious emotional and psychological consequences and effects on the body. Alcohol abuse is a disorder according to the DSM-III, distinguishable from use of alcohol for recreational purposes when there are no undesirable behavioral consequences. Pathological use of alcohol thus involves daytime intoxication or regular daily use, episodic or binge drinking, weekend drinking, inability to control one's drinking behavior, blackouts, personal injury to self and others, traffic accidents, occupational and interpersonal difficulties, and preoccupation with the question of obtaining and drinking alcohol. The DSM-III calls these behaviors alcohol abuse only if the foregoing disturbances have had at least one month's duration (although not necessarily continuously).

Alcohol dependence (according to the DSM-III) involves physiological need, evidenced by either tolerance or withdrawal. The term alcohol dependence is sometimes used interchangeably with alcoholism.*

Tolerance refers to the markedly increased amounts of alcohol that are now required to achieve the desired effect or to the markedly diminished effect with regular use of a socially acceptable amount.

Withdrawal is an alcohol-specific syndrome. Each substance (for example, heroin) has its own withdrawal pattern following cessation of or reduction of prolonged and heavy ingestion.

* The mechanisms behind physiological dependence are not entirely clear. The tolerance, for example, found in heavy, chronic drinkers, in which there are fewer (or more diminished) physical responses to alcohol than is the case for lighter drinkers, might result from the fact that heavy drinker may metabolize alcohol more quickly than the light drinker. This speculation has had some moderate (but not entirely consistent) evidence (Miller, 1976). It can also be that the tissues in the various systems of the body, for example, the gastrointestinal or cardiovascular systems, may adapt to the presence of alcohol.

If heavy, uncontrolled drinking continues, there are many severe consequences in addition to those already mentioned. These include impairment of memory and judgment, liver and gastrointestinal damage, hallucinations, psychotic episodes, and irreversible peripheral and central nervous system damage. And for many, of course, there is death—through accidents, disease, homicide, and suicide.

Table 16.1 presents some of the behavioral signs that enter into a diagnosis of alcoholism and Spotlight 16.1 describes the DSM-III's diagnostic criteria and classification system of disorders associated with alcohol abuse.

It should be stressed that despite common be-

Table 16.1 "Diagnosing" Alcoholism: Some Behavioral and Psychological Indicators

Signs in behavioral, psychological, and attitudinal areas, that, according to the National Council on Alcoholism, help to distinguish social drinkers from problem drinkers or alcoholics. The numbers after each sign mean:

1: a person who fits this criterion is definitely an alcoholic
2: a person who meets this criterion is under "strong suspicion" of being an alcoholic
3: these signs are common among alcoholics but do not constitute a diagnosis, since there are also medical and physicial criteria to consider.

Signs	*Rating*
Drinking despite strong medical contraindication known to patient	1
Drinking despite strong, identified social contraindication (job loss for intoxication, marriage disruption because of drinking, arrest for intoxication, driving while intoxicated).	1
Patient's subjective complaint of loss of control of alcohol consumption	2
Gulping drinks	3
Surreptitious drinking	2
Morning drinking	2
Repeated attempts at abstinence	2
Blatant, indiscriminate use of alcohol	1
Skid row or equivalent social level	2
Medical excuses from work for variety of reasons	2
Shifting from one alcoholic beverage to another	2
Preference for drinking companions, bars, and taverns	2
Loss of interest in activities not directly associated with drinking	2
Chooses employment that facilitates drinking	3
Frequent automobile accidents	3
Frequent change of residence for poorly defined reasons	3
Anxiety-relieving mechanisms, such as telephone calls, inappropriate in time, distance, person, or motive	2
Outbursts of rage and suicidal gestures while drinking	2
When talking freely, makes frequent reference to drinking alcohol, people being "bombed," "stoned," etc., or admits drinking more than peer group	2
Drinking to relieve anger, insomnia, fatigue, depression, social discomfort	2
Unexplained changes in family, social, and business relationships; complaints about spouse, job, and friends	3
Spouse makes complaints about drinking behavior, reported by patient or spouse	2
Major family disruptions: separation, divorce, threats of divorce	3
Job loss due to increasing interpersonal difficulties, frequent job changes, financial difficulties	3
Resentment, jealousy, paranoid attitudes	3
Symptoms of depression: isolation, crying, suicidal preoccupation	3
Feeling that one is "losing one's mind"	2

Source: Adapted from *The American Journal of Psychiatry,* 1978, *129*:2, 129–31. Copyright 1972, the American Psychiatric Association. Reprinted by permission.

Case 16.1 Mary: Alcoholism

Mary's drinking behavior began in high school. She would drink a little more at parties, feel a little worse the next day, and remember a little less than her friends did about how she behaved: seductive, "wild," boisterous, argumentative. Her mother was an alcoholic but had been abstinent for many years. Mary never knew who her father was and her mother was never sure. But even if fatherless, Mary felt secure with her mother, who worked tirelessly to support them both.

Mary dropped out of high school, she said, to help her mother by going to work. Instead, she stole money from her mother's purse for afternoon and evening drinks in the neighborhood tavern. Occasionally, she would "turn a trick" for money. This pattern continued for years.

Mary is thirty-five years old. She lives in a furnished room in a run-down building downtown. Although there are roaches and rusty water and she is thin and depressed, she no longer feels overwhelmingly hopeless. For she has finally stopped drinking. A bout with a liver ailment and bleeding ulcers had brought her to the city hospital and, when she was over the acute stage, to the office of a social worker in the hospital's clinic for guidance to "help her to reshape her life." For she had been frightened by the hospitalization and was beginning to feel suicidal, despairing of ever getting better.

Currently, Mary feels moderately hopeful. She is receiving some vocational training, is attending group meetings with other struggling alcohol abusers, and is building up her physical strength with diet and exercise. She also has a part-time job and soon will be looking for full-time work.

Mary claims that she very much wants to live and even looks forward to supporting her mother. She credits her strong motivation to participate in her own rehabilitation and her use of the social supports available to her, especially the group and individual counseling, for the changes in her life. Her future may be uncertain, but today she is struggling to "make it" in a world that is offering her some opportunities to do so.

lief, there is extreme variation in the way different problem drinkers go about the business of drinking as well as what becomes of them. Being "drunk," how socially acceptable or unacceptable one's behavior while drinking is, and even whether or not one is labeled an alcoholic are very much dependent on the drinker's social group and its social standards. The label "alcoholic" thus is frequently applied to a person whose pattern of drinking behavior deviates from the modal (or typical) pattern of his or her social group, rather than assigned on the basis of criteria intrinsic to the pathological process.

Is Alcoholism a Disease?

Whether or not to call alcoholism a disease has polarized the community of experts on alcoholism. Many say yes (the majority opinion); a smaller, but rather vocal, group says no.

There are distinct advantages in calling alcoholism a disease (see Jellinek, 1960), according to the "establishment"—the recognized authorities on alcoholism. For at one time alcoholics were viewed with disgust—as morally weak people who were a problem for the police and law-enforcement agencies. These psychologically infantile individuals were to be pitied, but not helped. The resulting guilt and shame associated with being an alcoholic or a member of his or her family prevented all concerned from seeking help. Today there is another view: Alcoholism is an addictive disease (not a moral problem), and like most diseases it can and should be treated (Schneider, 1978). It was this different view of alcoholism that not only encouraged alcoholics and their families to be open about seeking help, but that also permitted exploration of both treatment and prevention. This view took alcoholism away from the "do-gooders"—the watchdogs over the nation's moral stamina—and placed it in

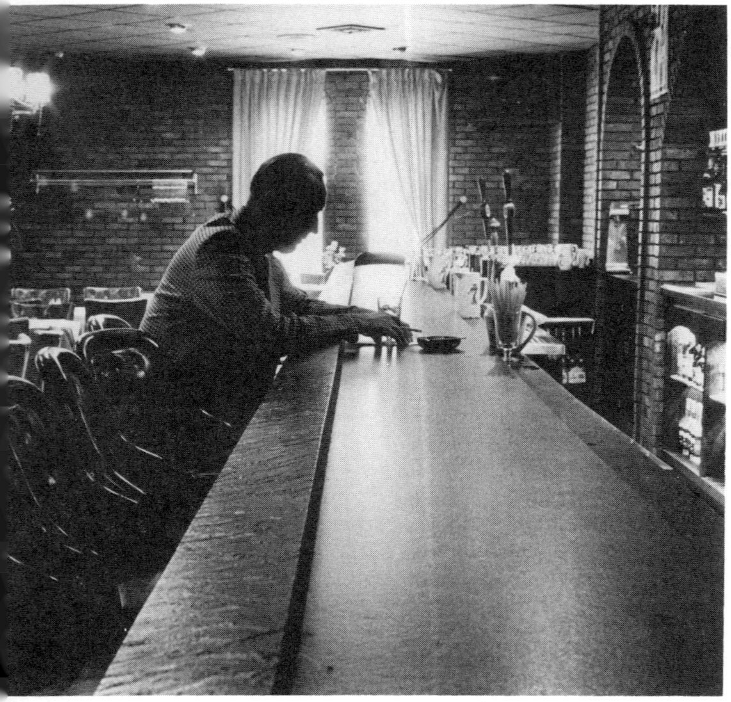

Why does a social drinker become a problem drinker? (© 1981 Ed Lettau/Photo Researchers)

the hands of researchers and clinicians so that its pattern, epidemiology, and correlates in physical, psychological, and social areas can be studied and its pathology treated.

Viewing alcoholism as a disease, however, especially as an addictive one, is now seen by many as having some distinct disadvantages. These include the widely held conviction that total abstinence is the only way an alcoholic can be "cured" (if indeed a cure is possible), that only one or two kinds of treatment strategies are effective, that all people become alcoholics for similar reasons, and that its course, as a disease, follows a progressive, predictable pattern. A disease approach not only assumes that alcoholism is a single unitary syndrome, but also is interpreted by some as implying that there is a recognizable prealcoholic personality with a consistent, definable set of personality traits that are intrinsic to the pathology. However, some of these assumptions have been challenged.

Those who view alcohol abuse as a "learned behavioral disorder" prefer to think in terms of "problem drinking" rather than alcoholism. Drinking problems can have a wide range of severity, it is claimed, with consequences that can be rather varied in content and significance to the individual and his or her life. Some problem drinkers may not have to give up drinking entirely, it is further claimed, but can learn to drink in a controlled, moderate way for social purposes. We will return to these considerations later in this chapter.

How Does Alcohol Do Its Work?

Alcohol is a chemical, a central nervous system depressant that slows down the responses of the brain and spinal cord. In the early phases of a drinking period, especially if there are others present in a friendly, social context, the individual may feel an "energizing" effect: an elevation in mood and a feeling of being witty, sharp, and outgoing. Soon, however, as the course of intoxication continues, the individual becomes sluggish and uncoordinated. The speech thickens; judgment becomes impaired. If the drinking continues, the by now heavily intoxicated person becomes sleepy and depressed. He or she may become comatose, and even die if the drinking is further continued.

Alcohol does not affect the individual until it is absorbed into the bloodstream. Food in the stomach delays absorption; water and carbonated drinks increase the rate of absorption. Once in the bloodstream, alcohol is distributed to all parts of the body, including the brain. Its main effects are on the brain, and the rate and quantity at which alcohol is consumed as well as absorbed and metabolized determine its influence. In other words, if drinks are consumed rapidly, the actual content of the alcohol level in the blood will continue to rise to extremely high levels until the individual "passes out."

In the bloodstream, alcohol is metabolized at a

fairly even rate—about three-quarters of an ounce of alcohol per hour. At this rate of consumption alcohol does not accumulate within the body and the drinker does not become "drunk." There is no known way of increasing the rate of metabolization of alcohol.

The amount of alcohol in the bloodstream is called blood alcohol content, concentration, or level (BAC) and is by convention presented as a percentage. Table 16.2 lists the typical BAC levels if an individual were to consume various amounts of alcohol within a two-hour period and the accompanying behavioral and physical consequences. If an individual stops drinking alcohol, the BAC drops about .02 per hour. If he or she continues to drink, however, BAC levels continue to rise until extremely dangerous levels are reached.

The BAC levels in Table 16.2 arise as a consequence of consuming pure alcohol. What are resulting BAC levels from ordinary alcoholic drinks? For a person weighing about 150 pounds, a three-and-one-half-ounce martini or manhattan results in a BAC of about .04; a three-ounce serving of wine, a BAC of about .02; and a mug of beer (about 12 ounces), a BAC of about .02. Thus, if a person orders two wines or beers for every martini a friend is ordering, that person's BAC levels will be about the same as the friend's.

Consequences of Alcohol Abuse: Some Hard Data

According to the National Institute on Alcohol Abuse and Alcoholism, long-term heavy drinking reduces an individual's life span by about 10 to 12 years. Here are some additional facts about alcohol abuse.

Cost. The 1979 Surgeon General's Report states that in 1975, the nation's losses as a result of alcohol abuse was 43 billion dollars, calculated in such terms as crime, fire, health and medical costs, ab-

Table 16.2 Typical Effects of Rising Alcohol Levels in the Blood

Amount of Pure Alcohol Consumed in Two Hours	*Percent of Alcohol in Blood (BAC)*	*Typical Effects*
3 ounces	.05	Loosening of judgment, thought, and restraint; carefree sensation and release of tension
4.5 ounces	.08	Tensions and inhibitions of everyday life lessened
6 ounces	.10	Voluntary motor responses such as hand and arm movements and gait are affected: incoordination, sluggishness; thickening of speech
10 ounces	.20	Severe motor and language impairment; person is "drunk": staggering gait, loud and boisterous behavior; incoherent speech; fighting; risk for traffic accidents is 100 times greater than for others
14 ounces	.30	CNS effects are widespread: various neurological signs are present; individual is going into stupor
18 ounces	.40	Individual is asleep, difficult to rouse; voluntary action is not possible
22 ounces	.50	Coma: involuntary respiratory and cardiac responses diminish and disappear; death

Source: Copyright © 1976 by Morris E. Chafetz. From the book *Why drinking can be good for you,* pp. 172–73. Reprinted with permission of Stein and Day Publishers.

senteeism, sick leave, compensation benefits, traffic accidents, and the cost of community facilities concerned with alcoholism.

A major health problem. The National Council on Alcoholism views alcoholism as the "most neglected health problem in the United States today," ranking it with cancer and heart disease. At least 30,000 deaths a year occur from cirrhosis of the liver, a frequent outcome of chronic alcoholism. As a matter of fact, one out of every ten deaths in this country is associated with alcohol abuse. In addition, the chronic alcoholic, after many years, may show serious mental dysfunctions such as memory impairment and general cognitive deterioration as a result of CNS damage. Although heavy alcohol ingestion is especially damaging to the liver, which is the prime detoxifier of alcohol, prolonged and chronic drinking can also affect the heart, lungs, gastrointestinal system, and the body's immune system (alcoholics, for example, are more susceptible to pneumonia) (Lelbach, 1974; Miller, 1976).

It was once thought that malnutrition was responsible for the many ailments of the alcoholic. It is true that heavy drinkers often eat poorly because of loss of appetite and motivation. But failure to eat a balanced diet is not the only reason for the severe malnutrition and vitamin deficiencies many alcoholics show. Chronic, heavy consumption of alcohol, many experts now believe, affects the degree to which essential foods and vitamins are used by the body. In other words, even if there is adequate food intake, the body is impaired in its ability to make use of the food's nutritional value.

Finally, the fetal alcohol syndrome should be mentioned again, with its high risk for mental retardation and other kinds of developmental disabilities, a result of the mother's alcohol consumption during pregnancy.

Alcoholism and violence. Many alcoholics die earlier than most people as a result of violence. The figures speak for themselves. In the United States, alcohol is thought to be a significant factor in 65 percent of murders, 55 percent of assaults in the home, 60 percent of instances of child abuse, and 35 to 50 percent of rapes (Facts on alcoholism, 1979; Rada, 1975). The suicide rate is 20 times higher among alcoholics than in the general population.

Alcoholism is a major cause of injury and death due to accidents. Fifty percent of all fatal traffic accidents, 80 percent of deaths due to fires, 65 percent of drownings, 77 percent of falls, and 44 percent of pilot accidents are associated with alcohol. Among teenagers and young adults, accidents that are alcohol-related are the leading cause of death (Facts on alcoholism, 1979).

Who Are the Alcoholics?

The typical picture of an alcoholic is an urban, single, low-SES male, with a spotty employment history and of ethnic minority background (although not among Jewish groups according to Cahalan, 1970). However, alcoholics are well represented among all SES, educational, and cultural backgrounds.

SES levels. In general, alcoholism is more frequently found on low-SES than on other levels, for most ethnic minority and age groups. Skid row alcoholism, however, accounts for only about 3 percent of the alcoholic population (Facts on alcoholism, 1979). Further, the consequences of alcoholism are strikingly different when SES groups are compared: joblessness, ill health, murder, accidents, and violent deaths are relatively more frequent among the poor than among the more affluent.

Ethnic and racial minorities. Epidemiological studies indicate that there are variations in alcoholism and alcohol-related deaths (for example, through cirrhosis of the liver) among different ethnic and racial groups (Zeiner and Paredes, 1978). Heavy drinking among rural black low-SES males is pervasive. This pattern is tolerated, even expected, as an indication of "manhood," and as a way to deal with loneliness and boredom (Benjamin, 1976). Urban black males

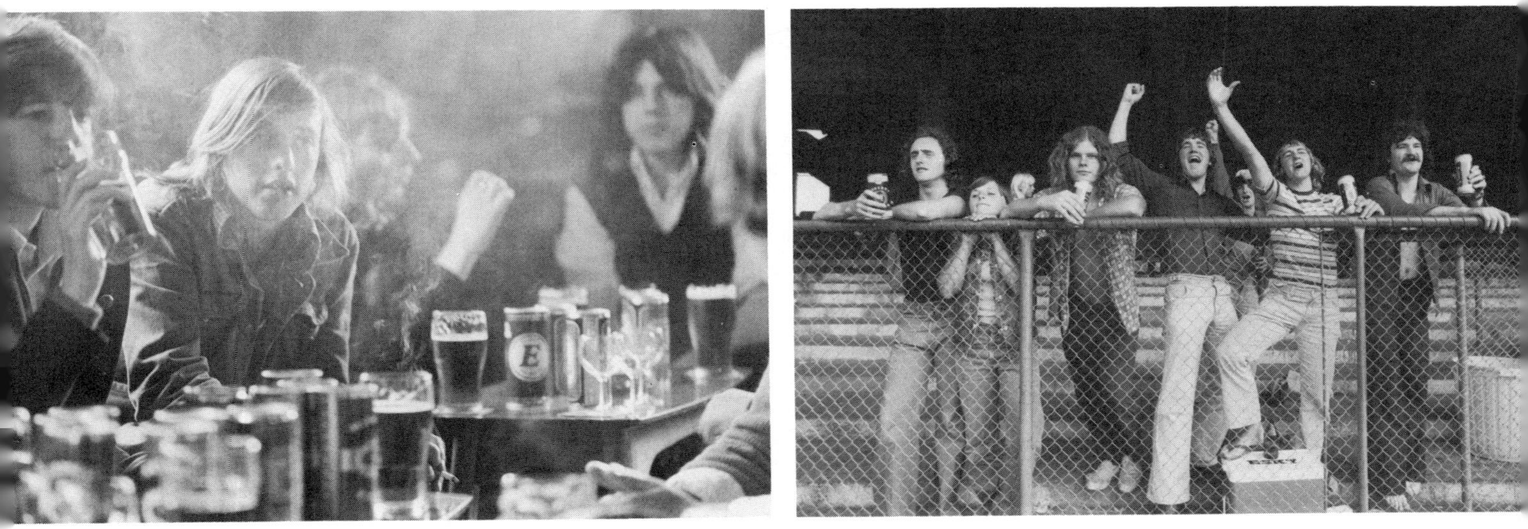

Heavy drinking and alcoholism among teenagers are known facts . . . and killers. (Left: Paul S. Conklin/Monkmeyer Press: Right: Rick Smolan/Stock, Boston)

also tend to have a high rate of heavy drinking and alcoholism (Bourne, 1976). The social consequences in terms of homocides, arrests, and assaults are higher for black than for white alcoholics, even though overall rates of alcoholism among black men are only slightly higher than those for white men.

In general, although black males are heavy drinkers, black females are not. As a matter of fact, black females not only drink less than white females, but they also abstain from drinking more than any other group (Wechsler, 1980).

Extremely high rates of alcoholism, alcohol-related diseases, and alcohol-related problems such as accidents, suicide, and homocide are found among certain native North American groups, for example, the Eskimos of northern Canada or some Indian societies in the United States. Generally, high prevalence rates tend to be found in those societies in which there are also high unemployment, a shift from the old economies (such as hunting or fishing), disruption of social and family ties, and a lack of group and individual purpose. However, studies also indicate that there is as much variation—from high incidence to virtually no incidence at all—within various ethnic and racial groups as between them (Zeiner and Paredes, 1978).

Young adults and teenagers. Drinking is on the rise among youth, with heavy drinking on the high-school level nearly doubling between 1966 and 1975. There seems to be a shift from drugs to alcohol on both the high-school and college levels (Saltman, 1973).

It is estimated that from one to over three million of the vast population of young drinkers (many of them offspring of alcoholics) show signs of later alcoholism by their pattern of alcohol abuse (Cohen, 1975; Facts on alcohol, 1979). Males in the 21-to-24-year age group have the greatest number of drinking problems, and about half of this problem group can be found in low-SES levels.

Gender. Throughout the world, men drink more than women. Estimates of problem drinking and alcoholism among males, compared to females, run about four or five to one. But the number of female alcoholics has doubled in the past twenty-five years, and the large gap between male and female rates is narrowing (Gomberg, 1979).

CAUSES OF PROBLEM DRINKING

Humans differ from animals in that they show a "persistent predilection for altering (themselves) and the world. . . . Our efforts to reshape our consciousness have resulted similarly in a number of experiments. . . . Among the best known and most widely used means of altering human consciousness is the ingestion of ethanol (alcohol)" (Heath, 1975, p. 1).

Why do people drink? Many experts believe that if we could answer this question, we might begin to understand why some people become problem drinkers. The general assumption is that the consumption of alcohol ranges along a continuum from social, nonpathological drinking to pathological drinking, and that the underlying mechanisms are the same for all types of drinking, problem or otherwise (Cahalan, 1970; Pattison, Sobell, and Sobell, 1977; Vuchinich, Tucker, and Sobell, 1979). For this reason the next sections explore some general considerations underlying drinking behavior as well as more specific aspects of problem drinking.

Psychological Benefits: "Feeling Good"

One general explanation as to why people drink can be conceptualized simply. People feel, or think they feel, better after a few drinks.

Tension-reduction hypothesis. Some of us tend to view alcoholic beverages as having some anxiety-reducing or tension-reducing function. This belief is also shared by many experts, with some going so far as to suggest that the primary function of drinking in all societies is the reduction of anxiety. According to Horton (1943), for example, the intensity of anxiety generated by a society, for example, the fear of witchcraft, or suffering because of hunger and poverty, or anxiety because of rootlessness as a result of social change, determines its alcohol consumption. Formally expressed in psychological terms, this hypothesis states that the lowering of anxiety or frustration levels ("aversive emotional states") tends to reinforce the consumption of alcohol (the tension-reduction hypothesis, Conger, 1956).

There is certainly some reason to believe that alcohol ingestion serves a tension-reducing function. People with tension, anxiety, or conflict may learn to continue their drinking behavior because of the reinforcing properties of alcohol. Alcohol can also be socially reinforcing—associated with good times at parties or with easing social interactions.

The trouble is that the validity of the tension-reduction model has not been consistently established, judging by a review of the experimental literature (Cappell, 1975). In one study, for example, the performance of socially anxious male subjects was actually *impaired* and they performed less skillfully on several experimental measures in a social situation after alcohol consumption than did the controls, who consumed a placebo (Keane and Lisman, 1980).

On the other hand, if alcohol is consumed in large enough dosages and if the stressful situation is real and intense, some experimental evidence does suggest that the magnitude of autonomic responses to stress tends to be dampened (Levenson et al., 1980).

Changes in affect and mood. Popular belief as well as some experimental evidence (see McCollam et al., 1980) also suggest that moderate amounts of alcohol enhance positive feelings, lift mood, and even contribute to feelings of elation. An interesting observation in this regard is that as blood levels of alcohol (BAC) increase, mood is energized and lifted, whereas decreasing BAC levels are associated with self-reports of depression and tiredness (Goldberg, 1966; McCollam et al., 1980). However, once again, evidence for the mood-enhancement hypothesis is not consistent (see, for example, Freed, 1978); and it has also been found that prior mood, setting in which the alcohol is consumed, and amount of consumption all affect self-reports of mood change.

Other psychological benefits. Additional explanations as to why people drink include overcoming feelings of loneliness or depression, handling excessive anger, dealing with various kinds of emotional pain (Ryback, 1974), and reducing neuroticism as measured by scores on the Eysenck Personality Inventory, especially among people who like to drink (Blackburn and Zeiner, 1979).

Another approach hypothesizes that drinking patterns and drunkenness are found more frequently in societies in which there is conflict over dependence and independence. This conclusion was drawn by Irvin Child and his associates after studying role expectations for adults and child-training patterns in 139 societies. Alcohol reduces anxiety levels, satisfies desires for dependence, and at the same time allows fantasies of achievement and assertiveness to occur (Barry, 1976; Child, Bacon, and Barry, 1965; Child, Barry, and Bacon, 1965).

Power. Power, as a motivation for drinking in men, is yet another hypothesis (McClelland et al., 1972). The feeling of being powerful is made possible through the physiological effects of drinking. In our society, this is a pleasurable, sought-after feeling in the light of role expectations for men for power, strength, and mastery. If there is failure to attain power, men will turn to drinking anyway to achieve a fantasy sense of power. Heavy drinking results in a vicious cycle, because under these drunken circumstances, men are even less likely to achieve the recognition they want.

Expectancy, Set, and Cognitive Labeling

People can often make of alcohol consumption what they wish to make of it. From observations of various social groups (see Spotlight 16.2) we have learned that the ways in which people become intoxicated and the reasons for their drinking are as diverse as the people themselves. In addition, we have learned that peer and social influences, even when there is no overt pressure, are also important determinants in how much people drink.

Social learning and social modeling aspects of drinking were explored in an experimental study of male college students using "confederate models." For example, in one study, subjects were exposed to a heavy drinking "model" and a moderate- or low-drinking "model." Subjects drinking in the presence of the heavy drinker drank significantly more alcohol—about twice as much—as the subjects drinking with the light drinker or in the "non-model" condition (Caudill and Marlatt, 1975). All measures of alcohol consumption, whether actual amount of wine consumed, number of sips taken, estimates of amount of alcohol in each sip, or level of alcohol in the blood, showed this pattern.

The social setting and the influence of social models may actually be mediated or do its work through various cognitive variables: what one expects, the labels one assigns, the beliefs about alcohol's effects may be of extreme importance in shaping patterns of drinking as well as their behavioral consequences.

In some of the literature that explores these cognitive factors, the term *expectancy* appears again and again. This phrase is generally taken to mean the anticipated consequences of alcohol use (Brown et al., 1980). Examples of expectancies include effects of alcohol consumption on sexual arousal (positive with moderate drinking, but inhibitory with heavy drinking), aggression (increased), sociability (increased), and so on. A recent factor analysis study of questionnaire responses administered to 440 social drinkers (the group was a heterogeneous one, consisting of black, white, male, female, and mostly single subjects of varying SES levels) isolated some of these expectancy factors (Brown et al., 1980). Listing 16.1 presents the independent factors that were derived from the subjects' responses and typical questionnaire items that illustrate these factors.

Listing 16.1 What Do People Expect of Alcohol? Independent Factors Extracted from an Empirical Study of Responses to a Questionnaire and Examples of Typical Items

Factor I—Alcohol Is a Global, Positive, Transforming Agent

- Drinking makes the future seem brighter
- Alcohol seems like magic
- If I'm feeling restricted in any way, a few drinks make me feel better

Factor II—Alcohol Enhances both Social and Physical Pleasure

- Having a few drinks is a nice way to celebrate special occasions
- Drinking makes me feel good

Factor III—Alcohol Enhances Sexual Experience and Performance

- After a few drinks, I am more sexually responsive
- I often feel sexier after I've had a few drinks
- I am a better lover after a few drinks

Factor IV—Alcohol Arouses a Sense of Power and Aggression

- After a few drinks it is easier to pick a fight
- I feel powerful when I drink, as if I can really influence others to do as I want

Factor V—Alcohol Increases Social Assertiveness

- If I have a couple of drinks it is easier to express my feelings
- A few drinks make it easier to talk to people
- Drinking gives me more confidence in myself

Factor VI—Alcohol Produces Feelings of Relaxation and Tension Reduction

- Alcohol enables me to fall asleep more easily
- Alcohol decreases muscular tension
- Alcohol can act as an anesthetic, that is, it can deaden pain
- Alcohol makes me worry less

Source: S. A. Brown, M. S. Goldman, A. Inn, and L. R. Anderson, Expectations of reinforcement from alcohol: Their domain and relation to drinking patterns, *Journal of Consulting and Clinical Psychology,* 1980, *48,* 419–26. Copyright 1980 by the American Psychological Association. Adapted by permission of the author.

The authors, in addition, sought to discover whether these beliefs or expectancies (factors) can in any way be related to the drinking patterns—light or heavy—of the subjects. They found that the moderate, light, or inexperienced drinkers tended to have global expectancies along lines of the first two factors, that is, alcohol was seen as a "magical" drug that is a "positive transforming agent" and as a "pleasure" enhancer in social and physical areas. Heavier, more experienced drinkers, on the other hand, tended to have responses that were reflected by more specific factors: expectations of "sexual enhancement" and "aggressive arousal."

Overall, there is little disagreement that each person has expectancies about what alcohol does for him or her. Do these expectancies affect people's behavior? Here are some typical research findings in this interesting area.

Alcohol as a pain-killer. Some people view alcohol as an "analgesic"—a pain-killer. And indeed, many people do claim that alcohol consumption "works for them" in just this way. Does expectancy enter in? If we assume that social drinkers and problem drinkers have a different network of beliefs, experiences, and expectancies concerning the effects of alcohol, then are there also differences in the effectiveness of alcohol as a pain-killing agent for these different subjects?

This question was explored in a study of 51 male volunteer subjects divided into problem drinkers (for example, on the basis of solitary, bar-room drinking) or social drinkers (Brown and Cutter, 1977). The subjects were administered pain stimuli (pressure to a finger, cold to a hand) before and after controlled amounts of alcohol consumption. It was found that the problem drinkers tended to report pain reduction as well as increased ability to deal with pain, whereas the social drinkers did not do so. The authors concluded that increased ability to cope with pain is a reflection of how alcohol is regarded by the individual, what it is expected to do. Problem drinkers believe in the salutary effects of alcohol and apparently turn to it when needed. Alcohol may well have an analgesic effect for certain types of drinkers, but not for others.*

Alcohol and aggression. Expectancy factors can also determine the expression of aggression. In one study, for example, subjects who believed that they were drinking an alcoholic beverage, regardless of what they were drinking (vodka and tonic or tonic alone), expressed significantly more (provoked) aggression than the subjects who believed that they were drinking nonalcoholic beverages, regardless of what *they* were drinking (Lang et al., 1975). That there are popular beliefs about an association between alcohol consumption and aggression was demonstrated in another study in which subjects who were allowed to express (provoked) anger against an experimental "plant" (confederate) consumed significantly less alcohol than subjects who were not allowed to do so (Marlatt, Kosturn, and Lang, 1975).

Alcohol and sexual arousal. Many people believe that moderate amounts of alcohol consumption increase sexual interest and arousal, whereas in males, *heavy* alcohol ingestion is thought to contribute to sexual dysfunction. What are the facts? Does expectancy play a role in these behaviors? Measurement of sexual arousal in both male and females that does not rely on subjective self-report has been made possible in the past several years by the development of methods that objectively measure and record penile tumescence and vaginal blood volume and pressure (penile plethysmograph and vaginal photoplethysmograph, respectively). Studies of blood alcohol levels and sexual arousal using these methods have shown that in both males and females there is a *decrease* of sexual arousal in response to erotic visual stimuli with increasing amounts of alcohol consumption in nonproblem drinkers (Briddell and Wilson, 1976; Wilson and Lawson, 1967a; Wilson, Lawson, and Abrams, 1978).

Because these results are not consistent with findings of other studies in this area, Wilson and Lawson (1976b) constructed a situation in which the subjects were told that they were drinking vodka and tonic or plain tonic (regardless of what they were drinking). In this situation, expectancy (cognitive set or cognitive labeling), what the subjects *believed* they were drinking was directly related to penile tumescence during the exposure of an erotic film depicting various scenes of explicit heterosexual and homosexual sex. Subjects were left to their own expectations as to the effects of alcohol. Those who thought they were drinking an alcoholic beverage showed greater sexual arousal than those who believed they were drinking a nonalcoholic beverage. The authors concluded that these results, along with those having to do with the expression of aggression, demonstrate "the importance of cognitive-mediating processes in alcohol's influence on behavior" (p. 594). Table 16.3 summarizes some of these findings.

An interesting postscript is that a rough duplication of this study with women social drinkers (who were told that they were drinking either

* An alternate possibility, still speculative, is suggested by some recent biochemical possibilities: problem drinkers and alcoholics may produce chemicals as a result of the way alcohol is metabolized that may have a pain-reducing, opiate-like effect on the brain.

Table 16.3 Mean and Maximum Percentage Increase in Penile Diameter for Experimental Groups Exposed to Erotic Films

	Film			
	Heterosexual		*Homosexual*	
Experimental Condition	*Mean*	*Maximum*	*Mean*	*Maximum*
Expect alcohol/receive alcohol	27.349	30.979	13.456	16.812
Expect alcohol/receive tonic	26.913	32.161	16.220	23.429
Expect tonic/receive alcohol	23.039	27.688	9.463	14.281
Expect tonic/receive tonic	19.166	17.931	3.549	3.942

Source: G. T. Wilson and D. M. Lawson, Expectancies, alcohol, and sexual arousal in male social drinkers, *Journal of Abnormal Psychology,* 1978, *87,* 358–67. Copyright 1978 by the American Psychological Association. Reprinted by permission of the author.

vodka or tonic regardless of the actual beverage) failed to confirm the findings with males as to increased sexual arousal in response to erotic films (Wilson and Lawson, 1978). All female subjects showed decreased sexual arousal during the erotic films after drinking alcohol, regardless of whether they thought they were drinking vodka and tonic or plain tonic. Expectancy seemed to have no effects on sexual arousal, nor did expectancy in combination with alcohol have any influence on arousal.

It can well be that a more valid test of sexual arousal for women would not involve erotic films, but other types of arousing stimuli—love scenes, for example, or "romantic" scenes from old movies. Women might be more sexually aroused by stimulation of fantasy rather than by explicit, visual sex scenes.

The general thrust of these studies has been confirmed in various replications with males: greater sexual arousal in response to erotic stimuli is reported by male subjects who think they are consuming an alcoholic beverage, whether in fact they are or are not doing so. However, there are individual differences in this effect. For example, male subjects who felt guilty about sex were even more aroused than other male subjects who had less guilt, under experimental conditions in which they thought they were consuming alcohol, regardless of what the actual drink contained (Lang et al., 1980).

Overall, the general hypothesis that people often make of alcohol what they wish to and then behave accordingly, is empirically supported. Each of us, it is suspected, carry in our heads some models as to what is allowable or permissible when "under the influence," expect alcohol to have certain effects, and then find or think we find that our expectations have been met. There are individual differences in resulting behavior patterns when intoxicated, however, apparently determined by subjective "self" variables, such as guilt, moral judgments, and social attitudes and standards regarding one's own as well as others' behavior.

Personality and Temperament

Predisposing personality factors. Clinical judgment tends to link personality variables and alcohol abuse. However, the predisposing traits in the literature are numerous and vague, and can apply to many pathological conditions. Traits include underlying hostility that later turns against the self in a destructive way; poor, fragile, generally unsatisfactory interpersonal relationships; limited control over impulsivity; denial as a major defense; low frustration tolerance, that is, inability to deal with having one's wishes thwarted; deprivation in early childhood; extreme dependency or dependence-independence conflict; inadequate personality; a high degree of love-hate ambivalence (the simultaneous presence of two conflicting opposite emotions, feelings, or drives—for example, self-love and self-hate); an excess of early pain and frustration within the family constellation; and overindulgence as a child (see Gomberg, 1968; Lisansky, 1960). These traits, it is presumed, form a core or a background for the development of alcoholism.

Unfortunately, evidence for a predisposing constellation of traits is only minimal, and is found, if at all, in white male samples primarily. Further, not all dependent, conflicted, inadequate personalities with poor self-control and low frustration tolerance become alcoholics.

An alcoholic personality? There is little agreement that alcoholism represents a unitary disease entity with a consistent set of symptoms such as loss of self-control. It cannot even be assumed that drinkers and nondrinkers differ in consistent ways on personality tests (Miller, 1976). Yet we tend to use the label "alcoholic" rather narrowly, as if it subsumes a common set of behaviors and traits. For this reason, it is of particular interest to inquire if there is evidence for an "alcoholic personality." By and large, the answer is: There is no common personal denominator (Miller, 1976).

1. *Personality assessment methods,* for example, the MMPI or projective techniques, generally yield inconsistent results, with no single personality type emerging as the alcoholic personality (Miller, 1976). As a matter of fact, a variety of traits are found. So many traits are involved that one is hard put to pick out any single type that can characterize the alcoholic. The list of traits contains contradiction after contradiction.

the major contenders are depression . . . dependency . . . power needs . . . neuroticism . . . homosexuality and schizoidness . . . and psychopathy. . . . One could conclude from this research that the average alcoholic is a passive, overactive, inhibited, acting-out, withdrawn, gregarious psychopath with a conscience, defending against poor defenses as a result of excessive and insufficient mothering (Miller, 1976, p. 657).

Does factor analysis help to clarify the picture? Using objective inventories such as the MMPI, various investigators have delineated not one but several alcoholic types. One study, for example, using a personality questionnaire, reliably delineated two distinct types of alcoholics in a group of low-SES white male inpatients: one group was characterized by high anxiety and introversion and the other by dependency and conformity (Nerviano and Gross, 1973).

Findings from another study based on responses of 366 male inpatient alcoholic veterans on several objective personality instruments, however, suggested that there are not two but several distinct subgroups of alcoholics (Nerviano, 1976)—at least seven. The personality types yielded by this study cover a wide gamut, for example, compulsive, impulsive, aggressive-paranoid, submissive, narcissistic psychopathic, and various schizoid types. These results further confirm the speculation that alcoholism is probably not represented by a single, homogeneous, personality diagnosis.

2. *Locus of control methods* (Rotter, 1966) attempt to measure how people perceive the major circumstances that control their personal behavior and problems. External locus of control characterizes those people who view personal events—and especially the rewards and reinforcements for one's behaviors—as being contingent on outside factors: I got my job through luck, chance, powerful people, unpredictable events. Internal locus of control, on the other hand, attributes these rewards and reinforcements to stable processes within the individual: effort, motivation, intelligence, imagination, drive. That is, some people perceive reinforcing factors as not entirely contingent on their personal actions but on fate or complex surrounding forces, whereas others perceive events as contingent on their own behavior or personalities.

Generally, external rather than internal locus of

control characterizes the heavier drinkers, with female alcoholics showing the highest degree of externality (Naditch, 1975c; Nowicki and Hopper, 1974; Rohsenow and O'Leary, 1978). Further, alcoholics with the greatest degree of pathology (as determined by MMPI scores) tend to have external locus of control and those with the least, internal locus of control (O'Leary, Donovan et al., 1976).

Although these studies do not yield entirely consistent results, they do suggest that the heavier drinkers, or those with the greatest degree of disturbance, may rationalize their drinking so that personal responsibility (internal locus of control) is not assumed. Treatment of alcoholics that stresses shifting over to internal locus of control, with an emphasis on personal responsibility, may therefore be effective. Reviews of the relevant research do indicate that during treatment alcoholics show higher internal locus of control scores, but whether or not this shift is related to eventual outcome of treatment (controlled drinking or abstinence) is not clear (Rohsenow and O'Leary, 1978).

Psychoanalytic Views

Once quite popular, psychoanalytic explanations of alcoholism, reformulated by dozens of writers, stressed conflict, immaturity, narcissism, and oral strivings and cravings (literally enacted in the ingestion of alcohol) of a regressed, dependent person. Some psychoanalytic writers have linked oral cravings to homosexual tendencies in creating the dynamic for alcoholism (see Lorand, 1945). Menninger (1938) saw alcoholism as a push toward suicide, a great need for punishment stemming from guilt because of rage against parental figures.

Fenichel (1945) hypothesized that most people drink heavily to deal with internal or external "miseries." When these "miseries" diminish, however, most people curtail this type of drinking. Those who persist are the alcoholics; they have "premorbid" predisposing traits such as orality and narcissism. Their families generated "specific oral frustrations" and, as a result, "oral fixations." In boys, such families also generate homosexual tendencies, which are repressed. Alcoholics thus can be characterized not only by oral impulses but also by unconscious homosexual impulses (Fenichel, 1945, p. 379).

The link between orality, oral conflicts, dependency needs, regressive defenses and "latent homosexuality" in the etiology of alcoholism has not been empirically demonstrated. To suggest that alcoholics in our society possess strong conflicts is to beg the question. Certainly, they are tortured, anguished individuals, filled with guilt and conflict. Retrospective, post hoc, piecing together of their oral childhoods, however, is another issue, not resolved by speculation. Long-range predictive studies—as with children at risk for schizophrenia—can supply us with more of the answers.

Patterns of Drinking Behavior Among Different Cultural Groups

People have consumed alcoholic beverages throughout the ages. It is probably the earliest "psychoactive" substance used by humans, and today it is probably still the most widely used. Perhaps one of the reasons for its enduring popularity is that alcohol is easily manufactured; low concentrations can be produced by a simple process of fermentation using fruit, berries, vegetables, grains, and various natural juices (Heath, 1975). Observers of the drinking behaviors of different groups of people are quick to note, however, that the ways in which people go about the business of getting drunk and the behaviors they display when drunk are impressively diverse.

Alcohol apparently serves a variety of functions for different groups of people, and its ingestion seems to be a cue that sets off behaviors that are not only permissible, but also expected, depending on the group. This signaling mechanism "triggers" behaviors, however, that are acceptable while drinking but not when sober (McAndrew and Edgerton, 1969). Social expectations and cultural variables thus are powerful shapers of patterns of

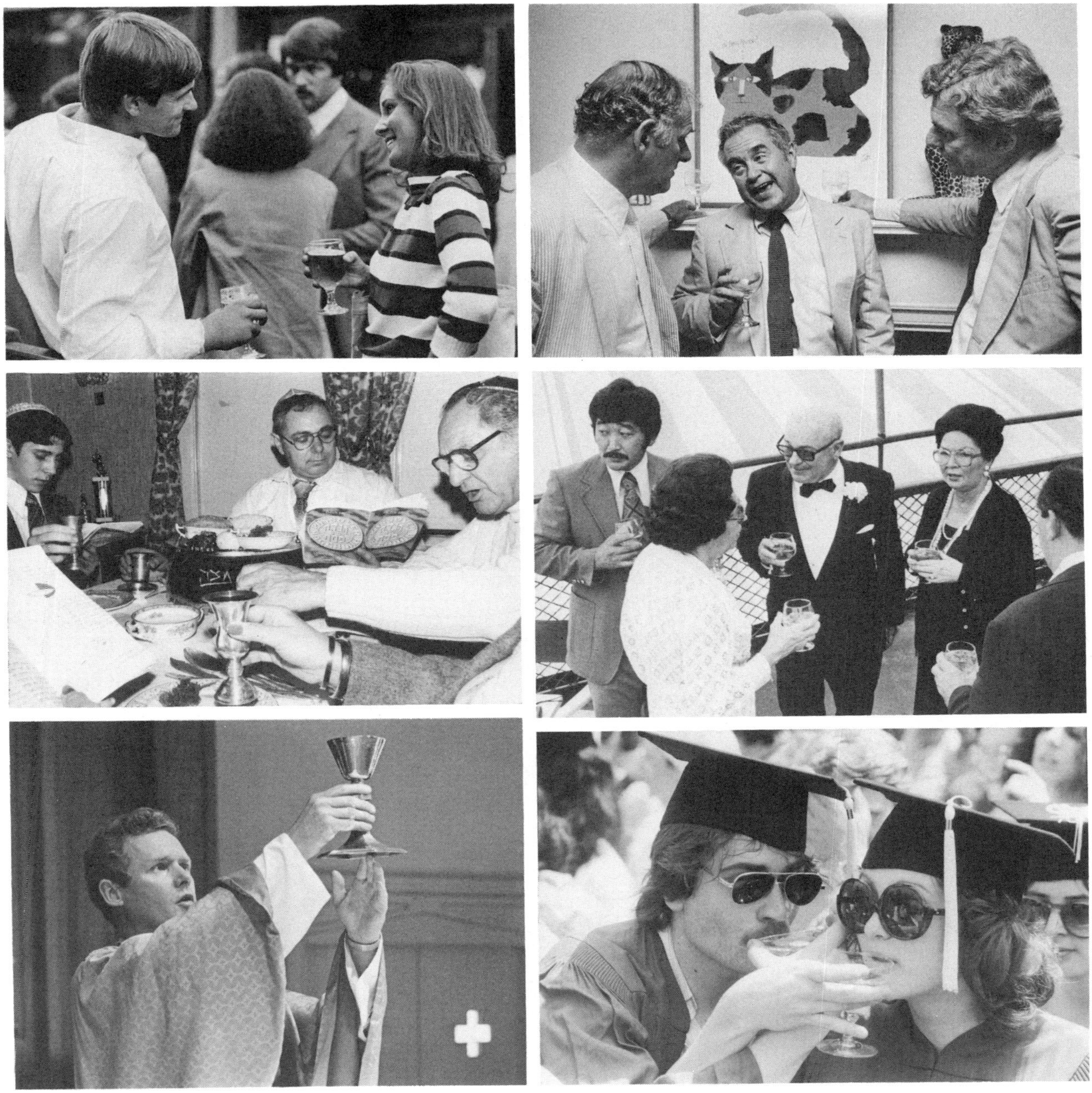

Drinking alcoholic beverages is socially sanctioned, whether it is at a singles bar, corporate get-together, wedding, graduation, or religious ceremony. But why do some people become alcoholics? (Clockwise, from upper left: Ellis Herwig/Stock, Boston; Richard Kalvan/Magnum; Tim Carlson/Stock, Boston; Owen Franken/Stock, Boston; Sylvia Johnson/Woodfin Camp; Ellen Pines Sheffield/Woodfin Camp)

drinking behavior. Spotlight 16.2 takes a closer look at some of the ways in which people in other cultures and in various subgroups within our own culture drink and get drunk.

Biochemical and Genetic Factors

Some researchers claim that even if we understood why people drink and why some of these people become heavier drinkers than others, we would still not understand why a small percentage of this group become alcoholics. These researchers suggest that there may be physiological differences between social drinkers and alcoholics. The evidence they point to generally comes from two sources: (a) differences in the rates in which alcohol in the bloodstream is metabolized or in various other biochemical levels among various ethnic groups or between alcoholics and nonalcoholics; and (b) data from familial studies that point to the possibility that there is a genetic predisposition to alcoholism.

Metabolic and biochemical differences. One hypothesis suggests that biochemical imbalances may characterize some people, placing them at greater risk for becoming alcoholic. These imbalances may include nutritional and vitamin deficiencies or a constitutional (bodily) tendency to metabolize alcohol in ways that create a quickened state of intoxication or a "craving" for alcohol as a rapid source of energy. It has also been proposed that as alcohol metabolizes, various chemical by-products are produced that in turn might have an addicting influence on the brain.

Acetaldehyde is a chemical released during al-

Spotlight 16.2 Cultural Variables in Alcohol Usage

"There is no universal use, meaning, or function for alcohol" (Heath, 1975). Social patterns determine how it is used. In some cultures, people drinking within a group drink only in sequence, determined by how old they are. In other cultures, everyone must drink simultaneously. Hundreds of studies of alcohol usage throughout the world and within our own culture have taught us that socially and culturally sanctioned aspects of drinking are embedded in the value system of the culture, with alcohol's effects shaped by these values and attitudes. The social setting of the drinking itself is a significant aspect of what happens. Attitudes toward intoxication also vary. In Western society, for example, overt female intoxication is viewed quite negatively (Gomberg, 1979), but we are more tolerant of covert drinking patterns.

Here are some more observations taken from many sources, especially Heath (1975), an anthropologist.

1. Alcoholism is rare in many cultures of the world, virtually unknown outside of Western culture, but becoming increasingly widespread with acculturation, with the impact of socialization and industrialization. However, there might be physiological variations among different groups in tolerance for and reactions to alcohol ingestion.

2. Crosscultural studies indicate that there is no relationship between consumption of alcohol and aggression. Aggression accompanying alcohol is often patterned by culturally expected behaviors—what the individual has learned is the normal outcome of drinking. Violent comportment with drinking seems to be more a stylized accompaniment to drinking under certain conditions than a necessary outcome.

3. Being drunk and behaving in a drunken way is patterned by a social and cultural learning process. For example, religious ritual requires alcohol ingestion among orthodox Jews, who rarely behave in a drunken fashion and who have a low rate of alcoholism. On the other hand, Irish males,

among whom there is a high rate of alcoholism, ingest alcohol for recreational, social, and "happy" purposes and will frequently behave in an intoxicated manner.

4. Young problem drinkers begin to drink early (many even earlier than high school), initiated by peers and family. Their pattern is one of serious, heavy drinking, with quick intoxication. They then becoming unruly and disruptive with consequent interpersonal and social problems, including fighting, drunken arrests, traffic accidents, and injuries to themselves and others (O'Gorman and Lacks, 1979). As a matter of fact, half of all traffic accident deaths in which alcohol is involved have something to do with teenagers (Do kids and alcohol mix? 1977).

5. In almost all societies there are striking differences in the drinking patterns of men and women (Gomberg, 1974). In our culture, many female alcoholics, especially those from middle-class backgrounds, "hide" in their homes, protected by their families. Women alcoholics begin heavy drinking at a later age than male alcoholics, and their drinking patterns tend to differ from those of men (Gomberg, 1974, 1979; Wechsler, 1980). For example, they tend not to be public drinkers, have solitary drinking patterns, and are arrested less often than men for drunken behavior. Even on skid row, drinking patterns differ. In one study of skid-row alcoholics, for example, 62 percent of the women, but only 26 percent of the men, were solitary drinkers; women were rarely members of "bottle gangs," as were the skid-row men (Garrett and Bahr, 1973).

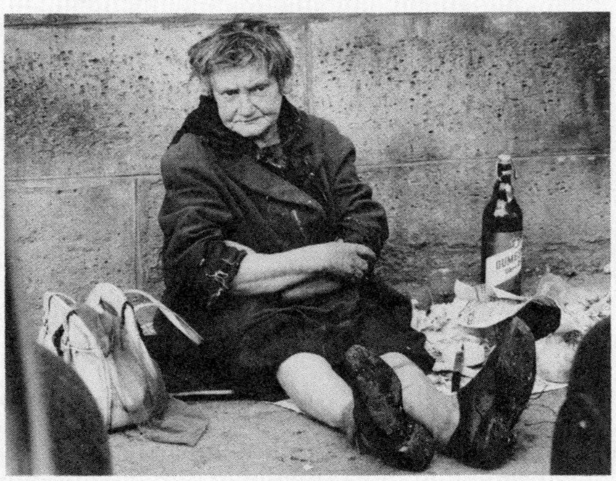

Most female skid-row alcoholics are solitary drinkers, whereas most male skid-row alcoholics drink with others in "bottle gangs." (Peter Martens/Nancy Palmer Agency)

6. There is evidence that the stereotype of the North American Indian as having little tolerance for "firewater" (that is, becoming easily intoxicated and requiring a long time to sober up) may be valid for some, but not all, Indian societies. Even so, this pattern is probably a consequence of socially acquired patterns. Many North American Indian tribes show little or no incidence of drunken behavior or alcoholism. For example, the Tarahumara Indians of Mexico show an extremely low incidence of alcoholism. It is of interest that the cultural habits, living style, and ritualized behaviors of this society are quite primitive, resembling those followed in pre-Columbian days (Zeiner, Blackburn, Stratton, and Paredes, 1978).

Social models, as mentioned, may be extremely important factors in accounting for the explosive drinking patterns of some Indian societies. For example, the Iroquois Indians' first contact with alcohol did not involve drunken brawling. Alcohol had initially been used in religious rituals, specifically in a quest for religious "visions." Later, however, in the eighteenth century, the Iroquois began to imitate the drunken behavior of the white traders and trappers with whom they were coming into frequent contact. By 1800, drunken brawls and unruliness became enmeshed in the social drinking patterns of the Iroquois, obviously a result of a cultural learning process.

Some Indians show a pattern of "blitz" drinking in the context of family and extended kin drinking parties. Convivial, gregarious peer-group drinking may indeed end in explosive, assaultive patterns. In some Indian societies, this is considered socially acceptable behavior, supported by the general attitude that when drunk a person is not responsible for his or her behavior (Andre, 1979).

cohol metabolism. It has been known for some time that levels of acetaldehyde, even after small doses of alcohol consumption, tend to be much higher in alcoholics than in nonalcoholics (Brody, 1975). This chemical, toxic to heart and liver tissues, also interacts with other chemicals within the body to produce alkaloids that interfere with certain nerve functions. The alkaloids, rather than the alcohol itself, may be the agent that causes harm to alcoholics. It is claimed that differences in level of acetaldehyde can explain variations among people in degree of adverse response to even minimal amounts of alcohol.

In any event, several explorations have focused on looking for differences in acetaldehyde and other chemical levels as well as differences in rates of alcohol metabolism in different groups of subjects. Some of these studies have reported such differences. For example, comparisons of various Chinese, Japanese, and some American Indian people with other samples show that they have higher rates for metabolizing alcohol, special sensitivities to small doses of alcohol, and higher levels of chemicals essential for alcohol metabolism (Cohen, 1979a; Hanna, 1978). Another study reported that twenty subjects who were "healthy young men" with an alcoholic parent or sibling had especially high levels of blood acetaldehyde concentration compared to a carefully matched control group after a moderate dose of alcohol. The researchers suggested that the former subjects may have a predisposition to alcoholism (Schuckit and Rayses, 1979).

A genetic predisposition to alcoholism? Adoption and various other types of family studies suggest that there may be inherited physiological mechanisms that predispose some people to alcoholism. For example, studies of several generations of offspring of alcoholics in a Swedish population found that the chances that the grandchildren of alcoholics are also alcoholics are "three times greater than are the chances for grandchildren of nonalcoholics (Kaij and Dock, 1975). Identical (MZ) twins in a Swedish population had a higher concordance (percentage agreement) for alcoholism than fraternal (DZ) twins, but the latter rates were higher than those in the population at large (Kaij, 1960).

Danish studies tend to support the same thesis (DeFries and Plomin, 1978; Schuckit, Goodwin, and Winokur, 1972). For example, one study found that of a large number of families with an alcoholic parent, twenty offspring were adopted away and raised by nonalcoholic parents (Goodwin et al., 1974). These adopted-away children had siblings who were raised by their alcoholic, biological parent. These reared-apart-from-each-other biological siblings were interviewed to ascertain whether the rates of alcoholism among them differed in any way. Both groups of offspring had the same rates of alcoholism, which were higher than those for the offspring of the nonalcoholic parents—a finding that was true essentially for the males.

On the other hand, it is becoming clear that social models and cultural patterns for drinking behavior play an extremely important role in the development of alcoholism. Further, biochemical sensitivities in the body's response to alcohol and variations in how alcohol is metabolized do not necessarily have a one-to-one relationship to alcoholism. For example, although genetic aberrations in the metabolism of alcohol have been suggested as underlying the low incidence of alcohol consumption among the Chinese and Japanese, rates of alcoholism in these populations are increasing. These data are explainable only by sociocultural factors, for genetic ones are presumably stable (Cohen, 1979).

TREATMENT OF ALCOHOLISM

Most experts, no matter what their beliefs are about the causes of alcoholism, agree that there is no one method of treatment that works equally effectively for all. But whether treatment services are offered in a private or public hospital, weekend or day hospital, clinic, halfway house, private clinician's office, community clinic, or nonprofessional group setting, for the long-term, chronic drinker, after a binge or otherwise, there may have to be a period of detoxification during which withdrawal symptoms may occur. This period is best handled in a hospital setting for many patients, who may require emergency health care and a generally supportive environment. Not all alcoholics require this kind of care, however. Whether or not the detoxification step is required, most alcoholics who wish to control their drinking problems will require attention to long-neglected physical and health problems that have arisen as a result of sustained injury to their bodies. Even if these steps are well-handled most experts agree that successful outcome depends in large part on the patient's ability to sustain a changed pattern of behavior in many areas, interpersonally, for example, not only in connection with drinking.

Above all, as is the case for most if not all interventive strategies, the key for successful outcome is not only the patient's recognition of the need to change, but also a strong motivation to embrace and to continue with the treatment program selected.

The goal of most therapeutic interventions is total abstinence, a view that is currently being challenged by some experts. We return to this issue shortly. Whether or not total abstinence is a criterion, the next section discusses the methods in current use in dealing with alcoholism.

Counseling, Psychotherapy, and Family Approaches

Traditional psychotherapeutic methods, in which there is a one-to-one verbal interchange, are still very popular (see Lynn, 1976). In psychotherapy, the alcoholic can "ventilate" or air the problems that led to heavy drinking and at the same time receive support and reassurance as he or she attempts to control the drinking pattern. In combination with other methods, counseling and psychotherapy—an opportunity to talk things over—can be crucial in providing a sense of support, hope for the future, and a hedge against the periodic failures that occur in the course of recovery.

Group methods are among the most popular of the "talking" therapies, probably because of their relative efficiency (cost per patient). Also, many clinicians believe that these methods can be of benefit to the patient because of the opportunity they provide for social and interpersonal interactions with other alcoholics and the consequent sharing of problems, frustrations, and experiences. Reassurance from others, especially former alcoholics, may be an important weapon, it is believed, in an alcoholic's fight for control. Many people assume, therefore, that group methods are highly effective. Yet there is only inconclusive support for this assumption (Baekeland, Lundwall, and Kissin, 1975).

Some clinicians use a family approach in dealing with alcoholism on an assumption that the veiled support of the problem drinking, the secrecy that shrouds the alcoholic, and the hidden family dynamics that have produced the alcoholic's problems can be best unraveled in a family context. Further, it is thought that seeing an alcoholic through the recovery period as he or she gains confidence and begins to feel more hopeful about the future is a family, rather than an individual, concern.

In general, most programs that deal with alcoholics directly or indirectly subscribe to the view that familial and interpersonal relationships are important areas of focus through the entire course of treatment. For example, there are many group programs (for example, Al-Anon and Alateen), for wives, husbands, and children of alcoholics to help them understand how to deal with their alcoholic relatives.

Vocational Counseling

Work and training programs, vocational rehabilitation, employment opportunities, and similar aids that generate opportunities for a former alcoholic to remain rooted in the community are essential to help him or her sustain controlled drinking or abstinence. These programs are often necessary accompaniments to the approaches described in this section, for they may make possible the transfer of what has been "learned" in the hospital or clinic to the natural life setting.

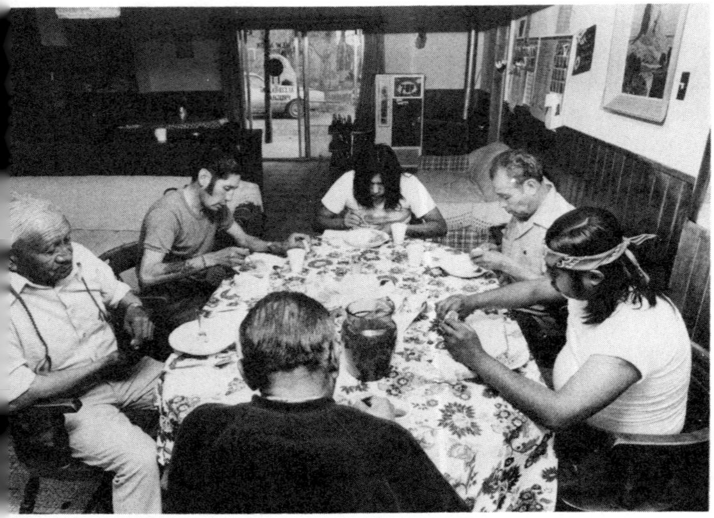

Halfway houses can provide important emotional supports and pathways to employment and sustained abstinence after detoxification. (Michael D. Sullivan)

Disulfiram (Antabuse)

Some alcoholics need help to stay away from alcohol, especially at the beginning of long-term treatment. This can sometimes be achieved through the daily ingestion of a drug, disulfiram (Antabuse), which in combination with drinking produces a violent reaction: severe nausea, constriction in the neck area, difficulty in breathing, headache, and flushing in the face, upper chest, and arms. These symptoms are often accompanied by intense anxiety.

Responses to the combination of Antabuse and drinking are so unpleasant that most people who voluntarily take this drug avoid alcohol—come what may. Antabuse works only with motivated alcoholics, for drinking can be resumed without these ill effects about forty-eight hours after the drug regimen has been terminated. For this reason, Antabuse therapy is not the treatment of choice for most alcoholics. In addition, there may be side effects, including psychotic reactions (Skopkova, 1973), as well as instances in which disulfiram is contraindicated, as when there are certain types of heart disease. Finally, this method does not offer a long-range approach to changing the drinking patterns, life style, and emotional needs of the alcoholic.

Aversion Therapy

Aversion treatment is an "old" form of conditioning therapy—used as far back as the 1920s—that links drinking with nausea and vomiting by having the alcoholic take an emetic when he or she desires a drink, or after smelling, tasting, and swallowing a drink. Conditioning sessions last 30 to 60 minutes, and there are usually several of them, administered over a period of many weeks. If the program is successful, then nausea or vomiting will occur whenever the alcoholic wants a drink. Eventually, distaste, indifference, and then complete abstinence should result. There are some physical dangers in this approach, which is rather unpleasant and unpopular for therapist and client alike. Nontheless, there are reports of some success with this method (Baekeland, Lundwall, and Kissin, 1975).

Electric shock has also been used as an aversive stimulus. This also is an extremely unpleasant procedure. A review of outcome of these and related methods indicates some success, but because they have been tried only on limited samples with limited follow-up, generalizations as to their effectiveness in the real-life situations of most alcoholics cannot be made (Baekeland, Lundwall, and Kissin, 1975). Moreover, many people have raised questions about the "humanity" and ethics of aversive procedures in the treatment of alcoholism, even when introduced on a voluntary basis.

Chemical Substitutes

Some therapists use psychoactive medications as a substitute for alcohol in an attempt to sustain the alcoholic without alcohol. The assumption is that most alcoholics suffer from anxiety, depression, and similar emotional difficulties. It is thought that treating these states directly through appropriate medications to help the alcoholic stay away from, instead of turn to, alcohol to feel better, might wean the alcoholic away from his or her usual drinking pattern. Although there is moderate evidence of some success with tranquilizers with some patients, most reviews indicate that these methods show little or no effectiveness (Baekeland, Lundwall, and Kissin, 1975). There are also some ethical objections to methods that substitute one drug for another (Bissell, 1975). Some people claim, however, that if the alcoholic is helped through substitute drugs and counseling to get back to work, reconstruct personal relationships, and build a more personally rewarding life without alcohol, perhaps the means do indeed justify the end.

Alcoholics Anonymous(AA)

Alcoholics Anonymous (AA)—acclaimed as the most successful treatment program—is a self-help, voluntary, loosely structured organization of people who have or have had problems with drinking. Its purpose is to have individuals with similar problems help one another to give up drinking entirely and to remain abstinent for all time. To accomplish this purpose, AA encourages frequent meetings that are open and free to anyone with a drinking problem. AA also offers unstinting availability of its members to those among them who are tempted to drink (for example, accepting an urgent three-A.M. telephone call). In addition, AA promotes an approach that encourages members to put their faith in a higher power while at the same time admitting that they are and always will be alcoholics, even when abstinent.

AA has no political or social beliefs and never opens its files and records (if indeed there are any) to scientists for study. But it does allow observers to attend open meetings at which there are testimonials. The atmosphere is social, friendly, and supportive, but at the same time, communicates the "evils" of alcoholism. In closed meetings members discuss their personal bouts with alcohol freely, providing a personal example or receiving needed support and reassurance.

AA, founded in 1935, claims more attendance than any of the other approaches. Up to a million alcoholics worldwide at any point in time go to AA meetings regularly. There are about 30,000 AA groups, supported entirely by contributions from their members.

What is AA's track record in dealing with alcoholism? Many experts question the applicability of AA's program to large numbers of alcoholics, for example from low-SES or skid-row groups or from certain minority groups such as some North American Indian or West Indian cultures (Heath, 1975; Jilek-Aall, 1978). The content and themes of AA meetings and the general program may be irrelevant to, or poorly understood by, alcoholic people in these groups, and the values expressed simply not absorbed. Many alcoholics in these subcultures may have a high rate of failure because they do not comprehend such concepts as "responsibility," "morality," and "sponsorship."

According to some experts, AA is rather successful with good "premorbids"—middle-class, educated men and women who are motivated to control their drinking and who have the family and social supports to help them (Baekeland, Lundwall, and Kissin, 1975). But available data indicate that AA is no more successful than a clinic approach that employs a combination of many methods. Low-SES people do not go to AA meetings, nor do isolates or those who find it difficult to accept AA's spiritual orientation. Outpatient clinics, on the other hand, treat a broad spectrum of patients and seem to have about an equal rate of success, probably because they generally employ a variety of approaches, including group, individual, disulfiram, behavioral, and vocational counseling methods.

In general, the effectiveness of AA is less than one would expect. According to one estimate (Ludwig, 1972), only 5 percent of the population of alcoholics participate in AA at any point in time, and only 7 percent of recovered alcoholics attribute their cure primarily to AA. These estimates may be more pessimistic than others, but they do not paint a rosy picture of AA's effectiveness. On the other hand, extremely high rates of success are reported for those who gravitate to AA and who *remain in the program,* probably higher than all other programs combined.

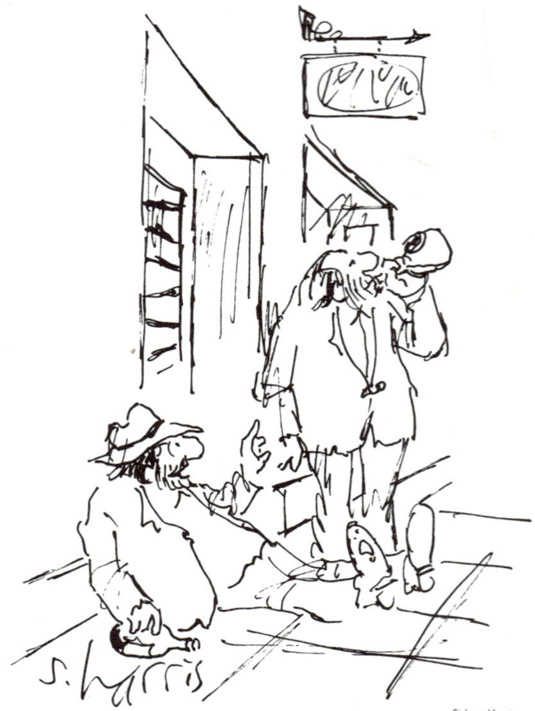

Sidney Harris

"THAT'S WHERE WE DIFFER. I CAN STOP WHENEVER I WANT."

CONTROLLED DRINKING

Many experts on the treatment of alcoholics believe that total abstinence is the only goal for alcoholics, because even one sip appears to set up the pattern for alcohol abuse all over again, characterized chiefly by loss of control. Alcoholism is considered to be an addictive, irreversible disease; and these experts maintain that there is no such thing as a cured alcoholic.

The goal of total and life-long abstinence has been the major thrust in most treatment programs offered to alcoholics. Many alcoholics agree, stating that their periodic lapses into social drinking eventually lead to heavy drinking, with all its negative consequences, not the least of which is a sense of deep failure, depression, and hopelessness.

A lively controversy has developed over this issue, with some experts suggesting that "controlled" drinking or moderate social drinking may in some instances for some people represent a more realistic and attainable goal than that of total abstinence. If the patient can control his or her drinking and work toward general family and occupational adjustment, interpersonal adequacy, and a workable life style, then the unattractive, and often unreachable, goal of total abstinence might be discarded for some alcoholics (Pattison, 1976).

The advantages of controlled drinking as a viable alternative to abstinence might not only attract a much wider sample of alcoholics who would thus be helped, but would also hold out promise for many alcoholics who have frequently failed in achieving the goals for total abstinence offered by so many programs (Lloyd and Salzberg, 1975).

Those who favor the exploration of possibilities held in controlled drinking programs also point out that the concept of craving—a physical or psychological feeling that one must have more alcohol following an initial sip—has not received empirical clarification and confirmation. Further, the feeling of craving is subjectively defined in different ways. Even so, some people who have reported feelings of uncontrollable craving have been able to learn to drink in moderate fashion without any treatment at all (Lloyd and Salzberg, 1975).

A further advantage lies in the possibility of controlling blackouts. That is, it might be possible to train the drinker to control the rate, amount, and style of drinking (not gulping, nor ordering straight drinks) so that the alcohol within the bloodstream is kept below the level at which blackouts take place. One method that employed avoidance conditioning, for example, not of drinking itself but of patterns associated with abuse (such as gulping, drinking straight drinks, or ordering more than three drinks), was successfully demonstrated in a study that had good follow-up results (Mills, Sobell, and Schaeffer, 1971).

In the forefront of the controlled-drinking approach are Mark and Linda Sobell (Sobell and Sobell, 1978), whose pioneer work early in the 1970s involved attempts to teach hospitalized male alcoholics to control their drinking through behavioral methods so as to not go beyond a certain level of consumption or display intoxicated behavior. Two-year follow-up results indicated that subjects with the controlled-drinking goal were functioning much better in their worlds (mostly abstinent or moderate drinking) than either a control group of subjects who had received no treatment at all, or a comparable group of subjects who had been trained with abstinence as a goal. Although there were many methodological flaws in this research, overall some empirical confirmation of this general approach was subsequently reported, suggesting that at least for some alcoholics, controlled drinking can be a reasonable goal.

As a matter of fact, proponents of a controlled-drinking approach feel that much work needs to be done regarding which of many possible approaches, behavioral or otherwise, represents the best procedure to train the subject. Some success has already been achieved with aversive methods, behavioral self-control training, and self-monitoring of blood alcohol levels with groups of problem drinkers (Miller, 1978; Miller, Taylor, and West, 1980).

However, continued research efforts demonstrate that the controlled-drinking versus total-abstinence controversy is not a clearly polarized, either-or issue that can be easily resolved, favoring one side or the other. In a recent report of follow-up status of 780 alcoholics—four years after an earlier report that had suggested that controlled or moderate drinking is not only possible but to be recommended for many alcoholics—the Rand Corporation (The course of alcoholism, 1980) has "softened" (but not modified) its original position. Although more than half of the original group still had serious drinking problems, about 28 percent were abstinent. About 18 percent of the follow-up sample, however, were drinking—some even quite a bit (more than four drinks a day) but without problems and negative social consequences. The Rand Corporation now feels that only certain types of alcoholics fare well with controlled or social drinking and that for most, total abstinence is the only viable goal. Apparently, subjects who were successful "targets" of controlled-drinking programs were under forty years of age and were less dependent on alcohol to begin with, judging by such symptoms as morning "shakes" and blackouts.

The most recent challenge to the controlled drinking approach has appeared in the form of a ten-year follow-up of the original twenty experimental subjects in the Sobell and Sobell study discussed earlier (Pendery, Maltzman, and West, 1982). This research demonstrated extremely disappointing results, with only *one* of the original subjects displaying a sustained pattern of controlled drinking and the majority returning to their old, destructive patterns of alcoholism.

Overall, the "established" treatment community continues to adhere to its position on total abstinence for all alcoholics. Continuing to observe the findings as they accumulate regarding this lively, significant, polarized issue will be of major importance in the coming years.

Treatment Failures: Relapses, Dropouts, and Other Dismal Data

The high refusal-of-treatment rate among alcoholics is further compounded by the fact that many alcoholics simply drop out of treatment. And those who remain to the end of a program show a high rate of relapse within a relatively short period of time. Obviously, a "successful" program is not truly successful if it has not modified the drinking patterns of large numbers of alcoholics—the dropouts and the relapsers. Identifying the characteristics of these "failures," and then (a) finding ways to motivate the dropouts to stay (were they offered an inappropriate service, for example?) and (b) helping the potential relapser to deal with his or her loss of control, are obviously most important areas for further study.

Fortunately, in the past several years, there has been some empirical exploration of the processes underlying the tendency to relapse, even among highly motivated subjects who have successfully completed a program. When relapse does occur, as has already been noted, there is a despondent, hopeless response that propels the client into total loss of control, a "full-blown" relapse. This pattern has been called the abstinence violation effect by Marlatt and Gordon (1978) in their attempts to understand and then deal with the problems faced by such people.

These researchers indicate that the responses to relapsing after a period of abstinence fall into a common pattern whether it concerns alcohol or other kinds of drugs. They examined the nature of these relapses (the crucial point occurs within 90 days after treatment termination) in terms of underlying mechanisms and discovered that relapse episodes are essentially responses to failures to cope adequately with negative inner emotions, social pressures to break down ("one little drink won't hurt you"), and interpersonal conflicts (Marlatt, 1979). If clients are helped to understand the abstinence violation effect and what the high-risk-for-relapse situations are, and are given opportunities to develop strategies for dealing with these situations, then perhaps they will be better able to cope with the tendency for a full-blown relapse to occur.

These researchers believe that those who successfully control their drinking possess certain "survivor skills" which, if understood completely, would be of enormous help in coping with relapse.

Treatment Success

One overall conclusion drawn from different outcome studies is that a combination of many approaches is more effective than any single approach, and that (as with schizophrenia) the outcome is generally more favorable with good "premorbids" than with poor "premorbids." As a matter of fact, the client, rather than the method, is probably the best predictor of outcome (Baekeland, Lundwall, and Kissin, 1975). Marital, residential, and occupational stability as well as SES level are all related to outcome, as are education and social stability. Low SES is generally related to poor outcome. High-SES people in stable social settings show the best progress. One can almost predict the success of a particular program by examining these client variables rather than the program itself.

Overall, successful programs like AA or some individual therapies work only for some people. Low-SES alcoholics require more direct methods. Above all, motivation for treatment is a crucial factor in determining the outcome of a particular treatment program.

The success of any method, of course, can be determined only after a reasonable follow-up period, after the client has lived for some time with the usual stresses of work and family. And it is here that practical help, family supports, vocational training and counseling, jobs, and other social assets really count. Chiefly, however, the client's expectations for himself or herself and faith or lack of it that he or she can really "make it" become dramatically relevant.

Who Are at Risk?

Finally, if we are interested in *prevention,* we might ask questions about the people who are at risk for later alcoholism. Of interest is that whether one believes in genetic predisposition, social learning, or complex interactions among many variables, the facts are clear: 25 to 50 percent of alcoholics have a parent or close relative who is also an alcoholic, and the offspring of alcoholic parents are twice as likely to become alcoholic as the offspring of nonalcoholic parents, according to a 1976 survey by the National Institute on Alcoholic Abuse and Alcoholism.

Retrospective studies point up the poor educational, familial, and social adjustment of young people who later become alcoholic. For example, among black, lower-class men, alcoholism is associated with prior school truancy and family disorganization (Harper, 1979). Similarly, prior history of 451 Vietnam veterans with heavy drinking problems include having become intoxicated at an early age, dropping out of school, truancy or expulsion from school, and a father with a history of alcoholism or arrests (Goodwin, Davis, and Robins, 1975). Important to note is that an entirely different set of risk factors would be involved were one to make predictions about people from other cultural groups—white, middle-class females, for example.

The point is that if we are to select high-risk individuals for intensive, preventive efforts, we should be concerned not only with the so-called genetic markers, but also with the cultural and social patterns, familial models, and psychological variables that are associated with alcohol abuse within that individual's social group.

SUMMARY

Chapter 16 surveyed alcoholism and alcohol abuse. Although it has been common to distinguish among alcoholism, alcohol abuse, and problem drinking, this chapter did not consider these labels as separate entities. The chapter described some of the signs that the experts employ to diagnosis alcoholism, the ways in which alcohol affects the individual, the consequences of alcohol abuse (for example, its relationship to violence, accidents, and death), and the association between alcoholism and SES levels, ethnic and minority status, age, and gender. It then considered the causes of problem drinking, including various psychological and psychoanalytic approaches, as well as biochemical and genetic ones. The chapter also discussed the powerful effects of expectancy and set in drinking behavior, the question of the relationship of personality variables to alcoholism, and some cultural determinants of patterns of drinking behavior in different cultural groups. The general conclusion was that social models and cultural patterns play a powerful role in the development of alcoholism. The chapter then described the different treatment approaches to alcoholism and discussed the possibility of controlled drinking (instead of total abstinence) as a goal for some alcoholics. The overall conclusion was that a combination of many treatment approaches is more effective than any single approach. The chapter concluded with a brief description of variables that predict risk for alcoholism.

Highlights

1. It is estimated that there are about ten million alcohol abusers in this country. The social, individual, financial, and physical consequences are of staggering degree, including the threat to babies born to alcoholics (FAS). There are many early signs of what has been traditionally labeled alcoholism, for example, the gulping of drinks or the undue interest in planning the next drinking occasion. Later, there may be blackouts. Severe problem drinkers complain of loss of control or of "craving." It is commonly agreed that in addition to psychological dependence, alcoholism is characterized by physical dependence, defined in terms of tolerance or an abstinence (withdrawal) syndrome. However, the chapter stresses that patterns of drinking behavior, the consequences of heavy drinking, and even the label *alcoholic* all are very much dependent on the drinker's sociocultural group.
2. Alcohol is a CNS depressant, despite the fact that initially the drinker may feel an elevation of mood and an increase in energy level. Alcohol does its "work" after it enters the bloodstream, which distributes it to all parts of the body, including the brain. The rate and quantity of alcohol that is ingested, absorbed into the bloodstream, and metabolized determine its effects, which can be lethal. Alcohol is metabo-

lized at a fairly regular rate—about three-quarters of an ounce per hour. Amounts of alcohol in the bloodstream that have accumulated too quickly for normal metabolization determines how "drunk" an individual becomes. Continued rises in blood alcohol content (BAC) produce severe motor, language, and judgment impairment and eventually various neurological events, including stupor, coma, and death.

3. Alcoholics are found in all SES, educational, and cultural groups. However, it is most frequently found (or diagnosed) on low-SES levels. Important to note is that the consequences of alcoholism, in terms of joblessness, ill health, and violence, are more severe on low than on high SES levels. Epidemiological studies also indicate that there are variations in alcoholism and alcohol-related deaths among different ethnic and racial groups. Heavy drinking is on the rise among teenagers, with an estimate from one to over three million of this large population of drinkers showing signs of potential for later alcoholism. Finally, throughout the world, the number of alcohol abusers among males is considerably higher than among females.
4. An understanding of why people drink alcoholic beverages might shed light on why some of them become alcoholics. Hypotheses as to why people drink generally allude to various psychological benefits, such as tension-reduction, lifting of mood, energizing and motivating effects, pain-reduction, achieving a sense of power, overcoming depression, feeling more confident and assertive, or becoming more sexually aroused. Although most of these purported benefits are not directly due to chemical action, studies were described that suggest that the powerful effects of expectancy and set might indeed produce some of these desired states.
5. The common presumption that there are predisposing personality factors or constellations of traits (alcoholic personality) associated with alcoholism and alcohol abuse is not empirically confirmed. However, locus-of-control methods, although not yielding entirely consistent results, do suggest that the heavier drinkers or those with the greatest degree of disturbance may rationalize their drinking so that personal responsibility (internal locus of control) is not assumed.
6. Various psychoanalytic views linking orality, oral conflicts, dependency needs, regressive defenses, and "latent homosexuality" in the etiology of alcoholism have not been empirically demonstrated.
7. Social expectations and cultural variables are powerful shapers of drinking behavior, which varies considerably from culture to culture and from group to group. Some cultural groups, for example, may permit,—even encourage—aggression and violence during intoxicated states. The so-called "blitz" drinking, involving brawls and unruliness, of some North American Indians may be derived from social models and socially sanctioned or permitted behaviors. Similar social variables probably account for the striking differences in the drinking patterns of men and of women.
8. Metabolic, biochemical, and genetic variables have been proposed as underlying the possibility that some people are at greater risk for alcoholism than are others. Although there is moderate evidence for the validity of some aspects of this and related approaches (for example, in one Swedish study, identical twins had a higher concordance for alcoholism than had fraternal twins), it has become increasingly clear that learning and sociocultural patterns also play a significant role.
9. In the treatment of alcoholism no one method seems clearly the most effective. The subject's motivation to change as well as willingness to continue with the treatment program is probably the best predictor of successful outcome. This chapter notes that the many methods of treating alcoholics include individual psychotherapy and counseling, group and family

methods, the daily ingestion of disulfiram (Antabuse), aversion therapy, and chemical substitutes. Described in detail is Alcoholics Anonymous (AA). Despite wide acclaim as the most successful of the treatment programs, many experts point out that AA's approach is not relevant to large numbers of alcoholics and that its success is based primarily on the good "premorbids" who remain within the program.

10. The goal of total abstinence for most treatment programs (the "establishment" position) has recently been challenged. There may indeed be advantages for controlled drinking as a goal for some alcoholics, but the chapter points out that there is still considerable controversy regarding the merits of either position.
11. Problems requiring research exploration include the high rate of relapse after treatment and the high rate of dropout from treatment.
12. Finally, the chapter describes several high-risk-for-alcoholism variables, especially in low-SES groups. In addition, it points out that 25 to 50 percent of alcoholics have a parent or close relative who is also an alcoholic, and that the offspring of alcoholic parents are twice as likely to become alcoholic as are the offspring of nonalcoholic parents. It also notes that specific predictors of high risk should take into account the cultural, social, and psychological variables associated with an individual's social group.

ISSUES AND QUESTIONS

1. *Brisbane's "139 Club," a drop-in center for the homeless, is described as an example of the self-help approach that could ameliorate the skid-row life style in Australia. Such a life style, as compared with its counterpart in the U.S., is distinguished by its lack of geographical definition. There are few buildings in Australia that provide skid row services; no special streets on which one can openly drink and panhandle, and no doorways or park benches that constitute unique sleeping facilities. The 139 Club plays an important role in helping the derelict to develop a sense of belonging. Needs of the skid row derelict are expressed in terms of an increased sense of group identity, the establishment of clearly defined home territories, and improved communication among those agencies that cater to the needs of homeless persons. In a postscript it is noted that the 139 Club on which this article is based has been closed down due to pressure from local businesses. 39 ref. (Abstract by National Clearinghouse for Alcohol Information of an article by J. Ward in the* Australian Journal of Social Issues, *1977, 12, 255–65: Towards being down without being out: self-help on skid row).*

   Do you believe that this ill-fated project for derelicts would have had some positive results if permitted to carry on? Should the Australians be envious of the skid-row panhandling and sleeping facilities in doorways we have in America? Do you go along with the businessmen's unwillingness to share some of their territory with Brisbane's skid-row alcoholics? What answers to this apparently universal problem would you come up with?
2. Low-SES alcoholics are generally poor-outcome subjects in treatment programs. They are not motivated for treatment, and even if participating, they drop out very quickly. And yet, some people claim, because they cause traffic accidents, are on welfare rolls, glut the city and state hospitals, and occupy the prisons, we should at least explore the possibility of enforcing treatment: detoxification, adequate physical and medical care, group counseling, and eventually, job rehabilitation. Remaining in treatment, of course, is necessary for a successful outcome. But can we impose this regimen, like a prison sentence, without robbing a low-SES or skid-row alcoholic of his or her civil rights?
3. In the light of what you have read in this chapter, should there be some control over the extensive advertising of the liquor industry? Should the government sponsor "equal time" for educational campaigns that promote a deeper understanding of the effects of heavy alcohol consumption?

4. There is much debate as to what the legal drinking age should be. In the past several years, several states have raised the minimum age—Georgia, for example, has raised it from eighteen to nineteen, with the exception of people in the armed services. Many say, however, that because eighteen-year-olds can vote as well as be drafted, it is hypocritical to deny them drinking privileges. Those in favor of raising the legal age point to the shockingly high rate of alcohol-related deaths in this age group. What is your position on this debate? Remember, young problem drinkers generally begin their drinking patterns earlier than at the age of eighteen.
5. Public drunkenness is a major problem in the United States. In 1980 there were about one million arrests for public drunkenness, usually on such charges as disorderly conduct. These people are released, but many are arrested again, on the same charge. Most states have decriminalized public drunkenness, and many provide "sobering-up" stations, and treatment facilities, rather than jail, as an alternative. Should a disorderly public drunk be arrested or brought into a special facility for "sobering up"? Should we provide treatment or punishment for the publicly intoxicated person? Is being noisily intoxicated at the country club different from being noisily intoxicated on Main Street?

SUGGESTIONS FOR FURTHER READING

Bourne, P. G., and Fox, R. (Eds.) *Alcoholism: Progress in research and treatment.* New York: Wiley Academic Press, 1973. This collection of papers may be of interest to those who want a close look at various aspects of alcoholism. The first two articles present the disease and social learning models of alcoholism. Additional articles discuss cross-cultural studies of alcoholism, treatment approaches, alcoholism and crime, and the family relations of the alcoholic. Of particular interest is an article by Leach that presents a careful evaluation of the effectiveness of one of the most popular and respected methods for treating alchoholism: Alcoholics Anonymous.

Marlatt, G. A., and Nathan, P. E. (Eds.) *Behavioral approaches to alcoholism.* New Brunswick, N. J.: Rutgers Center of Alcohol Studies, 1978. Paperback. This book is a collection of papers that address the problem of alcoholism from a behavioral perspective. The first section presents behavioral theories of alcoholism; the second section discusses behavioral observations and assessment of alcoholism; and the third section describes various behavioral treatment approaches to alcoholism. This is an excellent reference for an in-depth review of behavioral approaches to alcoholism, with chapters written by important experts in the field.

Pittman, D. J., and Snyder, C. R. (Eds.) *Society, culture, and drinking patterns.* New York: Wiley, 1962. Paperback available. This book, still a classic, focuses on the social and sociological aspects of drinking behavior. Articles by numerous experts include the relationship of drinking behavior to ethnic and religious affiliation and to such variables as age, gender, and social class. Social attitudes toward drinkers and drinking as they relate to ethnic patterns, crosscultural estimates of prevalence, and related sociocultural issues are also covered. This book will be of interest to those whose curiosity about drinking behavior goes beyond the case-history level.

Sandmaier, M. *The invisible alcoholics: Women and alcohol abuse in America.* New York: McGraw-Hill, 1979. Paperback available. Because men and women experience different styles of upbringing, with different social and role stressors, the factors that lead to their abuse of alcohol, the treatment they receive, and their personal experiences of alcoholism are different, according to this author. This book is addressed to the history and scope of alcohol abuse among women in the United States. It presents research data in a readable manner as well as the personal accounts of alcoholics who are housewives, working women, minority women, lesbians, teen-age girls, and women living on skid row. It is an interesting and informative presentation.

For further information about alcohol abuse and facilities for treatment, write to:

Alcoholics Anonymous
P.O. Box 459
Grand Central Station
New York, N.Y. 10017

Al-Anon Family Groups
115 East 23rd Street
New York, N.Y. 10010

National Clearinghouse for Alcohol Information
Box 2345
Rockville, Md. 20852

National Council on Alcoholism
733 Third Avenue
New York, N.Y. 10017

The National Institute on Alcohol Abuse and Alcoholism
5600 Fishers Lane
Rockville, Md. 20857

17

Abuse of Substances Other Than Alcohol

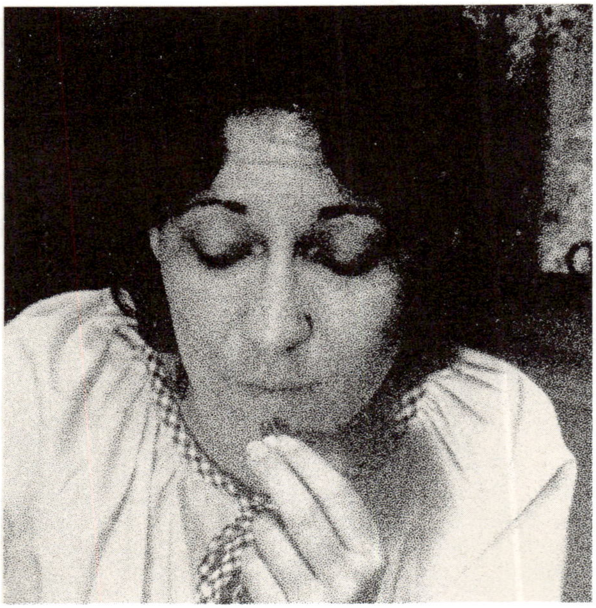

Half an hour after swallowing the drug I became aware of a slow dance of golden lights. A little later there were sumptuous red surfaces swelling and expanding from bright nodes of energy that vibrated with a continuously changing, patterned life. At another time the closing of my eyes revealed a complex of gray structures, within which pale bluish spheres kept emerging into intense solidity and, having emerged, would slide noiselessly upwards, out of sight. But at no times were there faces or forms of men or animals. I saw no landscapes, no enormous spaces, no magical growth and metamorphosis of buildings, nothing remotely like a drama or a parable. The other world to which mescalin admitted me was not the world of visions; it existed out there, in what I could see with my eyes open. The great change was in the realm of objective fact. What had happened to my subjective universe was relatively unimportant (A. Huxley, *The doors of perception and heaven and hell* [New York: Harper & Row, 1954], p. 16).

Truckin', got my chips cashed in,
Keep truckin' like the doo-dah man,
Together, more or less in line,
Just keep truckin' on.

Arrows of neon and flashing marquees
Out on Main Street, Chicago, New York, Detroit and
It's all on the same street.
Your typical city involved in a typical day dream,
Hang it up and see what tomorrow brings.

Sometimes the lights all shinin' on me,
Other times I can barely see.
Lately it occurs to me,
What a long strange trip its been.

What in the world ever became of Sweet Jane?
She lost her sparkle you know she isn't the same.
Livin' on reds, vitamin C, and cocaine,
All a friend can say is ain't it a shame.

Source: From "Truckin," a song performed by the Grateful Dead. Music by Jerry Garcia, Robert Weir, Billy Kreitzmann, and Philip Lesh. Lyric by Robert Hunter. Copyright 1971/1973 Ice Nine Publishing Co.

DRUG ABUSE—DEPENDENCE AND ADDICTION

This chapter is concerned with substances that have a potential for abuse. Drug or substance abuse can be defined as a pattern of using substances that "adversely affect(s) the user's interpersonal relations or cause(s) adverse physical, social, or economic consequences to others as well as to himself [sic]. . . . " (World Health Organization, 1969, pp. 6–7). The substances we will be considering have a wide range of subjective and physical effects. Many of these effects result not only from type and amount of drug ingested, but also on set, expectancy, social setting, and various other individual and situational factors.

These chemicals generally affect the central nervous system (CNS) producing various subjective states, mood changes, and alterations in thinking processes. Some people find many drug-related experiences pleasurable, especially in social situations. They may seek to repeat these experiences from time to time and suffer few adverse effects as a result. Such recreational and social use of substances is not our primary focus. On the other hand, there are persons who become so intensely involved in seeking and ingesting the substance(s) of their choice that they risk many serious consequences including interpersonal and financial difficulties, disruption of their lives, illness, and even death.* These are the drug abusers with whom this chapter is concerned.

Motivations for compulsive drug-seeking behavior vary for different people. Thus, although we may speak of dependence we are not necessarily talking about physical dependence or even implying that we know the reasons for an individual's pattern of drug-related behavior. At one time, it was assumed that compulsive drug-seeking, physical dependence, and addiction were, if not entirely synonymous, at least strongly overlapping entities. Today, more and more experts think that this is not the case. So-called addicting substances such as heroin do not necessarily produce compulsive drug-seeking behaviors in large numbers of users. And some drugs that are not associated with *physical* dependence (abstinence syndrome and tolerance; see Spotlight 17.1 for definitions) are so highly reinforcing (cocaine, for example) that some people become addicted to them. Further, if craving for a substance such as heroin is ascribed to physical dependence, how is it possible for many former addicts to experience craving and even undergo an abstinence syndrome months after their last dose when returning to their old haunts? I shall return to this question later in the chapter.

* There are costs to society, too. According to a National Institute on Drug Abuse report, drug abuse problems cost the United States over ten and a half billion dollars annually.

Drug-seeking behaviors are largely learned behaviors that are very much part of one's subculture, past history, and socially expected roles. The concept of physical dependence gets in the way of understanding these behaviors more completely, especially because we still know very little about the nature of physical dependence and its relationship to drug-seeking behavior (World Health Organization, 1978).

In this chapter, the term *dependence* refers to certain behaviors associated with drug abuse that are not necessarily explained by physical dependence. These behaviors often involve compulsive drug-seeking—an intense preoccupation with obtaining certain substances and the ritual involved in their use.

Later, during the discussion on heroin abuse, this chapter will use the terms *addiction* and *addict* because these are the frequently used, popular labels that many clinicians and researchers still use. By *addiction,* we will mean the behavior associated with the pattern of heroin abuse and dependence. *Addict* refers to a person who is unable to modify his or her compulsive, heroin-seeking, heroin-dependent behavior. Addiction and physical dependence are not necessarily interchangeable concepts; and terms like *addict* and *addiction* do not refer to well-identified, well-understood concepts.

Spotlight 17.1 DSM-III Categories of Disorders Associated with Substances Other than Alcohol

In the preceding chapter, Spotlight 16.1 described the DSM-III's distinction between alcohol-induced organic mental disorders and other kinds of disorders associated with alcohol use. The same general distinction applies to the substances described in Chapter 17. The DSM-III's classification lists (a) the organic mental disorders associated with various kinds of substances; and (b) other disorders associated with these substances. In this classification scheme, each substance does not necessarily give rise to all the possible organic conditions. For example, whereas only one organic state (intoxication) is associated with cocaine, several organic states (intoxication, delirium, delusional disorder, and withdrawal) can be induced by the amphetamines and related stimulants. The meanings of the various substance-induced organic disorders are the same as those described in Spotlight 16.1, for example, amnestic disorder or delirium. Withdrawal or abstinence syndromes, however, have characteristics that are specific to the substance under consideration. Alcohol or heroin, for example, each has a distinct set of typical behaviors and symptoms that arise after termination of long-term use.

The opposite page lists the substance-use disorders, which, according to the DSM-III, are classified as either substance abuse and/or substance dependence. Substance abuse refers to maladaptive behaviors associated with regular use of a substance. It is pathological, distinguished from nonpathological use for medical or recreational purposes, because its use is characterized by behavior patterns that interfere with social, interpersonal, and occupational functioning. For example, cocaine intoxication throughout the day, inability to cut down despite repeated efforts to do so, and financial troubles because of its expense can be called cocaine abuse. Substance abuse is not diagnosed unless the disturbance has been manifested at least one month.

Substance dependence, on the other hand, is characterized by the presence of either tolerance or withdrawal, defined in the usual way, as physiological dependence. Tolerance is evidenced by the increasing amounts of the substance required to produce the desired effect or by a markedly diminished effect with regular use of the same dose; withdrawal is defined as a substance-specific syndrome—abstinence syndrome—following cessation or reduction of regular, long-term use of the substance. Not all the substances, according to this classification, have potential for dependence defined in this physiological sense, but most have potential for psychological dependence because of their reinforcing properties.

Substance-Induced Organic Mental Disorders

Barbiturate or Similarly Acting Sedative or Hypnotic Substances *(Includes minor tranquilizers and hypnotics like chloral hydrate)*	Intoxication Withdrawal Withdrawal delirium Amnestic disorder
Opioid Substances (Heroin and Morphine) *(Includes synthetics with morphine-like action such as methadone)*	Intoxication Withdrawal
Cocaine	Intoxication
Amphetamine or Similarly Acting Sympathomimetic Substances *(Includes substances that have amphetamine-like action such as methylphenidate or "diet pills")*	Intoxication Delirium Delusional disorder Withdrawal
Phencyclidine (PCP) or Similarly Acting Substances	Intoxication Delirium Mixed organic disorder
Hallucinogen substances *(Includes substances such as LSD and mescaline)*	Hallucinosis Delusional disorder Affective disorder
Cannabis (Marijuana and Hashish)	Intoxication Delusional disorder
Tobacco	Withdrawal
Caffeine	Intoxication*

Substance-Use Disorders

Substance Abuse	*Substance Dependence (Tolerance or Withdrawal)*
Barbiturates and hypnotics	Barbiturates and hypnotics
Opioids	Opioids
Amphetamines	Amphetamines
Cannabis	Cannabis
Cocaine	No DSM-III diagnosis
PCP	No DSM-III diagnosis
Hallucinogens	No DSM-III diagnosis
No DSM-III diagnosis	Tobacco

*Caffeine intoxication, a rare condition, is characterized by such signs as restlessness, excitement, insomnia, cardiac arrythmia, psychomotor agitation, and even rambling thought and speech. This organic condition is not referred to again in this chapter.

Who Uses What—Some General Data

Age. Drugs are abused by a staggering number of teenagers. It is estimated that one in six adolescents have heavy drug-related problems, whereas one in eleven adults have such problems (Cummings, 1979). Teenage substance abuse often involves alcohol. Heavy alcohol users, as a matter of fact, are more likely to be abusers of other substances than are light drinkers or nondrinkers (Wechsler and Thum, 1973).

Gender. More males than females use and abuse drugs, but the gap is narrowing, especially among younger people. However, older women are more frequent abusers of barbiturate and sedative substances (mostly, these are prescription drugs) than any other group of people, forming a distinct subgroup not identified with the usual drug subculture (Mercer and Smart, 1974; Suffet and Brotman, 1976).

SES. Up to the early 1960s most drug abusers were found in lower SES groups. Abused substances were largely confined to the opiates, marijuana, and cocaine. With the rise of the "hippie" movement in the 1960s and the introduction of substances such as LSD, drug abuse rapidly spread to the middle classes (McGlothlin, 1975).

Ethnicity. There is a general tendency for black and Hispanic abusers of drugs to do so with heroin and the opiates, whereas white drug abusers tend to use more of the hallucinogens, barbiturates, and amphetamines.

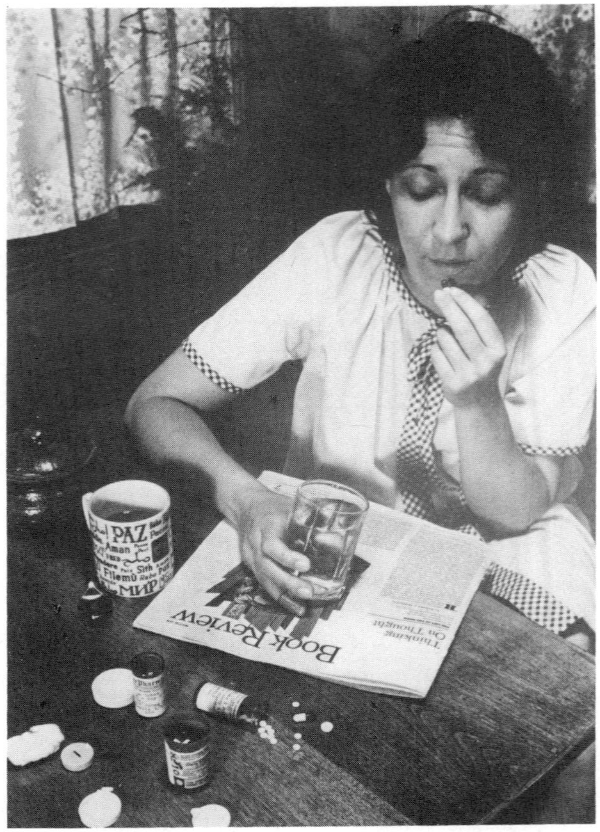

Substance abuse among older people who medicate themselves with "prescription" drugs (for example, barbiturates) is a more common practice than one would suspect, judging by the emphasis in the media on substance abuse by the young. (T. C. Fitzgerald/ The Picture Cube)

Patterns of Drug Abuse

Drug abuse is often *polydrug* abuse. That is, abusers tend to be involved with several substances at the same time, rather than just one. (Lenora, described in Case 17.1, is an example of a polydrug user.) Frequently, alcohol abuse is a partner to other substance abuse. Most heroin addicts before and after treatment are heavy users of alcohol, and about half the patients in alcohol treatment centers are already dependent on other substances (Wechsler and Thum, 1973). In the military, the pattern of polydrug use varies with different regions. For example, barbiturates flourish in Korea; heroin, methaqualone, and amphetamines in Germany; and in the United States it is LSD, cocaine, heroin, and PCP (Weinraub, 1978). Considerations such as these have led some researchers to question the validity of the DSM-III's classification of drug abusers by single substance only.

Are there distinct patterns of use that can be readily identified? One such classification suggests that there are basically three types of drug users: a small group of young people who use many different types of substances but especially the opiates; a larger group of young users involved with such street substances as marijuana, LSD, and cocaine; and an older, middle-class population who medicate themselves with "prescription" substances such as the barbiturates (Douglass, Khavari, and Farber, 1980). Whether such classifications are more meaningful than those based on substances depends on their usefulness in identifying abuser subsamples. Are there underlying differences in these groups in connection with drug-seeking behavior? Would intervention into patterns of drug abuse differ among these samples? Only further research will tell us the answers.

Spotlight 17.2 Commonly Abused Substances: What's In A Name?

Spotlight 17.2 is a classification of the commonly abused substances. The first column lists the generic, chemical names for various substances. The second column lists the natural source or brand or trade name—the pharmaceutical company's label for the substance. Only one brand name for each substance will be presented.

The generic chemicals and their trade names are known on the "street" by many different slang terms, examples of which are also listed here. For example, Tuinal, a trade name for a combination of the generic barbiturate drugs amobarbital and secobarbital, is known on the street, where it is distributed and sold for kicks, as "tooies."

The street glossary can never really be up-to-date or reflect the rich variation of terms that users, especially different subcultures of users (jazz musicians, for example, or suburban teenagers, or ghetto pushers), employ within their own social groups. Outsiders, nonusers, and special types of users (alcoholics, for example, versus heroin users), can even be objectively differentiated by the street words they know and do not know (Haertzen et al., 1979).

In addition to street names for specific substances, the drug subculture also uses a rich language that denotes procedures for getting high and various subjective states associated with substance use. An extremely limited glossary, illustrating some of these words, appears in Spotlight 17.3.

Class or Generic Name	Trade Name or Source	Street Names
Narcotic Analgesics		
opium	poppy plant	tar, black stuff, big O, pin yen, hop, wen shee
morphine	morphine sulfate, a constituent of opium	dope, M, cube juice, hocus, morpho, white stuff, Miss Emma, emsel
heroin	semisynthetic substance derived from morphine	H, hard stuff, horse, junk, shit, skag, smack, doojee, noise, TNT, boy, foolish powder, smeck, schmeck, Harry, pee, duet (also cocaine)
hydromorphone	Diluadid	lords
oxymorphone	Numorphan	blues
meperidine	Demerol	
methadone hydrochloride	Dolophine	dollies, amidone
pentazocine	Talwin	
tincture of opium	paregoric	PO, PG, licorice
cough preparations with codeine	elixir Terpin Hydrate Robitussin A-C	schoolboy, blue velvet, turp Robby, robe, robo, spaghetti sauce
hydrocodone	Hycodan	
oxycodone	Percodan	
Nonnarcotic Analgesics		
propoxyphene	Darvon	

Class or Generic Name	Trade Name or Source	Street Names
Anxiolytics		
chlordiazepoxide	Librium	
diazepam	Valium	
oxazepam	Serax	
chlorprothixene	Taractan	
Central Nervous System Stimulants		lids, uppers, ups, wakeups, eye openers, pep pills
d, di amphetamine	Biphetamine	black beauties, B-20s
amphetamine sulfate	Benzedrine	As, beans, bennies, cartwheels, crossroads, roses, peaches, jelly beans, hearts, whites
amphetamine sulfate/amobarbital	Dexamil	greenies
dextroamphetamine sulfate	Dexedrine	brownies, Christmas trees, spots, dexies, hearts, wakeups, oranges
methamphetamine hydrochloride	Methedrine	Cris, Cristina, bombit, bombida, crank, crystal, meth, speed, splash, crinic
methylphenidate	Ritalin	
cocaine	derived from coca leaves	bernies, Bernice, big C, Carrie, coke, flake, happy dust, ice, snow, lady, girl, gold dust, dream, Corrine, Cecil, nose candy, joy powder, big bloke, stardust, dust, Cholley, heaven dust
Drugs With Hallucinogenic Properties		
d lysergic acid diethylamide (LSD or LSD-25)	synthetic derivative (ergot fungus)	acid, squirrel, pink wedges, sandos, sugar cubes, yellow dimples, Hawaiian sunshine, strawberry field, peace, orange sunshine, California sunshine, domes, microdots, big D, white lightning, sunshine, grape parfait, cupcakes, black magic, chocolate chips, flats, chief, smears
psilocin/psilocybin	mushroom *Psilocybe mexicana)*	business man's acid, magic mushroom
dimethyltryptamine (DMT)	synthetic	DMT, DET, DPT, business man's trip
morning glory seeds	bindweed *(Rivea corymbosa)*	flower power, heavenly blue, pearly gates
mescaline	peyote cactus	barf tea, big chief, buttons, cactus, mesc
methyldimethoxy-ampthetamine (DOM)	synthetic	STP, peace, magic pumpkin, serenity, tranquility
myristicin	nutmeg	MMDA
muscarine	mushroom *(Amanita muscaria)*	fly

Class or Generic Name	Trade Name or Source	Street Names
phencyclidine	Sernyl, Sernylan	angel dust, killer weed, buzz, crystal flakes, crystal weed, cadillac, crystal, crystal joints, dust, hog, PCP, elephant, THC, tic, PeaCe Pills, superjoint, wobble weed, monkey dust, cyclones, goon, horse tranks, KJ, mist, ozone, peace weed, rocket fuel, scuffle, snorts, supergrass, superweed, surfer
Tetrahydrocannabis		
marijuana	cannabis plant (leaves, flowers)	grass, hay, joints, Mary Jane, pot, reefer, jay, boo, bush, Indian hay, Indian bay, griefo, rope, smoke, tea, weed, Acapulco gold, Panama red, dope, hot sticks, gage, stick, keif
hashish	cannabis plant, resin	hash, shit (poor quality), keif
Barbiturates		barbs, candy, dolls, goofers, peanuts, goofballs, GBs, sleepers, stoppers, downers, downs, idiot pills, King Kong pills
amobarbital	Amytal	blue angels, bluebirds, blue devils, blue heavens, blues, lilly, blue dolls, blue tips
pentobarbital	Nembutal	nibies, nebbies, yellow bullets, nembies, nemmies, yellow dolls, yellow jackets, yellow submarines, yellows, yellowbirds
secobarbital	Seconal	bullets, pink ladies, red devils, reds, seccies, seggies, pinks, red birds, red lillies, F-40s, Mexican reds, red dolls
phenobarbital	Luminal	phennies, purple hearts, feenies
amobarbital/ secobarbital	Tuinal	trees, double trouble, rainbows, tootsies, tooies, reds and blues, gorilla pills
Other Sedative Hypnotics		
chloral hydrate	Noctec	Peter, chloral, Mickey, Mickey Finn (mixed with alcohol)
ethclorvynol	Placidyl	
flurazepam	Dalmane	
glutethimide	Doriden	CIBAs, CBs, gorilla pills
methaqualone	Quaalude	sopors, ludes
methyprylon	Noludar	
paraldehyde	Paral	
scopolamine	Sominex	truth serum
Muscle Relaxants		
meprobamate	Miltown	mother's little helper

Class or Generic Name	Trade Name or Source	Street Names
Volatile Solvents and Gases		
benzine	gasoline	
toluol	glue vapor	
carbon tetra-chloride	cleaning fluid	
naphtha	cleaning fluid	scrubwoman's kick
amyl nitrite	amyl nitrite	amys, pears, snappers, poppers
nitrous oxide	nitrous oxide	laughing gas, nitrous

Sources: Adapted from the American Psychiatric Association, *A Psychiatric Glossary,* 1980; Claridge, 1970; Goredetzky and Christian, 1970; Kornetsky, 1976; and Wesson and Smith, 1977.

Spotlight 17.3 Words, Words, Words: Some Examples from the Drug Subculture

acid head heavy user of LSD

bad trip subjective sensations after LSD ingestion that are extremely frightening, panic-inducing

bhang a drink made from the leaves of the Indian hemp plant

coasting the light sleep that follows the immediate effects of heroin, often accompanied by "nodding"

crash, crashing after a "speed" trip or a high from cocaine, the coming down; the withdrawal into sleep, sometimes stupor or coma

cutting mixing a substance with other substances to make it stretch further, a procedure generally used with narcotics

dosing giving someone a strong substance without his or her knowledge

flash, rush generally, the immediate sensations following "mainlining" of a substance, generally a narcotic or stimulant, but also a barbiturate

flashback reappearance of LSD-induced experiences at some time—perhaps months—after the last dose (sometimes called "return trip")

huffing mouth inhalation of a volatile solvent

jag the initial, immediate effects of inhaling vapor from an organic solvent such as airplane glue or cleaning fluid

junkie addicted person, usually to heroin

mainlining intravenous injection of drug, usually heroin

O.D. overdose of a drug, causing coma or death

pot head heavy user of marijuana

pusher a person who sells drugs illegally

shoot, shooting injecting a drug directly into the vein

sniffing, snorting inhalation of a drug, usually cocaine

strung out exhaustion or stupor following excessive use of "speed"; also, addicted—usually to narcotics

trip subjective experiences of LSD ingestion

MARIJUANA

Marijuana, one of the leading recreational substances in this country (second only to alcohol), is comprised of the leaves, stems, and resin of the *Cannabis sativa* plant, which grows wild or is cultivated all over the world. If smoked in a joint (cigarette), marijuana produces a "high" that most people find rather pleasurable. There are hundreds of different kinds of chemicals in the cannabis plant and there are several species, each with different types and strengths of its chief psychoactive, intoxicating chemical—delta-9-tetrahydrocannabinol (THC).

Marijuana is absorbed by the tissues and organs of the body and is transformed into other chemicals (THC metabolites) that can be found in the blood and urine of people who have smoked it up to a week after it is smoked.
These and related chemicals can cross the placental barrier and can be found in mother's milk, although just how it affects fetal development is not entirely clear (Marijuana and health, 1980).

The percent of THC content in street marijuana is so variable that it is difficult to observe people in their natural settings and then draw conclusions about its effects on behavior. Tests of strengths of THC content in confiscated (street) samples indicate that the amount of THC content in street marijuana is increasing rapidly (Marijuana and health, 1980). In 1975, the average THC content was 0.4 percent to rarely more than 1 percent. In 1979, however, the average THC content was about 4 percent and there were samples as high as 5 percent. At one time, hashish ("hash"), another substance derived from the cannabis plant, was stronger than marijuana, with a THC content of about 2 percent. Today, street marijuana is stronger in its psychoactive ingredient than hash. Hash oil, a tarlike extract from the cannabis plant, which is smoked on tobacco in joints, or in glass pipes, contains about 28 percent THC.

Prevalence. Many observers regard marijuana smoking as "embedded" in the American culture (Grinspoon and Bakalar, 1977c; Jessor, 1979). Although 22 million people are probably current users, over 50 million Americans report having used marijuana at least once (For parents only, 1980; Maugh, 1982). Race, SES, and education are not significantly related to marijuana use (although use is slightly higher among the college-educated). Twice as many males than females use marijuana, but the gap is narrowing.

Marijuana is used most frequently in the young adult group (eighteen–twenty-five years), with three out of five people in this age category reporting some use (Marijuana and health, 1980). However, there is a trend for increasingly younger people to try marijuana, and many current users report having smoked marijuana regularly in grade school, before they were twelve years old (Marijuana and health, 1980).

How introduced. Most surveys reach similar conclusions: users report having been introduced to marijuana through social circumstances—social models and friendship patterns, in particular (Jessor, 1979; Kandel, 1974; Marijuana and health, 1980; O'Donnell et al., 1976). Close friends as well

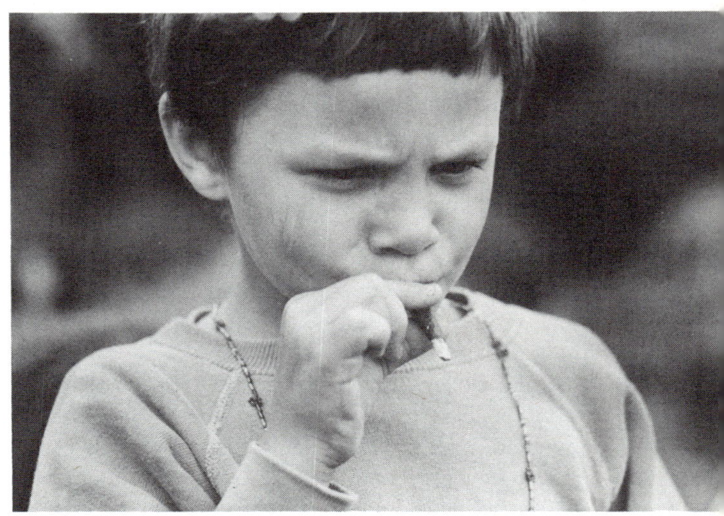

Many current users report having smoked marijuana regularly in grade school. (Nacio Jan Brown/Black Star)

as acquaintances who are admired and respected, or who fill the role of models are generally involved. These social "facilitators" provide reinforcement as well as controls and guidelines for using patterns. (Such social influences, of course, are also important determinants of dress, taste in music, and even sexual attractions.) Clinicians used to think in terms of poor parental models or poor parental controls when considering the question of initial use, but these family variables are probably less important than was once thought to be the case.

Effects. When smoked in moderate doses in "favorable" social settings, marijuana produces mild euphoria and feelings of relaxation, especially in situations in which the smoker is "set" to have a good time. Physical effects include increases in heart and pulse rates, body temperature, and appetite, as well as possible accompanying redness in the eyes and dryness in the mouth and throat. Many users report increased sensory and perceptual acuity as well as heightened sensitivity to music, food, and sex, but these effects have not been experimentally confirmed.

Although level of dose is important, there is evidence that many subjective effects of smoking marijuana depend on the user's expectations, the social setting, and what he or she "knows" about the drug's effects. Many users report, for example, that inexperienced smokers do not get a "high" initially. Only after learning has taken place (and after exposure to the "highs" of others) do some smokers begin to feel and enjoy the effects of smoking marijuana—often learning to discount any discomfort that ingestion of the drug may produce. Thus, seeing others become intoxicated and having fun affects the degree of intoxication that many smokers experience.

High doses of marijuana and long-term heavy use, it is now believed, produce some problems. However, there are some misconceptions concerning adverse effects. One is the presumed connection between marijuana and violence. A review of the empirical literature does not yield support for this association, and there is little evidence that the chemical agents in marijuana produce or increase crime and aggression among smokers (Abel, 1977; Grinspoon and Bakalar, 1977c). Some marijuana users may be violent, but so are some nonusers, and apparently in equal proportion.

A second area of misconception has been referred to as the amotivational syndrome—a pattern of apathy, disinterest, and sluggishness that supposedly arises as a result of heavy, long-term use. Most longitudinal and correlational data suggest that an amotivational pattern, manifested by poor grades, career indecision, and dropping out of school may *precede* heavy marijuana use (Grinspoon and Bakalar, 1977c; Jessor, 1979; Mellinger et al., 1976, 1978) rather than result from it. As a matter of fact, in other cultures—for example Jamaica—heavy users smoke marijuana to produce opposite effects: for energy, stimulation, and *raising* motivational levels.

The following adverse effects of heavy or chronic marijuana use have received some recent attention.

1. Strong doses of marijuana produce heightened levels of intoxication that are associated with lowered motor coordination, some perceptual and sensory disturbances, impairment in judgment, and a decrease in reaction time. For this reason, most experts now consider driving and piloting during acute stages of marijuana intoxication as involving risk to self and others.

2. High levels of intoxication may in some instances produce anxiety reactions, paranoid feelings, and fears of "going crazy." Such responses are rare and occur primarily among inexperienced users and under conditions of fear and negative expectancy (Grinspoon and Bakalar, 1977c). Similarly, people who attempt to "treat" depression or other problems through marijuana use often find that their problems are worsened rather than aided. In extremely rare instances, a psychotic episode can be triggered. Despite these possibilities, most experts agree that marijuana does not directly cause emotional problems.

3. During high levels of intoxication, there may be negative effects on cognitive performance. These areas include attention, thinking, judgment, controlled thinking, short-term (immediate) memory,

the formation of long-term new memories, and time estimation (Carlin et al., 1972; Grinspoon and Bakalar, 1977c; Loftus, 1980; Marijuana and health, 1980; Maugh, 1982). However, long-term users may compensate for or learn how to counteract these effects. This may explain the minimal consequences in these areas among heavy users in Jamaica, Greece, Costa Rica, and our own country (Loftus, 1980; Weckowicz et al., 1975). Moreover, there may be tolerance to long-term marijuana use.

Despite the foregoing, most investigators agree that there are few irreversible, long-term effects of heavy marijuana smoking on intellectual functioning, although there is as yet no conclusive evidence that this is the case (Marijuana and health, 1980).

4. As for physical health consequences of long-term heavy use, a review of evidence to date, despite earlier reports, does not indicate that such use causes chromosomal or brain damage. However, heavy daily use of marijuana does apparently involve some risk in other areas, including lung damage—some of it similar to that involved in tobacco smoking, although a link between cancer and heavy marijuana use has not been established—and some negative effects on reproductive capacities in both males and females, especially in young adults (Marijuana and health, 1980; Maugh, 1982; Reinhold, 1981). Heavy marijuana use is also not recommended for people with impaired heart functions or who are pregnant.

Some benefits. The government has approved of the manufacture of synthetic marijuana pills for use in controlling the nausea and vomiting of some cancer patients that may arise as a result of chemotherapy. At least one state, Connecticut, is allowing physicians to prescribe marijuana cigarettes for the same purpose (Connecticut allows . . . , 1981). It has been found, however, that the pills, which contain several times the amount of THC as does a single joint, are effective in only half or less than half of patients with such complaints, and there may also be some side effects, especially in older patients (Sun, 1980).

For patients with certain types of glaucoma, a disease that involves abnormal pressure within the eye and that can eventually lead to blindness, THC may offer some benefits. The eventual outcome—successful or unsuccessful—of smoking marijuana or applying THC as an eyedrop to reduce pressure in cases of glaucoma is still not absolutely clear, however, nor is it known whether immediate successes will be sustained over longer periods of time.

Tolerance and dependence. Despite most early claims, the literature has begun to indicate that with heavy, regular, long-term use there is tolerance to marijuana, that is, a lowered or diminished response to repeated dosages (Marijuana and health, 1980). Ordinary, social usage of marijuana yields no abstinence syndrome (almost all agree), and there are no reports of such signs even after heavy use (Dimijian, 1978); but the reinforcing qualities of marijuana may lead to compulsive drug-seeking behaviors. Some people feel thus that marijuana has a potential for dependence and abuse.

Decriminalization. For decades, in most states, there have been extremely harsh penalties for the possession of even small amounts of marijuana. Decriminalization—the legal process of reducing these penalties from a crime to a violation—has been adopted by many states. The idea was to make the punishment more commensurate with the crime. In states where there has been decriminalization, possessing small amounts of marijuana for one's own recreational use is considered only a minor infringement of the legal code, equivalent to a traffic violation. Generally, violations apply to amounts of less than an ounce. Punishment for the *sale* of marijuana is being reduced from a felony to a misdemeanor, but again, only if very small amounts are involved. In states where there has been decriminalization, there is no evidence that there has been a rise in marijuana use.

Overview. Although the view that marijuana use leads to serious drug problems such as heroin addiction—the "stepping-stone" hypothesis—is no longer held by many experts, there have been some changed attitudes regarding adverse effects among heavy, long-term users, especially in the light of the sharp increase of the strength of street marijuana.

There are still some contradictory reports of the so-called facts, however. The prevailing view is that moderate, occasional, recreational use of marijuana has negligible effects on physical or psychological health, and that marijuana is probably the least toxic of all the psychoactive drugs. But there is growing belief that people with heart and lung disease, pregnant women, "self-medicators" with emotional problems, and those with emotional disturbance or a history of a "bad" response to other drugs should probably avoid using marijuana, even in moderation (Marijuana and health, 1980; Schmeck, 1979). Yet, firm conclusions about the long-term effects of marijuana still cannot be drawn in the light of meager research evidence (Reinhold, 1982).

HALLUCINOGENS: LSD AND PCP

Some chemical substances have been called hallucinogenic, because subjective effects after using them have been likened to hallucinations. Actually, these effects, especially in early stages of intoxication, are not quite hallucinatory, but they do include various kinds of perceptual, sensory, and time distortions and changes in perception of self and one's own body. These distortions in awareness and perception of reality have generated descriptions of such drugs as "mind-altering," "mind-expanding," "mind-blowing," and "psychedelic."

The hallucinogenic drugs include not only LSD, but also mescaline, an alkaloid derived from the peyote cactus, which grows naturally in the southwest of the United States and parts of Mexico, and psilocybin (found in various types of mushrooms). Additional substances that fall into this category are certain types of synthesized amphetamine derivatives referred to by their chemical names, such as DOM (2,5-dimethoxy-4-methyl ampthetamine, also called STP*), DMT (dimethyltryptamine), MDA (methylenedioxyamphetamine), and DOET (dimethoxy-4-ethylamphetamine).

Pharmacological effects on the central nervous system are dose-related, but many subjective experiences, especially whether it has been a "good" trip or a "bad" trip (see the following discussion) are related to personality factors, expectancy, mood, and the social setting in which the substance is ingested.

* STP are initials taken from the logo, Scientifically Treated Petroleum, but is also said to symbolize: Serendipity, Tranquility, Peace.

LSD (D-lysergic acid diethylamide tartrate)

LSD, no longer a major substance of abuse, is a semisynthetic chemical that, along with several other substances, was first studied in the laboratory to further understand schizophrenia (a method now abandoned). It had been thought that its toxic action produced psychotic-like behaviors and states (hence the label psychotomimetic). Also, some clinicians felt that LSD might be useful in treating people under supervised and controlled conditions, in which it was hoped that inner layers of consciousness could be probed without the usual ego controls and defenses. Although there were some early reports of success in the treating of alcoholism with LSD, such treatment efforts were also abandoned because of unreliable and unsubstantiated findings.

LSD is derived from lysergic acid, which is obtained naturally from a fungus, ergot, found in the seeds of rye and other grass plants.* It is a colorless,

* LSD was first snythesized by A. Hoffman and a colleague in 1938, research chemists at the Sandoz pharmaceutical laboratories in Basel, Switzerland. The synthesis of LSD-25 meant nothing to Hoffman for several years (it had been tested only with animals), until 1943, when he accidentally ingested a small quantity of it and found that he experienced such a variety of sensations and perceptual distortions that he could not continue working. He experimented with doses of LSD a few days later, and then wrote extensively about his predominantly unpleasant experiences—visual distortions, choking sensations, problems in concentration, and other subjective states for which he was essentially unprepared. He found the perceptual distortions and alterations in awareness grotesque and frightening.

odorless, and tasteless powder, whose chemical actions within the central nervous system apparently influence the metabolism of certain neurotransmitters, with a consequent disruption of normal sensory-perceptual processing, especially within the visual processing system of the brain. Many of the bizarre subjective experiences with these and similar substances result from such distortion in the processing of sensory input. That some visual (afferent) sensory information is necessary for these effects is suggested by the fact that LSD apparently does not induce visual distortions in blind people, and blindfolded people experience fewer visual distortions than subjects who are not blindfolded (Tarshis, 1972).

Effects. LSD is usually ingested in tablet form with food or liquid (typically, a dose is from 50 to 200 micrograms; a microgram is 1/1000th of a milligram or 1/1,000,000th of a gram). Its effects, which last from four to ten hours after ingestion, begin to be felt in about forty minutes. Physically, there is pupillary dilation, rapid heart beat, a rise in blood pressure and temperature, tremors, incoordination,

Spotlight 17.4 A Quest for the New Consciousness—Turn On, Tune In, and Drop Out

Timothy Leary, an instructor at Harvard, began his LSD voyage on a legitimate scholarly basis in 1960, when he initiated an exploration of the effects of psilocybin—a hallucinogenic drug—on changing the values of prisoners in a Massachusetts facility. Soon he was experimenting with psilocybin and LSD with himself and a group of students as subjects. Harvard and the media, supported by the zeal of Leary and his followers, soon created a national figure of Leary, about whom an aura of messianic leadership developed. Leary was asked to leave Harvard in 1963, but he was already well established as a hero on campuses all over—as he and students sought answers to such questions as, "What is life all about?" and "What is our true essence?"

Leary's popular image was bolstered by flamboyant followers, many of whom were also dropouts from academia. One of these people was Richard Alpert, now known as Baba Ram Dass, whose transformation from a Harvard academic into a follower of the sacred life is summarized in his book *Be Here Now* (1971).

Alpert describes his first experience with psilocybin—in initiation into a turn in his life that ended with heavy LSD use—in this way:

Sweat broke out on my forehead. I wasn't at all sure I could do without being Richard Alpert. Did that mean I'd have amnesia? Was that what this drug was going to do to me? Would it be permanent? . . . As I looked down at my legs for reassurance, I could see nothing below the kneecaps, and slowly, now to my horror, I saw the progressive disappearance of limbs and then torso, until all I could see with my eyes open was the couch on which I sat. A scream formed in my throat. I felt that I must be dying since there was nothing in my universe that led me to believe in life after leaving the body. . . . The panic mounted, adrenalin shot through my system—my mouth became dry, but along with this, a voice sounded inside—inside what, I don't know—an intimate voice asked very quietly, and rather jocularly it seemed to me, considering how distraught I was," . . . but who's minding the store?"

When I could finally focus on the question, I realized that although everything by which I knew myself, even my body and this life itself, was gone, still I was fully aware! Not only that, but this aware "I" was watching the entire drama, including the panic, with calm compassion.

Instantly, with this recognition, I felt a new kind of calmness—one of a profundity never experienced before. I had just found that "I," that scanning device—that point—that essence—that place beyond. A place where "I" existed

independent of social and physical identity. That which was I was beyond Life and Death. . . . It was a voice inside that spoke truth. I recognized it, was one with it, and felt as if my entire life of looking to the outside world for reassurance . . . was over. Now I need only look within to that place where I Knew.

Seventh page of foreword, Be Here Now.

Alpert's search for "truth" brought him to India and into contact with holy men, Zen Buddhism, and his guru, Maharaj-Ji, leading him, he claimed, to a state of "cosmic consciousness." Many others followed his path, "dropping out" to look inward for important answers to important questions.

Today, LSD has lost its glitter—its power to influence life styles and to uproot people from their ordinary surroundings. It is no longer the medium sought by seekers of cosmic truths. What, if anything, is taking its place?

and sweating. LSD is metabolized within the body almost entirely and very little is excreted. There is no indication of either psychological or physical dependence, and there are few reinforcing highs or euphoric states created by this and similar substances.

The effects of LSD are experienced while the subject is fully alert and conscious and include various perceptual and sensory changes, as noted, such as overattention to details, distortions of body image, visual sensations that take on patterned, geometric qualities, synesthesias ("mixed" perceptions—for example, seeing colors when hearing certain sounds), and often a sense of depersonalization—being outside of one's own body, as if floating in space, away and apart from oneself. Although there might be some tactile and taste changes, there are few olfactory and auditory effects.

The "acid heads" of the 1960s who used LSD for "mind-expanding" purposes spoke of oneness with the world, loss of ego and body boundaries, increased understanding of cosmic issues about life, mystical ecstasy, and a sense of deep understanding of self. Users also proclaimed the brilliance and intensity of the visual and perceptual experiences this drug induced and of the great impact on one's aesthetic responses to one's world. Some users also talked of increased creativity, but there is little evidence for this (Grinspoon and Bakalar, 1979b)

No wonder then that such "psychedelic" claims were not sought by the poor in the ghetto. Here heroin, with its calm and its retreat from woe, continued to be king.

Some adverse effects: myth and reality. The history of LSD is closely intertwined with the hippie movement and the 1960s. The media, word-of-mouth, concerned parents, and the movement itself allowed many rumors about the effects of LSD to flourish. LSD was paired with heightened levels of consciousness and awareness, self-discovery, and mood expansion; also religious cults, Eastern religions, unrest among youth, and rock festivals. But its name was also associated with permanent personality change, brain damage, psychotic states, homicide, and genetic abnormalities. There were reports of suicides or accidental deaths during trips; of people jumping off roofs, or of staring into the sun and becoming permanently blind. There were also reports of intense panic reactions—fears of going insane—and of frightening "flashbacks" (see the following discussion).

It soon became clear that such reports were not only inconsistent but also not always reliable and that there were wide individual differences in tolerance for various subjective experiences during a trip. Although some people describe great feelings of discomfort, unpleasantness, or anxiety, others do not. Nevertheless, some generalizations about reported negative effects can be made:

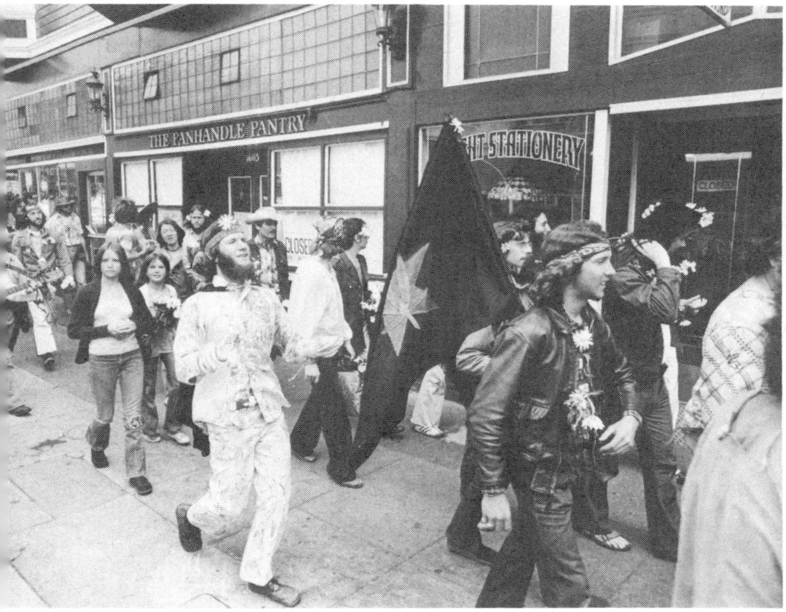

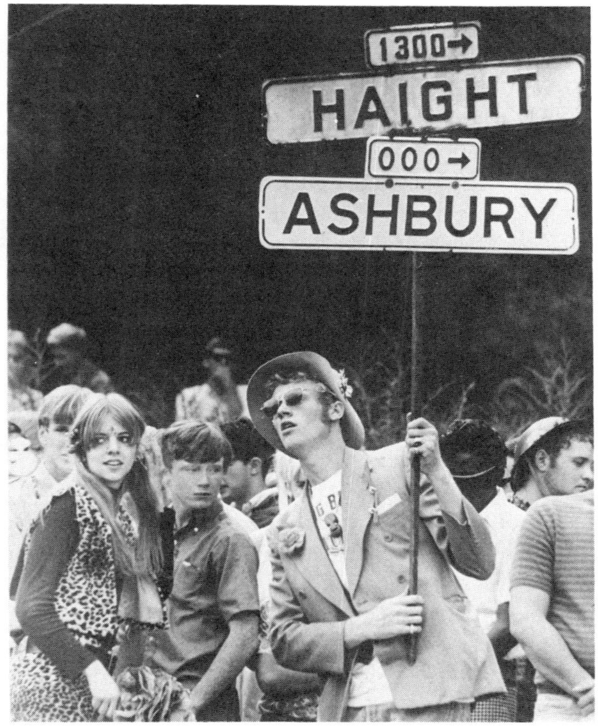

San Francisco's Haight-Ashbury area was a center for hippies, drugs, "flower children," costumes, and rock music in the 1960s and early 1970s. (Above: Gregg Mancuso/Stock, Boston. Right: Michael C. Hayman/Stock, Boston)

1. The most frequent adverse effect is that of anxiety, terror, and panic, accompanied by fears of "losing one's mind," or "losing control." Despair, depression, guilt, and strong and painful emotional responses are also reported. Clinical and empirical concensus is that poorly adjusted users are more likely to have adverse reactions than adjusted users (Barr et al., 1972; Naditch, 1975a,b). Individual differences in personality and adjustment are not the only influences in adverse responses, however, for the expectancy, setting, and dosage levels all interact with personality factors to produce the subjective experiences during an LSD trip.

2. Psychotic states produced as a transitory response to LSD ingestion—actual "breaks with reality" in the form of delusions or a manic or depressive episode—are rare. Can LSD trigger a long-term, chronic psychosis? Yes, but this too is quite infrequent. Most experts believe that such pathology occurs only in those who are predisposed to a psychotic "break" (Grinspoon and Bakalar, 1979b).

3. Suicide, accidents, and violence are extremely rare responses to the LSD experience, their frequency exaggerated by the media and street talk.

4. Evidence for genetic damage as a result of heavy LSD use is minimal: offspring of LSD users apparently show no more defects than offspring of nonusers and there is no evidence of chromosomal damage as a result of LSD ingestion (Dishotsky et al., 1971; Grinspoon and Bakalar, 1979b). However, there is still controversy in this area in the light of findings from studies with animals (Tarshis, 1972).

5. Some heavy users may show signs of mental impairment, for example, attention and concentration problems and difficulties in making abstractions; but most of the literature indicates that these differences disappear when heavy use ceases.

6. Flashbacks refer to the involuntary reap-

pearance of some aspects of an LSD trip weeks or months after the last dose. They can be extremely frightening, sometimes even causing panic reactions. Flashbacks are not due to the presence of LSD in the body, for all traces of this substance disappear within several hours after the last dose. It is estimated that up to one-fourth of heavy users experience flashbacks (Grinspoon and Bakalar, 1979b), but many claim that this overestimates actual incidence.

Flashbacks can be triggered by substances such as marijuana or by various emotional or bodily states (stress, medication, or anxiety, for example). They can be mild or intense, can disappear in a few seconds, or can last for hours.

There is still little understanding of why flashbacks occur. Explanations for flashbacks might lie in the pharmacological action in certain people in whom threshold for imagery is now lowered or attentional focus on certain stimuli now enhanced.

Other explanations are that flashbackers differ from nonflashbackers in various personal traits. For example, some studies have shown that flashbackers are "looser" in thinking strategies, less able to cope with stress, and more likely to have experienced acute adverse reactions while under the influence of LSD than nonflashbackers (Heaton and Victor, 1976; Naditch and Fenwick, 1977). One study found that flashbackers are more suggestible and tend to become more engrossed in role-playing than nonflashbackers (Matefy, 1980). This finding lends support to the hypothesis that flashbackers have a greater learned tendency than nonflashbackers to reenact their drug experiences when they are in situations that remind them of those that existed during their LSD trips.

In any event, the study of flashbacks and the reason for them opens up intriguing possibilities for further understanding certain perplexing subjective experiences related to drug use not "explainable" by the usual hypotheses.

Overall, personality factors, the substance itself and its chemical action, expectancy, and the social setting are now known to be determinants of the LSD experience. For some people, a trip can be extremely unpleasant. These may be the unstable people with "fragile" personalities and some predisposition to pathology. Because there are such risks, as well as some possible long-range effects that may still be unknown, most drug abuse experts do not favor the use of LSD except under well-controlled conditions or for a well-needed scientific purpose. An abstinence syndrome has not been reported for LSD, and although there is rapid development of tolerance, it disappears as soon as LSD is discontinued (Dimijian, 1978).

Phencyclidine (PCP)

PCP's reputation as a "horror" drug—the "ultimate monster drug"—paired with danger, violence, suicide, bizarre behavior, and psychosis, has been fed by word-of-mouth as well as by sensational stories in the press and other media. However, these presumed associations are probably based on extremely rare instances (Feldman et al., 1979).

History of PCP use. In the mid-1950s, one of the pharmaceutical companies began research with phencyclidine, a chemical that had been synthesized about thirty years earlier. It seemed to have potential as an anesthetic, for early animal work indicated that it had fewer side effects than the usual anesthetics. By the mid-1960s, however, the company that had been responsible for its development and subsequent experimental work with humans discontinued research with this chemical because of its profound psychological side effects with experimental post-operative patients (for example, delirium, hallucinations, agitation, and several other "schizophrenic-like" symptoms).

In the late 1960s, phencyclidine appeared in hippie communities (Haight-Ashbury in San Francisco and the East Village in New York City) as PCP—also known as PeaCe Pill or hog. According to Pittel and Oppedahl (1979), PCP was sometimes sold under more "acceptable" names such as mescaline or LSD, a so-called drug of deception. Many experts claim, however, that users were not truly being deceived. For, despite its bad reputation on the street, it soon became a drug of choice for many people—becoming quite popular in the early to mid-1970s as a matter of fact (Feldman et al., 1979).

Users of PCP. PCP users tend to be predominantly white, young, and from lower or middle-class backgrounds (Abelson et al., 1977; Feldman et al., 1979). Judging from data from one state, PCP use is fairly widespread. In 1977–78, about 15 to 18 percent of New York State's teenagers had tried PCP at least once; but only about one in 100 people older than twenty-six years of age reported having done so. Currently, there seems to be a decrease in new users, and because most regular PCP users eventually quit, there is an overall decline in its popularity (Abelson et al., 1977; Feldman et al., 1979; Molotsky, 1978; and Reinhold, 1981).

*Effects.** The method of ingesting PCP has changed since the early days, when it was swallowed as a pill. Today it is generally smoked (with parsley, tobacco, marijuana, or mint leaves), snorted, or put into beer. If there is oral ingestion, effects begin to be felt within an hour. Otherwise, effects are felt within a matter of minutes. Pharmacologically, PCP's effects on the body include elevated blood pressure, nystagmus (vertical and horizontal), numbness, higher threshold to pain, increased salivation and perspiration, incoordination in voluntary action, and difficulties in speech.

PCP's pharmacological properties apparently interfere with feedback from stimuli within one's own body (proprioceptive distortions) so that there are sensory disturbances while moving. These sensory and perceptual impressions create misperceptions and body image changes resulting in various bizarre, "out-of-body" sensations, a sense of estrangement and unreality ("losing one's identity"), and, as dosages increase, thought disorganization, hallucinations, inability to maintain a set, and speech and language difficulties. Some PCP users report that they are among the "living dead" or that they are dying. Although these effects are dose-related, set, expectancy, and the positive or negative social context—all familiar variables—play an extremely influential role in how all this is actually experienced, either as an exciting, "way-out" experience or as a terrifyingly bad trip with anxiety or extreme agitation.

The successive stages of intoxication are fairly well identified on the street. They are:

Buzzed refers to a mild euphoria, a "floaty" feeling, and disinhibition that nevertheless permits the user to put up a good front while attending school or working.

Wasted, according to some users, is the feeling of being invisible, isolated, with a body-wide anesthetic effect—a kind of numbness. Users speak of "shrinking legs" and, when walking, of a sensation that makes the ground feel spongy. The speech is slurred and overall coordination is impaired, but some users report that their thought processes are quickened. Many users also report "out-of-body" experiences. There are sensory and perceptual distortions such as sense of slowed time and synesthesias, and mood changes (for example, irritability, suspiciousness). In some instances, there may be agitation.

Ozoned describes the stage in which there is incoherence, muscle rigidity, immobility (catalepsy), or near stupor—but subjective reports are that there is still consciousness.

Overdosed applies to a level of drug ingestion in which there is loss of consciousness, perhaps convulsions, and a risk of death as a result of respiratory inhibition.

Burned out or *spacey* applies to the long-range effects of heavy, chronic PCP use in which users are incoherent and show disorientation, some memory loss, and thought distortions (Feldman et al., 1979). These states are not sought-after results and have low status among users.

Why is PCP used? Many PCP users are aware of PCP as a powerful "mind-blowing" drug with certain risks. Some experts claim that it is this very risk factor—the street reputation of danger—that lies behind the popularity of PCP in some of the big

* Much of the material in this section is derived from Domino and Luby, (1973); DSM-III; Feldman et al., (1979); Pittell and Oppedahl (1979), and Walters (1979).

cities. It is regarded as a "challenge" and if one can deal with it, one can achieve some status among one's peers as someone who can handle a powerful drug in a "macho" way—without becoming "ozoned," or overdosed, "burned out." These status-seeking maneuvers, nevertheless, have recently lost their glitter, according to Feldman et al., (1979), because PCP's risks are now recognized on the street. Today, PCP is often assigned a place (with polydrug users) among more "controllable" drugs that have a more palatable reputation (National Institute on Drug Abuse, 1978).

Even so, the extent of PCP's negative reputation, for example, in the media, surprises regular users, especially in connection with its association with violence (Feldman et al., 1979). Users believe that the powerful effects of PCP actually militate against violence and aggression. They claim that it is generally the *user* who is injured, rather than the outsider, possibly because of panic or an ensuing struggle when authorities try to restrain a user. Many experts also claim that if there is violence, it is because there is a pattern of aggression—a socially acceptable set of deviant behaviors—that precedes, rather than follows, PCP use.

The development of tolerance or the presence of an abstinence syndrome has not been reported in connection with PCP use (Dimijian, 1978).

STIMULANTS

Amphetamines

The amphetamines and related chemicals include a large class of synthetically produced central-nervous-system stimulant substances with many legally allowable uses (for example, as energizers, as antidepressants, or as appetite suppressants). The amphetamines—dextroamphetamines, methamphetamines ("speed"), together with methylphenidate (Ritalin)—fall into this class of drugs. These and similar chemicals are legally manufactured in pill form by the billions, for distribution through medical prescription. In 1967, 31 million legal prescriptions for stimulants were written and in 1971, eight billion pills were legally produced in the United States (Ellinwood, 1974).

Today, widespread medical use of the amphetamines has been challenged. Its potential for abuse is so well known that its production has been dramatically curtailed. Even so, only a few years ago, 5 million prescriptions for amphetamines were still being written, and over five million dosage units were stolen from pharmacies (Ellinwood, 1979).

Who uses amphetamines? Taken orally or intravenously for nonmedical purposes, amphetamines are second only to marijuana and alcohol as a leading drug of abuse (Johnson et al., 1977). The amphetamines are abused by many people who are not part of any special drug subculture, largely for self-medicating purposes to get through a boring day's work, stay awake for studying or crosscountry truckdriving, or for an "up" performance on the stage as a singer or actor. Fighting depression or energizing one's self rather than the recreational "feeling good" is the motivation among a large number of such users. In this group of self-medicating people, women of eighteen to thirty-four years of age are overrepresented (Chambers and Griffey, 1975; Ellinwood, 1974).

Among the relatively large number of amphetamine users (in the early 1970s, about six million people had used an amphetamine, according to one estimate, and in 1981, this number had increased appreciably, Chambers and Griffey, 1975; Reinhold, 1981), there is another abusing group, motivated chiefly by recreational purposes. This type of user was first "turned on" to amphetamines in the mid-1960s in this country and tended to come from a young, middle-class population with no criminal record or past history of narcotics abuse (Grinspoon and Hedblom, 1975). Today, a rising number of such abusers claim that they use amphetamines "to get through the day" or to "lose weight" rather than to get high (Reinhold, 1981), an interesting trend that should be watched.

Reinforcing effects. Users of amphetamines describe their effects as extremely reinforcing: a sense of well-being, alertness, euphoria, exhilaration, energy, and excitement, along with a lift from boredom, fatigue, and depression. There is also heightened activity, a sense of mastery, and an accompanying social aggressiveness. Amphetamines, like cocaine, are extremely reinforcing even among animals (monkeys or rats), who will voluntarily work (press a lever, for example) for indefinite periods until they die in order to ingest intravenously administered stimulants.

Patterns of abuse. As early as the 1960s, amphetamines were already used in a form other than pills—intravenously injected by the "speed freaks" who preferred its immediate effects ("rush" or "flash") to the longer-lasting energized high a slower acting pill produces. A speed freak might "shoot up" several times daily, and if on a binge or speed "run" of several days, there is little or no sleep or food. Such runs are followed by a "crash," during which the abuser may shoot up again, to avoid the anguish of "coming down."

Whether ingested orally or intravenously, many abusers tend to combine speed with other drugs, for example, some of the depressants and tranquilizers. Alcohol with or preceding amphetamine ingestion, or amphetamines as a pick-me-up after tranquilizers or alcohol is a common pattern of abuse. Another pattern is to "mainline" (inject intravenously) speed to supplement the effects of methadone or poor-quality heroin (Green et al., 1973).

Adverse effects. In extreme instances of abuse, there are many adverse effects which vary with manner of ingestion, level of dosage, and the frequency of ingestion. But even with moderate usage, amphetamines often provide a deceptive "high"—a feeling that there is great intellectual power, physical capacity, and personal charisma. Although performance actually might be improved on simple tasks, people high on speed often do poorly on more complex tasks because of anxiety, motor restlessness, and poor judgment.

Excessive amphetamine use can produce an acute toxic stage characterized by psychomotor agitation, grandiosity, loquacity, suspiciousness, aggressiveness, and impaired judgment. Physically, there is tachycardia (rapid heart beat), elevated blood pressure, and pupillary dilation; also, nausea and vomiting. There may be delirium or hallucinations that can last for several hours (DSM-III; Ellinwood, 1979).

Occurring less often is the so-called amphetamine psychosis which may arise as a consequence of excessive, chronic use of amphetamines by "speed freaks." Characteristic behaviors in this syndrome are rapid speech, religiosity, grandiosity, repetitive, meaningless activity, excitement, suspiciousness, paranoid ideation, and aggressiveness. These psychotic episodes occur less often than one might infer from descriptions in the literature, but related effects can last for years (Ellinwood, 1974).

There is some speculation that severe pathology such as an amphetamine psychosis can arise when there are dopamine, norepinephrine or other neurochemical imbalances (excesses and deficits) in the brain and that individual susceptibility to such states are reflections of variations among people in the nature of these biochemical systems (Grinspoon and Hedblom, 1975), hypotheses that offer exciting possibilities for future research.

The crash (or abstinence syndrome) after a run is a period of very intense suffering. Sleep may be required for a few days. Generally, people undergoing a crash experience severe depression, disturbed sleep with increased dreaming, exhaustion, and extreme irritability, resulting in part from the overactivity, overstimulation, and heightened responsiveness during the run. Observers of crash syndromes in one clinic categorized the dominant patterns into types: extreme anxiety; exhaustion syndrome; prolonged depression; a prolonged hallucinatory episode; and amphetamine psychosis.

A young man who had been introduced to amphetamines at college in the early 1970s described the crash in this way:

Of course, there's another very important negative factor about speed that comes whenever you use it, and that's the crash. Com-

ing off speed, or crashing, is one of the most uncomfortable, if not painful things I've ever gone through. It hasn't been too bad when I only take one dose, but if I continue to speed by taking more pills when the first wears off, when I finally do stop, it causes an intense crash that makes my body feel terrible and is emotionally trying. The crash can last several hours itself, and by that time I usually regret ever taking the speed at all and promise myself never to do it again. . . .

People I know . . . go through incredibly bad feelings coming off the drug after a long period of use. The time involved would probably average two days or so. The worst case of crashing that I knew of was a female friend of mine who would speed for long periods and go without sleep several nights in a row. When she finally crashed, she became almost impossible to be around, because her mood would become so bad. . . . The feeling of insanity, even in my case, never seemed very far away. Only a little more intensity, a little more pain, would seem to separate me from losing control over myself.

(Grinspoon and Hedblom, 1975, pp. 36–37)

The amphetamines have enormous capacity for abuse: there is physical dependence (chiefly tolerance effects, rather than an abstinence syndrome, according to Dimijian [1978]) as well as the immensely reinforcing properties that were previously described. Many experts claim that it is the latter, rather than the former, qualities that contain the abuse potential (see Ellinwood, 1979).

Cocaine

Cocaine, in purified form, has been isolated from the leaves of the coca plant,* grown in the Andes Mountains of South America, for only about 100 years. But the psychoactive (stimulant) properties in

* Not to be confused with the cacao tree from which the beverage cocoa is derived. Cocaine and cocoa are chemically unrelated substances.

Spotlight 17.5 Some Myths: The Amphetamines, Crime, and Sexuality

1. There is little empirical evidence that amphetamine abuse and criminal activity are linked causally, although not all are in agreement with this generalization (see Smith, 1969). By and large, these data—and they include Japanese and Swedish studies—indicate that young lower-class male abusers of amphetamines may tend to get involved in criminal activity, but that the pattern of antisocial behavior preceded the abuse. It has been suggested that amphetamine abuse and crime among abusers grew out of the similar social contexts such as poverty, social disorganization, delinquent or deviant life style, thrill-seeking patterns, and so on (Allen et al., 1975; Ellinwood, 1974; Greenberg, 1976).

In rare incidents, there may be an act of violence or aggression in the context of an amphetamine psychosis because of a "misinterpretation of the sensory flood" in the context of psychomotor stimulation (Grinspoon and Hedblom, 1975). This may be a response to some paranoid fantasy. In general, however, most of the empirical evidence suggests that even high dosages of amphetamine bear no relationship to aggressive or criminal activity (Greene et al., 1973).

2. Another myth is the presumed heightening of sexuality as a result of amphetamine use. Users' description of the acutely pleasurable "rush" after an intravenous injection of speed is sometimes described in sexual terms as a "total body orgasm," thus adding to the myth. In actuality, sexuality and sexual performance can either be increased or decreased because of expectancy and belief, rather than as a result of the pharmacological action of the chemical substance (Grinspoon and Hedblom, 1975).

the leaves have been recognized for centuries. Bolivian and Peruvian Indians have chewed or brewed the leaves of the coca plant for generations following long-standing cultural and religious traditions (DuPont, 1977). Today, millions of poor South Americans chew coca leaves for energy, a lift to fight fatigue (just as we drink coffee), and squelching hunger pangs. Pure cocaine, however is 50 to 100 times more powerful than the ingredient in the coca leaf.

The use of cocaine as a strictly recreational substance is relatively recent, as is its illegal status. Cocaine was found everywhere in the late nineteenth and early twentieth centuries—in soda pop or in patent medicines that were offered as a cure for practically everything, including loss of sexual desire (Grinspoon and Bakalar, 1976; 1977a,b). In the 1880s, cocaine was one of the ingredients in Coca Cola (banned after 1903). Even Freud, at about this time, experimented with cocaine, with himself and a friend as subjects. The friend was a morphine addict and Freud wished to treat him with cocaine. But Freud obviously enjoyed the exhilaration that he himself felt as he studied its possible use as an anti-depressant and as an increasor of energy (Byck, 1975).

Cocaine is sold as a white powder containing other ingredients, for example, sugar. It is a high-status, extremely expensive luxury drug with a "good reputation" of having few adverse effects. Cocaine is vigorously sniffed or snorted but can also be applied to the nasal membranes; more infrequently, it can be smoked or injected under the skin or into the veins (sometimes with heroin). Its chemicals can be absorbed directly into the bloodstream from the nasal membranes.

Cocaine is becoming one of the most popular of the recreational drugs, with a large number of drug users stating that it is their preferred substance (Reinhold, 1981). More than ten million people and about 20 percent of eighteen-to-twenty-five-year-olds have used cocaine at least once (Abelson et al, 1977). Adults report greater experience with cocaine than do younger people, probably because of its expense.

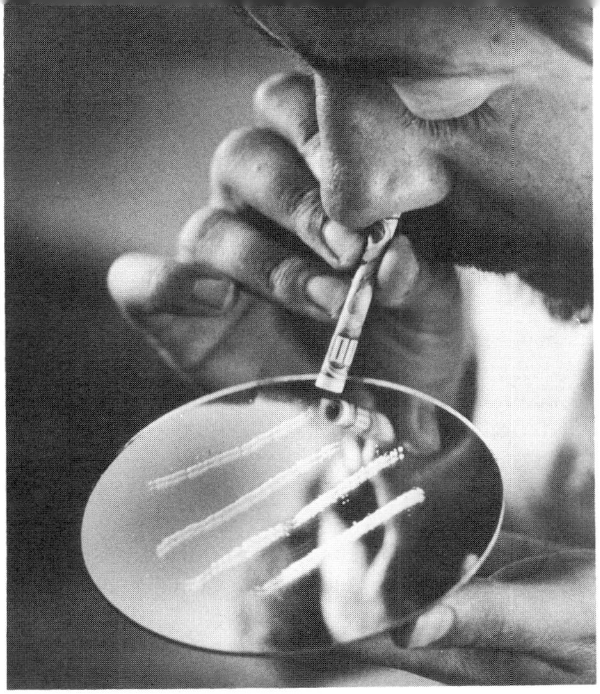

Snorting cocaine. (© Joel Gordon 1980)

Effects. Knowledge about the effects of cocaine is obtained from many sources, including clinical observations, experimental findings (frequently with animals), and reports from the "street" (see Table 17.1). Many reported effects are heightened or otherwise modified by expectancy factors and the social setting in which it is ingested (Van Dyke and Byck, 1982).

The subjective effects of cocaine are described as a short-lived surge of euphoria and heightened energy level, accompanied by feelings of power and mastery, adeptness, and confidence. Accompanying these extremely reinforcing subjective states are objectively recorded physiological changes that include rise in heart rate, blood pressure, respiratory rate, body temperature, and metabolic rate, dilation of the pupils, and constriction of peripheral blood vessels (Fischman et al., 1976; Grinspoon and Bakalar, 1979a; Resnick et al., 1977).

Cocaine leaves little tell-tale signs in the system. Its effects, which are not as long-lasting as is the case for the amphetamines, disappear fairly rapidly, so that another dose must be taken to continue the high. Heavy cocaine use irritates or otherwise damages the mucous membranes of the nasal passage and there is sometimes a runny or clogged

Table 17.1 Reported Effects of Cocaine and Source of Reports

Reported Effects	Source
Local anesthesia	Clinical, experimental, street knowledge
Heart rate increases	Clinical and experimental
Blood pressure increases	Clinical and experimental
Alertness increases; drowsiness decreases	Street knowledge
Sleep decreases	Case material and street knowledge
Appetite decreases	Case material and street knowledge
Creativity increases	Street knowledge
Mood is raised in normal people	Experimental, case material, street knowledge
Mood is raised, mood is lowered in depressed people	Clinical
There is a "crash" after heavy use	Case material, street knowledge
Physical performance enhanced in normals	Street knowledge
Physical performance enhanced if user is tired	Case material, street knowledge
Sexual performance and drive reported increased or decreased	Street knowledge
Aggression reported increased or decreased	Street knowledge
Cocaine is reinforcing—there is drug-seeking behavior	Clinical, street knowledge
There is no tolerance effect	Case material, street knowledge
There is no withdrawal syndrome	Street knowledge
There may be toxic effects such as arrhythmias (abnormal heart rhythm), convulsions	Case material
With abuse, there may be psychosis	Case material, street knowledge
With abuse, there may be perforation of nasal septum	Case material, street knowledge

Source: From Byck and Van Dyke, 1977.

nose that accompanies the irritation. Rarely, there may be actual perforation of the wall of cartilage between the nostrils. When snorted, cocaine produces a numbing sensation in the nose and reduces taste sensation.

Abuse and consequences of excessive use. Heavy, but intermittent, use generally yields few undesirable effects. However, the "coming down" or "crash" may be similar to that for the amphetamines: irritability, depression, extreme fatigue, or anxiety.

Daily, heavy use frequently affects eating and sleeping patterns, and can create interpersonal and financial problems. There may be difficulties in concentration, paranoid ideation, grandiosity, excessive loquaciousness and excitement, compulsive activity like scribbling ("graphomania"), mood changes (from extreme elation to anger and depression), and physical debilitation due to loss of weight, sleeplessness, and high level of autonomic nervous system activity.

With continued, chronic ingestion, hallucinations can occur along with hyperventilation (excessively rapid and deep breath), convulsions, coma, and death. These states are extremely rare, for cocaine use is mostly a recreational activity and its expense forces it to remain a drug with few daily, heavy users except among the very affluent (Byck and Van Dyke, 1977, Grinspoon and Bakalar, 1979a; Resnick et al., 1977; Siegel, 1977).

Street talk has it (as with amphetamines) that there is an increase of sexual interest and enhancement of sexual performance as a result of cocaine use. This is hearsay, not rooted in empirical evidence; but expectancy factors and the mystique of cocaine as the "aphrodisiac for the rich" may contribute to these purported effects. Heavy use, on the other hand, actually reduces sexual drive (Grinspoon and Bakalar, 1979a).

Tolerance and an abstinence syndrome are not associated with cocaine use (Dimijian, 1978). However, cocaine is one of the most reinforcing drugs we know in animals and humans (Petersen and Stillman, 1977). Animals will ingest unlimited intravenously administered cocaine on a voluntary basis until death occurs. Many people turn to cocaine again and again because of its extremely enjoyable qualities—the subjective sense of euphoria—to counteract lassitude, boredom, and depression that may arise after its effects wear off, even claiming they "crave" it. In this sense, then, we can speak of strong psychological dependence.

BARBITURATES AND SIMILARLY ACTING SEDATIVES OR HYPNOTICS

As for a general class, the barbiturate substances discussed in this section such as phenobarbital, seconal, and secobarbital, as well as nonbarbiturate substances such as chloral hydrate and methaqualone (Quaalude) are central nervous system depressants. They have been legally prescribed for decades for inducing sleep or relaxation, controlling seizures, or reducing anxiety (Wesson and Smith, 1977). Although in the early 1970s their effectiveness as sleeping aids was seriously challenged and their potential for inducing physical dependence acknowledged, barbiturates are still among the most frequently prescribed psychoactive drugs in this country. They are also among the most frequently abused substances: with or without alcohol—the former is often a lethal combination, for the drunk barbiturate user may forget how many "barbs" or how many drinks he or she has taken—barbiturate use has been associated with thousands of deaths each year as a result of overdoses or of deliberate suicide.

Barbiturate users, like stimulant users, fall into two categories. First there is a large group of over-thirty people, mostly females, estimated to number among the millions, who take these drugs with or without alcohol to deal with tension and anxiety, blank out the stresses of daily living, or reduce insomnia. This type of drug user often first become acquainted with barbiturates through a medical prescription. Such abusers rarely participate in the so-called drug subculture.

A second group of abusers is comprised mostly of males in their teens or twenties who use barbiturates to get "high"—for kicks and recreational, rather than self-medicating, purposes. Many of these people are polydrug users; often alcohol is the other substance. Sometimes, the barbiturate is used to offset the effects of a speed run, for example, agitation, insomnia, or paranoid feelings. Among this group are the "barb freaks" who intravenously inject ("mainline") these substances, dissolved in water, for the "rush"—an immediate, all-over, warm, relaxed feeling. The popularity of this method of ingesting barbiturates has waned, however.

How these substances work. If orally ingested, barbiturates are rapidly absorbed into the bloodstream; alcohol aids in the speed with which this happens (a synergistic effect). If injected, barbiturates cross the blood-brain barrier within one minute. The central nervous system is the primary site affected by barbiturates, and the essential effect is depression, a slowing down of responses. The extent of the depressant action depends on the substance, dosage, whether or not it was injected or orally ingested, and the chemical and emotional state of the user (Wesson and Smith, 1977).

Effects. Immediate effects are subjectively experienced as calming, relaxing, and reducing tension. The barbiturates can also induce euphoria much like that of alcohol, accompanied by "disinhibition." Disinhibition euphoria—a "high" of loquacity, openness, and sociability—is often the subjective effect sought after and is frequently obtained in social settings such as a party.

As ingestion continues, most of these substances result in a highly intoxicated state with slurred speech, incoordination, slowed-down responses, poor judgment, attention and memory difficulties, nystagmus, respiratory depression, and sleepiness. If ingestion is continued further, there is stupor, coma, and death.

How can a drug have seemingly opposite effects? How is it possible for drugs that are used to induce sleep, reduce anxiety, slow one down, and relax also to be sought for *opposite* effects such as euphoria and disinhibition? The answer lies not only in the substance's pharmacological action in the central nervous system, which indeed does produce some disinhibitory effects, but also in how a drug is perceived. If a pleasurable high is anticipated, others around us are behaving accordingly, and we are in an expectant, sociable mood, then disinhibition euphoria will be experienced. If a substance is used not for social, "partying" purposes to get high but as a self-medicating aid to fall asleep, then as millions of people will attest to, that is precisely the achieved effect (Wesson and Smith, 1977).

Table 17.2 Typical Signs of Withdrawal from Barbiturates in Adults and Infants

Adults	Infants
anxiety	high-pitched cry
irritability	tremors
restlessness	restlessness
sleep disturbances, including nightmares	sleep disturbances,
postural hypotension*	increased reflex action
delirium	excessive or insatiable appetite
excessively high fever	diarrhea, vomiting
major motor seizures	major motor seizures
autonomic hyperactivity	
amnestic syndrome	

Sources: From Wesson and Smith, 1977, p. 100; and DSM-III.

*Fall in blood pressure when patient goes into an upright position.

Physical dependence on barbiturates and similarly acting sedatives such as methaqualone (Quaalude) has been clearly established by an intense abstinence syndrome in long-term, heavy users and in infants born to such users. Infants often experience this syndrome after they have left the hospital, so that its nature is easily misdiagnosed. Similarly, convulsions in adults can occur several days after the last dosage (Wesson and Smith, 1977). Table 17.2 presents some typical signs in the barbiturate abstinence syndrome for adults and infants. Tolerance effects with heavy barbiturate use are also reported (Dimijian, 1978).

INHALANTS

There is a class of intoxicants whose acute effects can be easily confused with drunkenness from alcohol. These are the commercially marketed solvents such as cleaning fluid, paint thinner, model airplane glue, fingernail polish, and polish remover. The hundreds of different products falling into this class release vapors that are deliberately inhaled to provide a cheap, "legal" high. For this reason, chronic usage is often found among the very young (inhalants are more frequently used among elementary and junior high school than in high school or college) populations and among low-SES Mexican-Americans and American Indians (in contrast to whites, blacks, and middle-class youth). Although young middle-class, white youths are likely to try inhalants, they often proceed to alcohol or other drugs rather than remain with these substances as chronic users (Abelson et al., 1977; Cohen, 1979b).

Because some solvents are extremely toxic—are known poisons—they are no longer commercially available. But others that are legally sold are also dangerous. If inhaled quickly in large enough doses and in enclosed spaces (a plastic bag, for example), they can sometimes result in death.

One volatile chemical that has achieved some status with young adults as a presumed enhancer and prolonger of orgasm is amyl nitrite. Whatever the subjective effects are, they come about as a result of vasodilation of cerebral blood vessels almost immediately after inhalation. Ampules of amyl nitrite, known as poppers, pearls, snappers, rush, kick, bullet, and toilet water, are also sold in sex or "porno" shops (Cohen, 1979b).

Although about one in ten (mostly male) young people from twelve to about twenty-five years of age report having inhaled a volatile solvent at least once, less than one in a hundred older adults, it is estimated, report current use (Abelson et al., 1977). Physical dependence effects have not been reported for the volatile solvents.

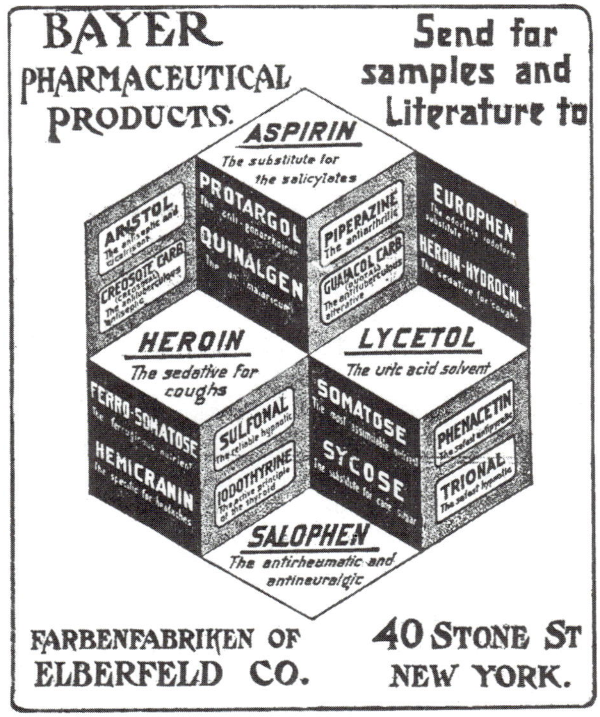

Heroin was not always an illicit substance, as shown by this nineteenth-century advertisement. (The Bettmann Archive Inc.)

NARCOTICS

The opium poppy plant flourishes in the Middle East and in the Southeast and Southwest Asian countries as well as other parts of the world if the climate and other conditions, such as soil, are right (for example, in some parts of Mexico). Each year this plant yields a whitish fluid that becomes gummy and darker when dried. When this substance is further dried and ground into a powder, it becomes the product known as opium of which both morphine and codeine are derivatives. Heroin—a semisynthetic substance—is derived from morphine by the introduction of other chemicals that alter morphine's chemical structure (Platt and Labate, 1976).

The sources and flow of narcotics into Europe and the United States change from decade to decade, sometimes from year to year, depending on the abundance of the crops, the availability of "routes," the market for sales, and various political considerations. Whereas Mexico and Turkey were once the major suppliers, Iran, Afghanistan, and Pakistan as well as the Golden Triangle countries of Indochina, Laos, Burma, and Thailand have become major sources of supply.

In the United States, the most common method for ingesting heroin is through "mainlining"—injecting it directly into the vein. When it reaches the brain it is metabolized to morphine. If injected in this way, heroin is absorbed by the brain more quickly than morphine, which is delayed by the blood-brain barrier. But it can also be taken orally, inhaled, or injected subcutaneously into tissue just under the skin. Morphine is rapidly absorbed by various organs of the body such as the liver, lungs, and kidneys. Physical effects include pupillary constriction, respiratory depression, and analgesia. Within twenty-four hours after the last dose, much of it is excreted (Platt and Labate, 1976).

The addict generally seeks heroin to avoid an abstinence syndrome and for a calming effect rather than for the euphoria or "high" of, let us say, the amphetamines, even though there might be a temporary "rush." Subjective reports are of peace, relief, and tranquility—of not being ruffled by events.

Heroin is sold on the streets in glassine envelopes—"bags"—that come in different sizes according to price and that can be called by a "brand" name that users learn to trust as an indicator of the quality of its contents. Often, however, users do not know how much pure heroin has been "cut" (mixed with quinine or other substances), nor can they be sure of the quality and purity of the bag's contents. Heroin sold on the street can be of extremely poor quality, with impurities that can be fatal.

Case 17.1 Lenora: Polydrug Abuser

Lenora was a thirty-year-old physician when she died—alone—in a hotel room. It was suicide, according to the coroner. Her friends and estranged family were not surprised. They had given up hope, as she had.

Lenora's two children were living with her husband, from whom she had been legally separated. There was also a lover who was in a mental hospital at the time of Lenora's death, with a diagnosis of alcoholism and schizophrenia. During their last harried telephone call, her lover had informed her that he had fallen in love with someone else and she was not to attempt to get in touch with him again. This announcement was probably one of the "precipitating" factors in her suicide. But there had also been a recent professional attempt to remove her from all drugs. The ensuing "crash" was too much for Lenora to deal with. During that final week, she could barely talk, walk, or interact with anyone. She refused hospitalization. Most of the people who had tried to help Lenora stated that she has been on a determined suicide course for years. But this time, she reached the end of the line.

Lenora's mother and father were alcoholics. She was an only child—brilliant, sensitive, high-strung. During college and medical school, she discovered drugs. She soon claimed that she could not live without them. Lenora was a polydrug user in the ultimate sense: in the course of a day she would ingest huge amounts of alcohol (occasionally Antabuse), cocaine, barbiturates, amphetamines, tranquilizers such as Librium or Valium (prescribed by various physicians who probably did not know about the other substances she was ingesting), marijuana, and occasionally, heroin. She would eat sparsely, if at all, but from time to time would pop an enormous number of vitamin pills into her mouth. Lenora was not physically dependent on these drugs, but her *psychological* dependence was as tenacious as any physical dependence could be.

After her internship, Lenora worked in a community clinic for a few years. In the past several years, however, she and the director realized she could not hold down her job. Because she was brilliant and because she still had a few compassionate professional friends, she was occasionally invited to do volunteer work at the clinic (mostly reviewing case material for a research project)—a job supervised by the assistant director, who found her work quite good. However, because she could not be counted on to show up each day, a regular job could not be arranged for her.

Lenora's early marriage ended in shambles, as might be expected. Her husband took the children away. Since that time, Lenora lived alone but her bed was almost always occupied by one stranger or another. For she was "on call" for money to support her massive need for drugs, which she claimed were required for pick-me-up, sleeping, reducing anxiety, facing the day, planning a meal, or even energizing herself to greet one of her "johns." In the past year, Lenora fell in love with one of her "johns," who supported her sufficiently well so that she could afford to sleep only with him. It was this man who dealt her the final blow.

Lenora had been hospitalized three times after three suicide attempts and had been in treatment for seven years up to the time of her death. She was gradually wasting herself, her mind, her body. She kept dropping out of treatment when "forced" to face the possibility that she was capable of changing her life style.

Lenora's childhood was characterized by fear, ambition, desire for approval, guilt over failure, and alcoholic parental models who did not prepare her for facing adult responsibilities. Her case history suggests that she had been a deeply depressed adolescent, but her academic brilliance and output overshadowed her emotional problems.

Could Lenora have been "saved?" Yes, but perhaps only temporarily, had she been willing to be hospitalized or to accept a daily, intense, clinic arrangement (a day hospital) with constant supervision, support, and concern. But she was not willing to do so. She was "dead weight," a "dead loss" to the others around her, who had long ago "given her up for lost." That figure of speech is now a reality. Should her family have hospitalized her against her will? Who was in charge of her life?

Case 17.2 Nancy: Heroin Addict

And on the other hand, Nancy is the twenty-two-year old daughter of two physicians. Her father is an alcoholic and she is a heroin addict. But her world is now supplying her with the supports and lifelines to overcome her dependence on heroin.

Nancy dropped out of college in her sophomore year. She had been introduced to heroin by a talented musician who lived near campus and with whom she was living. She became part of his drug culture so that she could keep up with him, his friends, his "hip" talk, and his "cool" life style. She sang a little with her friend's jazz group, but she did not have much talent. She was always a little strained with his friends and he in turn began to get bored with her. He sent her packing after her suicide attempt and she returned home.

Nancy's parents were compassionate, kind, worried, but insistent in their demand that she kick the habit. They supported her heroin needs but never let up with their demand. She left home several times. They always found her. They sent her into methadone treatment. She was detoxified but picked up her habit again a few months later. They put her in the hands of a new clinician, a different method to detoxify her. Today, Nancy is on methadone once again, from which she is gradually withdrawing, and is sharing a communal living arrangement with several ex-"junkies." She is completing her studies in a nearby college, earning money by teaching piano (she is a pretty good jazz pianist), and working very hard at rearranging her life. She is not depressed and looks forward to teaching music, taking singing lessons (opera, not jazz), kicking her habit, and falling in love.

Nancy's interpersonal world contains many reinforcements for her new life style. She had never felt abandoned or alone in her fight to save herself. She will probably make it.

Users and Addicts

It is difficult to estimate the numbers of heroin users and addicts in the population, except through indirect means, such as obtaining estimates of numbers of people seeking treatment or admitted to hospitals for hepatitis. For obvious reasons, surveys and questionnaires all underestimate street usage. However, most estimates agree that there is a general decline in the number of addicts as a result of extensive treatment facilities now available. It is estimated that there were about 400,000 addicts in this country by the end of 1980, compared to about 700,000 in 1970, with about half of these individuals residing in New York City (Goldman, 1980). In New York, the trend is for more young people (under sixteen years of age) to be involved than ever before.

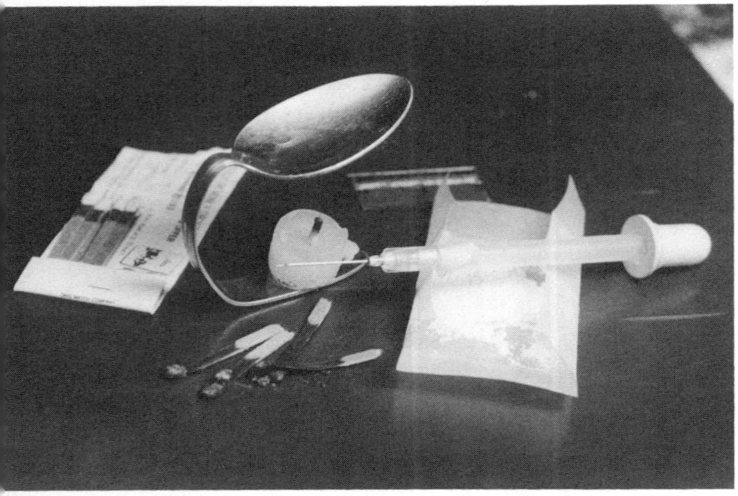

Paraphernalia for mainlining heroin. (Charles Gatewood/Stock, Boston)

Not all users are addicts. The foregoing figures do not include the sizable population (about 2 million people nationwide, it is estimated), who use heroin but who do not become addicted (McGlothlin, 1975). Thus, because there are about three times the number of users as there are addicts, it would appear that addiction is not an inevitable consequence of heroin use (Drug use in America, 1973; McGlothlin, 1975). In fact, many experts feel that the social and environmental context may be the crucial factor in producing heroin dependence.

In one study (Robins, 1973), it was found that in a sample of 451 enlisted men returning from Vietnam in 1971, almost half had used opiates and about one in five were addicted. About a year later, fewer than one percent of this group were addicted despite the fact that most had received no treatment. Further, many were still using heroin.

It has been suggested that, in addition to the social context, belief in the powerful effects of heroin, rather than the pharmacological action of the drug itself, "hooks" many users. This might explain the well-known observation that even after many months of abstinence, some former addicts will "crave" heroin when returning to old social environments. The explanation is also relevant to the observation just noted that most heavy heroin users in Vietnam were no longer addicted once they returned to the United States as well as the observation that some users can show "controlled" opiate use (say, weekends only), without becoming addicted (called "chipping" or "chippying") (Zinberg, 1979).

Effects and pattern of abuse. The immediate rush of injecting heroin may have a euphoric quality as noted, but this is soon followed by apathy, sluggishness, a general slowing down of responses, slurred speech, drowsiness, a raised threshold for pain (or other discomforts), and some cognitive and physical impairment (for example, in attention, memory, and judgment).

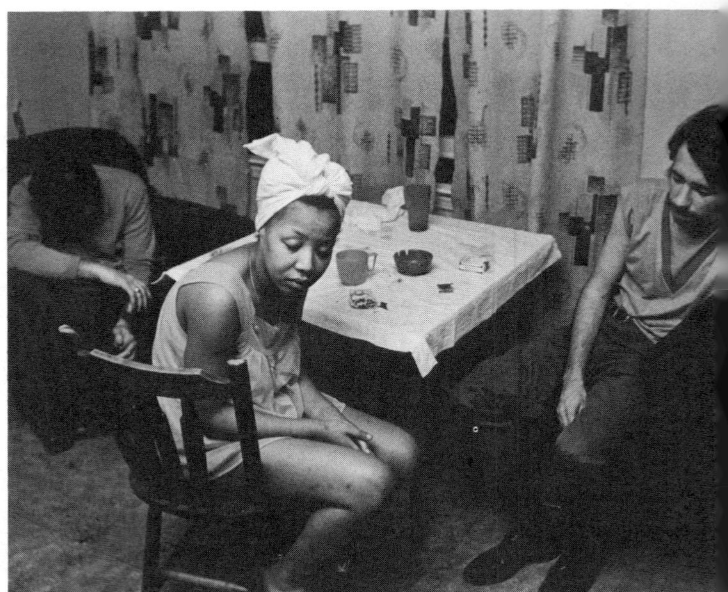

A group of heroin users. (© 1977 Michael Hanulak/Photo Researchers, Inc.)

Many addicts are on the fringes of society because of their preoccupation with obtaining heroin, an inability to stop or cut down, and its continued expense. These circumstances interfere dramatically with the social, occupational, and interpersonal performance of the dependent individual, who may find himself or herself totally embedded in a junkie subculture with no way out.

Crime and delinquency. Although there is a well-known relationship between heroin abuse and criminal activity (after all, heroin is extremely expensive), most experts are agreed that there is no pharmacological basis for assuming that heroin causes aggressiveness and crime. On the other hand, there is rather strong evidence that certain antisocial life styles tend to precede heroin abuse and that the same social conditions may give rise to both crime and heroin abuse (McGlothlin, 1979; Nurco, 1979; Winick, 1974). Although many junkies had engaged in criminal activity before their first experience with narcotics, there tends to be an increase in income-generating crime—burglary, for example—after narcotics dependence has been established (McGlothlin, 1979).

Neonatal withdrawal risk. In 1960 in New York City, one in 164 births were to narcotics-dependent women, whereas in 1972 this figure increased to one in 27 (Platt and Labate, 1976). Many of these offspring have high mortality rates because of poor prenatal care. About three-fourths of them undergo an abstinence syndrome within a few days after birth, manifesting such dysfunctional behavioral states as tremors, irritability, hyperactivity, hypertonicity (excessive body tone or tension), vomiting, eating, breathing difficulties, diarrhea, and fever, a high-pitched cry, and motor seizures (Dinges, Davis, and Glass, 1980; Platt and Labate, 1976). In addition, observation of sleep states of these infants, for example, amount of REM sleep, indicates that during neonatal withdrawal there is an alteration of nervous system integrity with such disturbances being particularly evidenced in infants whose mothers had long-term polydrug ingestion, rather than ingestion of opiates alone (Dinges, Davis, and Glass, 1980).

Physical complications and mortality. Among heroin-dependent people, not surprisingly, there are more deaths, and at younger ages, than for the general population (Platt and Labate, 1976). About one addict in every 100 dies because of heroin-related factors: physical complications, overdose, or a life style of violence. For both males and females in New York City, there were ten to fifteen times more narcotics-related black deaths than narcotics-related white deaths (Helpern and Rho, 1967).

Spotlight 17.6 Abstinence Syndrome: Three Narcotics

When narcotics are not available to addicts with well-established habits, physical and psychological manifestations follow a fairly predictable sequence that has been studied with many people. Specific symptoms and signs can be expected to arise with regularity after a certain number of hours have elapsed.

Opiate substances get from the bloodstream into the brain and work their effects—possibly—on neurons in the hypothalamus as well as on other CNS systems (Zimmermann and George, 1974). But the precise nature of these neurological and biochemical processes and the physiological mechanisms involved in the abstinence syndrome are not clearly understood.

The following table presents the expected

physical signs and their severity or intensity at various times elapsed since the last dose. Note that methadone, a narcotic frequently used to aid in either detoxification or in "maintenance" programs (see later sections) has its own withdrawal sequence. Methadone is rarely, however, associated with levels 3 and 4 of symptom severity or intensity.

Intensity Level		Hours After Last Dose		
		Morphine	*Heroin*	*Methadone*
0	"Craving," anxiety	6	4	12
1	Yawning, perspiration, secretion of tears, mucousy discharge from the nose, "yen sleep"	14	8	34–38
2	Level 1 signs become more intense, plus: dilation of the pupils, gooseflesh, muscle twitches, hot and cold flashes, aching bones and muscles, anorexia	16	12	48–72
3	Level 2 signs become more intense, plus: insomnia, increased blood pressure, temperature, respiratory rate, and pulse rate, restlessness, nausea	24–36	18–24	—
4	Level 3 signs become more intense, plus: feverish body surfaces, curled-up position, vomiting, diarrhea, weight loss (5 lbs. daily), spontaneous ejaculation or orgasm, and various chemical changes in the blood cells due to loss of plasma or water (hemoconcentration)	36–48	24–36	—

Source: Adapted from P. H. Blachly, Management of the opiate abstinence syndrome, *American Journal of Psychiatry*, vol. 122, p. 743, 1966.

Physical complications arising from chronic narcotics abuse include lung, heart, digestive, and circulatory problems, hepatitis, and skin infections if there is skin popping. Overdoses can be intentional or unintentional, for example, because of impure products in the heroin, inadequate notions of how potent the substance is, or lack of tolerance due to a period of abstinence. The physical indications of overdose include shallow and slow breathing, clammy skin, low blood pressure, cyanosis (bluish-purplish skin discoloration), low body temperature, and coma (Platt and Labate, 1976).

Dependence. Narcotic substances are associated with marked tolerance effects and an abstinence syndrome, which follows a fairly predictable course after there is cessation of regular use. A subjective feature often accompanying termination is anxiety in connection with obtaining more of the substance. The abstinence syndrome for morphine or heroin peaks on the second or third day and ends in seven to ten days, whereas the abstinence syndrome for methadone (another narcotic—see later sections) peaks in about two to four days, is relatively mild, and ends in ten to fourteen days (DSM-III).

THEORIES OF DRUG ABUSE

The large numbers of people who use substances such as marijuana without major personal consequences are not the concern of this section. Instead, I will focus on a smaller group of people who are drug abusers. Theories of narcotics dependence will receive special emphasis.

The basic question boils down to: In the light of the wide exposure and availability of drugs to a sizable population, why does only a small portion of users fall into the drug-abusing category?

Predisposing Personality Factors

Attempts to explain drug abuse and/or dependence in terms of personality and emotions tend to stress predisposing factors within the abuser while at the same time underplaying the role of sociocultural, environmental, and learned behaviors. Although these approaches vary among themselves, they explicitly or implicitly suggest that those people who become drug-dependent differ in aspects of emotional makeup from those who do not, especially in personality traits predisposing them to drug abuse. Researches that are designed to verify these approaches, however, are often unable to demonstrate personality differences among people who later do or do not become drug-dependent, because such demonstrations require longitudinal studies. Instead, studies designed to explore these and related hypotheses tend to seek differences between matched groups of drug-abusing and nondrug-abusing subjects in various personality traits (for example, in locus of control, or method of dealing with anxiety or hostility).

In general, although sometimes one and sometimes another of the following views receives occasional empirical support, most of the presumed personality correlates of drug dependence either cannot be adequately explored or studies have not yielded consistent or repeated, positive results.

Psychodynamic formulations. Some psychoanalytic approaches describe narcotics abusers as showing "orality"; they are viewed as generally infantile, dependent people who lack "meaningful object relationships." Other psychodynamic approaches imply that the addict has difficulty in dealing with aggressive feelings, turning to drugs as an escape from intensely uncomfortable feelings of anger (Nurco, 1979). Still other views stress conflicts concerning parental authority figures—with drug abuse reflecting rebelliousness against conventional restraints (society).

Problems in delaying gratification. A popular theme in the literature on the etiology of drug abuse is that drug-dependent people show impulsivity—an inability to delay gratification. They have a strong inner push toward getting immediate rewards. This inability to defer gratification may stem from any number of childhood factors, it is claimed, but it is sometimes likened to the impulsivity of the delinquent or antisocial personality (Nurco, 1979).

Sexual substitute. It has been hypothesized that addicts may turn to drugs as a substitute for genital sexual activities because of difficulties and fears regarding heterosexual relationships (Fenichel, 1945). Some street lore indeed suggests that heroin ingestion "wipes out" sexual desire (Nurco, 1979).

Deviation-proneness and sensation-seeking. It has also been proposed that addicts show a norm-breaking tendency well before a narcotics habit is developed (Nurco, 1979). Involvement in marginally acceptable behavior, that is, in behavior that deviates from traditional, mainstream patterns, may result from a need to escape from boredom. Sensation-seeking activity, as this pattern has been described, may lead to behaviors that depart from those expected by the mainstream norm.* The illicit status of drugs such as heroin may enhance the sensation-appeal associated with them, attracting young people who show deviation-proneness to experiment with them. Risk-taking behavior, sensation-seeking activities, defiance of the law, and an action-oriented pattern thus may all precede drug abuse (Nurco, 1979).

An addict personality? Some observers suggest that addicts are more disturbed, show more psychopathology than their nonaddict peers. Although there are difficulties in isolating specific traits that distinguish addicts from nonaddicts, some consistency is found in the empirical finding that there is more emotional disturbance among addicts than among their nondrug-dependent peers. There is equal consistency in the finding, however, that attempts to define the "addictive personality" have not been successful (Dole, 1980; Penk, Woodward, Robinowitz, and Parr, 1980; Platt and Labate, 1976).

Socially Oriented Views

Escape from poverty, pain, and crowdedness. Because drug dependence (and alcoholism) flourish in the slums and in poverty, some experts speculate that an escape from unbearable reality and from the pain associated with it is the major element in accounting for addiction. Although it is possible to demonstrate the association between poverty and addiction, it is not possible to explain the fact that most impoverished people do not become addicts despite the high availability of narcotics in their surroundings (Dole, 1980). Further, this approach does not account for the drug dependence of many individuals who come from more affluent backgrounds and neighborhoods.

Peer pressure and the drug subculture. Many experts agree that the most important and consistently found correlate of initial use of a substance and in the maintenance and continuation of a drug abuse pattern is social and peer pressure—group influence. Peers are also the most important source of information about drugs (Kandel, 1975; Mercer and Smart, 1974; Nurco, 1979). Thus, a drug-oriented subculture which sets the style and the manner of drug abuse and the individual's susceptibility to be influenced by this subculture emerge as fairly reliable correlates of both initial use and later drug abuse. Many experts believe, thus, that the life style of the drug subculture provides an opportunity for some abuse-prone people to structure their lives around the excitement, thrill, and peer acceptance that are now available to them—circumstances that may be highly reinforcing for people who would otherwise have very little rewards in daily living.

Learning and conditioning. Some people answer the question of why people abuse drugs—actually become dependent on them, as with heroin—by alluding to learning theory. Either classical or operant conditioning (see Chapters 6 and 20) has been invoked as an explanatory principle.

One learning paradigm suggests that drug abuse is "learned behavior that is acquired and maintained by a variety of internal and environmental stimuli" (Callner, 1975, p. 144). In this view, some drugs initially reduce tension or diminish unpleasant emotional states such as anxiety. If the drug is not ingested, tension levels build up once again, until relieved or reduced by drugs. Eventually, stimuli within or from the environment produce "withdrawal" symptoms associated with lack

* Although deviation-proneness may reflect a tendency to depart from the norm, much of what has been called deviant behavior is actually *appropriate* behavior, when the so-called deviant-prone person's peer group is considered.

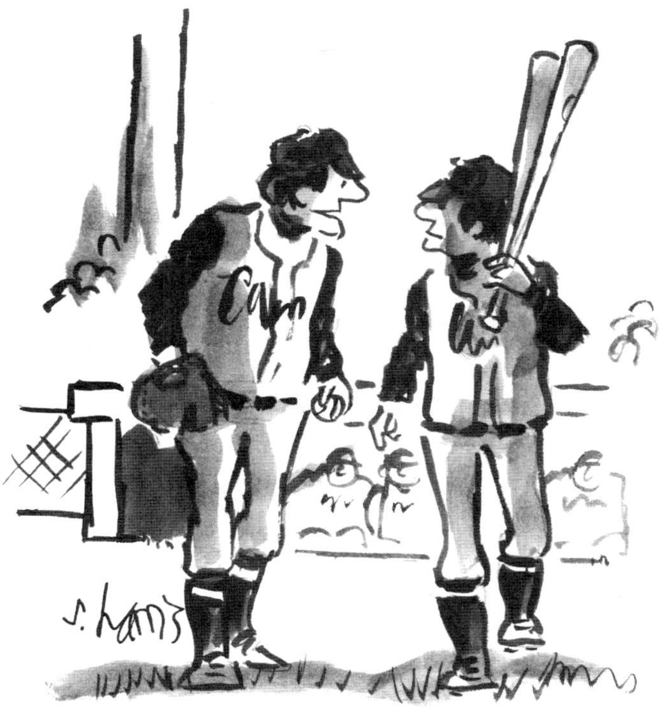

"ACTUALLY I TAKE ONE PILL FOR MY HITTING, ONE FOR MY FIELDING, AND ONE FOR A GENERAL EUPHORIA."

Sidney Harris

of drug intake, driving the individual toward more of the intake. Thus, social stimuli and various environmental cues such as drug-taking friends, old haunts, and certain kinds of music can produce craving and even physical symptoms well after the subject is abstinent (detoxified in the case of heroin addiction), implying that craving is not a strictly pharmacological or chemical drive (Dole, 1980; Wikler, 1973), a point already made. In learning terms, it can be said that certain manifestations of withdrawal syndromes can be conditioned to environmental cues, so that even after detoxification, when the body is presumably no longer in need of narcotics, these responses are evoked.

The contingencies that may reinforce the acquisition of a drug-taking response include the following (Callner, 1975): (a) reinforcement derived from peers, life style of drug or "street" subculture, excitement in connection with defying authority or in engaging in an illicit activity; (b) pharmacological reinforcement effects—euphoria, "flashes," anxiety reduction produced by physical properties of the drug itself; (c) negative reinforcement in that drug use may provide a means of escape from aversive environmental aspects such as boredom, hostile family life; (d) negative reinforcement in connection with reducing physical states associated with the abstinence syndrome.

Biochemical Approaches

It has been already noted that some recently discovered opiate-like chemicals, called endorphins, are produced naturally in the body. These chemicals have properties that resemble synthetic substances in their pain-relieving qualities, and it is thought that under certain circumstances, they are produced by the body to deal with extreme pain and stress. In the case of heroin-dependent individuals, it may be that endorphins are not produced in sufficient quantities to fend off or to ease the stress of the abstinence syndrome, "forcing" the individual to seek more heroin so as to avoid the extreme distress experienced. Prior knowledge that heroin can relieve the distress is of course essential, so that craving is not an entirely biological process.

The notion that there might be some chemical correlates of addiction is not new (see Bejerot, 1972). What is new is the search for explanations of the fact that among those who try narcotics, only a small percentage become dependent, including people who are given large doses of morphine for medical purposes, despite the presence of personality problems, poverty, and unfavorable family circumstances (Nurco, 1979). It could well be that along with learning and conditioning and peer and social pressures are genetic and biochemical substrates that distinguish the narcotics-dependent individual from those who do not get "hooked," despite the repeated experiences of both types of people with narcotics.

TREATMENT*

Many addicts die, but most "mature out"—gradually dropping their drug patterns by the time they are in their mid-thirties, generally in about nine years (DSM-III; Nurco et al., 1975). But even those who give up their habit are left with considerable damage, not necessarily in the physical sense, but with educational, vocational, and interpersonal disabilities that are frequently beyond repair. This may be especially true for low-SES people who have enormous difficulties in coping with their harsh worlds. It is easy to understand why so many of the programs described in this section are plagued with high relapse rates. It is perhaps for this reason that more than almost any other area of pathology, vocational and educational rehabilitation have become essential features of drug treatment programs. Helping the formerly drug-dependent person adopt a new life style that is reinforcing and economically self-maintaining is generally supplemented with attempts to reorient him or her away from his or her former drug subculture and social setting in which peer pressure, availability of drugs, and tensions and anxieties associated with drug abuse may cause relapse behavior.

Detoxification. These procedures involve the gradual reduction of all narcotic ingestion, usually with the help of other chemicals such as methadone, to lessen the intensity of the abstinence syndrome (see Spotlight 17.6). Gradually, the supplementary drug is also withdrawn. Therapeutic goals are complete abstinence, aided, as noted, by vocational and educational guidance and personal and social counseling. Although hospitalization is recommended for this program, it is not absolutely necessary. In 1974, there were about 130,000 people enrolled in detoxification programs in this country (DuPont, 1974).

The majority of addicts who are completely detoxified, with little pharmacological need for the substance, relapse—fall back into their patterns of narcotics use (Dole, 1980). Further, there is a high dropout rate from detoxification centers. But even among those who remain, there is much cheating (Hall, 1979).

Most experts now agree that the psychological aspects of drug-seeking behavior, the reinforcing aspects of life style, and the social and peer pressures for drug-seeking behavior (see earlier sections) prevent most detoxification programs from achieving their major purpose: to send heroin-free, former addicts into comprehensive rehabilitation programs so that they can remain abstinent while readjusting to society.

Therapeutic communities. Supervised, communal living arrangements—an extremely popular method of treating addicts—have proliferated throughout this country. They date back to 1958, when Synanon (now held in disrepute because of its cultlike status) was founded. In a typical communal program, such as Daytop Village, Odyssey, Phoenix House, and Gateway House, former addicts play supervisory and/or therapeutic roles. In addition, professionally trained staff members in the vocational guidance, medical, and mental health areas also serve as consultants or staff members. These residential self-help, drug-free communities employ techniques that promote personal responsibility. Such techniques may use group methods of confrontation, sometimes painful "encounter" and "rap" sessions with a general atmosphere of abrasive and aggressive interaction, all designed to return the former addict to the community with skills and a job plan. There is, however, a high dropout rate for the tens

* As in the preceding section on theories, emphasis in this section will be on narcotics dependence. However, many of the programs described are appropriate for other types of drug abuse.

of thousands of addicts who have tried the therapeutic community (De Leon, 1979); and to begin with, only a small percentage of addicts are ever "reached" by these services (Platt and Labate, 1976). Even among those who stay, success rates (future abstinence) are disappointing—about 30 percent.

Group methods. As in alcohol treatment programs, methods that employ some group interaction have been particularly popular in drug-abuse programs. The mainstay of the therapeutic community has been the "rap" session and direct group confrontation. Hospitals also lean heavily on group methods, which are regarded as superior to individual methods because they rely on peer pressure toward health. Many believe that the group provides the basic support in maintaining motivation to go "clean" (Cummings, 1979). The thinking underlying this approach is based on etiological considerations already discussed: peer pressure and a seeking out of certain types of life styles associated with drug-seeking behavior are as reinforcing, perhaps, as the substance itself. In turn, social systems and peer pressure might be equally effective in supporting and reinforcing abstinence.

Psychotherapy and family approaches. Individual psychotherapeutic methods have apparently not resulted in positive outcomes when used as the primary method of intervention (Callner, 1975; Kaufman and Kaufmann, 1979; Platt and Labate, 1976). Some of the psychodynamic approaches that employ largely verbal methods, it is argued, may not be relevant when applied to low-SES groups (which yield a large number of addicts). Moreover, etiological assumptions associated with the more traditional approaches ("orality" or "addictive personality") may simply not be valid. Further, many drug abusers are usually not motivated to continue in a treatment regime that extends over a long period of time.

However, despite the generally pessimistic view about some of these approaches, there are some claims that with appropriate modifications, individual therapy, as well as several family approaches, may offer useful possibilities. Confrontation, a realistic approach, and directive guidance might be successful on an individual basis (Platt and Labate, 1976), whereas family methods may be especially appropriate in drug-free outpatient programs* (Kleber and Slobetz, 1979).

It is of interest that while family approaches in the treatment of alcoholism have become increasingly popular—as adjuncts to AA, for example, or in the treatment of young alcoholics—drug abuse programs have traditionally stressed the removal of the drug abuser from the family, encouraging little or no family contact. This thinking has been challenged on the assumption that the possibility of veiled or even overt support for drug abuse within the family (as with alcoholism) should be explored; also, the family may be crucial in the maintenance of abstinence (Kleber and Slobetz, 1979).

Narcotics maintenance—heroin. Because many addicts who attempt abstinence repeatedly fail, some experts support the notion of simply supplying the addict with necessary narcotics. Advantages accrue not only to the addict, who can now satisfy his or her narcotics needs openly and legally, but also to society. For example, prostitution to support one's habits, pushing drugs, muggings, and burglaries that may stem from the expense of narcotics and the profits that can be made, might be reduced. Also, the worldwide drug trafficking that involves many millions of dollars might thus be dealt a major blow.

In England, where narcotics can be legally obtained, there was a vast rise in addiction after a narcotics maintenance program was introduced, as well as misuse of the program for profit by physicians as well as addicts who sold heroin illicitly. Today, many of these ills have been cured by a tighter system of controls over registration of addicts, physi-

* These are programs that offer neither chemical aids, for example methadone or narcotics antagonists (see the following discussion), nor twenty-four hour supervision as in a hospital or therapeutic community.

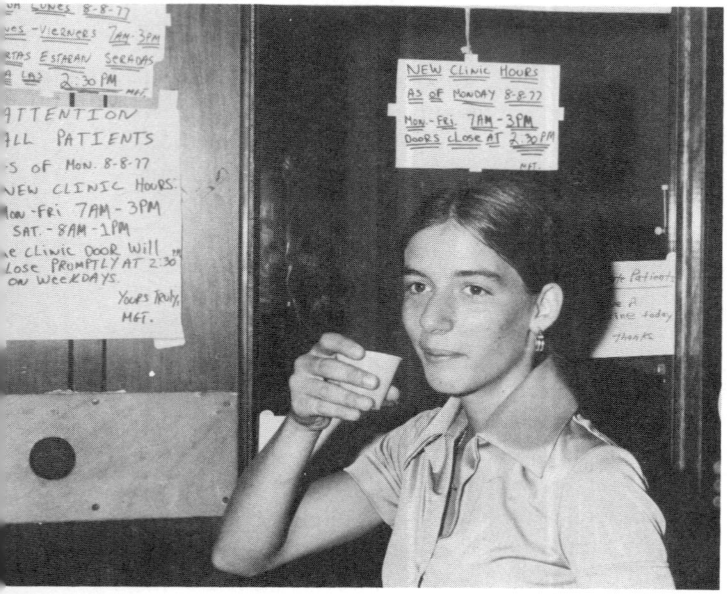

Methadone maintenance has become the major treatment approach to heroin dependence. (© *Eric Kroll/Taurus Photos*)

cians, and pharmacies where the substances are obtained.*

Narcotics maintenance—methadone. Methadone is a narcotic, chemically related to heroin, but with more benign consequences to the organism (Dole, 1980). Sufficiently high, daily doses of methadone (administered on an outpatient basis), if established over a period of time by gradual increases in daily amounts, can be stabilized so that narcotic (dulling, "spacey") effects are not only blocked but also, withdrawal symptoms eliminated. This leaves the narcotic-dependent individual alert, at ease, and in a relatively "normal" state—free to go about his or her work and to get involved in day-to-day interpersonal situations without craving heroin (Dole, 1980; Dole, Nyswander, and Warner, 1968). If administered in oral dosages, methadone does not result in the "rush" of injected narcotics, proponents of methadone maintenance programs claim, and therefore is not sought for its euphoric, reinforcing effects.

Methadone maintenance has become the major treatment program for heroin dependence. In 1974, there were about 80,000 methadone patients in this country (DuPont, 1974). Not all is rosy, however, in connection with methadone programs. Many great claims had been made for the success of methadone maintenance programs: high percentages of clients remaining in treatment; increases in employment among narcotics-dependent people; and a decrease in antisocial, criminal activities in the light of the free, legal availability of a heroin substitute (Dole, 1980; Platt and Labate, 1976). However, a large number of clients do not remain within the program and reports of large improvements in socialization and reduction of crime among those who do remain simply do not hold up (McGlothlin, 1979). Further, we need to know more about methadone's effects on pregnant women and their offspring as to the behavioral responses and growth of infants thus exposed.

Methadone and other maintenance drugs have great abuse potential. They are being sold on the street, pushed for profit, and introduced to new users through illicit channels. Abuse by administrators and clinic doctors is by now well-known. Most experts agree, however, that this most popular of programs has attracted and retained more addicts than any other form of treatment and that many negative individual and social consequences of the heroin problem have been reduced as a result, even if only moderately (McGlothlin, 1979).

Narcotic-blocking (narcotic "antagonist") drugs. There are some chemicals, for example, naloxone or naltrexone, that block the reinforcing effects of narcotics (for example, "relief," the blocking or reduction of the abstinence syndrome). In the treatment of heroin addiction, these drugs, which have no

* Most maintenance programs in England now employ methadone, not heroin, and it is injected rather than orally ingested (McGlothlin, 1975).

abuse potential (for they are not associated with dependence or reinforcing effects) would cause an abstinence syndrome if administered to one dependent on heroin or would "protect" the abstinent individual from becoming dependent were he or she to use heroin. The idea is that individuals thus "protected" can return to social environments associated with former use of heroin without becoming readdicted as a result of craving. Thus, if it were possible to block the reinforcing effects of narcotics through the use of antagonists, perhaps the narcotic-seeking behavior of addicts can be eliminated.

Although some success has been reported with narcotic antagonists under laboratory conditions, the true test is on the street, where it is hoped that drug-related behaviors would become extinguished under nonreinforcement conditions. It is too early to tell about the success of chemical antagonists in treating addicts. The main problem, it seems, even with chemically effective opiate antagonists, remains the psychological problem of motivation. For many addicts would probably continue to search for other drugs or for heroin itself, even if the reinforcing action of heroin had been successfully blocked. And most would probably not volunteer for treatment at all. Thus, the success of this presumably promising method of treating addicts is still largely unknown (Dole, 1980). Many experts continue to feel, in light of only moderate success with narcotic antagonists, that chemical blocking of narcotic effects would only work if accompanied by intensive programs of counseling and rehabilitation.

Treatment of Drug Abuse: Overview

1. Motivation to change is probably the single most important element in shaping the outcome of treatment programs.

2. Generally speaking, no single interventive approach seems to be the most effective. A combination of several approaches—group sessions, for example, with direct counseling and vocational training—would appear to be more appropriate than any one method.

3. Because a sizable portion of drug abusers are polydrug abusers, the search for a specific intervention appropriate to a specific drug is fruitless, as might be expected (Wesson and Smith, 1979).

4. One major objective of most treatment programs is to keep the client motivated enough to "stay with it," to remain in treatment. The prevention of relapse, not surprisingly is another major objective.* No wonder then, that these areas have become important foci for research explorations.

5. As already noted (see p. 482), it might be possible to select successful treatments on the basis of classifying drug abusers as to the function or purpose of their drug use as well as the type of user they are (Carlin and Strauss, 1977; Douglass, Khavari, and Farber, 1980). This classification acknowledges the general finding that some substance abusers are self-medicators, using drugs to counteract the effects of other drugs or to relieve stress and anxiety, whereas other drug abusers use drugs for hedonistic or recreational purposes, to feel good, get high, enhance sociability or sexuality (Carlin and Strauss, 1977). In addition, some users are "streetwise" (they participate in a drug subculture and they tend to be unconventional in dress, grooming, impulse control, and employment patterns), whereas other users are "straight" (they are not members of any particular drug subculture and tend to be older, more conventionally employed, groomed, and clothed than the "streetwise" users). Such classifications depart from the DSM-III's diagnostic framework based on substances. It remains to be seen, however, whether or not this typology leads to the development of appropriate treatment strategies with more successful outcomes, espe-

* According to some experts, three months after detoxification and counseling is the time of greatest risk of relapse for many addicts. Some particularly high-risk variables are: involvement in a heroin subculture and a community in which the substance is easy to obtain; low education, unemployment; and being, young, black, and unmarried (Robins, 1979).

Spotlight 17.7 Cigarette Smoking Is Hazardous to Your Health

Cigarette smoking is one of the top health problems in this country. It has been described as a key factor in lung cancer, emphysema, various heart ailments, and a host of other diseases. Over one-quarter of a million deaths each year in this country alone are directly linked to smoking. Yet despite public knowledge about these hazards, about 60 million people still smoke.* There are now more younger females who smoke than males and the rates for lung cancer for women are rapidly rising (Sobel, 1980).

Most heavy smokers find that they are unable to "kick" their habit easily, stating that they "crave" a cigarette when they try to do so despite the fact that there is no special high from smoking. Moreover, craving is described even when there are no reports of an especially intense abstinence syndrome.

Generally, a nicotine abstinence syndrome is relatively mild and of short duration (never more than a few days), and is not always present for all people; at its most intense level it consists of irritability and anxiety, stomach cramps, difficulties in concentrating, and subjective reports of craving. Because people who have been abstinent for weeks or months may report a deep sense of need for cigarettes and often relapse despite their best intentions, experts speak of strong psychological, rather than physiological, dependence.

Can we characterize the heavy smokers? Who are the people who can quit easily and how do they differ from those who cannot? Is there some physiological "addiction" center in the brains of some people that can account for differences between relapsers and nonrelapsers? These and other aspects of smoking behavior have recently come under the scrutiny of behavioral researchers. There are still no definitive answers. What may be of even greater importance is that despite considerable efforts, we still cannot say that we know how to get people to stop smoking and to remain abstinent. For even when there is success, judging by immediate results, followup yields predictable findings: after a period of time has elapsed, usually several months, the majority of people suffer a relapse (Yates, 1975).

What are some of the methods that have been used? Treatment programs cover a wide ground, including: aversive consequences for smoking or thinking about smoking (for example, shock, or nausea induced by a pill); mechanical devices, such as a special cigarette dispenser that is locked up for increasingly longer but specified periods so that the smoker becomes "desensitized" to his or her discomfort in not being able to smoke; direct advice or persuasion by a respected authority (Raw, 1976); positive reinforcement for abstinence rather than aversive methods for smoking; training in relaxation; the substitution of behavior incompatible with smoking; role-playing (assuming the role of a cancer patient, for example); hypnotic methods and self-hypnosis in particular (moderately successful but only for highly hypnotizable people [Spiegel, 1982]); hypnosis combined with behavioral methods (highly successful, according to Watkins [1976]), and so on.

A method that has elicited some interest involves "rapid smoking"—an aversive method that is regarded by some as one of the most powerful techniques to induce smoking cessation (Hackett and Horan, 1976). This method requires the subject to take "drags" on a cigarette every few seconds until it becomes impossible to do so. This single trial, which lasts for about five minutes, is followed by two or three additional trials, with several minute rest periods between each within each session. A program of treatment is comprised of eight to twelve sessions. Claims of excellent success have been made for this approach. Unfortunately, there are many physical hazards in this

* This number alone causes many people to question the inclusion of tobacco in the DSM-III's list of substance-induced organic mental disorders and substance-use disorders.

procedure, especially for those with heart conditions and related physical involvements, so that despite its presumed effectiveness, it is not a generally recommended procedure with universal application (Horan et al., 1977, 1980).

Overall, the more successful approaches to smoking reduction are those that combine several techniques, such as hypnosis, group methods, the signing of contracts, and various behavioral methods (especially aversive ones), with booster sessions and follow-up to maintain abstinence; accompanying programs in recreational and social areas also bear on successful outcome (Conway, 1977; Hunt and Matarazzo, 1973; Lando, 1977; Pederson et al., 1975).

Most important of all is the subject's motivation to quit. In addition, how one sees one's reinforcement contingencies may also be important in maintaining abstinence, judging by the results of one study in which subjects who were able to stop smoking were shown to have more internal locus of control than those who could not stop (Mlott and Mlott, 1975). Apparently, the degree to which one feels that one can shape one's own behavior through internal rewards is related to the ease with which one can stop smoking.

cially regarding relapse rates, than are reported for the current approaches.

6. Educational programs, school discussion groups, and media efforts to educate children and the general public as to the dangers of drug abuse are generally ineffective: they are regarded as of uncertain outcome, if not as failures entirely. A possible reason might be that teachers, counselors, and the authorities, unfamiliar with many aspects of the drug subculture, sometimes take a rigid position on the use of "softer" drugs such as marijuana; they might push for total abstinence, for example, thus losing the trust and respect of the "hip" users of more toxic substances (PCP or the opiates), the real targets of their educational thrusts (Feldman et al., 1979; McGlothlin, 1975). In any event, much research is needed to develop successful methods for employing the schools and the media in the battle against drug abuse.

7. Finally, the long-range outcome for drug abusers undergoing treatment in any one of thousands of treatment centers all over this country is largely still an unknown quantity and poses a formidable research challenge for the experts (Sobell, Sobell, and Ward, 1980).

SUMMARY

This chapter covered the abuse of substances other than alcohol. After defining drug abuse and considering some of the confusions in distinguishing between dependence and addiction, it briefly discussed the relationship of age, gender, SES, and ethnicity to drug abuse. It pointed out that because patterns of drug abuse vary, for example, many abusers are polydrug abusers, the usual classification of drug abuse by single substance only may be obscuring some important facts. The bulk of this chapter surveyed the major substances of abuse, describing for each of them such characteristics as patterns of use, prevalence, subjective effects, and consequences of heavy, long-term use. It considered marijuana, the hallucinogens such as LSD and PCP, the amphetamines, cocaine, the barbiturates and similarly acting sedatives, the inhalants, and narcotics. The effects of many of these substances, the survey noted, are very much related to expectancy, mood, and the social setting in which the substance is ingested. Described also were theories of drug abuse, with special emphasis on narcotics addiction, including hypotheses about predisposing personality factors; various socially oriented views (for example, peer pressure and learning and conditioning); and biochemical approaches. The chapter concluded with a summary of treatment approaches to drug abuse—again, with special emphasis on addiction to narcotics—and a Spotlight on cigarette smoking.

Highlights

1. This chapter stressed that addiction, drug dependence, and drug abuse are not clearly defined and differentiated terms, and that drug-seeking behaviors are largely learned behaviors that are very much part of one's subculture, past history, and socially expected roles. The concept of substance dependence, which generally refers to tolerance and the abstinence syndrome, gets in the way of understanding the nature of substance abuse that may not be based on *physical* dependence but that may nevertheless involve dependence, judging by behaviors that show an intense and compulsive preoccupation with obtaining certain substances as well as the rituals involved in their use.
2. As for patterns and groupings of drug abuse and abusers, the chapter notes that teenagers are heavily "into" drug abuse. More males than females use and abuse drugs, but the gap is narrowing, especially among younger people. Although low-SES groups were once identified with the heaviest drug use, this is no longer the case. There are distinct ethnic patterns in drug abuse. For example, black and Hispanic abusers tend to do so with heroin and the opiates, while white drug abusers tend to use other types of substances. Different subgroups among drug abusers have been identified: a young group of abusers of substances such as the opiates; a larger but also young group of users of substances such as marijuana, LSD, and cocaine; and third, an older, middle-class group of "self-medicating" abusers of such substances as the barbiturates.
3. Marijuana is one of the leading recreational substances in this country, with over fifty million Americans reporting having used it at least once. Social models and friendship patterns are probably the most important factors in understanding how marijuana is first introduced. When smoked in moderate dosages in favorable social settings, marijuana produces mild euphoria and feelings of relaxation. However, it has been shown that many of these subjective effects depend also on the user's expectancy about effects. Although high doses of marijuana and long-term heavy use produce some problems (for example, lowered motor coordination or some negative effects on cognitive performance), it is still not clear what the long-term effects are. However, heavy use is not recommended for people who have heart difficulties or who are pregnant. Although there is no evidence for an abstinence syndrome, long-term heavy use of marijuana is apparently associated with tolerance effects.
4. The hallucinogenic drugs include LSD, mescaline, and psilocybin. LSD, no longer a major substance of abuse, is a semisynthetic chemical that was first used in the laboratory to understand schizophrenia. Many of the bizarre subjective experiences associated with LSD result from distortions in the processing of sensory input. Claims of permanent personality change, brain damage, psychotic states, and genetic and chromosomal abnormalities as a result of LSD use have not been substantiated but reports confirmed by some people of flashbacks and extremely unpleasant experiences during a "bad trip" add up to a generally unfavorable view of LSD use. An abstinence syndrome for LSD has not been reported, and although there is rapid development of tolerance, it disappears when LSD ingestion is discontinued.
5. Phencyclidine, or PCP, is a synthetic chemical

once thought to have potential as an anesthetic with animals. Its reputation as a "horror drug," paired with mental derangement and violence, probably has little basis in fact. PCP users, who tend to be predominantly young, white, and from lower-or middle-class backgrounds, are aware of PCP as a powerful "mindblowing" drug with certain risks, including the possibility of convulsions and a risk of death with heavy use. Today, PCP use is probably declining and it is probably now used most often along with other more controllable drugs. There is apparently no tolerance or abstinence syndrome associated with PCP use.

6. The amphetamines include a large class of synthetically produced central nervous system stimulants with many legally allowable uses. These drugs are manufactured in pill form by the billions, for distribution through medical prescription. Taken orally or intravenously for nonmedical purposes, this class of substances, second to marijuana and alcohol, is probably the leading drug of abuse, especially by people who are not part of any particular drug subculture. A large group of amphetamine abusers, however, use them for recreational purposes. Effects of heavy use in this group are highly reinforcing, including a sense of wellbeing, alertness, joy, and excitement. "Speed freaks" inject amphetamines intravenously for their immediate effects and sometimes shoot up several times daily—even go on a binge or speed "run" that lasts for several days. Excessive amphetamine use can produce many toxic effects, such as elevated blood pressure, psychomotor agitation, grandiosity, and even an amphetamine psychosis characterized by great excitement, aggressiveness, and paranoid ideation. The "crash" after a speed run is particularly debilitating and emotionally draining. The amphetamines have an extremely high capacity for abuse because of their highly reinforcing effects. Physical dependence is characterized chiefly by tolerance effects.

7. Cocaine, an extremely popular recreational, high-status, expensive stimulant substance derived from the leaves of the coca plant, is reputed to have few adverse effects. If vigorously sniffed or snorted, its chemicals are absorbed from the nasal membranes directly into the bloodstream with highly reinforcing, immediate effects that are relatively short-lived. These include euphoria, heightened energy level, feelings of power, confidence, and mastery, and a sense of skilled sociability—much sought-after effects. Daily, heavy, long-term use can create many interpersonal, financial, and physical problems, however. The latter includes changes in sleeping patterns and physical debilitation after "coming down." The many myths about cocaine, for example, as an enhancer of sexual interest, drive, and performance, come from the street rather than from empirical evidence. Tolerance and abstinence syndromes are not associated with cocaine use.

8. Barbiturates and sedative substances such as Quaalude are CNS depressants that have been legally prescribed for decades. They are among the most frequently abused substances which, with alcohol, are responsible for thousands of deaths each year through accidental overdose or deliberate suicidal intent. Like amphetamine abusers, barbiturate abusers fall into two main classes—a group of older people, mostly women, who attempt to "deal" in this way with tension, anxiety, and sleeplessness and who are not part of any particular drug subculture, and a second group of younger people who use barbiturates (often with other substances such as alcohol) to get "high" for recreational purposes. Included in the latter group are "barb freaks" who intravenously inject these substances for the "rush." A mild relaxing, tension-reducing effect is the most immediate consequence of ingestion of this class of substances, which also frequently yield disinhibition euphoria—a "high" that is much sought after in social settings. If ingestion continues, toxicity is severe,

with many serious adverse effects, including incoordination, nystagmus, respiratory depression, and with continued use, stupor, coma, and death. An abstinence syndrome has been clearly established with long-term, heavy use of these substances, and has even been dramatically demonstrated in infants born to heavy users. Tolerance effects have also been reported.

9. Various commercially marketed volatile solvents—for example, cleaning fluid, paint thinner, and nail polish remover—are frequently inhaled for a cheap "legal" high, especially by young, lower-SES people of ethnic minority (but not black) background. Some of these toxic substances are so dangerous that if inhaled quickly in large enough doses, they can produce death. Physical dependence effects have not been reported for these volatile solvents (inhalants).
10. Heroin, a semisynthetic substance derived from morphine (a dried product of the opium poppy plant), is commonly "mainlined"—that is, injected directly into the vein—with immediate physical effects including pupillary constriction, respiratory depression, and analgesia. The user of heroin generally seeks it out to avoid an abstinence syndrome and for its calming effects of peace, relief from anxiety, pain reduction, and detachment from worldly worries rather than for the euphoria or "high" of other drugs. It has been estimated that there are almost one-half million "addicts" in this country but that about three times as many are regular users who are not "hooked." Many people think that belief in the powerful effects of heroin as well as the social context itself "hooks" heroin users rather than the pharmacological action of the drug itself, for many months of abstinence can be followed by intense craving when former addicts return to their old haunts.
11. Adverse effects of heroin use include impaired responsiveness, slurred speech, and lowered cognitive and motor performance. There is in addition a preoccupation with obtaining heroin that not only interferes with daily living routines such as work but also may cause the user to turn to crime, delinquency, and prostitution. Many experts believe, however, that crime-proneness and "deviation-proneness" *precede* heroin abuse rather than are caused by it. There is a high mortality risk for babies born to addicts, an abstinence syndrome, and a challenge to developmental health. Addicts die more frequently and at younger ages than other people, risk death through accidental overdose, and are frequently part of a subculture of crime and violence. In addition, many physical complications arise from chronic narcotics use, including lung, heart, digestive, and circulatory problems. Narcotics are associated with marked tolerance effects and an abstinence syndrome that follows a fairly predictable pattern.
12. Various psychological theories and hypotheses about drug dependence (especially narcotics abuse) include the presence of predisposing personality factors, common personality types, psychodynamic formulations, and specific hypotheses as to delaying gratification, heroin use as a sexual substitute, and deviation-proneness. In general, most of these hypotheses, although receiving occasional empirical support, have not been consistently confirmed. Socially oriented hypotheses about drug dependence were also touched on, and it was concluded that although drug dependence as an escape from the pain of poverty did not seem to be a valid hypothesis, approaches that stressed peer pressure and the drug subculture as well as various learning and conditioning models really held more promise. The possibility of biochemical correlates of addiction-proneness might explain the fact, it was noted, that some users of narcotics get "hooked" while others with equally frequent narcotics use do not get hooked.
13. Various treatment approaches to drug dependence focus on narcotics dependence. Treatment

methods include detoxification procedures, therapeutic communities, psychotherapy and family approaches, and narcotics maintenance through methadone (probably the most frequently employed and most successful of the approaches), as well as using narcotic-blocking drugs. Motivation to change is probably the single most important element in determining treatment outcome, and no single interventive approach seems to be the most effective one. Staying in treatment is an important goal of treatment programs; to achieve this end, awareness of the subculture and pattern of the abuser as a powerful interventive weapon was emphasized.

14. Finally, Spotlight 17.7 briefly reviewed a variety of programs and problems in connection with the cessation of cigarette smoking, one of the nation's top health hazards. Here also the subject's motivation to quit is of key significance.

ISSUES AND QUESTIONS

1. Many people have wondered about the ethics of substituting synthetic narcotics for heroin, as in methadone maintenance programs. They say that it is "dehumanizing" to treat individuals with chemicals so that although they continue to be drug dependent they adapt more placidly to society's expectations. Do you agree?
2. Controversy surrounds the issue of controlled heroin use, even though proponents claim that such use is possible. The experts feel that legally sanctioning controlled use would greatly increase the population of addicts in this country. What is your opinion?
3. Although decriminalization of marijuana is not legalization, there are claims that it amounts to a "go ahead" signal for drug abuse. Advocates of penalties for marijuana use do acknowledge the fact that Oregon, the first state to decriminalize, did not find an immediate increase in marijuana use. Yet, they contend the long-range effects of decriminalization, as with alcohol, will result in moral and social sanction of all drug ingestion. Should society encourage the use of *any* drug? they ask. What is your opinion about decriminalization?
4. In some countries, heroin addicts are maintained on heroin so that criminal activities in connection with obtaining it are reduced. Although heroin maintenance programs do not always work, the philosophy behind them, according to their proponents, is to help the addict move away from a "junkie" subculture, become more stabilized, become less involved with the procurement of an illegal substance, and allow him or her to feel less guilty, less alienated. Do you agree? If not, do you reject such programs philosophically or because you think they will not work?
5. People like Szasz (1974) feel that the persecution of drug users and the suppression in particular of certain types of drugs are reflections more of the historical and social times than of the adverse effects of the drugs themselves. Alcohol is *licit* and has deleterious effects on people and society. Marijuana is *illicit* but apparently has few dire consequences, they claim. They further claim that some drugs are feared or controlled during certain historical times because they are associated with social divisiveness (for example, alcohol and Indian uprisings, LSD and student protest). Society's legal and social attitudes reflect political considerations, rather than pharmacological or medical ones, they say.

   Should there be no restrictions on drug use? Should we be more lenient about such substances? Otherwise we tend to increase the profits of the black market distributors as well as help shape the subculture that makes drug use so attractive.
6. Members of the armed forces can sometimes obtain hard substances such as narcotics more readily than can other people. It has been pro-

posed that routine "sweeps"—random, involuntary urine tests—be employed to find the users. Controversy has arisen over this procedure. On the one hand, drug abuse has been increasing in the armed forces at an alarming rate and many feel, therefore, that our national security is being undermined. Critics, on the other hand, talk of invasion of privacy, boomerang effects such as great resentment on the part of our troops, and the fact that such a program would be doomed to failure anyway, because users would find ways to avoid being "caught." Where do you stand on this issue?

SUGGESTIONS FOR FURTHER READING

Brecher, E. M., and the Editors of Consumer Reports. *Licit and illicit drugs: The Consumers Union report on narcotics, stimulants, depressants, inhalants, hallucinogens, and marijuana—including caffeine, nicotine, and alcohol.* Boston: Little, Brown, 1972. Paperback available. This fascinating book presents an integrated historical review of the pharmacological, legal, and social effects of legal and illegal drugs. It distinguishes between the direct pharmacological effects of drug ingestion—which are fairly stable over time—and the indirect effects of laws, policies, and attitudes—which may vary considerably from decade to decade.

Feldman, H. W., Agar, M. H., and Beschner, G. M. (Eds.) *Angel dust: An ethnographic study of PCP users.* Lexington, Mass.: Lexington Books, 1979. This book presents an inside look at PCP users: who they are, when, how and why they use PCP. It also describes the drug culture "rules" that influence both the use of the drug and the nature of the drug experience. It is interesting to see that although there are certain commonalities among users, the PCP user is quite different for each of the four cities studied (see Chapters 5 through 8). For an interesting, relatively unbiased presentation of PCP use and its users, this book is highly recommended.

Gorodetzky, C. W., and Christian, S. T. *What you should know about drugs.* New York: Harcourt, Brace Jovanovich, 1970. This slim book is recommended for easily understandable, but good coverage if you want a quick survey of the drug scene. There are excellent illustrations that your little brother or little sister would probably enjoy seeing also.

Grinspoon, L., and Bakalar, J. B. *Cocaine: A drug and its social evolution.* New York: Basic Books, 1976. Paperback available. This book examines cocaine—including its history, botany, neurophysiological, psychological, and pharmacological effects, and its use in our culture—with an eye toward discussion of legal policy regarding its use. Written for the nonspecialist, it is largely anecdotal and quite readable. Although the authors have a generally favorable bias regarding legal policy, however, they do present some of cocaine's adverse effects.

Novak, W. *High culture: Marijuana in the lives of Americans.* New York: Knopf, 1980. Paperback available. This book, based on the self-reports of over 300 marijuana users and the author's own personal experience, presents various aspects of marijuana use: getting high for the first time, the experience of "double consciousness," and marijuana's effect on activities such as eating, listening to music, reading, sex, and driving. Although the approach of this book is basically pro-marijuana, the author does describe possible adverse effects. A frank discussion of marijuana use by people who are users, this book is both interesting and informative.

Szasz, T. *Ceremonial chemistry: The ritual persecution of drugs, addicts, and pushers.* Garden City, New York: Anchor Press/Doubleday, 1974. We meet Szasz again; this time, he is presenting his unconventional views about drug use. Szasz favors the lifting of all restrictions against drug use—stressing the black market profits to be made when there is restriction. He describes society's sanction of *legal* drugs as inconsistent with its harsh attitudes toward other drugs such as heroin. He also notes the "totalitarianism" of such social control—attempts to manipulate and mold others into conventional social contours. Again, Szasz stresses individual freedom and each person's right to determine and shape his or her own behavior. He suggests that drug use is a social and ceremonial behavior, and that drug "persecution" is a political, not medical, act, claiming that drug users in many societies are scapegoated in the same way as are members of certain religious and ethnic groups.

Wolfe, T. *The electric kool-aid acid test.* New York: Farrar, Straus & Giroux, 1968. Paperback available. This is a brilliantly written, dazzling narrative about Ken Kesey, the Merry Pranksters, acid trips, "acid tests" (turning on the world), and acid rock, back in the 1960s, mostly in California. The connection between the psychedelic movement and rock art, rock festivals, extravagant costumes, mixed-media light festivals, and bands like the Grateful Dead and the Mothers of Invention is probably not clear to you. Tom Wolfe's book clarifies all this. It is not only extremely enjoyable to read but is also an impressive illustration of a "marriage" between literary style and subject matter.

18

The Antisocial Personality and Violence, Aggression, and Crime

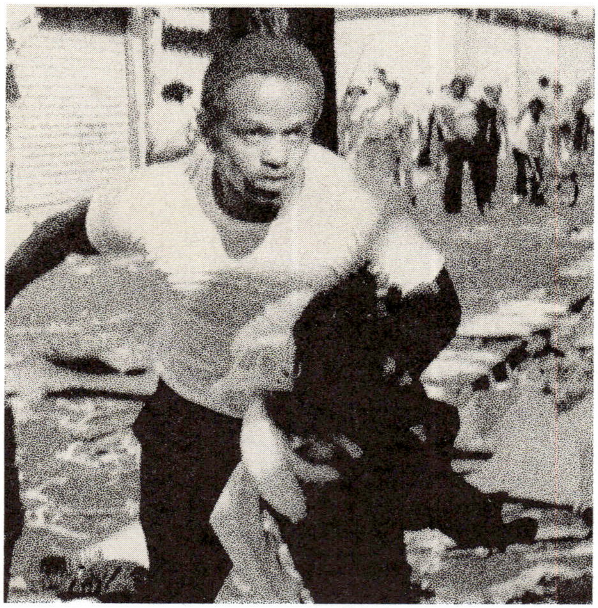

Tommy, an eleven-year-old from a New York City ghetto, was seen in Family Court six times in the past two years. He was arrested for the usual reasons: robbery, mugging, and beating up old ladies.

A senior vice-president of a large, successful investment firm is brilliant with numbers. He has been investing funds that do not belong to him for his own personal profit.

An eminent judge has repeatedly thrown out of court—for one legal reason or another—a suit brought against a certain real estate syndicate. He is a silent partner in that syndicate.

Two fifteen-year-old girls, one white, the other black, were picked up in two midwestern cities at about the same time for prostitution, dealing in drugs, and performing in pornographic movies.

A twenty-two-year-old woman is brutally abused by her boyfriends. In turn, she beats her young child mercilessly. This violent pattern continues until the child is twelve years old. Reasons for doctors' visits and hospitalizations for either her child or herself are shrouded in a veil of mysterious accidents and freaky falls.

A twenty-five-year-old man rapes and murders an elderly woman in the elevator of a low-cost housing project in an inner-city area.

What do these people have in common? That depends on your point of view. If you are looking at them from a legal stance, it is clear that all have broken some legal code. This is where the similarity ends. They are of different ages and SES backgrounds. They vary in color from the palest of flesh tones to very, very dark brown. Some will be apprehended by the police. Others will not. But even if caught in their criminal acts, they may or may not be convicted. So, though each is breaking the law, they do not have equal criminal status. Their outcomes and their lives unfold differently.

The eleven-year-old, Tommy, will have his arrest record sealed. He will commit many such offenses—perhaps twenty more—before he gets into "real" trouble and sentenced to imprisonment. The corporation executive and the judge will never be apprehended. The fifteen-year-old white girl will be placed in the custody of her middle-class parents and nothing much will happen. The fifteen-year-old black girl's mother is in a state hospital. She does not know who her father is. She will be sent to a special facility, where she will be raped by other women. Eventually, she will return to a life on the street—prostitution and drugs—just one step ahead of the law most of the time, but not always.

The child-abusing and abused mother will finally break out of the web of uncontrolled violence in which she is caught. But the ending is not a happy one. Her by-now-twelve-year-old child runs away from home to live out a marginally adequate, occasionally violent existence. The mother has turned to hard drugs and dies of an overdose.

In the meanwhile, the murderer-rapist is caught and sentenced to prison. He is still incarcerated. A few years ago, a similar charge against a similar offender was countered by a successful insanity defense; he was sent to a hospital for the criminally insane but may soon be released.

The point is: Legal, moral, and social codes are very complex and not uniformly applied across all situations. An eleven-year-old and a twenty-two-year old commit the same criminal act. The child is a juvenile offender; the older person is a criminal who goes to jail. The corporation executive gets away with his act. But the inner-city looter of a supermarket (12 cans of beer) gets thrown into jail—and remains there for quite a while before his case comes up.

Not only do legal and social codes differ for various people depending on their circumstances and who they are, but the legality or illegality of an act is also a social consideration. Depending on the historical context and the culture, specific behaviors can be designated at different times as acceptable or unacceptable, legal or illegal, or morally "right" or "wrong." As already noted, many sexual, political, and other behavioral deviances have been viewed through different lenses at various times. For example, smoking pot, homosexuality, sodomy, suffragette demonstrations, peace rallies, and strikes by municipal workers once were (and some still are) regarded as criminal acts.

The legality-illegality or social acceptance-nonacceptance of an act thus is not always a consensual designation. The *content* of the act is less important in these matters than one might think. Through the ages and across various cultures, child abuse and wife-beating, for example, have not always been regarded as punishable, nor have "crimes of passion" or infanticide. Indeed, killing and looting and raping during times of war and on foreign soil have not always been considered to be criminal acts at all, and they have either been condoned or ignored altogether by people in positions of power.

This chapter is concerned with several related but not entirely overlapping areas. It will be looking at the antisocial, or psychopathic, personality, a diagnostic label for people who consistently and flagrantly break the prevailing legal or social codes. As youngsters, they might have been (but not necessarily) juvenile delinquents or juvenile offenders (legal labels) who show conduct disorders (a psychological label). This chapter is also concerned with such behaviors as aggression and violence. These behaviors are not synonymous with crime and criminal behavior (legal and social constructs), which it will also touch on. It should be noted that not all antisocial personalities are criminals, juvenile delinquents, or violent and aggressive; and not all violent or aggressive people are criminals.

THE ANTISOCIAL OR PSYCHOPATHIC PERSONALITY

There are some people who consistently flaunt the standards of the group or the legal codes of the larger society in which they live. This propensity for violating social norms was once thought to stem

Spotlight 18.1 The DSM-III Classification of Antisocial Personality Disorder

The main characteristics of this diagnostic category are a history of fairly continuous antisocial behavior in which the rights of others are violated, with characteristic signs that existed before the age of fifteen years. The designation is generally applied to people eighteen years or older who fail to abide by social norms.* Generally, the DSM-III points out, the flagrant characteristics of antisocial personality disorders, such as sexual promiscuity, fighting, criminality, and vagrancy, begin to diminish after the age of thirty years.

Before the age of 15. There is a history of at least three of the following:

1. Truancy (at least five days per year for at least two years, not including the last year of school)
2. Expulsion or suspension from school for misbehavior
3. Delinquency (arrested or referred to juvenile court because of behavior)
4. Running away from home overnight at least twice while living in parental or parental surrogate home
5. Persistent lying
6. Repeated sexual intercourse in a casual relationship
7. Repeated drunkenness or substance abuse
8. Thefts
9. Vandalism
10. School grades markedly below expectations in relation to estimated or known IQ (may have resulted in repeating a year)
11. Chronic violations of rules at home and/or at school (other than truancy)
12. Initiation of fights

After the age of 18. The presence of at least four of the following:

1. Unstable employment history, for example, frequent job changes, long periods of unemployment, frequent latenesses and absenteeism, impulsive quitting of jobs
2. Irresponsible parenting behavior resulting in malnutrition, poor health and hygiene, and general neglect of child or children due to squandering of household money or parental absences from home

* The DSM-III also describes a childhood category which may in some instances be precursors to or the early stages of the antisocial personality, an adult diagnosis. These are the conduct disorders, described on pp. 529–32.

3. Repeated indications of unlawful or antisocial behavior such as thefts, illegal occupations such as pimping or prostitution, many arrests, or a felony conviction
4. Unstable sexual relationships as indicated by many divorces, separations, or desertion or promiscuity*
5. Repeated assaultiveness and fighting including physical abusiveness to family members
6. Financial irresponsibility, for example, defaulting on debts or not meeting financial obligations
7. Impulsivity and failure to plan ahead
8. Repeated lying, use of aliases, and "conning" others for personal profit
9. Recklessness, as in driving when drunk or recurrent speeding

* The DSM-III specifies that promiscuity refers to "ten or more sexual partners within one year."

from faulty superego development. For a long time, such individuals were called psychopaths, psychopatic personalities, and more recently sociopaths. Today, we speak of antisocial personality disorders.

According to Cleckley (1964), who has provided us with one of the most thoroughgoing descriptions of such people, the sixteen characteristics that distinguish a psychopath from other people are:

superficial charm and good intelligence; absence of delusions and other signs of irrational thinking; absence of "nervousness" or other psychoneurotic manifestations; unreliability, untruthfulness, and insincerity; lack of remorse or shame; inadequately motivated antisocial behavior; poor judgment and failure to learn by experience; pathologic egocentricity and incapacity for love; general poverty in major affective reactions; specific loss of insight; unresponsiveness in general interpersonal relations; fantastic and uninviting behavior with drink and sometimes without; suicide rarely carried out; sex life impersonal, trival, and poorly integrated; and failure to follow any life plan (pp. 362–63).

Most clinicians concur with Cleckley's model. Psychopaths have a low frustration tolerance. They desire immediate gratification of a need, finding it difficult to delay or put off their goal. They are impulsive, immature, unreliable; they form unstable relationships, if any, with others. They cannot be depended upon, and do not respond or adhere to the same moral code as the rest of us, such as keeping promises or paying bills. They do not necessarily modify their behavior with punishment, social humiliation, or censure. They show job instability and have a poor military record (for other than political protest reasons). And most of all, they seem to lack a sense of compassion, empathy, or pity for others. They are egocentric, callous, and flip. They show little guilt or concern for their acts and experience a minimum of worry and anxiety.

On the other hand, psychopaths do not show thinking disturbances. Although they may have poor interpersonal judgment, they have good memories and generally intact intellectual skills. Psychopaths are often charming, glib, fun to be with. They may be "con men" or swindlers. They are often liars, extravagant spenders. They may be attractive to others, even thought they do not show loyalty or consistency in their attachments. Sexually, they may be Don Juans with many Juliets rather than Romeos with only one.

In short, psychopaths do not have the same respect for others' rights and feelings that many of us have. They seem to live by values that most of us do not understand. Their limitations are moral, ethical, and social, rather than cognitive. Often they are in trouble with their jobs, marriages, the banks, and the law. Generally, they are not viewed as "mentally ill," legally insane, or incompetent to stand trial—at least in the eyes of the law (see the end of this chapter).

Antisocial personalities, according to most estimates, are more likely to be male than female—up to five times more likely (DSM-III; Freedman et al., 1972). The diagnosis is relatively common: about 3 percent among men and less than 1 percent among women.

Subclassifications

It has been common to distinguish two types of psychopaths or antisocial personalities (Cleckley, 1964; Hare, 1970; Quay, 1965). First there is the "classic" type just described, in which lack of certain emotional capacities such as compassion, the presence of "sensation-seeking" activities (see pp. 550–51), impulsivity, and low anxiety levels (underarousal) in the face of danger and risk are characteristic qualities. This type is sometimes referred to as the primary psychopath, or sociopath.

The secondary type may also indulge in antisocial activities, but here we find *high* anxiety levels (overarousal in the face of dangers and risks), inner conflicts, and severe emotional disturbance. This type is sometimes referred to as neurotic psychopath, neurotic character, or neurotic delinquent. It has been assumed that secondary antisocial types are motivated by the kinds of conflict-reducing defenses and behaviors (for example, setting fires to get attention of a rejecting parent) that are typical of psychoneurotics in general. It has also been assumed that primary and secondary psychopaths differ from each other in basic qualities (and some moderate evidence supports this assumption), for example, in the degree to which behavior can be modified as a result of such aversive consequences as punishment or a jail sentence (Fagan and Lira, 1980; Hare, 1970; Schmauk, 1970), and capacity for remorse, guilt, and empathy. As a matter of fact, some people claim that secondary psychopaths should not be labeled psychopaths at all (Hare, 1970).

Spotlight 18.2 Would You Answer This Ad?

We have learned much about so-called antisocial personalities from prisoners—an available sample. However, many antisocial personalities or psychopaths never get incarcerated. If you wished to study such people, how could a "true" population be obtained?

Widom (1977) was faced with this problem. She was interested in studying the kinds of antisocial people that Cleckley (1964) described. Such flamboyant, adventure-seeking, guiltless, often charming, impulsive, egocentric individuals, who form few loyal attachments to others, offer intriguing possibilities for clinical study. How would you collect a group of such subjects? Widom placed the following advertisement in a Boston counterculture newspaper in 1974 and 1975.

ARE YOU ADVENTUROUS?

Psychologist studying adventurous carefree people who've led exciting impulsive lives. If you're the kind of person who'd do almost anything for a dare and want to participate in a paid experiment, send name, address, phone, and short biography proving how interesting you are to . . .

A later version of the ad read:

Wanted charming, aggressive, carefree people who are impulsively irresponsible but are good at handling people and at looking after number one. Send name, address . . .

Of the seventy-three responses, a sample of twenty-three males and five females were chosen for further study. The others were eliminated because they did not seem to fit the diagnostic description of Cleckley and others as to psychopathic traits. The subjects were tested and observed in several ways: the MMPI, a biographical interview, delay of gratification situation, and various other tests including ones that measure empathy and social manipulation.

The results of this exploration did indeed indicate that an ambulatory, nonincarcerated sample can be obtained through a newspaper ad. The sample studied seemed more than adequately representative of a psychopathic group as measured by most of the instruments. In addition, even though they showed a high frequency of arrests, they did not show a high frequency of convictions. Apparently, they knew how to "get away with it."

Moreover, a high percentage among them met certain specific criteria (Robins, 1966) for sociopathy:

Some of Robins' Criteria	Percent of Widom's Sample
Poor work history	78.6
Single marital status	75.0
Excessive drugs	67.9
At least one arrest	67.9
Impulsiveness	57.1
Sexual promiscuity or perversion [sic]	50.0
Vagrancy (wanderlust)	46.4
Heavy drinking	46.4
Use of aliases	42.9
School problems and truancy	42.9
Meeting five or more of Robins's criteria	78.6

Source: Adapted from Widom, 1977, p. 679.

This method for locating antisocial personalities in the community-at-large, the author concluded, is a successful one, for many of the social, demographic, and test characteristics of more conventionally obtained antisocial groups were also found in her sample.

CONDUCT DISORDERS: ANTISOCIAL BEHAVIOR IN CHILDREN

The DSM-III distinguishes a childhood or adolescent category (under the age of eighteen years) characterized by behavior that violates the rights of others; also, there is a repeated pattern in which important age-appropriate social norms and rules are violated. Such antisocial behavior is more serious, according to the DSM-III, than ordinary mischief or pranks. These conduct disorders, especially the milder forms, do not necessarily culminate in criminal behavior; that is, the child with a conduct disorder does not automatically grow into a juvenile delinquent. Some other disorder, such as schizophrenia, may be involved.

Conduct disorders, according to the DSM-III, are much more common among boys than girls, with a ratio of 4:1 to 12:1. The undersocialized, nonaggressive type (see the following discussion), however, may be equally frequent for boys and girls. The DSM-III also points out that conduct disorders appear more often in children whose parents have antisocial personalities or who are alcoholics than in families without such disorders.

There are four basic subtypes of conduct disorders: undersocialized aggressive, undersocialized nonaggressive, socialized aggressive, and socialized nonaggressive, according to the DSM-III.

Undersocialized types of conduct disorder. In undersocialized types there is a minimum of normal social "bonding": that is, there are few, if any, relationships that include affection or empathy, a few friendships that last over several months, and infrequent "putting oneself out" for others without

Spotlight 18.3 The DSM-III Disorders of Impulse Control: A Related Diagnostic Category?

The DSM-III employs a diagnostic classification for behaviors that cannot be classified as antisocial personality disorders. These behaviors involve a special kind of impulsivity that is recurrent, often episodic, sometimes with disastrous consequences. There may or may not be voluntary resistance to these impulses.

Most impulse disorders tend to be characterized by mounting tension before the act and an experience of pleasure or release while committing it. Sometimes, there is guilt or self-reproach after the act is completed. We know very little about the etiology of such disorders.

Disorders of Impulse Control

	Prevalence	*Gender Distribution*	*Familial Incidence*	*Diagnostic Criteria*
Pathological gambling	No information	More common in males	Parents tend to show a pattern of alcoholism or gambling	Pattern of being unable to resist impulse to gamble; gambling disrupts family, vocational, and personal pursuits; at least three of: arrests for forgery and fraud, default on debts, interpersonal difficulties, borrowing of money illegally, absenteeism from work, calling on others to relieve a desperate financial situation
Kleptomania	No information	No information (although most apprehended people with this disorder are females)	No information	Pattern of being unable to resist impulse to steal objects of no immediate use and with no monetary value; increasing sense of tension before act; no planning or assistance from others
Pyromania	No information	More common among males	No information	Pattern of failure to resist impulse to set fires; increasing sense of tension before act; an experience of intense pleasure or release at time of committing act; no motivation, such as political action or monetary gain

Disorders of Impulse Control

	Prevalence	*Gender Distribution*	*Familial Incidence*	*Diagnostic Criteria*
Intermittent explosive disorder (*Isolated explosive disorder* is diagnosed when there is a single episode)	Very rare	More common in males	More common in family members than in general population	Several discrete episodes of extremely aggressive acts involving assault or destruction of property; act is grossly out of proportion to precipitating social or psychological stressor; no impulsivity or aggressiveness between episodes; no specific organic disorder such as brain tumor

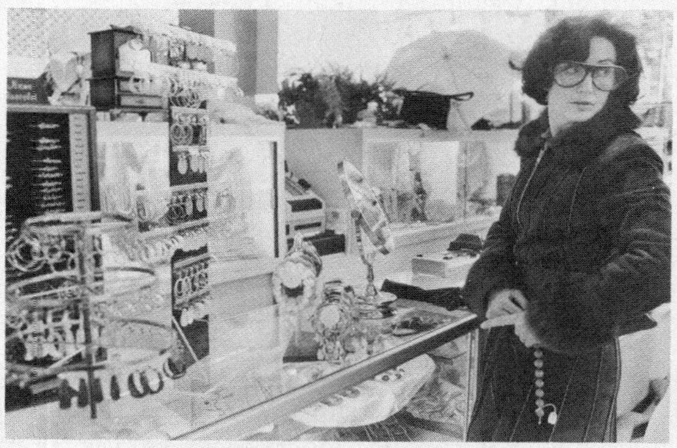

Is kleptomania—a pattern of being unable to resist impulses to steal objects, even if they have no immediate use or monetary value—related to the antisocial disorders described in this chapter? In actual fact, we know very little about the etiology of disorders of impulse control, such as kleptomania, pyromania, and pathological gambling. (Mimi Forsyth/Monkmeyer Press)

some personal advantage. In addition, undersocialized types show little evidence of guilt and remorse, there is little or no concern for the welfare of friends and companions, and if necessary, there is blaming, or informing on, friends.

Undersocialized aggressive conduct disorders, according to the DSM-III, are rather common. In addition to the faulty social bonding noted above, there is a persistent pattern of aggression that might involve physical violence against persons or property, for example, rape, mugging and assault, firesetting, breaking and entering, or thefts involving direct confrontation with victims—for example, purse-snatching or armed robbery.

Undersocialized nonaggressive conduct disorders are also characterized by limited or poor skills in social bonding, but without the physical aggression previously described. The rights of others or age-appropriate social norms are violated, but not in physically assualtive ways. For example, there may be repeated violations of important rules at home or in school such as truancy or substance abuse, a pattern of running away from home overnight, and repeated lying and stealing (without direct confrontation with the victim).

Socialized types of conduct disorder. In socialized types, evidence of greater capacity for empathy and friendships exists, such as feeling guilty or remorseful, showing concern for the welfare of one's friends, or extending oneself to others even when there is no immediate advantage. There also may be gang membership and gang activities with socialized conduct disorders.

Socialized aggressive conduct disorders involve the physically aggressive acts and the violation of the rights of others already noted.

Socialized nonaggressive conduct disorders are rather common according to the DSM-III, and apply to people who show some skills in friendship and social bonding (see above) and whose violation of age-appropriate norms and rules do not include physical assaultiveness or acts against property. These conduct disorders instead may involve persistent truancy, substance abuse, running away from home overnight, and lying or stealing (without direct confrontation with the victim).

CRIME: RATES AND RELATIONSHIP TO SOCIOCULTURAL VARIABLES

Antisocial personality disorders do not bear a one-to-one relationship to criminal behavior, crime, and juvenile delinquency, which are social and legal constructs. Nevertheless, people with antisocial personalities do commit crimes, and much of our theoretical and empirical understanding of them is derived from criminal populations. To understand the antisocial personality better and to explore the origins and nature of criminal activity, we will now briefly survey some relevant sociocultural data.

Many of us may talk about the extent of criminal activity in high crime areas without appreciating its proportions. For example, in 1976 in one high-crime area (New York City's borough of Manhattan) there were 13,459 victims per 100,000 people for such violent crimes as murder, rape, robbery, and aggravated assault (Blau, 1977); and every thirty-two seconds a violent crime is committed in the United States (Some violent statistics, 1978).

Nationwide, are there some trends in the overall picture that can help us to understand criminal behavior? Fortunately, crime data (a large number of criminal acts, according to most experts, are unreported and unrecorded) that are collected from the local police are summarized annually by the Federal Bureau of Investigation in the form of *Uniform Crime Reports.* These and similar summaries suggest that criminal behavior bears a strong relationship to sociocultural factors, and that the search for strictly psychological explanations for crime may be fruitless.

General trends. In this nation there has been a steady increase in violent crimes in the past decade, according to the Federal Bureau of Investigation's Uniform Crime Reports (1980). In 1980, overall crime rate, based on an index derived from all crimes, including violent ones such as murder as well as nonviolent ones such as car thefts, increased by 10 percent over 1979. Rates of *violent* crimes rose by 13 percent: murder by 7 percent, forcible rape by 9 percent, robbery by 20 percent, and aggravated assault by 8 percent.

Age. About three-fourths of all violent street crimes are committed by people who are twenty-five years of age or younger; this age group also accounts for almost half of all reported murders (Some violence statistics, 1978). As for nonviolent crimes, nationwide, most larcenies and thefts are committed by teenage males, age fifteen to nineteen years (Uniform Crime Reports, 1978).

Gender. More than half of violent crimes are committed by young (under age twenty-five) males. As a matter of fact, males have cornered the market on all types crimes (Uniform Crime Reports, 1978). However, the incidence of crime is increasing among women and is rapidly moving in the direction of greater "equality" with men. In the mid 1970s, compared to 1960, there was a 350 percent increase in larcency, 300 percent increase in robbery, and 200 percent increase in murder and aggravated assault among women. But despite increases, rates of violent crimes among women (homicide, assault, and armed robbery) continue to be low, whereas those for nonviolent crimes (such as embezzling and fraud) are relatively high (Crimes by women, 1978).

Are women less aggressive than men? The evidence that men tend to be physically more aggressive than women whereas women tend to show more indirect aggression than men is not consistent (Frodi, Macaulay, and Thome, 1977). On the other hand, most studies of aggression in young children (direct observation, ratings in projective methods, and experimental manipulation) do indicate that boys are more aggressive than girls (Feshbach, 1970). But whether or not there is a direct relationship of aggressive behavior to criminal and antisocial behavior later on is not clear.

Murder among intimates. Many researchers (Goode, 1969; Lystad, 1974, 1975; Wolfgang, 1956) point to data that indicate a close relationship (often relatives) between murderer and victim. Murder emerges in the context, in such instances, of antagonisms and hostilities that have been smoldering for years. The murderer is not always the past aggressor, but, on the contrary, has often been the passive or submissive partner—the one who has been teased, "pushed around," bullied. Finally, in an act of outrage, after a turning point, he or she murders the "aggressor." Thus, according to some writers, murder is an act of intimacy in which friends and relatives provoke, taunt, or in some way set the stage for the act. Almost one in four murders in the United States is committed within the same family (Gelles and Straus, 1979). About 80 percent of murderers and victims are of the same racial background (Half of 1976 murder victims, 1977). And about 80 percent of homicides are committed by either a relative or an acquaintance of the victim (Houts, 1970).

Of additional interest is the fact that murder victims are not necessarily "innocents" (described by Rollo May, 1972) who promote or underwrite the evil around them by their weakness and their refusal to recognize corruption or malevolence. As a matter of fact, about half of the 1,622 murder victims in New York City in 1976 had arrest records and at the time of death had measurable levels of alcohol, narcotics, or both in their bloodstreams (Half of 1976 murder victims . . . , 1977).

SES and ethnicity. The highest incidence and rates of crime are in black America and compared to whites, a relatively larger number of homicide *victims* are black (Coombs, 1974; Harper, 1976). Almost all experts, however, stress the belief that it is the strong association of poverty with ethnic minority status, rather than ethnic minority status alone, that makes the major contribution to criminality.

To repeat, slum residence, crowded living conditions, poverty, ethnic minority status, unemployment, and family disorganization have been clearly associated with high rates of crime and delinquency. This strong correlation obscures some important complexities, however. Many impoverished families of a variety of ethnic backgrounds do not produce delinquent children or adult criminals (Minuchin et al., 1967). Further, because crime in middle-class populations may be less lurid, less vividly expressive, and therefore less in the public eye than, for example, the brutality of the pimp's vengeance on the slum street, we tend to be more impressed with the strength of the relationship between slums and crime.

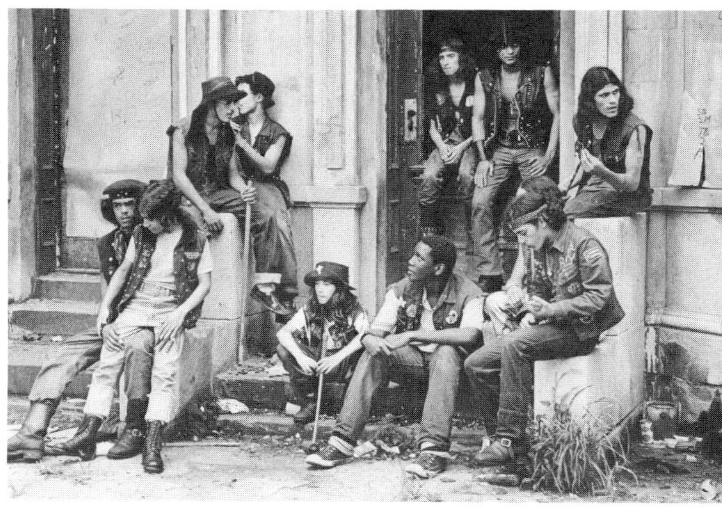

Slums and unemployment breed high rates of crime and delinquency. (J. P. Laffont/Sygma)

We are learning, however, that violence is not the exclusive property of the slum. One survey of family violence indicated that intact, "normal" middle-class families yield a staggering amount of physical violence—parents against children, siblings against siblings, and spouse against spouse (Violence is occurring in the best of families, 1977). Further, the experimental evidence is not at all clearcut or consistent that lower-class children are more aggressive than middle-class children, and that the latter are trained to curb the direct expression of aggression (Feshbach, 1970).

In short, crime, violence, and aggression appear to cut across all classes and all ethnic groups, even though the expression of violence—its quality, who the victims are, the suddenness of the aggression, and type of crime— probably does bear a relationship to ethnic and SES factors.

Antisocial personality disorders and crime. Many people with antisocial personalities commit crimes, but many do not. Can we predict who, among the psychopaths, will be particularly aggressive or commit crimes? According to recent hypotheses, it is not possible to predict violence from personality models alone (Heilbrun, 1979; Shah, 1978). This would be consistent with an approach that suggests that "person" variables in interaction with situational ones are the best predictors (see Mischel, 1973; Shah, 1978). An additional hypothesis suggested by a study of a white prisoner sample is that intelligence or cognitive variables as well as personality, in the light of a particular situation, might best predict violence or crime rather than any single variable, such as psychopathy, intelligence, or situation alone (Heilbrun, 1979). Heilbrun illustrates this model with a barroom brawl that might incite violence in psychopathic personalities with limited intelligence but not in those who are brighter or who are not psychopaths.

If we conduct research that looks at the criminal first, in a search for early, antecedent variables, another view is proposed: most or all hardened, long-term criminals are psychopaths. This is the position of Yochelson and Samenow (1976), whose long-term study of prisoners yielded the conclusion that violence-prone, "incurable" criminal repeaters (recidivists) who make up the bulk of high-security prison populations, are the "classic" primary psychopaths who begin criminal careers at an early age, are extremely difficult to treat, and possess the characteristics already described such as impulsivity, immorality, and lack of remorse.

THEORIES OF AGGRESSION, CRIME, AND ANTISOCIAL BEHAVIOR

As stated earlier, aggression, violence, criminal activity, and the antisocial behavior shown by the psychopath are only roughly related constructs. The following hypotheses sometimes apply to one and sometimes to another of these areas.

General Models for Aggression and Violence

Aggression can be defined as "an act which injures another person—that is (an) hostile, interpersonal, acting-out aggression (that) could be physical, verbal, acquisitive, or indirect" (Eron, 1980, p. 245). What are the causes of aggressive behavior?

We have already noted that some people view aggression as an inborn (instinctual) drive that all animals, including humans, possess (see Spotlight 18.4). This view is not shared by most psychologists, who tend to believe that although the biochemical, glandular, and behavioral mechanisms for the expression of aggression may indeed be within the organism's biological response repertoire, the socialization of the child—how he or she is raised, taught to behave, rewarded, punished—is a crucial factor in how aggressive that child actually becomes (see Eron, 1959, 1980).

Why are people aggressive? If aggression is learned, how does it first arise? Why are some people more aggressive than others? Researchers in the area of aggression are concerned with answering some, if not all, of these questions.

Spotlight 18.4 Are Aggression and Violence Inborn "Evils" That Culture and Society Must Curb?

Proponents of the view that aggression of human against human is instinctual and has always been present in one form or another point to cannibalism, tribal warfare, lootings, pillage, assassinations, massacres, ghetto riots, child beatings and killings, rape, murder, arson, kidnapping, skyjacking, piracy, destruction of property, large-scale wars.

Why does violence persist in such consistent ways through the ages and from culture to culture? Why is violence (and the more brutal and bloodier the more "appealing") so explicit, so frequently expressed in our own culture? Just look at our movies, theatre, plays, opera, animated cartoons, novels, mythology. Even in games and rituals that are culturally stylized and institutionalized—from the lions and the Christians, to jousting, car racing, and circus stunts—we see violence or potential violence (in death-defying risks).

Konrad Lorenz (1966), an eminent ethologist (a scientist who studies animal behavior in relationship to habitat and environment), is an outspoken believer in the inborn, instinctual nature of aggression and violence in humans and animals. The preservation of the species, the protection of the young and of one's own stake and property, and the search for food are all aided by aggressive instincts. An animal's or human's aggressive instincts are protections from the ravages of the natural or social world, preserving the organism's physical integrity so that propagation as well as protection of the offspring can ensure the species' survival. In these and related views, culture and society have developed complex ways of curbing, modifying, and controlling aggression—through ritual, family codes, and various social regulations—so that killing *within* the species is not a too-frequent occurrence.

Many observers of behavior, however, do not believe that there is an inborn, powerful aggressive drive. They conceive of aggression as learned behavior, which, like any other response or pattern of response, can be conditioned to a stimulus or modeled after the behavior of others.

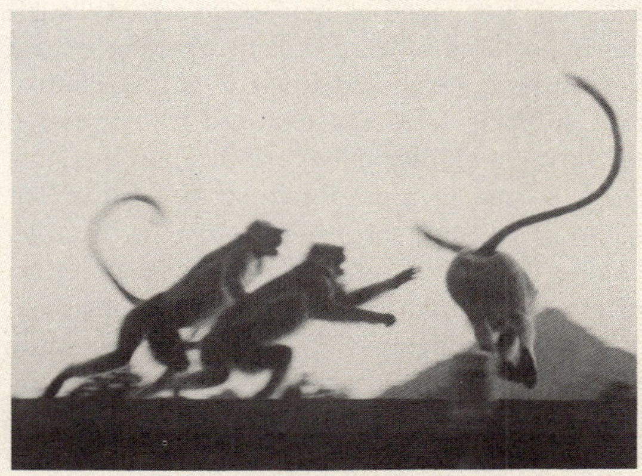

Animals' aggression—for example, to protect their young—may be inborn. Many researchers do not believe that there is a powerful inborn aggressive drive among humans, however. (Hrdy/Anthro-Photo)

The frustration-aggression approach. One early theoretical approach was the frustration-aggression hypothesis proposed by a group of Yale psychologists (Dollard et al., 1939). In this approach it was assumed that the organism possesses an unlearned capacity for aggressive responses that, under conditions of frustration and deprivation, will be spontaneously evoked. Aggression—attempts to harm an object or a person—is a direct response to a frustration; but many aspects of it can be modified through learning. It can be strengthened, reduced, or modified in various ways, such as displaced to another object, generalized to another person or situation, or turned against the self.

Modeling. What determines the nature, the content of the aggressive act? One approach that addressed itself to this question proposed that very young children learn aggressive responses by imitation (Bandura, 1973; Bandura and Walters, 1963). In the social learning approach (see Chapter 6, pp. 131–32), stress is placed on the role of observation, imitation, and modeling (a learned response that is acquired by imitating others such as a parent, teacher, or peer) in the development of aggressive responses. Even very young children learn to imitate aggressive responses, especially if performed by a respected adult model such as a teacher or parent.

In one classic study, three groups of children, while playing with toys and games, were exposed to either real models, the same filmed models, or cartoon characters engaged in aggressive activity, such as battering a large inflated doll or banging with a mallet (Bandura, Ross, and Ross, 1963). A control group of subjects were not exposed to aggressive models during a similar play period. Then the subjects were placed in a mildly frustrating situation: In a roomful of toys, they were told that the toys were being saved for other children. In the next step of the experiment, the subjects were observed and rated as to aggressive activity while they played. All experimental groups showed more aggressive play than the control subjects, with those exposed to aggressive real-life and filmed models showing the most aggression.

As the child develops, aggressive responses are shaped, maintained, and guided by exactly the same kinds of reinforcement (for example, a teacher's attention, parental soothing, getting other children to yield to one's behavior) that shape other kinds of behaviors. Thus, Bandura's social learning approach focuses on the *learned* aspects of aggressive responses rather than on its innate or unlearned origins that some theorists stress.

Early acquisition of aggressive traits. Early acquisition of aggressive responses that tend to persist much in the way a personality trait persists is stressed in the model proposed by Eron and his colleagues. This group of researchers formed these conclusions on the basis of a large-scale longitudinal study (Eron, 1980; Lefkowitz, Eron, Walder, and Huesmann, 1977) that involved careful observations of 875 eight-year-old children and a sizable follow-up: about half of the sample was reevaluated ten years later. Aggression, which could be physical, verbal, acquisitive, or indirect—as long as it injures someone else—was shown to be rather stable, durable, and predictable in this population. For example, subjects who had been rated as aggressive when they were young children were three times as likely to have been "entered on police records" later on as those who were not so rated.

Youngsters who are aggressive at home are aggressive in school and in the larger social environment; children who are physically aggressive are also verbally aggressive and indirectly aggressive; and there is predictability over at least a 10-year period from age 8 to age 18 and 19. Aggression is a behavior that is learned very early in life and is learned very well—the payoff is tremendous.

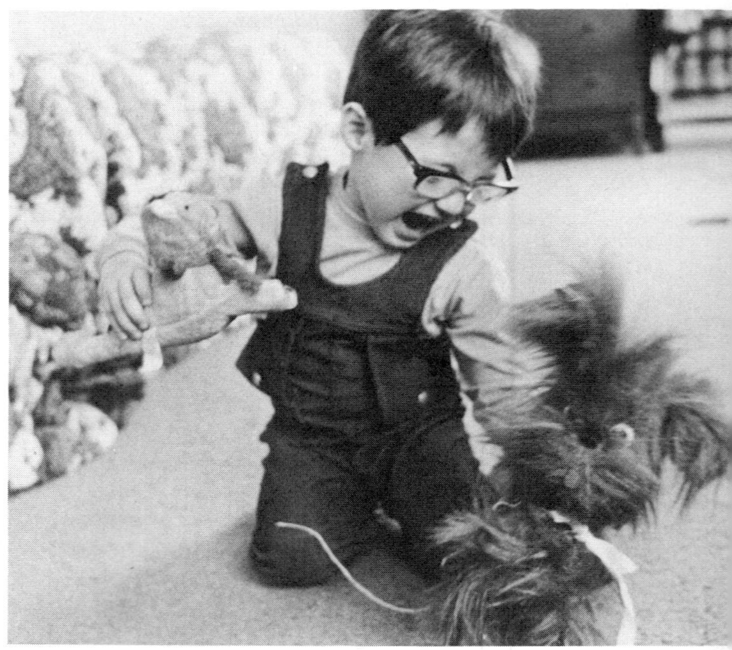

Some children are more aggressive than others. Psychologists are interested in exploring the antecedents of such behaviors. (Alice Kandell/Photo Researchers)

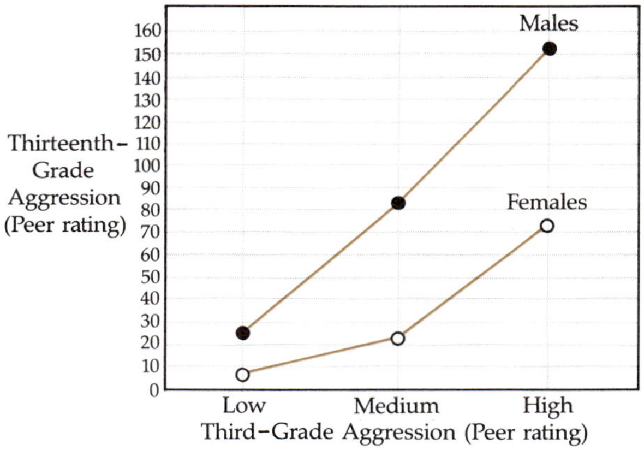

Figure 18.1 Consistency of aggression across time. (From L. D. Eron, Prescription for reduction of aggression, *American Psychologist,* 1980, *35,* 245. Copyright 1980 by the American Psychological Association. Reprinted by permission of the author.)

> *Thus aggression operates like a trait, and it is not easy, as we know, to eliminate or change traits—which is why we probably do not like to talk about traits or even admit that there are such things (Eron, 1980, p. 244).*

Interestingly, predictability of aggression is more striking and dramatic for males than for females, as Figure 18.1 illustrates. In Eron's large-scale longitudinal study, several variables were associated with aggression, especially watching TV violence among the eight-year-old boys. These and other "antecedent" variables are discussed later in this chapter.

Harlow's model. Another model derived from animal research may bear on the important question of individual differences in aggressivity. In Chapter 6, reference was made to Harlow's researches with monkeys. Harlow and his associates demonstrated that aggressive responses in monkeys were evoked if there were limited prior opportunities for contact with the mother, mother surrogate, or peers. Monkeys raised in isolation showed more aggression toward each other or to strangers than if there had been opportunities for social interaction with other monkeys. Also, in adults, aggressive responses toward their *own* children were evidenced if they (the adults) had had minimal play and contact opportunities when they themselves were young. Whether or not this approach can be applied directly to humans continues to be debatable, but there are many implications of this research that should be explored, especially as to the significance of social interactions with peers and age-mates in the production or modification of aggression (see Harlow's lecture, 1975).

Antecedents of Violence and Delinquency: A Search for Crucial Variables

The search for correlates and antecedents of violent and aggressive behavior may result in methods for predicting such behavior as well as point to possible directions for intervention. This reasoning was the backdrop for the extensive work of the Gluecks designed to identify those children at risk for delinquency. The large-scale attempts of these researchers to develop a method to predict delinquency yielded indices that would presumably alert researchers, for example, or staff members of various social agencies to the possible unfolding of delinquency later on.

The Social Factor Prediction Scale developed by the Gluecks (1950) focused on one set of variables—parental and familial factors—that characterized the delinquent population they worked with. Among the important variables that correlated with delinquent status were discipline of boy by father; supervision of boy by mother; affection of father for boy; affection of mother for boy; and cohesiveness of family.

The promise of the Gluecks' early, ambitious investigation was not fulfilled, for they were not able to successfully predict delinquency in individual children. One reason for this poor record of success might be that indices were derived from inner-city samples that were not representative of delinquent subcultures in many large urban areas. In the Gluecks' original research, for example, English, Irish, and Italian parentage represented 69 percent of their sample.

Spotlight 18.5 TV: Training for Violence?

Occasionally, an act of violence mimics a television or movie plot. For example, in the attempt to assassinate President Reagan in 1981, a specific film and actress in a film became intertwined in the confused and irrational fantasies of the would-be assassin. But murders of famous people are not daily occurrences nor are they always modeled on a film or television plot.

On the other hand, thousands upon thousands of violent acts—murders, armed robberies, rapes—occur annually in this country. Is it possible that some of these acts can also be traced to television or movie violence?

There is a continuing debate over this issue, especially as to the influence of television violence on the very young. A longitudinal study that is frequently cited by those who claim that there is a definite relationship between television violence and aggressive behavior did indeed demonstrate a strong statistical relationship between the viewing of violence in their very young sample and later aggressive behavior (Lefkowitz et al., 1977):

> *. . . television habits established by age eight-nine years influence boys' aggressive behavior at that time and at least through late adolescence. The more violent are the programs preferred by boys in the third grade, the more aggressive is their behavior both at that time and ten years later. This relation between early television habits and later aggression prevails both for peer-rated aggression and for self-ratings of aggression. Actually, these early television habits seem to be more influential than current viewing patterns since a preference for violent television in the 13th grade is not at all related by concurrent aggressive behavior, nor are early television habits strongly related to later television habits (Lefkowitz et al., 1977, p. 120).*

Why boys only? It has been suggested that because violence on television programs in the 1960s was portrayed by male actors primarily, boys could more readily identify with, and model their behavior along lines of, violent acts, than girls. Also, the authors conjectured, boys are trained very early to behave aggressively; as a result, they normally and quite naturally perceive aggression and violence on television in *realistic* terms. Because girls, on the other hand, are trained to seek fantasy and imaginal outlets for hostile impulses, they would tend not to perceive television violence in realistic, concrete terms or as a model for behavior.

Data from this study also suggest that early television viewing practices, rather than later ones, are related to aggressive behavior, much as if tendencies for aggression, once developed, do not require a current situational influence (that is, current television viewing of violence) to be maintained. Young boys, in other words, who watched and preferred physical violence on programs like *Kojak* grew up to be aggressive young men even if, as young adults, they tend to prefer programs like *Father Knows Best.**

Some psychologists believe that predispositional elements may be brought to the television set, influencing which programs are selected and how they are perceived and interpreted. In addition, the extent to which roles on many of these programs serve as models for behavior may also be based on predisposition toward violence. One need not have theoretical biases as to the physiological, hormonal, or learning components in such predispositions. The point is: some children may bring "violence-proneness" to their television viewing that in turn reinforces the already existing inclinations.

On the other side of the debate are those who claim that explanations for aggressive and violent behavior are rooted in a more complex set of variables than is contained in the simple hypothesis of television viewing. Violence in its varied forms, they say, such as war, pillaging, rioting, looting,

* Occasionally, the defense in a robbery or murder trial is built around the implicating of television violence as a strong influence on the defendant's behavior. Most of these defenses have not won in the courts, however.

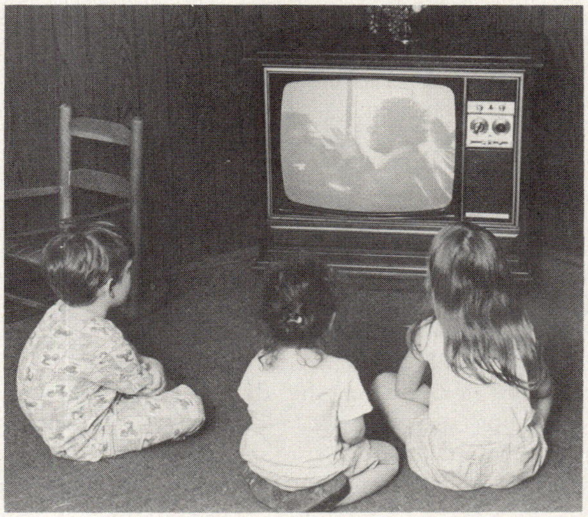

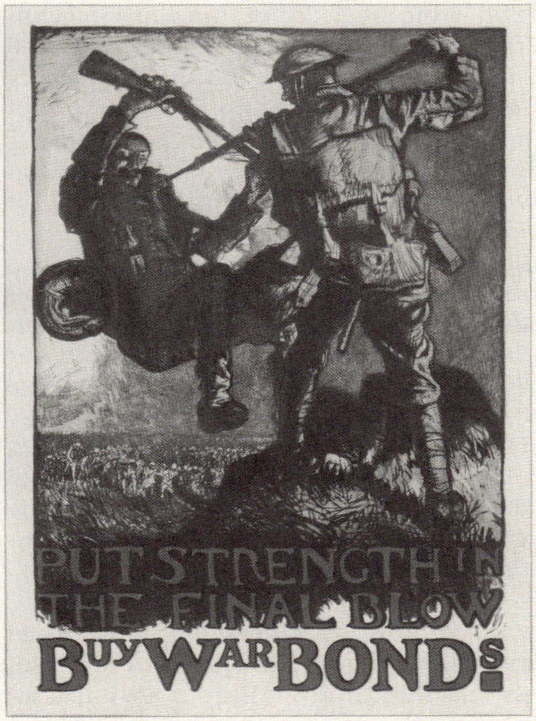

raping, murder, political terrorism, assassination, and capital punishment has been around for years. It is experienced by many on close, intimate, interpersonal levels—on the streets, in local taverns, and within families. Long before television, there was violence. Think of Dickens's London of the nineteenth century, how we won the West from the Indians, and our Civil War. Think, also, of the lynchings of slaves or of the cockfighting, bullfighting, and prizefighting values in many subcultures within our society. The point is that in eras long past as well as today, models for violence exist on many levels of our social fabric and within easy reach and perception of very young children on all social strata.

Selective viewing of and preference for violence on television may be an outgrowth of early, learned aggressive tendencies that, along with peer pressure, peer models, adult models, and cultural pressures and values, may create "person" variables which in appropriate situational contexts result in violence. But we need not invoke television violence alone, many people say, as the truly important influence in creating patterns of violence.

What are your thoughts about this debate?

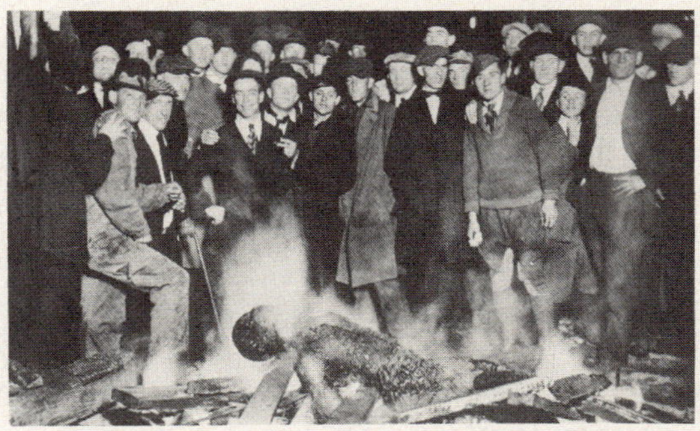

Television undoubtedly provides a model for violence for the children (and adults) who watch it, but models for violence have always existed. For example, is there a connection between the socially sanctioned, "patriotic" violence in this World War I poster and the violence of the St. Louis race riots of 1919? Notice the expressions on the faces of these men—and boys. (Above left: George Roos/Peter Arnold. Above, top and bottom: Culver Pictures)

Nevertheless, the search for variables that "hold up" in the prediction of delinquency continues. From these studies,* several antecedents and correlates of aggression, violence, and delinquency have emerged.

Physical punishment of the child at home as well as the witnessing of violence and physical aggression are associated with aggressive and violent behavior. Poor identification with the parent or parents, and lack of parental support, nurturance, and understanding (which reduces the effectiveness of discipline for aggressiveness), lack of parental supervision and discipline, broken and one-parent families, peer pressure, truancy, dropping out of school and the availability of models who display antisocial behavior are also associated with delinquency and aggression. In addition, criminal behavior and/or alcoholism in the parents is moderately predictive of later delinquency. Attentional difficulties and conduct disorders are thought to be precursors of antisocial personality disorders in adults, but evidence for this relationship has not been clearly established. Low SES is often correlated with aggression and violence, but there is not a one-to-one relationship between these variables, and middle-class backgrounds do yield delinquency.

What accounts for the fact that some family and social milieus (poverty, broken family, role models in the "street") do not necessarily produce delinquent children or extreme aggression. One answer may lie in a closer examination of certain family "climates" that might be breeding grounds of crime and delinquency. In this view, slums and poverty per se do not produce violence, even when role models and peer pressure are present. Instead, family disorganization, with limited or crude "rules" of communication and a chaotic atmosphere without structure and regulations might set the stage for the development of antisocial behavior in the children (Minuchin et al., 1967).

* Reports on which some of these generalizations are based include Eron (1980); DSM-III; Feshbach and Feshbach (1973); Lefkowitz et al. (1977); Rizzo (1975); Schaar (1977).

Important to remember is that no one of the above variables predicts delinquency or antisocial behavior. This is as much true for a broken home (death? divorce? abandonment?), a deprived, low-SES background, antisocial and alcoholic parents, as for the other single variables.

Sociological Approaches to Crime and Delinquency

The broad correlation of crime and delinquency to social factors such as poverty and class was a giant step forward in the direction of understanding crime and violence. Here is a brief summary of some major sociological approaches:

1. Durkheim (1938), an eminent sociologist, was responsible for a dramatic shift in thinking about crime. According to Durkheim, crime is prevalent in all societies. But a particular act is not intrinsically criminal. Each society determines its own morality. Because what is immoral and possibly punishable is determined by societal concepts of morality and of right and wrong, notions of "innate criminality" and the "criminal mind" fall by the wayside, for they imply a universality of meaning and behavior that cuts across all cultures—an implication for which there is little evidence.

2. Merton (1938, 1957), another sociologist, suggested that the basic values of a culture are related to the criminality that can be found within that culture in a very special way. There are some goals in a society that are common for everybody. In our society, for example, the enormous stress on acquiring wealth for social status is a common goal. For some individuals, however, there are few legitimate means to achieve these goals. Such people, according to Merton, will turn to illegitimate means to arrive at these same, common goals.

Differential access to the means for attaining these cultural goals among various groups leads to a high frequency of antisocial acts in groups with fewer opportunities, for example, those with low educational levels, of ethnic minority status, or from impoverished, slum situations. Merton notes that lack of opportunity, poverty, or poverty in the midst of plenty do not lead to crime by themselves. Differential access to a commonly shared goal, however, would. The goal of financial success cuts across all of our social classes, whereas the means for achieving this end are withheld from a large portion of our population. Thus, in our society, there is a higher association between poverty and crime than in some other societies in which a more rigid class structure is accompanied by different (rather than similar) goals and symbols of achievement from class to class.

It is the ill-balanced "social structure," according to Merton, that places pressure on some people to behave in deviant ways. The imperfect coordination between goals and means to goals within a society—for some people—leads to *anomie* (according to Durkheim, normlessness), an inability to implement or execute a goal by knowing how to get there, knowing how to "make it" through legitimate channels.

3. The differential association theory was proposed by Sutherland (Sutherland & Cressey, 1966) on the basis of an extensive review of the literature on the correlates of crime. Sutherland's approach is based on learning principles. Criminal behavior is learned behavior. Many sociologists, including Sutherland, have attempted to specify the mechanisms by which this learning takes place (for example, through principles of operant conditioning; Burgess and Akers, 1966).

The differential association theory, in brief, consists of the following: Criminal behavior is learned through association with other people, primarily within intimate personal groups, in communication processes that are both verbal and nonverbal. The "impersonal" mass media, therefore, are relatively unimportant with respect to the origins of delinquent behavior. This learning includes not only techniques for committing the crime, but also the attitudes, motives, and drives associated with the crime. The principles of "differential association" pertain to the actual contacts with or isolation from criminal patterns and these associations vary in frequency, duration, priority, and intensity. Finally, the general needs and values in a society do not explain criminal behavior, for noncriminal behavior is also derived from these same needs and values.

Overall, Sutherland's notions "explain" the paradox faced by those who are strict socioeconomic theorists: why does one slum child become delinquent and another not. Sutherland's approach underscores the possibility that even within the same locale—as on a ghetto street—opportunities for learning certain types of behavior may vary from individual to individual.

4. The delinquent subculture, in transmitting its values to its members, is thought to have a powerful influence on behavior. Although this view is relevant to gangs of delinquents and to groups of people who share a nonconformist, antisocial view, it does not explain the emergence of the individual psychopath or criminal who may never have been a member of a delinquent gang (Cloward and Ohlin, 1960).

Cohen (1955) attempted to examine this delinquent subculture from the point of view of

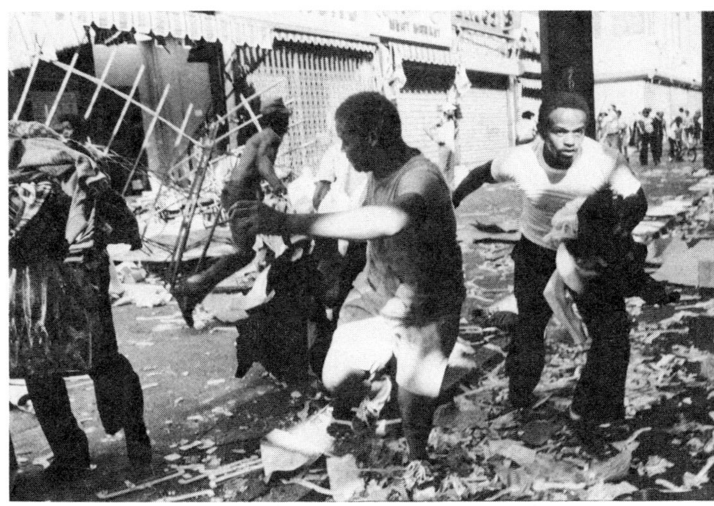

Looting during New York City's blackout several years ago. Does such antisocial behavior have the same causes as do crimes by individuals acting alone? (© Tex Fuller 1978/Woodfin Camp)

Sutherland's approach: special "styles" of living and values characterize the delinquent subculture. This style is unique to lower-class young males rather than delinquent females, delinquents from other SES groups, or adult criminals. The specific interpersonal dynamics within a family are not too relevant in the understanding of delinquency. To repeat, it is the delinquent subculture itself that transmits certain values and provides the rewards to maintain them.

According to Cohen, the delinquent subculture is nonutilitarian, "malicious," and negativistic. There is short-run hedonism, group autonomy, and group cohesiveness. Values and styles are unconcerned with middle-class ambitions of upward mobility or financial success (in this sense, Cohen disagrees with Merton). Instead, this subculture sanctions aggression, respects the stolen dollar, but not the dollar saved or earned, and sees little need for property ownership for its own sake other than the immediate gratification it can provide. Further, the subculture nurtures a strong drive for status in the eyes of other delinquents, resolved through achievements and exploits typical of a "macho" style.

Personality Theories of Crime and the Antisocial Personality

The psychoanalytic approach. Ego and superego interactions and balances play an important role in psychoanalytic theorizing about people with antisocial personality disorders. In brief, such people lack conscience and guilt as a result of faulty development in childhood. The child never develops beyond an impulse-ridden pleasure-principle level. Thus, in this arrested personality development, there is a disturbance of "libidinal balances," so that the adolescent and the adult are not governed by the usual checks and balances of superego controls and reality versus pleasure principle themes.

Psychoanalytic writers sometimes acknowledge the presence of strong guilt feelings in some criminal types. Such feelings may be unconscious and vague, but they propel the criminal to get caught and to be punished for his or her crime—thus allaying guilt. Even if the criminal is not caught, feelings of guilt can be reduced: "There is no reason why I should feel so guilty. I am not being punished. I am not so bad, after all." In such interpretations, impulsive characters and criminal types possess faulty, rather than no, superego development (see Fenichel, 1945). Identification with parental figures and internalizaton of their social values were somehow incomplete, interrupted, or weak and disorganized.* But superego is not lacking entirely.

In a related view, aggressive "acting out" in adolescents is not explained by weak superego development but rather by lack of superego in certain circumscribed areas. These specific areas correspond to those reflecting the parents' forbidden impulses. The antisocial child vicariously enacts the parents' own wishes as a result of their (the parents') conscious or unconscious permissiveness or inconsistency in these areas. In other words, the superego lacunae of delinquent children are derived from similar defects in their parents (Johnson, 1947).

Psychoanalytic writers sometimes link certain crimes with sought-after modes of sexual excitement—for example, "incendiarism" to problems in masturbation (Simmel, 1949). Fenichel's classic work (1945) is laced with such explanations. For example, with regard to pyromania (an obsessive concern and excitement over setting and watching fires), which the DSM-III calls a disorder of impulse control, Fenichel states:

> *Sexual excitement at the sight of fire is a normal occurrence in the children. It is not easy to explain. Analysis reveals the effectiveness of sadistic drives, which aim to destroy the object, and a cutaneous pleasure in the warmth of the fire. . . . Regularly a deep-seated relationship to urethral eroticism is to be found. Freud took this as a starting point for a speculative hypothesis about the origin of the cultural use of fire. . . . The pleasure in starting a fire (in reality or in fantasy) may become the indispensable condition for sexual enjoyment. In an incendiary perversion, intense*

* Such reasoning implies that the parents had "*good*" socially desirable values that somehow were not internalized by their delinquency-prone offspring.

sadistic strivings govern the sexual life, the destructive force of the fire serving as a symbol for the intensity of the sexual urge (Fenichel, 1945, p. 371).

In general, specific psychoanalytic concepts such as the broad linking of criminal behavior to behavior dominated by the pleasure principle have not received empirical confirmation. It seems more likely that the different crimes committed by different individuals are motivated by a wide variety of factors. In regard to the domination of the pleasure principle, for example, some antisocial people can be extremely reality-oriented: think of the disciplined and patient embezzler who waits for years to achieve his or her goal.

An overall evaluation of the contribution of psychoanalytic theorists to an understanding of delinquency and criminal behavior yields a negative picture. There is inconsistency of hypotheses and fuzziness of concepts and thus little direct empirical evidence to support the various psychoanalytic explanations. In addition, the psychoanalytic view conspicuously avoids dealing with matters of social group membership, subcultural values, and the realities of poverty and the slum as possible correlates of antisocial and criminal behavior.

Psychoanalytic stress on the individual delinquent or criminal as "sick" and in need of help, rather than "bad," however, has made a singularly important contribution to the development of more humane methods of treatment and punishment in our judicial and penal institutions and in the general climate of opinion about criminals, especially young ones. This view is currently shifting, however, a theme I will return to later in this chapter.

Spotlight 18.6 "I Have Achieved In One Day What It Took Robert Kennedy All His Life To Do": Sirhan Sirhan, Assassin

There is little evidence that criminals can be identified by personality type. There are some crimes, however, that are so spectacular in their political and social implications and in their national and international scope, that the search for a profile, or for some identifying characteristics of the criminal, becomes crucial in order to prevent—it is thought—future occurrences of the crime. Thus, after the attempts to assassinate President Reagan and the Pope in 1981, there was a flurry of interest in painting the portrait of the typical assassin. Unfortunately, the "base rate"—the number of actual assassins—is so small that it is difficult to describe more than some possible common denominators. To make matters worse, it is likely that the terrorist who assassinates a political figure for *political* reasons is probably different in personality and emotional makeup from the assassin who kills because of compulsion to act out private fantasy.

In America, assassinations of high-level leaders usually do not have the political motivation of European and South American assassinations. In the last century, there were about fifty assassinations and assassination attempts of powerful or celebrated people, in and out of government, including Abraham Lincoln, Robert and John Kennedy, Martin Luther King, George Wallace, Gerald Ford, and Ronald Reagan, not to mention John Lennon of the Beatles. Mostly these violent acts have not been the acts of a left or right political zealot, determined to get his or her ideological message across to the people.

A profile of these assassins, based on a crude composite picture, is beginning to emerge. This is an after-the-fact sketch, not especially useful in *predicting* an assassination. There are probably hundred of thousands of people who fit the bill, even to the purchasing of handguns.

The "typical" picture that emerges, then, is that of a young, white, single isolated male who feels sexually inadequate, unloved; he has been able to form few male and female friendships and attachments. There may be a dominant mother and a passive or absent father, but this is not always the family pattern. Typically, this man is a shy, well-behaved loner who did not get into trouble at school and even though described as a "model" child, conscientious and dutiful, was basically not liked by his peers.

The fantasy search for fame, for achieving celebrity, for leaving a lasting mark soon becomes an overwhelming, central preoccupation for this isolated man, who travels from city to city, sometimes even stalking his prey. There may be, also, an intense identification with either the victim or someone connected to the victim who also has notoriety—an actress or sports figure. Frequently, there is ambivalence about authority and strong "father" figures. Often, there is preoccupation with the purchase of weapons and in developing expertise regarding the weapon's use. Above all, the irresistable push from within—a planned, detailed execution—is consciously experienced as an act of ego, of fame, of establishing identity, and of making impact on the world-at-large and sometimes on some fantasy figure in particular.

Many agree that there is a "contagious" aspect to notorious assassination attempts that may remain in the headlines for days, flooding the TV images as well as the mind of the would-be assassin with motivation to act out a fantasy, a private, central preoccupation that might have been festering for years. Whatever the immediate provocation, it is doubtful whether screaming headlines *cause* the act, except in the most immediate sense of "*Now!* Now is the time for me to make world history."

A criminal personality? Psychologists have been intrigued by the possibility that criminal "types" can be identified by a set of special or unique personality traits. However, despite some limited success with objective personality instruments like the MMPI (see Joesting, Jones, and Joesting, 1975), there appears to be no one single diagnosis or set of traits that distinguishes criminals from people who are not (Henn et al., 1976). A major problem in much of this research is that the samples studied are drawn from apprehended or incarcerated populations, with those who are not caught forming a poorly identified group. Such bias in sampling procedures also characterizes many other clinical investigations that depend on available (generally institutionalized) populations.

In one large-scale study of 1,195 people accused of having committed crimes and referred for diagnosis by the courts, the most frequent diagnosis was some type of personality disorder (for example, explosive personality or antisocial personality) (Henn et al., 1976). However, there were also other diagnoses and these tended to be related to some aspects of the presumed crime. For example, many of the defendents accused of assaultive crimes were thought to suffer from brain involvements. When the criminal behavior appeared to arise from faulty thinking and cognitive problems of some sort, schizophrenia was the major diagnosis. In this and other criminal populations, alcoholism and drug abuse were also frequently implicated (Guze, 1976; Henn et al., 1976; Mayfield, 1976; Solursh, 1975).

Overall, although the search for diagnostic and personality correlates still continues, many experts no longer believe that criminals fall into any one simple diagnostic category. Further, many no longer believe that criminals are mentally ill (see Yochelson and Samenow [1976], who based this conclusion on data emerging from 70,000 hours of interviews with and 300,000 documents concerning 240 "hardened" criminals studied over a fourteen-year period).

Temporal orientation. In young offenders, inability to delay an impulse, that is, lack of or faulty impulse control, has again and again been related to delinquent status. Lack of impulse control, it is thought, arises from an orientation toward time that focuses on the here-and-now accompanied by a disinclination to be concerned about the future (Davids, Kidder, and Reich, 1962; McCord and McCord, 1964).

This hypothesis does receive some empirical confirmation. In one study, for example, subjects who stole from the experimenter during her absence were more "constricted" in use of temporal concepts in stories they made up than subjects who did not steal (Brock and Del Giudice, 1963). In another study, a group of twenty delinquent boys were assigned to either a control group of no treatment or a vocationally oriented treatment program (Ricks, Umbarger, and Mack, 1964). As measured by scores on a specially developed set of TAT cards (see Chapter 5), the authors reported that the successfully treated subjects compared to the controls did show significant increases in scores measuring prospective (orientation toward the future) time span and to a lesser extent, retrospective (orientation toward the past) time span.

In this connection, the Porteus Maze Tests should be mentioned (Porteus, 1933). This is a classic paper-and-pencil test that involves the timed ability to go through a series of printed mazes with a minimum of error. Many studies suggest that Porteus scores measure foresight, delay of impulsivity and gratification, planning ability, and future time perspective. Some researchers are thus intrigued with the possibility that scores on this test correlate with delinquent or antisocial behavior. In a review of the Porteus literature, Riddle and Roberts (1977) sought to discover whether such an association could be found for either quantitative scores (speed) or qualitative scores (based on apsects of task execution such as bumping into lines, lifting the pencil, and cutting across corners all contrary to instructions). In these studies, scores based on speed and time do not distinguish the delinquents from the nondelinquents nor are these scores correlated with recidivism. On the other hand, some of the qualitative scores do bear some relationship to delinquency; they distinguish those with "stronger" delinquent tendencies from those with "milder" tendencies, delinquents from nondelinquents, and recidivists from nonrecidivists.

Organic Approaches

An older view: physical types. Strictly physical explanations for criminality have a rather tenacious history. One early view explained criminal behavior as an "atavistic reversal," a throwback to "primitive man" whose features include lobeless, small ears, receding chin, and wooly hair (Lombroso, 1911). Because Lombroso provided some physical measurement of criminals to "prove" his views, the largely unscientific method he used (for example, small sample, no matched groups) were overlooked. Such physical explanations for criminal behavior held sway in the early nineteenth century. Since that time impressive evidence has been amassed exploding the theories of Lombroso and others of his genre: no physical stigmata characterize criminals nor are there basic physical differences between criminal and noncriminal people.

The search for physical criminal types (criminal anthropology) continues however, and was revived with Hooton (1939). Hooton studied over 13,000 male prisoners and a smaller noncriminal, nonprisoner group, "showing" that crime not only results from inherited biological inferiority ("organic degeneration") but also that specific types of crimes were associated with specific physical types. Moreover, he felt that different ethnic and racial groups have characteristic criminal patterns.

Hooton's recommendations of segregation and sterilization of these types logically followed from his hypotheses. As would be expected, his conclusions have been severely criticized, especially in the light of many serious methodological inadequacies of his work (narrow, unrepresentative sample, for example, or bias in defining inferiority; see Sutherland, 1939).

A more "respectable" attempt to relate personality and behavior to physical type was made by Sheldon (1949), who after somatotyping (classifying people by their body form) 200 "more or less" delinquent males, concluded that a relationship between physical type and a vague measure of delinquency existed. Glueck and Glueck (1956) partially confirmed Sheldon's findings in a large, better controlled study. Mesomorphs (athletic, muscular types) appeared twice as often among delinquents than nondelinquents, and there were fewer ectomorphs (tall, lean, delicately-boned types) among the delinquents than the nondelinquent youth.

Explanations other than strictly physical ones can account for these findings. For example, certain ethnic groups, even if characterized by distinctive physical types, might be overrepresented in delinquent or criminal populations—but because of *cultural,* not physical, reasons. Or mesomorphic boys might be "more easily stereotyped as delinquents" or "more likely to be rewarded for aggressiveness" than nonmesomorphic boys (Nassi and Abramowitz, 1976).

Overall, this avenue of research has not yielded consistent or conclusive findings nor has it led to further understanding of crime and delinquency.

Search for the biological correlates of criminal or antisocial behavior: behavioral genetics. Even the staunchest of behavioral geneticists will not hold to the strictly one-to-one relationship of genes to criminal behavior (see Spotlight 18.7, however, for a research

Spotlight 18.7 XYY Chromosomes and Criminal Behavior

In 1965 it was reported that in a group of 197 inmates of a Scottish maximum security installation for violent criminals, 7 had an abnormal chromosomal makeup: an extra Y chromosome (Jacobs et al., 1965). This is an unusually high incidence, for estimates of this chromosomal aberration run at the rate of about one in 1,000 to one in 3,000. XYY males are usually extremely tall (well over six feet) and often of borderline intelligence.

Since the original report, there was a flurry of interest in the possibility that unusually violent behavior could be a by-product of abnormal chromosomal makeup that produces extremely high levels of testosterone (male sex hormone). (It is of interest that little attention was paid to the large majority of violent criminals with *normal* chromosomal makeup.)

One approach to exploring this hypothesis is to karyotype (classify chromosomally) infants to determine whether they display XYY structures and to follow the development of those that do to see whether or not XYY chromosomes would be associated with aggressive criminality.

But labeling an infant as being at high risk for violent crime would affect his entire life. Further, stigmatizing the child and his family in this way might sabotage any positive findings, for parents would treat their XYY children differently from those who are chromosomally normal. Many agreed with this position, for professional and public controversy halted a Harvard University project that was attempting to screen newborn babies along these lines (Culliton, 1975).

Even supporters of the hypothesis of Jacobs and his colleagues generally agree that the XYY makeup cannot account for the overwhelming majority of violent crimes. The number of people with XYY chromosomes in the general population and in the criminal population is simply too small. Further, it has also been stated that the frequency of aggressive behavior in normal chromosomal males is about the same as in XYY males matched for social and economic backgrounds (Borgaonkar and Shah, 1974).

A study reported by Witkin et al. (1976) seems to have laid the issue to rest. All men born in Copenhagen in a four-year period in the mid 1940s who as adults were over six feet tall were studied.

More than 4,000 men were thus examined for chromosomal makeup. Intelligence and educational levels were also ascertained. Criminal registers were then examined to see whether or not a relationship existed between XYY (or XXY) men and crime—especially that of a particularly violent or aggressive nature.

An extremely small group of men with chromosomal abnormalities was found— twelve XYY and sixteen XXY men in the group of over 4,000. Five of the twelve XYY men did have some criminal records (about 40 percent) compared to about nine percent of the chromosomally normal XY men and about 18 percent of the XXY men. The XYY and XXY men, however, were of lower intelligence than the XY men. Further, the crimes committed by the XYY men were not of any more violent nature than those committed by the XY men; mostly, these were crimes against property such as automobile thefts. After a detailed analysis of the data, the authors concluded that the higher crime rate of the excessively small number of XYY men in the large general sample may be related to lower intelligence (as a result of which, perhaps, they were more easily apprehended because they were probably less crafty about their crimes) rather than to aggression associated with their chromosomal abnormality.

thrust that had maintained a "hard line" in this area). The view is more likely to be put forth that genetic structures, by some intervening process (for example, biochemical makeup or hormonal system), might in the long run play a role in the expression of behaviors that society labels as criminal or antisocial (Rosenthal, 1975b). Expression of behaviors—even if biological predisposition is involved—is very much influenced by environmental factors.

What is the evidence?

Twin studies do indeed indicate that concordance (agreement) in criminality between MZ (identical) twins is higher than that for DZ (fraternal) twins. However, the *discordance* (disagreement) in rates of criminality among MZ twins is so high as to suggest that genetic factors cannot truly "explain" or totally account for, criminality (Nassi and Abramowitz, 1976).

Using adoption data, some evidence points to the possibility that offspring of criminal mothers, even if adopted away, have a higher percentage of criminal records than does a group of matched controls (adoptees with noncriminal biological parents) (Crowe, 1972, 1974; Schulsinger, 1972, 1980).

Perhaps the most extensive attempts to explore genetic hypotheses were made in Denmark, which maintains a national register of adoptions, criminal records, hospitalizations, and related demographic data. In one exploration, 143 adoptees with criminal records were selected and the criminal histories of their adoptive and biological parents ascertained. The same information was obtained for a matched control group of noncriminal adoptees (Hutchings and Mednick, 1975). The results showed that adoptees with criminal records had a greater percentage of criminal biological fathers than did the noncriminal adoptees. Table 18.1 presents the same data in slightly different form (after DeFries and Plomin, 1978, p. 489).

These and other explorations of the Danish data (see Schulsinger, 1972) lend some support to the hypothesis that there may be a slight familial predisposition for criminal behavior. However, these findings tell us little about the nature of such predisposition.

A study of Table 18.1 suggests that there is considerable weight to "criminal milieus" (when there is a familial predisposition for criminal behavior). That is, adoptive criminal parents are more

Table 18.1 Criminality in Sons of Criminal and Noncriminal Adoptive and Biological Fathers

Noncriminal adoptive fathers and Noncriminal biological fathers	10 percent of adoptive sons show (registered) criminal behavior
Noncriminal adoptive fathers but Criminal biological fathers	21 percent of adoptive sons show (registered) criminal behavior
Criminal adoptive fathers but Noncriminal biological fathers	12 percent of adoptive sons show (registered) criminal behavior
Criminal adoptive fathers and Criminal biological fathers	36 percent of adoptive sons show (registered) criminal behavior

Source: Reproduced, with permission, from J. C. DeFries and R. Plomin, *Annual Review of Psychology*, Volume 29, p. 489. © 1978 by Annual Reviews Inc.

likely to raise criminal children if those children have biological parents with criminal records than if their biological parents had no criminal record. But Table 18.1 states that most adoptive sons, despite their parentage, did not show criminal behavior and that about 80 percent of adopted children with criminal biological fathers but with noncriminal *adoptive* fathers did not have registered criminal records. In other words, despite biology, most adopted-away children, if raised in noncriminal environments, turn out to live noncriminal lives.

Neurochemical and biochemical variables. Moderate evidence points to the possibility that some types of aggressive behavior, ranging from irritability to violence, may result from dysfunctions or imbalances in the body's neurochemical makeup (for example, in norepinephrine and serotonin levels, androgen levels, blood sugar levels, and other biological systems within the body—Moyer, 1976). However, most experts agree that there is no consistent evidence pointing to a one-to-one relationship between neurobiological variables and antisocial or criminal behavior (Nassi and Abramowitz, 1976).

An excess of prenatal or perinatal (conditions at the time of birth) exposure to androgens or to chemicals that "mimic" these hormones does result in increases in energetic and aggressive behavior in animals and humans according to recent evidence (Quadagno, Briscoe, and Quadagno, 1977; Reinisch, 1981). That this leads to violence or crime does not follow, however, because social learning makes a large contribution to the actual expression of antisocial, criminal behavior. Further, even if such relationships are sometimes found, it is not necessary to conclude that genetic variables play a role in creating them. For learning, culture, and environmental factors such as medication during pregnancy, diet, persistent stressors, malnutrition, and the presence of toxic factors in the environment can modify, even determine, many neurochemical systems within the body—for example, blood sugar levels that are sometimes associated with aggression and irritability (Moyer, 1976).

Neurological variables. There is moderate evidence that some instances of violent outbursts, sexual assaultiveness, or sudden, inexplicable crimes involving great rage may be associated with neurological dysfunctions. A study of about 100 delinquent boys divided into two groups depending on the violence of the crime (rape, or murder, for example versus fistfights) indicated that the more seriously violent offenders had more neurological signs and symptoms (for example, blackouts, epilepsy, EEG abnormalities) than the less serious offenders (Lewis, Shanok, and Balla, 1979a,b). In addition, case backgrounds indicated that the more violent delinquents tended to have suffered serious physical abuse from their parents that could have contributed to neurological impairment as well as other types of physical dysfunctions. The authors stated that some neurobiological dysfunctions can predispose a child to vulnerability to stress from the environment that, in turn, can be expressed as violence. They felt, however, that such behaviors can be controlled through interventions that include medication combined with psychotherapy and counseling.

Many studies do indeed indicate the presence of abnormal EEG patterns among "psychopaths" (Ellingson, 1954; Hare, 1970; Hill and Pond, 1952; Hill and Watterson, 1942; Stafford-Clark and Taylor, 1949). However, because different samples, age groups, and selection criteria (e.g., "motiveless crimes," "poor judgment and poor impulse control," "extreme violence") were used, the most that can be said by way of interpretation is that in some instances of extreme aggression some types of brain dysfunction may be involved (Rosenthal, 1971).

From time to time, there are reports of a relationship between temporal lobe epilepsy and violence. (According to Valenstein [1973] 60 percent of epilepsy is diagnosed as temporal lobe epilepsy.) The association between epilepsy and violence has been challenged, however, for estimates of the incidence of violence among epileptics is thought to be as low as 1 up to 4 percent (Coleman, 1974; Goldstein, 1974; Valenstein, 1973).

Finally, the episodic dyscontrol syndrome should be mentioned, for it has recently received some attention. It has been characterized as "paroxysmal" violent outbursts accompanied by an appearance of losing contact with reality. Typically, these behaviors are associated with acute alcohol intoxication. Also, there may be assaultive behavior toward family members, impulsive sexual violence, and a history of automobile accidents (Mark and Ervin, 1970). It has been hypothesized the "episodic dyscontrol" appears in conjunction with temporal lobe tumors (Moyer, 1976) or with other kinds of brain impairments because there is often a history of head injury, seizures, and positive neurological signs in people who display this pattern of violence.

Overall, then, there is moderate evidence that some instances of violent outbursts, criminality, and inexplicable aggression and rage may be associated with neurological dysfunctions. However, such associations do not help us to understand crime and criminal behavior in general, for even though a few individual instances of extreme violence may have neurological underpinnings, most crimes are not of this nature to begin with. Even if in some instances the strength of the association is convincing, there is no need to introduce genetic explanations, for malnutrition, severe physical abuse, drugs, birth injuries and anoxia, and various infectious states can underlie the impairment. Even proponents of the view that neurobiological factors are important in some types of violent acts (see Lewis, Shanok, and Balla, 1979a,b) point out that the presence of such signs is not a result of an inevitable unfolding of genetic factors but, as already noted, a vulnerability, a predisposition to respond with violence to environmental stressors that can probably be controlled or prevented through medical and psychological interventions.

Autonomic variables. In Chapter 9, studies on autonomic responsiveness were described in connection with anxiety and psychoneurotic subjects (see pp. 220–23). These explorations tended to suggest that anxiety subjects differed from other kinds of subjects in their heightened levels of arousal during stress and in maintaining these levels for longer periods of time (before returning to baseline levels). Can it be shown that psychopathic subjects have the opposite pattern? This might explain their failure to respond to stress, danger, or the anticipation of punishment in the same way that others do, and it would also help us to understand the lack of guilt or the amorality of the classic psychopath.

Reviews of relevant studies indicate that there is a tendency for psychopaths to respond on various autonomic indices such as skin conductance (electrodermal responses) on lower than normal levels while at resting conditions and to show smaller amplitude of these responses when there is stressful stimulation (Hare, 1970). Thus, it is possible that the psychopath does not experience the feelings of discomfort, tension, and subjective emotional unease that normals or neurotics experience in many types of situations that would normally elicit such arousal.

On the other hand, some experimental evidence suggests that although classic psychopaths tend not to learn to avoid shock in the manner of neurotic criminals or noncriminals (Lykken, 1957), punishment that involves *monetary* loss seemed fairly effective in a simple learning task (Schmauk, 1970). It may be that punishment that is appropriate to the psychopaths' values, or stronger-than-usual punishment, might be effective in dealing with their seeming lack of response to aversive stimulation (Hare, 1970). One study found, for example, that when levels of fear responses were raised by injections of adrenalin, psychopaths did indeed learn to avoid electric shock, much in the manner of nonpsychopathic subjects (Schachter and Latané, 1964).

Two Biosocial Hypotheses

Mednick's approach. Access to extensive Danish data on registered criminality made it possible to explore speculations that hard-core criminals are "different" from the rest of us as well as from other criminals. This difference may account for the fact that the hard-core criminals do not learn to fear the consequences of their antisocial acts (Mednick and Christiansen, 1977). How can we explain, Mednick and his colleagues wondered, that half of all the criminal offenses of a group of 30,000 men born during the same period of time in Copenhagen were committed by the same 1 percent of this group—over and over again.

Mednick and his colleagues demonstrated that hard-core criminals do indeed have a lower autonomic (electrodermal) responsiveness, as already indicated. But in addition, Mednick also found that "recovery" of these responses (that is, return to baseline levels) is slower than that for normals or other types of criminals. In other words, responses that generally accompany fear and emotionality not only are constricted, but also, they do not dissipate quickly. As a result, Mednick hypothesized that these physiologically "different" people, because they do not have a sharp reduction of fear to serve as reinforcement for avoidance, are at high risk for recidivism. They do not develop a conditioned fear response; that is, they have difficulty in learning to inhibit aggression, because the inhibition is not reinforced sufficiently by a reduction of autonomic responses.

Mednick's hypothesis connects physiological substrates with learning principles in a simple, even elegant way. But these speculations are based on limited physiological data and on an assumption that rapid autonomic (electrodermal) recovery rates form the basis for learning not to be antisocial. In addition, Mednick's approach tells us little about *most* crime and aggression. As a result, we are left with some intriguing possibilities for explaining the behavior of a small group of hard-core criminals, who, because of their physiological "apparatus," may have difficulty in learning to restrain or curtail aggression in response to punishment or other aversive consequences.

Sensation-seeking and underarousal. Which of the following items would you choose if you were forced to make a choice?

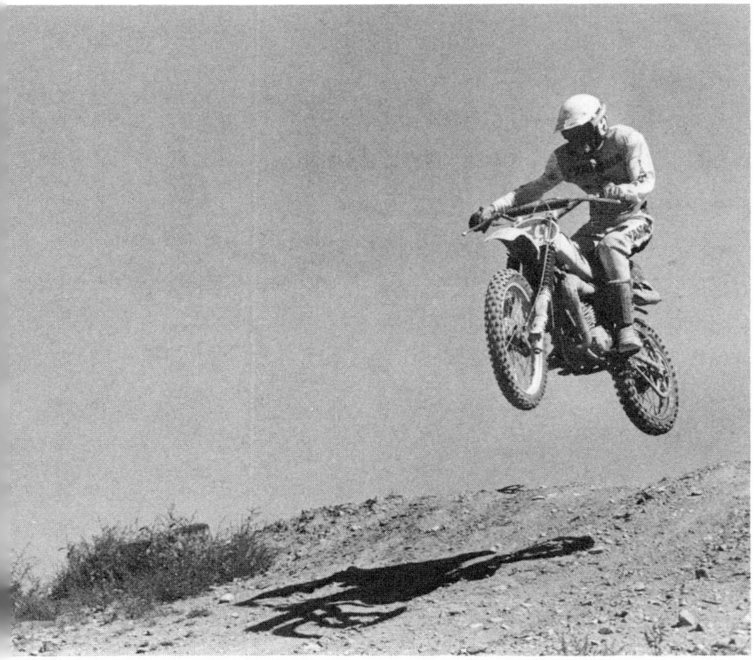

It is possible that risk-taking allays physiological discomfort by raising levels of stimulation. One hypothesis suggests that some juvenile offenders and psychopaths have chronically low levels of cortical arousal that require intense variation of stimulation for optimal functioning. (Mimi Forsyth/Monkmeyer Press)

a. having to cancel your vacation
b. standing on the ledge of the twenty-fifth floor of a building

On a specially constructed questionnaire that required subjects to indicate preferences for one of two paired items such as those above, psychopathic subjects tended to prefer the more dangerous, risk-taking items whereas "normal" subjects did not do so (Lykken, 1957).

Both observations and empirical evidence have led many researchers to hypothesize that people at risk for antisocial behavior, including juvenile offenders and psychopaths, have a chronically low level of cortical arousal that requires intense stimulation and variation of stimulation for optimal brain functioning and affective well-being (Quay, 1965). Such people, it is suggested, experience discomfort under conditions of normal stimulation, as a result of which they will seek excitement, thrills, new experiences, and risk-taking activities—all designed to allay this discomfort.*

One study compared antisocial, preadolescent children to groups of normal and neurotic children matched on several variables (Whitehill, DeMeyer-Gapin, and Scott, 1976). All subjects were tested in an experimental situation designed to be boring. They were asked to view a monotonous series of slides, controlling its rate of exposure. Viewing time was employed as a negative measure of stimulation-seeking (the lower the time, the higher the stimulation-seeking score) with the expectation that antisocial children would show the most stimulation-seeking, normals the next most, and neurotics, the least. The findings confirmed the authors' hypothesis. Antisocial children did show heightened stimulation-seeking and neurotic children the least. Normals were in an intermediate position. Figure 18.2 presents these data graphically.

The pathological stimulation-seeking hypothesis—that delinquents, psychopaths, and certain types of criminals are underaroused and seek increases and variations in sensory output for optimal functioning and for a sense of well-being—has been explored in many contexts (Chesno and Kilmann, 1975; Lykken, 1957; Whitehill, DeMeyer-Gapin, and Scott, 1976). In general, the thrust of these explorations—that delinquents and antisocial people actively seek to reduce "boredom" to heighten levels of physiological arousal—has received moderate confirmation.

* An interesting speculation is that the hyperactivity of some children as well as the "speed seeking" of some amphetamine abusers can also be explained by cortical and physiological underarousal. Similarly, the self-injurious behavior (called carving) displayed by incarcerated delinquent girls (Ross and McKay, 1979) which involves self-mutilation, for example, making deep incisions into arms or legs with a sharp instrument, may also result from a search to raise stimulation because of underarousal.

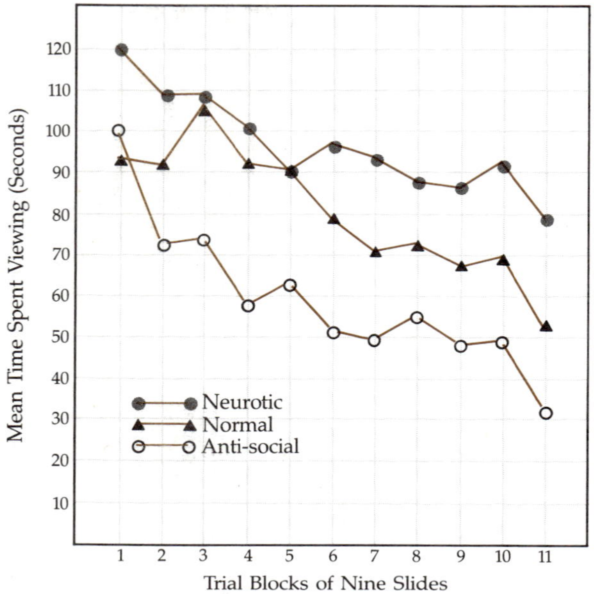

Figure 18.2 Mean group viewing times for successive blocks of slides in neurotic, normal, and antisocial children. (From M. Whitehill, S. DeMyer-Gapin, and T. J. Scott, Stimulation seeking in antisocial preadolescent children, *Journal of Abnormal Psychology*, 1976, *85*, 103. Copyright 1976 by the American Psychological Association. Reprinted by permission of the author.)

FAMILY VIOLENCE: A CLOSER LOOK

The ideal picture of the American family as a peaceful, harmonious unit has become blurred as we learn more about the patterns of violence contained within it (Adams, 1979; Lystad, 1975). Each year, well over a million children are abused in this country, with some estimates running even higher (Bybee, 1979; Gelles, 1973, 1977). I have already touched on this problem many times in this book, especially in connection with brain-damaged and developmentally disabled children and in the context of sexual assault.

It has been further estimated that nearly two million husbands and wives are physically abused by their spouses: kicking, hitting, beatings, and threats with, or actually using, a knife or a gun (Gelles and Strauss, 1979). In this frightening picture of physical violence, it is assumed that there are more serious consequences for the wife than for the husband. Why?

There are often strong cultural sanctions for women to remain within an abusive marriage and in some social settings, abusive behavior of this sort is even *expected* (Gelles and Straus, 1979). Men are freer to leave an abusive marriage and often do so while many women are silently tolerant of their own victim-role, sometimes because they are economically and psychologically dependent.

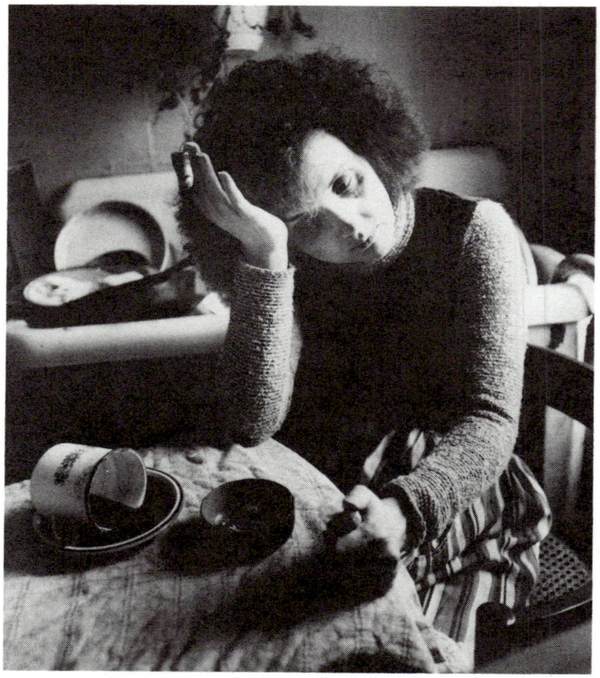

Many women suffer physical abuse silently, frequently because of financial and psychological dependence on their husbands and because of social expectations to remain within an abusive marriage. (Arthur Tress)

Another way of conceptualizing the abused woman's trapped behavior is through the learned helplessness model (see Chapter 10), which proposes that women become bound to their situations through helplessness, having learned that nothing they do can control, change, or modify the situation they are in (Walker, 1979). In this connection, an interesting fact emerges: homocides of husbands and wives by each other occur with approximately equal frequency for each sex. However, criminological studies indicate that women are *seven* times more likely to kill their spouses in self-defense than are the men (Wolfgang, 1956).

Family abuse, most data suggest, is very much related to education, income, and related SES variables (Gelles and Straus, 1979; Sweet and Resick, 1979). However, abuse occurs on all class levels, and some of the reported preponderance of abuse on the lowest SES levels may in part reflect the social machinery in which powerless and helpless low-SES abusers get "caught" more often by the courts and welfare agencies than do the middle-class abusers. As a matter of fact, although it is common practice to look for signs of abuse in the inner-city emergency room, the middle-class physician is probably less likely to suspect or report abuse in connection with his or her middle-class patient (Bybee, 1979; Newberger, 1977).

What are the correlates of family violence? From a maze of speculations and attempts to sort the evidence, it has become clear that no single trait, diagnostic category (such as alcoholism), or stressful life event (e.g., unemployment) is consistently associated with family violence. However, it is likely that the *interaction* of these variables with each other and with SES (for example, a family crisis in a poverty-stricken home) are better predictors of violence than any one of these factors alone (Egeland et al., 1980; Gelles, 1973; Gelles and Straus, 1979; Sweet and Resick, 1979). In this multicausal context, contributing variables include high anxiety, aggressiveness, poor skills in interacting with babies (Egeland et al, 1980), impulsivity (Spinetta and Rigler, 1972), low intelligence and/or education, aggressive role models, individual psychopathology, value systems in which aggression is condoned, and family disorganization characteristic of multiproblem families (Gelles, 1973).

It should be stressed that family violence has a self-perpetuating quality. For it is well known that experiencing or witnessing violence predisposes a child to repeat patterns of violence with his or her own children and spouse (Feshback and Feshback, 1973; Gelles and Straus, 1979). In addition, the practice of harsh physical punishment in child-rearing practices and the existence of polarized gender roles in which the husband is "allowed" to aggress against a wife who has overstepped her bounds (Gelles and Straus, 1979; Martin, 1976) also nurtures a pattern of family violence which is a model for future generations.

The elimination of poverty, intervention into cultural values that sanction violence and aggres-

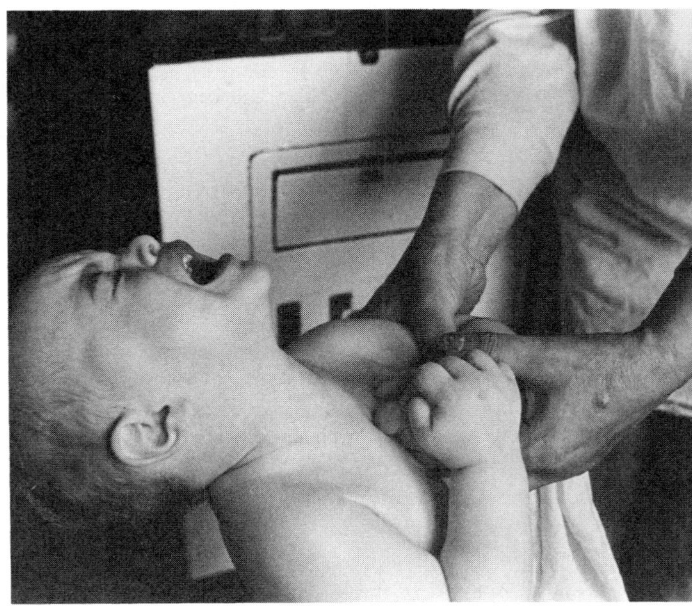

In the United States, well over a million children are abused each year, with some estimates running even higher. (© Eugene Richards/The Picture Cube)

sion, and the breaking up of polarized male-female patterns that permit physical violence between men and women might contribute to a social climate that reduces the incidence of family abuse. These ideal goals, however, are difficult to attain. More practical intervention includes educational efforts targeted at high-risk people that encourage them to use available facilities for group and individual counseling.

A more aggressive approach involves screening babies at risk for abuse, determined on the basis of family disorganization, poverty, and a history with the courts, as well as observations of the parents and children in pediatric clinics that suggest a potential for abuse (Kempe, 1976; Kempe and Helfer, 1972). It has been noted, for example, that it is often only one child in a family that is abused, and that *that* child is likely to be "special"—with problems that are bewildering to an immature, unstable, harrassed parent (Friedrich and Boriskin, 1976). These problems can range from mental retardation, physical or neurological impairment, and congenital birth defects to deviant behavioral styles such as unpredictable sleep patterns, persistent crying, or refusal to be cuddled or held. Yet, even when the clinician identifies the high-risk potential of some family contexts, is it ethical to "invade" this domain by compulsory health supervision in the form of monitoring and home visits? Should we thrust educational efforts and preventive measures on unwilling families?

INTERVENTION

The next sections touch briefly on measures that have been used to modify patterns of juvenile delinquency and crime. But first, a few words about prevention of aggressive behavior patterns. On an assumption that aggression is learned early, it has been proposed that we provide the same kinds of learning experience for our boys as we do for our girls (Eron, 1980). That is, if we wish to reduce male aggressive behavior in adult years, we might try to train our boys to be tender, cooperative, nurturant, and to seek nonaggressive solutions to problems. We might also try to reduce the violence on television, Eron continues, supervise our children's viewing, and help them distinguish reality from fantasy in the programs they watch.

*Traditional psychoanalytic and more eclectic psychotherapeutic approaches.** Psychotherapy has not been shown to be effective in the treatment of juvenile offenders or adult criminals. Failures, especially in regard to the so-called psychopath, are well known. Psychotherapeutic methods, in addition, are uneconomical and usually not attuned to the variables that seem relevant to some types of antisocial behavior such as sensation-seeking. Also, they rely on voluntary and motivated choices to seek help—conditions that are not always present in this particular population.

Broad social and community programs. In high-risk areas, it is common to introduce various types of social and community programs. These efforts include summer programs, day camps, jobs and vocational training, individual and family counseling, and medical attention. In one major long-range research project (known as the Cambridge-Somerville Youth Study), 500 delinquent-prone subjects were targets of an intensive community effort of the kind described, to prevent the inevitable unfolding of delinquency. Follow-up questionnaires thirty years later disclosed that more of the treatment subjects had criminal records and antisocial careers than did the control subjects, who had received no treatment at all (McCord, 1978). Although McCord's con-

* Psychoanalytic approaches to delinquency attempted to establish an intense, compassionate relationship between therapist and patient so that the superego processes that did not take place early in the life of the offender could now take place. Also encouraged was an abreaction of rage and destructiveness (see Aichorn's classic work, 1935). Abreaction is the process in which unconscious memories are brought to consciousness and the experiences associated with them relived, generally accompanied by a release of tension.

clusion that such social action programs "risk damaging the individual they are designed to assist" (p. 289) would be challenged by most people, many experts in the area agree that the usual community interventions have to be supplemented by more innovative techniques.

Group and family methods. These methods were considered excellent interventions on the assumption that attempts to modify an offender's behavior must recognize that antisocial value systems are reinforced in peer and family groups and in certain types of social "climates." Family and group treatment with all delinquents and criminals is not possible, of course. And by and large, these approaches have not stacked up an impressive record of success.

Structured and directive group methods. Challenge, confrontation, peer pressure, and stress on responsibility and the here-and-now are rather widely used in correctional facilities, training schools, and halfway houses (see Agee, 1979; Rachin, 1974; Ross and McKay 1979; Schmideberg, 1975; Yochelson and Samenow, 1977). These methods are sometimes abusive in their direct challenge of the offender's thinking and in their insistence on considering the consequences of and responsibility for one's actions.

In one such approach to hard-core criminals in which attending three-hour group sessions daily was required as a condition for probation, Yochelson and Samenow (1977) worked with 255 hard-core criminals over a fourteen-year period on an assumption that more compassionate rehabilitation does not work (an assumption that has received some confirmation—see later sections). In these sessions, subjects were told how "rotten" they were; they were confronted with their "ugly" childhoods and were harangued to maintain "impeccable" lives. Counseling was not concerned with feelings but with thought processes and the assuming of responsibility. Follow-up of about thirty people who had about 500 or more hours of such treatment indicates that about half were successfully "cured" (no further arrests and no "criminal thinking").

Convict counseling. Another widely publicized technique involves the enforced visits of teenagers to prisons in which hardened, tough criminals— many of them "lifers"—do convict counseling: they abuse, intimidate, and yell at juvenile offenders and delinquent-prone subjects about the harshness of prison life (being sexually assaulted, for example). This interventive effort was so popularly acclaimed that many states modeled similar programs on the one that was filmed at New Jersey's Rahway State Prison* in 1978.

But even here, despite the wide appeal of the Rahway "experiment," initial claims of huge success in preventing further offenses have been challenged (Waldron, 1979). As a matter of fact, almost half of the juvenile offenders who were part of the program committed offenses within six months, whereas only about 10 percent of a matched control group, who were not part of the program, got into trouble. As a result, the State of New Jersey is informing other state correctional programs that the claims made in the film—for example, that 80 to 90 percent of delinquents who go through the program "go straight"—were not substantiated.

Behavioral interventions. Especially with institutionalized subjects in prisons, special schools, and halfway houses, behavioral interventions (see Chapter 20) have also been employed. Although the ultimate goal of such interventions, as with other therapies, is to change an offender's behavior in the "real world," to date there is little evidence that this goal is being met in a significant way. However, behavioral interventions have been effective in maintaining smoothly running environments, for example, by managing the behaviors of difficult

* This documentary film *Scared Straight!* won an Oscar. It was written, produced, and directed by Arnold Shapiro, and is distributed by Pyramid Films, Santa Monica, California.

prisoners, or in maintaining high levels of mutual cooperation among inmates. An offender's change toward prosocial behavior in life outside of the institution, however, involves the extension of the principles of a "managed environment" to the offender's family and to the community itself (Khanna, 1975)—an exceedingly complex job of social and psychological engineering that is beyond the scope of current technical knowledge. However, there are interesting leads. For example, Little and Kendall (1978) have described interventions with adolescent delinquents that focused on developing the capacity to feel for other people (empathy)—presumably victims. It remains to be seen whether such attempts to modify antisocial behavior can generalize to the "real life" situation.

In sum, the control of violence and crime is far from being reached. Despite many innovative therapeutic interventions, community programs, and educational thrusts, the problems of crimes and delinquency, and of changing the behavior of hard core adults and delinquents are still very real ones. Further, we have yet to develop truly effective methods for modifying, or preventing the development of, the antisocial personality.

THE CRIMINAL JUSTICE SYSTEM: SOME RELEVANT ISSUES

"Enlightened" Views of Crime

According to Menninger (1968), punishing criminals for crimes is the real crime. *Treatment* should be offered instead. Menninger's admonition reflects a traditional, humanitarian view of criminals: they do what they do because they are twisted by psychosexual conflicts. Because we no longer punish mentally ill people but treat them, the reformists thought, we should do the same for criminals, who are really mentally ill.

This enlightened approach involved some attempts to detect high-risk individuals so that preventive methods could be introduced, the introduction of "softer" informal proceedings as a substitute for criminal trials, the handing down of indefinite sentences until the offender is pronounced cured (in a treatment center rather than a prison), and a view that regards incarceration as rehabilitative rather than punitive.

Thus, until quite recently, the major thrust of the newer criminology was to find the best therapeutic, educational, and rehabilitation methods that society could offer (Silber, 1974). Methods for training inmates to counsel other inmates or to lead inmate groups were developed in an attempt to improve the morale of prisoners. Efforts were directed in many prisons throughout the nation to involve the staff as well as citizens in the surrounding community to support mental-health programs within the prison walls (Hosford and Moss, 1975).

The past decade has seen a reluctant shift away from these humanitarian values in the light of hard data: crime rates of inmates who had received psychotherapy, behavior modification, vocational training, or other kinds of intervention were as high as the rates of those who received no rehabilitation attempts. These conclusions were reached by hundreds of separate studies (Monahan, 1977).

Connecticut, for example, which had spent millions on intensive rehabilitation programs that included indeterminate sentences, education, vocational training, and flexible parole programs, discovered that recidivism rates were not at all affected (Prison official's revisionism, 1976). Despite access of most of Connecticut's inmates to a variety of programs, 33 percent of released offenders were back in prison for new crimes in less than two years; in another Connecticut study, 75 percent of a group of 200 released prisoners were back in prison, most of them after parole was discontinued.

Generally, between 60 and 75 percent of released prisoners, after serving a full term or after parole, are rearrested within a four-year period, whereas in some urban areas, up to 90 percent are rearrested (Silber, 1974). In sum, the concept of treating criminals as patients may have been a good idea at one time, but because of its documented history of failure, it is gradually being abandoned.

Newer Views About Prisons and Punishment

Some of the changes in attitude and policy are so new that they are difficult to evaluate. This is what seems to be happening as a result of growing discontent with the ability of penal institutions to rehabilitate their inmates.

1. Many states are revising laws on indeterminate sentences and are returning to the idea of fixed sentences, eventually with a view toward abandoning the parole system (Indeterminate sentences. . . . , 1976). Indeterminate sentences until the prisoner "proves" he or she has changed (especially unjust, it is claimed, when the legal sentence for the crime is short), plea bargaining, early parole, time off for good behavior, and the generally wide variations in the length of prison sentences for the same crime are viewed with disfavor.

2. The medical model of crime as an illness that can be diagnosed, treated, and cured is gradually being abandoned. Criminals, it is thought, should not be treated as sick, especially because only a small percentage of them are actually diagnosed as mentally ill.

3. Forcing treatment or rehabilitation efforts onto a prisoner is also being abandoned. Imprisonment is punishment for an offense and is also, perhaps, a deterrent to others, not rehabilitation or treatment time. Treatment, job training, and educational opportunities are offered, but should be on a voluntary basis only, no longer tied in with parole possibilities. Voluntary enrollment in programs thus does not hold out a promise for early release.

4. Prison reform is essential, but is taking a different tack from the "treatment" days of yore: punishment, yes, but not in degrading, overcrowded, dehumanizing conditions. In some states, for example, the classification system is so bad that violent and nonviolent prisoners are housed together, with some prisoners actually seeking solitary confinement for protection. Prison reform thus now looks to an improved classification system, with supervised, well-guarded environments so that the rape, robbery, assault, and murder within the prison walls are controlled. Prisons should no longer be regarded as repositories for senile, infirm, brain-damaged offenders, long forgotten by their states.

5. As an approach to reducing crime, deterrence implies that the greater speed, certainty, and severity of punishment for a given crime, the more individuals will be deterred from enacting that particular crime (Gibbs, 1975). This view is based on the criminal-at-risk's perception of such variables and his or her knowledge about what the effects of a given criminal act will be or were. The possible offender, thus, must weigh the risks of punishment—how soon and how much and how certain—against benefits that the successfully completed criminal act will accrue for him or her. Although many criminologists are interested in deterrence theory, as yet little empirical research exists to implement this approach or to substantiate its efficacy in reducing crime.

6. Still being debated is the legal stance toward juvenile offenders. New York State has toughened its laws so that even thirteen-year-olds, if committing murder or serious injury, are treated by the law as adults and subject to serious punishment. These newer attitudes emerged from the fact that young offenders were arrested time and again for serious offenses but were typically returned to the streets until they reached an age when the legal machinery for adults could be applied, often too late to prevent rapes or murders committed in the interim.

The Insanity Defense

Daniel M'Naghten's acquittal of criminal charges (a shooting) in England in 1843 on the basis of "mental defect" has spawned almost a century and a half of legal precedence in the courts. In this country, most states still describe to the M'Naghten rule, which determines legal sanity or insanity: knowing right from wrong and knowing the consequences of the charges for the crime. In 1954, a broader interpretation (the so-called Durham rule) expanded the M'Naghten rule to include not guilty, by reason of mental disease or mental defect. The Durham interpretation requires expert testimony as to the presence of mental illness, that is, "mental disease" or "mental defect." Since that time, Judge Bazelson, who introduced the Durham decision, simplified his ruling to whether or not the accused is mentally capable of appreciating the illegality of his act (Miller, 1975).

As a result, many criminals who plead not guilty on the basis of insanity literally "get away with murder." For, if declared legally insane, the courts can remand the defendant to a mental institution for treatment until he or she is declared sane. In short, the insanity defense has been frequently used as a defense against serious charges, with a consequent avoidance of imprisonment.

Insanity as a legal concept is now being seriously challenged by many people who feel that such defenses in the courts are attempts by criminals to avoid punishment. Further, a related legal designation, being judged not fit to stand trial because of mental incompetence,* is also being challenged on the ground that it deprives the criminal of due process of law—an inalienable right.

The status of the insanity defense and judgments as to mental competence is being challenged throughout the nation (see Miller, 1975; Smith, 1978). Here are some of the points made by the challengers.

1. The insanity defense should be banished altogether. An act should be judged legally, as either criminal or noncriminal. Thus, in the eyes of the law, the person committing the crime is either guilty or not guilty. One recommendation is to use a defense of guilty, but mentally ill or not responsible by reason of mental disease or defect, in instances in which psychopathology was clearly responsible for the criminal act.

2. The courts and juries, not the so-called mental experts, should determine guilt and punishment. Punishment should be in prisons, not mental institutions.

3. In any event, judgments as to mental disease and mental competence are notoriously unreliable. There is little agreement as to what constitutes mental illness. Is a psychopath or an alcoholic mentally ill? Further, the adversary system does not work as far as judgments about sanity are concerned. For every expert on one side, one can get experts on the other side—and the jargon is often confusing to juries of lay people who cannot be expected to understand the issues and the disagreements.

4. Are some crimes *really* excusable in the eyes of the law? Is the insanity defense simply a ploy for criminals to avoid imprisonment?

5. In an instance of confinement to a mental institution for a series of bizarre murders (on the basis of being judged incompetent to stand trial or not guilty, on the basis of insanity), how long should the inmate (prisoner? patient?) remain in the hospital? Until judged cured? What about the dangers to society? Such indeterminate sentences may have some unjust consequences: some people may be released quickly, whereas others may be incarcerated for years for the same crime.

Dangerousness

Confinement to a mental institution by reason of mental disease or defect involves an eventual decision about release. For a defendant can and must be released back into the community when judged by

* The determination of mental incompetence is based on whether or not the accused can understand charges against him or her and participate in his or her own defense, specifically in cooperating with the defense attorney and in understanding the legal processes that are involved.

experts and the courts that he or she is no longer dangerous to himself or herself and to others. This eventuality and the granting of weekend passes and furloughs to inmates of mental institutions, raises an extremely important issue—the validity of our predictions or "diagnoses" of dangerousness.

Predicting dangerousness is riddled with uncertainty and unreliability, for there are few set criteria to judge and to predict an individual's dangerousness (Shah, 1978). It is important to remember that probabilities are involved, never certainties, when one predicts such future behavior. What should the level of certainty be? How many experts should be involved? What level of agreement among the experts should be sought?

There is not even consensus as to what constitutes dangerousness. A threat of aggression? A threat to kill? Does a designation of dangerousness deprive an individual of his or her civil liberties? Can we detain anyone because of a prediction as to *future* behavior? Finally, if someone is judged guilty, but mentally ill, and is confined to a mental institution, should he or she stand trial when no longer regarded as dangerous to himself or herself or others?

SUMMARY

This chapter focused on descriptions and hypotheses about the antisocial personality, violence, aggression, and crime. First it reviewed antisocial personality disorders, a term applied to people who consistently flout social norms and show low frustration tolerance and impulsivity. It then turned to antisocial behavior in children, sometimes called conduct disorders. Although a one-to-one relationship between these disorders and crime was not suggested, the chapter focused on crime and its relationship to different sociocultural variables, including age, gender, SES, and ethnicity. Theories of aggression, crime, and antisocial behavior discussed include general models for aggression (for example, the frustration-aggression approach); modeling; and the view that aggressive tendencies are acquired at an early age and tend to persist, much in the way a trait does, through life. The chapter reviewed the antecedents of, and sociological approaches to, crime and delinquency, as well as various personality theories of crime and the antisocial personality, including psychoanalytic views, a search for common personality denominators, and the "temporal orientation" hypothesis. After reviewing the older "organic" approaches to criminality, it described more recent attempts to find biological correlates of criminals or antisocial behavior, including the behavioral genetics model and neurobiological approaches. Two biosocial hypotheses were presented: Mednick's approach and the sensation-seeking (underarousal) model. The next sections looked more closely at family violence and its correlates and possible causes, followed by a brief review of interventive methods into crime and delinquency. Finally, concluding sections of this chapter focused on the criminal justice system, touching on newer views about crime, prisons, punishment, the insanity defense, and the concept of dangerousness as a criterion for conviction and/or punishment.

Highlights

1. Antisocial or psychopathic personality disorders have long posed a challenge to the experts. These sometimes intriguingly charming people flout social, legal, and moral codes, are irresponsible and impulsive, and form unstable relationships. They show no thinking disorders, it is thought, and are not generally regarded as "mentally ill." Yet in some ways they seem to be "missing the boat" as far as inner guilt, conscience, and a sense of responsibility to their worlds is concerned. They are more likely to be male than female, may or may not end up as "hardened" criminals, tend to

show little or no anxiety, and are not modified by the usual punishments of disapproval or later, perhaps, jail. These qualities characterize the *primary* psychopath or sociopath, usually differentiated from the *secondary* or neurotic psychopath, who, although "antisocial," is capable of showing high anxiety levels. Also described in these introductory sections were the DSM-III's related categories of conduct disorders among children of which several types, for example, undersocialized aggressive and socialized aggressive, were briefly described.

2. Trends in crime data indicate that there has been a steady increase in violent crimes in the nation and that about three-fourth of all violent street crimes are committed by young people, as are most nonviolent crimes. More males than females commit crimes, although the incidence of crime is rising among women. About 80 percent of murders and victims are of the same racial background and about 80 percent of homocides are committed by relatives or acquaintances of the victim. The highest incidence and rates of crime are in black America and a greater number of *victims* are black. Most experts concur that the strong association of poverty and ethnic minority status accounts for this statistical relationship.
3. Models for understanding the origins of aggression include the frustration-aggression model, modeling and imitation, and early acquisition of aggressive responses that function like traits. The Harlows' research with monkeys was also described. These demonstrated that aggressive responses in monkeys were evoked if there were limited prior opportunities for contact with the mother, mother surrogate, or peers.
4. Some of the antecedents of aggression, violence, and delinquency described include, in addition to criminal behavior and/or alcoholism in the parents (only moderately predictive), physical punishment of the child, the witnessing of violence and physical aggression, lack of parental supervision and discipline, peer pressure, truancy, and the availability of models who display antisocial behavior. Low SES is often associated with these behaviors, but a one-to-one definitive relationship with SES and violence and aggression has not been clearly established. There is continued controversy as to the relationship of early television viewing of violence as a causal variable for later aggression and violence.
5. Various sociological and personality theories of crime and the antisocial personality described include Sutherland's differential association theory, a broad social view, and a contrasting psychoanalytic position that focuses on the criminal or delinquent as "sick" or as displaying neuroses—a person in need of help. The search for a common criminal personality type has largely been fruitless, and most experts do not believe that criminals are mentally ill. Yet inability to delay an impulse—that is, a time orientation that focuses on the here-and-now—has been repeatedly noted (and moderately confirmed) in the literature as characterizing the young offender.
6. The search for common physical types among criminals has become an old, worn-out tradition in sociology and criminology. Even contemporary typological approaches of this sort, however, have yielded inconclusive findings. Also, a recent research thrust that attempted to link an extra Y chromosome in males to violence and crime has not been promising. On the other hand, Scandinavian adoption studies lend some support to the hypothesis that there might be a slight familial predisposition for criminal behavior. Moderate evidence points to the possibility that some types of aggressive behavior, for example, violent outbursts, may result from imbalances and dysfunctions in the body's neurochemical and neurophysiological makeup. Such associations do not help us to understand criminal behavior, however, for even if there are some instances of violence with neurological underpinnings, most crimes are not of this nature. It was also noted that,

judging by some autonomic indicators, psychopaths may not experience the same levels of emotional tension and anxiety that might be elicited in nonpsychopathic individuals under conditions of high arousal, such as severe punishment.

7. Two biosocial hypotheses that have received some confirmation attempt to explain the behavior of some types of hard-core criminals by connecting physiological substrates with sociopathic behavior. One is Mednick's hypothsis that certain people are physiologically different from others in their greater difficulty in establishing a conditioned fear response, thus having limitations in learning to inhibit aggression. The other model is a sensation-seeking hypothesis that states that certain juvenile offenders and psychopaths have a chronically low level of cortical arousal that requires intense stimulation and variation of stimulation for optimal brain functioning—resulting in daredevil risk-taking activities that raise levels of physiological arousal.
8. A closer look at family violence disclosed certain correlates, judging by the results of several studies. Although no single trait or diagnostic category or life event seemed crucial, an interaction of many variables (including SES) seemed better able to predict such violence. These included high anxiety, aggressiveness, poor skills in interacting with babies, impulsivity, low intelligence, individual psychopathology, aggressive role models, and family disorganization. It was stressed that family violence has a self-perpetuating quality that establishes a repeated pattern for the next generation.
9. Studies of interventive efforts have shown that individual psychotherapy is not particularly effective in the treatment of criminal offenders. Other methods briefly touched on include broad social and community programs, group and family methods, and methods of direct, harsh confrontation and challenge. Behavioral interventions were also described. The question of transfer of change to the real-life situation of the community and the street is of course the true test of effectiveness. This brief survey concluded that despite many innovative interventions, the problems of crime and delinquency and of changing the behavior of hard-core criminals are still very much with us.
10. Reviewed were the shifts in attitude of the judicial system toward prison rehabilitation in the light of growing discontent with the ability of penal institutions to rehabilitate their inmates. These changes include the revision of laws about indeterminate sentences (with a return to the notion of fixed sentences), changes in attitudes toward the medical model of crime as a reflection of illness or as regarding criminals as sick, posing questions about enforcing treatment and rehabilitation onto prisoners, and the rise of deterrence theory, which suggests that the greater the speed, certainty, and severity of punishment for a given crime, the more individuals will be deterred from enacting that crime. In addition, changes in attitudes toward the juvenile offender have resulted in new statutes that require that serious offenders, even if young, be tried, convicted, and sentenced in adult courts.
11. An examination of the status of the insanity defense and the use of judgments about mental competence to stand trial revealed many challenges to the old views. For example, many clinicians believe that a criminal act should be judged *legally,* not psychiatrically or by mental health experts and/or a jury, because judgments of this nature (sanity, insanity, mental competence, or incompetence) are notoriously unreliable. Further, a person committed to a mental institution on an indeterminate sentence may be quickly released, if judged cured, whereas someone else may be incarcerated for years for the same crime, obviously an unjust state of affairs.
12. The chapter concluded with a brief word about the prediction of dangerousness and the uncertainty and unreliability of such predictions.

ISSUES AND QUESTIONS

1. In most verified instances of child abuse, the battered child remains at home while the family receives treatment. The child is removed from the home by court order only after repeated abuse. The rights of the child, the parents, and the foster parents, as well as the state's obligation to treat the family as intensively as possible to avoid such removal are complex legal and ethical issues (Derdeyn, 1977). Is there an unqualified parental right to possession of a child? Who decides when such a "right" is no longer in the interests of the child?
2. Electrode implantation in, and surgical procedures on, the brain as well as direct chemical application to specific brain sites may reduce violence and rage (and the crimes associated with them) in a limited number of instances. Do you agree that "we would be in serious trouble if a number of influential people became convinced that violence is mainly a product of a diseased brain rather than a diseased society" (Valenstein, 1973, p. 353)? Or do you feel that as long as there is informed consent, implantation, surgical, and chemical procedures should be considered—if appropriate to the specific situation?
3. Some experts are convinced, in the light of prison rehabilitation failures, that only top offenses, such as those of personal violence, should receive prison sentences. In this view, the same crimes would receive the same punishment; judges would have less discretion in reducing or eliminating sentences. The focus would be on what the criminal *did,* not on what a judge or a panel of experts expects to happen in the future. This view reflects the waning popularity of indeterminate sentences, parole, probation, and other practices. What is your opinion?
4. A few studies have had success in predicting recidivism. For example, on the basis of intensive interviews with eighty-one eighteen-to-nineteen-year-old male offenders, "temporary delinquents" could be distinguished from those who continued to offend after the age of seventeen years (Knight and West, 1975). If a valid index of recidivism could be found that distinguishes the one-time offender from the hard-core repeater, should a sentence be determined by this knowledge? Do you agree that deciding a legal issue (such as the length of prison sentence) on the basis of risk for future criminality violates the offender's civil rights? Nevertheless, would not some offenses be prevented if the judge knew the past record of the offender?
5. Should the worst of the juvenile offenders be judged by the same standards as adult offenders, and given punishment appropriate to the offense, rather than to other considerations (for example, the availability of parental supervision or psychotherapy)? Some states, New York, for example, have lowered the age of responsibility for crimes such as murder. Under this system, even thirteen-year-olds can be tried and judged in the public adult judicial system, rather than in the private Family Court. Do you agree with this harsher view toward tough, violence-prone youngsters?
6. If you were a therapist and one of your patients told you of his intention to engage in a nonviolent crime for personal vengeance, should you inform the potential victim of the patient's expressed plan? Should you threaten the patient with termination of treatment if he acts on his plan? Remember that the patient expected the therapy sessions to be completely confidential. Remember also that the therapist's role is not that of moral advisor, teacher, or "authority." What would you do in this situation?
7. Does a therapist have the responsibility to notify the intended victim that a patient is planning to kill him or her? Should the police be notified? A famous case—Tarasoff v. Regents of the University of California—resulted in a decision in 1974 by the California State Supreme Court that bears on this question.

The court, while recognizing the general confidentiality of therapeutic content, ruled that "the public policy favoring protection of the confidential character of patient-psychotherapist communications must yield in instances in which disclosure is essential to avert danger to others. The protective privilege ends where the public peril begins." This decision understandably creates many problems in interpretation and implementation. In addition, it assumes that predicting violence is as objective, for example, as detecting an infection.

What would happen if whenever a therapist felt there was a possibility of violence, he or she notified the police or someone in the patient's family? Remember, a threat is not a crime, and predicting violence from a threat is often incorrect. Would patients stay away from psychotherapy because they would be afraid to disclose inner fantasies about violence?

8. Should prisoners be allowed to volunteer for behavioral interventions that employ aversive methods (for example, electric shocks or strong emetics)? Many people claim that voluntary consent is not truly voluntary in settings such as prison in which the inmate might feel it is to his or her advantage to "go along" with any procedure, no matter how aversive.

SUGGESTIONS FOR FURTHER READING

Cleckley, H. M. *The mask of sanity: An attempt to clarify some issues about the so-called psychopathic personality* (5th ed.). St. Louis: Mosby, 1976. This readable classic almost makes one wish we could go back to the "beauty" of the old-fashioned diagnostic system. Cleckley discusses the fine details of this clinical diagnosis as if it were a pure, consistent single entity providing rich illustrations of all the facets, features, and details—in short, a full composite portrait—of all the "psychopathic" people we have known. The psychopathic personality becomes palpable, real, and familiar, in the hands of this skilled and insightful writer.

Kempe, R. S., and Kempe, C. H. *Child abuse.* Paperback available. Cambridge, Mass.: Harvard University Press, 1978. This is a brief, sensitively written presentation of the problem of child abuse in our society. The first part of the book describes the abused child, his or her parents, and the disturbed interaction between them. Causes for child abuse are also explored. The second part is addressed to treatment issues and the rights of children. As an introduction to this disturbing and important topic, it is a book of great interest.

Lystad, M. *An annotated bibliography: Violence at home.* Department of Health, Education and Welfare Publication No. (ADM) 75-136, 1974. This impressively thorough, annotated list of almost 200 references provides an excellent survey of the correlates and possible causes of violence, murder, and aggression among family members: child abuse, violence between husband and wife, and violence between siblings. Theoretical excursions into family pathology and structure as they relate to violence are also included in this detailed bibliography. This publication is for sale by the Superintendent of Documents, U.S. Government Printing Office, Washington, D. C., 20402.

Monahan, J. (Ed.) *Who is the client? The ethics of psychological intervention in the criminal justice system.* Washington, D. C.: American Psychological Association, 1980. This paperback collection of short essays raises questions about ethical issues in connection with the psychologists' role in the courts, prisons, parole boards, and other judicial contexts. Should they be used as experts to predict dangerousness or determine competence to stand trial? Are psychologists concerned about the validity of their methods? Is it ethical to attempt to treat prisoners or do research on them without their consent? Are defendants and prisoners entitled to the same rights as the rest of us, for example, as to the privacy and confidentiality of their communications to a mental health worker? This book is a fascinating survey of these and related ethical questions facing mental health workers working within the judicial system. There are many concrete illustrations and examples of the issues involved from "real life," as well as an extensive reference list.

Silberman, C. E. *Criminal violence, criminal justice.* New York: Random House, 1980. Paperback. This book, written by a journalist, presents an excellent report and analysis of the current state of crime (as "American as Jesse James") in the United States today. The author's prose is easy to read and very understandable. A thorough index makes it possible for the book to be used as a reference. In addition to reportage and analysis, the author presents psychological and sociological theory as it relates to crime, violence, and the criminal justice system. He also discusses crime from the perspectives of the victim, the criminal, and law enforcement.

Part III

Interventions

Chapters 19–21

19

Psychotherapies: Individual and Group Methods

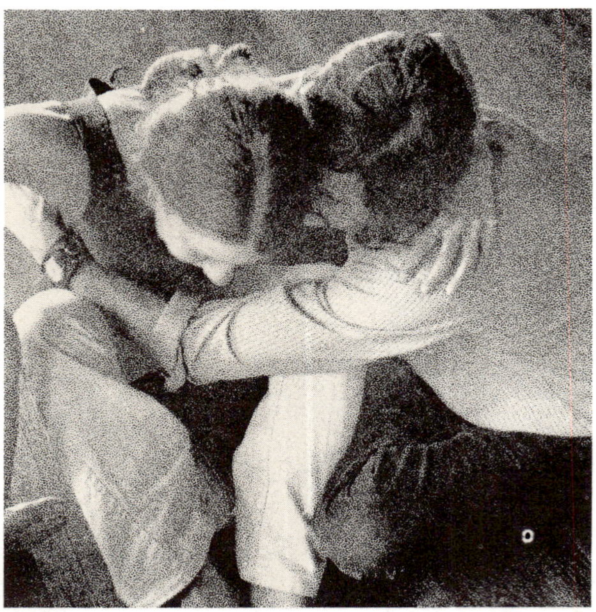

INTRODUCTION

Psychotherapy is taken to mean the informed and planful application of techniques derived from established psychological principles, by persons qualified through training and experience to understand these principles and to apply these techniques with the intention of assisting individuals to modify such per-

sonal characteristics as feelings, values, attitudes, and behaviors which are judged by the therapist to be maladaptive or maladjustive (Meltzoff and Kornreich, 1970, p. 6).

Similar definitions of psychotherapy assume that therapists use a common core of therapeutic techniques and that they are consciously aware of all the elements in this process. Another assumption is that there is a set body of psychological knowledge about how to change people's behaviors so that "informed" therapists can draw on this material. Still another assumption is that all forms of psychotherapy are practiced by equally qualified individuals with guaranteed levels of training and experience.

In actuality, psychotherapy is practiced by many different kinds of individuals, with many different kinds and degrees of training. Methods of psychotherapy are so varied that it is nearer to the truth to state that there is little or no agreement as to "established" procedures.* Further, many therapists are challenging the notion that the therapists' job is to change behaviors that they (the therapists) judge to be maladaptive or maladjustive. Judge? What is maladaptive or maladjustive?

Can psychotherapy be defined in a way that makes fewer assumptions? Yes, if the term is used in such a way that it applies to systematic methods, techniques, processes, interventions, and strategies that a professionally trained individual uses to help another person or a group of people to modify behaviors, feelings, or interpersonal relationships. The *specific* goals of therapy can vary quite dramatically: personal growth; making the unconscious conscious; achieving emotional maturity; symptom reduction; increases in self-confidence and self-esteem. Still other goals might be more concerned than are some of those just mentioned with altering cognitive processes: how one perceives, thinks about, or labels, one's conflicts.

Most definitions of psychotherapy imply a mutual "contract." The client willingly seeks and enters therapy. As a matter of fact, there is considerable agreement that when an individual seeking help shows some motivation to change, the conditions for effective therapy are at an optimal level. Later, I shall say a bit more about the effectiveness of psychotherapy.

Certain methods used for inducing change in people have already been described: the activities of Alcoholics Anonymous, for example, or some of the approaches to sexual dysfunctions. Later chapters will describe some of the "newer" methods, which employ hypnosis, biofeedback, medication, and various types of behavioral interventions. Some of these methods are not as new as one might think; and many of the more "traditional" methods described in the current chapter are basically new and innovative.

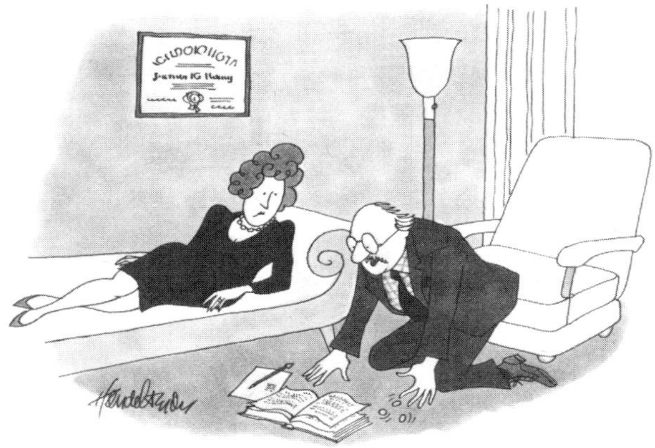

"The Electra Complex is always a toughie, and on top of that, you were born under Aquarius. Let's see what the I Ching says."

* Reviews of the literature suggest that there are from 100 to 140 "mainstream" schools of psychotherapy (Marshall, 1980).

Hooking. Intrinsic to most therapies, but not necessarily formalized as an aspect of any particular system, is an often unplanned process that has been referred to as hooking (see Cashdan, 1973). This process, when it takes place, occurs in initial phases of the therapeutic encounter and involves the client's early perceptions of the therapist as a caring, involved, trustworthy person who is offering the possibility of help. If the client accepts the therapist and therapy in such a trusting way, he or she develops a strong feeling of wishing to remain in therapy. If this feeling does not develop, the client tends to drop out of treatment.

Some advocates of particular systems of therapy might deny the presence of hooking effects. It is most likely, however, that almost all therapeutic processes and methods, explicitly or implicitly, involve hooking maneuvers: clients would otherwise simply not show up again. As a matter of fact, some of the beneficial effects of therapy might result from related elements that are generally referred to as placebo or nonspecific effects.

The placebo effect. Throughout the ages, people have been "cured" by a variety of techniques with the aid of chemicals, herbs, magic, and faith healing.

> *Patients took almost every known organic and inorganic substance—crocodile dung, teeth of swine, hooves of asses, spermatic fluid of frogs, eunuch fat, fly specks, lozenges of dried vipers, powder of precious stones, bricks, furs, feathers, hair, human perspiration, oil of ants, earthworms, wolves, and spiders, moss scraped from the skull of a victim of a violent death, and so on. Blood from every animal was prepared and administered in every way, and was used to treat every conceivable symptom and disease. Almost all human and animal excretions were used. . . . Throughout medical history patients were purged, puked, poisoned, punctured, cut, cupped, blistered, bled, leached, heated, frozen, sweated, and shocked (Shapiro, 1971, p. 441).*

Not all people have been helped by the foregoing, and not all such methods have worked. But some people have indeed been helped. The history of success in medicine, we are told, is very much related to belief in, and expectation of, success, rather than to tangible medical interventions. People have also subjected themselves to an amazing variety of psychotherapeutic methods, and many of these have actually worked (Chapter 2 discusses fads and fashions in treating deviant behavior). The admonition is appropriate: treat as many patients as possible with the new remedies while they still have the power to heal. For many therapies may work because people believe in them. When the popularity of a method wanes, so does its power to heal.

Placebo effects refer to the hidden, indirect healing powers in a method that are not explicitly or specifically designed or built into the process "as advertised." They are the unexpected or nonspecific ingredients that work surprisingly well, often better than the method explicitly offered. For example, the therapist-client, healer-patient, witch doctor-tribesperson relationship of trust, suggestion, and belief may be the true determinant of cure, not the medicine, family technique, or lizard liver actually prescribed.

Although many clinicians have known for a long time that placebo factors are important in successful psychotherapy (for example, through belief in the power of the therapist to "cure"—see Rosenthal and Frank [1956]), some experts believe that the reason psychotherapy works at all is because of its placebo effects only (Shapiro, 1971)!

Within the therapeutic context, many qualities of the therapist, the client, and the therapist-client relationship may be extremely influential in successful outcome, in addition to, or despite, or instead of, the formal interventive procedure. These placebo elements include, among other variables, the suggestibility of the client and his or her faith in the treatment; the therapist-client relationship; the arousal of hope by the therapist; the warmth and support the therapist expresses toward the client; and even the fame of the therapist. Therapists who are innovators of certain methods that may be named after them, or who have "celebrity status," or who show intense enthusiasm for the method they espouse, may be powerful determinants of "cure" (Strupp, 1973).* When such therapists accept a client for treatment, hope and the expectation of successful outcome become part of the therapeutic package and may indeed be responsible for a good part of the beneficial effects of the method.

The following sections describe many different approaches to psychotherapy; bear in mind that the success for some of them may have to do with the placebo effects, which are strongest when the therapeutic maneuver is new, innovative, and in current word-of-mouth vogue. Thus, the proverbial test of time is especially important in evaluating outcome. Do the positive effects last? For, as the client's expectations, perceptions, and cognitions about certain therapeutic procedures change, so, perhaps, will the overall effectiveness of these procedures. It takes great experimental know-how to separate out placebo effects of a particular method as practiced by a particular therapist from the more objective process of therapy. Or, as some will have it, perhaps this is not necessary at all, for charisma, like catharsis, confession, and positive cognitions, may do its own important work.

PSYCHODYNAMIC** THERAPIES

Psychoanalysis and Psychoanalytically Oriented Methods

Chapter 6 outlined Freudian theories of the development of the personality. In addition, some of the other chapters presented Freudian explanations for such pathologies as alcoholism, schizophrenia, or depression. The method of treatment developed by Freud—psychoanalysis—has not been specifically described, however.

Because many of the different techniques in psychotherapy are "spinoffs" from classical psychoanalysis, the best way to understand them is to describe in moderate detail traditional psychoanalytical methods. But remember, even the staunchest of Freudian traditionalists do not consistently adhere to the letter of Freudian technique. The purpose of psychoanalysis can be simply stated: psychoanalysis purports to be a method that mainly serves to make the unconscious conscious. To accomplish this goal, Freud developed elaborate techniques and principles (see Freud, 1963; Menninger, 1958).

1. Psychoanalytic method is offered as a "cure" for the neuroses. In this context, the analyst portrays his or her role as an omnipotent one—I know the cure and the path to it, if only you, the patient, would cooperate. Implicit in this approach, of course, is the notion that the neuroses (and other pathologies) are disease processes.

The aura of omniscience is enhanced by the fact that all applicants for help are not accepted for psychoanalysis. Potential patients are interviewed and often rejected as unsuitable for treatment. These individuals may be psychotic or borderline people. Or perhaps they are simply not verbal, educated, or able to understand the rules of therapy. As a result, many low-SES and ethnic-minority people are excluded as candidates for psychoanalysis.

2. Traditional psychoanalytic method calls for frequent analytic (therapy) sessions, perhaps four or five times weekly. The patient is asked to recline on a couch, facing away from the analyst, who sits outside of the patient's line of vision at an angle to the couch, near the patient's head.

3. The road to cure is through the unconscious—the mass of repressed feelings, conflicts, memories, attitudes, and desires that are not accessible to the individual and that must be uncovered. Much of the material has to do with the frustra-

* It has been suggested that the power of these placebo effects and of belief and expectation lies in increased action of certain biochemical processes within the body that reduce pain, for example, through the endorphin system. Research as to the relationship between placebo effects and the body's biochemistry is still in exploratory stages.

** *Psychodynamic* is generally intended to refer to therapeutic approaches that place emphasis on the patient's drives, motivations, and, frequently, unconscious processes.

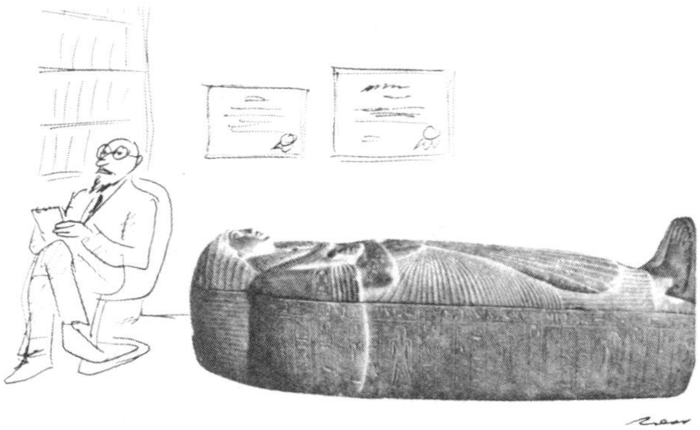

Drawing by Ross; © 1979 The New Yorker Magazine, Inc.

tions, conflicts, and difficulties arising as a result of the clash of infantile sexual strivings and id impulses with the requirements of the "real world." The real world is largely represented by the roles and behaviors of the mother and father, especially the mother, in ministering to the basic needs of the child. Because the neurosis emerges from conflicts experienced at early developmental levels, a cure is effected by uncovering those unconscious conflicts from the past that are considered to be the source of the neurosis.

4. The basic rule in psychoanalysis is to follow the path to the unconscious through free association, that is, saying whatever comes to mind without censorship. This is the royal road to forbidden, repressed mental content. The analyst asks for dreams, and the patient is encouraged to associate to his or her dreams. Later, interpretations of dreams—their manifest (overt, obvious) and latent (hidden) content—is an important aspect of the analytic process. Freudian symbolism plays an important role here. For example, dreams about pencils, implements, or horses are symbolically phallic; dreams of rooms, caves, or mouths are symbolically vaginal or uterine.

5. During this time—and this period may take a year or two—the patient follows the rule of free association while the therapist follows the rule of silence. He or she (the analyst) does not respond to pleas for support, sympathy, or even to the anger expressed by the patient in need of reassurance or symptom relief.

Phillip Roth's novel *Portnoy's Complaint* (1967) is an elaborate, anguished outpouring of first-person free-association material in the presence of a silent, fictional analyst. The book thus tells a loose story about masturbation, guilt, sexual hang-ups, forbidden desires, and adolescent fantasies, dreams, and wishes.

The book ends after 273 pages of Portnoy's distress: verbal anguish, yelling, crying, and suffering. His final fantasy is about GUILT. After removing a mattress tag that says, "Do Not Remove Under Penalty of Law," his fantasy continues:

"This is the police speaking. You're surrounded, Portnoy. You better come out and pay your debt to society." "Up society's ass, Copper!" "Three to come out with those hands of yours up in the air, Mad Dog, or else we come in after you, guns blazing. One." "Blaze, you bastard cop, what do I give a shit? I tore the tag off my mattress—" "Two." "—But at least while I lived, I lived big!"

Aaaaaaaaaaaaaaaaaaaaaaaaaaaaaaaaaaaaaaaaaaaa aaaaaaaaaaaaaaaaaaaaaaaaaaaaaaaaaaaaaaaaaaaaaaa aaaaaaaaaaaaaaaaaaaaaaaaaaaaaaaaaaaaaaaaaaaaaaa aaaaaaaaaaaaaaaaaaaaaaaaaaaaaaaaaaaaaaaaaaaaaaa aaaaaaaaaaaaaaaaaaaaaaaaaaaahhhh!!!!!

PUNCH LINE

So (said the doctor). Now vee may perhaps to begin. Yes?

(Excerpted from Philip Roth, *Portnoy's Complaint* [Random House, 1967], p. 274.)

Portnoy's analyst was obviously obeying the rules.

6. Perhaps one of the most important aspects of the analysis is the interpretation of transference: an emotional response to the therapist as if he or she is playing some significant role in the patient's past—mother, father, feared older brother, for example. The transference, with all of the early feelings, fear, problems, desires, and wishes on the part of the patient reflected in it, plays a key role in traditional psychoanalysis. The analyst interprets the irrational responses to the analyst (love, hate, anger, dependency) as being reflections of past emotional

events in which feelings toward significant figures *then* are being expressed to the analyst *now*. The goal is for the patient to perceive the nature of his or her early relationship needs in order to understand how they are shaping his or her current emotional needs.

Psychoanalysts talk of the transference neurosis as assuming dominance over the symptom neurosis. For at this stage, the symptoms with which the patient entered analysis are less significant than the form of the interpersonal conflicts—between patient and analyst—that emerges.

The analyst is also trained and expected to focus on his or her feelings of countertransference—the emotions experienced by the analyst toward the patient that can restrict personal growth of the patient or actually interfere with the analytic process.

7. The analyst looks for—and interprets to the patient—resistance: blocks to free pathways to the unconscious. Not paying bills, coming late, skipping appointments, failure to free-associate, not bringing in dreams, or acting-out (behaving "poorly" in the "outside world"—criminal activity, promiscuity, self-destructive behavior) probably reflect resistance to the attempts on the part of the analyst to get the patient to open up with unconscious material. Things have become "too hot to handle."

8. Eventually, the analyst becomes even more active in the interpretative process. Together, therapist and patient examine the story of the neurosis and its development. Soon, the patient is encouraged to take more and more responsibility for interpretations as the analysis proceeds, and will, if the analysis is successful, continue to so after the analysis is completed. The patient presumably learns the origins of his or her conflicts and symptoms and can trace it back to infantile psychosexual struggles.

The interpretations and insights achieved at this stage are employed in another context before the analysis is regarded as completed. This is called the working-through stage. The analyst actively helps the patient review the same conflicts, symptoms, or problems again and again until its origins in unconscious processes are understood. Presumably, this helps in the dissolution of the unwanted symptoms or conflicts and aids in the solution of problems in the daily life of the patient. But education for change in the patient's real world is not the ultimate assumed goal of a successful analysis. It is sufficient for the therapist to feel that there is an understanding of early infantile conflicts. There is less focus on the patient's problems in the real world in traditional analysis than in other kinds of therapy.

Neo-Freudian approaches. In Chapter 6, when some of the socially and culturally oriented approaches to personality development were described, people like Karen Horney and Harry Stack Sullivan were mentioned. These analysts, and others like them, Erich Fromm, for example, introduced some important variations in analytic treatment methods. The newer movements tended to move away from the biologically oriented tenets of Freud: culture, society, and current interpersonal forces bear a more important relationship to anxiety, conflict, and the development of the neuroses than had been previously thought to be the case.

The methods of the neo-Freudians are not summarized here, but it should be noted that their therapeutic procedures, like Freudian psychoanalysis, tend to serve verbally oriented, middle-class people who had time and money. These methods also stress curing the psychoneuroses rather than other forms of disturbance.

The work of the neo-Freudians was nevertheless important in significant ways. It led to the consideration that not all Freudian theory was sacrosanct—that the rules were not inviolable (lying on the couch, for example, or the silence of the analyst), and it set the stage for more eclectic, flexible psychotherapies, which, if still owing a great debt to Freud insofar as theory and general principles are concerned, made it possible for many more people with crises and problems in their personal worlds to seek and to receive help.

*Evaluation of psychoanalysis.** Almost all agree: Freudian theory has made an enormous intellectual contribution to the twentieth century, with inestimable influence on the arts, literature, education, and psychology. Its scope includes almost all of people's activities and its stress on the complexity of human motivation and on the significance of the unconscious has influenced us all. Chapter 6, however, noted that empirical results have failed to validate most aspects of Freudian theory. Even dedicated Freudians will acknowledge the difficulty in putting all of the theory to the test, and what little evidence does exist is not that convincing.

In addition, most surveys as to therapy outcome indicate that psychoanalysis is not any more successful than the other forms of therapy (see, for example, Fisher and Greenberg, 1977; Luborsky, Chandler, et al., 1971; Luborsky, Singer, and Luborsky, 1975; and Luborsky and Spence, 1971). Overall, the picture is somewhat bleak. Outcome research regarding traditional psychoanalysis is quite sparse, with very little to be extracted as to relationship of specific analytic method to specific outcome. Most of the empirical research in psychoanalysis focuses on what happens to patients *within* the treatment, such as changes in frequency of self-observations, ability to free-associate, and general verbal productivity (Luborsky and Spence, 1971).

Eclectic Psychodynamic Methods

As traditional classical and neoclassical psychoanalysis declined, the eclectic therapies arose (see Hollender, 1965; Weiner, 1975). These are the methods probably practiced by the majority of therapists today. It is impossible to summarize their precise nature—for they differ in many practical aspects—but some general common denominators among them will be outlined.

One common denominator is that culture, society, interpersonal conflict, and the here and now are important themes in therapy and in therapeutic exploration. Current crises in the client's real world are not avoided. And even though it continues to acknowledge the importance of the unconscious in determining behavior, therapeutic technique is less strenuously committed to seeking paths to the unconscious. Yet the significance of the unconscious and of infantile sexuality, or at least of some kind of conflict-producing early family drama, the importance of the past in the understanding of the present, the use of some kind of dream interpretation, and the belief in concepts such as transference and resistance continue to be aspects of principles and strategies in many of the eclectic psychodynamic therapies.

The psychodynamic eclectic psychotherapies differ from classical psychoanalysis in these important ways.

1. Therapy sessions can be held as infrequently as one or two times weekly.
2. The course of psychotherapy is of shorter duration and the client is generally informed of this expectation (classical psychoanalysis may take up to five or six years). Often, client and therapist agree to jointly evaluate how the therapy is proceeding.
3. The therapist more actively interprets, analyzes, confronts, and questions the client.
4. The rule of free association is not strictly adhered to.
5. There is often cognitive help (see later) in regard to identifying and examining irrational elements in what the client says or does.
6. There is greater encouragement on the part of the therapist to help the client to get by in his or her world with regard to assertiveness, jobs, marital problems, child-rearing problems, sexual dysfunctions, and reality crises. That is, the therapist does not avoid dealing with the client's present-life problems.
7. Intense transference is not generally encouraged; at times it is nipped in the bud, even discouraged.

* Overall evaluation of therapy outcome is described at the end of this chapter. However, comments about some of the schools of therapy are presented as the discussion proceeds, if appropriate.

8. If necessary, the therapist offers reassurance and support to the client, for example, in instances of severe anxiety or depression.
9. Rigid conformity to the rules is not a dogmatic necessity. For example, psychoactive medication is not ruled out, if appropriate; or behavioral interventions, hypnosis, or biofeedback might be recommended (see Chapter 21).
10. Overall, there is a greater tendency to stress the social and interpersonal origins of conflict and stress—including those that arise from cultural and economic considerations.

HUMANISTIC APPROACHES

This section reviews several general approaches to psychotherapy that emphasize the capacity of people to develop, change, and exercise choices in their lives (see Chapter 6, pp. 122–24).

Client-Centered Therapy

The views of Carl Rogers (1942, 1951, 1961) have played a major role in some of the newer therapeutic approaches of the past few decades (for example, encounter groups).

Chapter 6 briefly touched on Rogers's views about the development of personality—of the self. These hypotheses emerged from the Rogerian approach to counseling and psychotherapy, which emphasizes the view that knowledge of motivation, drives, symptoms, or diagnoses is not essential to the counseling process. The therapist's role is simply to show understanding of the feelings expressed by the client and to indicate that understanding by "reflecting" the client's feelings back to him or her. Rogerian therapists do not express judgment, hold opinions, or offer advice and guidance, for it is assumed that they do not know what is best for the client. Instead, it is understood that each client contains within himself or herself the capacity to grow, to develop, and to change. Rogerians hold that these growth processes will take place in circumstances in which the therapist acknowledges the client's feelings, accepts them entirely, and allows them to be expressed openly and freely.

In this approach, dream interpretation, transference, long-term treatment, and dwelling on the past are cast aside. Short-term therapy (for example, 20 sessions) as opposed to long-term traditional Freudian analysis is encouraged. And the stress in therapy is on what the client brings into the session. Generally, these are current, present-day problems that the client faces in real life.

The client, not the doctor, contains the "formula" that will help him or her flower into a fuller, more mature individual, provided that some therapeutic circumstances exist. These circumstances are simple. They involve listening skills on the part of the therapist, who can reflect back to the client what his or her feelings are, and also empathic skills, with complete acceptance of the client as a person. The therapist indicates "unconditional positive regard" for the client and communicates his or her ability to see the world as the client sees it, through the subjective frame of reference that is unique to the client. Spotlight 19.1 presents illustrations of client-centered interactions.

Goals of Rogerian therapy include (a) increasing self-awareness of feelings and (b) becoming fulfilled. The fulfilled client is less defensive about himself or herself, is open to new experiences, and has high self-regard.

The fully functioning person, a Rogerian ideal, can grasp the meaning of the "good life" (Rogers, 1961). Such a person is not necessarily without tension—in a state of homeostasis—nor is such a person necessarily always happy or contented. The person who is in the process of "becoming himself or herself" is reaching toward the good life. That person has complete psychological freedom to make choices, to move in various directions. The process of "becoming a person" involves several dimensions. One of these is becoming more open to feelings one experiences: to be aware of and to sense hatred, love, awe, affection, anger, desire, or embarrassment. It would follow that such people are less defensive.

Spotlight 19.1 I Really Feel Miserable! You Are Really Feeling Miserable

In the 1940s, "hip" graduate students, exposed to the work of Rogers, joked about his methods in psychotherapy, smirking about the directionless reflection of feeling that Rogers espoused in his approach. Wisecracks were rampant.

Student (desperately): Doctor, help! Where is your nearest bathroom?
Doctor: You have to go to the bathroom badly.

Decades later, there were fewer wisecracks. Even a computer could be programmed to show empathy, reflect feeling, and elicit a genuine opening up to and an emotional involvement with it. Here is an excerpt from a program called DOCTOR, modeled after Rogerian-type responses.

Client: *Men are all alike.*
Computer: IN WHAT WAY
Client: *They're always bugging us about something or other.*
Computer: CAN YOU THINK OF A SPECIFIC EXAMPLE
Client: *Well, my boyfriend made me come here.*
Computer: YOUR BOYFRIEND MADE YOU COME HERE
Client: *He says I'm depressed much of the time.*
Computer: I AM SORRY TO HEAR YOU ARE DEPRESSED
Client: *It's true. I am unhappy.*
Computer: DO YOU THINK COMING HERE WILL HELP YOU NOT TO BE UNHAPPY
Client: *I need some help, that much seems certain.*
Computer: WHAT WOULD IT MEAN TO YOU IF YOU GOT SOME HELP
Client: *Perhaps I could learn to get along with my mother.*
Computer: TELL ME MORE ABOUT YOUR FAMILY
Client: *My mother takes care of me.*
Computer: WHO ELSE IN YOUR FAMILY TAKES CARE OF YOU
Client: *My father.*
Computer: YOUR FATHER
Client: *You are like my father in some ways.*
Computer: WHAT RESEMBLANCE DO YOU SEE
Client: *You are not very aggressive but I think you don't want me to notice that.*
Computer: WHAT MAKES YOU THINK I AM NOT VERY AGGRESSIVE
Client: *You don't argue with me.*
Computer: WHY DO YOU THINK I DON'T ARGUE WITH YOU
Client: *You are afraid of me.*
Computer: DOES IT PLEASE YOU TO BELIEVE I AM AFRAID OF YOU
Client: *My father is afraid of everybody.*
Computer: WHAT ELSE COMES TO MIND WHEN YOU THINK OF YOUR FATHER
Client: *Bullies.*
Computer: DOES THAT HAVE ANYTHING TO DO WITH THE FACT THAT YOUR BOYFRIEND MADE YOU COME HERE

(From *Computer power and human reason: From judgment to calculation* by Joseph Weizenbaum [W. H. Freeman and Company], pp. 3–4. Copyright © 1976.)

Although the computer appears to be empathic and is certainly not expressing opinions or judgments about the client's responses, some clinicians feel that the quality of its programmed responses differs from those of a real live therapist. Compare the foregoing, for example, with the following excerpt from an eighth interview between Rogers and Mrs. Oak (T and C, respectively) in which some very powerful feelings are beginning to emerge:

C: *You know over in this area of, of sexual disturbance, I have a feeling that I'm beginning to discover that it's pretty bad, pretty bad. I'm finding out that, that I'm bitter, really. Damn bitter. I—and I'm not turning it back in, into myself . . . I think what I probably feel is a certain element of "I've been cheated."* (Her voice is very tight and her throat chokes up.) *And I've covered up very nicely, to the point of consciously not caring. But I'm, I'm sort of amazed to find that in this practice of, what shall I call it, a kind of sublimation that right under it—again words—there's a kind of passive force that's, it's pas—it's very passive, but at the same time it's just kind of* murderous.

T: *So there's the feeling, "I've really been cheated. I've covered that up and seem not to care and yet under-*

neath that there's a kind of a, a latent but very much present bitterness *that is very, very strong."*

C: *It's very strong. I—that I know. It's terribly powerful.*

T: *Almost a dominating kind of force.*

C: *Of which I am rarely conscious. Almost never . . . Well, the only way I can describe it, it's a kind of murderous thing, but without violence. . . . It's more like a feeling of wanting to get even. . . . And of course, I won't pay back, but I'd like to. I really would like to.*

(Excerpted from Carl R. Rogers, *On becoming a person,* p. 92. Copyright © 1961 by Houghton Mifflin Company, One Beacon Street, Boston, Mass. 02108. Used by permission.)

This theme is not explored again until much later, when in the thirty-first interview, the client is trying to describe a feeling that is deep within her:

C: *I have the feeling it isn't guilt.* (Pause. She weeps.) *Of course I mean, I can't verbalize it yet.* (Then with a rush of emotion) *It's just being* terribly hurt!

T: *M-hm. It isn't guilt except in the sense of being very much wounded somehow.*

C: (Weeping) *It's—you know, often I've been guilty of it myself but in later years when I've heard parents say to their children, "stop crying," I've had a feeling, a hurt as though, well, why should they tell them to stop crying? They feel sorry for themselves, and who can feel more adequately sorry for himself than the child. Well, that is sort of what—I mean, as though I mean, I thought that they should let him cry. And—feel sorry for him too, maybe. In a rather objective kind of way. Well, that's—something of the kind of thing I've been experiencing. I mean, now—just right now. And in—in—*

T: *That catches a little more the flavor of the feeling that it's almost as if you're really weeping for yourself.*

C: *Yeah. And again you see there's conflict. Our culture is such that—I mean, one doesn't indulge in self-pity. But this isn't—I mean, I feel it doesn't quite have that connotation. It may have.*

T: *Sort of think that there is a cultural objection to feeling sorry about yourself. And yet you feel the feeling you're experiencing isn't quite what the culture objected to either.*

(Rogers, 1961, p. 93)

The differences between the computer and the therapist in expressing and reflecting the client's feelings are rather striking. But yet, it is conceivable that one day a computer can be programmed (and this can include memory for preceding sessions as well as for background material) to reflect feelings and emotions in a nonjudgmental way and with as much empathy and sensitivity as did Rogers. But can a computer show "unconditional positive regard" for the client? Can a computer respond to affective facial cues or to gestures or to glances the way a real live therapist can? What is your opinion?

Another dimension of the process of becoming a person concerns a growing ability to live completely and fully in the here and now, in the moment. At the same time, such people become increasingly accepting of themselves, their experiences, and their judgments. They feel they can trust their ability to respond, to feel, and to size up situations. They make increasing use of their feelings, abilities, and bodies to live out each moment without fear. Such people are truly free, according to Roger's interpretation of the good life, to make choices and to use their own free will to decide their own courses of actions. Psychotherapy, if successful, thus enriches the individual to live creatively, with less constriction and fear of being controlled from without.

Overview. Rogerian methods are among the most important influences in the history of psychotherapy (Garfield, 1981). The contribution of this general approach lies not so much in the rigor of its hypotheses or in its record of success (see Lambert,

DeJulio, and Stein, 1978), but rather in creating new perspectives in a domain long dominated by the mystique of psychoanalysis. The overthrow of the large superstructure of Freudian theory and methods is in in large part due to the simple methods proposed by Rogers, which, combined with the stress on brief therapy (for example, twenty or thirty sessions on a once-a-week basis), the questioning of the expertise and aura of the doctor, and the proposition that people contain within themselves the seeds to get better all add up to freshness and innovation in approaches to helping people. People in counseling deserve respect, their rights are to be protected, and they can determine their own options and goals.

Two additional contributions can be traced back to Rogerian hypotheses. One is the budding notion that flowered into skepticism as to whether or not the disease model is helpful in diagnosing and treating people with problems in everyday living. The other has to do with the methodology of conducting research in an area that previously had not lent itself to rigorous dissection. For example, recording the content of sessions, establishing reliable methods for assessing the progress of a client in counseling, and making evaluations of outcome a matter of public record—these were all becoming areas of focus after years of neglect. Psychology was beginning to assume a sense of legitimately concerning itself with psychotherapy, long considered a discipline of medicine.

Gestalt Therapy

The Gestalt Prayer
I do my thing, and you do your thing.
I am not in this world to live up to your expectations
And you are not in this world to live up to mine.
You are you, and I am I,
And if by chance, we find each other, it's beautiful.
If not, it can't be helped.

Fritz Perls

Gestalt therapy, like Rogerian methods, is also an extremely influential force in many of the newer therapeutic approaches (see Fagan and Shepherd, 1970; Perls, 1971, 1973; and Polster and Polster, 1973). Its principles depart radically from most of the psychodynamic and psychoanalytic therapies. The latter methods rely heavily on techniques to delve into the past in order to understand conflict. Gestalt therapy, on the other hand, stresses the here-and-now. It shares some common ground with existential approaches in therapy, which not only stress the here-and-now but also regard personal awareness and subjectivity (phenomenology) as the only reality.

According to Perls (1971), people in their natural, undisturbed states will "self-regulate." They will be aware of their most pressing needs, and they will seek to satisfy those needs. Pathology occurs when people cut themselves off from thoughts and feelings that are unacceptable to themselves and/or to others. Then, because "You do not allow yourself—or you are not allowed—to be totally yourself. . . . Your ability to cope with the world becomes less and less. . . . " (p. 11). The purpose of Gestalt therapy is to help people become aware of all aspects of themselves—of their real needs at each moment—so that they will be able to self-regulate.

Because self-awareness, especially of feelings, is regarded as curative and beneficial in its own right, much of the Gestalt movement (and the human potential movement discussed later) is concerned with ways to encourage, to set the stage for, the individual (in a one-to-one situation or in groups) to get in touch with, to become aware of, and to establish contact with the self and with his or her feelings. In this way, reaching toward and achieving one's potential is developed.

Interpretations, examinations of the past, discussions of the future tend to be avoided by many Gestalt therapists, who prefer not to use words like "why" and "because." There is no emphasis, as in Freudian treatment, on bringing unconscious, repressed memories into consciousness. One's current experience is stressed. People can change and grow as a result of being fully aware of what they are experiencing. As a result, therapy sessions are often dramatic and appealing (to therapist and client alike), especially to those who feel that there is a thanklessness in theorizing, conceptualizing, and hairsplitting.

Sessions are most typically workshops in which the therapist works with an individual in a group situation, often using various tasks (such as "dreamwork"—see later) to accomplish one essential purpose: to help the client become aware of the here-and-now and to block any attempt to avoid this awareness. Therapists use direct, active methods designed to help people become more directly aware of their feelings and of what they are experiencing in the here-and-now.

Below are a few methods and tasks that some Gestalt therapists use:

The hotseat. A willing participant in the group sits in the hotseat and the therapist and individual then engage in a series of tasks, maneuvers, and exercises designed to help the individual become aware of true feelings.

Person in dialogue with self. Gestalt therapists may use an empty chair when wishing the patient to have an "encounter," a dialogue, with parts of the self. For example, a client might be requested to carry out a "dialogue" between perceived polarities within himself or herself. Here is an excerpt from such a "dialogue" expressed by a woman who oftens puts on a cheerful efficient facade (Big) to hide her lack of confidence (Little).

Little: (crying) I feel so little . . . I feel helpless and weak . . . I need somebody to take care of me. I don't *want* to be big and have to take care of somebody else. They always want me to watch over someone, and I'm too little!

Big: Come on, don't be like that. You don't have to be like that. I'm big and I can do things. I'm able to get things going.

Little: I don't *want* to be big . . . I'm little . . . I'm only 3½ and . . . I'm watching my little brother and . . . he falls off the porch! I'm too little to watch him. I feel so bad!

Therapist: Sounds like a big job for a little girl.

Little: It *was* . . . I shouldn't have been doing it . . . it was too much to expect. I've always been asked to act big and do things and I'm little. (pause)

Now I feel bigger . . . I'm 11 years old and I'm asked to go to Cape Cod and watch my cousins. And I worry about who will watch my baby sister . . . there's a river in front of our house and I'm afraid she'll fall in and nobody will see her.

Therapist: So it's *you or nobody.*

Big: That's baloney!

Therapist: What's baloney?

Little: Somebody will watch . . . it doesn't *have* to be me! (crying) I want to be little and have somebody *hold* me. (curls up into a ball on the couch . . . stretches out her hand.)

Therapist: What do you want now?

Patient: Oh, I don't know . . . I feel like a baby! It's silly!

Therapist: What you want is silly? (long pause)

Patient: Could you . . . could you hold me?

So I sat next to her on the couch, took her onto my lap and held her. She continued to cry, and little by little the tension and stiffness drained out of her. After about five minutes I asked her just to experience what it was like to be held. After about five minutes more, I asked her what she was aware of.

Patient: I feel more relaxed right now than I have ever been.

Therapist: Do you feel *big* or *little* right now?

Patient: I don't feel little . . . I don't feel like a baby. But I don't feel big either. I mean, I don't feel like I have to act big and pretend I don't want to be held . . . I . . . *That's* the baloney! I can be big and still want to be held!

(Polster and Polster, 1973, pp. 250–51)

Enactment. Acting out feelings, unfinished business from the past, roles and events in dreams, or characteristics of oneself or others (being tied up in knots, for example, or being at loose ends, or behaving like a bull in a china shop, or sliding on thin ice) is an important device in Gestalt sessions. Presumably, these gamelike tasks heighten self-awareness.

Dreamwork. Dreams are not interpreted but are acted out. The client becomes the vampire, or the child being thrown off the cliff, or the angry mob, or the person about to be eaten alive. Indeed, many different parts are acted out by the client, not just the parts of the protagonist. In addition, feelings are acted out. Spotlight 19.2 illustrates dreamwork in a session with Perls.

Spotlight 19.2 Perls's Dreamwork

This excerpt provides the flavor of a Gestalt therapy session. It is a dialogue between Fritz Perls and a client (F and M, respectively) who is being actively encouraged to act out aspects of a dream she is reporting. Note how active Perls is in the therapeutic contact and how consistently the awareness of what one is experiencing is stressed, as opposed to conceptualizations about it.

F: *. . . I think we are ready for the dream now, so let's have the dream.*

M: *I was home, and I'm—I'm with my sister, and—and we have a lot of fun together.*

F: *In the dream? /M: Yeah. /What kind of fun?*

M: *We talk together, we do things together, we—*

F: *What do you do together? You see, I can't understand abstract language. I must have something real to work with.*

M: *We—we escape together, we—*

F: *You escape together.*

M: *We escape from people, and—*

F: *I don't understand the word "people." From whom do you escape?*

M: *From my parents.*

F: *Ah. And that's fun.*

M: *It's fun. And we understand each other. I can tell her—I can take out my hostility on her, I can scream at her, and pick at her. I can't do that to my parents. All I can do is be just—just lifeless with them, just listen to them.*

F: *Okeh. Have an encounter with your sister.*

M: *You're a bum. You're no good. I'm better than you are . . .*

F: *Change seats. What does she answer?*

M: *I don't like being called a bum. F: Say this again. (louder) I don't* like *being called a bum. /F: Again./ (animated) I don't* like *being called a bum! F: Again. I'm sick and tired of you calling me a bum all the time!*

F: *Now you sound real. Do you hear it?*

M: *I don't like you for it, (high petulant voice) and I hate you, I don't—*

F: *I don't believe the hate. "I hate you." I didn't hear* any *hate in there. You're talking literature again.*

M: You're *the bum.*

F: *Ah! Say this again.*

M: You're *a bum,* you're *a bum, I'm not the bum.* You're *the bum.*

F: *Change seats . . . What do you experience now?*

M: *I—I feel like I would like to tear her apart. I'd like to tear her clothes off, and her legs off, and I'd just like to smash her to pieces.*

F: *Now do it—dance this. Act it out.*

M: *I can't act it out.*

F: *Do it! Don't give me that crap . . . You could squeeze me very nicely. Do we have anything she could tear apart? (someone gets some newspapers) And breathe when you do this, and make noises. Make noises.*

M: I can't *tear you apart, Norma . . . I would like to but—*

F: *Yah? What's your objection?*

M: *I—I—You're not the one I'm really angry at.*

F: *Ahah.*

M: *I don't want to hurt you.*

F: *How don't you want to hurt her? (laughter)*

M: *You're not the one—I don't want to kill you. I don't want to tear you apart. I don't wanna—to make a* vegetable *out of you. Not kill you physically, but I don't wanna—*

F: *Whom do you want to kill?*

M: *(softly) I'd like to kill my father.*
F: *Okeh. Let's call Papa in. (Fritz whistles) You know, of course, parents are* never *good, parents are* always *at fault. If they are tall, they should be small. If they are that, they should be this. So, tell him off. How does he not fit your expectations? What should he be like?*
M: *He should let me alone.*
F: *Say this to him.*
M: *(petulant, complaining) Let me alone, Dad. Go away from me. Let me alone. Let me live my own life and just stop interfering, and leave me alone.*
F: *Does he hear you?*
M: *No.*
F: *So try again. Get communication.*
M: *I—I feel very sad—when I tell you this.*
F: *Say this to him.*
M: *I feel sad when I tell you this, because I really don't want to hurt you. I feel guilty when I try to hurt you.*
F: *We translate the word "guilty" in Gestalt Therapy by* resentful, *so let's try this on for size. How do you call him?*
M: *Dad.*
F: *"Dad, I resent this and this—I resent this and this."*
M: *Dad, I resent—I resent your trying to make me—fill your needs—*

(Excerpted from F. S. Perls, *Gestalt therapy verbatim* [Real People Press, Box F, Moab, Utah 84532], pp. 143–46.)

Shuttling. The therapist uses a directed task called shuttling—requesting that the client use and feel his or her mental energies by going from "here" (what is being experienced) to "there" (fantasy content) and then coming back to "here." This method supposedly sharpens one's awareness of the current here-and-now of one's experiences.

The goal of Gestalt therapy, then, is to help clients achieve maturity, a continuing process of personal growth that involves increasing one's awareness of one's inner self and its various parts. It is difficult to assess the success of the Gestalt approach because it is not possible to define and measure either its goals or its methods with any degree of objectivity. However, many clients tend to favor both its methods and its overall goals because of their dramatic appeal and "commonsense" qualities.

The Encounter Movement: The Human Potential Explosion

"The most important social invention of the century is the encounter group" (Rogers, 1968, p. 29). The encounter group is the vehicle of the human potential movement, which is dedicated to the goal of developing human potential. What does this potential consist of? What were the goals of the encounter movement when it reached its peak? Supporters of the movement (see Schutz, 1973) speak of personal growth and self-expression, developing trust, openness with others, increasing one's capacity to relate to others, recognizing and defeating self-deception, getting to know and like oneself, becoming responsible for oneself, emerging from despair and loneliness, and developing sensual awareness.

The paths to these goals are generally through the emergence of awareness of one's feelings and body as encouraged through a variety of group experiences that can be very intense and take different paths as a result of methods introduced by the leader.

Many encounter programs call for the meeting of a dozen (more or less) people in a group situation for a few hours over several sessions, often in close sequence. A weekend in one continuous encounter is a marathon group. Sometimes sessions can last for an entire day, or for an afternoon and evening. All groups have a leader whose chief function is to encourage members to interact with great intensity with one another.

Acting out feelings—doing something rather than talking about it—is one of the mottos of encounter programs. But interest and activity may lag. The leader at such times introduces tasks, exercises, and structured activities. Activities that have given encounter its special notoriety have included various kinds of rhythmic exercises such as clapping, jumping, massaging, dancing; or eyeballing-to-eyeballing; and holding, hugging, touching. The exercises can also involve nudity, exploring each other's bodies, or physical closeness. Whatever these tasks, exercises, and rituals may be, presumably they are not encouraged for their own sake but to help induce feelings of joy, spontaneity, closeness, intimacy, anger, and assertiveness, or to increase expressiveness (as in screaming exercises, for example). These techniques are presumably employed to get people to open up with honest feelings about themselves in a direct, nondeceptive way.

The marathon group encourages a continuous, intense group experience that can last anywhere from eighteen to forty-eight hours. These sessions focus on the group itself, so that everything else loses importance. Many people report that extremely intense emotional experiences arise as a result of the forced intimacy and emotional sharing that goes on in such a continuous session. The dropping of pretenses, the trying out of new behaviors, and the "charged" group atmosphere that an extended group experience permits—and these include experiences that some participants describe as intense and "beautiful"—may or may not affect behavior in the real, "outside" world of Sunday night and Monday morning. Many supporters of the marathon movement believe that it usually does, however, at least in terms of inducing greater belief in oneself or in acceptance and understanding of others (Mintz, 1971). These expectations, however, have not been empirically confirmed.

An interaction in an encounter group. (Paul Fusco/Magnum)

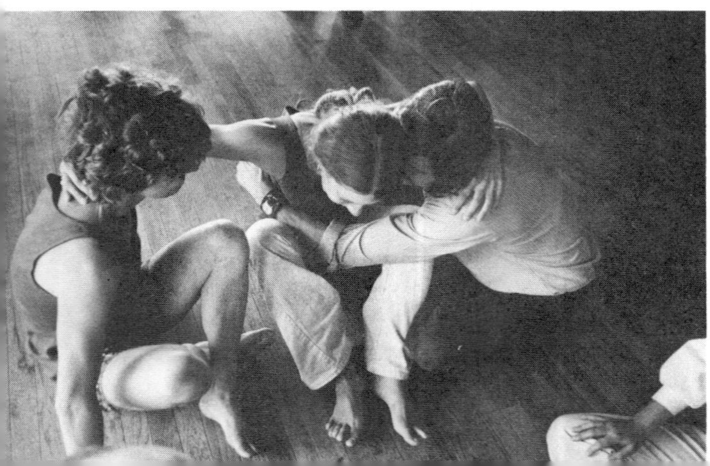

Evaluation. Dissatisfaction with the encounter movement is by now widespread enough so that even defenders admit that its popularity has diminished considerably. What are some of the criticisms? Some negatives concern the bandwagon effect that swept the media and many lay groups, lending greater credence to the claim of beneficial effects than was warranted. Many critics question the "quickie" training programs—the push of the movement that permits the feeling that everyone can be a leader. Others point to the use of the prepackaged, structured exercises by untrained nonprofessionals that lends an air of pseudoscientific validity to the encounter group. Szasz calls the use of such gimmicks *scientism,* and likens it to the "healing power" of the primitive ritual or magical practice.

Other criticisms concern the strong possibility that the appeal of the movement—and its potential benefits—is relevant essentially to middle-class, educated groups who can afford the time, luxury of introspection, and great expense involved. After all, critics say, a jobless ghetto mother of four who is marginally adjusting to life does not need enhanced self-awareness nor the opportunity to learn to drop social pretenses. The needs of the poor, some say, are met by social solutions, but not of the encounter type (Schur, 1976).

Many researchers object that the movement is antiscientific: its proponents do not encourage evaluative methods despite its many claims (Harper, 1975; Lieberman, Yalom, and Miles, 1973; Maliver, 1973; Yalom and Lieberman, 1971). Still other criticisms are leveled at the risks that may be present when the defenses of unstable people are removed. To reports of such "casualties" the movements's most trenchant defense is: We always say, come at your own risk; you can choose your own options within the group; no one, including even the most blunt or confronting of leaders, can force you to do anything you do not wish to do; you must assume full responsibility for yourself.

What is the empirical evidence, if any, as to the effectiveness of the encounter movement or the validity of the criticisms leveled at it? Are there changes as a result of the encounter experience? A review of forty-five investigations (most were based on "normal" college volunteers and employed a variety of evaluation methods, generally of a questionnaire type, administered immediately following or a few weeks after the encounter experience) yielded the conclusion that there was not even "modest support" for positive findings despite some temporary group effects (Kilmann and Sotile, 1976). These authors noted a common difficulty in generalizing from these studies: there was methodological crudity in many of the investigations, including poor reliability of the assessment procedures, lack of uniformity among the studies in time elapsing between encounter experience and evaluation procedures, and wide differences from study to study in key elements, such as the evaluation procedures employed, the experiences within the group itself, and leader differences.

The difficulties involved in evaluating effectiveness are difficulties inherent in many psychotherapeutic methods—including some very respectable ones (see later sections of this chapter). Even assertions that leaders do not rate participants validly or that they tend not to do what they said they do within the group (Lieberman, Yalom, and Miles, 1973) can be said to apply equally well to many different kinds of psychotherapists practicing within the fold of many different schools of therapy.

What are the casualty rates? Definitions of casualty vary but many include psychotic episodes, reports of increases of anxiety, or negative attitudes about the experience. Relevant information about casualties are obtained from a number of sources through questionnaires immediately after the encounter sessions or through follow-up procedures (Hartley, Roback, and Abramowitz, 1976).

Casualty rates vary from almost none at all to a figure as high as almost half of the participants. Why? A review of the literature suggests that variables associated with high casualty rates were poor preexperience adjustment, expectations being too high, poor self-image, leader variables (inability to recognize some conflicts, for example), and harsh experiences such as extreme pressure to participate in the group or to expose one's feelings (Hartley, Roback, and Abramowitz, 1976).

It was suggested that casualties can be reduced by applying screening methods for participants (in attempts to exclude psychotics, for example, or to watch out for psychotic potential), preparing participants for group experiences by some prediscussion, and creating certification procedures for leaders of the groups. The latter, however, would be particularly offensive to the spirit of the encounter movement, for it generally tends to oppose authority, institutional regulation, and autocratic control.

The conclusions of the most extensive, well-controlled study of encounter groups are by now fairly well-known: they are generally pessimistic. In this study, Lieberman, Yalom, and Miles (1973) randomly assigned over 200 Stanford University undergraduates to one of ten different "encounter" group experiences. Each series of groups met for about 30 hours in contexts determined by the particular group approach, which included, among others, the Gestalt and transactional approaches (see later section), the Esalen eclectic approach, and the psychoanalytic approach. There was also a control group of 69 students.

One of the major conclusions of this research was that of the subjects who underwent group experience, a high proportion (16 out of more than 200) suffered psychological damage as determined by subsequent evaluations. This result appeared to be related not to the group approach or purported principles involved, but to the style of the leader. Casualties consisted of psychotic episodes, need for treatment, or subjective sense of distress. More moderate negative effects were also reported.

Those who appeared to benefit (one-third seemed to benefit, one-third appeared to manifest only moderate change, and one-third seemed to show no change at all) came from groups whose leaders were empathic and supportive, and who occasionally approached problems from a cognitive point of view (see later discussion). Some groups, as a matter of fact, had no casualties at all. Groups with a high proportion of casualties were led by leaders who challenged, confronted, were very active, and created a highly charged emotional atmosphere.

The encounter movement began as an inspirational explosion, attracting not only "giants" like Carl Rogers, but also some of his peers, such as Fritz Perls and Abraham Maslow. With the Esalen Institute at Big Sur on the Pacific coast serving as the geographical and spiritual haven for the movement (a startlingly beautiful site), and in the light of the media's fascination with anything new (especially if it suggests an underlay of psychology, nudity, and the occult), it is easy to understand the contagious spread of the movement. It was embraced with open arms because of significant other reasons, too. There was dissatisfaction with the authoritative "know-it-all" attitudes of the power structure within the domain of psychotherapy and especially psychoanalysis, with its over-conceptualizing, deification of the analyst, stress on *talking* about things, and dismal history of poor success. Has the movement fulfilled its promise? The answer, unfortunately, is no.

GROUP AND FAMILY METHODS

Group Therapy

Group therapy is a general term that refers to a variety of different methods with a common denominator: helping people to modify their behavior, attitudes toward themselves or others, and feelings through participation in regularly scheduled meetings (sessions) in which other clients are also present. Group methods, because they are not comprised of individual, one-to-one therapist-client sessions, were at first especially popular in hospitals, prisons, and other institutional settings because of their economic feasibility. Soon, however, it became apparent that they offered many other advantages in addition to strictly economic ones that will be described later on in this section.

Because each group therapist has his or her own method, manner of forming groups, and principles that govern the focus of the sessions, set rules and procedures for "running" groups do not exist.

Group composition. Groups can be homogeneous or heterogeneous with regard to age, sex, marital status, and problems. Some groups are created from a clinician's private practice. Sometimes they are formed with clients who seem to have stopped makirg progress in the individual sessions. At other times, they are chosen as the primary treatment method. Some groups are specifically focused around problems: drug addiction, alcoholism; obesity; marital problems; phobias; sexual problems. Or they can be aggregates of people in similar life circumstances: single-status parents; parents of retarded children; about-to-be-divorced males. Groups can be comprised of four or five up to twelve or more people who meet regularly.

Logistics. A group can meet in a client's home or in the therapist's office; the therapist may see some or all of the group members in individual sessions; and group sessions can be held once or twice weekly with or without the leader.

Role of the leader (therapist). The leader can be active: he or she can interpret, confront, defend, take sides, stir up. Or, at the other extreme, he or she can be entirely silent during the meeting. The leader of a group may or may not encourage transference. Sometimes he or she is the focal point, the polarized center against which everything bounces or to

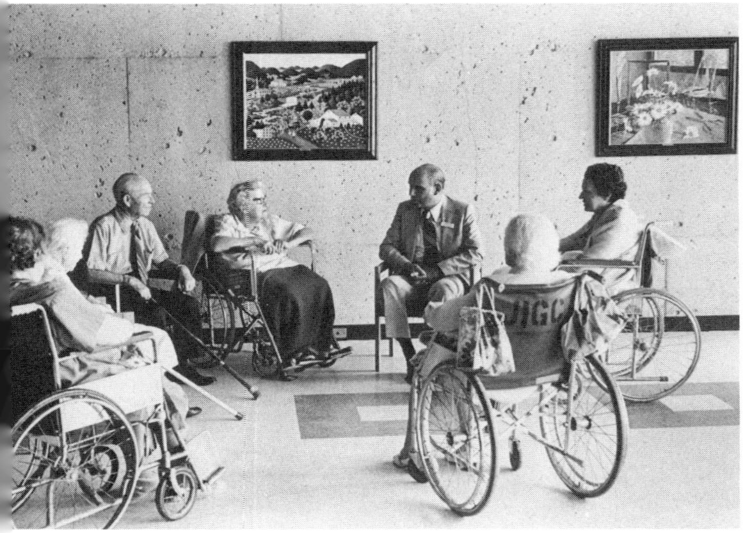

A group-therapy session with disabled patients. These people can provide mutual support for one another, as well as share solutions to common problems. (© Joel Gordon 1978)

which everything is directed. At other times, he or she may be entirely passive, intervening only when too much anxiety has been engendered in a group member.

Mechanical aids. Some group sessions are videotaped, recorded, transcribed. Sometimes the leader or observers will take notes, perhaps on the basis of viewing group events on closed-circuit television. The purpose of these recording aids might be to collect data for research; or the leader might wish to feed back to the group members some of the events that took place as a jumping-off point for discussion or for increased awareness of some of the interactions.

Evaluation of group methods. There are many different ways of running groups. As a result, progress in measuring the effectiveness of group methods has not been rapid, nor have results been uniformly open to inspection. In general, although it is difficult to compare outcome of different group methods because the goals of group therapists differ among one another rather widely (see Rosenbaum and Berger, 1975; Yalom, 1975), group methods have many advantageous common denominators. They provide an opportunity for the member to see himself or herself in a social setting, and to experience and perceive what the effects of his or her behavior are on others. In turn, groups permit other group members to provide feedback to, interact with, and confront, a group member. Thus, awareness of one's behavior in interpersonal contexts is sharpened to a degree that is not possible in the face-to-face therapist-client situation. One group member, for example, who was particularly argumentative and yet easily hurt and defensive when others argued back, learned after many painful confrontations to perceive himself more accurately. At first he was hurt, bewildered, and confused when he perceived how much anger he elicited from others. Now he understands that he *provokes* many of these responses and that by modifying his behavior he can accordingly reduce the intensity of the arguments leveled at him.

Groups also permit the member to expose psychological problems to others, and at the same time to see that one's inner feelings can be accepted by them; or that others describe similar feelings; or that people can provide support, understanding, and compassion. Groups also permit the trying out of certain behaviors—of testing them in real-life situations. Thus taking social risks and testing the reactions of others are made possible in groups. Further, these behaviors can be observed and discussed by other group members, the therapist, and group member himself or herself. For example, feared behavior—such as speaking up, expressing anger, disclosing affection for another, or revealing one's self directly to others—can be tried out in a relatively "safe" setting.

Groups also permit the therapist to see the client *in vivo,* in a real-life social and interpersonal context, so that his or her responses, interactions, and patterns of behavior that would normally have to be talked about away from real life are displayed directly and in the here-and-now. Group processes thus provide the opportunity for development of interpersonal and social skills, for support from others, for feedback and confrontation, and for directly becoming aware of how one behaves in interpersonal situations. They provide an opportunity, also, for lonely, alienated, isolated people to feel part of a larger process. Group membership is concrete enough to be "grabbed onto"—for example by uneducated or nonverbal people who do not understand the relationship of introspection, talking about oneself and one's feelings, and relating of past events to gaining a solution to one's problems.

Group therapy has other advantages. It is economically feasible—in terms of time and money and staff—for large numbers of people. Thus it is a very popular therapeutic method in hospitals, prisons, and other institutions operating on a controlled budget.

Groups do not provide intense individual focus on deep psychological problems. This might be a real handicap to the individual in an acute period of emotional turmoil; such individuals also may not be prepared for the lack of attention allocated to them by the group. Another disadvantage lies in the possibility that some groups are very rough on some of its members, who may be scapegoated and scorned, and who may emerge with crushed egos and a heightened sense of inadequacy. Most therapists would not permit such group processes to go this far, however. Finally, many group members report rapid deterioration effects: that is, the "good" outcomes that members report immediately after group experiences tend to fade rather rapidly.

Family Therapy

Chapter 12, when theories about the etiology of schizophrenia were discussed, noted the significance of the family unit in producing (and maintaining) pathology in a particular family member as well as the communicational breakdowns, confusion, scapegoating, double-bind messages, and alliances that can be observed in family interactions. Although family therapy, one of the newer approaches to treatment, makes use of some of the notions first observed in the study of schizophrenic families, it actually draws on many theoretical approaches and is comprised of many different techniques (see Ackerman, 1966; Haley and Hoffman, 1967; Minuchin, 1974; Minuchin et al., 1967; and Satir, 1967). But these methods share a common view: individual symptoms, motivations, and behaviors are less important for therapeutic change than was once thought to be the case. Further, family balances, imbalances, communication patterns, and transactions are probably the most important target for change and become the chief unit for observation, intervention, feedback, and interpretation. Only when the family patterns change, it is felt, is it possible for family members to change on any enduring basis.

Family sessions can run over a two-hour period once or twice a week. Therapists can be active or simply passive observers. Sometimes they make home visits so that actual interactions in real-life situations are observed. At other times, tasks, games, and problems might be introduced so that family members are observed as they go about

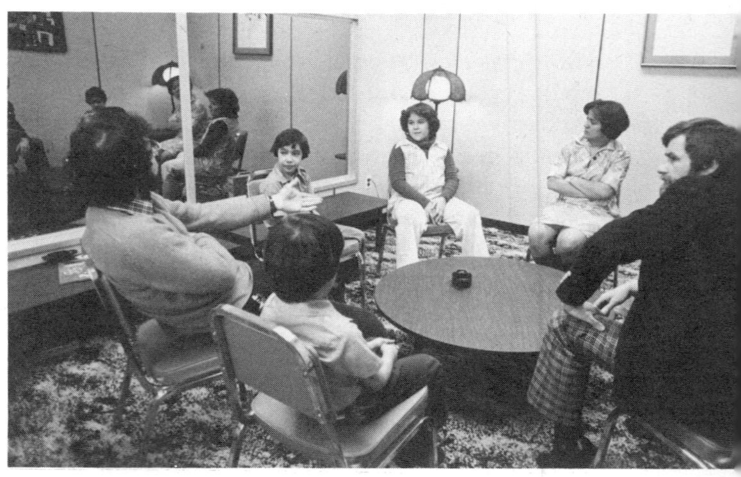

A family-therapy session. The family members are being observed through a one-way mirror on the left. (© Linda Ferrer 1981/Woodfin Camp)

solving the problems before them. Individual complaints and content are generally of less significance than what is actually happening: the kinds of communications, who blocks whom, disruptions, power plays, and alliances within the group.

Who pushes for the decisions? Who remains passive? Who straddles the fence, or is off in a fantasy world detaching himself or herself entirely? Who is the scapegoat? Who is the "executive?" These questions may get some answers if the family-in-interaction is observed. Often, material that is a complete surprise to the family members may emerge. (Videotaped sessions, later shown to family members, often have dramatic impact on some members.) The passive, shy, silent mother who seems to offer very little according to the other family members, may actually show up to be rather controlling—by a look, a disapproving gesture, avoidance of a question or an appeal for help, or by never sitting next to or looking at the disapproved-of family member. The disruptive angers, movements, and motions—who sits near whom, who avoids eye contact, what sort of physical contact there is—all emerge as significant "facts" that the therapist, whether observing or actively participating, may interpret back to the family members.

Family treatment does not depend on individual insight, on introspection about motives. On the other hand, it does make an attempt to interpret the family system and its unique methods of maintaining equilibrium. Cover-up, retreats, passive acceptances, fighting behaviors, bullying—these all maintain the family in a way that must be disrupted, shaken up, and unbalanced so that it becomes palpable to the family and to observers watching it. The assumption behind all this is that families engender and nurture conflicts, and even support maladaptive solutions to problems that so many people who seek help come in with. Individual family members, thus, are not regarded as clients, no matter what their symptoms are. On the contrary, the entire family (including even very little children) are encouraged to come in for sessions; it is the family "system" that requires help.

Family treatment methods are becoming very popular in clinics and hospitals throughout the nation. Lower-class people especially, uncomfortable in the one-to-one, introspective, verbal middle-class psychotherapy relationship, can also profit from this approach, it is thought. Further, it is claimed that almost all forms of pathology (from anorexia nervosa and delinquency to schizophrenia) can be helped or at least approached through family treatment.

There is little doubt that family approaches have "caught on" in many professional circles. Its advantages, like those for group methods, lie not only in economic feasibility, but also in opportunities to expose the many complex ways in which family members interact with one another, often nurturing, rather than remediating, pathology. Evaluation of outcome of these methods (as well as of marital therapy) is so beset with methodological difficulties, that at best, it can be said only that family methods show promise but not yet hard evidence as to effectiveness (Gurman and Kniskern, 1978).

SOME NEWER APPROACHES

Transactional Analysis (TA)

Transactional analysis (TA), a method for understanding and helping people that was developed by the psychoanalyst Eric Berne (1961; 1964; 1966), is a set of psychotherapeutic procedures that focuses on the patterns of interactions of two or more people. For this reason it is conducted in group sessions, which generally take place weekly over a period of months.

Transactions, according to Berne, consist of the things people say and the responses people elicit from others. One of the goals of TA is to increase the awareness of our roles in such interactions and to have insight into how people may manipulate or be manipulated by others in them. If patients are able to transcend their habitual modes of entering into transactions by recognizing these modes, then

TA will have accomplished one of its important purposes.

There are several stages in transactional analysis. In structural analysis, an early stage, the patient is helped to become aware of the three ego states—the basic units within the personalities of each of us that enter into all of the transactions in which we engage: these are Parent, Child, and Adult.

When a person is in his or her Parent ego state, he or she feels, acts, and thinks as though he or she were a parent. The parent is that part of all of us that is authoritative, has set attitudes about how things "should" be, and is judgmental of ourselves and others. Our Parent state reflects aspects of our own parents that we have internalized and accepted—almost without awareness. Our Parent can be nurturing, too. For example, when we see other people who are upset, we may feel the urge to run to their rescue, regardless of whether sympathy or "rescue" is needed.

The Child ego state is a carryover from one's own childhood. When a person is in his or her Child state he or she feels dependent and compliant, withdrawn and shy, or self-indulgent and rebellious. Often it is this state that creates the difficulties that bring someone into therapy. For when the Child dominates the individual may behave in maladaptive, self-destructive ways.

Finally, the Adult ego state is that "reasonable" part of us that calculates probabilities, that plans actions and sees them through. When a person's Adult is in control, that person reacts to reality as it actually *is* rather than as his or her Child or Parent would have him or her believe it to be. TA aims to educate and strengthen the Adult so that it will be more in control of a person's behavior.

Once TA patients are able to identify their own Adult, Child, and Parent ego states, TA proceeds to the next stage: transactional analysis. The analysis of transactions (the verbal exchanges among two or more persons) involves identifying the ego states of the persons involved in the transactions. If the ego states are complementary (for example, Child to Child, or Child to Parent, and Parent, in turn, responds to Child), the transaction will proceed smoothly. Crossed transactions, which often cause interpersonal conflict or discord, occur when the ego states are not complementary (for example, the Adult of one person speaks to the Adult of another, but the Child of the second person responds as if the Parent of the first had spoken).

Still other transactions involve ulterior motives, for example, when someone who knows that another person who is on a diet had a cream puff for lunch inquires, "How's your diet going?" Ulterior transactions occur when one person appears to be speaking as an Adult, but, in fact, has an ulterior motive: to elicit the Child or the Parent in the other.

The next stage of TA is game analysis. A game is a series of ulterior transactions that generally result in a hidden payoff (Berne, 1966). Spotlight 19.3 illustrates game analysis.

Game analysis is essential for achieving social control, the major goal of TA.* With social control the Adult is able to hold onto the role of executive (the chooser of options, the decision-maker)

> *in dealings with other people who may be consciously or unconsciously attempting to activate the patient's Child or Parent. This does not mean that the Adult alone is active in social situations, but it is the Adult who decides when to release the Child or Parent, and when to resume the executive. Thus one patient might think: "At this party, in contrast to last night's formal dinner, I can afford to take a few drinks and have some fun." Later he might think: "Now I'm beginning to get sloppy, so I'd better stop drinking and simmer down, even though they're all trying to encourage my clowning" (Berne, 1961, pp. 90–96).*

Only the most advanced TA groups get as far as stage four: script analysis. A script is an unconscious plan for living life absorbed by a person between the ages of three and seven years. Some scripts (for example, "I have to please Mommy and Daddy, so I'll become a doctor") can be adaptive.

* There are other goals of TA that are not described in this section, for example, the development of the capacity to interact at the level of intimacy. According to Berne, people have a need to structure their time. He calls this structure hunger. People can structure their time with fantasy, rituals, work, pastimes, and games. However, only intimacy, which involves open and honest interactions between Adults, is truly satisfying.

Spotlight 19.3 Games: Hidden Weapons?

A GAME *is an ongoing series of complementary ulterior transactions progressing to a well-defined, predictable outcome. Descriptively it is a recurring set of transactions, often repetitious, superficially plausible, with a concealed motivation; or, more colloquially, a series of moves with a snare, or "gimmick." . . . Every game . . . is basically dishonest, and the outcome has a dramatic, as distinct from merely exciting, quality (Berne, 1964, p. 48).*

The following game, "Why Don't You—Yes, But," according to Berne, was the original dialogue that stimulated game analysis. Most of us probably recognize the familiar pattern in the following game, in which the payoff is the complete stymying of people who are trying to be helpful. The other people are frustrated in their Parent role—into which they have been cast—whereas the person who is in need of help (but rejecting it) plays the Child role, unable to find a way out of a frustrating situation. Note that the Child does not wish, really, to receive solutions to the problem she is facing.

White: *"My husband always insists on doing our own repairs, and he never builds anything right."*
Black: *"Why doesn't he take a course in carpentry?"*
White: *"Yes, but he doesn't have time."*
Blue: *"Why don't you buy him some good tools?"*
White: *"Yes, but he doesn't know how to use them."*
Red: *"Why don't you have your building done by a carpenter?"*
White: *"Yes, but that would cost too much."*
Brown: *"Why don't you just accept what he does the way he does it?"*
White: *"Yes, but the whole thing might fall down."*

(Berne, 1964, p. 116)

However, when scripts are "tragic," people often seek help. An example of a tragic script is that of a man who married one alcoholic after another in order to fulfill his rescue fantasies. Through script analysis, it is hoped that the Adult patient can alter the tragic script.

One criticism lodged against TA is that it focuses on conscious activities and interactions rather than on deeply felt feelings and emotions. Another criticism arises primarily because of TA's popular appeal to people—therapists and patients alike—who are intrigued by its streamlined, contemporary language and its game-like, "TV-show-like" group activities. There are thousands of TA therapists who have been attracted to TA, for example, many of whom do not meet the standards of professional training that most professional groups expect for therapists. But these criticisms matter less than the major one, which, after all, is not so different from the criticism leveled at many other therapies: Beyond the level of testimonial, there is little evidence for the long-range success of transactional analysis.

Cognitive Therapies*

In Chapter 10, when depression was discussed, Beck's work was briefly noted in connection with a special approach: Depression can be understood as a cognitive defect in that depressed people view the events around them, their futures, and themselves negatively. They label and interpret events incorrectly and irrationally in support of their hopeless outlook. This theoretical approach is closely related to a major shift in the direction of assigning more

* See Chapters 6 and 20.

weight to such cognitive factors as attention, self-appraisal, attitudes, verbal habits (in labeling behavior, for example), and judgments when attempting to modify people's behavior. As a matter of fact, some proponents of cognitive approaches in therapy go so far as to suggest that the cognitive aspects of psychological functioning underlie all the therapies—no matter what is claimed for each one of them. The way the client perceives, labels, and views his or her problem—the meaning assigned to that problem—is the core substance that requires therapeutic intervention. Feelings and emotions occur as an aftermath of, rather than a precursor to, such substance. Already, some experimental evidence is beginning to suggest that there is some degree of validity in working with the client's way of thinking.

Thus the approaches of Beck (1976) and of rational-emotive therapy (RET) (Ellis, 1973; Ellis and Grieger, 1977) assume that an individual's problems arise chiefly from irrational views and thoughts about reality, incorrect premises, and distortions in judgments. Further, the disordered behavior is maintained by the continued irrationality of that individual's thoughts. Cognitive models of disordered behavior include many different forms of pathology: from obsessional states and fears to uncontrollable rages or severe panic.

Cognitive approaches differ from one another in the procedures used for changing beliefs. But first steps generally involve helping clients to see the illogical ways in which they distort reality, and how, in holding onto irrational judgments, they maintain maladaptive behavior (emotions, symptoms). Therapists employ many different methods to challenge the client's ideas, including combining cognitive with behavioral methods (see Chapter 20). Eventually more rational beliefs are substituted and the behavior (emotions, symptoms) changes.

The paths to making the distortions conscious involve hard-headed, direct, active interventions aimed to change people's behavior through conscious analysis of their erroneous, self-defeating notions, often followed up by firm therapeutic insistence that clients try on for size new forms of behaving in their real worlds. For example, direct confrontation, role-playing, challenges from the therapist, and "homework assignments" are used—all directed toward the goal of substituting more rational thoughts and labels for the cognitive content on which the client has been relying.

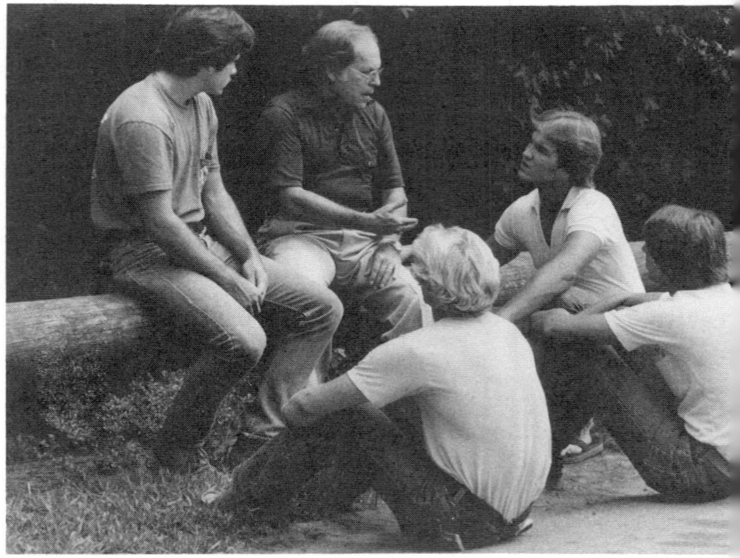

Some therapeutic methods employ direct persuasion and advice. (Meri Houtchens-Kitchens/The Picture Cube)

Cognitive approaches thus depart from traditional therapeutic procedures that stress delving into the past, free association, and psychodynamic explanations of symptoms and conflicts. Instead, clients are "reeducated" to relinquish old ways of thinking and to try out new ways of perceiving themselves, others, and their worlds.

Cognitive methods, especially those advocated by Ellis, have been used in marriage counseling, sex counseling, and in individual and group therapy with considerable effectiveness, according to many followers. But the empirical evidence for the effectiveness of cognitive approaches is only now beginning to emerge, with the result that there is not much evaluation-research literature to review.

Some critics decry the lack of focus on interpretative understanding and past history in this therapeutic approach. They also suggest that the verbal ability, skills in introspection, and high-level intelligence that are necessary for cognitive therapy to be effective eliminate many potential clients from consideration for treatment. These client attributes need not necessarily be requisites for successful cognitive therapy, however. For, depending on the ingenuity of the interventive methods, it is conceivable that changing one's irrational views can be achieved by simple, even elementary methods of challenge and feedback.

Reality Therapy

Reality therapy—a term associated with William Glasser (see Glasser and Zunin, 1973; Bassin, Bratter, and Rachin, 1976)—is often described as a directive, reality-oriented therapy with a moral approach to right or wrong in which clients are urged to assume responsibility for their actions, judge the quality of their behavior, and use various value judgments in assessing their actions. Reality therapy can best be placed within the framework of education—but of course, not classroom education. Reality therapy is largely associated with incarcerated populations, for example, prisoners.

Reality therapy makes very few assumptions about people. There is even a denial (along with Szasz) that mental illness exists. One basic assumption of this approach, however, is that everyone has an intense need for a sense of self, for an identity. The achievement of this overall goal is made possible by means of two paths: being loved and loving; and developing feelings of self-esteem. In the therapeutic context, changes can take place only if the therapist provides the patient with a sense of acceptance, warmth, and self-esteem. Besides a trusting relationship between client and therapist, reality therapy rests on an even more important assumption: people can change their behavior, can make choices, and can assume responsibility for themselves and for their fates by making conscious decisions.

In reality therapy sessions, clients are allowed to talk about whatever they wish. Transference is discouraged: clients are encouraged to relate realistically to the therapist as well as to their personal worlds. Client and therapist discuss goals for the present and for the future as well as why the client is not achieving his or her own goals and how he or she may succeed in reaching them. They review options open to the client and explore alternatives not previously taken by the client. But above all, the therapist insists that the client make choices and then assume responsibility for acting on these choices. Client-responsibility for one's actions, therapist-confrontations and arguments concerning moral principles, and a refusal to accept rationalizations and justifications for failures to act upon one's options and choices are all aspects of the reality therapist's approach.

Reality therapy is gradually gaining some approval among professional therapists. An overall evaluation based on objective evidence is not yet possible, however. For many types of pathologies—drug abuse, for example, or certain kinds of impulse disorders—it may turn out to be an extremely effective intervention that has the advantage of making few untested assumptions. On the other hand, because the effectiveness of this method, as the others, often depends on the client's motivation

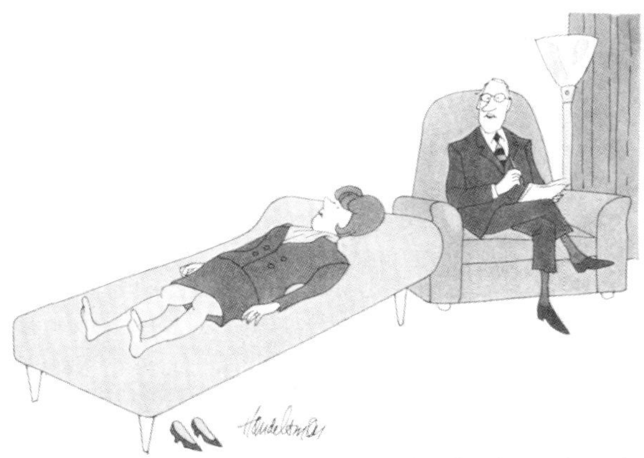

"After all these years, you still feel guilt? You should be ashamed of yourself."

for help, one wonders how many people from such target groups—especially if forced to seek help—will be reached by it.

BEYOND THE FRINGE: OTHER APPROACHES TO HELPING PEOPLE

All of us are aware of the many "therapeutic" fads and fashions that blossom and then fade away, each promising panaceas and cure-alls. During their actual flowering, many followers do indeed proudly point to success. Whether success is measured by personal testimonial or by "objective" observation, impressive reports are circulated—reports that lure others to try out the new methods. Testimonials ("My life has changed as a result of my experiences at . . . "), even sophisticated behind-the-scenes promotion, go a long way to enhance the placebo effects that probably do exist.

Research on long-range outcome (see next section) is rarely undertaken. As a matter of fact, it is not even necessary. For time and deterioration effects (initial success followed by gradual failure) take their toll. A new fad, in any event, begins to assume prominence, and as a general rule gradually creates enough of its own excitement to pull attention away from the old.

Many of the helping movements use the jargon of science, psychological or otherwise (computer jargon, for example). Common-sense methods of self-help, psuedoscientific phrases, sincere promises, "pop" paperbacks on bestseller lists, and dedicated authors willing to make personal appearances in department stores and on TV panels all help. Some of the fringe movements are spinoffs from the human potential movement and the ideas developed at Esalen. Others emerged from an amalgam of advertising tricks, religious exhortation methods, marathon exercises, brainwashing and sensory deprivation techniques, mass persuasion methods, and plain-talking, old-fashioned, common-sense psychology.

est

One popular amalgamation of many methods is called est (an acronym for Erhard Seminars Training) (see Fenwick, 1976) that has been described as having "trained" well over 100,000 troubled people. Est does not claim to be psychotherapy. Instead, in two consecutive weekends (of about eighteen hours a day for each of four days), it purports to hammer into the minds of its several hundred participants that they are responsible for the course of their own lives and can determine their own fates. Many of the hungry, shut-in people who emerge from this intense group experience in which they are cursed at, shouted at, insulted, and also allowed to talk about their own problems, do claim to have been through a rather moving experience. Indeed, most participants are very enthusiastic about their est weekends, insisting that their lives have dramatically changed for the better. The purpose of est—inducing dramatic changes in personal belief systems and helping people to take charge of themselves—they say, has been accomplished.

Most professionals doubt that any long-range effects exist. Further, despite est's disclaimers that it does not offer therapy and that it discourages those with deep emotional problems from participating, many professionals feel that it can actually do some harm, creating panic in unstable people or precipitating a psychotic break with reality. There is no doubt, however, that in the short run est is not only a vast commercial success but also has probably even helped many people in short-term ways, possibly because these people were highly motivated to receive help.

Janov and the Primal Scream

Some therapeutic approaches do not reach the standards set by the "establishment" and are rejected from mainstream consideration, sometimes for very good reasons. This is often the fate of methods that are zealously touted (as the only

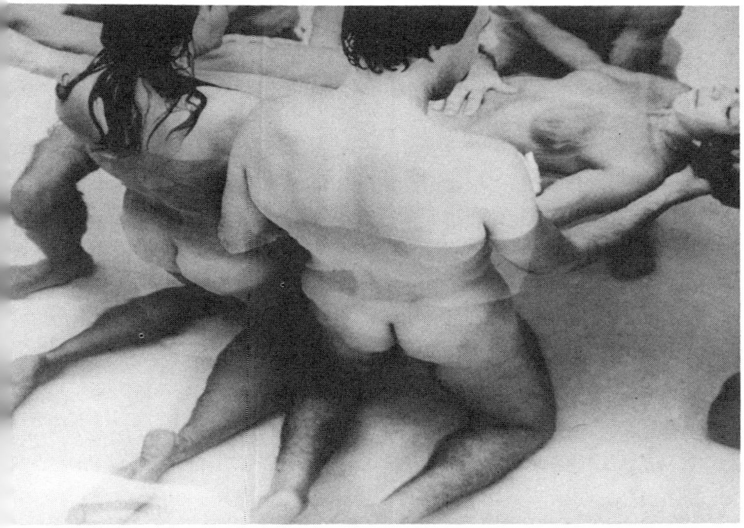

Beyond the fringe: Rebirthing—yet another approach to helping people with emotional problems? (Dan McCoy/Black Star)

"true" cure) by their proponents (frequently in best-selling books) before the scientific community has had a chance to systematically evaluate successes and failures or to differentiate subjective testimonial from fact. Janov's primal therapy is an example.

According to Janov (1970), the Pain which all of us endure as we are growing up will always hold us back. We spend most of our lives in defending against this Pain; as a matter of fact, our neurotic defenses are based almost entirely on an intense need to ward off the primary core of Pain. Janov's therapy, aimed at creating "post-primal persons" depends largely on helping people to fully reexperience such Pain. The method he uses, it is claimed, is the only system that permits the possibility of reliving the Primal Trauma—the feeling and realization that our parents did not love us.

In other words, casting off the neurosis is not achieved by being aware of current feelings nor by being in "touch with oneself." The neurosis is "cured" only when the primary pain is reexperienced in its full intensity. With the breaking down of all defenses against this pain in primal therapy, the neurosis (and symptoms) disappears.

In Janov's approach, the therapist sees no other client during the first three weeks of therapy. The client is asked to live in a hotel room with no supports such as drugs or recreational facilities. The client drops his or her regular routine such as job or school. During this time, the client and therapist have long, several-hour sessions in which the therapist helps in every way possible to get the client to express his or her feelings toward the parents. There is no other goal of therapy. Attitudes toward the therapist, real-life problems, dreams, fantasies—these are not the content of the primal sessions. Eventually, the client does indeed experience intense anguish—feelings that emerge with great suffering along with yelling and screaming.

After the three-week intense, focused sessions, the client returns to his everyday routine but continues therapy in a primal group for about six more months in which similar abreactions take place.

A major criticism of Janov's approach is lodged at his fervor about the validity of his understanding of the neurosis and of its "cure." Most researchers know the story of such ardor: eventual failure. Further, the easy, facile training of his primal therapists, the "cult" aspects of the movement itself, and its overall popular appeal has alienated most serious investigators. As with many other approaches, there is lack of substantial evidence of long-lasting changes that are beneficial to the client, despite the fact that some immediate claims of anxiety-reduction and changes in physiological measures of tension during the three-week intense period have been reported (Harper, 1975).

Perhaps the most severe criticism of the approach is directed at the post-primal client Janov describes as cured. One wonders if the flat, dull, passive person who has little ambition or concern about goals and who is indifferent to social struggles and issues is after all a picture of a "healthy" individual who is freed of neuroses (Harper, 1975; Kovel, 1976).

MISCELLANEOUS THERAPIES

Crisis Intervention

Acute stress in some life situations (for example, death of a close person, impending major surgery, or life-threatening forcible rape) can affect some people so acutely that they are unable to handle their lives at that point—they are unable to continue with their ordinary routines of living. Immediately available help is often an urgent necessity. Crisis intervention, which this help is often called, is an amalgamation of techniques and orientations designed to help "normal" people (in contrast to maladjusted people) experience and handle such periods of great stress (Korchin, 1976).

Crisis-intervention methods, such as those described in connection with suicide, involve short-term contacts in which help is immediately available, often, but not necessarily, through telephone contacts. Sometimes, sessions with entire families may be involved. Generally, various choices and options facing the individual are explored. The individual-in-crisis is encouraged to assess and to use community and family supports and lifelines. The therapist or counselor is active, enlists the aid of community resources, and stresses the real world of the immediate crisis, rather than deep psychological interpretations of conflict.

The active, short-term, interventive methods of the crisis counselor include many of the techniques already described such as support, reassurance, appraisal of choices and options, encouragement to be responsible for one's actions, assessment of the client's resources and coping skills, provision of information about community supports (for example, obtaining appropriate medical supervision), arranging for group discussions, scheduling family meetings, or making himself or herself (the counselor) available for around-the-clock telephone contacts (especially effective for suicidal individuals).

Evaluation studies of what actually takes place in crisis interaction and of outcome—in regard to the immediate crisis or long-range effects—are rather sparse (Korchin, 1976). And most studies of effectiveness fail to provide adequate outcome measures and often do not have control groups. Thus, in an evaluation of outcome research of crisis intervention methods, Auerbach and Kilmann (1977) described several studies with so many methodological problems that despite the appearance of positive results, they concluded that the benefits of crisis intervention (if any) could not properly be ascertained. Yet who would question the moral necessity of lending a helping hand during moments of crisis? This is one interventive area in which few would suggest any delay in helping the drowning person because hard data from well-designed research has not yet filtered in.

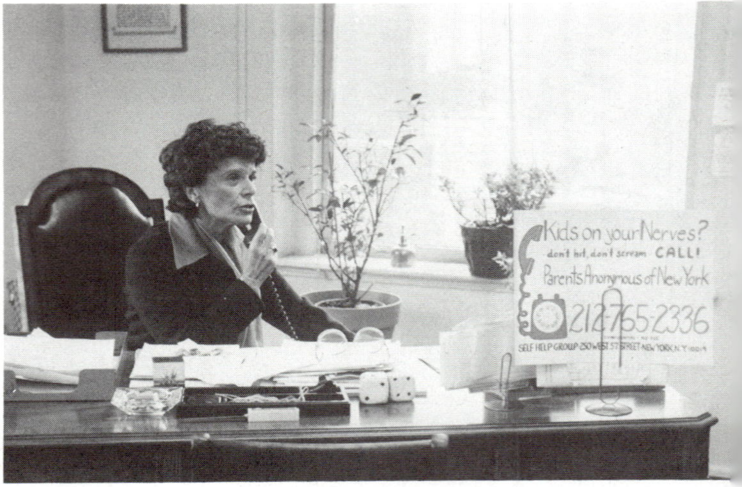

A crisis counselor at work. Crisis-intervention methods generally involve short-term contacts, often with the help of the telephone. (Joan Menschenfreund/Taurus Photos)

The Lively Arts as Therapy

Creative and expressive behaviors are often encouraged as therapeutic devices, in hospitals, clinics, or individual practice. Methods employed range from art expression with clay, fingerpaints, oils, and water colors, to mask-making, puppetry, dancing, rhythmic exercises, miming, poetry creation, and music performance. These individual or group expressive methods are thought to be ways of gaining access to unconscious conflicts or providing an opportunity for release of tension or anxiety in children and nonverbal individuals. Thus they serve a cathartic (releasing) purpose as well as an opportunity to provide the therapist with raw material for interpretation. Advantages are also said to lie in the group experience—if indeed a group is involved—as well as in the rewards and reinforcements that derive from producing a tangible, admired product as a result of one's efforts.

Although some of the foregoing methods might seek to disclose underlying, unconscious conflicts through art expression, such goals are not always necessarily an aspect of the therapeutic intent of the art or music therapist. These methods may be used as an opportunity to establish trusting bonds with the client or simply to provide him or her with an opportunity to "open up." There is little rigorous outcome research with regard to evaluating the effectiveness of these therapies. In any event, they are more often than not used as adjuncts to, rather than as substitutes for, other forms of therapy.

Psychotherapy with Children

There is no one method or "school" of psychotherapy that is exclusively relevant to work with children (Barrett, Hampe, and Miller, 1978), except perhaps play methods which arose from the spirit of the projective movement in testing (see Chapter 5) which purported to provide opportunities to disclose innermost feelings and conflicts through expressive behavior (Axline, 1947; Levy, 1938). Play methods also owe a debt to the Rogerian nondirective approach, which makes few assumptions about "treating people" except that it is possible to grow and change under permissive, accepting conditions. Play methods do not presume introspective skills or verbal ability, nor are they introduced under the essentially "artificial" and formal climate of a patient-doctor interview. Instead they encourage, in nondirected free situations, expressive activities with clay, darts, toys, fingerpaints, water pistols, peppets, and various mechanical objects that can be reconstructed or pulled apart. Some therapists have even worked with specially constructed dolls that can be "mutilated" and put together again to provide release for anger and tension (Levy, 1938). Play therapy methods have been thought to be especially useful with autistic, isolated, or withdrawn young children or with those with limited skills in verbalization, for they permit the acting out of fantasies, conflicts, deeply repressed feelings, frustrations, anger, and need for release that might be at the root of the problem.

Psychoanalytic methods with children were very popular for many years (Anna Freud, 1946b; Klein, 1960). When employed in classical form, techniques included dream interpretation, free association (sometimes through play rather than words), and the interpretation of transference. In more eclectic form, general psychodynamic principles are used in more flexible fashion (Cooper and Wanerman, 1977).

A third general thrust in helping children with

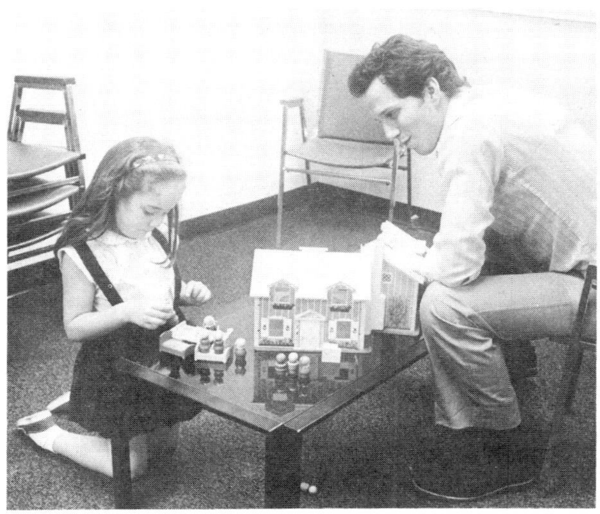

Psychotherapy with children often involves play methods that do not presume introspective skills or verbal ability. (Sybil Shelton/ Peter Arnold)

emotional problems comes from conceptualizations about groups and group therapy methods. As a matter of fact, the idea that "problem children" (for example, those with conduct disorders) could be helped in peer settings such as day centers, clubs, or special residences has a long history in the field of childhood psychopathology (Slavson, 1943). Some of the principles that guided work with such children made use of Rogerian-type thinking that minimized the importance of interpretation and direction. Instead, productive group and work experiences were by themselves thought to possess "curative" value. Today peer interaction—even without direct psychotherapeutic intervention—for example, with withdrawn children, continues to be viewed as an effective aid in developing more open interpersonal and affectional relationships (Mehl and Peterson, 1981).

Although tangible successes cannot be said to characterize many of the approaches to treating children described in the current chapter, this may in part be due to the failure to state methods and goals clearly so that objective evaluation of outcome is possible. On the other hand, behavioral methods, described in the next chapter, permit more objective criteria for judging improvement and tend to employ procedures that are at home in the laboratory.

In conducting psychotherapy with children, it is usually the parent or an "outsider" (teacher, school psychologist, or pediatrician) who asks for therapy, not the child. Explaining psychotherapy or some other intervention (and the accompanying diagnostic or assessment session that may precede it) to a child is often a difficult procedure. For this reason, child therapists sometimes spend several sessions with the parents, often before the child is even seen, not only to obtain background material but also to help pave the way for the child.* It is for this very reason, also, that some family therapists claim superiority over individual interventive methods.

* It should be noted that early in the history of the "child guidance movement" it was common to handle a child's problem by dealing almost entirely with his or her parents, sometimes after a diagnostic session with the child.

PSYCHOTHERAPY AND SOME SPECIAL SOCIOCULTURAL CONSIDERATIONS

SES and Ethnic Variables

The empirical literature shows that there are social-class differences in diagnosis, expectations for therapy, length of therapy contact, and nature of therapy offered (Aronson and Overall, 1966; Hollingshead and Redlich, 1958). In other words, who you are, where you come from, and what you can afford often determine what happens in therapy. Moreover, clients from lower educational and SES levels tend to drop out more frequently that those who come from higher levels (Garfield, 1971; 1977). There is less delivery of psychotherapeutic services to lower-class groups despite the fact that most pathological conditions described in this book were shown to have the greatest incidence among the lower social classes. This is especially so for clinics that offer individual psychotherapy: therapy is sustained for shorter periods of time, or it is more likely medication than verbal therapy that is offered to lower-SES, compared to higher-SES, patients. Psychoanalytically oriented clinics and clinicians in particular tend to screen patients, choosing the more intelligent, motivated, verbal, and educated patient for treatment, but this failure to deliver services is changing with the waning popularity of psychoanalysis.

An important problem that many therapists face when attempting to help lower-class people is that expectations for psychotherapy may differ from those of more sophisticated, educated groups (Goldstein, 1973). It may be assumed, for example, that one goes to a clinic to get "fixed up," made better, or healed, and that this can be accomplished fairly quickly. Talking about one's problems with a view toward getting better (rather than being "fixed up" from the outside) over a period of time rests on many assumptions: one of these is that the client understands the relevance of dredging up and using words to describe his or her feelings. Verbal therapies that require dealing with concepts, use of symbolic language, psychological interpretation and insights, introspective skills, and long-term therapeutic contacts may not appeal to or be appropriate for some uneducated patients, who may simply drop out of treatment if such methods are offered or who may insist upon other less verbal or shorter-term types of treatment. In any event, long-term verbal therapies have not been particularly successful with most clients from lower educational and SES backgrounds (Garfield, 1971; Minuchin et al., 1967).

It has been pointed out that the foregoing picture may be less valid than was once thought to be the case, and that the therapists themselves, with negative expectations and a certain amount of discomfort, not the low-SES client, are responsible for the poor outcome picture and high dropout rate. As a matter of fact, reviews of several studies suggest that the so-called unsuitability of low-SES patients for verbal psychotherapy is a stereotype (Gomes-Schwartz, Hadley, and Strupp, 1978). It may also be that the newer methods of verbal psychotherapy—more eclectic, flexible, shorter-term, and reality oriented—may in part account for this changing picture.

As for ethnic status, it appears that some therapists tend to more often terminate a black or Hispanic low-SES client than a white client (Cole and Pilisuk, 1976). But this may not reflect antiminority attitudes so much as cultural differences that may have led to misunderstanding or misinterpreting the needs of the client or failure to identify with his or her problems. Such patients, in turn, tend to terminate after a few sessions anyway because they sense that their problems are being ignored.

For some time, there has been a running argument in some of the literature as to the possible prejudices of white therapists (the majority of therapists are white) toward their black or Hispanic clients. One suggested solution is to assign clients so that there is racial similarity between therapist and client; this might promote a willingness to continue treatment (Banks, Berenson, and Carkhuff, 1967). However, some practitioners have voiced disagreement as to the relevance of this solution; they have suggested that the problem is a sociocultural one rather than a racial one, for a middle-class, educated black therapist may be as misperceiving of a lower-class black client as is a white therapist.

The problems that might arise in therapeutic relationships in which the therapist is white and the client black have been emphasized by many researchers, for example, Jones and Seagull (1977), who feel that such prejudice should disqualify a therapist from doing therapy with black clients—perhaps with all clients. The position expressed by Jones and Seagull is that most white people have some hidden reserve of bias, even if it is just that black people are different from themselves. Some white clinicians might view black clients as nonverbal, concrete, or nonintrospective—as poor risks for therapy, or as culturally deprived and culturally disadvantaged—stereotypes that are most certainly ethnocentrically derived.

Countertransference, the therapist's own feelings that may alter the course of therapy, may be very much involved in interactions in which there are unconscious, not fully understood biases and expectations regarding minority clients. Such feelings may include guilt on the part of the white clinician. Therapeutic activities motivated by guilt might result in overzealousness, fear of failure, fear of using confrontation or challenge, overly deferential or compassionate attitudes, or similar responses that have no place in the therapeutic interaction.

It has recently been suggested, despite the above, that most evidence indicates that appreciable biases in diagnosis and therapeutic intent and practice do not exist among white clinicians regarding their black patients (Abramowitz, 1978; Abramowitz and Dokecki, 1977). Once again, future research will provide us with more of the answers.

Psychotherapy and Sexism

The past decade or two has witnessed a keen awareness of the possibility that psychotherapists—both male and female—employ sex-role stereotypes toward their patients. For example, a therapist might hold a skeptical attitude toward a woman's desire to assert herself or to achieve success in a so-called "male" profession such as engineering. Or another therapist might have an unconscious bias against extremely intelligent, achieving, articulate women, who are seen as "castrating," controlling, masculine. A third therapist might feel that those women who do not see motherhood as their principal role in life are basically unfulfilled, "off," emotionally immature; this therapist might support only those behaviors and attitudes in women that are passive, dependent, compliant, and conforming.

That such attitudes have permeated the climate of many psychotherapeutic interactions has received some confirmation as incidents, illustrations, and actual data filter into the professional literature. For example, empirical evidence showed that psychologists had a "double standard" for mental health in that criteria for emotional health were applied basically to men but not to women (Broverman et al., 1970). Conversely, that standard dictated that emotionally healthy women (but not men) should be sensitive, submissive, passive, and characterized by "feminine" attributes of dependency and compliance. It had become apparent that many female patients internalized such standards, felt guilty about their assertiveness or intelligence, and strove to achieve "femininity" at all costs, less they be considered "deviant." Finally, more open acknowledgement was made of specific practices: sexual advances to and seduction of female patients.

Sexist attitudes, it became clear, also permeated therapists' attitudes toward one another: for example, negative biases toward unmarried female therapists or a tendency to refer male clients to male therapists or assign children to female therapists.

Allegations that professional therapists harbor many gender-linked stereotypes provided strong incentives for the establishment of official professional guidelines so that therapists can become aware of their biases in attitudes and behavior and become concerned about developing insights and skills relevant to women's problems in the areas of role, work, family, childbearing, sexuality, achievement, and assertiveness. Spotlight 19.4 presents the thirteen official guiding principles for nonsexist therapy adopted by the American Psychological Association as well as some illustrative accompanying material.

Spotlight 19.4 Guidelines for Nonsexist Therapy

An American Psychological Association Task Force on Sex Bias and Sex-Role Stereotyping in Psychotherapeutic Practice set out to establish some guidelines for nonsexist practice. To do so, it first attempted to discover how sexism in psychotherapy can be defined and illustrated. They surveyed many women psychologists as to this issue, finding that these psychologists' responses fell into four main themes. Sexist therapist attitudes were manifested by

1. fostering traditional sex roles
2. bias in expectations and devaluation of women
3. sexist use of psychoanalytic concepts
4. responding to women as sex objects, including seduction of female clients (Guidelines . . . , 1978, p. 1122).

From these general categories, thirteen principles were developed for guiding and maintaining ethical, nonsexist clinical practice. These are presented below along with several verbatim clarifying illustrations.

1. The conduct of therapy should be free of constrictions based on gender-defined roles, and the options explored between client and practitioner should be free of sex-role stereotypes. Women have complained

that they could not continue in therapy because the objective seemed to be for them to learn to adjust better to their roles as wives, mothers, daughters (underlings of one kind or another), and they needed to become free persons.

2. Psychologists should recognize the reality, variety, and implications of sex-discriminatory practices in society and should facilitate client examination of options in dealing with such practices.

3. The therapist should be knowledgeable about current empirical findings on sex roles, sexism, and individual differences resulting from the client's gender-defined identity.

Surprisingly, many colleagues (male and female) still define maturity in women as the capacity for vaginal orgasm. My feeling is that women who do not experience or report this are seen (and therefore treated) as emotionally disturbed.

4. The theoretical concepts employed by the therapist should be free of sex bias and sex role stereotypes.

5. The psychologist should demonstrate acceptance of women as equal to men by using language free of derogatory labels.

6. The psychologist should avoid establishing the source of personal problems within the client when they are more properly attributable to situational or cultural factors.

7. The psychologist and a fully informed client mutually should agree upon aspects of the therapy relationship such as treatment modality, time factors, and fee arrangements.

Female psychiatrist asked me if I had my husband's agreement for me to see therapist twice a week. (I earn more money than he, and am capable of making that decision with or without his agreement.)

8. While the importance of the availability of accurate information as to a client's family is recognized, the privilege of communication about diagnosis, prognosis, and progress ultimately resides with the client, not with the therapist.

I've seen child therapists who were concerned that a mother is not appropriately handling her child, tell the husband about this concern, without confronting the mother herself.

9. If authoritarian processes are employed as a technique, the therapy should not have the effect of maintaining or reinforcing stereotypic dependency of women.

Have recently tried to work as a co-therapist with a male psychiatrist who believes that all females need *to feel they are adjunct to the male; his idea of solving most marital problems is to manipulate the female into a subordinate position and convince her that she likes it.*

10. The client's assertive behaviors should be respected.

Tendency to label healthy assertive behavior as "castrating" or "phallic" in a derogatory manner.

11. The psychologist whose female client is subjected to violence in the form of physical abuse or rape should recognize and acknowledge that the client is the victim of a crime.

A psychoanalytically oriented male therapist, with some agreement from some of the other males [therapists], insisted that there was no such thing as rape—that the woman always "asked" for it in some way.

12. The psychologist should recognize and encourage exploration of a woman client's sexuality and should recognize her right to define her own sexual preferences.

My male therapist at ______ who was a clinical diplomate told me I was too aggressive sexually, that I should put up a good show, every man likes a challenge, but go down gracefully in defeat.

13. The psychologist should not have sexual relations with a woman client nor treat her as a sex object.

In my years as a psychotherapist, many women have come to me with stories of seduction and sexual intimacies with male therapists. In most instances the patients were deeply disturbed by these relationships, saw them as exploitative (although sometimes they justified the therapists' role and protected them), and sometimes resulted in psychotic breaks. This is the ultimate of sex-role bias: the rationalization of the therapist that his exploitation of the doctor-patient relationship for his gratification could be construed as therapeutic "for a woman."

Source: Extracted from Task Force on Sex Bias and Sex Role Stereotyping in Psychotherapeutic Practice (Annette M. Brodsky and Jean C. Holroyd, Co-Chairs), Guidelines for therapy with women, *American Psychologist,* December 1978, *33,* 1122–23.

Allegations of sex-role stereotyping in the profession stimulated a flurry of research that sought to explore in systematic, objective ways whether therapists indeed shared lay steroeotypes about women, and if they did, evidenced biases in the direction of distorted judgments about the mental health of women and a double standard in the therapy goals that are set for them. These researches tended to find little or no empirical evidence that this was the case (Smith, 1980; Stearns, Penner, and Kimmel, 1980; Stricker, 1977; and Whitely, 1979). The lack of recent positive findings might stem in part from the changing attitudes of therapists in recent years—a shift away from the stereotypes manifested a decade or two ago. It is further suggested that lack of evidence for sex-role stereotyping might arise from the methods used: determination of bias is not based on the implicit goals, interactions, and subtle cues provided *within* the therapy session, but rather, on surveys, questionnaires, checklists, and self-reports of subjects volunteering for the various studies. One wonders whether such investigations, essential as they are, disclose the actual expression of such biases, which often emerge as hidden cues and tacit assumptions. Future research in this area, as attitudes shift, should demonstrate that the failure to find evidence for bias is a valid reflection of changed attitudes among therapists, not an artifact of data collection.

PSYCHOTHERAPY OUTCOME RESEARCH

Is psychotherapy effective? What are the records of success accruing to the different methods? Such questions are more easily asked than answered. To answer them, it must be assumed that (a) there have been reliable and valid investigations of outcome; (b) it is possible to explore systematically outcome for each of the approaches; and (c) similar evaluation procedures and criteria for success are used for the different studies, making it possible to present objective records of "hits" (success rates) for the different therapies. Spotlight 19.5 lists some of the difficulties in establishing the veracity of these

Spotlight 19.5 Problems in Getting to The Bottom Line: Does It Work?

Is treatment successful? Which ones? And for what problems? What aspects of psychotherapy actually work? With whom? We are a long way from being able to make statements about the effectiveness of the different therapies (Albin, 1977). We are more likely to be faced with now-you-see-it-now-you-don't effects. For it should be clear by now that the research paths directed to shedding light on such questions are beset with problems. I have touched on some of these problems throughout this book. Here are a few of them:

Criterion measures. How is therapy success defined? through test scores? subjective opinion such as degree of personal satisfaction? objective measures, such as return to school or job or reduction of anxiety level? disappearance of symptoms?

Temporal variables. At what point during treatment or how long after termination of treatment does the researcher assess its success? Remember, a great number of alcoholics and drug addicts, as well as other types of clinical populations, return to their problems within months after termination. Assessing therapy during or immediately after termination does not constitute the whole story. Is short-term therapy as effective or perhaps more effective than long-term therapy—and if so, what kinds of therapies and with whom?

Therapeutic processes. Many clinicians do not know why they are successful. Often their theoretical reasons may have nothing to do with what they actually do or why they are (or are not) successful. There is failure to objectify what it is that the therapist actually does in his or her sessions—what actually goes on. And further, it is apparent from the literature that clinicians who all claim to be using method A—for example, nondirective therapy—are in fact each doing different things.

Therapist variables. Successful treatment often depends on the therapist. Therapist variables should be assessed whenever success of treatment is evaluated, for some special feature of the clinician (warmth? empathy?) may be indirectly related to successful treatment. Some "successful" clinicians may gravitate toward some types of clients or types of therapy, lending an appearance of greater success to the method itself than is warranted.

Client sample: nature of disturbance and level of motivation. Different treatment approaches are differentially successful for different kinds of problems and disturbances. Defining success should take into consideration the question of treatment for whom: verbal psychotherapy for chronic schizophrenia, for example, may be unsuccessful, but highly successful for someone with a psychoneurotic depression. A related variable is client motivation to get help—often one of the most significant determinants of success in that no matter what the treatment, once a client has decided to get help and gets it, he or she may show more improvement than those who are not motivated to get help.

Client sample: sociocultural variables. The empirical evidence points quite clearly to an association between ability to derive beneficial effects from various kinds of treatment and educational, SES, and ethnic variables. Evaluation studies that do not consider these important variables are failing to control for significant influences on outcome findings.

Client-therapist interactions and "matches." Are ethnic, educational, and SES differences or similarities between client and therapist important in determining outcome? Is the personal interaction (warmth, trust, frequency of dialogue) between therapist and client of significance in determining outcome?

Staying in or dropping out. Evaluation of outcome of particular methods is not complete unless some consideration is given to the dropouts and the failures to "reach" a sizable group. Who are the dropouts? This is a formidable question with no easy answers.*

---

* A comprehensive review of many studies indicates again and again that certain variables are associated with dropping out. These include age (younger people); sex (more females than males); low SES; social isolation and social instability; aggressive, passive-aggressive, or antisocial personality traits; low motivation; low "psychological mindedness"; low suggestibility; and some therapist qualities such as disinterest, boredom, or dislike of clients (Baekeland and Lundwall, 1975). Higher levels of anxiety are associated with remaining *in* treatment, however.

assumptions. I shall try, nevertheless, to find some pathways through this tangled maze in the following discussion.

Relative effectiveness of different therapies. Again and again, outcome research demonstrates that there is little difference in outcome among the different therapies, such as among psychoanalytic, client-centered, or common-sense, eclectic counseling (a combination of several methods) as judged by objective measures (for example, the MMPI) or subjective ratings (Albin, 1977).

In one review, almost 400 separate controlled investigations of different therapy methods were evaluated along objective, uniform lines to determine whether or not therapy was more effective than no therapy and whether there would be demonstrable differences among several different kinds of treatment methods (Smith and Glass, 1977). These included the different behavior therapies as well as the nonbehavior therapies (Rogerian, traditional, eclectic, rational-emotive, etc.). The results definitely suggested that *any* therapy was superior to no therapy. However, no differences among the methods were found. Although there is controversy regarding the validity of the method these authors used to summarize conclusions from many disparate studies, it should be noted that their conclusions are generally confirmed by others.

I shall return to the general question about whether or not psychotherapy works at the end of this section. As for the effectiveness of one method over another, it is becoming increasingly apparent that some methods and techniques work better for some people and some problems than do others. A more sophisticated research challenge for the future is to determine, given the kind of person presenting which problem, what methods are most effective.

Client variables. Among the most important variables that predict outcome of psychotherapy are those pertaining to the characteristics of the clients themselves, for example, the level of motivation to become involved in the therapeutic process, the adequacy of personal functioning at initial phases of therapy (Albin, 1977; Luborsky, Mintz, and Christoph, 1979; Mintz, Luborsky, and Christoph, 1979), and capacity to "collaborate actively" with the therapist (Gomes-Schwartz, Hadley, and Strupp, 1978). The higher these levels, the more successful the outcome.

This connection to outcome may appear obvious, but its significance was not always known. A series of early researches (Luborsky, 1962) highlighted the possibility that *patient* variables, rather than what psychotherapists offer to patients in the way of treatment, are significant determiners of outcome. By uncovering the significance of personality variables that characterized patients at the beginning of long-range therapy (particularly, psychoanalysis), Luborsky and his colleagues pointed the way to later discovery that such variables as intelligence, premorbid status, SES background, motivation, and educational level are fairly good predictors of successful treatment.

Therapist variables. It is by now a well-known finding that therapist variables are of extreme significance—perhaps of the greatest significance—in predicting or in determining the success of any therapeutic endeavor. Reviews of many studies and conclusions reached by careful scrutiny of findings by scientists indicate that many verbal therapeutic interventions in the hands of experienced, stable, wise therapists tend to work; the same methods tried by inexperienced, inept, or unstable clinicians tend not to work or may even be harmful (Bergin and Lambert, 1978; Strupp, 1980). On the other hand, sheer warmth, empathic ability, and genuineness are not sufficient qualities by themselves to predict successful outcome (Gomes-Schwartz, Hadley, and Strupp, 1978).

That the treatment presumably offered may be less important than the characteristics of the therapist was not always a known and accepted insight. Some early researches on therapist-personality variables and their relationship to outcome helped to point the way (Betz, 1962; Whitehorn and Betz,

1954, 1960). These studies showed that the personality of the therapist bore a crucial relationship to outcome of treatment of schizophrenic patients.* It was specifically shown that the improvement in schizophrenic subjects could be predicted on the basis of whether or not the therapists could be classified as Type A therapists or Type B therapists. Type As, who were associated with a higher proportion of improved patients, were characterized as persuasive, articulate, and active in their therapeutic attitude, whereas Type Bs were more passive, permissive, and interpretative.

Since these early studies the search for clarification and confirmation of A versus B types and their significance to outcome has not yielded consistent findings. As a result, many researchers are no longer following this particular line of conceptualization. On the other hand, other therapist qualities as well as various therapist-client interactions are now judged to be of more significance.

Therapist-client variables. In the Whitehorn and Betz researches, it was probably the interaction between the subject and the therapist that determined outcome, rather than the personality of the therapist alone. It seems increasingly clear that the "collaborative relationship" between therapist and client is of extreme importance in determining outcome (Strupp, 1980). Therapists' qualities and clients' responses to these qualities apparently transcend the specific treatment or method offered in accounting for the success or lack of success of any particular method. Many of these interactions in connection with placebo effects have already been described: the trust, faith, and expectation of support and success that permeates the therapeutic climate. Some of these effects may arise only in certain contexts but not others, for example, only when there is a mutual liking or when the therapist seems to understand the patient's problems.

An interesting research area is whether the "match" of the therapist and the client along personality and/or demographic lines, such as marital status or gender, influences outcome. In one study, moderate ability to predict success was found in the match between the client's and the therapist's marital status. Apparently, similar status (neither had ever been married or both were married) made possible the kind of understanding and insights that can be offered more effectively than if this sharing of experience is not possible. On the other hand, the effectiveness of matching female patients with female therapists has not been clearly established (Gomes-Schwartz, Hadley, and Strupp, 1978), and there is only moderate evidence that shared values influence therapeutic outcome.

Treatment variables. The strong possibility that no one treatment method shows superiority to the others, judging by outcome studies, has already been noted (Strupp, 1980). Is it possible to isolate strategies, techniques, and interventions within various therapeutic endeavors sufficiently well so that we can say more specifically that this tactic (for example, maintaining long periods of silence) works better than another (for example, confrontation, being verbally active)?

Unfortunately, we probably know less about what goes on within psychotherapy sessions than we do about the other sorts of variables we have discussed. This may in part arise from the reluctance of many clinicians to have the privacy of their sessions invaded. However, with the advent of film and video methods and the systematic application of reliable observation procedures, it is now possible to find out more about what takes place during the therapy session and to formulate hypotheses about their relationship to outcome than was once the case.

Treatment sessions contain not only events and interactions but also take place over a period of time. The empirical evidence indicates that tempo-

* It should be stated, however, that training schools in psychoanalysis for many years stressed the emotional adequacy, empathic skill, successful personal psychoanalysis, and general mental health of all candidates for psychoanalytic training on an assumption that only special "types" of therapists would become successful analysts.

ral variables (number of sessions or length of treatment over time) bear a relationship to successful outcome. Moreover, this variable may be one of the few predictive variables that hold up in regard to predicting outcome of psychotherapy (Lorr et al., 1962; Luborsky, Mintz, and Christoph, 1979).

Overview: Does Psychotherapy Work?

For a long while, many experts agreed that the pessimistic views of Eysenck (1952b, 1966) were probably true. On the basis of a review of a large body of outcome literature, Eysenck had concluded that although about two-thirds of neurotic patients who enter therapy improve in a two-year period, an equal percentage of such patients improve (spontaneous remission rate) without the benefits of therapy in an equivalent length of time.

This pessimistic picture—that after decades of promise, contemporary psychotherapeutic procedures have failed to accomplish anything more than would the natural passing of time—is not so willingly accepted these days (Erwin, 1980).

The more commonly held view, emerging in review after review of outcome studies, is that psychotherapy, no matter of what type, is better than no psychotherapy (Bergin, 1971; Bergin and Lambert, 1978; Frank, 1979; Marshall, 1980; and Strupp, 1980). Margins of this success vary according to different reports, ranging from slightly better to claims of vastly better results than no treatment (see Bergin and Lambert, 1978; Luborsky, Singer, and Luborsky, 1975; and Tramontana, 1980). However, most of these reviews stress that type of treatment is less important than the client variables just described (for example, motivation of the client), the therapist variables just described (for example, the experience of the therapist), and the interaction between the two. As for those subjects who do not receive treatment, some do indeed get better; but the percentage who do is now claimed to be much smaller than the two-thirds claimed by Eysenck (Bergin and Lambert, 1978; Erwin, 1980).

How can intervention be extended, with more meaningful results, to larger numbers of people? More specific, tangible, measurable, short-term methods described in subsequent chapters have indeed become the direction of many current therapies, and some of these are highly effective with some types of problems, for example, phobias, obesity, compulsions. It is still a moot point, however, whether their effectiveness levels—culled from outcome research—will present a rosier picture than the one presently painted.

That some therapists are doing something "right" raises an interesting direction for research. Perhaps, indeed, some therapists are powerful shapers of behavior. Can we isolate and articulate just what they do so we can test its effectiveness with other therapists? Or is it just the old placebo effect that depends on the charisma and promise held out by the therapist? Is it the witch doctor, the herbs, or the client's expectations about both that work? Or do clients themselves bring with them, when they enter treatment, the seeds that flower into successful outcome?

SUMMARY

This chapter surveyed the traditional therapies that generally employ verbal exchanges between therapist and client. After loosely defining the term psychotherapy, it presented some common denominators including hooking and placebo effects. The chapter then described psychodynamic therapies, including psychoanalysis, psychoanalytically oriented methods, and various eclectic approaches, and humanistic approaches, which rest on assumptions that differ from those of the psychodynamic methods—for example, regarding client-therapist relationships or the role of the unconscious and the past in the therapeutic context. The humanistic approaches discussed in this section were client-centered therapy, Gestalt therapy, and the encounter movement. It next described group and family methods, transactional analysis, cognitive approaches, and reality therapy, followed by two therapeutic approaches that were described as "beyond the fringe": est and primal therapy. The survey of psychotherapeutic approaches continued with a brief presentation of additional, miscellaneous approaches to helping people, such as crisis-intervention methods and expressive methods in the arts. Finally, a brief section on psychotherapy with children stressed the fact that there is no one method or school of psychotherapy that is exclusively relevant to work with children. After touching on the relationship of certain psychotherapeutic variables to SES and ethnic variables, some problems in connection with sexist attitudes in the therapeutic encounter were raised. The chapter concluded with a detailed overview of the effectiveness of psychotherapy and the general problems involved in evaluating outcome.

Highlights

1. Psychotherapy, which is practiced by many different kinds of individuals with many different kinds and degrees of training, is a general term which applies to methods, techniques, interventions, and strategies that a professionally trained individual uses to help another individual or group of individuals to modify behaviors, feelings, or interpersonal relationships. Many therapies imply a mutual "contract" between client and therapist, and although not necessarily formalized, there are other hidden processes, such as "hooking," which involves the client's early perceptions of the therapist as a caring, trustworthy person. Placebo effects, which are extremely important aspects of the therapeutic encounter, may be powerful determinants of "cure." These effects, for example, the client's faith in the treatment or the word-or-mouth fame of the therapist may be more important than the method as formally advertised.
2. Psychoanalysis is a method that purports to make the unconscious conscious. Many of the techniques in the psychodynamic therapies are spinoffs from analytic methods. But most current methods no longer adhere to the classical rules that were described in some detail, for example, the reliance on free associations, several sessions weekly, the "rule of silence" on the part of the analyst, and resistance and transference as therapeutic devices. Overall, outcome studies for classical analysis are sparse and results not too impressive for most of the pathologies. The newer Freudian methods as well as the more eclectic psychodynamic therapies depart from some of the rigid rules described in this chapter. There is greater stress on current problems of the patient, less grudging acknowledgement of cultural forces in the development of conflict, and increased flexibility of techniques, including more active intervention on the therapist's part.
3. Rogerian approaches to therapy stress the capacity of the client to grow and to change without active intervention by the therapist. Therapists are nondirective; they are encouraged to show "unconditional positive regard" for the clients and to reflect feelings in a permissive, accepting way. Goals for therapy are never established by the therapist and the course of therapy tends to be of relatively short duration. Rogerian methods played an important role in permitting other types of therapy to emerge after decades of dominance by the Freudians. In stressing simple and objective hypotheses, questioning the disease model of mental health, accepting problems in day-to-day living as relevant, and acknowledging the importance of establishing reliable methods for evaluating outcome, the Rogerians have made an enormous contribution to the field of psychotherapy.
4. Self-awareness, especially of feelings, is regarded as curative in its own right in some of the newer approaches, which include Gestalt therapy and the encounter movement. These

approaches deemphasize past history and the unconscious and stress current experiences and feelings through the use of various therapeutic maneuvers (for example, dreamwork) to encourage the "actualization" and growth of the individual. Although Gestalt therapy is interesting and appealing to both therapists and clients, and has gathered support from a sizable group of therapists, much criticism has been leveled at the encounter movement because of its wide, unprovable claims, "trendy" adoption by lay people, and failure to deliver its inspirational promise.

5. Group and family methods, described in moderate detail in this chapter, are attractive, economical alternatives to the more traditional, individual methods. For this reason they are widely used in hospitals, clinics, and other mental health programs and institutions throughout the nation. Group and family techniques vary considerably from one another in method, assumptions, and interventive principles. But most experts agree that they permit therapist and client alike to see behaviors in real-life situations. Family approaches, in particular, do not stress content and dynamics of family interactions but rather the social and interpersonal climate and communicational systems that induce pathology in individual members. Working with family members to change this climate has provided imaginative clinicians with opportunities for many innovative interventions that depart radically from the usual methods of psychotherapy. Evaluation of both group and family methods is beset with methodological difficulties so that hard evidence as to effectiveness with different clinical groups is not available.

6. Additional approaches to helping people described in this chapter include TA or transactional analysis, crisis intervention, and expressive methods that employ artistic activities. Also touched on were different techniques to helping children, which, in addition to family treatment, range from analytic methods to play and behavioral approaches. Work with children involves a special problem: it is usually the parent (or teacher or other authority—for example, a judge) that requests help, raising some ethical as well as psychological problems—for example, the child's motivation and willingness to receive help.

7. Cognitive approaches to working with people cover a wide variety of methods that have a common assumption: a person's beliefs, judgments, perceptions, and expectations are crucial ingredients in not only emotional difficulties but also their remediation. First steps in many of the cognitive methods are often concerned with helping clients to understand their irrational beliefs and the ways in which they distort reality.

8. As for sociocultural variables, there seem to be differences in expectations for therapy, length of therapy contact, and nature of therapy offered. Further, clients from lower educational and SES backgrounds tend to drop out of treatment more frequently than those who come from higher ones. There are suggestions that white therapists might be biased in their attitudes toward black clients, but this has not been fully substantiated, and, as a matter of fact, has even been refuted by some empirical evidence. There is a keen awareness that psychotherapists, both male and female, may harbor sexist attitudes and employ sex-role stereotypes in their therapeutic interactions. Spotlight 19.4 presents guidelines for maintaining ethical and nonsexist clinical practices.

9. Is psychotherapy effective? Is one particular therapeutic method superior to the others? Which client and which therapist variables best predict outcome? The concluding sections of this chapter explore these and other cogent questions; Spotlight 19.5 delineates the many methodological problems in conducting research in this area. Even so, an overall conclusion is that there is little difference in outcome among the different therapies. A more specific conclusion is that among the most im-

portant variables that predict outcome are those that pertain to the clients themselves—for example, level of motivation, or personal adequacy at initial phases of therapy. Therapist variables and therapist-client variables are also crucial in predicting outcome. Finally, the empirical literature suggests that psychotherapy—no matter of what type—is better than no psychotherapy at all, even though margins of success vary according to different reports.

ISSUES AND QUESTIONS

1. The question of disclosing the content of presumably voluntary and confidential psychotherapy sessions raises some interesting issues, for most clients assume that some version of the Hippocratic Oath, which guarantees the silence of the clinician even under extreme pressure is maintained (Everstine et al., 1980). The confidentiality of records and of a client's intent to harm society or self may not always be desired, however—for example, when assassination or suicidal fantasies or intent are revealed. In such instances, do the rights of society outweigh those of individuals? Should therapists inform their clients that under "crisis" conditions, they may be in touch with the family or police? Should the therapist's position on these matters be discussed in initial phases of the therapy or only after the client has learned to trust the therapist?
2. Should therapists have implicit goals for emotional health despite, or contrary to, the client's goals? For example, a woman wants to have more fun with her husband, who is "into" drug use and group sex, or at least that is what she claims. Actually, her husband has persuaded her to agree to go for therapy. If you were the therapist, how would you handle her request? Would your own sexual preferences and drug use or nonuse influence your approach? Is it a question of "anything goes" in that the therapist should be regarded only as an engineer or technician employed by an individual to achieve his or her goals?
3. Therapy is usually imposed on a child from without, and most often, there is no choice or voluntariness. When should we impose therapy? Should we ever do so? Are there exceptions that are in the long-range interests of the child? Who is to make this decision, and by what standards?

   Another issue in psychotherapy with children concerns its confidentiality. If the parent of a young child who is in trouble (for example, a child who is constantly stealing from other children) arranges and pays for therapy sessions, is the parent entitled to confer with the therapist about the child's progress? Remember, most therapists believe that trust is essential in achieving results in therapy.
4. Many therapists not only carry to the therapy situation their own implicit and explicit goals but also those that the culture engenders. For example, some popular methods focus on being "open"—being able to drop one's defenses and to experience intimacy with others. A few people are beginning to suggest, however, that some personal controls and defenses may be appropriate in day-to-day living. Further, outgoingness may not be for everybody. Getting along with the group, being popular with one's peers, and possessing certain social skills may be necessary for politicians, for example, or teachers, or group therapists. But what about a scientist who has spent ten years in the laboratory and wishes to spend the next five writing up his or her results? Are social skills and ability to get "close" necessary for everyone? Why or why not?
5. Not many would disagree with the generalization that women in our society have very special problems. They have for generations been scapegoated by men, society, even other women who may wish to preserve the status quo. Do you feel that specially trained women are the most appropriate therapists for women?

Why do you think so? Should there be black therapists for black people? Lesbian therapists for homosexual women? And elderly therapists for elderly people? Before you decide, consider some positive outcomes that might result from such matches. Perhaps a schizophrenic in remission would be of considerably more help to an anguished, confused schizophrenic than someone who has never been "ill."

6. An extremely small percentage of therapists engage in sexual relations with their patients: More male therapists than female therapists do so and most report that sexual contacts are more than a one-time affair (Holroyd and Brodsky, 1977). Females are more often sexually approached than males. Implicit in such contacts (as well as in so-called nonerotic ones—for example, affectionate touching, holding, kissing, and hugging) may be a power relationship between therapist and patient. That is, these contacts generally involve exploitation of someone who is powerless to do anything about it.

   Most therapists ascribe little positive value to such contacts. On the contrary, they believe that the patient can be severely hurt as a result. Further, many clinicians believe that therapists who initiate sexual contact do so because of their own sexual needs, power motives, and loneliness. How could you discourage such contacts? What do you think about nonerotic physical contacts—for example, with a depressed patient or a deprived child in need of affection?

SUGGESTIONS FOR FURTHER READING

Beck, A. T., Rush, A. J., Shaw, B. F., and Emery, G. *Cognitive therapy of depression.* New York: Guilford Press, 1979. This excellent, readable book provides a detailed picture of depression and of cognitive therapy. Case histories and transcripts of actual therapy sessions are used to teach the reader about cognitive techniques.

Berne, E. *Games people play: The psychology of human relationships.* New York: Ballantine, 1978. Paperback. This best-selling book presents a brief description of transactional analysis, structural analysis (of Parent, Adult, Child roles), and the use of games and rituals in our lives. It then goes on to its main purpose, which is to present an annotated list, with illustrations of actual dialogues, of the games that people play in their transactions with each other. This book covers, in popular terms, the games we play in life and the "payoff" we expect to get from them.

Ellis, A., and Grieger, R., with contributors. *Handbook of rational-emotive therapy.* New York: Springer, 1977. Paperback available. This book comprises several chapters written by psychologists who have been influential in the area of rational-emotive therapy. In addition to Ellis' ideas, various applications and approaches are described. This book is recommended for the student who wishes to know more about the various contemporary forms of cognitive therapy.

Hollender, M. H. *The practice of psychoanalytic psychotherapy.* New York: Grune & Stratton, 1965. This slim, extremely readable book is an excellent, understandable, undogmatic description of psychoanalytically oriented psychotherapy. It presents a description of the therapeutic process from beginning to end, reflecting the psychodynamic eclectic therapies practiced in offices and clinics all over the country.

Papp, P. (Ed.) *Family therapy: Full length case studies.* New York: Gardner, 1977. The papers in this book were written by prominent family therapists. Each is a presentation of a family therapy case from the initial interview through termination. Although not all types of treatment methods are represented, there is sufficient diversity among the therapists and the family problems (for example, alcoholism, psychotic disorganization) to provide the reader with a good sense of the breadth of family techniques.

Perls, F. S. *Gestalt therapy verbatim.* New York: Bantam, 1971. This paperback book is based mostly on taped materials from Perls's seminars at Esalen Institute. It is enjoyable, relatively easy reading that provides illustrative material from actual dialogues and interactions between therapist (Perls himself) and client. As a result, the flavor of Gestalt therapy, its focus, and some of its methods are portrayed to the interested student.

Rogers, C. R. *On becoming a person: A therapist's view of psychotherapy.* Boston: Houghton Mifflin, 1961. This is a collection of fascinating, sensitive, touching essays on Rogers's views on psychotherapy, the "good life," and fully functioning people. These essays highlight Rogers's conviction that people are trustworthy, worthwhile, and potentially creative. Rogers's writings also show how person-centered therapy stresses unconditional positive regard for the client through careful listening, empathy, and complete acceptance of the client's values and frame of reference.

Prochaska, J. O. *Systems of psychotherapy: A transtheoretical analysis.* Homewood, Ill.: Dorsey, 1979. This book provides a very complete but concise overview of a dozen therapeutic approaches. For each approach, a biographical sketch of the main theorist, the underlying personality theory, the theories of psychopathology and therapy, and the major criticisms are given. All this is presented in an interesting, readable style.

20

Behavioral Interventions

(in collaboration with Karen M. Simon*)

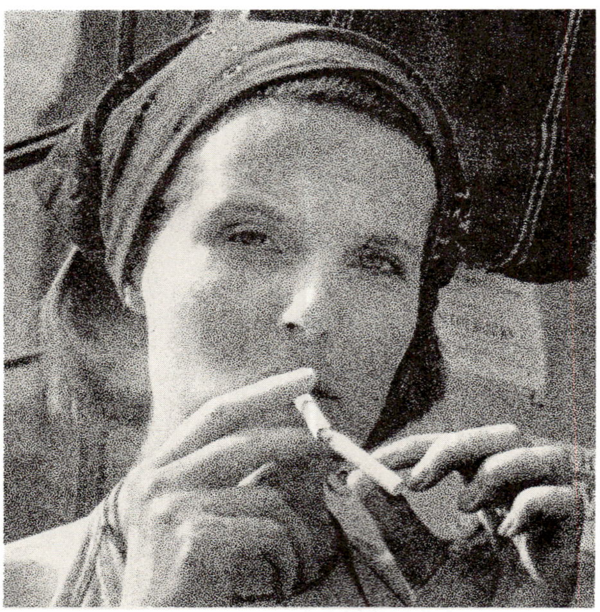

INTRODUCTION

As more and more evidence has accumulated regarding the ineffectiveness of traditional therapies, profound changes have taken place in the practice of psychotherapy. Some of the expensive and time-consuming "talking therapies" have been replaced by approaches that attend to immediate needs—actual problems in the client's life—and that stress pragmatic results rather than theoretical issues.

In retrospect, it seems logical that these changes would be accompanied by a rapid rise of interest in behavioral interventions. In fact, more books, articles, self-help programs, journals, and vi-

* Department of Psychology, University of Pennsylvania.

deotapes have been based upon behavior therapy since 1960 than upon any other single therapeutic approach (Hoon and Lindsley, 1974; Yates, 1975).

But before going any further, we need to define what we mean by the term *behavior therapy*. Originally, a distinction was made between the terms *behavior therapy* and *behavior modification*. Behavior therapy was reserved for those interventions that were based upon classical conditioning. Behavior modification was applied only to those interventions that were based upon operant learning. Although some therapists still make this distinction, most no longer do. Thus, this chapter will use the term behavior therapy to refer to any intervention derived from research in the experimental psychology of learning that is used to alter behavior. As discussed in Chapter 6, there are at least three basic learning paradigms—classical conditioning, operant learning, and social learning. Each of these paradigms has formed the basis for several behavioral interventions. This chapter considers the relationships between these learning theories and their corresponding therapies.

Some Important Features of the Behavioral Approach

The behavioral approach rejects the medical model of psychopathology (see for example, Eysenck, 1960b). Thus, terms such as etiology, prognosis, and mental illness are not used. The behavioral model states that because most deviant behaviors, and especially the neuroses, are learned, learning principles can also be used to eliminate the behaviors associated with the neuroses. Furthermore, even if certain deviant behaviors are not learned, they can still be altered through learning. For example, when physical injury causes brain damage, we do not need to (and indeed, cannot) physically repair the brain damage in order to help the paralyzed patient to recover impaired skills. We can use behavioral interventions to teach new skills or to eliminate old ones.

According to the behavioral approach, it is the *behavior*, not the person, that is maladaptive or undesirable. Thus there is less chance of stigmatizing the client than is the case in traditional diagnostic procedures. Furthermore, the behavioral interventions can be used without knowing the original cause, the etiology of the problem. This is useful because, more often than not, it is claimed, we can do nothing about biochemical, physical, and genetic origins of behavior—if indeed they did help cause the deviance. We can, however, teach people the skills necessary to remedy their deficiencies.

The behavioral approach does not deal with such considerations as what is normal or abnormal. It is not concerned with labels and diagnoses. It does not deal with past history, unconscious motivation, or inner conflict.

Behavioral interventions have other advantages for the client: they usually take much less time than do traditional therapies. As a result, they are also much less expensive. But perhaps most important, treatment goals can be set explicitly at the beginning of therapy by mutual agreement between the therapist and the client. These goals are measurable by objective and reliable standards that can be directly observed and evaluated by both the client and the therapist. As a matter of fact, clients are often encouraged to chart their own progress as a built-in reward system for change.

Behavioral approaches tend to stress self-mastery, independence, and self-help—a do-it-yourself orientation that promotes the client's sense of strength and power over his or her own fate. Many of the traditional psychotherapies, on the other hand, encourage the client's dependence on the therapist for long periods of time. Furthermore, the behavior therapist does not impose his or her own values, implicit beliefs, or conceptions about mental health on an unsuspecting client, for it is the client who sets his or her own goals and makes them explicit at the outset.* Finally, in the view of many scientists, the greatest advantage of all is the ease with which one can evaluate the effectiveness of these interventions.

Unfortunately, there have been some instances in which unscrupulous and untrained people have presented themselves as behavior therapists but have not followed these guidelines. Unwilling children, hospital inpatients, prisoners, and retardates have sometimes been recruited for participation in behavior change procedures without their consent. Also, there have been instances in which treatment goals have been vague and unclear, even to the therapist. In general, however, most of these problems have been corrected through the actions of conscientious behavior therapists and through regulatory legislation. Thus, according to many therapists, the advantages of behavioral interventions—the ease of evaluation, the saving of time and expense, and the demystification of therapy—appear to outweigh the problems.

Historical Background

Decades ago, Watson and Rayner (1920) demonstrated how a phobic reaction can develop and become generalized through classical conditioning. They worked with an eleven-month-old boy, Albert, who was unafraid of white rats. In this study, Albert was allowed to play with a white rat. Whenever he attempted to reach for the rat, however, the researchers made a loud, frightening noise. After five trials, Albert was visibly frightened when he saw the white rat. This fear soon generalized to a rabbit, a short-haired dog, and a sealskin coat. One month later, Albert continued to avoid the rat.

A few years later several experimenters proposed the use of conditioning methods to countercondition children's phobias. One of these early experimenters was Jones (1924), a student of Watson's. She demonstrated this approach with Peter, a three-year-old who had a rabbit phobia as well as a great fear of similar animate and inanimate furry objects. In this study, a rabbit was shown to Peter while he was playing enjoyably with other children. In addition, whenever the rabbit was introduced, a tasty piece of food was given to Peter. Gradually, Peter became less afraid of the rabbit and it could thus be brought closer and closer to him. Finally, the rabbit could roam freely in the play area without causing Peter to be afraid. Eventually, the boy would even play with the rabbit. A follow-up assessment indicated that the phobia did not recur.

Other early experiments used avoidance conditioning as a treatment for certain problems. For example, Mowrer and Mowrer (1938) devised treatment for enuresis—bed wetting. Their procedure required the enuretic child to sleep with a pad between his body and the bed. When the child started to urinate at night, wetting the pad would close a circuit and set off a loud alarm. This taught the child to wake up and use the toilet when his bladder was full, rather than wetting the bed.

Fear of furry animals can be easily "counterconditioned," as shown by early experiments in classical conditioning. (Margaret Thompson/The Picture Cube)

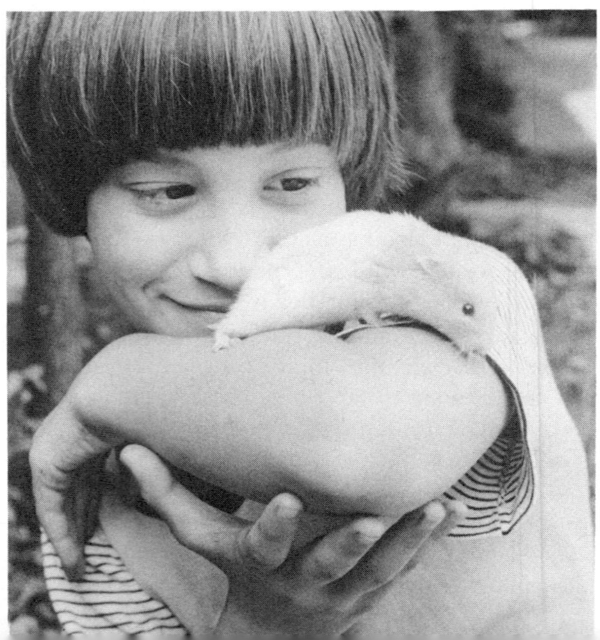

* Most well-trained practitioners of verbal psychotherapy, it should be noted, are similarly careful not to impose their values and beliefs on unsuspecting clients.

More than a decade later, there was a widespread increase of interest in the use of conditioning, counterconditioning, extinction, and inhibition to alter people's emotional reactions, especially intense fears (Salter, 1949; Wolpe, 1948). It took another decade of interest in psychotherapeutic methods for researchers to suggest the sweeping possibility that learning principles could account for improvement in *all* forms of psychotherapy (Bandura, 1961; Eysenck, 1960b) and that it was not necessary to invoke the Freudian mechanisms of resistance, transference, or insight to explain some people's improvement in therapy.

Bandura (1961), for example, noted that many of the successful methods in psychotherapy, such as permissiveness, are in fact unlabeled behavioral interventions that derive validity from experimental principles (in this case, extinction). Bandura went on to point out that some types of patients (the psychopath, for example) are probably not amenable to the usual treatments because the behavior to be reinforced is simply not in their behavioral repertoires. Furthermore, he noted that in traditional therapy, the therapists' approval may serve as reinforcement to aid in the acquisition and maintenance of increasingly socialized behavior.

As a matter of fact, many early demonstrations of therapeutic change used principles of extinction, reward, punishment, or modeling (Bandura, 1961). Behavioral interventions in current use thus have a long history in psychology. What is new is the wide variety of interventions available as well as the popularity of these interventions among clinicians.

BEHAVIOR THERAPIES BASED ON CLASSICAL CONDITIONING

Systematic Desensitization

Systematic desensitization is a technique that is often used to treat phobias. It uses counterconditioning to establish an association between feelings of relaxation and stimuli that previously elicited fear and anxiety. This therapy requires the client to gradually and systematically imagine increasingly aversive stimuli while he or she maintains a relaxed state with the help of drugs, hypnosis, or previously trained relaxation exercises.

One commonly used exercise for inducing relaxation is the Jacobson (1929) technique. In this procedure, clients are first taught to discriminate tension from relaxation in various muscle groups. For example, a client might be instructed to clench her hand into as tight a fist as she can, to hold this position for one or two minutes, and then to relax her hand. When the client can distinguish between muscle tension and relaxation, she then practices relaxing without first tensing.

Although desensitization is a behavioral treatment, it has some very traditional aspects. For example, the use of imagery (fantasy) is an integral aspect of systematic desensitization. Another traditional aspect of this method is that case history taking is essential. For, in addition to relaxation training, systematic desensitization requires the therapist and client to construct a hierarchy of the client's fears. This is a list that progresses from the least frightening to the most frightening instances of the feared situation. An example of such a hierarchy is given in Spotlight 20.1.

Systematic desensitization employs the notion that in a state of relaxation, the least aversive stimulus in a hierarchy will elicit very little anxiety because the relaxation will inhibit it. After a certain number of trials, the client will signal the therapist that he or she no longer experiences any anxiety. The client is then ready to proceed to the next image, which is only slightly more anxiety producing than the previous one. With practice, relaxation will take the place of anxiety as the client's response to the imagined stimulus. And so, in systematic steps, the client practices relaxing in the presence of each item in the fear-producing hierarchy. Finally, the client is able to imagine the situation that previously was most intolerable and still remain calm.

Spotlight 20.1 presents a case in which systematic desensitization was used to treat dream-induced anxiety.

Spotlight 20.1 Systematic Desensitization as a Treatment for Nightmares

An unusual application of systematic desensitization was described by Cavior and Deutsch (1975). Their client was a sixteen-year-old inmate at an institution for juvenile offenders who told the therapists that he had been repeatedly having a nightmare in which his father murders his mother.

The dream goes as follows:

The subject is sitting in his bedroom when he hears his father enter the house. His mother then begins to shout at her husband for being drunk; an argument ensues which leads to a physical battle. Finally, the subject "hears" his father pick up a knife . . . from the kitchen table and threaten to kill his wife. The subject runs out to the living room where he sees his father holding the knife to his mother's throat. At this point, the subject wakes up (Cavior and Deutsch, 1975, p. 433).

The content of this nightmare came from the client's own experience. His mother and father fought frequently (but there had been no murder). He reported that whenever he had the dream he would wake up and be unable to fall asleep again. This caused him to be extremely drowsy and irritable the next day, leading to trouble with the staff. These dreams occurred about once a week for over a year. The therapists and client decided that their goal would be to eliminate the anxiety that the nightmare elicited. A modified form of systematic desensitization was used.

The nightmare was first broken up into twelve hierarchical steps (steps 9–11 were introduced during the second session):

1. Hears father coming into the house drunk
2. Mother yells at father for returning home drunk
3. Father shouts back at her
4. Mother and father begin to argue
5. Father hits mother
6. Mother hits father back
7. Both parents are fighting
8. Subject "hears" father pick up knife from kitchen table
9. Father shouts, "I'll kill you"
10. Mother begins to scream
11. Subject runs into living room and actually sees parents fighting
12. Subject sees father with knife at mother's throat, ready to kill her

(Cavior and Deutsch, 1975, p. 434)

The Jacobson relaxation technique was used. When the subject was completely relaxed, the therapist described step (1) in the dream hierarchy, asking him to visualize it with closed eyes. The client was instructed to open his eyes if he felt any anxiety at all. The type of systematic desensitization used in this study was different from the usual type in that the client went through the relaxation training only once at the beginning of the session, instead of stopping after every step to relax again. The therapist merely said, "You are still very relaxed," before and after each step of the dream hierarchy.

The client stayed relaxed throughout treatment until step (12), the last step (steps 9–11 were not introduced in this session), in which his mother was about to be killed. At that point, he got very upset and the first session was ended.

In the second session, all twelve steps were used so that the increase in anxiety would be much more gradual. The client found it easy to visualize each step in the dream. He was even able to imagine step (12) for two minutes without being overcome by anxiety. Therapy was terminated after the third session, but the client was encouraged to practice the procedure at home.

Follow-up interviews after one, two, and six months indicated that the client continued to have the dream, but without anxiety. He reported that he was able to fall asleep again almost immediately, even though the dream woke him up. As a result, he was less irritable during the day after the dream and had fewer difficulties with the staff.

Although desensitization was used originally to treat phobias (Wolpe, 1961), clinical evidence soon began to indicate that it could be used to treat an enormous range of human problems (Kazdin and Wilcoxon, 1976). These problems include not only fears of social interactions, enclosed spaces, open spaces, animals, disease, and death, but also nightmares, stuttering, anorexia nervosa, excessively frequent urination, depression, anxiety, seizures, and compulsive, ritualistic behaviors of various kinds. Desensitization has also been used with some success for impotence and frigidity (Glick, 1975).

Although there is little question as to the effectiveness of systematic desensitization (Franks and Wilson, 1976; Yates, 1975), there is much question as to why it is effective (Bandura, 1977; Kazdin and Wilcoxon, 1976; Yates, 1975). Some indication of the problems associated with the counterconditioning explanation follows: first, relaxation training is not necessary for desensitization to occur. Second, the use of hierarchies based upon anxiety intensity is not necessary either. Third, massed, as opposed to spaced, trials may be quite effective in reducing fears. And fourth, hierarchies can go from the highest to the lowest intensity, rather than the reverse, and still be effective. These exceptions to the rules of systematic desensitization caused many observers (for example, Yates, 1975) to look for explanations other than counterconditioning to account for the effectiveness of desensitization. One explanation is that placebo effects and other cognitive factors, such as expectancy, are responsible for its success. (Lick and Bootzin, 1975).

Although the poor methodology of many studies prevents us from determining whether such factors did account for desensitization's effectiveness (Davison and Wilson, 1972; Kazdin and Wilcoxon, 1976; Slutsky and Allen, 1978), great care is currently being taken to control for placebo and expectancy factors (Franks and Wilson, 1976). In addition, care is being taken to improve the effectiveness of systematic desensitization, regardless of its theoretical basis. For example, some researchers are exploring the use of vicarious desensitization procedures—such as having the client watch someone else being treated for the same fear that he or she has. Other researchers are exploring the effectiveness of self-administered desensitization programs.

However, the best improvement on systematic desensitization is probably the use of graduated exposure to actual rather than to imagined fear-producing situations. The effectiveness of this variation—called contact desensitization—has been dramatically shown in several studies. In one of these studies (Bandura, Blanchard, and Ritter, 1969), all but one of the subjects receiving contact desensitization were completely cured. However, the subjects receiving systematic (imaginal) desensitization could only perform a little more than half the items on their hierarchies after treatment.

Because treatment effects do not completely generalize to activities unlike those used in the actual treatment, many persons continue to avoid real-life threats even though the imagined threats no longer make them fearful. (Barlow, Leitenberg, Agras, and Wincze, 1969). Thus, the use of situations that involve actual rather than imagined stimuli is generally preferred. Unfortunately, this is not always possible—for example, in the case of certain sexual interactions or intensely feared situations that the client will take great pains to avoid.

Flooding and Implosion

As noted, it is not always necessary to progress through a desensitization hierarchy from the least to the most feared situation for treatment to be effective (Hogan, 1968). In flooding and implosion, the client is immediately placed at the highest—the most feared—level of the hierarchy and "flooded" with anxiety. The flooding approach involves direct and prolonged exposure to aversive stimulation of high intensity. For example, a claustrophobic might be locked in a small, stuffy closet; or a compulsive handwasher might be required to handle filth and be subsequently prevented from washing. Implo-

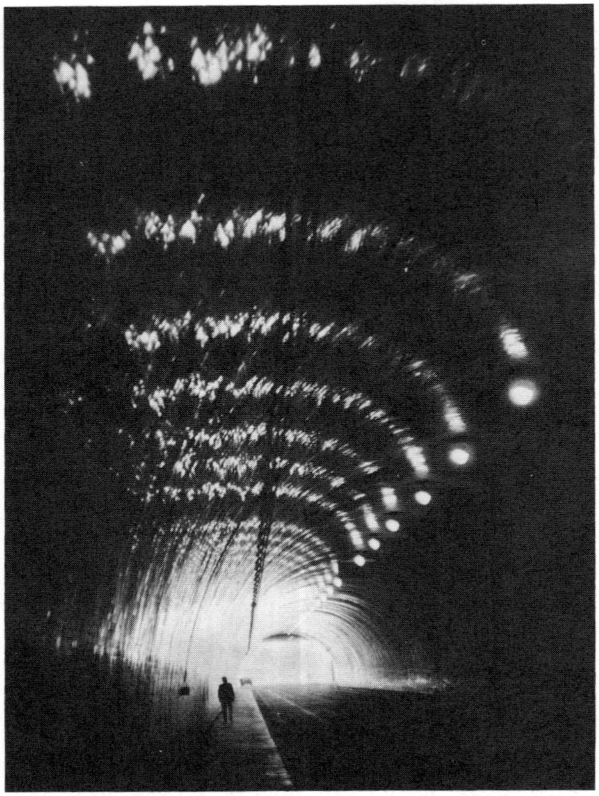

This person is attempting to confront his phobia directly by exposing himself to the most intense level of anxiety—walking through a long tunnel. This behavioral method is called "flooding." (George Gardner)

sion therapy, on the other hand, involves imagined rather than actual situations. The client is often given homework assignments, such as imagining specific, highly feared, aversive scenes for extended periods of time. Although homework is regarded as successful in reducing fears by itself, clinicians using implosion report that the therapeutic results often do not generalize to the real-life situation.

Unlike the other interventions discussed in this chapter, implosion is based upon psychodynamic, as well as upon learning theory. According to psychodynamic theory, anxiety responses are essential to the maintenance of a neurotic symptom (the symptom acts to reduce anxiety). Thus, if anxiety can be extinguished in the face of stimuli that usually elicit it, then the neurotic symptom will also disappear. The person will no longer find it necessary to rely upon the symptom.

Note that according to this approach, the goal of therapy is to elicit and sustain a high level of anxiety. This is very different from the goal of systematic desensitization, which is to prevent *any* occurrence of anxiety. As one might predict, Wolpe does not approve of either flooding or implosion because the client frequently experiences panic—extreme, acute, and disorganizing anxiety. In fact, some clinicians (for example, Nathan and Jackson, 1976) report that these methods are not useful at all with phobic patients because of excessive anxiety. However, implosion apparently does work with many kinds of clinical problems.

Aversive Counterconditioning

Aversive counterconditioning (Rachman and Teasdale, 1969) involves the principles of classical conditioning, using a punishing or aversive event so that the client learns a response incompatible with the one that is being counterconditioned.

Here is an example: An adult male client who seeks treatment for pedophilia (see Chapter 15) might be shown photographs of undressed young girls followed immediately by an electric shock. After repeated pairings of these stimuli, pictures of young girls will elicit anxiety and avoidance, rather than sexual arousal. Another application of this procedure is the counterconditioning of alcoholism through the administration of the drug Antabuse as discussed in Chapter 16.

A wide range of aversive stimuli have been used to countercondition undesirable responses. They can be chemical (for example, Antabuse or curare), electrical, or even imaginal. In covert sensitization, the client is asked to imagine a nauseating or anxiety-producing scene in combination with the maladaptive behavior (Cautela, 1966, 1967). Spotlight 20.2 describes the application of covert sensitization to a case of sadistic fantasy. It appears that almost any unpleasant event can be used in aversive counterconditioning.

There are certain ethical issues that must be addressed regarding the use of aversive counterconditioning, especially when they are used to treat incompetent or incarcerated people who cannot control what happens to them. Some people believe, however, that when a client is self-injurious or injurious to others (a rapist, for example), or when a client desires to change a socially undesirable habit, aversive counterconditioning should not be ruled out. These important issues will be discussed more fully when aversive techniques are described in the section on contingency management procedures later in this chapter.

Spotlight 20.2 Covert Sensitization With a Case of Sadistic Sexual Fantasy

Davison (1968) has reported a very interesting case study suggesting that covert sensitization can be used effectively to alter the content of deviant sexual fantasies. In this case, a twenty-one-year-old male college senior became quite concerned over the fact that he could become sexually aroused only by sadistic fantasies. He sought therapy after reading a Freudian explanation of sadomasochism, which had greatly upset him because it mentioned that this "illness" had a poor prognosis. The client had avoided dating and marriage because of his concern about his fantasies.

There were four elements in Davison's treatment of this man. First, because the client was so upset by the Freudian interpretation of his problem, Davison reinterpreted it in learning-theory terms. He mentioned that clients often found it liberating to think about their maladaptive behavior in terms of "normal" psychological processes rather than as the result of an incurably "diseased" mind.

The second step in treatment was designed to increase the client's ability to become aroused by nonsadistic fantasies. In the privacy of his room, the client was to obtain an erection in whatever way possible, probably with a sadistic fantasy. Then he was to masturbate while looking at a picture of a nude woman. He was to conjure up his sadistic fantasy to regain the erection, if he began to lose it. However, he was told that it was crucial that he focus on the picture of the nude woman at the moment of orgasm.

Although he improved in his ability to reach orgasm with nonsadistic fantasies, the client was reluctant to give up his sadistic fantasies entirely. Therefore, covert sensitization was used as the third step in treatment. To use this technique, it was first necessary to find an imaginal scene that the client found revolting. Thus, Davison described several scenes to the client in order to find one that was effective. The scene that worked best—as indicated by the client's "grimaces, contortions, and groans"—was "a large bowl of 'soup,' composed of steaming urine with reeking fecal boli bobbing around on top" (Davison, 1958, p. 86).

With his eyes closed, the client was instructed to imagine a pretty girl struggling to free herself while tied to stakes on the ground. Then, for the following five minutes, he was to imagine drinking from the bowl and getting nauseous while peering at the girl over the floating debris. Within two weeks the client reported that he was unable to become aroused by a sadistic fantasy, even when he tried.

The final step in this treatment was to increase the client's normal interactions with women. For example, he was instructed to spend time looking at women, to ask a woman out for a date, and so on.

One month after the end of treatment, the sadistic fantasies had still not returned. However, sixteen months later, he reported that he had "premeditatedly" resumed his sadistic fantasies six months after the end of treatment,

> *. . . resolving to enjoy my fantasies until June 1, and then to reform once more. This I did. On June 1, . . . right on schedule, I bought an issue of* Playboy *and proceeded to give myself the treatment again. Once again, it worked like a charm. In two weeks, I was back in my reformed state, where I am now. . . . I have no need for sadistic fantasies. . . . I have [also] been pursuing a vigorous (well, vigorous for* me*) program of dating. In this way I have gotten to know a lot of girls of whose existence I was previously only peripherally aware. As you probably know, I was very shy with girls before; well, now I am not one-fifth as shy as I used to be. In fact, by my old standards, I have become a regular rake! (Davison, 1968, p. 89)*

In addition to the ethical questions raised by the use of painful procedures, there are other drawbacks to aversive methods. There is, for example only moderate experimental or clinical evidence for their effectiveness. Also, even when treatment is successful, relapses are more likely to occur after aversive counterconditioning, than certain other interventions, such as systematic desensitization, for example. Another serious disadvantage is that aversive methods can make the client angry, fearful, and anxious. Thus, the client may avoid therapy altogether. As a result of such drawbacks, most psychologists rarely, if ever, use aversive counterconditioning, and then only in extreme instances.

BEHAVIOR THERAPIES BASED ON OPERANT LEARNING

Contingency Management Procedures

Reinforcement and extinction techniques. Some people feel that operant learning enters into all therapies—even the traditional ones. For example, in systematic desensitization, when the client masters each level in the hierarchy, the therapist ordinarily will signify approval by nodding, or by simply saying "That's fine" to the client. In this example, the therapist can be viewed as providing social reinforcement for therapeutic progress (Krasner, 1971).

Some of the earliest attempts to translate experimental learning theory into therapeutic procedures arose from efforts to modify the behavior of psychotics in hospital settings (see Lindsley and Skinner, 1954). Although these early efforts did not cure schizophrenia, they did demonstrate that therapeutic gains can be achieved even by people with this severe disability.

Soon, the feasibility of a behavioral model of psychopathology arose. By moving away from a disease concept and by conceptualizing "mental illness" as a collection of undesirable behaviors, it was possible to change the various "deviant" behaviors by providing reinforcement (money, food, privileges, etc.) for desirable behaviors while withholding reinforcement (extinction) for undesirable behaviors. This is not as easy as it sounds. For example, a psychotic may not know how to perform behaviors that are important constituents of a desirable behavior pattern. And, how can a behavior be reinforced—by candy, or a smile, or a cigarette—if it is never emitted?

As was described in Chapter 6, behavior therapists use such methods as shaping to gradually train the client to achieve closer and closer approximations of the complex behavior by mastering, with the aid of reinforcements, the simpler component behaviors. It was later recognized that other techniques can be used to circumvent the painfully slow method of successive approximations. For example, the therapist could use modeling (see later in this chapter) to demonstrate the desired behavior to the client.

Today contingency management is used, often in combination with other behavioral interventions, with many kinds of people. One application that has had much promise combines the use of operant and other techniques with autistic children (see Spotlight 20.3).

Token economies. Earlier chapters have mentioned token economies, in which operant methods are used to alter the behavior of people in self-contained social settings, such as classrooms, prisons, and hospital wards. Token economies are employed as methods by which deviant behavior can be shaped into more socially desirable behavior.

In order to implement a token economy, the

Spotlight 20.3 Behavioral Interventions for Infantile Autism

Contingency management strategies have produced dramatic changes in the behavior of autistic children. Because most of these strategies can be taught to the parents of these children, there is the added advantage of utilizing the parents themselves as therapists for their own child. The gains of therapy are thus maintained, because home and clinic are indistinguishable.

In Chapter 14, some special features of autistic children were described. These included mutism, echolalia, self-mutilation, temper tantrums, violent behavior, lack of social behavior, and similar problems. Margolies (1977) has reviewed some remarkable clinical illustrations of the various skills that have been successfully taught to otherwise "unreachable" autistic children. Although these are moving instances of the effectiveness of the behavioral methods, the success of the procedures does not—nor is it meant to—attest to the validity of any particular theory about the *etiology* of autism. Contingency management can improve the functioning of these children without addressing this issue.

In much of the work with autistic children, the selection of an appropriate reinforcer is essential. Music or kaleidoscopic displays of light may be more reinforcing to them than verbal approval. A nod or a smile may be completely meaningless events to an unsocialized child who makes no eye contact. Furthermore, some reinforcers may be too distracting; they may divert the child from the task at hand. For, as with brain-damaged children, the avoidance of distracting extraneous cues and sudden changes in the learning environment is essential.

Some of the behaviors that have been targets for treatment include toileting, making eye contact, speaking and language usage, self-injurious behaviors, temper tantrums, aggression, disruptive behaviors, and repetitive self-stimulation, such as rhythmic rocking, spinning and twirling of objects before one's eyes, prolonged staring into lit bulbs, etc.

Margolies (1977) cites many illustrative studies. Here is one such study of toilet training.

Marshall (1966) treated a nonverbal autistic boy who defecated in his pants approximately 95% of the time. This child was kept in diapers until age 4½, stopped bed-wetting at age 6, and stopped wetting during the day at 6½. Treatment consisted of shaping the appropriate behavior by reinforcing its component parts (e.g., approach to the toilet, removal of clothing, proper body posture, straining). In addition, punishment in the form of a slap on the buttocks was employed, contingent upon soiled pants. By the end of therapy, the rate of soiling was reduced to 30% of the time. The child's mother was trained to continue treatment after termination and was successful in completely toilet training her son (Margolies, 1977, p. 255).

Verbal training of autistic children is a difficult task in which considerable success has been demonstrated. In speech training for mutes, shaping based on vocalization is employed. Thus methods for inducing vocalization must be introduced.

But even before this, the child must learn to focus on the task at hand.

To reduce bizarre inattentive behavior, the therapist may have to sit very close to the child so that he or she is forced to be aware of the therapist's responses. The child is not permitted to ignore or to withdraw from the task or to resort to "psychotic" activities (Lovaas, Freitas, Nelson, and Whalen, 1967).

These initial maneuvers are followed by arduous one-to-one training sessions. Margolies (1977) describes an effort by Hewett (1965) to teach verbal skills to a four-and-a-half-year-old mute autistic boy. An entire week was devoted to developing an association of the teacher with positive reinforcement and to allow the child to feel comfortable in the special learning situation.

A month followed in which imitation skills were developed. Speech training lasted 6 months; verbal imitation was shaped until the child had acquired a 32-word vocabulary and was capable of answering a variety of questions. The final 8 months were devoted to maximizing generalization; newly learned words were required to be used properly in various social settings with a number of individuals besides the teacher. The child's vocabulary grew to 150 words (Margolies, 1977, p. 257).

In much of the work with autistic children, therapy "packages" are employed. That is, several behaviors are concurrently targeted for change. Furthermore, one therapist might attempt to shape verbal skills, toilet behavior, and reduce the tantrums of an autistic child, while another might choose to work with an entirely different set of behaviors.

Although the studies reviewed do not indicate that autistic children become "normal" after treatment, there is now some evidence that this may be possible. At the UCLA Autism Project, Lovaas and his colleagues identified a large number of autistic children who were under 30 months of age. Half the children received intensive behavior therapy, half did not receive this treatment. After about one year, approximately 50 percent of the children who received behavior therapy could be placed in regular classrooms, whereas only about 1 percent of the control children were considered to be normal (Lovaas, 1976). Thus, if these children are identified while they are still very young, and if they are given comprehensive behavioral treatment, they have a good chance of behaving more normally.

therapist must first specify the desirable behavior or behaviors—for example, learning not to interrupt, to focus on a task, to clean floors, or to defecate in the toilet rather than on the floor. A program is then instituted in which the subject receives reinforcement for performing these desired behaviors.

The reinforcement given does not have direct value to the subject, however. Instead a token, chip, piece of plastic, or any other object that can be exchanged for "real" reinforcers is used. These real, or backup, reinforcers vary too. They can be food, money, candy, movie passes, privacy, time off hospital grounds—whatever it is that makes for the "good life" of an individual. Clearly, the desirability of the backup reinforcers will be an important determinant of the effectiveness of a token economy. People will work only for tokens that can be used to "buy" commodities and privileges that they value. Thus the therapist must assess, for the individual with whom he or she is working, what these valuables are.

Early demonstrations of the token economy were generally in closed-ward mental hospitals (see Ayllon and Azrin, 1965, 1968). These studies provided powerful evidence that the rate of appropriate behaviors can be increased and maintained by imposing token reinforcement systems and that the rate of inappropriate behaviors can be reduced when reinforcement was withheld. Some of the target behaviors were self-care, work activities, social interactions, and aggressiveness. Today, token economies are used in many settings. They are employed in classrooms and nursery schools for normal, retarded, and brain-damaged children. They are also used in halfway houses for juvenile delinquents and in day hospitals for certain kinds of patients.

As a result of this widespread use of token economies, the courts have begun to clarify the rights of institutionalized patients. Thus, there are certain reinforcers that cannot be withheld from an individual in a token economy. These include the right to a comfortable bed and the right to nutritional meals (*Wyatt* v. *Stickney,* 1972). In addition, many people agree that what goes on in institutions should be subject to review by community boards to ensure that the rights of the individuals within them are protected. Record-keeping, supervision of the economy, and preparation of a manual in which all the rules are explicit and open to question is essential, not only to run an effective economy, but also because ethically, such programs should be subject to independent scrutiny.

There is no question as to the effectiveness of properly designed token economies (see Kazdin and Bootzin, 1972). Although people with severe brain damage and chronic psychoses are not completely "cured," their level of functioning is greatly improved—many are able to be discharged from the hospital. But what happens when these people are released from the institutions? Do they continue to function well in the community?

In spite of the many demonstrations of the effectiveness of token economies, there has been very little research on whether behaviors taught in the hospital generalize to the community. However, what research there has been indicates that behavior rapidly deteriorates if not reinforced in the new environment. Thus, generalization should be planned for rather than "hoped for."

Several techniques have been used to increase generalization of treatment gains (Kazdin and Bootzin, 1972). The most frequently used procedure is to teach only those behaviors that will continue to be reinforced after training (Ayllon and Azrin, 1968). Only behaviors that will come under the control of naturally occurring reinforcers in the subject's environment should be reinforced in a token economy—anything else will be quickly forgotten after discharge.

A second procedure is to decrease token reinforcement gradually while substituting social approval, privileges, and other "normal" reinforcers. The idea here is to make reinforcement conditions within the institution indiscriminable from those outside.

A third procedure, which is probably the most promising of all, is to train adaptive behaviors in the actual settings to which generalization is desired. Fairweather and his colleagues (Fairweather, Sanders, Maynard, and Cressler, 1969) pioneered this approach by demonstrating that self-help lodges can be a viable alternative to hospitalization. In their lodge, patients were taught the skills necessary to make them self-sufficient and self-supporting, for example, they were taught how to shop, cook, manage money, and start a business. Then the training staff withdrew and the patients took over the lodge. They became completely independent of the hospital and were able to live successfully as a group within the community.

Thus, it is clear that treatment effects can be maintained outside the therapeutic setting. However, it is not a magical occurrence—"generalization should be programmed, rather than expected or lamented" (Baer, Wolf, and Risley, 1968, p. 97).

Aversive techniques. On occasion, aversive events are presented as a consequence of undesirable behavior. Thus, a person may have to pay a fine, temporarily lose a privilege, or be isolated from positive reinforcers (time-out), or may even be electrically shocked. Shock, of course, is almost always reserved for severe problems that have failed to respond to other, less drastic treatments.

Some people think that it is always wrong to use physically aversive events, but most realize that there are instances in which it is justified. Take the following case study, for example. Two behavior therapists (Lang and Melamed, 1969) were consulted to treat a nine-month-old boy who was starving to death because he vomited every time he was fed. Since the problem began at the age of five months, the infant had been hospitalized four times for medical tests and treatments—but he continued to lose weight. In fact, he weighed only twelve pounds at the beginning of the behavioral treatment.

For the first two days, the behavior therapists observed the infant before and after meals. They also measured the muscle activity (EMG) in the boy's throat in order to be able to predict when he was about to vomit. Starting on the third day, whenever the infant's EMG indicated that he was beginning to vomit, he was shocked on the leg. And the shock continued until muscle activity ended. Treatment sessions were given once a day for one hour immediately after a meal.

By the third session, the child had learned to suppress his vomiting and was rarely shocked. By the sixth session, the child had stopped vomiting altogether. After three more shock-free sessions, treatment was discontinued. However, two days later the boy vomited again and was given three additional treatment sessions to make sure he was cured. Five days after the last of these sessions, the infant was discharged from the hospital weighing sixteen pounds. Five months later, the child had

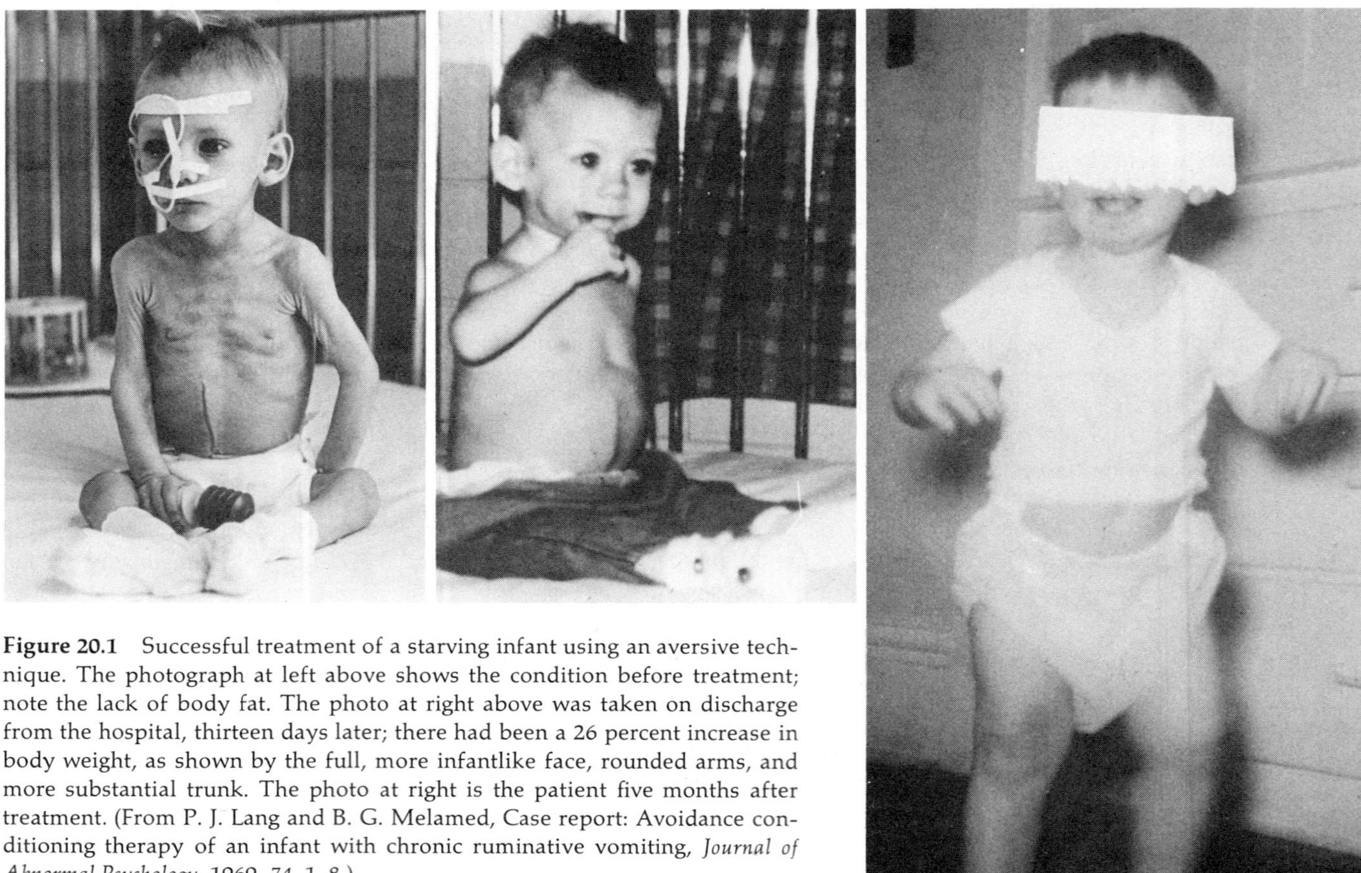

Figure 20.1 Successful treatment of a starving infant using an aversive technique. The photograph at left above shows the condition before treatment; note the lack of body fat. The photo at right above was taken on discharge from the hospital, thirteen days later; there had been a 26 percent increase in body weight, as shown by the full, more infantlike face, rounded arms, and more substantial trunk. The photo at right is the patient five months after treatment. (From P. J. Lang and B. G. Melamed, Case report: Avoidance conditioning therapy of an infant with chronic ruminative vomiting, *Journal of Abnormal Psychology,* 1969, *74,* 1–8.)

gained another ten pounds and had not vomited at all (see Figure 20.1).

When confronted with a choice between allowing a child to die and applying a painful but nonlethal stimulus, few persons would consider punishment unethical. Another example of the use of punishment is given in Spotlight 20.4.

Note that these treatments were dramatically successful even though the therapists did not know the original causes of the problems. Furthermore, there was no evidence of symptom substitution following the treatments, as some psychodynamic theories would predict. In fact, the infant who was treated by Lang and Melamed became much more responsive to adults, smiled more frequently, and became more interested in toys and games than he had been before treatment.

This is not to say that punishment always has the desired effect on behavior. Sometimes there is little or no change; on occasion the punished response is even strengthened (Church, 1963). Thus, punishment does not always suppress behavior.

Spotlight 20.4 Aversive Contingency Management versus Extinction as Treatments for Self-Destruction

Lovaas and his colleagues have presented some of the most systematic investigations of the therapeutic use of aversive stimulation with human subjects (see Bucher and Lovaas, 1968). They came to use such extreme measures as a result of trying to treat children with a formidable disorder—infantile autism.

At the UCLA Autism Project, most of the children engaged in self-destructive behavior. Among those children who were self-destructive, headbanging was the most frequent behavior. The children hit their heads against sharp edges of objects, and against walls, and some also punched themselves in the face. The Autism Project was located in a state hospital that did not have sufficient staff to implement a program to reinforce behaviors incompatible with self-destruction. Therefore, these researchers were faced with a choice between two workable treatment alternatives—extinction and aversive contingency management. The following example illustrates their rationale for concluding that aversive contingency management is more ethical than extinction in treating severe self-destruction.

John was a seven-year-old boy, diagnosed as retarded (IQ 25), with psychotic-like behaviors. He had been self-injurious since he was two years of age, a behavior which necessitated his hospitalization one year prior to his being studied at UCLA. During that year he had to be kept in complete restraints (legs, waist, and with a camisole to restrain his arms) on a 24-hour-a-day basis. When removed from restraint he would immediately hit his head against the crib, beat his head with his fists, and scream. He looked extremely frightened when removed from restraints. He was so unmanageable that he had to be fed in full restraints; he would not take food otherwise. His head was covered with scar tissue, and his ears were swollen and bleeding (Bucher and Lovaas, 1968, p. 86).

Although John was studied under several conditions, only two are relevant here. These are the extinction and the punishment conditions. In the extinction condition, John was simply left to himself in his bed without restraints, with no attention given to his self-destructive actions. This was done for one and one-half hours on each of eight days. Extinction of his self-destructive behavior was slowly achieved. The rate fell very gradually from the first day, when John hit his head 3,000 times, until the eighth day, when he hit himself only 15 times. Although this behavior eventually did extinguish, he had hit himself over *10,000* times and the staff was very much concerned about damage caused by edema of his ears. Furthermore, extinction in bed did not generalize to other places in the house, the living room, for example.

The decline in self-destruction brought about

by the use of contingent electric shock (see Figure 20.2) is markedly different from the extinction data above. The first fifteen sessions were preexperimental, and showed that self-destruction had neither increased nor decreased. In session 16 John started to receive shock for head-banging. He earned punishment only twelve times over the next fourteen sessions. As the figure shows, head-banging was much more quickly suppressed by the aversive contingency than it was by extinction. Thus, John hurt himself much less.

Some additional results of this study are interesting. The first relates to generalization across experimenters. During the first twenty-nine sessions John was punished only by Experimenter 1. The reduced rate brought about by Experimenter 1 generalized only partially to the other three experimenters. By sessions 25, 26, and 27, John's rate of self-destruction with these other experimenters had greatly increased. However, when Experimenter 3 punished John on the thirtieth session, the effects generalized across all the other experimenters.

In addition, treatment effects generalized to a wide variety of other behaviors: as self-destruction decreased, John avoided adults less and cried less. He also began to enjoy running, playing in the tub, and he acted more normal in other respects. Thus, there were no negative side effects of treatment. The authors were quick to point out, however, the possibility that other children might experience negative side effects.

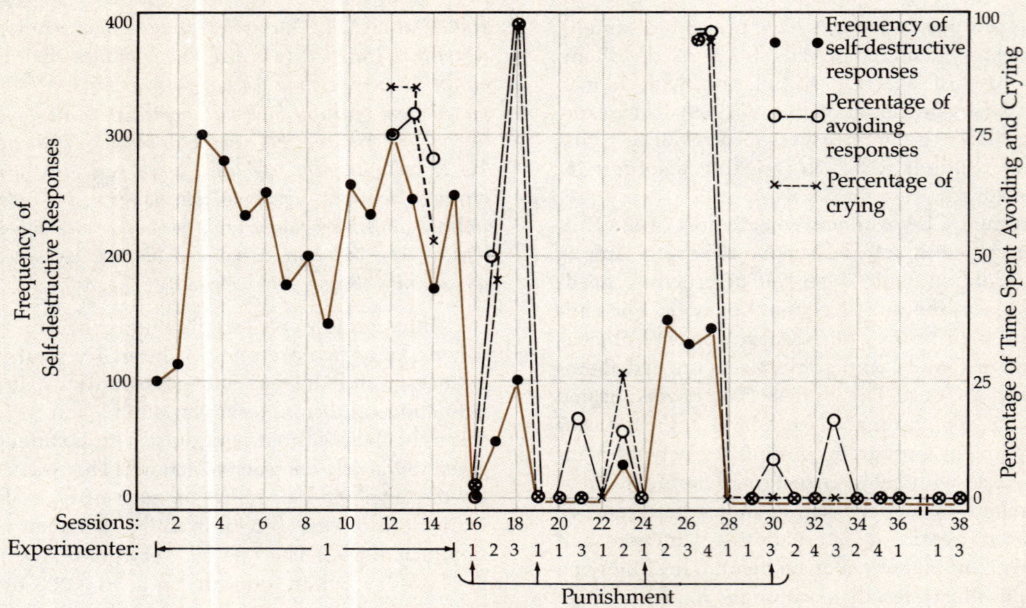

Figure 20.2 Reduction in head-banging as a result of electric-shock treatment. The graph shows John's behaviors in the living room. The vertical arrows below the horizontal axis indicate when shock was given; note that all responses were ultimately reduced to zero. (From B. Bucher and O. I. Lovaas, Use of aversive stimulation in behavior modification, in M. R. Jones (Ed.), *Miami Symposium on the prediction of behavior, 1967: Aversive stimulation* [Coral Gables, Fla.: University of Miami Press, 1968], p. 88.)

Often it causes the person to try out other behaviors—some of which may be no more constructive than the original activity. Of course, when a therapist uses punishment, the intention is for a more constructive behavior to take the place of the punished behavior. Thus, for treatment to be effective, the therapist must provide the client with a desirable alternative behavior. Some researchers are convinced that one of the most powerful methods for eliminating extremely undesirable behavior is to punish it while consistently reinforceing the desirable alternative behavior (Martin and Pear, 1978; Stolz, Wienckowski, and Brown, 1975).

Apart from the issue of effectiveness is the issue of ethics: When is it ethical to use aversive methods?* Most people will agree that the two cases presented in this section (Bucher and Lovaas, 1968; Lang and Melamed, 1969) represent ethical applications of aversive methods. On the other hand, some people say that the use of punishment is always unethical with certain types of subjects—prison inmates for example—even when they are merely denied privileges, a point raised earlier in this book.

Extremely aversive procedures are in fact rarely used (see Wallace, Burger, Neal, van Brero, and Davis, 1976). When they are used, it is usually to reduce life-threatening behavior or to alter the behavior of extremely violent persons. Most people would probably agree that such uses are ethical. However, aversive treatments should be administered only by professionally trained personnel under carefully monitored conditions, especially with the helpless and with the incompetent.

Stimulus Control Procedures

Often a maladaptive behavior is not completely or always maladaptive. Sometimes a behavior is a problem because it occurs at inappropriate times

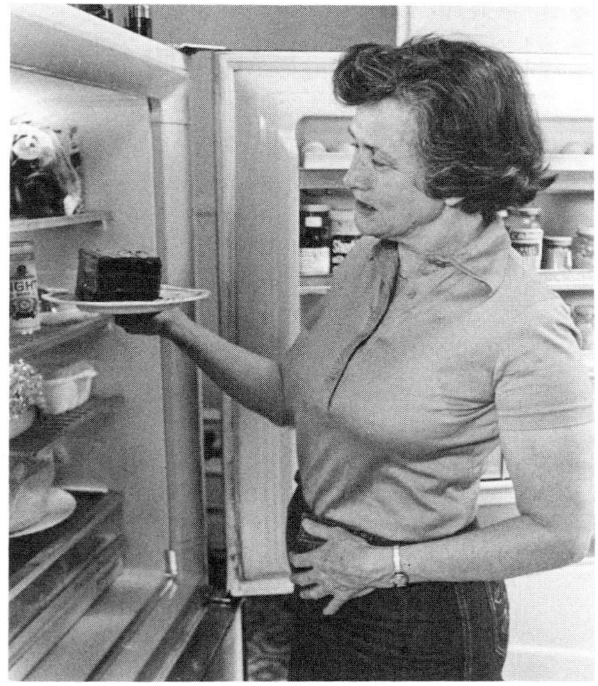

Interventions that employ stimulus control procedures attempt to eliminate specific undesirable responses, such as "sneaky" eating, rather than to modify all *eating responses. (Jean Boughton/The Picture Cube)*

and places. For example, wakefulness is a problem only for the person who is lying in bed in a dark room wishing to fall asleep. When this happens, it is called insomnia and may prompt a person to seek psychological help. The client certainly does not want to eliminate wakefulness completely, but just under certain stimulus conditions. Thus, the interventions used are called stimulus control procedures (see Chapter 6). For example, what would be the goal of a treatment for insomnia based upon a stimulus control paradigm? In Bootzin's (1972) study, the goal was to make the bed and bedroom the occasion for sleep rather than for worry—which is what insomniacs often do in bed. The instructions that Bootzin gave his subjects were:

* This term includes both aversive counterconditioning and aversive contingency management procedures.

1. *Lie down intending to go to sleep* only *when you are sleepy.*
2. *Do not use your bed for anything except sleep; that is, to not read, watch television, or eat in bed. Sexual activity is the only exception to this rule. On such occasions, the instructions are to be followed afterwards when you intend to go to sleep.*
3. *If you find yourself unable to fall asleep, get up and go into another room. Stay up as long as you wish and then return to the bedroom to sleep. Although we do not want you to watch the clock, we want you to get out of bed if you do not fall asleep immediately. Remember the goal is to associate your bed with falling asleep* quickly! *If you are in bed more than about 10 minutes without falling asleep and have not got up, you are not following this instruction.*
4. *If you still cannot fall asleep, repeat step 3. Do this as often as is necessary throughout the night.*
5. *Set your alarm and get up at the same time every morning irrespective of how much sleep you got during the night. This will help your body acquire a consistent sleep rhythm.*
6. *Do not nap during the day.*

(Bootzin, 1978)

How effective was this treatment? Over the course of the study, the subjects using this procedure decreased the time it took them to fall asleep by about seventy-four minutes. This was two to five times more effective than the other treatments used, including relaxation training, and placebo and waiting list controls.

In actual practice, a therapist would most likely use stimulus control procedures in combination with one or more other interventions. Spotlight 20.5 describes a multidimensional program for the treatment of obesity. Note that the problem in obesity is that the person eats too much and at inappropriate times and places. Unlike treatment for drug addiction or smoking, treatment for obesity cannot have as its goal the complete elimination of the problem behavior. Thus a stimulus control technique is very appropriate.

Spotlight 20.5 Behavioral Control of Overeating Using Stimulus Control and Contingency Management

Several studies have suggested that obese persons tend to eat in response to environmental cues rather than to internal, physiological cues (see Chapter 8). Thus, an obese person will be likely to have lunch when the clock says 12:00 o'clock (Schachter and Gross, 1968), whereas a nonobese person will be likely to eat when he or she experiences hunger pangs (Stunkard, 1959). So Stuart (1971) thought that to have an effective weight loss program, he would have to establish firm control over the food-relevant cues in his subjects' environments in addition to reducing the amount of food they ate.

In order to accomplish this, he used three types of intervention. First, he sought to eliminate or suppress cues that had been associated with overeating. For example, he had subjects prepare and serve only small amounts of food, eat in only one room, and do nothing except eat during mealtimes. Also, he had subjects chew their food slowly, swallow food already in their mouths before adding more, and eat with utensils. In addition, Stuart altered the consequences of overeating and normal eating. For example, he had subjects display the caloric value of food eaten daily as well as their weight changes. Furthermore, he arranged to have the family and friends of the subjects applaud diet success but ignore failure. In this way, he sought to increase the likelihood of desirable eating habits and decrease the likelihood of undesirable habits. Second, a balanced dietary program was prepared for each subject on an individual basis. And third, an individualized exercise program was also planned for each subject, based primarily on walking.

How effective was this program? Stuart found that the subjects lost about a pound a week for all thirty-five weeks of treatment. Furthermore, they were still losing weight at follow-up sessions six months after the termination of treatment.

Additional evidence was obtained in this study by using a control group. During the first fifteen weeks in which the experimental group received Stuart's three-dimensional program, a control group was given the same diet planning and exercise instructions that the treatment group was offered. However, they were merely told to practice "self-control," but were not told how to do this. Not only did this group fail to lose weight, but also, they gained about five pounds in those fifteen weeks. When, at the end of that time, they were given the three-dimensional program, they began to lose at approximately the same rate as the experimental group.

BEHAVIOR THERAPIES BASED ON SOCIAL LEARNING

Psychological Modeling

Many socially desirable behaviors, such as altruism, are learned through observation. Moreover, observational learning can be most easily accomplished if the model (for examples, mother, father, teacher, or therapist) has prestige, high status, competence, and is interpersonally attractive (Bandura, 1971). Thus, some improvement that occurs in traditional therapy may be the result of having a prestigious model—the therapist—unintentionally provide cues and values that patients adopt.

Modeling can be used for three distinct purposes (Bandura, 1965). First, it can be used to teach new skills (didactic). Therapists do not have to employ elaborate shaping procedures—waiting for the chance emission of a particular response and then reinforcing it. Through modeling, complex patterns of behavior can be learned by the observer in a relatively short time. For example, an extremely insecure person can learn to stand up for her rights by observing videotapes of assertive individuals coping with excessive demands.

Second, modeling can be used to strengthen or weaken the observer's tendency to act in a certain way by imparting information about the probable consequences of the behavior (vicarious reinforcement). If the model is punished for acting in a particular way, observers may draw the conclusion that they would receive the same treatment for the same behavior. So they will be much less likely to perform the action than if they had observed the model get rewarded or if the model was neither punished nor rewarded. Thus a child who observes a playmate get severely reprimanded for hitting a smaller child will be less inclined to hit other children.

Third, modeling can have a facilitating effect upon behavior (cuing). This means that it can act as a stimulus for similar, already learned behavior to occur even though the model does not get reinforced for the action. Thus, a person will be more likely to assist someone in distress if he or she has recently observed a model do so.

Enactive modeling. In this type of modeling a live model—most likely the therapist—demonstrates appropriate behavior. It is easy to see how this technique can be used. If an extremely violent child is brought in for treatment, the therapist can model aggression or nonaggression in the form of play activity using dolls. At the same time, the consequences of these actions—punishment or reward—are modeled for the child. If this modeling procedure is following by appropriate reinforcement in the child's home and school, the greatest reduction in aggression will probably be obtained.

Symbolic modeling. In this procedure filmed or videotaped models are used. Thus, a therapist can expand his or her treatment effectiveness to cover many kinds of problems. For example, symbolic modeling has been used to reduce the anxiety of

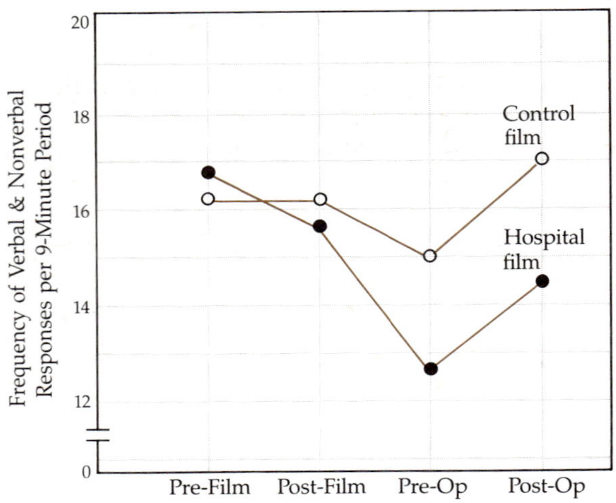

Figure 20.3 Anxiety in children facing surgery. The graph shows the frequency of observed verbal and nonverbal anxiety responses for the experimental and control groups during four different sampling periods. (From B. G. Melamed and L. J. Siegel, Reduction of anxiety in children facing hospitalization and surgery by use of filmed modeling, *Journal of Consulting and Clinical Psychology,* 1975, *43,* 518.)

children about to undergo various kinds of surgical procedures. In one study, children were either shown a film about a child being hospitalized for surgery or a control film about a child on a nature trip in the country (Melamed and Siegel, 1975). Those shown the nature film showed significantly more anxiety in the hospital than those shown the film about surgery, as illustrated in Figure 20.3. Furthermore, parents reported a significant increase in behavior problems three to four weeks after surgery in the group of children who had not seen the hospital film.

Covert modeling. In covert modeling the client *imagines* one or several models performing the behavior that is being learned. Cautela (1971) has demonstrated that covert modeling can be effective in reducing some kinds of avoidance behaviors and in remedying other behavior deficits. Covert modeling is, of course, easier and less expensive that enactive or symbolic modeling. However, the use of imagery always poses certain problems, such as ensuring that the image is indeed what the therapist thinks it is and in measuring it (imagery is a subjective process, after all). Another problem is that actual mastery experience is not provided in covert modeling.

Participant modeling. When using this technique, the therapist models the desired behavior, and in addition, employs a variety of induction aids designed to get the clients to actually try out the behavior themselves. For example, in the treatment of snake phobia, the therapist would provide aids sequentially from a preestablished hierarchy to enable the client to perform the feared activities successfully. Intimidating performances would be

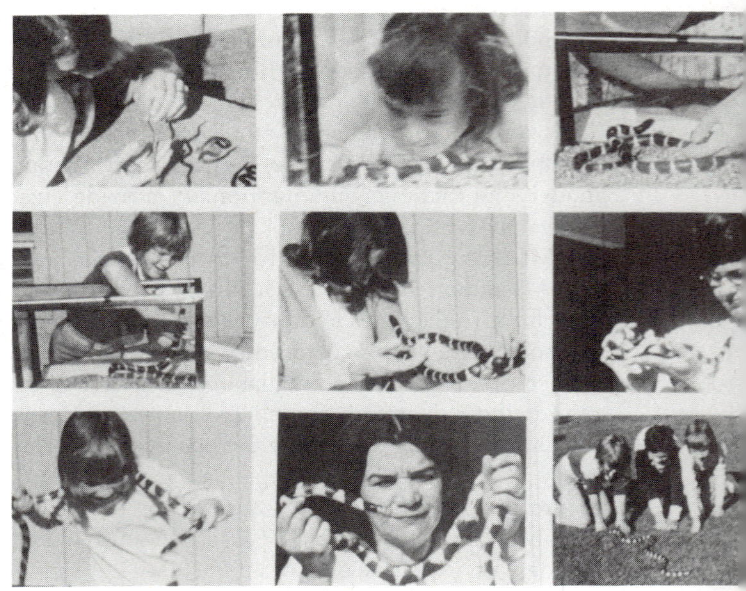

Figure 20.4 Children and adults modeling various levels of intensity of fear-arousing interactions with a king snake. (From A. Bandura et al., Efficacy of desensitization and modeling, *Journal of Personality and Social Psychology,* 1969, *13,* 179. Copyright 1969, American Psychological Association. Reprinted by permission).

broken down into easily mastered steps of increasing difficulty ranging from (a) looking at, touching, and holding the snake; (b) placing open hands in front of its head as it moves about; (c) holding the snake in front of their faces; (d) allowing the snake to crawl freely in their laps; to (e) letting the snake loose in the room and retrieving it (Bandura, Jeffery, and Wright, 1974).

This "stepwise induction of skills" in snake-touching is designed to gradually induce the subject to try out the feared behavior without the assistance of the therapist. Providing this sense of personal mastery has been empirically found to be extremely effective in reducing phobic behavior and in generalizing the new skills to nonexperimental situations (Bandura, Jeffery, and Gajdos, 1975; Bandura, Jeffery, and Wright, 1974).

Self-Regulation

Some exciting possibilities have arisen with the relatively recent investigations into self-regulation. It seems that almost any behavioral intervention that can be effectively used by a therapist, can be successfully self-applied by the client. Thus a person can develop a hierarchy of fear-producing scenes, and use self-desensitization to eliminate anxiety (Wenrich, Dawley, and General, 1976). Or a person can provide positive self-reinforcement for desirable actions and self-punishment for unwanted actions (Bandura, 1977b).

Although many different techniques can be self-administered, the process of self-regulation has three constituent parts. First, the relevant aspects of the problem behavior (for example, frequency, quality, rate) must be self-monitored to determine their baseline level. Second, once a reliable record of the behavior has been obtained, the person must set a goal specifying the desired posttreatment rate or quality of that behavior. Finally, a person must self-reinforce when and only when he or she attains that goal. Self-reinforcement can be as varied as reinforcement provided by others. It can consist of the opportunity to go out for dinner or to a movie, or it can be self-evaluative—when a person feels self-approving for outstanding achievements, or self-critical for substandard performances (Bandura, 1977b).

The most difficult aspect of self-regulation for many people is withholding the self-reinforcement until meeting the goal that they have set. One technique that has been used to make this more likely is the self-contract. This is a document that specifies the target behavior, the method of data collection, and the reinforcers to be used, among other information, which is dated and signed by the client and at least one witness.

Cognitive-Behavioral Interventions

The significant contribution of cognitive factors in emotional states such as depression (see Beck, Rush et al, 1979; Seligman, 1975) and in producing changes in behavior has already been noted. As a matter of fact, much of the preceding material suggests that many positive results in therapy research might in part be due to such cognitive factors as set and expectation of success or improvement. In addition, many treatments use the powerful effects of cognitive abilities on emotion and behavior.

Thus, we are beginning to see a merging of models and paradigms that were once seemingly irreconcilable—for example, the multimodal behavior therapy of Lazarus (1976, 1977). In fact, several of the interventions described in Chapter 19 might just as easily have been included in this chapter. For example, Ellis's (1962) rational-emotive therapy and Beck's (1976) cognitive therapy are probably just as accurately described as cognitive-behavioral interventions.

Bandura provided much of the impetus and rationale for incorporating cognition into behavior theory. His studies have led him to conclude that behavioral interventions are the most effective treatments, but that they produce their effects by altering relevant cognitions—especially self-efficacy, as discussed in Chapter 6 (Bandura, 1977a).

An illustration of the combined use of cognitive and behavioral strategies in controlling anger was described by Novaco (1977) who used a stress inoculation procedure, a skills-oriented approach in behavior modification that increases clients' coping skills through education, rehearsal, and the development of insight into the anger, anxiety, or other feelings the client has difficulty in controlling (Meichenbaum and Turk, 1976). Such cognitive strategies as using logic or humor, assessing other

Spotlight 20.6 Cognitive-Behavioral Interventions: An Illustrative Study

Cognitive approaches are becoming so popular that there are almost as many cognitive methods for producing therapeutic change as there are behavioral methods. Many of these interventions, when used in combination with behavioral procedures (cognitive behavior modification or CBM) are powerful tools for helping people to change. CBM methods include problem-solving and self-instruction training, problem relabeling, coping skills training, and correcting of irrational self-statements in combination with one or more of the behavioral interventions already described (Ledwidge, 1978).

An exploration of the effectiveness of a combined cognitive-behavioral approach with children follows. In an attempt to train impulsive children to stop and think before acting, Kendall and Finch (1978) made use of Kagan's work (1966) regarding the reflective-impulsive dimension. The reflective dimension refers to the ability to delay and to consider alternative behaviors when uncertain as to how to respond. Children with high reflectiveness tend to make correct choices under these conditions. The impulsive dimension, on the other hand, is characterized by impulsive and quick responses. Children with high impulsiveness tend to make incorrect choices. The MFF (Matching Familiar Figures Test; Kagan, 1966), which is scored for errors as well as for speed of response (latency), was designed to measure the reflective-impulsive dimension among children. The basic task of the MFF is to choose from an array of six variations one picture that is identical to the standard picture.

In the Kendall and Finch study, the first step was to select impulsive children from the new admissions to a children's treatment center on the basis of the MFF and to assign them randomly to one of two conditions. All children were given six training sessions. The subjects in the control condition received training in conceptual thinking, attention, recognition of details, and visual-motor reproduction.

The subjects in the experimental group received verbal self-instruction training through modeling: the therapist-model demonstrated how to talk out loud about possible ways of performing the task. The subject was then instructed to do the same. When the subject could do this, the therapist modeled self-instruction again—but whispered this time. Again the therapist encouraged the subject to do the same. Finally, the therapist "demonstrated" nonaudible self-instructions and the subject did the same (presumably). Furthermore, the experimental subjects also had to give up one of ten chips when they made errors. At the end of each session whatever chips remained could be used by the subjects to purchase a reward, such as candy.

The experimental group showed improved classroom performance as measured by less impulsive behavior, as well as by higher latency scores (more delay) and by lower error scores on the MFF test. The authors concluded that combined cognitive-behavior methods for altering impulsive behavior is more effective than traditional training methods. However, they did not determine whether self-instruction training or punishment (losing chips) alone would have been as effective as the combination.

options for coping and problem-solving, relabeling inner feelings in more constructive ways, and recognizing the beginnings of sequences that are likely to end in outbursts of anger, are combined with behavioral interventions such as relaxation training, desensitization, and modeling.

Cognitive-behavioral techniques have been applied not only to anxiety and anger problems, but also to obesity, alcoholism, depression, sexual dysfunction, fears, phobias, and other problems. Spotlight 20.6 presents another illustration of the use of cognitive training in combination with behavioral methods—this time in an attempt to increase the "reflectiveness" of impulsive children.

Already a great deal of empirical work has accumulated highlighting the importance of cognitive variables in therapy. And the cognitive-behavioral combination seems especially powerful. However, some therapists (see Ledwidge, 1978) remain unconvinced that cognitive-behavioral interventions are superior to behavioral interventions alone. The next ten years will probably see considerable attention to this issue.

BEHAVIORAL ASSESSMENT

Behavioral assessment is a general term for various procedures used to identify the behavioral target for change and to evaluate the subsequent effectiveness of the interventions (see Goldfried and Kent, 1972; Kanfer and Saslow, 1969). The traditional diagnostic categories—for examples, paranoid schizophrenia—say little about how to select, treat, or measure problem behaviors. Similarly, they do not tell what such individuals' lives are like, how they act in different situations, or how their families and friends respond to the maladaptive behaviors. This information is important to the behavior therapist. Therefore, behavioral assessment differs in these important ways from traditional assessment.

1. The problem behavior must be specified objectively. It is not sufficient that a client identify his or her problem as an "identity crisis," or even as "depression." The behavior therapist would try to assess the actual behaviors, feelings, and events that the client is labeling as "depression." These may include feelings of apathy, an inability to get out of bed before noon, and an avoidance of social situations.

2. Problem behaviors should be "counted"—that is, objectively recorded as having occurred by peers, teachers, parents, observers, or by the clients themselves. This is necessary so that a baseline of their occurrence can be established from which changes or improvement can be judged.

3. Generally, it is also necessary to identify any events that tend to occur just before and after the unwanted response so as to understand the immediate circumstances that tend to maintain its occurrence. For example, a client may experience intense anxiety that appears only when he or she enters an empty elevator alone; that same client may feel little anxiety when others are present. (This bit of information is only one of many necessary to establish a hierarchy of fears.) The therapist would also want to know the consequences of the behavior. For example, does a mother "give in" to her daughter's temper tantrums, and therefore reinforce them?

4. Data should be taken during treatment and at various times afterwards. In behavior therapy, assessment procedures are used to determine whether or not the therapeutic gains have been have maintained and whether or not they generalized to the client's day-to-day life.

5. If contingency management interventions are used, it is also necessary to ascertain the circumstances, behaviors, and events that are reinforcing to the individual so that they can be used in treatment. One person may find privacy reinforcing; another may find socializing reinforcing. The therapist must have this information.

Here is an example showing how behavioral assessment is used. A therapist would like to use cognitive-behavioral methods in order to decrease the amound of food that an obese person consumes so that this person will lose wieght. The therapist first must decide whether weight loss or change in eating habits is the primary goals. If change in eating habits is the focus, special data collection is necessary to keep track of where, what, when, how, how often, how much, and with whom the person eats. The conditions under which the eating took place would have to be recorded (for example, "alone in a cramped kitchen late at night, at which time a quart of ice cream and a pound of cookies were hastily eaten and all evidence of the binge removed; eating was 'normal' during the day"). Such material would have to be collected before, during, and after the behavioral program had ended in order to determine whether or not eating habits had changed. Thus, simply weighing the client would not yield sufficient data for a program of this sort.

Another example of behavioral assessment concerns a case of public-speaking anxiety. The therapist would first want to know when anxiety is experienced and how strongly it is felt. Does a large audience elicit more anxiety than a small audience? If the therapist if using systematic desensitization, he or she would want to construct a hierarchy of the client's fears, from the least to the most terrifying. He or she would probably also want to obtain several measures of anxiety and determine a baseline for the speaking behavior itself, so that changes in it can be assessed.

In attempts to modify behavior (for example, breaking a chain-smoking habit), it would be important to determine the circumstances that tend to maintain it—one of the goals of behavioral assessment. (Michael Weisbrot/Stock, Boston)

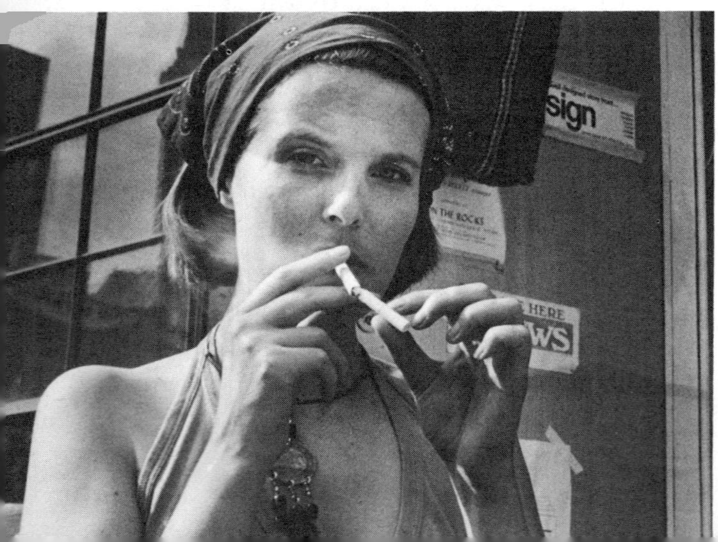

It is obvious that the content of assessment procedures varies widely. Furthermore, sources used for obtaining information are just as diverse: on one occasion, a therapist might make direct observations in a real-life situation; on another occasion, he or she might make observations in a laboratory setting, or observe responses in role-playing situations; on still another occasion, the client might supply the required information through self-report in a questionnaire (Goldfried, 1976).

It should be clear by now that there are important differences between traditional psychological assessment and behavioral assessment. Behavioral assessment does not result in global, "dynamic" personality descriptions or diagnostic categories. It is focused, specific, and generally based on objective evaluations.

Behavioral assessment yields baselines of behavior so that both the therapist and the client will have unambiguous information as to whether or not improvement has occurred. Above all, considerably fewer inferences are made about the "meaning" of responses and scores on behavioral assessment devices than is the case, for example, with Rorschach ratios or MMPI scores (see Chapter 5). But there are problems in behavioral assessment procedures, some of which are shared by traditional tests.

1. Self-ratings, questionnaires, observer ratings, and the establishment of hierarchies (as in desensitization) are all subject to the problem of reliability. How stable are self-reports over time? Do different observers of the same behavior arrive at the same assessment?

2. Observations in vivo—in real-life, naturalistic situations—are obviously desirable, because the goal is to alter behavior in the real world. But this may not always be possible with such behaviors as sexual arousal, deviant sexual behavior, or "sneaky" eating or drinking. How does one get self-report data that are accurate? Perhaps a role-playing situation or an imaginal process can elicit information otherwise difficult to obtain. But how valid are indices obtained from analogue situations such as in role-playing? Is imagining a feared situation the same as confronting the real thing? This needs to be

studied, but the answer is probably "no."

3. When using measurement, the therapist often has to deal with the possibility that the measurement device or procedure itself changes the behavior being measured, possibly in unknown ways. Measures of penile size in the treatment of sexual disorders and measures of blood pressure and breathing rate are all examples of methods that might affect the behavior being measured.

4. Sampling problems also exist. If one wishes to assess eating behavior through observation, one has to make sure to observe a representative sample of those situations in which the subject eats. (For example, does the subject eat alone? in restaurants? with friends? on weekends? during examination week? on a date?)

One also must make a decision regarding "time sampling." If, for example, the goal is to reduce a child's aggressive classroom behavior, the observer would want to be sure that he or she has picked a representative sample of time units during which to observe that child in the classroom. How often should the observer take measurements? Should he or she spot check at random times, or observe the child continuously for, perhaps, five minutes at the end of each hour? The time sampling procedure must allow the observer to determine how long the aggressive behavior lasts. It must also allow him or her to observe the antecedents and consequences of the aggression: is the aggression unprovoked? Is it in response to the teacher's goading or another child's aggression? Thus, just because behavioral assessment is objective, it is by no means without difficulties.

OUTCOME AND EFFECTIVENESS OF BEHAVIORAL INTERVENTIONS

It is possible to determine the effectiveness of behavioral interventions more reliably than most other methods. Because the goals of behavioral treatment programs are specific, public, and often contractually agreed upon, behavioral interventions are less open to the criticism noted in the last chapter regarding evaluation of the more traditional methods. Even so, there are some problems. Questions regarding the reliability of observations, self-ratings, and other measures continue to exist. Choice of appropriate control groups and of the appropriate length of follow-up periods after termination of treatment is still a problem. Furthermore, the importance of nonspecific placebo effects as possible underlying mechanisms for effective cures remains unresolved, as was discussed in Chapter 19 (Gomes-Schwartz, Hadley, and Strupp, 1978).

Nevertheless, there is an impressive amount of empirical evidence (Ledwidge, 1978; Stolz et al., 1975) that behavioral methods are effective in dealing with compulsions, insomnia, various kinds of sexual dysfunctions, some kinds of medical problems (such as asthmatic attacks), phobias, anxiety, speech disorders, self-mutilation, stealing, disruptive behavior in children (tantrums, fighting, screaming, etc.), dysfunctional language in retardates and psychotics, and various kinds of motor, cognitive, and social language skills in children at both preschool and school ages. Token economies have also been shown to be fairly effective in changing various kinds of behavior. In addition, promising results have been found with the use of counterconditioning methods with drug abusers, despite the many methodological problems of studies in this area (Callner, 1975).

But behavioral interventions are not consistently successful with certain problems, for example, alcoholism, smoking, tics, seizures, obesity, and rehabilitation of prisoners (Stolz et al., 1975; Yates, 1975). With many programs, treatment gains are not maintained at follow-up. One such area is weight control. Short-term control of food intake and concurrent weight loss are often followed by the usual finding: a return to pretreatment levels on follow-up evaluations.

However, the short-term positive findings with overweight patients are sufficiently encouraging as to provide an incentive for exploring possible methods for producing long-term results. One empirical finding, for example, suggests that the maintenance of immediate weight loss might be enhanced through the social pressures within group behavior therapy rather than individual behavior therapy (Kingsley and Wilson, 1977). Furthermore, there is a growing belief that the dependency that often develops in the therapist-client relationship can be avoided by placing greater reliance on self-regulatory procedures (Carter, Rice, and DeJulio, 1977). In fact, a recent study (Bandura and Simon, 1977) on self-regulated weight loss provides suggestive evidence that weight loss can be maintained by having clients self-monitor their weekly weight change and reimposing treatment on themselves when their weight goes above a certain predetermined level.

Are behavioral methods superior to psychodynamic methods when the same type of client is treated? Many studies have attempted to compare behavior therapy to psychodynamic therapy in a systematic way; one of these efforts is described in Spotlight 20.7. The results of investigations such as these show that behavioral interventions tend to be more effective than psychodynamic therapies. However, these studies also show that often any treatment is better than no treatment, with the implication that nonspecific effects are powerful ingredients of therapeutic change.

Despite the positive results of many outcome studies of behavioral interventions, psychodynamically oriented psychologists insist that be-

Spotlight 20.7 Behavior Therapy versus Psychodynamic Therapy: Is There a Winner?

All other things being equal, and with the best possible intent and delivery of services, which of the two general orientations, behavioral or psychodynamic therapy, produces the better results? This was the question asked by a team of investigators determined to arrive at an answer in a systematic, controlled way (Sloane, Staples, Cristol, Yorkston, and Whipple, 1975a,b).

The 90 subjects were clinic patients (mostly white females between the ages of eighteen and fourty-five years) with anxiety neuroses or personality disorders. These subjects were randomly assigned to one of three groups: four months on a waiting list (control group), four months of behavior therapy, or four months of psychodynamic therapy. Treatment sessions took place once each week.

In decreasing order of frequency, the subjects' symptoms were generalized anxiety, interpersonal difficulties (particularly with the opposite sex), low self-esteem, generalized worry, and bodily complaints. Excluded from the study through initial interviews were patients thought to be psychotic, mentally retarded, brain damaged, or in need of medication. All assessment was done independently of the actual treatment itself.

The six therapists (three for each of the two orientations) were experienced professionals. The control group was given the same assessment procedures but did not receive treatment. However, they were called every few weeks to remind them that they were on a waiting list and would soon be seen for treatment. All ratings were made by judges blind to the subjects' experimental condition.

During the initial interview, the patient and the assessor outlined three major target problems. The severity of each was rated. Additional ratings were also made, such as of work adjustment and social adjustment. The independent assessors rated these areas at the end of four months as well as one year after the first assessment.

Attempts were made to evaluate the status of the waiting-list group by inquiries of close friends or relatives.

This list of some of the guidelines drawn up by the research team for their therapists' techniques presents some differences in treatment.

Contrasting Elements	Behavioral therapy	Psychodynamic therapy
Frequent specific advice given	yes	no
Interpretation of transference	no	yes
Interpretation of resistance	no	yes
Interest in dream reports	no	yes
Explicit training in relaxation	yes	no
Use of desensitization procedure	yes	no
Practical retraining	yes	no
Explicit training of assertiveness	yes	no
Use of aversive methods	yes	no
Role training	yes	no
Practice in new skills	yes	no
Childhood memories as focal point	no	yes
Direct treatment of problems ("symptoms")	yes	no
Common Elements		
Biographical history taken	yes	yes
Formulate the problem	yes	yes
Seek original cause of problem	yes	yes
Seek current causes of problem	yes	yes
Try to produce beneficial change	yes	yes

Source: Adapted from Sloan et al., 1975a, pp. 237–40.

What were the results? After four months, the two treated groups improved significantly more than the nontreated group on target problems. However, all groups, including the waiting list group, improved. There were no significant differences between the two treatment groups in the actual amount of improvement.

Four months after treatment, however, a global, overall rating of improvement showed that 93 percent of the behavior therapy group improved, whereas only 77 percent of the psychodynamic therapy and waiting-list groups improved. Furthermore, even though all the groups showed significant improvement at the one-year assessment, only the behavior therapy patients showed significantly more improvement than the waiting-list patients. Thus, although both behavior and psychodynamic therapy seemed equally effective immediately after treatment, behavior therapy promoted greater overall improvement in functioning as long as one year after the termination of therapy.

It is important to remember, however, that all groups—even the waiting-list group—improved. Perhaps one of the reasons for this is that patient self-efficacy expectations can be changed in diverse ways and that this improved self-efficacy is responsible for clinical improvement, as Bandura (1977a) has proposed.

havioral methods are generally less appropriate than theirs for vague problems of alienation, despair, existential neurosis, loneliness, marital difficulties, antisocial behavior patterns, and similar difficulties. But the proponents of behavioral interventions tend to disagree: there are few problems, they assert, that cannot be approached through one behavioral method or another or some combination of interventions.

OVERVIEW: PROS, CONS, AND ISSUES

Because behavioral interventions are still controversial to many people—especially nonpsychologists—this section will comment on the status of the area. What are some of the problems facing it? What directions will it take in the future?

Behavior modification's bad name. Behavior therapists worry about the bad name of this field in the media and with the public. Some even blame themselves for using mechanistic terms like "social engineer," "behavior control," or "behavioral programmer" (Wilson and Evans, 1976). Beyond this, however, the public and press have often confused behavioral techniques with psychosurgery, electronic brain control, electroshock therapy, and chemical or pharmacological control of unwilling and unsuspecting people (Asher, 1974). However, none of these are behavioral interventions. Behavior therapists never use electronic, chemical, electrical, surgical, or any other type of brain intervention.

Since the earlier years of behavior therapy, the public has become more accepting of it. The testimonials of those who have been treated successfully have certainly helped to bring about this change in attitudes.

Informed consent and competence to judge. Almost all would agree that informed consent should be given by the client before any treatment is given. No problems with this policy arise when the client and therapist plan a treatment based upon a mutually agreed-upon goal. But problems often do arise when one applies the informed-consent criterion to very young children, to autistic children, or to extremely retarded individuals. These people may be informed, may consent, but may not, really, want to be treated. What does voluntariness or informed consent mean to someone who wants only to please those in authority or who is afraid to say no? Are these individuals freely choosing from among alternative options? Helpless people may feel that resisting the offer of treatment may prompt retaliation or disfavor on the part of the people in power. But there is another issue that has to do with the competence of an individual to judge what might be good for him or her. An incompetent individual may require a lay advocate. But how about competent minors? Should not they be allowed to make the decision for themselves?

What should one do with an *incompetent* minor? Should a parent make the decision? But some parents may themselves be incompetent to judge. What if consent of parents and of a special review board were required?

The vast number of legal briefs being written on this issue outlines the significance of these questions. One proposal suggests that a Human Rights Committee be formed in each state to help determine such weighty matters (Friedman, 1975). In that proposal, clients' consent would be weighed against clients' competence to judge. There are six possible situations, all yielding a decision as to whether or not to introduce a psychological procedure. For example, if a client says "no" to a procedure but his or her mental competence is uncertain, the committee would vote "no" to the procedure. A competent client who says "yes" is given the "go-ahead" sign. All clients, competent or otherwise, should be guided by a legal or lay advocate in reaching a decision.

Philosophy of behavior methods. An elusive criticism of behavior methods concerns its general philosophy: by reducing deviations, differences that are displeasing, or that make people uncomfortable, or make life difficult, are we leveling off individual differences in society (Kittrie, 1971)? What is the advantage to society of having people without deviances from the group standard? Do therapists mechanize people or dehumanize them by the use of behavioral interventions?

A reply to this criticism is that societies have always attempted to decrease deviations through many means quite independent of behavioral psychology—through laws, traditions, education, religions. And many insist that with regard to dangerous criminals, such as murderers and rapists, society has the right to protect itself for the common good. Therefore, the use of any method that will work toward controlling antisocial activity such as extreme and intractable violence, for example, is for the common good and therefore socially, morally, and ethically appropriate. Furthermore, if therapists fail to provide treatment, they are failing to meet their responsibility in settings in which the right-to-treatment issue has already been established—in state hospitals, for example.

Beyond these issues, however, all therapies exist in order to assist people in solving their difficulties, in making their lives more satisfying in some way. Thus, if behavior therapy is guilty of reducing the amount of variation in our society, so are the therapies described in Chapter 19. For example, many practitioners of orthodox psychoanalysis assume that a heterosexual marital relationship is an important treatment goal; cognitive therapy has a goal for its clients to become more logical and less "automatic" in their thinking than they were before therapy. In actuality, behavior therapy may be less susceptible to this criticism than some other approaches. Because the clients themselves define the goals of therapy, they can use the therapists' expertise to help them develop the competencies they value, rather than to be taught to conform to some predetermined norm.

Behavior therapy and psychotherapy. Behavior therapy apparently works. *Why* it works, however, is not yet clear (Yates, 1975). There is growing belief among behavior therapists that such factors as therapist characteristics, and relationship variables may contribute significantly to therapy's effectiveness. In fact, many behavior therapists (see Wilson and Evans, 1976) stress the significance of nonspecific factors in therapy and are joining their traditional, psychodynamic colleagues in talking about empathy, rapport, and suggestion as powerful ingredients in effecting therapeutic change.

Furthermore, as previously described, there is increasing evidence that cognitions, such as self-efficacy expectations, may be the medium of change in therapy—that behavioral (and traditional) interventions change behavior by altering clients' thoughts about what they can and cannot do.

Thus we can see that behavior theory and therapy has become much less radical since Skinner first defined operant learning. Behavioral and traditional therapists have more of the same concerns—cognitions, inner standards and evaluations, self-directed behavior, and interpersonal skills of the therapist. In fact, they are also using more of the same techniques. As a large body of literature has accumulated on the effectiveness of behavioral interventions, many traditional therapists have incorporated them into their practice. It is not unusual for a neo-Freudian to use systematic desensitization, for example. We can see, therefore, that the ideas of the traditional and behavioral therapists are converging in many ways. It should be kept in mind, however, that many of their assumptions about personality and abnormal behavior and the explanations for a particular technique's effectiveness are drastically different, as should be apparent from the descriptions in Chapters 19 and 20.

SUMMARY

This chapter discussed the characteristics and history of the behavioral interventions for abnormal behavior. It noted that the behavioral approach rejects the medical model of psychopathology and considers much deviant behavior to be modifiable through structured learning experiences (therapy). These therapeutic experiences can be classified into those that employ classical conditioning, operant learning, and social learning. The chapter described many types of behavior therapies and presented the types of problems to which they can be applied, case illustrations, and research results. It also addressed various issues involved in behavior therapy—for example, the philosophy that underlies it and the evidence regarding its effectiveness.

Highlights

1. Among the most important techniques based upon classical conditioning are systematic desensitization, flooding, implosion, aversive counterconditioning, and covert sensitization.
2. Systematic desensitization, flooding, and implosion are employed to decrease a client's anxiety regarding, and avoidance of, a harmless but feared object or situation.
3. Aversive counterconditioning and covert sensitization are employed to increase a client's anxiety regarding, and avoidance of, an inappropriate desired object or situation.
4. Among the important strategies based upon operant learning are contingency management and stimulus control procedures.
5. Contingency management procedures alter the frequency of behaviors by modifying their consequences. These procedures include reinforcement, extinction, token economies, and aversive techniques.
6. Stimulus control procedures are employed when the target behavior is not always maladaptive. It is used to alter the number and type of situations in which the behavior occurs.
7. Social learning techniques—such as modeling, self-regulation, and cognitive-behavioral methods—are designed to teach the client new cognitions as well as new behaviors.
8. Behavioral assessment differs in some important ways from traditional psychological assessment. Above all, behavioral assessment is more focused, specific, and objective than are the more "global" methods of projective tests such as the Rorschach technique and the Thematic Apperception Test.
9. There is an impressive amount of empirical evidence that behavioral interventions are effective in dealing with a wide variety of disorders.

ISSUES AND QUESTIONS

1. As mentioned in this chapter, there has been considerable discussion among psychologists as to ethical guidelines for therapists. The Association for the Advancement of Behavior Therapy has developed a checklist designed to evaluate the ethicalness of treatment. The eight general sections on this checklist are:

   a. Have the goals of treatment been adequately considered?
   b. Has the choice of treatment methods been adequately considered?
   c. Is the client's participation voluntary?
   d. Does the therapist refer the clients to other therapists when necessary?
   e. Has the adequacy of treatment been evaluated?
   f. Has the confidentiality of the treatment relationship been protected?
   g. Is the therapist qualified to provide treatment?
   h. When another person or an agency is empowered to arrange for therapy, have the interests of the subordinated client been sufficiently considered?

   (Stolz, 1978, p. 72)

   Do you think that such a checklist would adequately protect the rights of clients? Can you think of a better set of guidelines?
2. One of the differences between behavioral and traditional therapies is in what the participants are called. What do you think would be the ramifications of calling a person a "client" rather than a "patient?" What would be the ramifications of calling the therapist by his or her first name, rather than "Doctor?" Which would you prefer?
3. If you had a problem that you could not solve for yourself, would you consider seeing a therapist? If so, which type of therapist would you prefer—a behavioral, psychodynamic, cognitive, or some other type of therapist? Would the nature of your problem make any difference?

4. There are certain behavioral interventions whose theoretical bases are still controversial.
   a. In one of the procedures—time-out—the subject is removed from a reinforcing environment contingent upon emitting an undesirable behavior. Thus, a violent child might be put alone in an empty room for three minutes whenever he kicks or punches another child. Do you think this is an instance of extinction, aversive contingency management, or some other process?
   b. In another procedure—overcorrection—the subject not only corrects an undesirable situation that he or she has caused, but also *over*corrects it. For example, a patient in a mental hospital who overturns a bed in a dorm might be required not only to right that bed and make it up again (correction), but also to straighten the bedclothes on all the other beds in the dorm (overcorrection). How would you explain the effectiveness of this technique?
5. Does therapy perpetuate the status quo? Does it provide for social change to accommodate the needs of people? Or does it merely provide for personal change to accommodate the needs of society? Is there a difference among the various therapeutic models in this regard?

SUGGESTIONS FOR FURTHER READING

Lovaas, O. I., and Bucher, B. D. (Eds.) *Perspectives in behavior modification with deviant children.* Englewood Cliffs, N.J.: Prentice-Hall, 1974. This book is a collection of articles by eminent people who work with deviant children in the domains of self-help and social skills, language behaviors, childhood fears, parental control, school behavior, self-injurious behavior, and stimulus control techniques. It is a useful and informative book for advanced undergraduates, graduate students, teachers, and parents.

Mahoney, M. J. (Ed.) *Psychotherapy process: Current issues and future directions.* New York: Plenum, 1980. This is a scholarly book for the advanced undergraduate, graduate student, and professional who is interested in pursuing many of the current controversies within the field of psychotherapy. A wide range of topics—such as specifying "nonspecific" factors, "decontrolling" cognitive control, biomedical psychology, imaginal processes, and many others—are presented in a format that allows for consideration of the pros and cons of many important issues.

Mahoney, M. J., and Thoreson, C. E. *Self-control: Power to the person.* Monterey, Calif.: Brooks/Cole, 1974. The first part of this interesting, readable book gives the social learning theory of self-control, describes self-assessment procedures, outlines the use of stimulus control and contingency management techniques for self-control, and provides a basis for "behavioral humanism." The second part of the book consists of fourteen readings on self-control by eminent people in the field. Anyone new to the area of behavioral self-control should find this book helpful.

Rimm, D. C., and Masters, J. C. *Behavior therapy: Techniques and empirical findings* 2nd ed. New York: Academic Press, 1979. This is a scholarly book explaining various types of behavioral interventions, such as contingency management, systematic desensitization, modeling, and self-control. It also provides case histories and experimental evidence regarding the various techniques. This excellent book may be useful for many people who desire to change their behavior, as well as for people who would like more information about the many behavioral techniques and their uses.

Stuart, R. B., and Davis, B. *Slim chance in a fat world: Behavioral control of obesity.* Condensed edition, revised. Champaign, Ill.: Research Press, 1978. Paperback. This very practical and readable book represents a behavioral approach to weight management. It takes the reader through the steps of defining the problem behaviors, choosing the interventions, and implementing them. Numerous appendixes provide valuable nutritional and health information as well as prototypes of assessment forms.

Wenrich, W. W., Dawley, H. H., and General, D. A. *Self-directed systematic desensitization: A guide for the student, client, and therapist.* Kalamazoo, Mich.: Behaviordelia, 1976. Paperback. This is a very clear and amusing guide to the history, relationale, and implementation of self-desensitization. Examples of commonly employed hierarchies and detailed instructions for the Jacobson relaxation exercises are given.

21

Other Interventions and Mental Hospitals

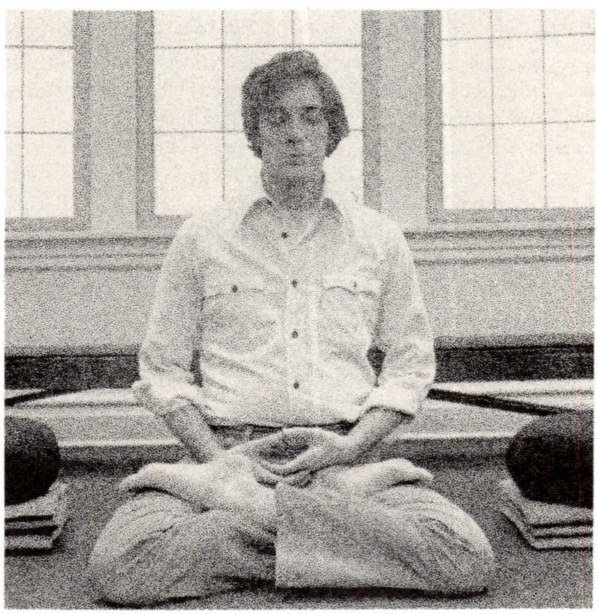

The traditional psychotherapies and the different behavioral interventions are not the only methods that are used to help people with emotional and mental problems. This chapter makes our survey more complete by describing (1) some additional nonphysical therapies such as biofeedback and hypnosis; (2) some physical therapies, especially pharmacological interventions; (3) mental hospitals and some relevant considerations; and (4) interventions in other countries.

SECTION I: SOME ADDITIONAL NONPHYSICAL THERAPIES

BIOFEEDBACK

Description and Clinical Uses

When people practice throwing darts, shooting baskets, or putting golf balls, they evaluate their progress by seeing if they are on target—or if not, by gauging how much off they are. They see the results of their efforts: failure, success, almost-on-target. The awareness of the consequences of their acts helps them in shaping future acts—a process termed feedback. All people need feedback so that with practice they can adjust their aim. If they were blindfolded, however, and there were no one around to tell them the outcome (consequences) of their acts, there would be no feedback. They could go on aimlessly shooting darts without correcting their movements. If someone were watching that performance, however, and evaluating it in the light of the goal—too high, too much to the left, too much energy in the shot—that evaluation would be feedback.

It has always been assumed that feedback could aid in the adjusting of voluntary responses only, as in throwing darts, whereas *involuntary* responses, such as heart rate or skin temperature, could not be modified in this way. How could feedback help people to control blood pressure, for example, if the people are unaware of and thus do not control these responses to begin with? So-called visceral responses, it was thought, could not be controlled by the methods of operant conditioning. Developments in biofeedback methods have altered this assumption dramatically.

Biofeedback is the term for a number of different methods designed to help people learn to modify various bodily responses, of which they are generally unaware, through the use of instruments that monitor and simultaneously provide information to the subject about these responses as they are occurring. The purpose of biofeedback is thus to help the subject become aware of hitherto inaccessible information so that eventually he or she can learn to voluntarily modify responses, especially those thought to be "abnormal," for example, higher than normal blood pressure, or irregular heartbeat (cardiac arrhythmia).

In other words, if we measure heart rate, heart rhythm, brain waves, blood pressure, galvanic skin responses, muscle tension, or skin temperature and display in some simple way an immediate, continuous, understandable record of these bodily processes while the subject is "hooked up," we can inform him or her—through a signal—when the internal response (for example, brain waves, heart rate) is within the desirable (normal, healthy, physically adaptive) range.

The refinement of measurement devices, recording apparatus, and computerized methods for transforming data has made much of the progress in biofeedback possible. In particular, biofeedback makes use of instruments that amplify or enlarge small changes in the system that is being measured. A display system signals when these changes bring the response into the desired area. Clicks, lights, buzzes, colored lights—any display, visual or auditory—that can communicate or signal when the desired responses are reached are essential so that the subject is "informed" of whether he or she is on target.

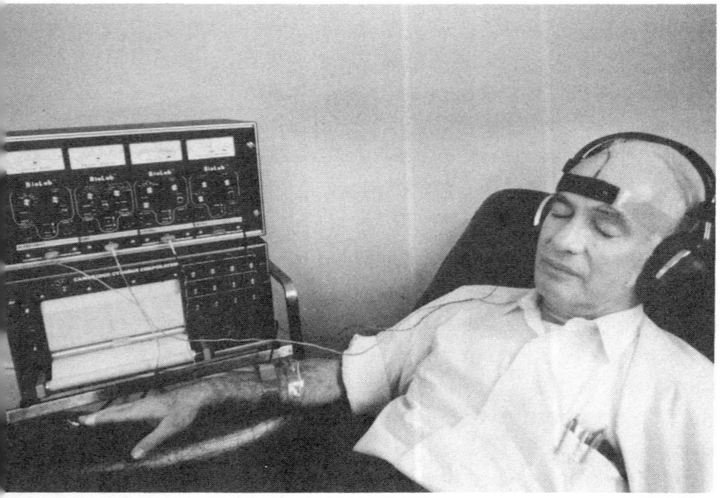

A biofeedback "hookup." (*Owen Franken/Stock, Boston*)

In just a few trials, it has been found that subjects are able to maintain many of these responses within a desirable range. They have voluntarily controlled a biological function without willing it or consciously attempting to manipulate it. As a matter of fact, trying too hard often makes biofeedback control more difficult to achieve than unselfconscious trying. That is, if subjects wish to produce internal controls or changes, he or she must relax to allow the control to occur. Subjects are often given training in relaxation responses prior to actual biofeedback trials.

Biofeedback methods have a respectable history in the experimental laboratory (Miller, 1969). Early in the 1960s, there was a report (Razran, 1961) of some Russian work with humans demonstrating that subjects learned to avoid electric shock by vasodilation (enlarging or widening of blood vessels) as a result of watching continuous records of their vasomotor activities. At about this time in America, Neal Miller was reporting success in the conditioning of certain autonomic responses in rats. Soon there began to trickle into the experimental literature many demonstrations that humans could regulate (control and modify) their internal systems through use of monitoring and signals that keep them informed as to what is going on internally.

One area of early feedback research that caught the public eye had to do with brain wave (EEG) activity. Alpha-wave activity is a special kind of rhythmic electrical brain activity that can be increased or decreased through biofeedback training. Because it was observed that people who were meditating (see pp. 648–50) showed increased alpha activity, it was thought that enhancing alpha activity could produce the states of relaxation thought to be a product of meditation. It was soon believed that alpha waves were associated with a level of alertness or consciousness that could be characterized by a pleasant, relaxed, "nonflappable" mood or state (Brown, 1970, Kamiya, 1969).

The media soon popularized alpha activity beyond its importance. People thought that the little machine attached to electrodes on the head was *doing* something to induce relaxation or decrease anxiety. But after the flurry of popular and professional interest, objective research indicated that the hopes placed on the significance of alpha activity in inducing a pleasant, nonanxious state were empty. For many controlled studies indicated that an increase in alpha does not compensate for sleep deprivation or provide restorative or recuperative rest; further, it interferes with cognitive efforts, does not reduce acute or chronic anxiety (and is often not incompatible with anxiety), and can even be rather unpleasant for some people (Miller, 1978).

Biofeedback methods designed to reduce pain, especially headache, have fared somewhat better. One of the many different types of headache is the tension headache, induced by muscle tension of the frontalis, a rectangular layer of muscle extending from the eyebrows to some distance up the forehead and to the sides of the head. Learning to control muscle tension, it was thought, could be an important therapeutic device.

Electromyograph (EMG) methods record muscle contractions and relaxations through measures of electrical discharges from the muscle fibers.

When there is less muscle activity, there is lower electrical activity. Biofeedback procedures amplify this electrical activity and display it to the subject. Under these conditions, it has been found that many subjects can voluntarily reduce the muscle tension sufficiently so as to modify or eliminate the pain experienced.

Another common headache is the migraine type described in Chapter 8, which in classic form is thought to be caused by dilation of the cranial blood vessels. Dilation is probably triggered by some irregularity in the autonomic nervous system in response to various internal cues, such as certain foods or the body's stress response. Treatments that have employed medications to produce vasoconstriction have had moderate success. Psychoanalytic and psychodynamic therapies, on the other hand, have been somewhat unsuccessful in the treatment of migraine (Adams, Feuerstein, and Fowler, 1980).

Biofeedback methods, it was thought, held out much promise for controlling migraine, especially with people for whom other treatments were contraindicated. The idea was to increase blood circulation in the peripheral system by helping the subject to increase the temperature of the fingers, which in turn, would reduce cerebral circulation and thus the headache (Sargent, Green, and Walters, 1972).*

Although claims for great success with this method were initially made—as high as 50 to 70 percent improvement, according to Orne (1979)—a review of the relevant experiments indicated that the relationship between finger temperature and migraine is not clear (Turk, Meichenbaum, and Berman, 1979). Further, there have been few demonstrations that patients can control the relevant physiological systems to reduce migraine headaches when they are separated from the continuous feedback of the monitoring system (Adams, Feuerstein, and Fowler, 1980). Most studies, as a matter of fact, demonstrate only small finger-temperature changes, with greater *decreases* than increases achieved (King and Montgomery, 1980).

* Actually, early peripheral temperature control combined biofeedback methods with autogenic training that helped people to relax by verbal self-instruction such as "I feel calm and my fingers are heavy and warm."

Evaluation

What is the picture of success with biofeedback? In addition to the successful use of EMG methods in inducing general muscle relaxation and relieving tension headaches and pain that come from the tightening of muscles in forehead and neck, EMG methods also have been successfully used in subvocal speech while reading, and in controlling fine motor movements, as with cerebral-palsied individuals or in rehabilitation after facial surgery (Blanchard and Young, 1974; Brener, 1974; Brown, 1974; Fuller, 1978; Miller, 1978).

Moderate, but encouraging, results have also been achieved with regulating cardiac arrhythmias, reducing frequency of some types of seizures, lowering blood pressure in essential hypertension, reducing bruxism (clenching and grinding of teeth), controlling incontinence, and reducing symptoms of Raynaud's disease (pathological constriction, as in frostbite, of peripheral blood vessels) by control of volume of blood flow to peripheral areas such as finger tips.

Despite these reported successes in the clinical application of biofeedback, the method has some problems that should be mentioned:

1. A major assumption of biofeedback is that after training, the patient is able to transfer the learned control over his or her internal responses (whatever that system is, for example, blood pressure) to conditions outside of the laboratory and that these effects will endure over a period of time (Miller, 1978). This generalization or transfer of learning has not been adequately demonstrated (Turk, Meichenbaum, and Berman, 1979).

2. The specific methods by which biofeedback has demonstrated some learned control over involuntary systems may be due to placebo effects and various cognitive factors in the same way that

expectation of successful treatment is a powerful determinant of success of other forms of treatment (Lazarus, 1976; Meichenbaum, 1977; Plotkin and Rice, 1981; Schwartz, 1973; Turk, Meichenbaum, and Berman, 1979). Does the personality of and confidence in the therapist affect results? Are there individual differences in ability to be trained? Does the impressiveness and charisma of the procedure—for example, the elaborate instrumentation—affect the results? Probably yes, according to Miller (1978). Further, because biofeedback methods have often been used in conjunction with other methods such as relaxation training, it could be that the *specific* effects of biofeedback are still unknown (Miller, 1978).

3. Also, many patients seek help when acutely ill. Acute problems, such as a sudden rise in blood pressure or migraine headaches, tend to return to a normal state even if there is no treatment. The general picture, thus, is bound to improve, with or without biofeedback. As a matter of fact, biofeedback procedures should not be recommended indiscriminately or viewed as a cure. They may be unnecessary or even contraindicated for some people, as in some types of high blood pressure, for example. The "undesirable" system may be an expression of a disease process requiring a knowledgeable decision as to its desired range and purpose in modifying it (Fuller, 1978; Miller, 1978).

4. Overall, detailed evaluations of biofeedback methods indicate that the picture is not as promising as had initially been claimed. Problems in evaluating reports of success as well as confusion as to why biofeedback works challenge the "super claims" as to its effectiveness (Miller, 1978; Winer, 1977; Yates, 1980). Thus, statements that biofeedback promises new forms of communication between mind and body with limitless possibilities for control over visceral or internal functions and that *any* "centrally" controlled internal system that can be measured in some way can be brought into voluntary control should be taken with a grain of salt, despite evidence that biofeedback is moderately successful in controlling some internal systems.

HYPNOSIS

Is hypnosis something more than a flamboyant demonstration of some mind-altering experience under the control of someone who has special powers to put the subject into a trance-like state, or is it a legitimate demonstration of the complex capacities of the human brain that we do not completely understand? The answer is probably the latter.

What is hypnosis and what are the mechanisms that underly it? First, hypnosis is probably best conceptualized as a heightened response to suggestion, especially in cooperating with the suggestions of the hypnotist (Spanos and Barber, 1974), for example, in not feeling pain (hypnotic analgesia). Hypnosis can also be conceptualized as an intense, heightened state of concentration and attention in which peripheral, extraneous cues and stimuli are minimized if they contradict the "central framework" provided by the hypnotist. Such heightened, focused concentration can be induced by signals from within or without. Hypnosis, thus, is a state of extreme concentration in which virtually all stimulation other than the ones relevant to the hypnotic period are ignored while the suggestions of the hypnotist are unconditionally accepted (Spiegel and Spiegel, 1978).

Other definitions stress the notion that the hypnotic state represents a special type of awareness and consciousness—an "altered state of consciousness" in which there is "divided" awareness. We will return to these considerations shortly, because there is some controversy regarding the merits of each of these models.

What Hypnosis Can Do

1. Hypnosis is often introduced as an adjunct to other treatment modalities (Kihlstrom, 1979), for example as an aid in remembering early experiences or in inducing relaxation and imagery in the context of a behavioral intervention such as desensitization. It has been used in connection with

Spotlight 21.1 Myths About Hypnosis

Misinformation about hypnosis abounds. Some people view hypnosis as a strange, occult phenomenon used primarily by entertainers or quacks. In stage demonstrations, it is believed, people from the audience are "made" to do silly things for the amusement of others. Others sometimes view hypnotized subjects as fakers. Or highly hypnotizable subjects are viewed as weak-willed or unintelligent.

Actually, many researchers indicate that "good" hypnotic subjects are often more intelligent and strong-willed than "bad" hypnotic subjects. Further, hypnosis is not a "pathological" state and hypnotizable subjects are not emotionally disturbed (Kihlstrom, 1979). Here are some popular myths:

Hypnosis is sleep. Hypnotized subjects often close their eyes while in a "trance" and breathe quietly and regularly, causing some people to assume that hypnosis is a form of sleep. In addition, hypnotists sometimes use sleep terminology to induce the hypnotic state (for example, "you are getting sleepy"). Although hypnosis, like sleep, is characterized by a reduction in peripheral awareness, that reduction is caused by a focusing of attention and concentration rather than by the dissolution of attention that occurs in sleep. Also, EEG patterns in the two states differ markedly. Alpha waves often increase during the hypnotic state, but not in the sleep state.

Hypnosis is projected onto the subject. According to this myth, hypnosis is forced upon, or "induced" in, the subject. Actually, the hypnotist offers the opportunity for the subject to become hypnotized only if there is motivation to do so. Even highly hypnotizable subjects, if unwilling, cannot be hypnotized. Further, posthypnotic suggestions are not carried out by the subject against his or her will.

Hypnosis occurs only when there is a hypnotist. The "trance" state can and does occur spontaneously in everyday experiences in many people with trance capacity. The "trance" state can in fact be voluntarily self-induced through learned self-hypnosis techniques.

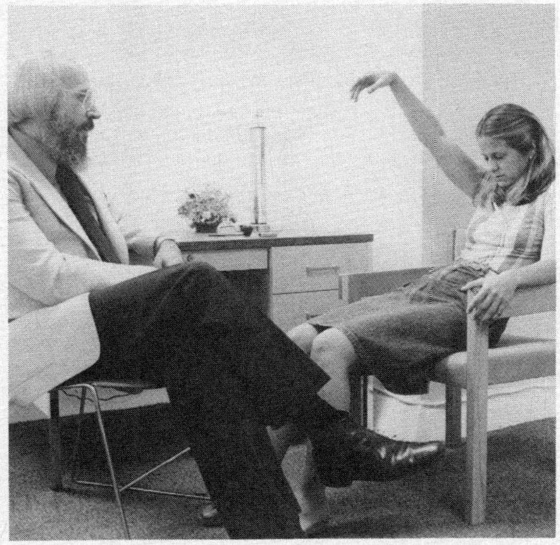

Hypnosis is not an occult phenomenon, and the hypnotist, despite the common belief to the contrary, has no special powers to control the mind of the subject. (Ken Buck/The Picture Cube)

Hypnosis is dangerous. There is no evidence that hypnosis is dangerous. In fact, it is regarded by many clinicians as an extremely useful technique. A word of caution, however: because hypnotic subjects are especially sensitive to suggestions provided by the hypnotist, they might pick up an inexperienced hypnotist's anxiety or fear. Hypnosis, thus, should be practiced only by an experienced, responsible hypnotist.

Hypnosis is therapy. The hypnotic state can be used as an aid in a therapeutic situation, but it is not, in itself, therapy.

A hypnotist must be charismatic to get results. Contrary to this myth, most hypnotists have no special, unique characteristics or particular personal charisma. In fact, peculiarities in a hypnotist may actually inhibit his or her ability to facilitate the hypnotic state, for subjects must be accepting and trusting of the hypnotist before allowing themselves to be hypnotized.

Women are more hypnotizable than men. This statement, which apparently developed out of the sex-stereotyping that holds that women are more passive, suggestible, and dependent than men, is simply, statistically, untrue.

Source: Adapted from Kihlstrom, 1979; Spiegel and Spiegel, 1978.

lowering anxiety and fears (for example, of flying or of public speaking), substance abuse, eating disorders, and insomnia (De Piano and Salzberg, 1979; Kihlstrom, 1979; Spiegel and Spiegel, 1978).

Of special interest is the use of hypnosis with psychosomatic and psychogenic ailments such as skin disorders, headache, and asthma, based on controlling various autonomic nervous system variables such as rate of blood flow. An extensive review of relevant research, as a matter of fact, concluded that hypnotic methods have shown moderate usefulness in treating skin disorders, such as psoriasis and boils, and headache, but that the most promising results have been with asthma (De Piano and Salzberg, 1979).

2. Under hypnosis, if asked to regress to a younger level (for example, to the age of three years), some subjects report compelling experiences that are of a more intense nature than are those reported by subjects simulating hypnosis (Schofield and Reyher, 1974). Subjects in these states, called age regression, behave—talk, think, function—as if they were at the regressed level. Some behave in developmentally "valid" ways, for example, demonstrating fears and emotional responses appropriate to an earlier childhood level; these subjects remember experiences long ago forgotten or use fluently a foreign language of their early years (Kihlstrom, 1979). Most experts agree that although there is not an actual return to childhood modes of functioning, there is a genuine age-regression phenomenon that is not "faked" or simulated (Nash, Johnson, and Tipton, 1979).

3. It is perhaps in the hypnotic reduction or elimination of pain in the dentist's chair, childbirth, or surgery, or with chronic pain, that hypnosis demonstrates its greatest effectiveness.

Why Does Hypnosis Work? Some Contrasting Views

Hypnosis played a major role in Freud's "discovery" of the unconscious and in explaining symptoms of conversion hysteria (Kihlstrom, 1979). In hypnotic states, it was thought, there is a divided awareness in which splits from the conscious level can occur, so that two levels of consciousness simultaneously can influence and guide behavior without the levels being in communication with each other. These "splits" are sometimes referred to as dissociations. In hypnosis, dissociation is illustrated by hypnotic analgesia or posthypnotic suggestions* (for example, amnesia for certain events), and in psychopathology, by conversion symptoms (so-called hysterical symptoms of blindness or deafness) and multiple personality syndromes described in Chapter 9.

This splitting or dissociation in awareness helps us to understand hypnosis, according to Hilgard (1973, 1977), who proposes that people do indeed experience divided awareness—an involuntary

* Suggestions made to the subject under hypnosis that are carried out by the subject in the posthypnotic state, generally without the subject's knowing why.

Spotlight 21.2 Chronic Pain Patients: Some Treatment Approaches

It is said that over 50 million people in this country complain of chronic or recurrent pain. This pain may have an organic basis, as in certain kinds of headache, cancer, or orthopedic injuries. But also, the pain may have no diagnosable physical basis. In such instances of psychogenic pain (see Chapter 8) as well as in many instances of organically-based pain, pharmacological and surgical interventions often prove fruitless. Chronic pain patients may go from doctor to doctor dutifully paying bills, eliciting sympathy (at first) from families, quitting jobs and eventually dedicating their lives in endless quest for *the* medicine, treatment, surgical procedure, or gimmick which can relieve their agony. Eventually, their lives become a continuous drama: decisions about which doctor, what medication, and what appointment become enmeshed with their complaints, sleeplessness, anger, and preoccupation with self. Clinicians who use traditional medical or psychological interventions, such as verbal psychotherapy, with pain patients often experience similar frustration. However, a new specialty offers promise to both patient and clinician, a specialty devoted to treating the pain patient independently of the underlying causes, in attempts to modify the pain—or the perception of pain—itself (Holden, 1977; Sternbach, 1974).*

Some interesting findings have emerged from work with pain patients. For example, a surprisingly large number of patients respond to placebo, to expectation of improvement, and to several methods addressed to the handling of anxiety. Cognitive factors are apparently of great significance in handling pain patients, especially those having to do with the therapist-patient relationship, expectancies concerning pain relief, and belief in the method used. The severity of the physical problem is often not related to the intensity of the suffering. And anxiety in connection with pain is a significant variable in the suffering experienced.

Further, because the perception of pain occurs in the brain (pain associated with phantom or nonexistent limbs is a good example of the brain's role in the subjective experience of pain), it should come as no surprise that many psychological methods are effective in reducing or alleviating chronic pain—headache, for example. In pain clinics all over the country, many different interventions, singly and in combination, have been employed to help chronic pain patients, often without any search for causes, emotional or physical. These methods include behavioral interventions, for example in reinforcing behaviors associated with being well rather than those having to do with pain, or by eliminating reinforcers that maintain the pain response, such as medication or the attention or pity from family members (Fordyce, 1976). Other methods include biofeedback, hypnosis, training in relaxation, and use of placebo and suggestion.

In this chapter, some of Hilgard's views about hypnosis as a special dissociative state are described. Hilgard arrived at these hypotheses through his interest in hypnotic analgesia, the reduction of pain experiences during hypnosis (Hilgard and Hilgard, 1975). In some experiments, Hilgard discovered that many hypnotic subjects demonstrate *two* levels of awareness—the hypnotized level and another level that is continuously monitoring and experiencing awareness of what is happening under hypnosis, the so-called hidden observer (Hilgard, 1973, 1977).

For example, under hypnosis, one of Hilgard's

---

* The discussion of psychogenic pain in Chapter 8 mentioned the role of recently discovered neurochemicals, the endorphins and the enkephalins. These chemicals, produced by triggering mechanisms within the body, are probably related to the blocking of pain perception. There are several methods of pain suppression not discussed here that probably block pain signals by stimulating neural pathways to release these chemicals (Liebeskind and Paul, 1977). These methods include the electrical stimulation of specific brain areas, cutaneous electrical stimulation of regions of the skin near painful areas, and acupuncture (which involves the insertion of very fine needles into specified body locations and manually twirling them or passing through them a low-voltage electrical current for brief periods of time).

subjects was able to hold her hand in ice water for several minutes, an experience that is excruciatingly painful under normal conditions, but that she claimed was painless. At the same time, however, another hand was writing a message that claimed that she was experiencing the pain with great intensity. Hilgard's work with many subjects in hypnosis confirms his view that there is a split in consciousness—with two levels of awareness during hypnosis, one that the hypnotized subject reports directly and overtly and the other that is deeply covert within him or her. The covert level can actually report pain through the "automatic writing" noted above, or through pressing a key, or raising an index finger while there is no awareness at all of pain on the other "conscious" level.

Whether a special "split" in awareness is involved, or, as others suggest, only a heightened suggestibility on a continuum with normal awareness (Stam and Spanos, 1980), there is little doubt that hypnotic methods are playing an increasingly important role in dealing with chronic pain.

parallel processing of streams of information on different levels. These levels are not in touch with each other. The hypnotic subject, according to Hilgard, is willing to relinquish or to delimit the role of the conscious "central executive and monitoring system" (p. 277), thus allowing other usually hidden levels to exert their influence more readily, even to surface when the conditions are appropriate, as in age regression, but without conscious awareness that this is happening. In other words, concealed experiences on deep levels are presumed to parallel the *conscious* experiences of the subject. It is in demonstrating the presence of some of these concealed experiences that Hilgard's ingenious experiments with pain are concerned (see Spotlight 21.2).

Hilgard's assumptions that hypnosis involves special instances of divided or split-off levels of awareness—dissociative states of the types involved in instances of multiple personalities, fugue states, or conversion symptoms—are challenged by Barber and his associates, who do not view hypnotic phenomena as reflections of a special state but rather as part of a continuum of normal mental processes involving intense imagery. As a matter of fact, these experimenters have been able to explain most "dissociative" hypnotic phenomena, for example, with regard to memory or pain perception, on the basis of set, suggestion, and imaginal processes. Expectancies, beliefs, motivation, suggestibility, and a general responsiveness to the "demands" of the hypnotic situation all enter into hypnosis, which

> *involves a shift in set or orientation away from the pragmatic one that governs our everyday transactions to one that involves imagining. This shift in orientation appears to involve at least two interrelated components: (a) a tendency to carry out and also to elaborate imaginings consistent with the suggestions that are administered, together with (b) a tendency to simultaneously ignore or reinterpret information that contradicts the imaginings (Spanos and Barber, 1974, p. 503).*

As a matter of fact, so-called hypnotic phenomena can be induced by an experimenter *without* hypnotic induction, according to many experimenters (see Barber, Spanos, and Chaves, 1974; Spanos and Barber, 1974). Cognitive aspects are thus stressed in many conceptualizations about why hypnosis is effective. Such models of hypnosis permit the possibility that a hypnotist's suggestions work because of placebo factors and that symptom alleviation after hypnosis may be based on motivation to change rather than on a special "ingredient" intrinsic to the hypnosis itself (Kihlstrom, 1979).

A third view proposes that highly hypnotizable subjects possess special attentional skills: they are better able to focus, and to attend to an instruction regarding the presented task despite difficult or distracting conditions (Karlin, 1979). Still another view proposes that hypnosis is nothing more than placebo and trust. Most experts agree, however, that processes in addition to placebo effects are brought into play in hypnosis, and that even though a skilled hypnotist will "maximize" placebo-related variables like trust and belief, some additional process seems to be involved (Kihlstrom, 1979).

Hypnotic Susceptibility*

It is well known that susceptibility to being hypnotized is a relatively stable characteristic; about 10 to 15 percent of the general population are highly hypnotizable; about 70 to 80 percent, moderately hypnotizable; and about 10 to 15 percent, not hypnotizable (Spiegel, 1974b). Highly susceptible subjects respond easily to hypnotic induction and various posthypnotic suggestions.

Are there personality differences between highly hypnotizable subjects and poor hypnotic subjects? Poor hypnotic subjects are described as fearful of ambiguous situations and of losing control over themselves. They distrust the hypnotist and the hypnotic situation. What are highly hypnotizable (susceptible) subjects like? One description, based on thousands of clinical cases, is that although showing excellent memory, these subjects are influenced primarily by cues from the present situation while ignoring or minimizing critical judgment based on past experience. They are suggestible and trusting and therefore "go along" with unfamiliar or unexpected explanations, metaphors, and incongruities. Susceptible subjects also have a capacity for intense and focused concentration and can "affiliate" or identify with new events (Spiegel, 1974b). High hypnotizable subjects are also described as especially creative and imaginative, as being able to think effortlessly and in a wholistic manner, much as if the nondominant cerebral hemisphere is involved (Bowers, 1979).

A few experts are so taken with the striking differences between susceptible and nonsusceptible subjects that they even wonder whether or not some genetic determination or some early imprinting (more or less permanent learning that occurs early in life) accounts for susceptibility or lack of it (Spiegel and Spiegel, 1978). However, most clinicians believe that hypnotic susceptibility is at least partially learned and can be increased moderately with appropriate training procedures (Kinney and Sachs, 1974).

Overall, then, good subjects do not contest or critically evaluate the validity of suggestions, situations, or imaginings generated by the hypnotist through verbal suggestion or even visual suggestion. Most investigators agree that under hypnosis, awareness of realities, experiences, and logic that contradict these imaginings is minimized, reduced, not acknowledged through the intense focus on and attention to the suggested experience (J. R. Hilgard, 1970; Sarbin and Coe, 1972). We all have experienced some form of such intense focus when we "lose ourselves" entirely in a book, or while watching a movie or play.

* Measuring hypnotic susceptibility rests on the demonstrable differences among different people in capacity to become hypnotized. Tests of susceptibility generally measure some form of response to suggestion. One much used measure is the Stanford Hypnotic Susceptibility Scale (SHSS—Weitzenhoffer and Hilgard, 1959). A more recent measure is Spiegel's Hypnotic Induction Profile (HIP—Spiegel, Aronson, Fleiss, and Haber, 1976). The HIP is a quick (five to ten minutes) test that includes, among other tasks, the "eye-roll" measure of suggestibility (ER) which, according to these authors, has an extremely high correlation with hypnotizability in a nonpsychotic "normal" population in which there are no neurological deficits or history of drug abuse (Spiegel, 1972; 1974a). The ER measure requires the subject to look upward (up-gaze) while closing his or her eyes (roll) and then asking the subject to open his or her eyes, letting them come back into focus. ER measures the amount of white showing in the eyes. According to these authors, the more white visible between the lower eyelid and the lower edge of the cornea, the more hypnotizable is the subject. In 2,000 consecutive cases of psychotherapy, the ER measure predicted hypnotic capacity in three out of four cases. The higher the roll capacity, the higher the "trance" capacity.

Evaluation

Hypnotic phenomena are best viewed as reflections of the remarkable range of cognitive behaviors of which the human brain is capable, for example, capacity for vivid imagery or intense attentional focus, rather than as an "occult" or mystical anomaly or quirk of some human minds. Moreover, as a short-term change agent, hypnotic methods can sometimes be more effective than most long-term psychotherapies (for example, in controlling overeating, as an aid to smoking cessation, or in reducing chronic pain). On the other hand we have a long way to go before we understand why some people are highly hypnotizable and just what happens in hypnotic suggestion such as age regression, analgesia, or posthypnotic amnesia. Obviously, the answers lie somewhere in the future when we know more about the intriguing capacities of our brains, personalities, and motivations to alter and to modify our perceptions about ourselves and the world around us.

MEDITATION METHODS AS THERAPY

In recent years, Eastern religions and philosophies have been explored, even embraced, by some Americans, especially young Americans interested in retreating from "establishment" values and practices. No attempt will be made to explore how some practices in these religions such as hatha (exercise) yoga and meditation are used to achieve religious insight or "liberation" from worldly cares. Instead, certain aspects of meditation and some of the claims made about its benefits will be described.

Meditation techniques have been learned by thousands of Americans of diverse life styles and ages. Some claim that as a result they experience an altered state of consciousness with such desirable qualities as sharp clairvoyance or ecstasy. Many practitioners of meditation are more reserved, however, but still claim that meditation has provided them with an easing of tension—generating feelings of relaxation, peace of mind, and a reduction of anxiety and worldly worry. Are these claims valid? Are meditation methods successful in reducing anxiety, providing a sense of well-being, and helping some people solve personal problems?

Many different types of meditation methods are practiced in this country, particularly Transcendental Meditation (TM), a simple, nonreligious technique developed by the Maharishi Mahesh Yogi and brought to this country in 1968. Most of these methods require the meditator to choose a quiet, not too brightly lit place or special room or area, and to sit in the lotus position, generally on the floor. The position, however, is not essential. Rather, it is the mental state and activities of the meditator that is the active ingredient in meditation methods. Most meditation methods also require cognitive focusing—enlisting the concentrated attention of the meditator on something such as a word or phrase (mantra) that is constantly repeated. The focus can also be on an internal visual image (such as a mandala), a prayer, or a bodily process such as pulse, heartbeat, or breathing. Frequently required is a passive attitude in which thoughts and awareness of what is going on in and outside of the meditator are allowed to pass gently through the mind—a kind of quiet observation of all mental content and experience and awareness. Many meditators meditate for about twenty mintues twice a day, in the morning and in the evening.

The beneficial effects claimed for meditation methods range from fear and anxiety reduction, reduced heart rate and oxygen consumption, increased alpha wave activity, reduced blood pressure (not only during meditation, but also throughout the day), and control of hypertension (Benson, 1975; Shapiro and Zifferblatt, 1976; Wallace, 1970). It is also claimed that meditation can ease recovery from stress (Goleman and Schwartz, 1976) and that it is correlated with a decrease in self-reported anxiety (Thorpe, 1977), improved performance on a complex perceptual-motor test (Blasdell, 1974), improved refinement in auditory discrimination (Graham, 1974). In addition, retrospective accounts from over 1,800 meditators showed a significant decrease

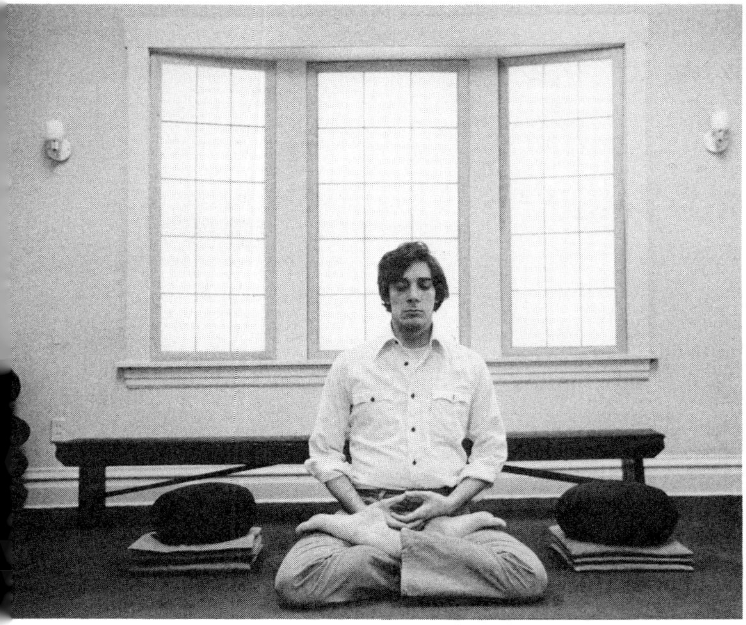

A meditator in the lotus position. (Jean-Claude Lejeune/Stock, Boston)

in drug use accompanying the practice of meditation (Benson, 1975).

One large-scale study of these claims (Benson, 1975) used volunteers who had been practicing meditation for two to three years. In the observation session, after thirty minutes had elapsed (during which time the subjects were expected to adjust to the presence of several monitoring instruments), measurements were recorded during alternate periods of sitting quietly and during meditation. Results showed that during meditation, oxygen consumption, heart rate, respiration, and blood lactate were lowered while alpha waves increased in amplitude and regularity. These findings suggest that while meditating there is a decreased activity of the sympathetic nervous system accompanied by a state of restfulness and relaxation (Relaxation Response).

Such responses, it was thought, represent the physiological opposite of the "fight-or-flight" response—an arousal response characterized by increased muscle tension, palmar perspiration, heart rate, adrenalin secretion, and brain wave activity.

> *Modern society has forced us to evoke the fight-or-flight response repeatedly. We are not using it as we believe our ancestors used it. That is, we do not always run, nor do we fight when it is elicited. However, our body is being prepared for running or for fighting, and since this preparation is not always utilized, we believe anxieties, hypertension and its related diseases ensue. The Relaxation Response offers a natural balance to counteract the undesirable manifestations of the fight-or-flight response (Benson, 1975, p. 173).*

Other explorations into the effects of meditation, however, yield less optimistic findings. For example, numbers of migraine headaches were not reduced; and the practice of meditation is not more effective in reducing anxiety than are some forms of sitting or other nonmeditation procedures (Boswell and Murray, 1979; Smith, 1977); in a minority of subjects, there is even an increase in anxiety and depression (Otis, 1974).

Evaluation

Some of the reported physiological responses during meditation occur in ordinary states of resting, relaxation, and sleeping. That meditation offers a special, unique state of consciousness cannot be confirmed, for apparently many meditators actually go through different stages of sleep while meditating (Pagano et al., 1976). It may well be that the long-term, positive effects of continued meditation practice may be oversold, because personality change does not take place with its continued use (Zuroff and Schwarz, 1978).

Moreover, the presumed spiritual effects of meditation ("freeing," "liberating"), as in Eastern religions, may actually result from the prestige and charisma of the guru or instructor, rather than from factors intrinsic to meditation. In this sense, psychotherapy and meditation may have much in common, for belief, expectancy, and placebo effects having to do either with the guru or the method

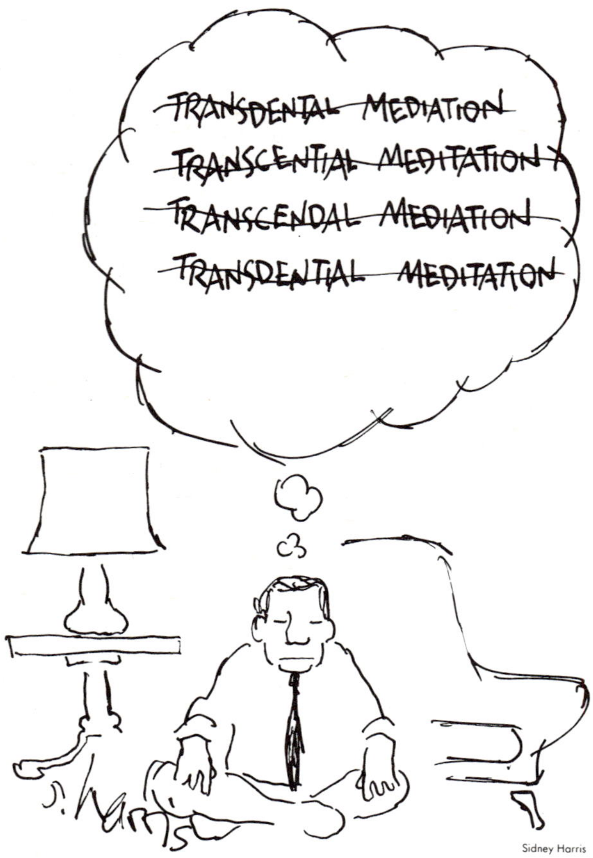

may play a large part in reducing anxiety and tension and increasing peace of mind (Watts, 1961). As a matter of fact, some experts believe that behavioral self-control methods and meditation have a large common core (Shapiro and Zifferblatt, 1976).

Many hold that meditation in combination with other procedures such as biofeedback or psychotherapy can be extremely helpful in reducing anxiety and tension. Meditation methods, however, are neither a cure-all or panacea for emotional ills, even though learning to relax through various techniques can be extremely helpful in the handling of stress and tension.

SECTION II PHYSICAL THERAPIES

PHARMACOLOGICAL INTERVENTIONS

Since the 1950s, the proliferation of drugs for soothing feelings, getting through the day, falling asleep, studying for an examination, lifting mood, or reducing tension has reached alarming proportions. A few hundred million prescriptions for minor tranquilizers (for example, Valium, Librium, Miltown) are written each year. Even a decade or so ago, the figures were staggering: In 1970, drugstores in the United States filled 214 million (new and refill) prescriptions. Almost half of these were for antianxiety drugs. In the same period, a survey indicated that almost one-third of American adults used one or more psychotherapeutic drugs (prescription or over-the-counter), with Valium alone being used regularly by 15 percent of this population (Lyons, 1979). Most of the prescriptions were written by general practitioners. Women took considerably more tranquilizers and sedatives than did men (Mellinger et al., 1974).

More data: According to the American Chemical Society, there are 4,039,907 distinct chemicals, of which 33,000 to perhaps 60,000 are probably in daily use (Maugh, 1978). Thousands of these are drugs developed for treating emotional problems. Of "nonorganic," chronic mental patients, it is estimated that 87 percent were "maintained" on drugs (Lentz, Paul, and Calhoun, 1971). We are indeed a drug culture. The pharmaceutical companies are profiting. Are the patients?

Psychotropic (also called psychotherapeutic, psychoactive, neuroleptic, or ataraxic) drugs refer to a class of chemicals that are prescribed for the treatment and control of emotions, mood, and psychotic ideation. These chemicals generally "bind" or lock into certain cells of the brain that have the appropriate structures, called receptors, to receive them. Psychoactive drugs are used in or out of hospital settings, often in conjunction with other methods of treatment. They are conventionally classified as the antianxiety drugs (minor tranquilizers), the antidepressants, and the antipsychotic drugs (major tranquilizers). In addition, there is lithium, used in the control of certain types of affective bipolar disorders and related syndromes. How are they used? What is their track record?

Antianxiety Drugs

As a group, the benzodiazepines are among the most widely used tranquilizers for daily living, with millions upon millions of prescriptions written each year for Valium and Librium alone, not to mention meprobamate (trade names of Equanil, Miltown) and Dalmane (the most frequently prescribed sleeping pill). Prescriptions for their use are written routinely by physicians when confronted with many problems they do not feel equipped to deal with, such as anxiety, insomnia, tension, phobias, restlessness, and general unhappiness. Sometimes these medications, when used sparingly and under supervision, can be helpful in the handling of minor anxiety, occasional sleeplessness, or in meeting a situational crisis or specific stressor. They can even be helpful in easing agitated patients into a counseling or treatment situation, be it behavioral, psychodynamic, or family, or they can be used as adjuncts to some of these treatments.

Scientists only recently have begun to explore the reasons for the drugs' actions, that is, how those substances produce the subjective and behavioral effects experienced as reduction of anxiety, muscle relaxation, and sedation. Laboratory evidence, based largely on animal research, has accumulated in that past few years that points to the strong possibility that the benzodiazepines' receptors in the brain bear a close relationship to neurotransmitters in the GABA system as well as to other naturally occurring substances in the brain (Kolata, 1979b; Tallman et al., 1980). Neurotransmitters in the GABA system perform a major CNS inhibitory and anticonvulsant action, and it may be that the benzodiazepines achieve their effects by interacting with chemicals with this inhibitory quality.

Most of these so-called minor tranquilizers are potent drugs with many side effects of which millions of users are unaware. High or even moderate dosages over a period of time are associated with tolerance and abstinence syndromes. Termination of chronic usage, for example, may result in convulsions and other major physical symptoms. These drugs are synergistic (have a combined effect) with alcohol and are CNS depressants; they are often used incorrectly to relieve a depressed mood. Overdosing with or without alcohol—especially with Valium—is well known in hospital emergency rooms, as a matter of fact.

There are additional problems. Infants born to women who used these drugs during the first six weeks of pregnancy have many more birth defects than do newborns whose mothers do not use drugs (Milkovich and van den Berg, 1974). Other side effects, even with light use, include impairment of motor skills, drowsiness, and decrease of judgment so that their use is not recommended when operating machinery, driving, or piloting planes.

Antidepressant Drugs

Although some types of depressions (the so-called psychoneurotic ones) do not respond to medications and are probably more effectively treated by other approaches (for example, Beck's cognitive therapy), many depressions of the so-called endogenous variety, which may have biochemical underpinnings, do seem to "lift" with the carefully supervised administration of drugs, especially of the tricyclic type (Akiskal and McKinney, 1975; Depue and Monroe, 1978).

The MAO (monoamine oxidase) inhibitors represent a large group of antidepressant drugs that were first employed for mood-elevating purposes after the discovery, early in the 1950s, that several chemically related drugs used for treating tuberculosis created mood-elevating effects in some patients. These drugs were soon to become unpopular, however, because of their many side effects. For example, the chemicals in them interact poorly with certain types of aged cheeses, chocolate, and chicken liver, resulting in increases in blood pressure to dangerously high levels in some patients and in others causing extreme agitation, jaundice, or convulsions.

Tricyclic drugs (for example, Elavil and Tofranil) were gradually favored over the MAO inhibitors because of their fewer physical risks and more impressive record of results. A review of 93 experimental, double-blind, placebo-controlled studies of tricyclic drugs, for example, indicated that about 65 percent of the investigations reported success in reducing depression (Morris and Beck, 1974). Other reports of researches (specifically of imipramine—Tofranil) indicated even higher success rates (Berger, 1978; Cole, 1970). Side effects, however, continue to be a problem for these drugs. These include dry mouth, urinary difficulties, constipation, excessive sweating, slow heartbeat (tachycardia), weakness, and fatigue, and even the possibility of myocardial infarctions (heart attacks).*

The beneficial effects of these medications are not felt immediately (a few weeks may be required). As a result, there may be an extremely stressful period for some patients, even a risk of suicide, unless there is intervening help in the form of social supports and individual therapy. Although biochemists appear to be getting closer to understanding the brain chemistry responsible for mood levels and for the "lifting" or elevating of those levels, they are a long way from understanding precisely how these drugs work. There appear to be large individual differences in response to medications: with some people, depression is lifted, whereas with others there appears to be little or no effect. Thus, there is often much trial and error in any individual situation before an effective medication regime is established.

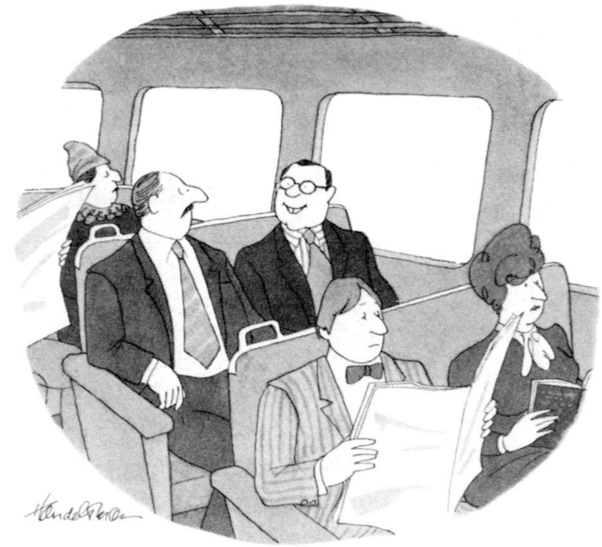

"Your tale is very sad, Ben. I'm almost sorry I took an anti-depressant."

Overall, psychotherapy is often a necessary adjunct to medication not only for the above reasons, but also so that the patient's pessimistic views about himself or herself, the world, and the future are modified and the sense of helplessness and powerlessness that is so characteristic of depressed people is challenged.

Lithium

J. F. J. Cade, an Australian physician, introduced lithium as a possible treatment for manic states on the basis of some success with a limited number of patients (1949). Since that time, it has been consistently confirmed that lithium carbonate, a natural salt or ion, is about 80 percent effective in the control and prevention of manic episodes in people with a diagnosis of manic-depressive illness. Lithium's impressive record of effectiveness in con-

* New drugs that have fewer side effects are constantly being tested in this country and abroad. Some of these are related to the tricyclic drugs, chemically speaking, and others are not so related. One recently introduced rather promising drug, now marketed in this country is Ludiomil, and another, not yet marketed, is Mianserin.

trolling manic episodes, manifested by poor judgment, racing mental and verbal activities, and excitability, is common knowledge here and abroad (Tosteson, 1981).

Of more recent discovery is the effectiveness of lithium salts in reducing the severity of and frequency of depressive swings in instances of manic-depressive (bipolar) depression (Dunner, 1975; Akiskal and McKinney, 1975; Depue and Monroe, 1978). But lithium is apparently effective only with certain types of depressive patients, and its use must be carefully monitored as to blood levels.

The use of lithium salts to limit the frequency or severity of manic episodes is not as simple as it sounds, for the euphoria and heightened sense of importance and power manic patients experience often cause them to resist medication. With depressed patients there may be similar resistance, not only because the patient is unwilling to accept the fact that he or she must rely on medication to get better, but also because of the necessity for routine monitoring of chemical levels within the body.

Overall, lithium has fewer side effects than do many other psychoactive medications and although its use depends on careful diagnostic appraisal of its appropriateness, it offers much promise to sufferers of bipolar affective disorders (see Chapter 10).

On the other hand, the unreserved enthusiasm for lithium displayed by some of its research pioneers in this country (see Fieve, 1975) with its implications of panacea for all depressions, has been seriously criticized by scientists and clinicians as too sweeping and as raising false hopes for many depressed people for whom lithium is inappropriate.

Antipsychotic Drugs

The discussion of treatment approaches to schizophrenia in Chapter 11 noted the relative success of the phenothiazines compared to other methods, for example, psychotherapy. Perhaps no other achievement in the field of mental health has had such a dramatic effect on the treatment of mental patients as did the development of the antipsychotic drugs. How did all this come about?

Antipsychotic drugs were developed as a result of interest in rauwolfia, a natural root used in India over a period of many years, which seemed to have many interesting effects on people. In the early 1950s reserpine, derived from rauwolfia, soon came into widespread use in the treatment of high blood pressure. But it was also noted at that time that reserpine had several side effects, such as dramatic decreases in anxiety, tension, and insomnia. As a result, researchers became interested in the possibility of deriving other chemicals that could have similar beneficial effects.

At about this time, in the early 1950s, French scientists were synthesizing chlorpromazine, one of the phenothiazines, which seemed to be showing dramatic promise in curtailing some of the flagrant symptomatology of some schizophrenic patients. Chlorpromazine was soon to be widely distributed in Europe (largely known as Largactil) and in the United States (Thorazine). The initial promise of success stimulated a flurry of activity in the laboratory to develop other chemicals in the phenothiazine family. By the mid-1950s, phenothiazines had been synthesized, and the use of antipsychotic drugs had begun to be viewed with favor by many clinicians.

In addition to the phenothiazines, the properties of other chemical families, and their effectiveness as "major" tranquilizers, were also explored. Table 21.1 lists some of these generic drugs and some of the brand names associated with them. Each has special qualities and differing degrees of effectiveness with patients depending on chronicity, age, and other variables.

What do these drugs do? In many schizophrenic patients, these drugs do all the things we want them to do: they control disorganized thinking, increase social and interpersonal skills, reduce delusions and hallucinations, reduce or eliminate bizarre behavior, and counteract agitation, excitement, and violent impulses. Unfortunately, these drugs also produce many side effects in initial phases, such as drowsiness and sleepiness and impairment of perceptual and motor functions, espe-

Table 21.1 Psychoactive Drugs

Representative Antianxiety Drugs

Generic Name	Brand Name
Benzodiazepines*	
Chlordiazepoxide	Librium
Diazepam	Valium
Oxezepam	Serax
Propanediols	
Meprobamate	Equanil, Miltown
Tybamate	Solacen
Miscellaneous	
Azacyclonol	Frenquel
Benactyzine	Suavitil
Phenaglycodol	Ultran

Representative Antidepressant Drugs

Generic Name	Brand Name
Monoamine Oxidase (MAO) Inhibitors	
Isocarboxazid	Marplan
Phenelzine	Nardil
Nialamide	Niamid
Tranylcypromine	Parnate
Pargyline	Alkaloids
Tricyclics	
Imipramine	Tofranil
Desipramine	Pertofranc, Norpramine
Amitriptyline	Elavil
Nortriptyline	Aventyl

Representative Antipsychotic Drugs

Generic Name	Brand Name
Rauwolfia Alkaloids	
Reserpine	Serpasil
Phenothiazine Derivatives	
Chlorpromazine	Thorazine
Promazine	Sparine
Triflupromazine	Vesprin
Thioridazine	Mellaril
Trifluoperazine	Stelazine
Perphenazine	Trilafon
Prochlorperazine	Compazine
Carphenazine	Proketazine
Acetophenazine	Tindal
Fluphenazine	Prolixin, Permitil
Butyrophenones	
Haloperidol	Haldol
Thioxanthene Derivatives	
Thiothixene	Navane
Chlorprothixene	Taractan

Source: Adapted from C. Kornetsky, *Pharmacology: Drugs affecting behavior* (New York: Wiley, 1976), pp. 111, 106, 88. Reprinted by permission of the publisher.

*One of the most frequently prescribed of the benzodiazepines is flurazepam, with the trade name of Dalmane. Promoted as a nonaddicting, effective substitute for the barbiturates as an aid to induce sleeping, millions of people are prescribed this drug with the further instruction that it is "safe" for 28 days. It is now known that these earlier statements were misleading (Smith, 1979). Along with the barbiturates, Dalmane does not break up the pattern of insomnia. Further, Dalmane accumulates in the body with an increasing build up of side effects that include problems in motor coordination, tolerance, and a synergistic interaction with alcohol. Dalmane and alcohol, as a matter of fact, can be a lethal combination. In short, Dalmane's "good" reputation appears to be unwarranted.

cially in moderately ill people. With chronic patients, however, many experts insist that there is no improvement of cognitive, perceptual, or motor skills. However, who is to know what the initial levels of performance of these patients were?

How do these drugs work? Chlorpromazine and its chemical cousins, according to one early hypothesis, curtail and limit the flooding of sensory input—afferent stimuli from within and without—that is so characteristic of the dramatic symptomatology of schizophrenia. Just in the way LSD (see Chapter 17) was thought to mimic the schizophrenic response by a flooding of afferent input, so, it was thought, the phenothiazines reversed this process by specific chemical action at relevant sites such as the reticular system of the brain that focuses and controls attention and regulates sensory input.

A hypothesis that has gained more recent favor is that the phenothiazines block the actions of dopamine, a neurotransmitter. This hypothesis—that antipsychotic drugs lock into and block dopamine receptors in the frontal cortex, which is the "seat" of thinking and cognition—is favored by many scientists in the light of accumulating laboratory and clinical evidence (Berger, 1978; Iversen, 1975).* Supporting this general view is the recently publicized fact that many of the phenothiazines induce Parkinson-like symptoms (involuntary muscle actions such as face twitching, gait and motor dysfunctions, and posture disturbances) in patients who ingest large dosages. By blocking dopamine activities, which reduce the symptoms of Parkinson's disease, clinicians are increasing the chances that there will be Parkinson-like symptoms in patients, especially those in hospitals, who take large quantities of these medications.

These symptoms, referred to as tardive dyskinesia or involuntary movement disorder, probably reflect a neurological dysfunction that will one day be responsive to treatment. For example, it has been discovered that tardive dyskinesia is associated with low levels of a certain chemical (acetylcholine) in the brain (Kolata, 1979a). But until then the presence of this syndrome—said to range from 0.5 to 41 percent, depending on the patients studied (Nasrallah, 1979)—presents a serious challenge to the wholesale use of the phenothiazines.

Reviews of the literature that consider only controlled studies indicate that the antipsychotic drugs have clearly established their success with all subtypes of schizophrenics at all stages of their disease, on all age levels, and throughout the world (Berger, 1978). Overall, in contrast to other kinds of treatment with schizophrenia, medication has also proved to be superior to psychotherapy—psychoanalytic or supportive—in follow-up studies (May, 1968).

However, questions have been raised as to whether or not prolonged maintenance on drugs is justified. There are many side effects with long-term use such as liver damage, drowsiness, and lowering of blood pressure. In addition, it is difficult to draw definite conclusions from what has been described as methodologically flawed studies as to the effects of prolonged drug use (MacDonald and Tobias, 1976; Tobias and MacDonald, 1974). However, one review indicates that there were almost twice as many relapses among long-term placebo patients than among long-term maintenance drug patients (Davis, Gosenfeld, and Tsai, 1976). Important to note, of course, is that not all placebo patients show relapse and that maintenance drugs do not always prevent relapse. Further, it is not possible to predict which patients will show what pattern (Berger, 1978).

However, despite the many disadvantages about the use of medication with schizophrenics, many researchers feel that the phenothiazines, particularly in combination with social supports and rehabilitation efforts, offer excellent promise for positive outcome with schizophrenic patients (Kornetsky, 1976).

Evaluation: Drugs as Therapy

The use of psychoactive medications has made possible the wholesale release of patients from mental hospitals and the relief of much suffering and anguish. Their widespread use, however, negative side effects, and the trial and error involved in their administration raise many serious questions. New research is continuing to highlight the dangers of some of the psychotropic medications. Many drugs, for example, have effects on the developing fetus,

* As a matter of fact, some scientists are beginning to wonder whether or not the schizophrenic disease is caused by a dysfunction of brain dopamine metabolism (Berger, 1978). Evidence in support of this promising hypothesis is still forthcoming, however.

especially some of the depressants (barbiturates and opiates), minor tranquilizers, and antipsychotic drugs (Milkovich and van den Berg, 1974). Most of these drugs do not mix well with each other, and abrupt termination is dangerous. Further, people metabolize drugs in different ways depending on their biochemistry, mood states, symptoms, previous or current drug ingestion, and nutritional status. Obviously, there is a need for considerable research in this area, especially regarding diagnostic subtypes and their response to medication. We await these findings eagerly in the light of the promise these medications are beginning to show.

Above all, as already noted, drug administration without psychotherapy, support, and encouragement from a therapist risks the possibility of failure, for many patients discontinue medication for a variety of reasons, ranging from a desire to make it on their own without reliance on "crutches" to obsessive fear of taking *any* substance because of concern over loss of control or body injury. It should be noted, finally, that the precise nature of specific drug and therapy combinations for specific patient groups is still not entirely clear (Hollon and Beck, 1978), a research area that is badly in need of attention.

PSYCHOSURGERY AND ELECTROCONVULSIVE THERAPY

Psychosurgery

Psychosurgery can be broadly defined as direct intervention into brain tissue with the specific purpose of modifying the behavior or emotional state of the patient. Psychosurgical intervention, in this broad definition, includes removal or destruction of brain tissue through surgical means, implantation of electrodes, laser beams, or the direct application of chemicals into brain tissue. Currently, only several hundred of these procedures are performed each year in the United States. There has been a gradual decline in their use with the advent of chemotherapy and the rise of strong public opinion against such interventions.

This section briefly touches on these procedures, beginning with the more drastic interventions that entail extensive destruction of brain tissue through surgical means. It has been estimated that over 40,000 such procedures have already been performed in the United States alone. How did the use of these methods come about to begin with? Have they had any history of success?

The surgical procedure of lobotomy or leucotomy developed from pioneer work of a Portugese surgeon, Moniz (later to win a Nobel prize), who experimented with severing the pathways between the frontal lobes and the thalamus of certain types of chronic, intractable (unmodifiable, resistant to treatment) mental patients, on an assumption that the thalamic-frontal pathways contain the seat of intense emotions.

Experimental work had already demonstrated that animals showed reduced temperamental behavior and excitement under conditions of frustration after frontal lobe surgery that severed connections between the frontal cortex and thalamus. In 1942, Freeman and Watts reported controlled laboratory findings with humans that further supported the hypothesis that severing this pathway helped to make less acute the emotion attached to unusual, bizarre, or "abnormal" thinking (Freeman and Watts, 1950).

In the decade to follow, this kind of psychosurgical procedure gained wide favor, especially with patients with severe symptomatology that was not eased through other means, such as paralyzing, intractable obsessions and fears, acute agitation or depression, and great subjective suffering in which the emotional disability prevented the patient from daily functioning. It was found after surgery that although the patient's ideas and impulses remained the same, his or her subjective suffering decreased. Further, patients no longer felt compelled to act out their impulses. However, this seemed to be accompanied by a general blunting of emotions, and sometimes postoperative status was also characterized by poor judgment and lack of foresight.

Since the 1950s, there has been a dramatic reduction in the frequency of these extensive surgical procedures. Earlier reports of favorable outcome with thousands of patients in whom pre-frontal lobotomies were performed were being challenged. For example, one systematic investigation of a large number of operated patients (Columbia-Greystone project) demonstrated neither significant deficits nor improvements in patients following surgery (Mettler, 1949).

More restricted, precise methods of psychosurgery in which extremely small areas of brain tissue are destroyed has elicited less disfavor. A cingulotomy, for example, creates small lesions severing a bundle of nerve fibers that connect the frontal lobes to the limbic system—the presumed "seat of the emotions." This is made possible by precision procedures for measuring exactly where the surgical or electrical instrument is penetrating the brain and exactly what small area of tissue is destroyed. These procedures are called stereotaxic methods. Most clinicians object to these procedures because they think they are based on an erroneous and oversimple hypothesis—that there is a one-to-one relationship between tiny portions of the brain and specific behaviors (Trotter, 1974). However, these procedures are still being performed today, for the kinds of patients previously described.

It is still not exactly clear why these methods are helpful. It is possible that psychosurgery affects the biochemistry of mood states and behavior or that minor surgically induced impairments actually help some patients to be less ruminative or obsessive.

Another explanation for the success of some of these methods rests on the possibility of placebo effects; that is, the patient's expectations for post-operative success are major influences in his or her subjective state following surgery. Many of the operated patients would have improved anyway, even without surgery.

Overall, because many of these procedures are performed privately with little or no controlled research or publication of follow-up results, it is difficult to conduct a systematic evaluation of these explanations. The debate continues, both with regard to uncontrolled studies as well as the many moral and ethical problems that such irreversible procedures entail (see Chorover, 1979; Valenstein, 1980).

Electroconvulsive Therapy (ECT)

Electroconvulsive therapy, first described as a method of treating schizophrenia, induces bilateral tonic-clonic grand-mal seizures in the subject by passing an electric current (anywhere from 70 to 150 volts) through electrodes attached to both temples for a duration of 0.1 up to one second.* The seizure phase lasts for about one minute. There is loss of consciousness as soon as the current is transmitted and no pain or recall of the events during the seizures. Subjects slowly recover consciousness (in approximately ten minutes) and there is, generally, confusion lasting one or two hours. Treatments are given several times a week for a period of several weeks, depending on the course of the improvement, and can range up to 20 sessions. Some patients, however, have been given hundreds of treatments over a period of only one year (Scovern and Kilmann, 1980).

ECT has reportedly had some success with severe endogenous depression, especially when accompanied by delusions (Scovern and Kilmann, 1980). But other kinds of depressions have not responded with improvement, and there is little evidence to support the notion that it prevents future episodes of depression in manic-depressive syndromes.

Up until fairly recently, it was not too well understood why or how ECT "worked," but it has become clear that it influences the levels of many neurochemicals, including dopamine, serotonin, norepinephrine, and the endorphins, and that its ef-

* In actual practice, there are many variations of procedure, including unilateral stimulation of only the nondominant hemisphere.

fects are not dissimilar to those of the antidepressant medications (Chiodo and Antelman, 1980).

Today the popularity of ECT has waned considerably. Nevertheless, it is estimated that at least 100,000 patients each year are receiving treatments, mostly in private hospitals (Breggin, 1979). The many side effects, including the possibility of fractures and memory loss for preceding events up to months prior to the treatments, patients' frequent reports of anxiety in connection with the treatments, and, the lack of evidence that in controlled studies ECT does better than placebo in modifying symptoms of schizophrenia and most depressions and in preventing suicide, have prompted many clinicians to conclude that as an alternative to other forms of treatment, ECT is a poor choice (Breggin, 1979). Finally, in the light of the success of various psychoactive drugs in the treatment of depression, even many physical-treatment-oriented clinicians are disinclined to introduce as drastic and risky procedure as ECT.

The use of the physical procedures described in this section, and of the chemotherapies previously described, especially if introduced without informed consent, raises many moral and ethical problems. But, even when consent is obtained from people such as prisoners or voluntarily and involuntarily confined patients in mental hospitals, there is still a potential for serious abuse, a point made many times in this book. This is true even when subjects are informed of risks, for many subjects will cooperate with a suggested procedure for a variety of reasons, including lack of competence to judge its risks and consequences, and desire to win the favor of the relevant authority.

Peer review, advocacy, and strict controls over such procedures (have all alternative measures been exhausted?) are strongly advised for these dramatic interventions. As a matter of fact, many people believe that such interventive methods should be eliminated entirely from the repertoire of procedures designed to modify behavior and emotions (Chorover, 1979; Valenstein, 1980).

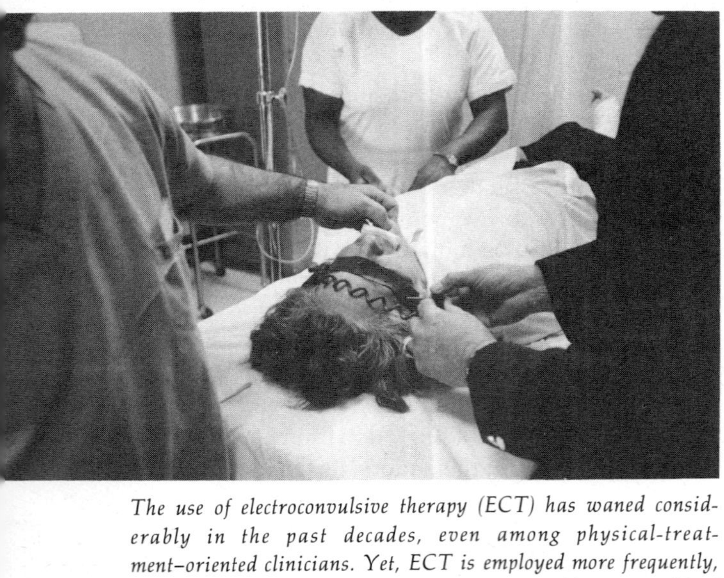

The use of electroconvulsive therapy (ECT) has waned considerably in the past decades, even among physical-treatment-oriented clinicians. Yet, ECT is employed more frequently, especially in private hospitals, than one would suspect. (Paul Fusco/Magnum)

SECTION III
MENTAL HOSPITALS AND ALTERNATIVE APPROACHES: AN OVERVIEW

Mental hospitals were alluded to many times in this book. What is their status today? What becomes of patients who need intensive care and who have no community ties and connections to support them as they obtain this care? This section reviews the remarkable decline of the large state institutions that dotted our countryside, examines some of the reasons for this decline, and raises some issues and alternatives that are intrinsic to these circumstances.

Deinstitutionalization

The long-standing tradition of isolating and incarcerating mental patients has fallen by the wayside. State hospitals are no longer looming, monolithic, threatening prisons, and they are changing their functions and their image. Nowadays they are used as short stopovers for intense emergency treatment, with a view to releasing the patient back into the community as soon as possible. At one time, however, they were long-term repositories for chronic patients or places in which patients were kept in isolation or restraint.

Unfortunately, until quite recently, the opinions of the patient about being hospitalized were only minimally considered. And once hospitalized, patients became "dehumanized," victimized, and powerless (see Spotlight 21.3). For the sad fact is that most often, one of the chief reasons for hospitalizing a patient was that there was nobody around to care for him or her—there was no one at home, no job, no community supports. Our society tends to "warehouse" its isolates and the people who behave differently from the rest of us. They are public eyesores, guilt-givers, reminders, like some of the infirm and the elderly, of what could happen to us.

Fortunately, the picture has changed dramatically. Involuntary commitment of patients is actually employed rarely, and only if the patient is judged to be dangerous to himself or herself or others.* Alternative paths, such as outpatient services and community care, are being followed.

* This is by no means a petty issue. Up until only a few years ago, at any one time there were hundreds of thousands of people involuntarily committed to mental institutions. The United States has committed more people than any other country, and one of every 300 people in this country was involuntarily committed to a mental hospital as recently as the late 1950s (Stone, 1978).

Spotlight 21.3 Of Dehumanization and Helplessness in Hospitals

Loss of freedom in a mental hospital, whether through voluntary admission or involuntary commitment, frequently results in alienation and dehumanization of the incarcerated patient. The fact of being institutionalized in a regimented world closed from the outside world leaves its mark on the inmate. Many hospitals are still poorly run or unsupervised, isolation is still used; there is overuse of medication; and nonprofessional or poorly trained staff members often supervise group or individual therapy. The process by which inmates of "total institutions" such as prisons and mental hospitals become dehumanized has been of great interest to social scientists (see Goffman, 1961).

In one demonstration of this process (see Spotlight 4.2), eight normal subjects "faked" their way into mental hospitals (Rosenhan, 1973). These "pseudopatients" then carefully observed the steps involved in the "depersonalization" that took place. The pseudopatients were never detected by the staff as "phonies," partially because of the enduring qualities of the label assigned to them (their diagnosis) and the aura it created around them. That is, the label (diagnosis) persisted even after the "patient" showed no symptoms and had done nothing bizarre. I have already alluded to the problem of diagnostic labels in earlier chapters.

According to the "sane" patient-observers, the patient's socialization to dehumanizing conditions in large mental hospitals is accomplished by the following: (a) inmates develop a sense of overwhelming powerlessness; (b) they are victimized by the staff; (c) they are deprived of many of their legal rights; (d) their movement is restricted and often confined; (e) they cannot initiate contact with a member of the staff but must wait until they are contacted; (f) they lose personal privacy—open bathroom stalls or physical examinations in the view of others; (g) their sense of private ownership is diminished (their personal possessions can be examined by any staff member, for example); (h) they are subordinate to anyone on the "other side," even aides or volunteers; (i) their case histories and personal data are available to anyone on the staff; (j) and the staff treats them as invisible or as unseeing (Rosenhan cites as an example a nurse who adjusted her bra in front of male inmates as if they either were "not there" or could not comprehend what was happening, even if they were).

What can be done about this process?

Recommended are changes within hospitals and institutions that encourage structured, close interpersonal roles and interactions among patients with clearcut responsibilities in a less overwhelmingly institutional setting. Smaller numbers of people on wards help, as well as attention to the climate and social atmosphere of the setting. Milieu methods, for example, which stress the total atmosphere of a hospital in which aides, nurses, therapists, physicians, and the patients themselves become involved in the administration of their own setting, may offset the dehumanizing process described. This community approach *within* a hospital goes beyond the one-to-one patient-doctor relationship by emphasizing the atmosphere of the entire therapeutic community. Patients participate in planning the activities for, and in the administration of, the hospital community in ways that provide them with a sense of power and control. Usually helpless patients in autocratic hospital atmospheres never or rarely experience such power. In the milieu approach, the hierarchical structures of the typical hospital begin to fade.

In this newer approach, individual choices are given to each patient, who is informed of the risks involved in the treatment that is offered and given a sense of control over his or her destiny. In addition, because patients are told that their civil rights are protected, including the right for counsel and representation, protection of their funds and private property, and a right for review of their situation for discharge, the overwhelming sense of loss of freedom and its accompanying feeling of helplessness that so many mental patients have described may be becoming more and more obsolete.

Why has this picture changed so dramatically? The release of large numbers of patients from mental hospitals became a discernible trend in the mid-1950s, spurred by the wholesale administration of psychoactive medications to patients. In the past decade, an additional boost to this trend was provided by a landmark Supreme Court decision in 1975 (*O'Connor* v. *Donaldson*), which held that it is unconstitutional to confine a nondangerous individual in a mental institution against his or her will unless adequate treatment is provided.

Here are some figures that attest to the decline in patient population.

In the nation as a whole, there was approximately a 2 percent increase each year in number of mental patients in hospitals, peaking with 550,000 in 1955. In 1978, there were only about 150,000 patients in these institutions (Altman, 1979b). New York State alone discharged 120,000 patients in a

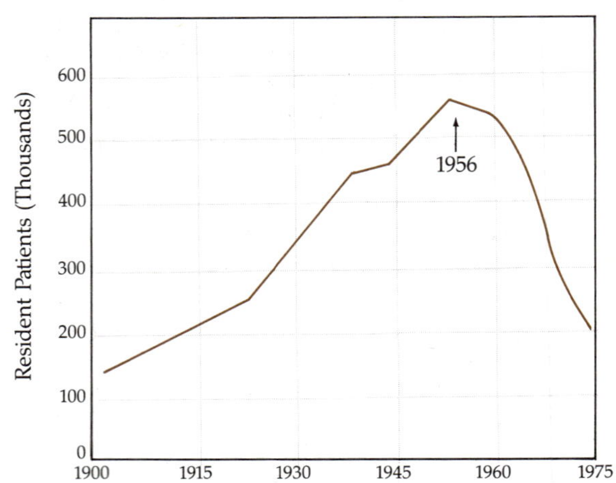

Figure 21.1 The patient population in public mental institutions, 1900–75. (From E. L. Bassuk and S. Gerson, Deinstitutionalizat on and mental health care, *Scientific American*, February 1978, *238*, 46. Copyright © 1978 by Scientific American, Inc. All rights reserved.)

twenty-year period (Sullivan, 1977) and in 1981, there were only about 23,000 people in New York's state hospitals. A continuing trend is that although admission rates are increasing (better diagnostic methods? more adequate screening?), there are more people being discharged from mental hospitals than admitted (Bassuk and Gerson, 1978).

Most people applaud these trends.* There are some who disagree, however, pointing to the large numbers of readmissions of discharged patients—the "revolving door" described later in this section.

Court Decisions

Item: On January 30, 1975, Martha Nelson died at the age of 103 years after having been confined to an Ohio state mental hospital for a century. One newspaper noted:

> *Miss Nelson received national attention last year when it became known that she had been hospitalized almost a century and no one knew why. She had no known family and her name became a rallying cry for persons seeking to reform the treatment of the mentally retarded. . . . State officials said they were still not sure why Miss Nelson was confined all her life . . . (Miss Nelson. . . . , 1975, p. 30).*

Miss Nelson's plight was not uncommon. By the early 1970s, civil rights groups were becoming interested in people like Miss Nelson, and were beginning to challenge and to confront these issues in the courts.

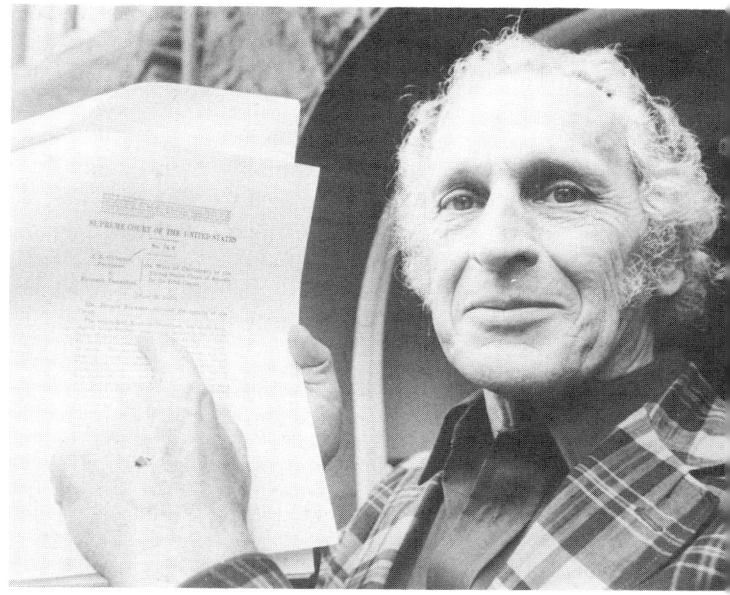

Kenneth Donaldson, who had been institutionalized against his will in a Florida state hospital, won a landmark decision by the United States Supreme Court in 1975. (Wide World Photos)

By 1974, in Montgomery, Alabama, the United States Court of Appeals for the Fifth Circuit ruled that "mental patients as a class have a Federal, constitutional right to adequate treatment when they are committed against their wills to state institutions and Federal courts may determine those standards" (A Mental Patient's Rights to Adequate Care Upheld, 1974). In 1975, the Supreme Court of the United States decided in favor of Kenneth Donaldson, who had been petitioning for his release from a state hospital in Chattahoochee, Florida since 1957, when he had been committed by his parents at the age of 48 years. Donaldson's suit was against a physician, O'Connor, who, he claimed, had kept him locked up against his will.

This landmark decision was accompanied by a related series of lower court interpretations of constitutional law that generally expressed the view (already described in Chapter 14) that the "right to treatment" for mentally retarded and mentally ill people should take place in the "least restrictive

* An exception already noted (see page 295) is a view that some patients—perhaps only a very limited number—might lose contact with the remaining social support system open to them if they are discharged. Such people are unable to establish or maintain any community contact for any length of time. If discharged, they would soon be floundering on the streets, isolated and helpless. The freedom to be "sick, helpless, and isolated" on the streets is not really freedom according to Rosenblatt (1974), who states that some patients should remain in a hospital setting for keeps, if they wish to stay. Maintaining them as custodial patients may actually guarantee their "rights" for care and protection, whereas discharging them into a world with which they cannot cope may be a violation of their rights for society's protection.

setting." An individual's liberty, in other words, cannot be curtailed, except in the "least drastic" way.

In these actions, the core issues concerned whether or not society can deprive an individual of his or her freedom, presumably to provide treatment, and still not offer it; or if treatment is offered, to do so inadequately and ineffectually. Moreover, being mentally ill—by itself—is not sufficient reason for involuntary commitment. Patients cannot be incarcerated indefinitely, even if they are thought to pose a risk for the future, or simply because they show socially undesirable, nonconforming, or even bizarre behavior.

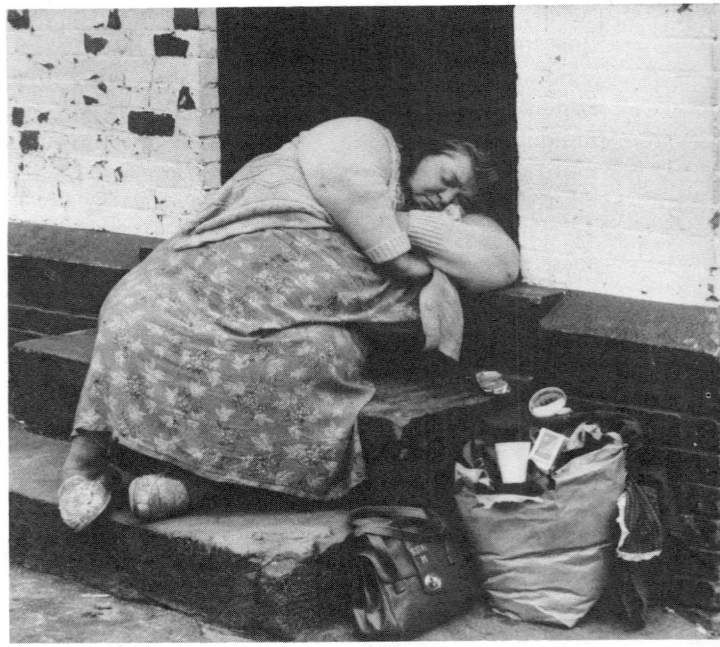

Deinstitutionalization, unless accompanied by appropriate community facilities and strong social supports, may result in a "revolving door" for many former mental patients. (Peter Simon/Stock, Boston)

Community Care and Revolving Doors

Because of the Supreme Court and other lower court rulings about treatment in least restrictive settings, mental hospitals have been releasing patients as quickly as possible, back into the communities from which they came, creating problems that were not entirely anticipated.

Many communities lack facilities and programs for the care of ex-mental patients who need jobs, social supports, and housing. Such people, it is claimed, find their way into run-down "single-room occupancies" in the inner-city hotels in the large cities. They become drifters and vagrants, and eventually have to receive welfare or other financial aid. Finally, they get into trouble in their communities and end up in a state institution once again—the revolving door that so many people find objectionable. Critics point to an occasional news item of a murder or rape committed by a just-released patient, and describe the fright of the communities that neighbor on the single-room-occupancy areas. They also mention the waste of the taxpayers' money. Until the communities provide adequate care for such released patients, it is claimed, their premature release is not warranted.

About 7 to 10 percent of "dumped" patients need to be readmitted because of lack of good community supports, according to a study of 500 discharged patients in one community in New York State (Rule, 1978). Most estimates are considerably higher, however: it seems that over 50 percent of hospital admissions are repeaters (Roberts, 1978).

Almost all agree that the revolving-door situation reflects not misguided motivation but the inadequacies of the community to provide rehabilitation programs, half-way settings, and counseling facilities for the readjustment of the ex-patient into life. Actually, the emptying of the large state facilities reduces the taxpayers' burden toward their support, thus releasing funds that can be used not only for developing refined screening and diagnostic methods (both at the point of hospitalization and discharge) but also for creating effective facilities for the rehabilitation of former patients within the community.

What can be done about discharged ex-patients floundering in nursing homes, rooming houses, or single-room welfare hotels, who exist marginally, without medication or supervision or job training?

If care in the least restrictive setting is a legally mandated goal, community support systems, some claim, should provide for a case aide or manager for each patient so that flexible programs for living, working, and getting by can be arranged and supervised on a completely individual basis. Group counseling, individual guidance, job training, and supervision of medication should be made available for all—but designated on an individual basis. Similarly, living contexts require more than a bed and mattress. Day hospitals, day centers, sheltered workshops, crisis-intervention centers, community residences, foster and/or boarding homes, halfway houses: these are all possibilities that should be carefully weighed for any individual patient.

Further, according to some specialists, rehabilitation, rather than treatment, should be the goal (see Anthony, 1977). Rehabilitation should involve assessment and special testing so that a subject's skills—both deficits and assets—could be evaluated. Skills training should be offered in a variety of areas: for employment, and for interpersonal, recreational, and social living. Job placement, after comprehensive skills training, would be the ultimate goal.

There are some who propose that such community support systems can actually be generated in one center, a kind of "psychosocial rehabilitation center" (of which there are only a few hundred in the country) that are like halfway houses for former mental patients. They could offer job training, living and sleeping arrangements, and counseling under one roof. Is there any evidence that this could work? Yes, according to Roberts (1978), who noted that former patients who are at these centers are rehospitalized at much lower rates than those who are not.

Former patients are as much in need of help, as are acutely ill people. Society tends to forget about people when their flagrant symptomatology subsides. Have we come up with the answers?

SECTION IV
INTERVENTIVE METHODS IN OTHER PLACES

It was noted earlier that cultural frames of reference play an influential role in diagnostic and treatment practices all over the world. I return to this theme with regard to therapy in three advanced contemporary societies: Japan, the People's Republic of China, and the Soviet Union. Doing do demonstrates once again that a society's pervasive philosophy and value system are important determinants of its approach to treating mental illness.

Japan

Prior to World War II, less than 5 percent of people with serious mental problems were in hospitals. The family traditions of Japan resulted in keeping mentally ill people at home, often without treatment. Since World War II, Japan has built many hospital facilities for the mentally ill, with an emphasis on using nonmedical personnel (Murakami, 1979). One widely practiced hospital approach to helping people is Morita therapy (see Kora, 1965)—named after a Professor Morita who worked in a Tokyo hospital over half a century ago. This method reflects the Japanese Zen orientation. Interpersonal goals are not stressed in Morita therapy. Rather, therapeutic goals encourage patients to "achieve acceptance of their positions within nature."

Morita treatment is provided in a hospital setting, rather than in a one-to-one office setting, and combines many elements that appear similar to our milieu therapy (a focus on a total therapeutic environment), directive therapy, cognitive and behavioral methods, and occupational therapy (helping the patient through meaningful, supervised work).

In the Morita method, patients suffering from psychoneuroses are admitted to a specialized hospital for several weeks. They remain in total isolation during the first phases of treatment. This period, in which there is bed rest and no activity other than toileting or eating, presumably forces the patient to face his or her problems, goals, and life patterns directly. Patients are encouraged to accept their lives and their symptoms and to allow their emotions to flow freely through them. This is followed by several other phases, each of which is designed to guide the patient through individual therapy, group counseling, positive self-appraisal, diary-keeping, and eventually reading and arts and crafts. Patients learn that to do nothing is boring. They are encouraged not to focus on their symptoms. To move in the direction of positive goal construction, the patient is not permitted any interaction with people other than staff members during the first few phases of treatment, but in the third phase they enter into a period of strenuous physical activity such as gardening or road repairing. The final phase of Morita treatment involves gradually increasing the interactions with nonstaff personnel and directive guidance designed to shape the patient's behavior in his or her real-life situation.

In sum, then, action and behavior are stressed throughout, with achievement of personal goals the focus rather than symptom reduction. Patients are helped to become less preoccupied with their symptoms and to focus on goal-directed activity through directive, cognitive, and persuasive approaches and organized interactions with others as in sports or dancing at first, and later, in working.

The People's Republic of China

Chinese interventive methods stress the group, community, and social unit as the prime focus of concern. On the level of children's disorders, for example, the "deviant" child is absorbed into group activities and involved in many adult-child and child-child interactions. Through constant activities in which group, rather than individual, goals are stressed, and cooperation rather than personal strivings are modeled, the socialization and molding of the child take place (Hsiao, 1977). In these early years, friendship and mutuality are stressed and the children are constantly being socialized into socially oriented, group-involved behavior patterns in which individual maladjustment is rare.

With regard to adult mental illness, schizophrenia is the most common diagnosis (Bazar, 1979). During the "cultural revolution" the slogan "revolutionary optimism" was described as the key to an understanding of the Chinese treatment approach (Sidel, 1973). Recently, however, it has been proposed that because internal and social forces create mental illness, there is no cure; however, treatment is aimed at restructuring the patients' thinking and attitudes so that they can return to their routine daily activities (Lee, 1979). Goals for treatment, thus, are practical rather than theoretical; they are not based on some abstract view of emotional organization or personality development (Bazar, 1979; Lee, 1979). Return to the work and family setting, rather than a more abstract goal of "adjustment" or mental health is sought.

The methods employed to achieve this end are diverse and eclectic in nature, ranging from "heart-to-heart talks," group methods, Western chemotherapy and medicines, and acupuncture, to direct counseling of family members and colleagues at work (Lee, 1979; Sidel, 1973). Peer supports and a "buddy" system (in which a sicker patient is paired with a healthier patient) are often introduced. Cognitive methods in rearranging one's life on the basis of a change in values are also stressed (Lee, 1979). Understanding of the illness is encouraged, with both the patient and the patient's family.

When patients are hospitalized, their employment status remains the same and they receive full salary for six months. During this time, they are regarded as "full-fledged members of society" (Lee, 1979). As a result, the pressures and stigma of a lengthy hospitalization are reduced. Hospitals and their routines are modeled on the "outside" community, with work and relatively normal lives within the hospital compound emphasized.

In the heart-to-heart talks and the verbal, educational methods, elements of persuasiveness and self-control techniques dominate. Patients are actively encouraged to understand their illness, to correct their mistaken thinking, and to participate in the solution of problems facing them. The patient's direct involvement in examining his or her problems is thus an important aspect of treatment, with the patient being given a sense of power over—to feel in charge of—his or her destiny and environment. Throughout, support and reassurance are provided as well as the feeling that the doctor really cares for the patients and is truly involved in their lives. Motivation to get better is also generated from without: the patient should want to get better not only for personal reasons but also for the sake of the group, his or her colleagues, and the family.

Suggestions that getting well is for "the sake of the group" are conveyed through persuasion and education that orient the patient to be thinking about the community as being larger and more important than the individual, which "gives meaning and joy to life" (Bazar, 1979; Lee, 1979).

Although the Chinese culturally were not "open" to studying Western methods until recently, some current interest has focused on the clinical use of hypnosis, biofeedback, and behavioral methods in treatment approaches (Ching, 1980). Psychopharmacology, however, is apparently not a well-developed treatment approach in China.

The Soviet Union

In the Soviet Union, treatment approaches reflect a rather complex amalgam of psychology and social and political philosophy. On the one hand, in the various therapeutic approaches can be found the generally rosy, optimistic approach already described: a socially oriented viewpoint in which the individual's aloneness is submerged and his or her relationship to the group, the community, and the social system is stressed. As with the Chinese, cognitive approaches that stress self-help and the individual's power to change his or her environment are important aspects of the different therapies. And here, as in China, suggestion, persuasion, placebo, and expectancy factors play an important, planned, built-in role.

On the other hand, the strict social or environmental determinism that one might expect from a society such as theirs (Marxist) is not found. Social and cultural factors do not cause all pathology. As a matter of fact, the Soviet approach to behavioral disorders stresses brain function and neuropsychology, in keeping with the precedents established by the laboratory research of over a half century ago (McLeish, 1975). Dysfunctions of the brain are the primary cause of severe emotional disorders such as schizophrenia, and even though the Soviets' view of a person is that of a physical, material organism interacting with the environment, primary methods for treatment have been the somatic and physical ones. Only in the past few decades has psychotherapy, as we more traditionally think of it, received wider recognition (Winn, 1961; Ziferstein, 1976). As might be expected, however, the psychoanalytic, Freudian view of the neuroses and of treatment never did get a foothold in Soviet academic or clinical settings.

By and large, the neuroses and the psychoses are generally thought of as separate entities requiring different treatments. With the schizophrenias and the depressions (but also with other problems), therefore, chemotherapy is in wide use. But other somatic therapies such as electroshock methods and sleep therapy (the patient is medicinally aided to sleep for long periods, say up to 20 hours a day over a period of a week or more) are also in use (Bieliauskas, 1977; Winn, 1961). Electrosleep therapy is also employed. This involves producing a state of relaxation or sleep in the patient (generally, there are half-hour daily sessions for a few weeks) by passing a mild electric current through the brain. However, even with the schizophrenias, support and reassurance—for example, through providing counseling for patients and their families—are frequently supplied. Less severe problems, presumably not based on organic causes, involve "re-educational counseling," which tends to be brief and supportive (David and David, 1962). Neurotic individuals are often given explanations as to why they learned to think and behave as they do so that they perceive their problems as not only curable, but also as resulting from cause-and-effect relationships that are understood scientifically (McLeish, 1975).

Hypnosis is in widespread use with individuals and groups, and hypnotic suggestion is frequently used to cure psychosomatic ailments. With alcoholics, hypnosis in combination with medication is frequently used, as is counterconditioning or conditioned reflex therapy.

Group methods are sometimes employed, generally beginning with "lectures" by the therapist and followed by group discussions to support the patient so that individual therapy is made easier. "Heart-to-heart" talks (using direct suggestion and persuasion) are also in use and here the power, prestige, mutual trust and respect, and authority of a caring therapist is very much built into the therapeutic technique. The approach to the neuroses is often through behavioral methods, and relaxation methods are frequently introduced, even stressed in the case of the phobias (Winn, 1961; Ziferstein, 1976).

In short, although the labels and theoretical underpinnings differ considerably from ours, many of the methods evolved in the Soviet Union bear a strong resemblance to those employed in our country. Surprising is the great stress on hypnotic methods, cognitive methods, group methods, directive and persuasive approaches, and on the placebo effects of trust and prestige of the therapist. We tend to regard the latter as "accidents" of design we wish to avoid but Soviet clinicians weigh these heavily as potent, therapeutic aids. Less surprising is the popularity of the behavioral approaches (Pavlov, after all, was a Russian) and the somatic approaches (Pavlov and his followers believed strongly in physiology and the brain as determinants of pathological behavior).

SUMMARY

This chapter surveyed and evaluated the effectiveness of several physical and nonphysical therapies not discussed in previous chapters. It described biofeedback methods, found to be moderately but not entirely useful in treating certain conditions; hypnotic methods, for highly hypnotizable subjects, effective in handling pain as well as aiding in other areas for example, smoking cessation; and finally, meditation as a therapeutic aid, useful in reducing tension and anxiety, but not because of any unique or special "power" that other methods do not possess. The next section of this chapter considered some specific physical therapies, including the widely used pharmacological interventions (the antianxiety, antidepressant, and antipsychotic drugs) and the less frequently used psychosurgical and electroconvulsive procedures. The text evaluated the limitations, problems, and research evidence on the effectiveness of these procedures. The third section of this chapter took a close look at mental hospitals, the history of deinstitutionalization in this country (for example, some of the court decisions that figured in this process), and some of the problems created by this historical trend. Finally, the chapter briefly described interventive methods in other countries, specifically those in Japan, the People's Republic of China, and the Soviet Union.

Highlights

1. Biofeedback methods help people to learn to modify various bodily responses, of which they are generally unaware, through the use of instruments that monitor and simultaneously provide information to the subject about these responses as they are occurring. A review of the relevant research concluded that although there is moderate clinical application of biofeedback methods (for example, in relieving tension headaches or in regulating cardiac arrhythmias), overall results using these methods are probably less promising than was initially thought to be the case.
2. Hypnosis, about which there are many myths (see Spotlight 21.1) can be conceptualized as an intense, heightened state of concentration and attention in which peripheral, extraneous cues and stimuli are minimized if they contradict the "central framework" provided by the hypnotist. Other definitions stress the notion that the hypnotic state represents a special type of

awareness and consciousness. Some theoretical controversy has developed over these explanatory thrusts. Some clinicians claim that highly hypnotizable subjects may possess unique attentional skills that less hypnotizable subjects do not possess; others believe that hypnosis can be explained almost entirely on the basis of placebo effects and trust. Although explanations for hypnosis vary, it is generally agreed that hypnotic states are "real" behavioral and attentional states, not just demonstrations of some occult powers on the part of the hypnotist.

3. About 10 to 15 percent of the general population is highly hypnotizable; about 70 to 80 percent, moderately hypnotizable, and about 10 to 15 percent not hypnotizable. There is considerable interest in attempts to define differences between highly susceptible and nonsusceptible subjects. As a short-term change agent, hypnotic methods can sometimes be more effective than many long-term psychotherapies with some types of problems—for example, in the control of overeating.
4. The widespread claims of believers in the powers of meditation as a special state of consciousness to help deal with different types of clinical problems are probably not empirically substantiated. However, meditation methods, along with other therapies, may be effective in inducing relaxation and reducing moderate forms of anxiety.
5. The minor tranquilizers—the so-called antianxiety drugs—are among the most widely prescribed of the psychoactive substances. They are recommended almost indiscriminately for dealing with the everyday problems of anxiety, insomnia, tension, and situational stress. Most of these medications have many side effects, especially with long-term use, and are associated with tolerance and abstinence syndromes as well as risk of birth defects in children born to users during the first six weeks of pregnancy.
6. The MAO inhibitors and the tricyclic drugs are widely used antidepressant drugs that are not necessarily effective with all types of depression. Another drug, lithium, which had stacked up an impressive record regarding its ability to control manic episodes in bipolar affective disorders, is also showing promise in controlling certain types of depressions associated with the major affective disorders. The unreserved enthusiasm for lithium as a medication for all depressions, however, appears to be unwarranted. Lithium has fewer side effects than many of the other psychoactive substances, but it requires careful monitoring of certain chemicals within the body. The use of most of these substances requires simultaneous psychotherapy as an adjunct to their administration, for a variety of reasons—for example, to help alter the patient's views of hopelessness and despair as well as to support motivation to continue with the recommended regime of medication.
7. The development of the phenothiazines—the antipsychotic drugs—has had a dramatic effect on the treatment and care of schizophrenic patients. These major tranquilizers often achieve important symptomatic changes in disturbed patients; for example, they can control disorganized thinking, reduce delusions and hallucinations, and limit bizarre behavior. Unfortunately, long-term and unsupervised use may produce many serious side effects, including tardive dyskinesia, an involuntary motor disorder.
8. Scientists are not entirely clear as to how or why the foregoing substances achieve their effects on behavior, but they are forming a more orderly (but far from complete) picture of these neurochemicals and how they interact with others in the brain. Several relevant hypotheses were briefly summarized, for example, the relationship of the phenothiazines to dopamine, a neurotransmitter.
9. Effectiveness research indicates that the phenothiazines have clearly established their success with all subtypes of schizophrenics at all stages of their disease, and on all age levels, especially if used in conjunction with psychotherapy, social support systems, and rehabilitation efforts.
10. The wholesale, widespread use of psychoactive

substances has many negative consequences; this is so, it should be stressed, even for the minor tranquilizers. These include serious side effects, high risk for developing fetuses, the sometimes dangerous, even lethal effects of using several medications at the same time, and the problems resulting from abrupt termination. In addition, there is the ethical question of sedating patients without focusing also on their day-to-day emotional problems. These issues are among the many raised by those who view the widespread use of such substances critically.

11. Invasive and directly physical methods for controlling behavior include psychosurgery and electroconvulsive treatments (ECT). These methods have generally declined in use not only because of the rise in pharmacological interventions but also because of public protest against their inhumanity. In addition, earlier reports of favorable outcome with different clinical groups were being empirically challenged. Even so, limited success is reported with controlled use of some of these methods for some types of pathological conditions (for example, ECT is reported to be successful with severe types of endogenous depressions that are accompanied by delusions).
12. The decline of the large state mental hospitals that once dotted the nation's countryside was attributed not only to the rise of effectiveness of the psychoactive substances that permitted patients to get by, even if marginally, in the "outside" world, but also to the gradual legal challenges to their loss of freedom and civil rights. In many of these actions, the core issues concerned whether or not society could deprive an individual of his or her freedom, presumably to provide treatment, and still not offer it; or if treatment is offered, to do so inadequately and ineffectually. It was pointed out that the "dumping" of patients has created its own problems—for example, the readmissions ("revolving doors") that reflect the communities' inadequacy to provide sufficent support and rehabilitative measures for ex-patients.
13. Interventive methods in Japan, the People's Republic of China, and the Soviet Union demonstrate that cultural frames of reference play an influential role in the kinds of diagnostic methods used and treatments employed in these places. For example, some of the methods used in Japan reflect a religious-philosophical orientation in which patients are encouraged to "achieve acceptance of their positions within nature." The People's Republic of China, on the other hand, approaches mental problems through a stress on responsibility to the community and the group, and therapy methods often rely on persuasion and education, rather than on more elaborate theoretical concepts.

ISSUES AND QUESTIONS

1. In the past several years, there has been some legislation to control the use of hypnosis for entertainment purposes. The law prohibiting "stage hypnosis" in Oregon was the first in the country to do so, and its constitutionality was tested and upheld several years ago. The assumption that there can be risks for the subject (for example, "mind-influence" for suggestible subjects) obviously underlies legislation of this sort. But should *therapeutic* use of hypnosis also be controlled for the same reason?

   A related issue concerns the use of hypnosis to jog the memory of witnesses for trial purposes. Such procedures may serve a socially and legally useful purpose—for example, in preparing evidence for convicting a rapist by helping a victim or a witness to recall the suspect's facial disfigurement. Many are contending, however, that use of hypnosis in criminal investigation procedures should be eliminated. They cite the danger of "memory contamination": witnesses giving testimony in an actual trial may be recalling false cues, suggestions, and information subtly provided to them during a hypnotic session. Do you agree that there should be careful control over the use of hypnotic procedures in criminal proceedings even though important, "true" information might be obscured?

2. Are we becoming a society of prescribed (or over-the-counter) drug abusers? Who benefits, the pharmaceutical houses or the patients? Many people are concerned that so-called normal people are becoming increasingly dependent on drugs to handle the tensions, inconveniences, and discomforts of everyday life—boredom, an examination, a fight with one's boyfriend, occasional insomnia, overweight. Are we becoming "soft" in meeting our responsibilities? Chapter 14 has already described the use of drugs with children, especially to calm down hyperactive children. Is this use ever justified? Should only major problems be handled with medication? Who is to decide what is major? How can this situation, with its many risks and dangers, be controlled?
3. There are so many issues concerning mental hospitals that only a few can be raised here. One issue is in connection with the right to treatment—with treatment being defined as adequate or appropriate care. Who decides what adequate or appropriate care is? Is our knowledge about mental illness so precise that we can construct criteria to which legislative bodies, the courts, and the facilities themselves can refer? Can minimum standards be defined? How would you go about tackling this problem?
4. A patient's right to treatment may violate other rights. For example, if voluntary consent is required at all times before a treatment procedure is introduced, some patients may abrogate their rights for treatment by refusing to give consent. Should a clinician ever be allowed protect a patient's right to treatment by insisting on medication, psychosurgery, aversive conditioning, or electroshock *without* consent?
5. Certain states (for example, Massachusetts and Ohio, among others) have upheld the rights of mental patients to refuse antipsychotic medication, even if they were once dangerous (but pose no threat to themselves or others currently). This precedent presumably holds for other drastic treatment methods also, psychosurgery or electroshock therapy, for example. Do you agree with this legal and ethical decision? What if there is an emergency such as an act of violence against staff members? Would this circumstance represent an exception to the general principle of right to refuse treatment?

   I have elsewhere discussed the question of the competence of some people to judge the merits of an offered treatment, for example, severely retarded or very young children. Who would say no for such people? Who would say yes, for that matter? Their parents? An outside review board?
6. The parents' "right" to commit their minor children to a state mental institution, provided that there is independent agreement by the hospital's medical staff, was upheld by the United States Supreme Court in 1979. The high court ruled that "adversary" hearings in which the parents' judgment is explored or challenged is not necessary before committing the child. What are your thoughts on this matter?
7. The right to informed consent and the right to treatment are not the only rights of patients in hospitals. Rights also include those for privacy, and individual dignity. How can patients' situations be reviewed and overseen so that their rights are protected? One solution lies in having patient "advocacy" as a built-in protection of the patient so that he or she is always represented—legally, civilly, psychologically. Do you agree that instituting outside advocates or representatives for all patients within hospitals might make some inroads into guaranteeing patients' rights?
8. It has been pointed out many times that informed consent is meaningless for many patients who do not fully comprehend what the treatment is or what its risks might be. Would all patients (and their families), for example, understand what psychosurgery is and what its risks are? Should informed consent be supplanted by a contract system between patient and clinician (Schwitzgebel, 1975)?

   Generally speaking, contracts would legally

bind the therapist to offer the most appropriate treatment the hospital context allows. The clinician's liability would then be determined within the boundaries of this broad commitment. Legal advocates or "contract managers," according to Schwitzgebel, would oversee the contractual arrangement, protecting both therapist and the patient. In this way, the patient could also demand as many options open for treatment as permitted or possible within the hospital setting. What are your thoughts on this matter?

9. In the case of involuntary commitment to a mental hospital, should there be liability on the part of the committing doctor so that patients can sue if they later feel they were unfairly dealt with? Should there be liability despite the claim of the professonal that he or she was acting in the "best interests" of the patient? Who sets up standards for determining what these best interests are?
10. Retaining patients in large institutions against their wills when they are not dangerous to themselves or others is now illegal. If such patients are "dumped" back into your community with no facilities for their care and you feel threatened, what alternative actions would you adopt—and why? Would you petition for the return of the ex-patients to the hospital? Would you support community action for more adequate care? What if adequate care is not immediately forthcoming?

    The vast majority of ex-patients do not tangle with the law—they are not rapists, criminals, or violently assaultive. However, there are rare exceptions. Let us say that an ex-patient in your community got involved in crime, and the release-of-patients issue thereby gained some notoriety in your local paper. Would you feel, on the one hand, that although you are on the side of humanity, justice, and civil rights for patients, that, on the other hand, if your own neighborhood or neighbors were involved you would take an opposite view? How does one resolve the issue of moral responsibility and ethical commitment when one's own immediate safety is involved?

SUGGESTIONS FOR FURTHER READING

Baldessarini, R. J. *Drugs and the treatment of psychiatric disorders.* In A. G. Goodman, L. S. Goodman, and A. Gilman (Eds.), *Goodman and Gilman's The Pharmacological Basis of Therapeutics.* 6th ed. New York: Macmillan, 1980. This chapter, in a classic, encyclopedic work, describes the chemical properties of most of the psychoactive drugs, their effects on the central nervous system, how they are used, and their benefits and risks. The material is concisely presented and up-to-date.

Barber, T. X., Spanos, N. P., and Chaves, J. F. *Hypnosis, imagination, and human potentialities.* New York: Pergamon Press, 1974. These authors take issue with the commonly held view that hypnotic behaviors represent a special state of consciousness often referred to as the "hypnotic trance." They hold, rather, that subjects comply with hypnotic suggestions because they are positively motivated to do so. This book not only presents an alternative explanation of hypnotic phenomena, but also it is of particular value to the student of hypnosis because it presents in a concise, simple manner the basic findings of many experiments on hypnosis. This is a scholarly, well-written book well worth reading by anyone interested in hypnosis.

Benson, H. *The relaxation response.* New York: Morrow, 1975. This book is simply written (it was a best seller, in fact) and presents an objective account of the research conducted at the Harvard Medical School and Boston's Beth Israel Hospital into the effects of meditation. Concentrating on hypertension, the book first reviews theories and research into hypertension, stressing simply physiological explanations. It then explores the "relaxation response" brought about by meditation. Finally, it describes a simple technique that "anyone can use" to elicit the relaxation response.

Bowers, K. S. *Hypnosis for the seriously curious.* Monterey, Calif.: Brooks/Cole, 1976. Paperback. This book differs in its approach to hypnosis from the approach described in the book by Barber and his colleagues mentioned above. It also addresses the question, "Is hypnosis an altered state of consciousness or simply a state of heightened suggestibility?" Unlike Barber, Bowers concludes that the hypnotic trance is a real phenomenon that exists concomitantly with heightened suggestibility. Bowers also presents experiments on hypnotically induced insensitivity to pain, hallucinations, and amnesia as well as clinical uses of hypnosis.

Brown, B. B. *Stress and the art of biofeedback.* New York: Harper & Row, 1977. Paperback available. This book describes the procedures that are used by biofeedback therapists in the treatment of various disorders including headache, anxiety, cardiovascular tension, insomnia, and gastrointestinal problems. It is popular in approach and easy to read. But be warned: the author views biofeedback methods as a "cure" for many ills, despite much evidence to the contrary.

Golann, S., and Fremouw, W. J. (Eds.) *The right to treatment for mental patients.* New York: Halstead Press, 1976. For the student or professional seriously concerned with the right to treatment issue in all of its complexity, this book is a must. The chapters are based on a conference held in 1973 and are supplemented with more current references. The material covered describes the history of the right to treatment issue and legal decisions concerning it. The ramifications of this issue for patients, communities, and the mental health field in general is also discussed. An appendix containing verbatim reports of several key court decisions provides the reader with first-hand exposure to the process of legal reasoning and judicial decision in this important area.

Goffman, E. *Asylums: Essays on the social situation of mental patients and other inmates.* New York: Doubleday, 1961. Paperback. This is an impassioned, well-written series of essays about "total" institutions such as jails and mental hospitals and the ways in which inmates of these systems are gradually but completely stripped of their freedom and privacy. The process of becoming dehumanized is the essential substance of this brilliant classic, which attempts to generalize several striking principles to all total institutions.

Jonas, G. *Visceral learning.* New York: Viking, 1974. Paperback. This is a readable, informative book about visceral learning and behavioral learning theory in general. It centers on the research and work of the renowned psychologist, Neal Miller, with particular emphasis on Miller's pioneering work in the area of learned control of functions of the autonomic nervous system. The author also discusses briefly and succinctly many other topics relevant to visceral control and learning including the history of learning theory from Pavlov through Hull and Skinner, the control of the viscera by Eastern yogis and Zen Buddists, the Western scientific analysis of these phenomena and bodily changes during meditation, and the current use of biofeedback techniques to facilitate visceral learning in Western culture. In addition, the author discusses briefly the social uses of behavioral learning techniques as proposed by Watson and Skinner. An excellent introduction or review, this book is highly recommended to the advanced and novice student alike.

Miller, K. S. *Managing madness: The case against civil commitment.* New York: Free Press, 1976. This book provides a well-written, well-researched discussion of civil commitment. Miller presents interesting case and legal material as well as epidemiological data in support of the position he takes, which argues against involuntary confinement of the mentally ill in all but "dangerous" cases. He points up the biases that are perpetuated and the abuses that result from the use of civil commitment and suggests several reforms. This book is recommended as a thought-provoking presentation of an important social and legal issue.

Sheehan, S. *Is there no place on earth for me?* Boston: Houghton Mifflin, 1982. The author, a journalist, presents with meticulous attention and great compassion, the anguishing experiences of Sylvia Frumkin, a pseudonym for a real person who has been in and out of mental institutions since she was sixteen years old with a diagnosis (but not always) of schizophrenia. The author has observed and talked and visited with Miss Frumkin and her family and doctors over a period of years; as a result, she has pieced together a vivid, moving, and frightening story of the misdiagnoses, abuse of medical prescriptions, and harried lives within large mental institutions. Above all, you will learn about and be deeply moved by society's failure to keep Miss Frumkin in the community for any length of time.

22

Epilogue: The Broad Picture

In this chapter, we step back a few paces to get a broad picture of the scene surveyed in the pages of this book. Are there discernible thrusts and trends in the field? Will these themes fade or will they become influential paradigms for the future? The following are just a few of the areas that represent emerging patterns of great interest among psychopathologists.

Theory

The traditional view that the different scientific disciplines have distinct and meaningful boundaries is fading rapidly. Many psychopathologists no longer jealously guard their domains, defending them against intrusive forces from without. They seem more willing to openly display their interest in genetic, physical, neurobiological, and neurochemical variables in their attempts to explore the origins and modification of abnormal behavior; nor must they look sideways, it would seem, lest they be caught staring, at sociological, familial, and cultural variables as they seek etiological understanding. Apparently, the field approach of this book is being embraced by many scientists interested in the enigma of such presumably diverse entities as schizophrenia, depression, substance addiction, certain types of antisocial behavior, and various manifestations of developmental disabilities—for example, infantile autism.

Diagnostic Procedures and Frameworks

Diagnostic systems, especially the DSM-III, are being carefully scrutinized and evaluated from the point of view of reliability and validity. Classifiers in the field of abnormal psychology seem eager to clarify various subtypes *within* categories—for example, the depressions or schizophrenia or substance abuse. Using computer systems, it might be possible to employ many simple, reliable indices drawn from biological, sociocultural, and familial domains in addition to the usual ones in order to pinpoint the pathological process accurately, so that valid inferences about appropriate interventions can be made. Many people are stressing the need to clarify the diagnosis of childhood disorders, an area in which great confusion abounds. For example, in addition to fuzziness in defining the categories of childhood schizophrenia or "minimal brain damage," the current classification of mental retardation often obscures the distinctions among the etiologies and thus the interventions that might be introduced. A good example is the need to diagnose the risk of psychosocial retardation early enough, so that aggressive preventive efforts can be instituted.

Assessment

It appears that assessment procedures are being increasingly tied in with methods for treatment, skills training, and behavior change rather than with the more traditional exploration of psychodynamic variables. Thus, whether the assessment is concerned with a search for reinforcers and rewards, assets and deficits after brain injury, or with level of skills for independent living in a schizophrenic about to be discharged from an institution, assessment for its own sake seems to be employed less frequently these days.

One emerging assessment need is to identify high-risk individuals—that is, the so-called "vulnerables"—for such eventual "unfoldings" as mental retardation, schizophrenia, developmental disabilities, alcoholism, addiction to heroin, endogenous depression, or suicide. Assessment of risk in these areas would most certainly be based on a complex patterning of many biological, cultural, familial, prenatal, perinatal (for example, nutritional), and personality variables as well as "triggering" circumstances for any given individual (see Zubin [1980] for this view regarding chronic schizophrenia). Once again, computers and sophisticated programs make this more than a remote possibility.

Diagnosis, Assessment, and Treatment—A Single Framework?

Projecting from current interest, there is a possibility that diagnostic and assessment schemes will be embedded within a single system that is almost entirely *treatment* oriented, circumventing many complex considerations that are too unwieldy and unreliable to include within any one framework. Thus, for example, it may be less important to determine the precise subclassification of substance abuse, let us say, or schizophrenia, that the patient presents, than the methods and their combinations that would be required to alter the behavioral picture. Should there be medication, hypnosis, or a combination of these with behavioral/cognitive procedures? What is the level of motivation and education of the patient, chronicity of the maladaptive behavior, and attitude toward the therapist and the offered treatment? Should less stress be placed on verbal interchanges and more on the powerful influences of placebo and trust for a particular patient? Or should the powerful tools of self-control and mastery be stressed with another patient? We would want to know ahead of time that although prescribed medications might clear up the delusions and hallucinations for a third patient, all available information indicates that the patient would refuse to ingest any psychoactive substance. In other words, we are beginning to learn a great deal about the effectiveness of treatment methods in relationship to hidden and no-so-hidden variables other than the "advertised" formal method. Perhaps assessment and diagnostic methods of the future will help us to pinpoint the best road to change in the light of this knowledge for *any given individual.* In this type of evaluation, availability of social support systems, level of motivation to change, premorbid status, the values of the individual and his or her family, SES and educational levels, and similar variables might assume equal status with the presence of delusions and hallucinations, for example, in determining the most effective treatment approach.

Therapy

The exciting trends that were described in the last chapters of this book point to the convergence of hitherto disparate views about helping people to change. Specifically, proponents of psychodynamic, behavioral, and cognitive approaches have begun to recognize the significance of each other's position in helping people to change. Further, the interactional aspects of therapist-patient relationship and variables such as placebo, expectancy, trust, and motivation to change are recognized as being of importance in *all* therapeutic endeavors. In addition, of crucial significance is the client's own perceptions and appraisal of what he or she wants, expects, achieves, or does not achieve in these therapeutic interactions. Finally, many therapists are now willing to give more than just lip service to the realization that the true test of therapeutic effectiveness lies not in the clinician's office or in the laboratory but in the day-to-day life of the patient.

Prevention

There is increasing focus on *primary prevention,* defined as embracing activities that prevent the development of mental illness in large groups of people, rather than its amelioration or remediation in smaller groups or in individuals (see Albee and Joffe [1977] for a classic volume in this area). Goals of primary prevention have to do with broadly based social change that makes inroads into poverty, unemployment, poor coping skills, family disorganization, and inadequate role models. Such thrusts would be concerned with attempts to change personal and social values and to bring potentially isolated people into contact with social support systems.

Primary prevention also attempts to change conditions that create nutritional deprivation in pregnant women and their unborn children as well as to reduce other types of prenatal and perinatal dangers. Such thrusts are aimed at modifying the circumstances that produce community models like the pimp, prostitute, junkie, pusher, and mugger. This broad-band approach involves efforts to change attitudes toward scapegoated people like the elderly or members of some ethnic minority groups while at the same time helping people from these populations to form positive self-images. Primary prevention thus involves interdisciplinary efforts aimed at reaching high-risk individuals and families with regard to, for example, alcoholism, drug abuse, delinquency, child abuse, family violence, rape, birth defects, developmental disabilities, schizophrenia, or psychosocial retardation. Many people believe, however, that the scope and goals of primary prevention represent Utopian ideals that are of great value but of limited practical usefulness in terms of reducing the incidence of psychopathology.

High-Risk Intervention

Even if we were able to reliably identify high-risk individuals for, let us say, schizophrenia, alcoholism, or relapse after heroin abstinence, many people are beginning to recognize the importance of developing strategies for interventions appropriate to the specific vulnerability. How does one work with the identified "vulnerables" in order to prevent the so-called inevitable from happening? How do we train vulnerable children for coping and for competence in their lives or for dealing with the possibility of relapse in an adolescent who has been heroin-abstinent for many months? How do we reduce patterns of family abuse and violence? The answers are not easily forthcoming but unless we come up with some, the seeds of vulnerability will bear bitter fruit.

The Invulnerables

An intriguing area for study concerns the so-called invulnerables, the people—especially the children—who despite the cards stacked against them, be it for schizophrenia, alcoholism, a life of violence or criminality, or psychosocial retardation, "make it," sometimes with flying colors. Where do their strengths come from? How do they deal with the stressors in their lives? Is there something about their biochemical makeups or their perceptions of themselves and their futures that differ from those who break down? We have much to learn about strength, hope, mental health, and, by inference, psychopathology, from studying the invulnerables.

The Neurosciences

Exciting developments in the neurosciences are beginning to have tremendous impact on models for understanding psychopathology. The body's (and especially the brain's) role in controlling, modifying, and causing disordered behavior is being acknowledged by many psychologists who are now conceding that there may be neurobiological underpinnings to diverse pathological conditions. For example, susceptibility to alcoholism, heroin addiction, recurring depressions, schizophrenia, or chronic pain may arise from biochemical imbalances in the brain. Endogenously produced opiates and various other neurochemicals may underlie many conditions hitherto thought to emerge from strictly psychological factors—for example, unexplainable shifts of mood or constant preoccupation with body aches and pains. Slow-growing viruses may speed up the aging process or be implicated in Alzheimer's disease. Trancelike states, dissociative phenomena, out-of-body experiences, and the cult follower's brainwashed passivity may arise from special states and levels of awareness, consciousness, and attentional focus induced by unusual types of brain involvements, for example, right-hemisphere takeover under certain types of experiences. Similarly, deviation proneness and sensation-seeking characteristics of some people may arise from states of underarousal that are neurobiologically produced. It could also be that motivation, hope, and a sense of control and mastery, even if induced by verbal counseling, belief, or placebo are ultimately effective because they stimulate the production of certain neurochemicals. Either way, there may be many promising pathways for changing disordered emotions and behavior.

Availability of New Clinical Populations

Hitherto unavailable or inaccessible groups may be available for study as techniques as well as attitudes toward volunteering for research change. The narrow base rates as well as the veiled and "hidden" nature of many clinical populations—for example, rapists, victims of rape, suicide attempters, members of sexual minorities, and abused family members—have presented researchers with serious problems. Some of these problems may be surmountable as motivation to volunteer for study and the availability of computerized central information services increase and as new research methods for exploring such clinical samples are developed.

Community Facilities

Psychologists and other mental health practitioners are becoming increasingly involved in what had seemed to them to be *social* rather than psychological problems—for example, the question of "revolving doors" and the social networks necessary to prevent the continual return of ex-patients to the hospital. The community's responsibility (and ability) to sustain all kinds of people within it, including the less strong, the less intelligent, and the more vulnerable, is probably not just of social concern but also, many believe, falls within the domain of the psychopathologist.

Attitude Change

Finally, it seems as we look around, that we are all becoming more tolerant and less rigid in our views and attitudes toward mental illness, deviance, and people who behave differently from those in our own groups. Indeed, what can be more fitting than to close this book by focusing on the same theme with which we opened it? Upon rereading the first pages of Chapter 1, in which the rigid labeling and stereotypes about the mentally ill are described, it becomes apparent that many changes have taken place since those pages were written. Many of us have become more tolerant, more accepting, even more able to appreciate the uniqueness and differentness of others. We are acknowledging and even absorbing into our own lives the changing status among men and women as their roles and perceptions of roles become more flexible. Perhaps we recoil less when faced with the frailties of others, mental retardation, sexual practices other than our own, or strange ways of dress and styles of living.

In the end, we are left with a deep awareness of the human organism's amazing will to survive, to change, and to hope and plan for a future that contains promise for a better life. This resilience and capacity for positive outlook, despite the day-to-day disappointments in life, present a constant challenge and sense of wonderment to the psychopathologist.

Appendix A

DSM-III Classification: Axes I and II Categories and Codes*

Disorders Usually First Evident in Infancy, Childhood, or Adolescence

Mental retardation
- Mild mental retardation
- Moderate mental retardation
- Severe mental retardation
- Profound mental retardation
- Unspecified mental retardation

Attention deficit disorder
- with hyperactivity
- without hyperactivity
- residual type

Conduct disorder
- undersocialized, aggressive
- undersocialized, nonaggressive
- socialized, aggressive
- socialized, nonaggressive
- atypical

Anxiety disorders of childhood or adolescence
- Separation anxiety disorder
- Avoidant disorder of childhood or adolescence
- Overanxious disorder

Other disorders of infancy, childhood, or adolescence
- Reactive attachment disorder of infancy
- Schizoid disorder of childhood or adolescence
- Elective mutism
- Oppositional disorder
- Identity disorder

Eating disorders
- Anorexia nervosa
- Bulimia
- Pica
- Rumination disorder of infancy
- Atypical eating disorder

Stereotyped movement disorders
- Transient tic disorder
- Chronic motor tic disorder
- Tourette's disorder
- Atypical tic disorder
- Atypical stereotyped movement disorder

Other disorders with physical manifestations
- Stuttering
- Functional enuresis
- Functional encopresis
- Sleepwalking disorder
- Sleep terror disorder

Pervasive developmental disorders
- Infantile autism
- Childhood onset pervasive developmental disorder

Specific developmental disorders—coded on Axis II
- Developmental reading disorder
- Developmental arithmetic disorder
- Developmental language disorder
- Developmental articulation disorder
- Mixed specific developmental disorder
- Atypical specific developmental disorder

Source: The American Psychiatric Association *Diagnostic and Statistical Manual of Mental Disorders,* Third Edition, 1980. Used by permission of the American Psychiatric Association, Washington, D.C.

* Unless specified, it is assumed that Axis I represents the principal diagnosis. Subjects are coded on both axes. When there is no diagnosis or a deferred diagnosis on Axis II, this must be noted. Unless indicated, the categories in this list are all coded on Axis I.

Organic Mental Disorders

Dementias arising in the senium and presenium

Primary degenerative dementia, senile onset
- with delirium
- with delusions
- with depression
- uncomplicated

Primary degenerative dementia, presenile onset

Multi-infarct dementia

Substance-induced

Alcohol
- intoxication
- idiosyncratic intoxication
- withdrawal
- withdrawal delirium
- hallucinosis
- amnestic disorder
- dementia associated with alcoholism, mild, moderate, or severe

Barbiturate or similarly acting sedative or hypnotic
- intoxication
- withdrawal
- withdrawal delirium
- amnestic disorder

Opioid
- intoxication
- withdrawal

Cocaine
- intoxication

Amphetamine or similarly acting sympathomimetic
- intoxication
- delirium
- delusional disorder
- withdrawal

Phencyclidine (PCP) or similarly acting arylcyclohexylamine
- intoxication
- delirium
- mixed organic mental disorder

Hallucinogen
- hallucinosis
- delusional disorder
- affective disorder

Cannabis
- intoxication
- delusional disorder

Tobacco
- withdrawal

Caffeine
- intoxication

Other or unspecified substance
- intoxication
- withdrawal
- delirium
- dementia
- amnestic disorder
- delusional disorder
- hallucinosis
- affective disorder
- personality disorder
- atypical or mixed organic mental disorder

Organic brain syndromes whose etiology . . . is either noted as an additional diagnosis to foregoing or is unknown
- delirium
- dementia
- amnestic syndrome
- organic delusional syndrome
- organic hallucinosis
- organic affective syndrome
- organic personality syndrome
- atypical or mixed organic brain syndrome

Substance Use Disorders (continuous, episodic, in remission)

Alcohol abuse

Alcohol dependence (Alcoholism)

Barbiturate or similarly acting sedative or hypnotic abuse

Barbiturate or similarly acting sedative or hypnotic dependence

Opioid abuse

Opioid dependence

Cocaine abuse

Amphetamine or similarly acting sympathomimetic abuse

Amphetamine or similarly acting sympathomimetic dependence

Phencyclidine (PCP) or similarly acting arylcyclohexylamine abuse

Hallucinogen abuse

Cannabis abuse

Cannabis dependence

Tobacco dependence

Other, mixed or unspecified substance abuse

Other specified substance dependence

Unspecified substance dependence

Dependence on combination of opioid and other nonalcoholic substance

Dependence on combination of substances, excluding opioids and alcohol

Schizophrenic Disorders: Code each as subchronic, chronic, subchronic with acute exacerbation, in remission, or unspecified

Schizophrenia
- disorganized
- catatonic
- paranoid
- undifferentiated
- residual

Paranoid Disorders

Paranoia

Shared paranoid disorder

Acute paranoid disorder

Atypical paranoid disorder

Psychotic Disorders Not Elsewhere Classified

Schizophreniform disorder

Brief reactive psychosis

Schizoaffective disorder

Atypical psychosis

Neurotic Disorders: These are included in Affective, Anxiety, Somatoform, Dissociative, and Psychosexual Disorders. . . . the DSM-II terms are included separately in parentheses after the corresponding categories

Affective Disorders

Major affective disorders

(a) Code major depressive episode in remission; with psychotic features; psychotic features as mood-congruent or mood-incongruent; with or without melancholia

(b) Code manic episode in remission; with or without psychotic features; psychotic features as mood-congruent or mood-incongruent

- Bipolar disorder
  - mixed
  - manic
  - depressed
- Major depression
  - single episode
  - recurrent

Other specific affective disorders
- Cyclothymic disorder
- Dysthymic disorder (or Depressive neurosis—DSM-II)

Atypical affective disorders
- Atypical bipolar disorder
- Atypical depression

Anxiety Disorders

Phobic disorders (or Phobic neurosis—DSM-II)
- Agoraphobia with panic attacks
- Agoraphobia without panic attacks
- Social phobia
- Simple phobia

Anxiety states (or Anxiety neuroses—DSM-II)
- Panic disorder
- Generalized anxiety disorder
- Obsessive compulsive disorder (or Obsessive compulsive neurosis—DSM-II)
- Post-traumatic stress disorder
  - acute
  - chronic or delayed
- Atypical anxiety disorder

Somatoform Disorders

Somatization disorder

Conversion disorder (or Hysterical neurosis, conversion type—DSM-II)

Psychogenic pain disorder

Hypochondriasis (or Hypochondriacal neurosis—DSM-II)

Atypical somatoform disorder

Dissociative Disorders (or Hysterical Neuroses, Dissociative Type—DSM-II)

Psychogenic amnesia

Psychogenic fugue

Multiple personality

Depersonalization disorder (or Depersonalization neurosis—DSM-II)

Atypical dissociative disorder

Psychosexual Disorders

Gender identity disorders (indicate sexual history, asexual, homosexual, heterosexual, unspecified)
- Transsexualism
- Gender identity disorder of childhood
- Atypical gender identity disorder

Paraphilias
- Fetishism
- Transvestism
- Zoophilia
- Pedophilia
- Exhibitionism
- Voyeurism
- Sexual masochism
- Sexual sadism
- Atypical paraphilia

Psychosexual dysfunctions
- Inhibited sexual desire
- Inhibited sexual excitement
- Inhibited female orgasm
- Inhibited male orgasm
- Premature ejaculation
- Functional dyspareunia
- Functional vaginismus
- Atypical psychosexual dysfunction

Other psychosexual disorders
- Ego-dystonic homosexuality
- Psychosexual disorder not elsewhere classified

Factitious Disorders

Factitious disorder with psychological symptoms

Chronic factitious disorder with physical symptoms

Atypical factitious disorder with physical symptoms

Disorders of Impulse Control Not Elsewhere Classified

Pathological gambling

Kleptomania

Pyromania

Intermittent explosive disorder

Isolated explosive disorder

Atypical impulse control disorder

Adjustment Disorder

with depressed mood

with anxious mood

with mixed emotional features

with disturbance of conduct

with mixed disturbance of emotions and conduct

with work (or academic) inhibition

with withdrawal

with atypical features

Psychological Factors Affecting Physical Condition

Specify physical condition on Axis III

Psychological factors affecting physical condition

Personality Disorders—coded on Axis II

- Paranoid
- Schizoid
- Schizotypal
- Histrionic
- Narcissistic
- Antisocial
- Borderline
- Avoidant
- Dependent
- Compulsive
- Passive-Aggressive
- Atypical, mixed, or other personality disorder

Conditions Not Attributable to a Mental Disorder That Are a Focus of Attention or Treatment

Malingering

Borderline intellectual functioning

Adult antisocial behavior

Childhood or adolescent antisocial behavior

Academic problem

Occupational problem

Uncomplicated bereavement

Noncompliance with medical treatment

Phase of life problem or other life circumstance problem

Marital problem

Parent-child problem

Other specified family circumstances

Other interpersonal problem

Additional Codes

Unspecified mental disorder (nonpsychotic)

No diagnosis or condition on Axis I

Diagnosis or condition deferred on Axis I

Appendix B

DSM-II (1968) Categories and Codes

Mental Retardation

Borderline

Mild

Moderate

Severe

Profound

Unspecified

Following or associated with:

Infection or intoxication
Trauma or physical agent
Disorders of metabolism, growth or nutrition
Gross brain disease (postnatal)
Unknown prenatal influence
Chromosomal abnormality
Prematurity
Major psychiatric disorder
Psycho-social (environmental) deprivation
Other condition

Source: The American Psychiatric Association *Diagnostic and Statistical Manual of Mental Disorders,* Second Edition, 1968. Used by permission of the American Psychiatric Association, Washington, D.C.

Organic Brain Syndromes (OBS)

A Psychoses

Senile and pre-senile dementia
Senile dementia
Pre-senile dementia

Alcoholic psychosis
Delirium tremens
Korsakov's psychosis
Other alcoholic hallucinosis
Alcohol paranoid state
Acute alcohol intoxication
Alcoholic deterioration
Pathological intoxication
Other alcoholic psychosis

Psychosis associated with intracranial infection
General paralysis
Syphilis of central nervous system
Epidemic encephalitis
Other and unspecified encephalitis
Other intracranial infection

Psychosis associated with other cerebral condition
Cerebral arteriosclerosis
Other cerebrovascular disturbance
Epilepsy
Intracranial neoplasm
Degenerative disease of the CNS
Brain trauma
Other cerebral condition

Psychosis associated with other physical condition
Endocrine disorder
Metabolic or nutritional disorder
Systemic infection
Drug or poison intoxication (other than alcohol)
Childbirth
Other and unspecified physical condition

B Non-Psychotic OBS
Intracranial infection
Alcohol (simple drunkenness)
Other drug, poison, or systemic intoxication
Brain trauma
Circulatory disturbance
Epilepsy
Disturbance of metabolism, growth or nutrition

- Senile or pre-senile brain disease
- Intracranial neoplasm
- Degenerative disease of the CNS
- Other physical condition

Psychoses not attributed to physical conditions listed previously

- Schizophrenia
  - Simple
  - Hebephrenic
  - Catatonic
  - Catatonic type, excited
  - Catatonic type, withdrawn
  - Paranoid
  - Acute schizophrenic episode
  - Latent
  - Residual
  - Schizo-affective
  - Schizo-affective, excited
  - Schizo-affective, depressed
  - Childhood
  - Chronic undifferentiated
  - Other schizophrenic

Major affective disorders

- Involutional melancholia
- Manic-depressive illness, manic
- Manic-depressive illness, depressed
- Manic-depressive illness, circular
- Manic-depressive, circular, manic
- Manic-depressive, circular, depressed
- Other major affective disorder

Paranoid states

- Paranoia
- Involutional paranoid state
- Other paranoid state

Other psychoses

- Psychotic depressive reaction

Neuroses

- Anxiety
- Hysterical
- Hysterical, conversion type
- Hysterical, dissociative type
- Phobic
- Obsessive compulsive
- Depressive
- Neurasthenic
- Depersonalization
- Hypochondriacal
- Other neurosis

Personality Disorders and Certain Other Non-Psychotic Mental Disorders

Personality disorders

- Paranoid
- Cyclothymic
- Schizoid
- Explosive
- Obsessive compulsive
- Hysterical
- Asthenic
- Antisocial
- Passive-aggressive
- Inadequate
- Other specified types

Sexual deviation

- Homosexuality
- Fetishism
- Pedophilia
- Transvestism
- Exhibitionism
- Voyeurism
- Sadism
- Masochism
- Other sexual deviation

Alcoholism

- Episodic excessive drinking
- Habitual excessive drinking
- Alcohol addiction
- Other alcoholism

Drug dependence

- Opium, opium alkaloids, and their derivatives
- Synthetic analgesics with morphine-like effects
- Barbiturates
- Other hypnotics and sedatives or "tranquilizers"
- Cocaine
- Cannabis sativa (hashish, marijuana)
- Other psycho-stimulants
- Hallucinogens
- Other drug dependence

Psychophysiologic disorders

- Skin
- Musculoskeletal
- Respiratory
- Cardiovascular
- Hemic and lymphatic
- Gastro-intestinal
- Genito-urinary

Endocrine
Organ of special sense
Other type

Special symptoms
Speech disturbance
Specific learning disturbance
Tic
Other psychomotor disorder
Disorders of sleep
Feeding disturbance
Enuresis
Encopresis
Cephalalgia
Other special symptom

Transient situational disturbances
Adjustment reaction of infancy
Adjustment reaction of childhood
Adjustment reaction of adolescence
Adjustment reaction of adult life
Adjustment reaction of late life

Behavior disorders of childhood and adolescence
Hyperkinetic reaction
Withdrawing reaction
Overanxious reaction
Runaway reaction
Unsocialized aggressive reaction
Group delinquent reaction
Other reaction

Conditions Without Manifest Psychiatric Disorder and Non-Specific Conditions

Social maladjustment without manifest psychiatric disorder
Marital maladjustment
Social maladjustment
Occupational maladjustment
Dyssocial behavior
Other social maladjustment

Non-Specific conditions
Non-specific conditions

No mental disorder
No mental disorder

Non-Diagnostic Terms for Administrative Use

Diagnosis deferred

Boarder

Experiment only

Other

Appendix C

Major Differences and Comparisons Between DSM-II and DSM-III Listings*

DSM-II	DSM-III
Mental Retardation	Mental Retardation
Borderline mental retardation	*No longer regarded as a mental disorder*
Mild mental retardation	Mild mental retardation
Moderate mental retardation	Moderate mental retardation
Severe mental retardation	Severe mental retardation
Profound mental retardation	Profound mental retardation
Organic Brain Syndromes	*Organic Mental Disorders*
Senile and presenile dementia	*Dementias arising in the senium and presenium*
Senile dementia	*Primary degenerative dementia, senile onset*
Presenile dementia	*Primary degenerative dementia, presenile onset*
Alcoholic psychosis	*No listing*
Delerium tremens	*Alcohol withdrawal delirium*
Korsakov's psychosis, alcoholic	*Alcohol amnestic disorder*
Other alcoholic hallucinosis	*Alcohol hallucinosis*
Alcohol paranoid state	*Alcohol dependence and a paranoid disorder*
Acute alcohol intoxication	*Alcohol intoxication*
Alcoholic deterioration	*Dementia associated with alcoholism*
Pathological intoxication	*Alcohol idiosyncratic intoxication*
Psychosis with cerebral arteriosclerosis	*Multi-infarct dementia*
Psychosis with child birth	*No listing: can be called atypical psychosis*
Non-psychotic Organic Brain Syndromes	*No listing*
Non-psychotic organic brain syndrome with alcohol (simple drunkenness)	*Alcohol intoxication*

*Adapted from Appendix C, pp. 371–87, DSM-III (1980) *Manual of Mental Disorders*. Italics highlight differences between DSM-II and DSM-III.

DSM-II *(continued)*	DSM-III *(continued)*
Non-psychotic organic brain syndrome with circulatory disturbance	*Multi-infarct dementia*
Non-psychotic organic brain syndrome with senile or presenile brain disease →	*Primary degenerative dementia, senile onset* *Primary degenerative dementia with presenile onset*
Psychoses Not Attributed to Physical Conditions Listed Previously	*No listing*
Schizophrenia	*Schizophrenic Disorders*
Schizophrenia, simple type	*Schizotypal personality disorder*
Schizophrenia, hebephrenic type	*Schizophrenia, disorganized type*
Schizophrenia, catatonic type* Schizophrenia, catatonic type, excited Schizophrenia, catatonic type, withdrawn →	*Schizophrenia, catatonic type* *Bipolar disorder, manic**
Schizophrenia, paranoid type	Schizophrenia, paranoid type
Acute schizophrenic episode →	*Schizophreniform disorder* *Brief reactive psychosis* *Schizoaffective disorder*
Schizophrenia, latent type →	*Schizotypal personality disorder* *Borderline personalilty disorder*
Schizophrenia, residual type Schizophrenia, schizo-affective type Schizophrenia, schizo-affective type, excited Schizophrenia, schizo-affective type depressed →	Schizophrenia, residual type *Major affective disorder (depressed or manic) with psychotic features* *Schizophreniform disorder* *Brief reactive psychosis* *Schizophrenia with superimposed Atypical affective disorder* *Schizoaffective disorder*
Schizophrenia, childhood type →	*Infantile autism* *Childhood onset pervasive developmental disorder*

*The DSM-III points out that some previously diagnosed cases of Schizophrenia, catatonic type would probably today be diagnosed as having an Affective Disorder.

DSM-II *(continued)*	**DSM-III** *(continued)*
Schizophrenia, chronic undifferentiated type	*Schizophrenia, undifferentiated type*
Major Affective Disorders	Major Affective Disorders
Involutional melancholia	*Major depression, single episode with melancholia or with psychotic features*
Manic-depressive illness, manic type	*Bipolar disorder, manic*
Manic-depressive illness, depressed type	*Major depression* *single episode* *recurrent*
Manic-depressive illness, circular type manic depressed no listing	*Bipolar disorder* manic depressed *mixed*
Paranoid States	*Paranoid Disorders*
Paranoia	Paranoia
Involutional paranoid state →	*Paranoia* *Atypical paranoid disorder*
No listing	*Shared paranoid disorder*
No listing	*Acute paranoid disorder*
Psychotic Depressive Reaction	*Major Depression (single episode), with psychotic features, with coding of severity of psychosocial stressor on Axis IV*
Neuroses	*No Listing*
Anxiety neurosis →	*Panic disorder* *Generalized anxiety disorder*
Hysterical neurosis	*No listing*
Hysterical neurosis, conversion type →	*Converison disorder* *Psychogenic pain disorder*
Hysterical neurosis, dissociative type →	*Psychogenic amnesia* *Psychogenic fugue* *Multiple personality* *Sleepwalking disorder* (childhood section)
No listing	*Phobic disorders*
Phobic neurosis →	*Agoraphobia with panic attacks* *Agoraphobia without panic attacks* *Social phobia* *Simple Phobia* *Separation anxiety disorder* (childhood section)

DSM-II *(continued)*	**DSM-III** *(continued)*
Obsessive compulsive neurosis	*Obsessive compulsive disorder*
Depressive neurosis →	*Major depression, single episode or recurrent, without melancholia* *Dysthymic disorder* *Adjustment disorder with depressed mood*
Neurasthenic neurosis	*No listing*
Depersonalization neurosis	*Depersonalization disorder*
Hypochondriacal neurosis	*Hypochondriasis*
No Listing	*Somatization disorder*
No Listing	*Post-traumatic stress disorder* *acute* *chronic or delayed*
Personality Disorders	Personality Disorders
Paranoid personality	*Paranoid personality disorder*
Cyclothymic personality	*Cyclothymic personality disorder*
Schizoid personality →	*Schizotypal personality disorder* *Schizoid personality disorder* *Avoidant personality disorder*
Explosive personality	*Intermittent explosive disorder*
Obsessive compulsive personality	*Compulsive personality disorder*
Hysterical personality	*Histrionic personality disorder*
Asthenic personality	*No listing*
Antisocial personality	*Antisocial personality disorder*
Passive-aggressive personality	*Passive-aggressive personality disorder*
Inadequate personality	*No listing*
No listing	*Narcissistic personality disorder*
No listing	*Borderline personality disorder*
No listing	*Dependent personality disorder*
Sexual Deviations	*Paraphilias*
Homosexuality (replaced in 1973 with Sexual orientation disturbance)	*Ego-dystonic homosexuality*
Fetishism	Fetishism
Pedophilia	Pedophilia
Transvestism	Transvestism
Exhibitionism	Exhibitionism
Voyeurism	Voyeurism
Sadism	*Sexual sadism*
Masochism	*Sexual masochism*
No Listing	*Psychosexual Dysfunctions*
	Inhibited sexual desire
	Inhibited sexual excitement

DSM-II *(continued)*	DSM-III *(continued)*
	Inhibited female orgasm *Inhibited male orgasm* *Premature ejaculation* *Functional dyspareunia* *Functional vaginismus*
No Listing	*Zoophilia*
No Listing	*Gender Identity Disorders*
No listing	*Transsexualism*
No listing	*Gender identity disorder of childhood*
Alcoholism	*Alcohol Abuse and Dependence* (included within Substance Use Disorder)
Episodic excessive drinking	*Alcohol abuse, episodic*
Habitual excessive drinking	*Alcohol abuse, continuous*
Alcohol addiction	*Alcohol dependence*
Drug Dependence	*Substance Use Disorders*
Drug dependence, opium, opium alkaloids, and their derivatives Drug dependence, synthetic analgesics with morphine-like effects	→ *Opioid abuse* *Opioid dependence*
Drug dependence, barbiturates Drug dependence, other hypnotics and sedatives or "tranquilizers"	→ *Barbiturate or similarly acting sedative or hypnotic abuse* *Barbiturate or similarly acting sedative or hypnotic dependence*
Drug dependence, cocaine	*Cocaine abuse*
Drug dependence, Cannabis sativa (hashish, marijuana)	→ *Cannabis abuse* *Cannabis dependence*
Drug dependence, other psychostimulants (amphetamines, etc.)	→ *Amphetamine or similarly acting sympathomimetic abuse* *Amphetamine or similarly acting sympathomimetic dependence*
Drug dependence, hallucinogens	*Hallucinogen abuse*
No listing	*Phencyclidine (PCP) or similarly acting arylcyclohexylamine abuse*
No listing	*Tobacco dependence*
No listing	*Dependence on combination of opioid and other nonalcoholic substance*
No listing	*Dependence on combination of substances, excluding opioids and alcohol*

DSM-II *(continued)*	**DSM-III** *(continued)*
Psychophysiologic Disorders	*Psychological Factors Affecting Physical Conditions*
Special Symptoms	*No listing*
Speech disturbance	*Stuttering*
No listing	*Specific Developmental Disorders*
Specific learning disturbance	*Developmental reading disorder* *Developmental arithmetic disorder* *Developmental language disorder* *Developmental articulation disorder* *Mixed specific developmental disorder*
No listing	*Stereotyped Movement Disorders*
Tic	*Transient tic disorder* *Chronic motor tic disorder* *Tourette's disorder*
Disorders of sleep	*Sleepwalking disorder* *Sleep terror disorder*
No listing	*Eating Disorders*
Feeding disturbance	*Anorexia nervosa* *Bulimia* *Pica* *Rumination disorder of childhood*
Enuresis	*Functional enuresis*
Encopresis	*Functional encopresis*
Cephalalgia	*No Listing*
Transient Situational Disturbances	*Adjustment Disorder*
Adjustment reaction of infancy → Adjustment reaction of childhood Adjustment reaction of adolescence Adjustment reaction of adult life Adjustment reaction of late life	*with depressed mood* *with anxious mood* *with mixed emotional features* *with disturbance of conduct* *with mixed disturbance of emotions and conduct* *with work (or academic) inhibition* *with withdrawal*
Behavior Disorders of Childhood and Adolescence	*Disorders Usually First Evident in Infancy, Childhood, or Adolescence*
Hyperkinetic reaction of childhood or adolescence	*Attention deficit disorder, with hyperactivity*
Withdrawing reaction of childhood (or adolescence) →	*Avoidant disorder of childhood or adolescence* *Schizoid disorder of childhood or adolescence*
Overanxious reaction of childhood (or adolescence)	*Overanxious disorder*
Runaway reaction of childhood (or adolescence)	*Conduct disorder, undersocialized, nonaggressive*
Unsocialized aggressive reaction of childhood (or adolescence)	*Conduct disorder, undersocialized, aggressive*

DSM-II *(continued)*	**DSM-III** *(continued)*
Group delinquent reaction of childhood (or adolescence) →	*Conduct disorder, socialized, aggressive* *Conduct disorder, socialized nonaggressive*
No listing	*Attention deficit disorder, without hyperactivity*
No listing	*Attention deficit disorder, residual type*
No listing	*Reactive attachment disorder of infancy*
No listing	*Elective mutism*
No listing	*Oppositional disorder*
No listing	*Identity disorder*
No Listing	*Factitious Disorders*
	Factitious disorder with psychological symptoms
	Chronic Factitious disorder with physical symptoms (Munchausen syndrome)
No Listing	*Disorders of Impulse Control Not Elsewhere Classified*
	Pathological gambling
	Kleptomania
	Pyromania
	Isolated explosive disorder
Conditions Without Manifest Psychiatric Disorder and Non-Specific Conditions	*No Listing*
Social Maladjustments Without Manifest Psychiatric Disorder	*Codes for Conditions Not Attributable to a Mental Disorder that are a Focus of Attention or Treatment*
Marital maladjustment	*Marital problem*
Social maladjustment	*Phase of life problem or other life circumstance problem*
Occupational Maladjustment	*Occupational problem*
Dyssocial behavior →	*Adult antisocial behavior* *Childhood or adolescent antisocial behavior*
No listing	*Malingering*
No listing	*Academic problem*
No listing	*Uncomplicated bereavement*
No listing	*Noncompliance with medical treatment*
No listing	*Parent-child problem*
No listing	*Other specified family circumstance*
No listing	*Other interpersonal problem*
Non-specific conditions →	*Unspecified mental disorder (nonpsychotic)* *Atypical psychosis*
No mental disorder →	*No diagnosis or condition on Axis I* *No diagnosis on Axis II*
Diagnosis deferred →	*Diagnosis or condition deferred on Axis I* *Diagnosis deferred on Axis II*

Glossary*

abnormal A broad range of behaviors—in such areas as *mood,* thinking, judgment, *motor* activities, and dress—that deviate from the *norm* in ways that are thought to reflect *psychopathology.*

abnormal personality A pattern of *temperament* or distribution of *traits* that deviates from the *norm* to a marked degree, probably reflecting *psychopathology.*

aberration A deviation from *normal* behavior.

abreaction In *psychoanalysis,* the process by which *unconscious* memories are brought to *consciousness* and relived, accompanied by a release of tension.

absence A momentary lapse of *consciousness,* lasting up to about 30 seconds, that occurs in some types of *seizure disorders;* see *petit mal seizures.*

abstinence Total refrainment from using a substance, such as alcohol or *heroin,* on which the subject has become dependent.

abstinence syndrome The *mental* and *physiological* state, sometimes lasting for days, that occurs after abrupt termination of an ingested substance, such as alcohol or heroin, on which the subject has become dependent or *addicted;* sometimes called withdrawal or withdrawal syndrome.

abstract attitude A *cognitive* approach, the opposite of the *concrete attitude,* which permits the formation of categories, the handling of symbols, the solving of *mental* problems, and the flexible use of ideas; presumably, this mental facility becomes impaired with certain types of brain injury.

acting-out The expression of *anxiety* and *conflict* through actions and behavior, generally without *conscious* awareness of *motivation.*

activity centers Places in the community in which recreational and training programs are offered to severely retarded individuals.

acupuncture An ancient Chinese method of pain suppression, which most frequently involves the insertion and twirling of needles into specified body locations.

acute Rapid and sudden onset of a disorder, usually of short duration.

adaptation The *physiological* tendency of a response to a repeated *stimulus* to become reduced in amplitude and intensity.

adaptive behavior Effective coping with one's environment and environmental demands.

addict One who is physically dependent on a substance, especially *heroin;* see *addicted, addiction.*

addicted, addiction A general term for heavy, uncontrolled substance *dependence*—for example, on heroin or alcohol; more specifically, these terms describe the *tolerance* or withdrawal effects that accompany long-term use of such substances as alcohol or heroin.

adrenal medulla The central part of the adrenal gland that produces *epinephrine* and *norepinephrine,* important *hormones* that regulate behavior.

adrenalin See *epinephrine.*

affect An individual's feelings, *emotions,* and *mood,* and the outward manifestations of these.

affective disorder Major disturbances of *mood* and feelings; see *major affective disorders.*

afferent apraxia A *neurological* disorder characterized by loss of ability to perform certain skilled *motor* acts because of disturbances in receiving impulses from one's own body.

afferent system The *neurological* system that receives and sends *sensory* signals from the skin, joints, and muscles to the brain.

age regression A state induced in *hypnosis* in which the subject seems to return to a younger level in speech, thinking, mannerisms, and other behaviors.

aggression Verbal, symbolic, or physical behavior directed toward other people that is designed to harm or hurt them.

agnosia A *neurological* disorder characterized by loss of ability to recognize objects.

agoraphobia *Irrational* fear of and avoidance of public places, generally characterized by inability to leave one's home.

* Words in italics are defined elsewhere in this glossary.

agraphia A *neurological* disorder characterized by loss of ability to write spoken words.

alcohol abuse Behavioral and interpersonal difficulties resulting from heavy, chronic ingestion of alcoholic beverages.

alcohol dependence The psychological or physical need for alcohol—the latter evidenced by either *tolerance* or *abstinence syndromes.*

alcohol hallucinosis A disorder—characterized chiefly by extremely unpleasant auditory *hallucinations*—that frequently appears following the cessation or reduction of alcohol ingestion in a chronic, heavy drinker.

alcohol withdrawal See *abstinence syndrome.*

alcohol withdrawal delirium A condition that may appear within the first few days after termination or reduction of heavy drinking in a person with a history of chronic drinking; characterized by *autonomic hyperactivity, delusions, hallucinations,* and agitation.

alcoholism A disorder of *alcohol abuse* or *alcohol dependence,* characterized by chronic, heavy, long-term alcohol use; interpersonal, social, and physical difficulties; and marked difficulty in remaining *abstinent.*

alexia A *neurological* disorder characterized by loss of ability to understand the written word.

alpha wave A pattern of *electroencephalographic* brain rhythm that characterizes an alert, wakeful, resting state.

alternate-form reliability A method of estimating test *reliability* by correlating the scores of subjects on two sets of equivalent tests.

Alzheimer's disease A degenerative, presenile brain disease that has symptoms similar to those of *senile dementia,* such as disorientation and confusion, memory loss, and general physical and intellectual deterioration.

ambisexuality A sexual orientation that is characterized by sexual attraction to partners of either sex.

ambivalence The simultaneous presence of contradictory and conflicting emotions, feelings, attitudes, and *drives* regarding the same person, situation, or circumstance.

ambulatory schizophrenia One of the labels for *borderline* syndromes.

amenorrhea The cessation of the normal menstrual cycle.

amnesia Partial or complete loss of memory as a result of an organic or psychological cause or both; see *continuous amnesia, generalized amnesia, localized amnesia, psychogenic amnesia,* and *selective amnesia.*

amnestic syndrome, amnestic disorder A condition generally associated with chronic alochol use, characterized by memory impairment; see *Wernicke's disease* and *Korsakoff's disease.*

amniocentesis The procedure by which a small amount of amniotic fluid is withdrawn from the uterus of a pregnant woman so the *chromosomal* and/or other disorders of the developing fetus can be detected.

amniotic fluid The fluid in the amniotic sac which contains the developing fetus.

amphetamine psychosis An *acute, toxic, pathological, mental* state characterized by heightened suspiciousness and *paranoid delusions* induced by excessive *amphetamine* use.

amphetamines A group of synthetically produced *central nervous system stimulants,* often abused by people seeking their reinforcing effects of euphoria and heightened energy.

anaclitic depression The deep sadness and withdrawal of an infant when separated from the mother, characterized by physical, *cognitive,* and other *developmental* delays.

anal character In *psychoanalytic* theory, a pattern of personality *traits* characterized by excessive neatness, orderliness, and stinginess.

analogue experiment See *experimental analogue.*

anal phase In *psychoanalytic* theory, the *psychosexual* stage in which the young child is preoccupied with the pleasurable feelings associated with the anus and bowel activity.

anal-sadistic phase In *psychoanalytic* theory, a period in early childhood in which *psychosexual* development is characterized by *erotic* focus on the anal area accompanied by an *unconscious* desire to hurt others—for example, the mother.

androgyny Possessing both male and female sexual structures; *hermaphroditism.*

angiography A method that permits the visual depiction of blood vessels by injecting a non-*toxic* fluid, opaque to X-rays, into them.

anhedonia The inability to experience pleasure.

anomie An inability to pursue a goal because of not knowing the paths to it; also, loss of values or purpose in a person; alienation.

anorexia nervosa An eating disorder characterized by excessive weight loss due to refusal to eat; associated with *amenorrhea* and *irrational* distortion of body image.

anoxia Severe oxygen deprivation with risk of harm to brain tissue.

Antabuse (disulfiram) A substance used in the treatment of *alcoholism* that produces extremely unpleasant responses—for example, nausea and vomiting—if there is alcohol in the body.

antisocial personality A disorder characterized by chronic problems in conforming to social and legal codes; individuals with this disorder generally experience a minimum of guilt and are shallow and unfeeling; see *psychopath.*

anxiety A distressing *emotional* state characterized by high levels of *autonomic* arousal (for example, rapid heart beat) and strong feelings of tension, apprehension, and dread, often of an *irrational* nature.

anxiety attack An *acute* episode of *anxiety.*

anxiety disorder One of several psychoneurotic or *neurotic* conditions characterized chiefly by *symptoms* arising from maladaptive ways of handling *acute* or *chronic anxiety.*

anxiety neurosis A non*psychotic* disorder characterized by generalized, *chronic anxiety, anxiety attacks,* or episodes of *panic.*

anxiety state See *state anxiety.*

anxiety trait See *trait anxiety.*

aphasia A *neurological* disorder characterized by loss or impairment of ability to use or produce language and verbal symbols.

aphonia A *neurological* or psychological disorder characterized by loss or impairment of ability to produce speech.

apraxia A *neurological* disorder characterized by loss of or impairment in ability to perform skilled voluntary *motor* acts.

arrhythmia An *abnormal* heart rhythm.

asthenic A tall, lean physique associated with certain types of *temperament* and *mental illness,* according to Kretschmer.

asthma A *psychophysiological* disorder, with *etiology* that is not entirely clear, that is characterized by severe difficulties in breathing—often called bronchial asthma.

asymptomatic Free of *symptoms.*

ataraxic A class of *psychotropic* substances that produce a state of tranquility and/or lowered *anxiety.*

ataxia In *neurology,* an incoordination and impairment in use of voluntary muscles, as in walking or reaching for objects.

atherosclerosis An accumulation of deposits on the walls of blood vessels that cause *circulatory* difficulties.

athetoid, athetosis A syndrome of *motor* difficulties—generally of *cerebral-palsied* individuals—that is characterized by involuntary, slow, wormlike movements of the fingers, toes, and hands.

athletic A muscular physique associated with a certain type of *temperament* and *mental illness,* according to Kretschmer.

attention The responsiveness of an organism to a portion of the *stimuli* impinging on it, accompanied by a decrease or absence of responsiveness to other (wider) portions of that stimulation.

attention deficit disorder A childhood *syndrome,* with or without *hyperactivity,* that, according to the DSM-III, is characterized by inattention and impulsivity but not necessarily *cognitive* difficulties; sometimes referred to as MBD, or minimal brain dysfunction.

aura A subjective sensation (for example, a strong, unpleasant smell) that often precedes onset of a *migraine headache* or convulsion.

autism A state in which there is excessive daydreaming accompanied by interpretation of reality based primarily on personal and subjective needs; see *infantile autism.*

autoerotic See *masturbation.*

automatism An act performed without *conscious* intent, as in some types of *epileptic* states.

autonomic, autonomic nervous system (ANS) The *physiological* system within the body that controls involuntary functions such as digestion, heart rate, and breathing responses; the ANS consists of two parts, the *sympathetic nervous system* and the *parasympathetic nervous system.*

aversive Punishing, painful, noxious.

aversive counterconditioning In *behavior therapy,* a method that pairs a punishing or *aversive* stimulus with an undesirable response, so that the client learns a new response incompatible with the one that is being *counterconditioned.*

aversive techniques In *behavior therapy,* procedures in which punishing, negative, or *aversive* events are presented as a consequence of a person's undesirable behavior.

avoidance-avoidance conflict A *conflict* in which both available choices are equally *anxiety*-producing.

avoidance conditioning In learning *experiments,* the pairing of a stimulus with an *aversive* one so that the previously neutral one is now avoided.

avoidant disorder of childhood or adolescence A *maladaptive* pattern of behavior characterized chiefly by extreme avoidance of strangers, including peers.

avoidant personality disorder A disorder characterized by hypersensitivity to rejection, avoidance of relationships, low self-esteem, and a strong desire for affection.

axon A part of the nerve cell (*neuron*) that may project a great distance, sometimes several feet, in order to transmit signals to other neurons.

barbiturate A commonly used and abused synthetic drug that acts as a *central nervous system* depressant.

base rate The "true," or actual, frequency or incidence of an event or trait in the population.

behavior modification Methods of treatment that use principles of learning, as in *behavior therapy,* to induce changes in behavior.

behavior therapy Methods of therapy that use *interventions* derived from *experimental* research in learning.

behavioral assessment The various procedures used to identify the behavioral target for change, and the conditions and *reinforcements* associated with the desirable or undesirable behavior; behavioral assessment also refers to methods used to evaluate the effectiveness of the *interventions* employed.

behavior theory The various theories about *normal* and *abnormal personality* that view much of human *psychopathology* as acquired through learning.

bell-shaped curve The shape of the *normal* frequency *curve.*

bilateral Having or pertaining to two sides or halves.

biofeedback The procedure by which people are helped to learn to modify some physiological processes—for example, blood pressure—through use of instruments that provide information to the subject about these processes as they are occurring.

biopsy The removal of tissue from a living body for *diagnostic* study.

bipolar affective disorder A major disorder of *affect* in which there are both *manic* and *depressive* episodes; formerly called *manic-depressive psychosis,* circular or mixed type.

bisexuality A sexual orientation that is neither exclusively *homosexual* or exclusively *heterosexual*—a condition in which there can be sexual attraction to both males and females; see *ambisexuality.*

blackout Memory loss for events during a drinking bout.

blood alcohol content (BAC) The amount of alcohol in the bloodstream.

blood platelets Greyish bodies found in the blood that are important for clotting.

blunted affect A disturbance in which the intensity of emotional expression and responsiveness is unusually reduced.

borderline A syndrome that is not flagrantly *schizophrenic* and about which there is considerable *diagnostic* confusion.

borderline personality disorder A *maladaptive* personal style characterized by unstable and unpredictable patterns in such areas as sexual activity, *substance abuse,* interpersonal relationships, and the handling of anger.

borderline schizophrenia See *borderline.*

brain equipotentiality The hypothesis that different parts of the brain possess equal capacity for learning and training.

brainstem The part of the nervous system that connects the brain with the *spinal cord.*

Broca's area A small area of the *frontal lobe* in the left *cerebral hemisphere* associated with speech.

bronchial asthma See *asthma.*

bruxism The clenching and grinding of teeth during sleep or *unconsciously* while awake, creating dental problems; may reflect *anxiety* and tension.

bulimia Episodic, *compulsive* binge eating often followed by self-induced vomiting.

Cannabis sativa The plant from which *marijuana* is derived.

"carving" Self-injurious behavior, sometimes practiced by incarcerated delinquent girls.

castration anxiety In *psychoanalysis,* the fear or *fantasy* of losing or injuring one's genitals.

catastrophic reaction The global *emotional response,* experienced by some brain-damaged patients, to awareness of their limited ability to cope with the ambiguities and confusion of their worlds.

catatonic stupor One of the many bizarre manifestations of *schizophrenia,* in which the patient may sit, lie, or stand in one position for hours or days, often in awkward, strained, peculiar postures.

catatonic subtype, schizophrenia A form of *schizophrenia,* less prevalent today, characterized by disturbances in *psychomotor* behavior, such as *stupor, mutism,* and *waxy flexibility.*

CAT (computed axial tomography) scan A technique that "summarizes" or integrates X-rays taken from many different angles to yield cross sections of living tissue that provide precise localization of hitherto undetected or unlocalized defects.

catharsis In *psychotheraphy,* the "talking out" of emotions with a consequent release of tension.

central nervous system (CNS) The brain and its various subparts and connecting sections, such as the *brainstem* and *spinal cord.*

cerebellum The section of the brain found in the back of the head that is generally responsible for maintaining balance, posture, gait, and equilibrium.

cerebral cortex The outer layer of the *cerebrum,* responsible for speech, thinking, and other related cognitions; "gray matter."

cerebral dominance The *cerebral hemisphere,* either the left or the right, that is most influential in controlling behavior and *mental* contents.

cerebral hemisphere One of the two halves of the *cerebrum.*

cerebral lobe One of the four main sections of the *cerebrum.*

cerebral palsy A disorder arising from injuries sustained at the time of birth, which result in *developmental* defects in the *motor* area—for example, in reaching, walking, talking, and maintaining posture.

cerebral thrombosis A blood clot in a cerebral artery, which blocks the flow of blood to nearby brain tissue, causing serious problems such as paralysis and speech loss.

cerebrovascular Pertaining to the blood supply to tissues of the brain.

cerebrum The largest part of the brain, made up of two *hemispheres,* or halves.

character disorder See *personality disorder.*

character neurosis See *personality disorder.*

childhood onset pervasive developmental disorder The DSM-III term for *childhood schizophrenia.*

childhood schizophrenia A childhood disorder, with onset before puberty, characterized by behavior that is bizarre and inappropriate but, unlike the adult form of *schizophrenia,* does not involve *delusions* or *hallucinations;* this disorder is usually distinguished from *infantile autism* and its *etiology* is not entirely clear.

"chipping" or "chippying" Occasional use of *narcotics* without becoming *addicted.*

choreic Referring to the jerky, involuntary motions of the face and extremities that characterize *Huntington's disease.*

chromosomal "error" An *abnormal* or unusual mix in the forms and structures of the *chromosomes,* resulting in many types of *pathological* conditions.

chromosomes, chromosomal Structures, found in the nucleus of the cells, that carry the *genes.*

chronic Referring to a condition that persists over time.

cingulotomy A method of *psychosurgery* in which the nerve fibers that connect the *frontal lobe* of the brain to the *limbic system* are severed.

circulatory Pertaining to any of the functions of the *vascular* system of the body; having to do with the circulation of the blood.

classical conditioning The type of learning in which a natural response (*unconditioned response*), such as salivation to sight of food, comes to be elicited by an "unnatural" *stimulus (conditioned stimulus*), such as a bell, after repeated pairing of the "unnatural" stimulus with the natural one; the *unconditioned response* now becomes the *conditioned response* because it is elicited by the *conditioned stimulus.*

claustrophobia An *irrational* fear of small, enclosed spaces.

client-centered therapy A type of brief, verbal *psychotherapy* in which the therapist expresses no goals or directions for the client because it is assumed that each client contains within himself or herself the capacity to grow and to become *self-actualized.*

clonic phase The phase in a *grand mal seizure* characterized by extreme jerking of the body as a result of alternating muscle contraction and relaxation.

CNS See *central nervous system.*

cognition, cognitive The higher *mental* processes of "knowing," thinking, understanding, reasoning, judging, remembering, and verbal/symbolic problem-solving.

cognitive behavior modification (CBM) A general term for *psychotherapeutic* approaches that combine *cognitive* and *behavior therapy* to produce changes in people.

cognitive focusing In *meditation,* a technique in which the meditator concentrates his or her attention on a word, phrase, body sensation, or image.

cognitive therapy One of several *therapeutic* approaches that makes use of reasoning, judgment, and other *mental* processes to achieve *emotional* and personal change.

coitus Sexual intercourse.

colitis Inflammation of the colon.

coma A state of *unconsciousness* that can last for a few hours, several days, or even months, during which there is no response to *stimulation;* can arise from disease, *trauma* to the head, or other *insults* to the brain.

commonality A term referring to the shared or overlapping ground between or among *variables.*

community support systems Networks of community facilities designed to help ex-hospital patients and isolated and/or disturbed individuals to cope more competently with the pressures of day-to-day living.

compensation A *defense mechanism* in which there is an excessive or exaggerated development of a behavior, trait, or interest to avoid the feeling of inferiority, pain, or *anxiety* associated with the subjective sense of limitation.

competence The level of ability to use one's resources and aptitudes to get along in life.

compulsion An irresistible, involuntary repeated act that seems to occur without *conscious* intent.

compulsive Characterized by the presence of *compulsions* in a generally orderly, organized, neat person.

compulsive personality disorder In adults, a long-term pattern of rigid behavior that involves limited ability to express warmth and an excessive preoccupation with details, rules, schedules, and lists.

computed axial tomography See *CAT scan.*

concordance In *genetics,* similarity or agreement in selected subjects (for example, twins) regarding a characteristic, trait, behavior, or *pathological* process.

concrete attitude or concrete reasoning A term describing certain types of brain-damaged people, in which there is limited ability in thought processes to make abstractions, generalize, and reason with symbols; contrasts with *abstract attitude.*

concurrent validity The *validity* of a test, as determined by the *correlation* of its scores with those obtained for the subject on other measures during the same general period of time.

concussion A temporary injury to the brain as a result of a blow on the head that creates a brief disruption of *mental* processes.

conditioned response A *response* that, through training, is elicited by an "unnatural" *stimulus.*

conditioned stimulus A *stimulus* that, through training, elicits an "unnatural" response.

conduct disorder A childhood or adolescent *syndrome* characterized by antisocial behavior.

confabulation A *pathological* process in which an individual, when questioned, relates fictitious, unlikely events to fill in severe memory gaps; often accompanies certain types of brain impairment.

conflict An *emotional, motivational,* or *mental* state in which there are two opposing *drives.*

congenital Existing at birth, but not *inherited;* usually applied to a defect, deformity, or disability.

conscious Aware of one's *mental* contents.

consciousness The state of being aware of one's *mental* contents; an aroused, responsive state.

constitution, constitutional In contrast to environmental, the traits and behaviors thought to arise from *inherited* endowment.

contact desensitization A variation of *systematic desensitization,* a procedure in behavior therapy, that makes use of graduated exposure to actual fear-producing situations, in contrast to imagined ones.

contingency management Methods in *behavior therapy,* based on the *reinforcement* control of behavior that alter the problem behavior by altering the consequences of that behavior.

continuous amnesia A type of *amnesia* in which the individual cannot recall events or identity from a specific time in the past to the present.

conversion disorder (formerly hysterical neurosis, conversion type) A disorder in which there is a specific loss of a physical function—for example, hearing or sight—for which there is no physical explanation.

conversion symptom A physical dysfunction for which there appears to be no physical cause, found in *conversion disorders.*

convulsive disorders See *seizure disorders.*

corpus collosum The group of fibers that connects the two hemispheres of the brain.

correlation The extent to which two *variables* are related.

correlation coefficient The quantitative reflection of *correlation* between two *variables,* ranging from -1.0 (negative) to +1.0 (positive).

cortex See *cerebral cortex.*

cortical Pertaining to the *cerebral cortex.*

counterconditioning The use of the principles of *classical conditioning* to introduce a response incompatible with the undesirable one; see *aversive counterconditioning.*

countertransference In *psychoanalytic psychotherapy,* the feelings, positive or negative, that a therapist has toward the patient that could interfere with the course of *therapy.*

covert modeling In behavior therapy, the imagining of one or several *models* performing the behavior that is to be learned.

covert sensitization A technique in *behavior therapy* in which the client is asked to imagine a nauseating or *anxiety*-producing situation in combination with *imagery* of the undesirable behavior that is the target for modification.

crash The marked *depression, anxiety,* and/or fatigue that may follow heavy use, generally of a *stimulant* substance; the *abstinence syndrome* following the abuse of certain drugs.

craving The subjective sensation, reported by many substance abusers, of an irresistible need for more of the substance.

cretinism A condition, appearing at birth, characterized by physical and *mental retardation* arising as a consequence of extreme insufficiency of the *thyroid hormone.*

crisis intervention A group of diverse techniques and orientations designed to help people who are experiencing a period of great stress (for example, after a rape).

criterion keying A method used in test construction to determine which test items (from a group of items) will comprise a scale or subpart of the test, usually determined *empirically.*

crosscultural studies Research that systematically compares and contrasts different *cultures* along specified dimensions.

cross-gendered identity See *gender identity disorder.*

cue The *stimulus* for a response.

cuing In social learning theory, the observation that a *model* can act as a *stimulus* for already learned behavior, even though the model's behavior may not be *reinforced.*

culture The sum of the values, child-rearing practices, habits, taboos, and social myths and beliefs of a society or a subgroup of a society.

cyanosis A bluish-purplish discoloration of the skin resulting from an insufficient amount of oxygen in the blood.

cyclothymic disorder A *mood* disturbance characterized by periods of *depression* and *hypomania* that are not as severe as those in the major *bipolar affective disorders.*

death instinct In Freudian theory, the basic *drive* or *instinct* that involves a push toward death, with a return to the inanimate, as the ultimate goal of living.

defense mechanism An *unconscious* process (for example, *compensation*) by which the *ego* curtails, guards against, or *represses* painful or shameful *mental* and *emotional* material (for example, *anxiety*) or guilt-ridden memories of experiences that lower self-esteem.

deinstitutionalization The policy by which patients from mental hospitals are discharged as rapidly as possible; the trend toward treating mental patients and the *mentally retarded* in the least restrictive setting—generally interpreted to mean the community.

delinquent See *juvenile delinquent.*

delirium An *acute mental* condition characterized by confusion, *hallucinations,* lowered attentional skills, and perceptual disturbances.

delirium tremens (DTs) An *acute mental* condition frequently appearing after termination of long-term, excessive *alcohol abuse,* characterized by *hallucinations, delusions, hyperactivity,* and fear.

delusion A persistent false belief.

dementia A general decline in or loss of intellectual abilities, especially memory, as in *senility.*

dementia paralytica See *general paresis.*

dementia praecox An older, now rarely used, term for *schizophrenia.*

demography The study of the vital statistics, such as age, education, and marital status, of a human population.

dendrites Branchlike, weblike nerve endings that transmit *neural* impulses to other neurons.

denial A *defense mechanism* that involves forgetfulness, *repression, amnesia* or detachment from the act, *emotion,* or memory of a painful event.

dependence, dependency The state or *trait* of needing someone for support and for general well-being; if excessive, can be *maladaptive;* also, habitual use or abuse of substances such as alcohol or heroin, as in *addiction.*

dependent personality disorder A long-term *maladaptive* behavioral pattern characterized by submissiveness, an avoidance of independent actions, and the allowing of others to assume responsibility for major decisions and actions in one's life.

dependent variable In an *experiment,* the variable that is affected by the manipulation of the *independent variable.*

depersonalization The feeling of not existing, of watching one's self from without, of having no identity or sense of self.

depersonalization disorder Feelings of unreality that persist over a period of time (at least a half-hour, according to the DSM-III) that are recurrent and frequent, and that interfere with daily functioning.

depersonalization neurosis See *depersonalization disorder.*

depression An inability to experience pleasure or to obtain *reinforcement* through pleasurable activities, in which the predominant *mood* is one of sadness, hopelessness, or despair.

depressive A general term for an individual who is prone to *depression.*

depressive neurosis *Nonpsychotic depression* arising from *conflict* or an acutely stressful situation, not *endogenous* in nature.

derailment A loosening of the flow of ideas so that they seem to go off onto another track that may be only minimally related to the main idea; frequently one of the qualities of the thought disorder found in *schizophrenia.*

deterioration effects In *psychotherapy* outcome research, the tendency for initial positive findings of effectiveness to diminish with time.

deterrence theory In criminology, the *hypothesis* that the greater the speed, severity, and certainty of punishment for given crimes, the greater the likelihood that potential criminals will restrain themselves from acting out their criminal intent.

detoxification The procedure, often used in medical settings, in which a heavy *substance abuser's* physical and psychological health is restored to a normal level.

developmental Pertaining to growth and the maturing process.

developmental reading disorder Sometimes called *dyslexia;* the DSM-III's category for various types of *reading disability.*

developmental scales *Psychological tests* that are especially designed to measure the growth of the infant and young child insofar as the expected growth patterns are evidenced—for example, in walking, talking, jumping, throwing, and use of number concepts.

deviation-proneness The tendency of an individual to be involved in behaviors and to have values that differ significantly from those of the mainstream, or the majority *culture.*

diagnosis The classification or labeling of a disease, disorder, or *pathological* process.

diathesis-stress An interactional model of *mental illness* (*schizophrenia* in particular) that proposes that predisposition to a disorder in conjunction with severe *stress* and psychological deprivation are necessary prerequisites for the disease to manifest itself.

differential diagnosis Classifying a disorder as distinguishable from other possible disorders by ruling out alternative possibilities.

dimorphism The existence of two different structures and forms in the same type of plant or animal.

discordance The degree of disagreement or difference between selected subjects (for example, twins) with regard to a trait, behavior, or disease.

disease model An approach that defines *abnormality* as a medical or physical illness with specific *symptoms* and causes that are *diagnosable* and treatable, in contrast to models that more heavily acknowledge social and psychological causes that are less specifically pinpointed.

disordered thought processes Disturbances in judgment, reasoning, and other *cognitive* processes that are exhibited by some types of *psychotic* patients.

disorganized subtypes, schizophrenia See *hebephrenic subtype, schizophrenia.*

displacement A *defense mechanism* in which a painful or unacceptable drive, wish, or *emotion* is *unconsciously* transferred to another person or object so that it becomes more acceptable and less painful.

dissociation A state of *consciousness* in which there is a loss, modification, or dramatic change in awareness; a state in which the individual no longer functions as a whole unit.

dissociative disorder One of several types of related *syndromes* that have in common problems in relationship to self-awareness, *consciousness,* and *mental* "wholeness"; examples include *psychogenic amnesia, fugue, multiple personality,* and *depersonalization disorder.*

disulfiram See *Antabuse.*

dizygotic (DZ) twins Fraternal twins born as a result of the fertilization of two ova by two sperms.

DNA (deoxyribonucleic acid) The basic protein of life, in which all the *genetic* information is coded.

dominant gene The unit of *heredity* with a fixed location on a given *chromosome,* which takes precedence over its partner in that it determines the form a particular *trait* will take by masking other possible forms.

dopamine A *neurotransmitter* thought to play an active role in the development of various disorders, such as *schizophrenia* or *Parkinson's disease,* through excessive or diminished chemical action on other neurotransmitters and brain sites.

double bind Communications, messages, and interactions between two people that contain contradictory demands or requests that are not possible to meet simultaneously.

double-blind method A research strategy in which neither the experimenter nor the subject knows the group—experimental or control—to which the subject has been assigned.

Down's syndrome A *chromosomal abnormality* resulting in a special type of physical and *mental retardation;* formerly called *mongolism.*

dream interpretation In some forms of *psychotherapy,* especially *psychoanalysis,* the technique in which the therapist and patient explore the meaning of the patient's dreams.

dreamwork In Gestalt therapy, the *therapeutic* procedure in which the patient is asked to act out his or her dreams.

drive A basic urge or *motive;* a strong inner (sometimes outer) *stimulus* that energizes behavior, causing the organism to do something to reduce its intensity.

drug abuse The use of a substance, sometimes but not always, for recreational purposes, in such a way that it adversely affects the user's everyday adjustment.

DSM-III The third Diagnostic and Statistical Manual of Mental Disorders, the official classificatory scheme of the American Psychiatric Association, published in 1980.

dualism In philosophy, a set of beliefs that subscribes to the view that people have two separate, parallel systems, the mind and/or soul (generally good, divine) and the body (generally bad, evil).

dyad A close couple in a interpersonal or social system, like mother and child, sometimes treated as a unit in some types of research investigations.

dyslexia The general term for a variety of reading disorders, some of which may have *neurological* causes.

dysplastic A term in Kretschmer's approach that refers to a mixed physical type not fitting the usual types he claimed were related to specific mental illnesses.

dyspnea Difficulty in breathing.

dysthymic disorder The DMS-III's term for *depressive neurosis.*

echolalia The senseless and involuntary repetition of a phrase, word, or sentence spoken by another.

ecology The study of the relationship of organisms to their environments.

ectomorph In Sheldon's system that attempted to relate *temperament* to physique, a tall, lean body type.

EEG See *electroencephalography.*

effector A nerve that transmits impulses to an organ, muscle, or gland.

efferent motor aphasia The loss of control over voluntary movements due to *lesions* in the *motor cortex.*

efferent system The *neurological* network involved in transmitting the brain's signals to muscles, organs, and other structures that are involved in *motor* activity.

ego The facet of the mind and *personality* that is the seat of the sense of *consciousness,* self, identity, decision-making capacity, and contact with and awareness of reality; in *psychoanalytic theory,* the structure of the mind that enables the individual to meet with and integrate *responses* to the *id, super-ego* and reality.

ego-alien Thoughts, attitudes, states, impulses, or behaviors that are seen as unwanted, unacceptable, and repugnant to the person experiencing them.

ego-dystonic See *ego-alien.*

ego-dystonic homosexuality According to the DSM-III, a *psychosexual* disorder characterized by a great desire to change sexual orientation from *homosexuality* to *heterosexuality* because of intense underlying *anxiety* and/or other dissatisfactions.

Electra complex In *psychoanalytic* theory, the attraction that a little girl has for her father; more commonly called the *Oedipus complex.*

electrocardiogram (EKG) A recording of the electrical activity produced by the muscular contractions of the beating heart.

electroconvulsive therapy (ECT) Electroshock *therapy;* the administration of electrical impulses to the brain to induce *seizures* used to treat major *depressions* and other mental disorders.

electrodermal See *galvanic skin response (GSR).*

electroencephalography (EEG) The procedure by which electrical activity of the brain is recorded through the use of electrodes placed on the scalp.

electrolytes Chemicals that influence the activities of the *neurons* in the brain.

electromyogram (EMG) The record of electrical changes produced by muscle activity.

embolism The obstruction of a blood vessel by any foreign matter, such as a blood clot or air bubble.

EMG See *electromyogram.*

emotion *Affect;* a strong subjective feeling (for example, rage, love, or fear), usually accompanied by *physiological* changes.

emotional lability Rapid shifting of *mood* and feelings.

empathy The capacity to understand the feelings and *emotions* of others.

empirical Based on observation or actual experience.

enactive modeling A type of *modeling* in which appropriate behavior is demonstrated by a live model (most likely the therapist).

encephalitis Inflammation of the brain.

encounter group A form of group activity and group experience employed in the *human potential movement.*

encounter movement See *human potential movement.*

endocrine system The complex group of glands that send *hormones* into the blood stream, chemicals that control and modify *mood, emotions,* and many *mental* and behavioral events.

endocrinological Pertaining to the *endocrine system.*

endogenous Arising in response to internal, rather than external factors, in contrast to *exogenous.*

endorphins A group of *neurochemicals* that are naturally produced *opiates* that may play a significant role in pain control, the *addictions,* and other psychological dysfunctions; chemically related to the enkephalins.

enkephalins See *endorphins.*

epidemiology The study of the frequency of occurence of various types of diseases and disorders in different populations.

epilepsy A general term for many different convulsive disorders, characterized by various types of *seizure* states.

epinephrine A hormone secreted by the *adrenal medulla,* one of the glands of the *endocrine system* that raises blood pressure and produces effects similar to those of the *sympathetic nervous system;* also called *adrenalin.*

episodic dyscontrol syndrome Behaviors characterized by sudden, unexplainable, explosive, and violent outbursts accompanied by an appearance of losing contact with reality; associated with *acute* alcohol *intoxication.*

erotic Referring to sexuality or to sexually arousing *stimuli.*

E-S interactions Experimenter-subject or therapist-patient interactions.

essential hypertension High blood pressure with no apparent physical *etiology.*

ethnocentric Interpretations, perceptions, and beliefs that are based on assuming the superiority of one's own group.

etiology The causes or origins of a disease or disorder.

eugenics A system of moral and ethical beliefs that proposes the sterilization of people thought to have "bad" or undesirable *genetic* endowment.

evoked potential A research method that measures and records electrical activity in the brain produced in response to *stimulation.*

exacerbate To increase the severity of, aggravate; usually applied to a *symptom* or disorder.

excitement In the language of sexual behavior, the initial stage of arousal in the sexual response cycle of men and women.

exhibitionism A sexual deviance, mostly in males, that involves a *compulsive* need to show one's genitals to an unwilling observer who is usually taken by surprise.

existential anxiety A state of *chronic anxiety* engendered by a sense of powerlessness and helplessness in the face of life's pressures, demands, and crises; see *existential neurosis.*

existential neurosis A common *maladaptive* condition in which the individual feels alone in the world, separated, disconnected, and aimless, with no sense of purpose or ideals; see *existential anxiety.*

existential therapy One of the schools of verbal *psychotherapy* which stresses free will, an active control over one's destiny, the making of choices, and the solving of problems in daily living.

exogenous An influence, cause, or *variable* that arises from events and circumstances outside of the individual; contrast with *endogenous.*

exorcise The use of rites and rituals to drive out or expel an evil force (for example, the devil) from an individual; a popular strategy for dealing with behavioral *aberrations* in some primitive societies.

expectancy A *cognitive* state having to do with one's beliefs, perceptions, and interpretations in regard to one's actions and the actions of others; an anticipatory belief.

experiment The controlled observation of the effect that the manipulation of one *variable* has on another—a powerful tool for testing *hypotheses* in the sciences.

experimental analogue The construction of a laboratory equivalent or parallel to test a *hypothesis* of a real, but overly complex nature, too difficult or unethical to explore experimentally; for example, a *hallucinatory* experience or impulses to rape.

experimental neurosis In laboratory research with animals, the creation of *conflict* by training the animal for two opposing *drives* or incompatible behaviors, with extremely disruptive consequences.

expressive movements Body movements and postures (for example, in gait or bearing) that differentiate one person from another and that seem to be consistent features of one's personal "style."

expressivity The degree or severity of the manifestation of a trait or behavior associated with a particular *gene.*

external locus of control A term for the tendency or *trait* some individuals possess to view personal events as being contingent on outside factors; opposite of *internal locus of control.*

extinction An *experimental* procedure in which repeated trials no longer elicit a *conditioned response*—accomplished by withholding the *reinforcement* or *stimulus* with which it is usually paired.

face validity A form of test *validity,* not overly stringent, that is based on appearances and surface assumptions.

factitious disorders States in which patients consciously and voluntarily simulate and "fake" actual physical and *mental* disorders.

factor analysis A *statistical* method that analyzes a large group of *correlation coefficients* obtained from testing the same group of people with different *psychological tests* in order to derive common dimensions that could account for the wide variations in their responses.

family therapy A group method of treatment in which different family members meet with the therapist at the same time; despite variations in techniques, family methods generally assume that the family unit plays an important role in producing *pathology* in a particular member.

fantasy A mental image, as in a daydream, sometimes of a *wish-fulfilling* nature.

feral Developing with a minimum of cultural and personal contact with other humans, generally living in a wild state.

fetal alcohol syndrome (FAS) *Developmental* and *congenital* defects of infants born to alcoholic mothers, frequently characterized by poor growth, physical deformities in the head and cranium, behavioral difficulties, and *mental retardation.*

fetal therapy Recently developed methods for treating some defects of the fetus *in utero.*

fetishism A sexual variation in which there is a preferred, persistent habitual reliance on objects or things for sexual arousal, *excitement,* and discharge.

fetoscopy A method that allows parts of the fetus to be viewed directly by bringing light into the uterus with specially developed optical instruments.

field approach A model of *abnormal behavior* that assumes that many forces within and outside the organism are affecting it at any given time, and in order to understand the cause of *abnormal* behavior, one must look at the interaction of those forces.

fixation In *psychoanalytic* theory, the arrest of *personality* development at a particular *psychosexual* stage.

flagellation The use of whipping for purposes of sexual arousal in either the victim or the aggressor.

flashback In the experience of some *substance* (especially *LSD) abusers,* the reoccurrence of some of the *sensory* distortions and subjective experiences some time, even many months, after the last dosage.

flatness of affect The inability to respond with any *emotion,* or tendency to respond only with constricted emotion, to situations in which emotional responses are appropriate and called for.

flight of ideas Uninhibited, illogical, excited verbal flow of ideas based on association rather than on coherent, logical thought processes; a *symptom* typical of *acute manic* states.

flooding In some types of *behavior therapy,* the direct and prolonged exposure of an individual to a feared *stimulus* or situation in order to produce extremely high levels of *anxiety* with the eventual goal of eliminating the anxiety response.

folie à deux A condition in which two close people—for example, husband and wife—share the same *pathological, irrational* beliefs.

folie du doute A form of *obsessive* thinking characterized by an inability to make decisions.

forced-choice method In *psychological testing,* the presenting of the client with two equally desirable or undesirable choices to eliminate the tendency most people have to pick the most socially approved item from a pair of items.

fovea The point of sharpest vision on the retina, the lens of the eye.

fragmentation Lack of connectedness or logical flow of ideas found in some forms of *thought disorders.*

free association In *psychoanalysis,* the therapeutic technique of having the patient say whatever comes to mind without censorship; this method is thought to help bring *unconscious* material to *consciousness.*

frigidity A loosely defined term that refers to several vaguely related sexual dysfunctions in women—for example, failure to become sexually aroused or to achieve *orgasm.*

frontal lobe The front sections of each of the *cerebral hemispheres* involved in planning, intent, foresight, and problem-solving.

frontal-lobe syndrome A group of related disabilities that emerge from injuries to the *frontal lobes* so that the *abstract attitude* is diminished, as are *cognitive* functions having to do with foresight, planning, goal-directed behavior, and judgment.

frontalis A rectangular layer of muscle extending from

the top of the eyebrows to some distance up the forehead which plays a significant role in *tension headache.*

fugue A disorder that involves *amnesia* for a previous life, an adoption of a new identity and a new role, and, often, a flight to a new locale; may or may not arise from *organic* causes.

functional autonomy In Allport's approach to *personality,* the persistence of an enduring *trait* without reward or *reinforcement* from the environment.

functional disorders The major *psychopathologies* that are believed to have no physical origin; for example, *schizophrenia* was once thought, and still is by many, to be one of the functional psychoses.

functional dyspareunia In women, a condition characterized by pain during intercourse.

functional vaginismus A condition characterized by involuntary spasms of the vaginal muscles, which prevent penile penetration.

GABA (gamma-aminobutyric acid) An important inhibitory neurochemical that probably plays a role in suppressing excessive neural activity, as in some *seizure disorders.*

galactosemia An inborn metabolic disorder in which there is an inability to metabolize glucose, leading to *mental retardation* if not corrected in early infancy.

galvanic skin response (GSR) Changes in the electrical resistance of the skin (generally as a result of *anxiety*) through the actions of the *autonomic nervous system.*

gamete A reproductive cell; a sperm or egg; a mature germ cell.

gametic mutation A change in the *genetic* material of an organism.

gay A colloquial expression for *homosexual;* a term now in common use among people of all sexual orientations.

gender A person's sex, male or female.

gender anomaly An unusual mixture of male and female sexual structures as a result of *abnormal chromosomes* and/or abnormal hormonal "mixes" during fetal development.

gender identity The *subjective* feeling and private sense of being male or female.

gender identity disorder A *pathological* state arising from the discrepancy between one's actual anatomic sexual structures and one's sense of being male or female; sometimes called cross-gendered identity or transsexualism.

gender role One's social and public behavior that identifies one as male or female.

gene The basic unit of *heredity,* consisting of a *DNA* molecule, which is contained in the *chromosomes* and which provides, with other genes, the program for the development of the individual.

general adaptation syndrome (GAS) According to Selye, the body's attempt to adapt to and deal with excessive demands (for example, a disease or strong *emotions*) and which itself may produce other diseases, some of them *psychosomatic.*

generalization The tendency of a learned response to be elicited by *stimuli* similar to the one with which it was originally paired.

generalized amnesia A type of *amnesia* in which the individual cannot recall any aspects of his or her life.

generalized anxiety disorder A disturbance characterized by persistent feelings of *anxiety;* also called *anxiety neurosis.*

generalized set According to Shakow, the goal or purpose that determines and controls most of our behaviors and that forms the backdrop to them; failure to maintain generalized *sets* may account for some of the difficulties *schizophrenics* display.

general paresis Another term for the avanced phase of *syphilis* (neurosyphilis), which involves *central nervous system* degeneration, *dementia,* and eventually death, unless treated.

genetic Pertaining to the *genes;* inherited.

genotype The inherited characteristics of the individual, determined at conception by the *genes; constitution;* compare with *phenotype.*

Gestalt therapy A form of *psychotherapy,* developed by Fritz Perls, that stresses the here-and-now, feelings, self-awareness, and personal growth.

grand mal seizure A disturbance caused by *abnormal* firing of *neurons* that produces loss of consciousness and violent convulsions, followed by confusion, disorientation, and *depression* in the immediate, post-seizure period.

grandiosity A trait and/or behavior characterized by an overestimated, exaggerated view of one's abilities and powers.

Grave's disease An *endocrinological* dysfunction associated with excessive production of the *thyroid hormone,* which produces *anxiety, hyperactivity,* and *mood* disturbances.

grief reaction An extended, intensive period of despair, guilt, and *depression* following the death of a loved one, more intensive than normal mourning.

group therapy A general term for several different methods used to modify people's behavior through group sessions that meet once or twice weekly.

habituate The *physiological* tendency for a *response* to a repeated stimulus to diminish in amplitude or intensity.

hallucination A *sensory* or perceptual experience with no basis in reality.

hallucinogen A general term for substances of abuse (for example, *LSD*) that produce sensory distortions and/or *hallucinations.*

hallucinosis An *abnormal* state in which there are *hallucinations* but no clouding or fuzziness of *consciousness.*

hebephrenic subtype, schizophrenia A form of *schizophrenia* characterized chiefly by incoherent speech, inappropriate *affect,* and silliness; called the *disorganized* subtype by the DSM-III.

hematuria A condition of blood in the urine.

hemodialysis A procedure in which the patient's blood is cleansed using special equipment.

heredity A general term for the *genetic* endowment within each individual; the transmission of genetic structures from parents to offspring.

heritability The degree to which a *trait* or characteristic is determined by *genetic* factors.

hermaphroditism A condition in which the sexual anatomical structures and the *chromosomal* makeup are in contradiction.

heterosexual, heterosexuality Sexual attraction to and sexual practices with members of the opposite sex.

histrionic personality disorder A long-term *maladaptive* pattern of behavior characterized by self-dramatization, self-centeredness, *emotional* instability, and attention-seeking.

homeostasis The body's striving for maintaining a steady *physiological* state.

homosexual, homosexuality Sexual attraction to and sexual practices with members of one's own sex.

"hooking" An informal term for the process by which the client comes to believe in and trust the therapist as a healing agent; many believe that this process is essential for *psychotherapy* to work.

hormones Chemicals transmitted to the bloodstream by glands of the *endocrine* system that have important regulatory functions in a wide number of areas, such as growth, sexual development, and *mood.*

hospitalism A pattern of extreme apathy observed in infants who are separated from their mothers or *mother-surrogates* for a prolonged period of time.

hotseat A term for a technique used in *Gestalt therapy,* in which a willing individual from the group participates in an exchange with the therapist involving tasks and exercises designed to help the individual become aware of his or her true feelings.

human potential movement A general view about helping people that relies on the *encounter group* as a primary method; this approach stresses the development of each individual's capacity for love, trust, and sense of personal responsibility for his or her actions.

humanistic approaches In *psychotherapy,* the general orientation of several methods—for example, those of Carl Rogers or Fritz Perls—that emphasize the individual's capacity to grow, learn, change, and to exercise choices and controls over his or her life.

Huntington's chorea See *Huntington's disease.*

Huntington's disease (Huntington's chorea) A rare inherited disorder associated with *irreversible* damage to the *central nervous system,* resulting in *dementia, motor* dysfunctions such as jerking movements, helplessness, and eventually, death.

hydrocephalus A *congenital* defect in which an excess of cerebrospinal fluid in the head exerts pressure on the brain; usually associated with *mental retardation.*

hyperactive, hyperactivity Excessive *motor* activity.

hyperacusis An *abnormal* condition of heightened acuteness of hearing.

hypermotility See *hyperactive.*

hyperthyroidism A *pathological* condition in which there is an excessive amount of *thyroid hormone* in the bloodstream, characterized by increased *metabolism, emotional* distress, jitteriness, and tension.

hypertonicity Excessive body tone or tension.

hyperventilation A state of rapid and deep breathing, usually brought on by *acute anxiety,* that reduces the level of carbon dioxide in the blood.

hypnagogic Pertaining to visual images that are sometimes experienced while falling asleep and upon awakening.

hypnosis A heightened, intense, focused *attentional* state that is associated with increased suggestibility and, some say, an altered state of *consciousness.*

hypnotic analgesia A state of reduced awareness of pain brought about by suggestion during *hypnosis.*

hypnotic induction The process by which an individual accepts the suggestion of the *hypnotist* to become hypnotized; also, the method used by the hypnotist to put the subject into a hypnotic state.

hypnotic susceptibility The degree to which an individual accepts the *hypnotist's* suggestion to become hypnotized.

hypnotist A person specializing or trained in the use of *hypnosis.*

hypochondriasis A disorder characterized by *chronic* and excessive preoccupation with one's physical health, disease, and with the possibility of becoming afflicted with illness.

hypoglycemia A physical condition in which there is an extremely low level of sugar in the blood, often associated with mood difficulties such as irritability, anger, and *depression.*

hypomania An *abnormal mood* state somewhere between high spirits and euphoria and *manic* excitement.

hypotension A condition of abnormally low blood pressure.

hypothalamus The part of the brain, underneath the *cortex,* that controls or is indirectly involved with many regulatory functions of the body—for example, the *visceral, autonomic,* and *endocrine* systems.

hypothesis In the science, the statement about the relationship among experimental variables that is tested in an *experiment.*

hypothyroidism A condition characterized by an insufficiency of the *thyroid hormone,* resulting in *cretinism* in children, unless treated.

hysteria A once-popular term referring to conditions found in *histrionic personality disorders;* also, sometimes used in conjunction with *hysterical disorders* or *conversion disorders.*

hysterical disorder A popular term for *conversion disorder* and for *dissociative disorder.*

hysterical personality style One of several patterns of *temperament,* not necessarily a disorder, that contains many elements similar to those found in *histrionic personality disorders*—for example, *attention*-seeking behavior and *emotional* changeability.

id In *psychoanalytic* theory, the structure of the mind that consists of *innate drives* and *instincts,* and the *unconscious;* the other parts of the mind are *ego* and *superego.*

ideas of reference One of the qualities found in *paranoid* thinking, in which the person interprets remarks and events as being directly related to himself or herself.

ideational Referring to the *mental* content of ideas and inner thoughts.

idée fixe An obsession; a powerful, recurrent thought that is difficult to relinquish and often *irrational;* see *delusion.*

identification One of the *defense mechanisms,* in which the individual *unconsciously* identifies with or *models* himself or herself after another, possibly feared, person, in order to reduce *anxiety.*

identity disorder A DSM-III category of disturbance, primarily of childhood or adolescence, in which there is severe distress in such areas as long-term goals, sexual orientation, and moral values.

idiographic Unique and singular qualities and *traits* of an individual.

idiopathic Of no known cause, as in idiopathic *epilepsy.*

idiosyncratic, idiosyncrasy Odd, peculiar behavior that deviates from the *norm.*

idiot savant A special type of *mental retardation,* typically with a pattern of unusually developed capacity in an extremely narrow area, such as memory for long strings of numbers, accompanied by generally limited or below average skills in most other areas.

imagery *Mental* pictures and likenesses, as in daydreaming, imagining.

implosion In *behavior therapy,* the method of having the client imagine, for extended periods of time, situations and circumstances that are extremely *anxiety*-producing, with the goal of eventually eliminating the *irrational* fear; see *flooding.*

impotence An inability to maintain and sustain an erection during intercourse.

imprinting The process of which a behavior is rapidly acquired through learning, usually at an early, critical stage of development.

impulse An urge to act, a striving; sometimes used interchangeably with *instinctual* urge.

impulse control disorder or impulse disorders Usually, a pleasurable, nonpsychotic difficulty in which there is poor control over *impulses.*

inappropriate affect An *emotional* response that is inappropriate to the situation.

incest Sexual relations between close relatives—for example, between siblings, or between father and daughter.

independent variable In an *experiment,* the *variable* that is manipulated so that it effects on the *dependent variable* can be measured or observed.

induction aid A technique used in *modeling* methods in *behavior therapy,* by which the therapist gradually helps the client to perform a desired behavior.

infantile autism A rare, early-childhood disorder, occurring more often in males than females (not to be confused with *childhood schizophrenia*) characterized by such *symptoms* as aloneness and aloofness, limited use of language for communication, avoidance of eye contact, and general "differentness" in posture, behavior, and *attentional* focus; this disorder is probably not of *genetic* origin but may be due to various environmental and biological circumstances.

inhalants Chemical solvents, often *toxic* (for example, cleaning fluid), that release vapors that are deliberately inhaled for a "high."

inherited *Traits* and structures that are transmitted from parents to offspring through the *genes.*

innate *Traits* and patterns of behavior that are fixed at birth through *heredity.*

insanity defense A legal argument used by some criminals that invokes the plea of not guilty because of *mental illness* at the time of the criminal act.

insomnia, persistent Recurrent and *chronic* periods of difficulty in falling or remaining asleep.

insomnia, temporary Short, brief-term period of difficulty in falling or remaining asleep.

instincts, instinctual A person's inner core of energy and inborn *drives.*

insult A blow, injury, or *trauma* to physical tissue, to the body.

intellectualization One of the *defense mechanisms,* in which the individual denies or covers up a strong, unacceptable *drive* with *rational, cognitive* activity such as reasoning and debate, in order to avoid high levels of *anxiety.*

intelligence *Mental* abilities; intellectual capacity or potential for learning, reasoning, and solving problems.

intelligence test One of several individually administered or group tests that attempts to measure *intelligence.*

intelligence quotient (IQ) The ratio obtained by dividing an individual's *mental age* by his or her chronological age multiplied by 100; the general numerical term reflecting intellectual capacity as determined through *psychological testing,* with approximately 90 to 110 taken to be the average range.

intermittent explosive disorder A rare *pathology,* more common in males than females, that involves several discrete episodes of extreme aggression, such as assault against someone or destruction of property; these acts are grossly out of proportion to the provocation.

internal locus of control An individual's perception of events as being caused by or linked to his or her own behavior and *personality* rather than to outside circumstances; opposite of *external locus of control.*

inter-rater reliability The agreement or disagreement between experts in *diagnosis* or ratings, as determined by *correlational* methods.

intervention In treatment and *psychotherapy,* any method, technique, or procedure introduced to modify, alter, or stop the course of a behavior, *symptom,* or *pathological* process.

intoxication A condition arising from the ingestion of noxious substances that adversely affect the *central nervous system.*

intractable Unmodifiable, resistant to treatment; usually referring to a *symptom* or *pathological* state.

introjection A *defense mechanism* in which the individual incorporates the characteristics, qualities, and *traits* of a closely related person to avoid the possible *anxiety* engendered by separation from that person.

introversion The opposite of *extraversion;* having to do with a predominately inner-oriented *temperament* that is less concerned with others, social activities, and outside events than with oneself, one's thoughts, and one's own actions.

introversion-extraversion An extremely important dimension of *temperament* in several major theories of *personality;* the behaviors and attitudes that have to do with one's relationship to the outer world of people and events or the inner world of one's own *moods,* mind, and feelings.

in utero Not yet born; in the uterus.

IQ See *intelligence quotient.*

involutional melancholia A once-popular *diagnostic* category, no longer in use, in which acute *depression* in middle-aged women was (erroneously) thought to arise from *menopausal* changes.

irrational A *cognitive* and *mental* condition characterized by poor judgment, lack of reason, and deficient logic.

irreversible A course of a *pathological* process that cannot get better, even with treatment, as in some types of advanced *neurological* conditions.

isolation A *defense mechanism* in which the individual retreats or withdraws from an *emotion,* experience, or memory having to do with an unacceptable *impulse* or *drive.*

junkie, junky Slang for a *heroin*-dependent person; an *addict.*

juvenile delinquent A legal designation for young people who engage in criminal activities or antisocial activities; age limitations and offenses vary according to changing legal codes.

karyotyping The procedure by which the classification of the *chromosomal* makeup of cells is achieved; the use of a photomicrograph in which the number, size, and shape of the chromosomes are displayed.

kleptomania An *impulse control disorder* that is characterized by repeated inability to resist the urge to steal an object of no immediate use and no special monetary value.

Klinefelter's syndrome A *chromosomal* sex-related disorder in which the male is born with 47 chromosomes instead of the usual 46 (there is an extra X chromosome); features include the development of breasts, slim body build, and underdeveloped penis and testes.

Korsakoff's disease The former name for *amnestic syndrome,* a condition frequently associated with serious vitamin deficiency; it often is the consequence of prolonged, heavy alcohol use and is characterized by *CNS* impairment and significant memory loss.

la belle indifférence The bland, neutral, nonworrying attitude displayed by many patients with *conversion disorders.*

labeling theory A model that holds that the labeling process affects the labeler's as well as the labeled person's judgments and interpersonal behavior.

lability A fluctuation of *moods* and *emotions* with no apparent reason.

latency In *reaction-time experiments,* the period that elapses between a stimulus or signal and the response to it.

latency stage In *psychoanalytic* theory, the phase in *psychosexual* development in which sexual and *libidinal* drives become *repressed* and inactive.

latent content In *psychoanalytic* theory, the hidden meaning of a dream used as a path to the *unconscious;* contrasts with *manifest content.*

latent schizophrenia One of the labels for *borderline* syndromes.

lateral dominance The right- or left-sided preference of the body, as in handedness.

lateralization The differences in function between the right and left *cerebral hemispheres.*

laws In science, the broad general "truths" about the relationships between and among phenomena in the real world.

learned helplessness The condition of having acquired the belief that no matter what one does, the undesirable situation cannot be modified; the "giving up" that has been learned after many "no win" experiences that is said to characterize *depression.*

lesion Any physical damage to living tissue.

leucotomy A form of *psychosurgery* in which the pathways between the *frontal lobes* and *thalamus* are severed.

libidinal Referring to the *libido.*

libido In *psychoanalytic* theory, the *drive* for life; sexual energy and sexual *instincts.*

lie detector See *polygraph.*

limbic system Structures in the brain that regulate behavior having to do with basic survival (for example, fighting or fleeing); also, the seat of the *emotions,* such as fear and rage.

lobotomy Surgical sectioning of certain tissues of the brain; see *leucotomy.*

localized amnesia One type of *psychogenic amnesia,* in which there is inability to remember anything after an extremely stressful event, such as a flash flood.

locus The position or site of a *gene* on a *chromosome.*

locus of control A *personality* dimension that bears on how one assigns causality for one's behavior, problems, and conflicts—that is, to either external events and causes or to internal ones.

longitudinal A type of research design that follows the progress of a group of subjects over a period of time—often years—in order to test a *hypothesis.*

longitudinal fissure The gap that separates the right and left *cerebral hemispheres.*

LSD (D-lysergic acid diethylamide tartrate) An *hallucinogenic* substance of abuse.

Lysergic acid diethylamide See *LSD.*

mainstreaming The teaching of *mentally retarded* children in regular classrooms, as opposed to special classes or separate facilities.

major affective disorder A general term for serious *mood* and *affect* disturbances that include *bipolar affective disorders* and major *depressions.*

major set See *generalized set.*

maladaptive Behaviors that interfere with a person's ability to cope, solve problems, and get by in life.

malingering A *conscious* and voluntary act in which an individual fakes an illness in order to avoid or shirk an obligation or duty.

mania A *psychotic* state of agitated excitement with *flight of ideas,* poor judgment, *grandiosity,* restlessness, and sleeplessness.

manic An excited, high, extremely talkative state—a *mood* swing in contrast to the *depressed* side of *bipolar affective disorder.*

manic depressive disorder, illness Another (older) term for *bipolar affective disorder.*

manifest content The overt, obvious, realistic meaning of a dream, in contrast to its *latent content.*

mannerisms A peculiar, purposeless, repeated stereotyped movement, posture, or facial expression that is often associated with *schizophrenia.*

mantra In *meditation,* a word or phrase that is concentrated on and constantly repeated by the meditator.

MAO (monoamine oxidase) inhibitors A large group of anti*depressant* drugs.

marathon group In the encounter movement approach, an intense group experience that takes place over a concentrated, extended, uninterrupted time period (for example, a weekend).

marijuana An illegal substance, comprised of the leaves, stem, and resin of the *Cannabis sativa* plant, that is used for recreational purposes to get "high."

masturbation Genital self-stimulation.

medical model An approach to *abnormal behavior* that regards it as a disease process that has a specific cause and *diagnosis,* a best method of cure, and a concrete, definable *prognosis;* see *disease model.*

meditation A general term for a relaxation method that involves quiet isolation and intense concentration on a simple phrase or image for a period of time with a consequent reduction, it is claimed, of tension and *anxiety.*

melancholia Severe depression, generally of the *endogenous* type.

meningoencephalitis Inflammation of the membranes of the brain or spinal cord.

menopause The phase in life, usually between 45 and 50 years, during which the menstrual cycle ceases.

mental Having to do with one's thoughts, ideas, and any other activity or response of the mind.

mental age (MA) The level of development of intellectual functions, expressed in years and months; originally, a score derived from the Binet *intelligence* scales, which was used in deriving the *IQ* score.

mental competence A legal term for the ability of defendants to stand trial—to understand the charges against them and participate in their own defense.

mental health A non*pathological,* stable state of *emotional* functioning that allows an individual full use of resources to cope with life and to engage in gratifying personal relationships.

mental illness Mental disease; mental disturbance; *psychopathology;* usually used in the *medical model* of *abnormal* behavior; contrasts with *mental health.*

mental retardation A general term for significantly below-average *intelligence,* with limited skills in *adaptive behavior.*

mentally retarded One who shows *mental retardation.*

mesmerism An early term for *hypnosis;* derived from the name of Anton Mesmer, who popularized it.

mesomorph In Sheldon's theory, which attempted to relate physique to *temperament,* an athletic, muscular type.

metabolic, metabolism Having to do with the rate at which the body transforms ingested food into complex chemicals and complex substances into simpler ones to produce energy.

metaphysics A branch of philosophy that attempts to explain the origin and structure of the universe, of existence, and of being.

methadone A synthetic *narcotic* substance, less *addictive* than *heroin,* used as a substitute for heroin in order to aid in the achievement of *abstinence.*

microcephaly A small, peculiarly shaped skull, frequently associated with *mental retardation,* that may arise from many circumstances, including excessive alcohol intake during the mother's pregnancy.

migraine headache A severe, incapacitating head pain, often accompanied by dizziness, nausea, and blurred vision, thought to be caused by the dilation of cranial blood vessels.

mild retardation A *mental retardation* category that accounts for 80 percent of the retarded population, with an IQ range of roughly 50 to 70; regarded as educable.

milieu methods An approach to *therapy* that emphasizes the atmosphere of the entire facility.

minimal brain dysfunction (MBD) See *attention deficit disorder.*

Minnesota Multiphasic Personality Inventory (MMPI) An extremely popular, well-constructed paper-and-pencil test of *personality.*

mixed lateral dominance Inconsistent left-right preference—for example, in handedness.

MMPI See *Minnesota Multiphasic Personality Inventory.*

model A teacher, parent, or therapist, who because of prestige and status, can provide examples of complex patterns of behavior that a subject can learn in a relatively short period of time by observation of the desired behavior.

modeling The ability to learn by watching someone

else (a *model*) perform the activity; the procedure by which the learned response is acquired by *imitating* others such as teachers, parents, or peers.

moderate retardation *Mental retardation* with an *IQ* range of roughly 35 to 49; regarded as trainable.

mongolism An obsolete term for *Down's syndrome.*

monozygotic (MZ) Twins developed from a single fertilized *ovum;* identical twins.

mood State of mind and feelings; affected by one's *emotional* condition.

mood-congruent psychotic features A rating of the *psychotic* features of a major *manic* or *depressive* episode that indicates consistency between the delusions and the dominant *mood.*

mood-incongruent psychotic features A rating of the *psychotic* features of a major *manic* or *depressive* episode that indicates lack of consistency between the *delusions* and the dominant *mood.*

Morita therapy A Japanese treatment that reflects a Zen orientation, in which interpersonal goals are not stressed; instead, goals encourage individuals to accept their positions within nature.

Moro reflex The startle response found in normal infants, in which the extremities of the body are extended in *response* to a sudden, loud *stimulus.*

mother surrogate A substitute or replacement for the mother in terms of *nurturing* and parenting behaviors toward the offspring.

motivation, motivational *Drives, instincts,* or energizers of behavior that push, incite, or impel the organism toward a goal.

motive A *drive* or *instinct* that incites to action; includes feelings and *emotions.*

motor Pertaining to movement and motion of, but also within, the body—for example, the motor impulse that activates a muscle.

motor cortex The part of the brain responsible for voluntary movement.

multi-infarct dementia According to the DSM-III, a rare form of *dementia* resulting from the cumulative effect that a series of cardiovascular accidents can have on brain tissue.

multiple personality A *dissociative disorder* in which two or more dramatically different personalities co-exist in the same person.

Munchausen syndrome See *factitious disorder.*

mutation In *genetics,* a sudden or dramatic variation from the previous generation, in contrast to gradual, evolutionary changes.

mutism A voluntary or involuntary inability to speak, sometimes found in certain *psychopathological* conditions—for example, some types of *schizophrenia.*

myocardial infarction A "heart attack."

narcissistic personality disorder A long-term pattern of *maladaptive* behavior and *temperament* characterized by feelings of *grandiosity* and self-importance, preoccupation with *fantasies* of success and power, and constant need for admiration.

narcolepsy A disorder in which the patient experiences sleeping attacks during the daytime.

narcotic One of several drugs—for example, *heroin* or *opium*—with strong *addictive* potential, that produces lethargy and frequently has a powerful pain-relieving effect.

narcotic antagonist (narcotic-blocking drug) A chemical that blocks the reinforcing effects of *narcotics,* used in the treatment of *heroin addicts.*

narcotic-blocking See *narcotic antagonist.*

neo-Freudian A follower of the *psychoanalytic* model who introduced innovations into Freudian theory—for example, in underplaying the biological causes of *psychopathology* while stressing social conditions, *culture,* and socially induced *conflict* in the development of the *neuroses.*

neologism A coined or manufactured word frequently found in the speech of *schizophrenics.*

neoplasm A tumor, an *abnormal* growth.

nerve A *neural* grouping or pathway that consists of a dense clustering of specialized *neurons.*

nervous system The network of *nerves, neurons,* and tissues that transmit signals to and from the brain to all parts of the body and from the sensory organs to the brain.

neural Pertaining to a *nerve* or the *nervous system.*

neurochemical A general term for a chemical substance that influences the actions of the nerve cells.

neurocutaneous dysplasia A *CNS hereditary* disorder frequently associated with *mental retardation.*

neurofibromatosis An *hereditary* disorder, frequently associated with *mental retardation,* involving multiple growths in the *peripheral* and *central nervous system* and "cafe au lait" spots on the surface of the skin.

neuroleptic See *psychotropic.*

neurological Pertaining to the *nervous system.*

neuromodulator A chemical substance that increases or decreases *neuronal* activity.

neuron, neuronal A *nerve* cell, the basic unit of the *CNS.*

neuropsychiatric Pertaining to behavioral abnormalities related to *organic* disturbances of the *nervous system,* primarily the brain.

neuroregulator See *neuromodulator.*

neurosis A non*psychotic* emotional disorder, generally of a mild nature.

neurosyphilis See *general paresis.*

neurotic Pertaining to symptoms, conflicts, or behaviors associated with any of the *neuroses.*

neurotic character A secondary type of *psychopath;* an individual involved in antisocial behavior in whom there is high *anxiety,* the presence of inner *conflict,* and other *emotional* disturbances.

neurotic character disorder An early term for *personality disorder;* a long-term maladaptive personal style that is extremely troublesome and distressing to the individual.

neurotic delinquent See *neurotic character.*

neurotic depression See *depressive neurosis.*

neurotic psychopath See *neurotic character.*

neuroticism The personality *trait,* according to Eysenck's views, that arises from a tendency to respond to stressful situations with high *autonomic* arousal.

neurotransmitter A *neurochemical,* released at the *synapse,* that carries signals from one neuron to another.

nightmare A terrifying dream occurring during *REM* sleep.

nominal aphasia A type of *aphasia* in which the patient has difficulty in naming an object though he or she understands what it is.

nomothetic method In research, the study of groups of individuals to discover general laws, in contrast to the *idiographic* method.

nondynamic approaches In *psychotherapy,* the views that stress the here-and-now, are more direct or persuasive, and/or do not focus on *unconscious conflicts,* the past, or on insight into and understanding of one's *personality.*

norepinephrine A *neurotransmitter,* released by *nerve* cells of the *sympathetic nervous system,* that stimulates and controls many *visceral* organs of the body.

norm The standard set by the majority in a group of subgroup.

normal Usual; conforming to standards found in the majority; not *abnormal; emotionally* and *mentally* healthy; not deviant.

normal curve In *statistics,* a bell-shaped graphic representation of the frequency of a behavior or *trait,* in which the greatest frequency occurs around the center or average, with a gradual and symmetrical reduction of frequency to either extreme, above and below the average.

normal frequency curve See *normal curve.*

normal personality Generally, a *temperament* or pattern of *traits* that does not contain *psychopathology* or *neurotic* or *psychotic* features.

normalization The social, educational, and legal doctrine that promotes and encourages the *mentally retarded* to live their lives as *normally* as possible, in terms of jobs, family, marriage, and community life.

norms In *psychological testing,* the summaries of the test performances of a group of subjects; the standards by which any particular individual's performance is judged.

nosology A systematic classification of disorders; a *diagnostic* framework.

NREM sleep Sleep stages that are not characterized by *REM* (rapid eye movement) patterns; nondreaming sleep.

nuclear family The primary family unit that typically, in Western culture, includes mother, father, and children; in other cultures, it can also include aunts, uncles, grandparents.

nurturant, nurturing In close relationships, as between mother and child, a supportive, *emotionally* permissive, and giving pattern.

nystagmus Involuntary, rapid oscillation of the eyeballs.

objective, objectivity In research terminology, the quality of being nonbiased, nonsubjective, and impersonal in making ratings, observations, and judgments; contrast with *subjective,* subjectivity.

obsession An unwanted persistent, frequently *irrational* thought, idea, or image that enters into one's *consciousness.*

obsessional Referring to a *personality syndrome* that is characterized by the presence of *obsessions.*

obsessive compulsive disorder A *neurotic* disturbance characterized by the presence of *obsessions, compulsions,* or both—that is, by the intrusion of unwanted, *irrational* ideas, thoughts, urges, and *impulses* into one's *mental* content and behavior.

obsessive compulsive neurosis See *obsessive compulsive disorder.*

obsessive compulsive personality A *personality style,* not a disorder, characterized by extreme orderliness, perfectionism, self-control, neatness, thrift, and *emotional* aloofness.

Occam's Razor In theory- or hypothesis-making, a

maxim that states that simplicity is desirable.

occipital lobe The part of each *cerebral hemisphere,* at the back of the head, that specializes in vision.

occupational therapy *Therapy* that helps the client through job activity, training, and related activities.

Oedipus complex In *psychoanalytic* theory, the stage of *psychosexual* development in which *fantasies* of a sexual and/or romantic nature are focused on the parent of the opposite sex; at one time, the term characterized the feelings a boy had for his mother, but currently the term also applies to the feelings young girls have toward their fathers.

operant learning A training method that tries to modify a response by altering the consequences of it.

operant response Any *response* that produces some effect on the environment.

operational definition A definition of a behavior, *trait,* or concept in terms of the procedures by which it is observed or measured.

opiate Any substance containing *opium.*

opium A derivative of the poppy plant used to manufacture *narcotic* substances—for example, *heroin.*

oppositional disorder A *DSM-III* childhood *diagnosis,* similar to the *passive-aggressive personality disorder* in adults, characterizing children who are unable to express anger openly and resort instead to hidden ways of doing so, especially in relationship to parents and other authority figures.

oral character In *psychoanalytic* theory, describing people who are preoccupied with oral satisfactions; they tend to be talkative, dependent, childish, and submissive, and may become dependent on substances such as alcohol; a person *fixated* at the *oral phase* of development.

oral phase In *psychoanalytic* theory, a *psychosexual* stage of development in which the infant is primarily concerned with oral preoccupations, such as sucking and feeding.

organic Pertaining to physical and bodily variables, in contrast to *emotional* or psychological ones.

organicity A quality of *pathological* behavior that results from physical factors, especially of the *CNS.*

organic personality syndrome A constellation of *personality traits* that are presumed to be typical of many individuals with brain damage; see *frontal lobe syndrome.*

orgasm The pleasurable climactic phase in the sexual response cycle of men and women.

overanxious disorder A DSM-III label for a pattern found in children, characterized by worry about future events, overconcern with competence, and excessive need for reassurance.

overcorrection A behavioral *intervention* in which the subject not only corrects an undesirable situation that he or she caused, but also overcorrects for it.

overinclusion A thinking style that involves overresponsiveness to external *stimuli* found in some types of *schizophrenics,* especially the *paranoid* subtype.

ovum The egg or reproductive cell of the female; the *gamete.*

panic A sudden state of intense *autonomic* activity of an acutely distressing nature; extreme *anxiety* and a subjective sense of having to flee.

panic disorder A disorder characterized by recurrent episodes of *panic,* usually with no clearcut external cause.

paradigm A model or theoretical scheme that attempts to account for most of the available facts about a given topic.

paranoia An extremely rare *pathological* condition in which the entire life style and *cognitive* functions of an individual is dominated by a thoroughgoing *delusional* system; yet there is seemingly intact functioning in all other areas.

paranoid Referring to *delusions,* feelings, or thoughts that one is being persecuted.

paranoid disorder The general DSM-III term for *paranoid* (but not *schizophrenic*) conditions that include, among other states, *paranoia.*

paranoid ideation Thoughts and ideas of *persecution* or of *grandiosity* that characterize some types of disturbances, especially *schizophrenia.*

paranoid personality disorder A disorder characterized by suspiciousness, mistrust of others, and a tendency to take offense quickly; regarded, generally, as neither a *psychosis* or *neurosis.*

paranoid schizophrenia A *psychotic* condition in which *delusions* of *persecution* dominate the *symptom* picture.

paraphilias Sexual practices that deviate from those of the majority.

parasympathetic nervous system A subsystem of the *autonomic nervous system* that in many ways produces bodily responses opposite to those of the *sympathetic nervous system,* such as the slowing of heart rate and respiratory responses.

paresthesia An *abnormal* sensation such as prickling, burning, or tingling of the skin, without apparent cause.

parietal lobe The part of each *cerebral hemisphere,* at the side and top of the head, that is involved in such functions as organizing complex spatial information.

Parkinson's disease A progressive, degenerative, deteriorating disease whose *symptoms* include involuntary *tremors* of the arms and legs and a masklike, expressionless face.

participant modeling A behavioral *intervention* that is a variation of the *modeling* procedure, which requires the therapist to model the desired behavior while also using *induction aids,* in order to help the client to try out the desired behavior.

passive-aggressive personality disorder A disorder, neither *neurotic* or *psychotic,* that is characterized by a long-term pattern of inability to express anger openly, using, instead, hidden ways of doing so; the consequences of this pattern are found in many areas, including ineffective, confusing interpersonal relationships.

pathological, pathology Pertaining to disease, usually in the physical sense, but currently applicable also to *emotional* and psychological disorders.

pathological gambling An *impulse control disorder* in which the individual is unable to resist the urge to gamble and to take money risks, often with disastrous consequences.

pavor nocturnus See *sleep terror disorder.*

PCP (phencyclidine) Also known as "angel dust"; a synthetic *hallucinogen* with a bad street reputation, formerly used as an analgesic substance for animals.

pedophilia A recurrent, *compulsive* need to achieve sexual arousal and discharge with children as objects.

penile plethysmograph A method used for research purposes that measures and records the tumescence (swelling) of the penis during sexual arousal.

penis envy In *psychoanalytic* theory, the much-disputed notion that young girls are angry and frustrated because they do not have a penis; in older females, the unconscious wish for unfulfilled, "masculine" women to have a penis.

peptic ulcer An erosion or *lesion* of the lining of the stomach or duodenum (the portion of the small intestine near the stomach) caused by excessive flow of gastric juices, and thought to be of a *psychophysiological* or *psychosomatic* nature.

percentile A test score that indicates the percentage of the sample tested falling below that particular score.

perinatal Circumstances, conditions, and events affecting the infant at the time of birth—for example, an insufficient supply of oxygen.

peripheral nervous system The *neural* pathways to and from *sensory* areas and musculature outside of the *CNS.*

persecution Frequent *delusional* content in many types of *pathological* conditions, involving *irrational* thoughts of being harressed, victimized, followed, and unfairly treated.

personality Distinctive, enduring pattern of *traits* and style of behavior that form the core of how each individual relates to others and to his or her world; the unique pattern of characteristics of an individual, as perceived by others.

personality disorder A *maladaptive,* long-term pattern of distinctive personal characteristics, neither *neurotic* or *psychotic,* that is disruptive, troublesome, and distressing to the individual and to those who are involved with that individual.

personality inventory A paper-and-pencil, *objective psychological test* used to measure some aspect of *personality* and *temperament.*

pervasive developmental disorder A DSM-III term for severe childhood disturbances that include *infantile autism* and *childhood schizophrenia.*

perversion An old term, now regarded as judgmental, for any sexual preference or practice that departs from the usual genital, heterosexual interaction.

petit mal seizures One of the milder *epileptic* or *seizure* disorders involving a momentary lapse of *consciousness* that lasts up to about 30 seconds, characterized by twitching of the eyelids or head, loss of muscle-tone, pallor, and a dreamy look.

phallic phase In *psychoanalytic* theory, the *psychosexual* level that focuses on the genital area in terms of *fantasies* and *masturbatory* activities.

pharmacological Pertaining to the actions, influences, and effects of chemicals and drugs on the body and on behavior.

phenocopy An environmentally determined *trait* or characteristic that resembles one that has a *genetic* cause.

phenomenological, phenomenology Pertaining to a philosophical and psychological model that holds that an understanding of the *personality* and experiences of an individual can be known only to that individual.

phenothiazines A group of anti*psychotic* medications that have been used, with considerable success, to control many of the *symptoms* of *schizophrenia.*

phenotype The appearance of a trait or characteristic that arises from the individual's *genetic* makeup in interaction with his or her environment.

phenylketonuria (PKU) A *hereditary,* metabolic disorder that, if not treated, produces *mental retardation.*

phobia An avoidance *response* or pattern of responses arising from an *irrational* fear of social or interpersonal situations, activities, or things.

phobic disorder A phobic *neurosis,* dominated by a pattern of avoidance of an *irrationally* feared social or interpersonal situation, activity, or thing.

phrenology An old-fashioned (though considered "scientific" when it was popular) view that proposed a direct relationship between particular areas of the skull and various personal *traits.*

physiological Pertaining to the structures, processes, and functions of the tissues, organs, senses, muscles, and various systems (for example, the *CNS*) of the body.

Pick's disease A degenerative, presenile brain disease that has *symptoms* similar to those of *senile dementia.*

placebo A substance or condition having no specific, intended effect on the subject, but that the subject believes to be important in the treatment, nevertheless.

placebo effect A phenomenon in which a substance, condition, or treatment, though having no direct effect on the subject because of its inherent properties, in fact has an effect merely because the subject accepts it as a viable treatment.

play methods In *psychotherapy* with children, the use of play and games to elicit the expression of *conflict,* release tension, and disclose *unconscious* themes.

pleasure principle In *psychoanalytic* theory, the guiding framework of the *id,* which seeks to release tension through the expenditure of *instinctual* energy.

pneumoencephalography A medical procedure that forces air into the cavities of the brain to locate, through X-ray methods, possible structural problems.

polydrug abuse *Dependence* on and overuse of several drugs at the same time, a frequent pattern in *substance abuse.*

polygenic In *genetics,* the involvement of several, rather than one *gene,* in the development of a *trait* or disease.

polygraph An instrument that simultaneously records various *autonomic* indices; when used in certain types of interviews, it has been called a "lie detector."

posthypnotic suggestion A suggestion given by the *hypnotist* to the subject under *hypnosis* that is carried out by the subject when he or she is no longer in the hypnotic state.

postpartum Following childbirth.

post-traumatic stress disorder A group of *symptoms* that arises after an extremely *traumatic* experience, such as combat or rape, that is characterized by severe anxiety, suspiciousness, and *insomnia.*

postural hypotension A sudden drop in blood pressure when an upright position is assumed; also called orthostatic hypotension.

precipitate To cause or to trigger, in the immediate sense, a *symptom* or *pathological* condition.

precursor An event, circumstance, or condition that exists prior to the onset of a disturbance that may or may not be causally related to it.

predictive validity The degree to which a score, test, or rating predicts the occurrence of a behavior or another score.

prematurity With humans, a gestation period (length of time in the womb) of less than 37 weeks; usually indicated by birthweight, rather than length of pregnancy.

premorbid Referring to the conditions and characteristics of an individual— for example, occupational or marital status—before the onset of the *pathology.*

presenile psychosis A general term pertaining to *dementias* similar to *senile dementias* with onset before age sixty-five (for example, *Alzheimer's disease*).

primal scene The *fantasies* or recollections of patients of having witnessed their parents having sexual intercourse.

primal therapy Janov's controversial approach to *psychotherapy.*

primal trauma In Janov's *psychotherapeutic* model, the overwhelming feeling or realization that one was not loved by one's parents.

primary areas (projection areas) The terminal points of excitation in the brain, beginning with nerve fibers from the *senses* that transmit signals to the brain.

primary gain The psychological rewards and consequences an individual obtains from his or her *symptom* or illness (for example, *anxiety*-reduction or the *repression* of severe *conflict*); contrast with *secondary gain.*

primary prevention *Intervention* into the possible social, economic, and biological causes of *pathology* before onset, so that the disease process does not take place; see *secondary* and *tertiary prevention.*

primary processes In *psychoanalytic* theory, the mass of *unconscious* material—for example, forbidden wishes, pushes, conflicts, and *fantasies* not bound by logic, *rational* processes, and the limits of reality that sometimes pushes to the surface of behavior and *consciousness.*

primary psychopath See *antisocial personality;* contrast with *secondary psychopath* or *neurotic character.*

problem drinking Excessive drinking leading to interpersonal and social problems; usually regarded as a *precursor* to *alcoholism.*

process schizophrenia A type of *schizophrenia,* in contrast to *reactive schizophrenia,* in which there is a long history of poor *premorbid* adjustment; onset is gradual and *prognosis* poor, with a chronic, *progressively* worsening pattern of illness.

prodromal A warning signal, a premonitory *symptom* before actual onset of an illness.

profound retardation *Mental retardation* in people with IQs below 20, regarded as being responsive only to limited training.

prognosis The forecasting of the probable course and outcome, for better or for worse, of a disease.

progressive A worsening pattern of *symptoms* and/or the disease itself in terms of severity and/or complexity.

projection A *defense mechanism* in which one attributes to others one's own unacceptable wishes, desires, thoughts, and *fantasies.*

projection areas See *primary areas.*

projective methods Any of several methods—for example, the *Rorschach* test—in which an individual is asked to respond to ambiguous *stimuli* (for example, inkblots), in order to reveal the innermost aspects of his or her *conflicts, personality,* and *emotional* makeup.

prosopagnosia A type of *aphasia* characterized by an inability to recognize faces.

prototype approach A model for a *diagnostic* system that proposes to construct categories that contain all or most of the features that experts attribute to a diagnosis.

pseudomutuality A surface illusion of stability and equilibrium that hides the *pathology* of some families.

psychiatry The medical specialty of diagnosing and treating *mental illness.*

psychoactive Referring to chemical substances prescribed for the control and treatment of various *mental* and *emotional* disorders.

psychoanalysis A method of treatment primarily of the psychoneuroses, based on the theoretical principles of Sigmund Freud.

psychodynamic Generally referring to models of *abnormal* behavior and/or to *psychotherapy* that stress hidden drives, *unconscious motivation,* and past history in the formation of *symptoms.*

psychogenic Physical *symptoms* or diseases having, in large part, psychological and *emotional* origins.

psychogenic amnesia A sudden inability to "retrieve" personal information from one's memory that is more dramatic than ordinary forgetfulness and is not due to any physical disturbance.

psychogenic fugue A *dissociative disorder* characterized by the assumption of a new identity, and frequently a new location, with no physical basis for this condition.

psychogenic pain Pain, often persistent, occurring with no apparent physical cause.

psychological androgyny The freedom from viewing oneself with rigid, either-or, gender-stereotyped perceptions as male or female.

psychological tests Devices or instruments designed to measure individual differences, especially in the area of *personality, intelligence,* aptitudes, and *emotions.*

psychomotor Pertaining to *mental* and *motor* activities.

psychomotor retardation Diminished *mental* and physical activities in certain types of *depressed* people.

psychomotor seizures One of the *seizure disorders,* similar to but longer-lasting than *petit mal seizures,* and characterized by repetitious, automatic movements, such as chewing.

psychoneurosis See *neurosis.*

psychopath An individual who is amoral, antisocial, impulsive, and *emotionally* shallow; someone with an ingrained pattern of antisocial behavior who shows little guilt or conscience.

psychopathic personality See *antisocial personality.*

psychopathology *Mental* pathology; pertaining to diseases of the mind.

psychopharmacology The study of the effects of prescribed drugs on *mood, emotions,* behavior, and *mental* states.

psychophysiological Pertaining to the interactions and interrelationships of *mental* and biological processes; also, another term for *psychosomatic.*

psychosexual In *psychoanalytic* theory, the different stages of development from infancy on, dominated by the chief method of deriving erotic and *libidinal* pleasure; more generally, the interrelationship among *mental, emotional,* and sexual *responses.*

psychosexual dysfunction One of several disturbances in the human sexual response cycle not due to physical origin.

psychosis Severe mental disorder, often, but not always, involving *delusions, hallucinations,* bizarre thought processes and/or deep mood disturbances—for example, *mania* or severe *depression.*

psychosocial retardation *Mild retardation,* thought to be due to social, cultural, and economic deprivation; a category into which about 80 percent of the *mentally retarded* population falls.

psychosomatic Physical or bodily dysfunction with *emotional* and psychological origins.

psychosurgery A general term for several operative procedures that remove or destroy brain tissue through surgical means for the purpose of modifying the behavior and *emotional* state of the patient.

psychotherapy, psychotherapeutic A general term for different methods, frequently verbal, used by a trained person to help another person change his or her behavior, feelings, *symptoms* and/or interpersonal relationships.

psychotic Having the qualities of a *psychosis* or a person who is *diagnosed* as having a *psychosis.*

psychoticism In Eysenck's approach to understanding *abnormal* behavior, a major dimension of *personality* that reflects an individual's awareness and contact with reality; see *neuroticism.*

psychotomimetic Referring to substances that induce *psychotic*-like behaviors and states.

psychotropic Generally referring to drugs that have an effect on the mind, *mood,* and *emotions;* see *psychoactive.*

pursuit system The visual system in which a moving object is perceived smoothly and on target by a coordinated relationship between the eye and the object.

pyknic In Kretschmer's outdated classification system for body types, a short, heavy body, tending to roundness; the attempt to link physique with certain types of *mental illness* proposed that this type tended to develop *manic-depressive* disorders.

pyromania An *impulse control disorder* characterized by inability to resist the *impulse* to set fires; the individual experiences great pleasure at the time of the act.

radiological Pertaining to X-ray methods.

random sample In research, subjects selected for study completely at random from another, larger group, so that theoretically the results obtained can be extended to the larger population from which they were drawn.

rational Logical, reasoned *mental* processes.

rational emotive therapy (RET) A *cognitive therapy* that assumes that an individual's problems arise from *irrational* views and thoughts about reality; the approach aims to get the individual to substitute these for more *rational* views.

rationalization A *defense mechanism* in which the individual assigns a *rational* or plausible explanation for a *motive,* behavior, or activity to cover up the true reason or motive, which may be *unconscious.*

Raynaud's disease Excessive constriction of peripheral blood vessels in response to cold.

reaction formation A *defense mechanism* in which a hidden wish or taboo thought is transformed into its opposite.

reaction time The time, generally measured in fractions of a second, that it takes for an individual to respond to a *stimulus;* a frequently studied *variable* in *psychopathological* research.

reactive attachment disorder of infancy A DSM-III category characterized by apathy and nonresponsiveness in children below the age of 36 months who have been separated from the mother or *mother surrogate.*

reactive schizophrenia A type of *schizophrenia* characterized by moderately good *premorbid* adjustment and favorable *prognosis* in contrast to *process* schizophrenia; onset in this type is sudden, *symptoms* are *acute,* and frequently, there is *remission* in a short period of time.

reading disability A general term for difficulty in learning to read; can be due to many causes, including limited learning opportunities, *neurological* dysfunctions, or psychological *conflict;* see *dyslexia.*

reality principle In *psychoanalytic* theory, the awareness of reality and its demands that the *ego,* in contrast to the *id,* possesses.

reality-testing The individual's ability to assess the qualities and demands of the real situation surrounding him or her.

reality therapy A method of *psychotherapy,* involving persuasion and direct guidance, in which the individual is urged to assume responsibility for his or her actions.

recessive gene A form of a *gene* that is not expressed in an individual unless it is paired with another gene "copy."

recidivism A pattern of recurring criminal offenses, even after repeated punishment.

reciprocal determinism A model that holds that behaviors, environments, and *cognitions* have interlocking, continuous influences on one another.

regress, regression A return, because of unresolved *conflicts,* to an earlier *psychosexual* level.

reinforce To reward a desired *response.*

reinforcement The reward for or consequence of an act that tends to be associated with the continued evoking of that response.

reinforcing stimulus A *stimulus* that increases the rate, intensity, or likelihood of occurrence of a *response* it follows.

reliability The consistency with which a test measures what it is supposed to be measuring; the amount of agreement between raters.

REM, REM sleep The stage of sleep characterized by rapid eye movements, during which dreaming occurs.

remission A *symptom*-free stage, usually temporary, of an illness.

replicate, replication In research, to duplicate an *experiment* or study to check for consistency of results.

repression A *defense mechanism* in which the *ego* places forbidden or shameful thoughts or wishes into the *unconscious* to avoid *conscious* awareness and therefore pain.

resistance In *psychoanalysis,* the reluctance of the patient to produce painful, *repressed* material; manifested by silence, failure to keep appointments, and similar obstacles to getting better.

response Any behavior, inner or outer, that occurs as a consequence of *stimulation.*

response generalization In learning theory terms, the tendency of *responses* similar to the *reinforced* response to be evoked by a *stimulus* unless it is punished.

reticular activating system (RAS), reticular formation The network of *neural* structures that is concerned with arousal and *attention.*

reticular inhibition A *neurological* process that limits or controls an over-aroused or over*attentive* state, permitting focus on limited aspects of the *stimuli* surrounding an individual.

retrospective A research design that studies data that had already been collected by the time of the study—for example, past school records.

Rorschach A *projective method,* consisting of ten inkblots, that requires the individual to assign meaning to what is perceived in order to reveal deep, hidden layers of *temperament* and *personality.*

rubella (German measles) A contagious viral disease that can result in fetal abnormality if the mother contracts the illness early in pregnancy.

rumination Preoccupation with repeated, unwanted ideas and thoughts; *obsessional* thinking.

rush (also, "flash") The immediate effects caused by the injection of illicit substances; found by some to be highly pleasurable.

schismatic family A type of family organization that is presumably associated with the development of *schizophrenia* in one of its members; these families are characterized by parental divisiveness and the imposing of contradictory values on their children.

schizoaffective disorder A *diagnostic* category, not in the DSM-III, that is applied to conditions in which *manic* or *depressive syndromes* are mixed with *schizophrenic* syndromes.

schizoid disorder of childhood or adolescence The childhood or adolescent form of *schizoid personality disorder,* characterized by isolation, inability to form friends, great reserve, and seclusiveness.

schizoid personality disorder A long-term pattern of maladaptive behavior characterized by few close friends, inability to form interpersonal relationships, lack of social skills, and difficulty in expressing *emotions.*

schizophrenia A group of *psychoses* characterized by gross disturbances in thinking and perception, peculiarities in behavior, and *hallucinations* and *delusions.*

schizophreniform disorder A *psychotic* condition of brief duration accompanied by *delusions, hallucinations,* and disorganized behavior; onset is sudden, *symptoms* are acute, and *prognosis* is good.

schizophrenogenic Referring to conditions or variables that tend to produce *schizophrenia,* as in some types of *pathological* families.

schizotaxia A *genetic* endowment for *schizophrenia,* which may or may not be expressed, observed, or manifested in the lifetime of the individual.

schizotypal personality disorder A long-term, ingrained pattern of maladaptive behavior characterized by oddness and peculiarity in language and thinking, social isolation, and suspiciousness and aloofness; it is similar in some respects to *schizophrenia,* but generally the disturbance is not severe enough to warrant a *diagnosis* of schizophrenia.

school phobia Intense avoidance and fear of school.

secondary gain The support, attention, and *rewards* that an individual achieves from a symptom, above and beyond the *primary gain.*

secondary prevention Early detection of the beginnings of an *emotional* or *mental* disorder accompanied by attempts to intervene into its further development by some form of treatment; see *primary* and *tertiary prevention.*

secondary processes Reality-based thinking processes that modify *primary process* material so that it becomes compatible with the demands of reality.

secondary psychopath A person with an antisocial personality who experiences *anxiety,* guilt, *conflict,* and *neurotic* problems; contrast with primary psychopath.

segmental set According to Shakow, responsiveness to minor, sometimes irrelevant aspects of a situation, typical of the behavior of most *schizophrenics;* see *generalized set.*

seizure disorder Any of the various disorders, sometimes called *epilepsy,* characterized by convulsions or temporary *absences.*

selective amnesia One type of *psychogenic amnesia,* characterized by an inability to recall only certain events.

self-actualization The growth of the individual toward fulfillment, self-acceptance, and full use of his or her capacities.

self-contract A document signed (and witnessed) by the client who is trying to *self-regulate* his or her behavior.

self-desensitization A behavioral *intervention* in which the client develops his or her own hierarchy of fears and uses *systematic desensitization* procedures to eliminate *anxiety.*

self-efficacy A person's appraisal of how well he or she has performed.

self-fulfilling prophecy The phenomenon that if one perceives a situation in a certain way or expects a certain outcome to occur, it is likely that that outcome will actually occur.

self-punishment A behavioral *intervention* in which the client self-administers punishment for unwanted actions.

self-regulate The application of behavioral *intervention* by the client, himself or herself, without the aid of a therapist.

self-reinforcement A behavioral *intervention* in which the client self-administers rewards for desirable actions.

senile, senility A *pathological* decline of abilities in old age.

senile dementia A *chronic, progressive, abnormal* brain condition associated with aging that involves a deterioration of *cognitive* functions, especially memory.

sensation-seeking Tending to find excessive sources of stimulation, as in risk-taking, to avoid boredom; this may have some *physiological* basis.

senses, sensory The faculties, in or outside of the body, such as sight, balance, and smell, by which *stimuli* are received and experienced as sensations.

sensorimotor Pertaining to the perception, control, and regulation of *sensory* and *motor* impulses and their interactions.

sensory deprivation The lowering or monotony of stimulation to a level below that which is desirable for normal functioning.

separation anxiety disorder A DSM-III *syndrome,* relatively common in children and adolescents, characterized by extreme fear or *panic* in situations that involve separation from a close individual—for example, a parent.

serotonin A *neurochemical,* concentrated in the *hypothalamus,* that has been implicated or associated with some *pathological* conditions.

SES An index of an individual's socioeconomic status based on several *variables* (for example, income and education).

set A state or orientation of preparation, expectation or readiness for a stimulus that may predispose the subject to perceive an event in certain ways.

severe retardation *Mental retardation* with an IQ range of roughly 20 to 34; regarded as moderately trainable.

sex linkage Referring to a *genetically* caused condition determined by a *gene* appearing in a sex *chromosome.*

sexual dysfunction Any one of several difficulties in maintaining levels of sexual arousal or in experiencing orgasm.

sexual masochism Sexual arousal and discharge through the experience of suffering as a result of being humiliated, bound, whipped, and hurt by one's partner.

sexual sadism The need to abuse, hurt, and humiliate one's partner to achieve arousal and discharge.

shaman A person who functions as both priest and doctor, using tribal customs, myths, and beliefs to effect cures; a "medicine man."

shape, shaping Procedures *behavior therapists* use to gradually train the client to achieve closer and closer approximations of a desired response by mastering, with the aid of *reinforcements,* small components of the desired behavior.

shuttling A technique in *Gestalt therapy* that encourages clients to sharpen awareness of their current feelings by requiring them to go from what is being experienced in the here-and-now to *fantasy* content and then back to the present, once again.

simple phobia In contrast to *social phobia,* an *irrational* fear and avoidance of specific objects, activities, or situations—for example, furry animals, knives, or enclosed spaces (the latter is called *claustrophobia).*

simple subtype, schizophrenia A *diagnostic* category no longer contained in the DSM-III, characterized by apathy, *emotional* shallowness, and gradual withdrawal from others; *delusions* and *hallucinations* are not present.

skewed family A type of family organization that may be related to a *schizophrenic* disorder in one of its members, in which values, viewpoints, and regulatory functions revolve around one of the parents only, usually the mother, with the rest of the family passively accepting this distortion.

sleep terror disorder (pavor nocturnus) A disorder characterized by recurrent episodes of sudden awakening from *NREM sleep,* usually with *panicky* screams and intense *anxiety;* there tends to be complete *amnesia* for these events.

sleepwalking disorder (somnambulism) Recurrent episodes of rising from bed during *NREM sleep* and walking about the room or house with an expressionless face; there is usually complete *amnesia* for these events.

social desirability The degree to which a test item reflects an approved-of behavior or value; see *forced-choice method.*

social phobia An *irrational* fear and avoidance of certain types of interpersonal or public situations (for example, speaking or eating in public).

social supports A person's family, friends, community facilities, social groups, and enduring ties.

socialization The process by which a child learns to think, value, and behave like other members of his or her *culture.*

sociopath See *psychopath.*

sodomy Anal penetration in sexual interactions.

somatic Pertaining to the body; physical.

somatization disorder A *neurotic* disorder characterized by vague, chronic, and shifting medical complaints, with little or no physical basis.

somatotyping A system of classifying people by their body form.

somnambulism See *sleepwalking disorder.*

spastic A *motor* difficulty characterized by rigidity, tension, and paralysis of affected areas, as in some individuals with *cerebral palsy.*

sphygmomanometer An instrument that measures blood pressure.

split-half reliability A method of determining the *reliability* of a test, in which the scores on the odd-numbered items are *correlated* with the scores on the even-numbered items; a perfectly reliable test would show a correlation of 1.0 of scores from the two halves.

spontaneous recovery The occasional recurrence of a *response* that has undergone *extinction.*

standardization The procedure used in the development of *psychological tests* to establish *norms* and baselines by which an individual's test performance can be judged.

standardization sample The group of subjects that formed the study population for developing *norms* for the test.

state anxiety The current *anxiety* experienced by an individual in the situation at hand, frequently observable and measurable; contrast with *trait anxiety.*

statistics, statistical The mathematical and computational procedures used to collect, summarize, organize, and compare research data.

statistical model An approach to defining *abnormal* behavior that holds that behavior that conforms to the *norm* is equated with *mental health,* whereas behavior that deviates from the norm is equated with *mental illness.*

statutory rape Sexual relations with a female youngster below the age of consent; the actual age varies from state to state.

stereotaxic Pertaining to the use of an apparatus that allows precise insertion of electrodes into specified areas of the brain for surgical and *experimental* purposes.

stereotype The assignment of the commonly, often invalidly, perceived attributes of a group to an individual.

stimulant A general term for substances that heighten *CNS* activity, increase arousal, and occasionally, induce euphoria.

stimulus, stimuli Anything that incites, evokes, or produces a *response* in the organism.

stimulus control A behavioral *intervention* used when

the *response* to be eliminated or controlled is undesirable only in some, but not all, situations.

stimulus generalization In learning theory terms, the tendency of *reinforced responses* to be evoked by *stimuli* similar to the original one.

stress In Selye's approach, the body's emergency response to unusual impact on it, in the form of injury, disease, or an intense external stimulus; see *stressor.*

stress inoculation A behavioral *intervention* that increases the client's coping skills—for example, in controlling angry outbursts—through education, rehearsal, and the development of insight.

stressor Any extremely intense or severe stimulation or event that has an impact on the individual.

stupor A state or condition in which there is only a minimum of *conscious* awareness and *mental* focus.

subjective Pertaining to content that exists in one's own mind and concerns one's *moods,* feelings, and perceptions.

subjectivity The quality of being *subjective* and biased in judging, perceiving, or rating others, in contrast to *objectivity,* which is based on definable, external criteria.

sublimation A *defense mechanism* by which, in Freudian terms, a sexually desired object, activity, or *fantasy* is suppressed and substituted with a nonsexual, usually more socially acceptable, activity.

substance abuse *Maladaptive* behaviors associated with the regular use of a substance (licit or illicit) that results in adverse consequences in terms of social, interpersonal, and occupational functioning.

substance dependence Excessive need to use licit or illicit drugs; characterized by the presence of an *abstinence syndrome* and/or *tolerance* when there is physical dependence; also, *emotional* and psychological need for a substance, even if there is no established physical dependence.

superego In *psychoanalytic* theory, one of the three parts of the psyche or mind; it is concerned with conscience and moral and social values; see *id, ego.*

symbiosis, symbiotic An extreme, emotionally interdependent, *maladaptive* closeness between two people—for example, mother and child or husband and wife.

symbolic modeling Pertaining to the use of filmed or videotaped *models* in behavioral *interventions.*

sympathetic nervous system The subdivision of the *autonomic nervous system* that prepares the organism for an emergency by releasing *physiological* energizers of various types, so that the organism can best protect itself against injury, attack, or other *stressor;* various *responses* are produced, which may also appear in *anxiety states.*

symptom A behavioral, observable sign or pattern of *responses* that suggests or reflects the presence of *pathology.*

synapse The gap or functional connection between *neurons,* across which the transmission of messages or signals from one neuron to another occurs.

syndrome A group of connected or interrelated *symptoms* that comprises or characterizes a particular disorder or disease.

synergistic Having a combined effect that is more than additive; for example, when two substances are ingested at the same time, one may increase the effects of the other.

synesthesia A sensation in one modality (for example, color) when the *stimulus* is in a different modality (for example, sound).

syntactical aphasia A type of *aphasia* in which there is difficulty in placing words into their usual sequence.

syphilis An infectious disease, usually transmitted through sexual contact, that can produce serious *CNS* damage if not treated.

systematic desensitization In *behavioral therapy,* a method used to treat *phobias* that requires the subject to gradually and systematically imagine increasingly aversive levels of the feared situation while at the same time maintaining a relaxed state.

tachycardia Rapid heart beat.

tardive dyskinesia An involuntary movement disorder characterized by facial twitches and various gait and posture disturbances, sometimes brought on by excessive use of the *phenothiazines* in treating the *symptoms* of *schizophrenia.*

Tay-Sachs' disease A *genetically* transmitted *neurological* disorder resulting from inborn *metabolic* errors always associated with *developmental* retardation and childhood death.

taxonomic, taxonomy Referring to classification systems.

temperament A general term for the presumably stable sum total of a person's personal *traits,* behavior patterns, inclinations, *mood* level, and natural disposition.

temporal lobe The lateral lobe of each *cerebral hemisphere,* primarily associated with auditory perception.

tension headache A headache induced by muscle tension and continued contraction of the *frontalis,* a rectangular layer of muscle on the forehead.

teratogen Any condition or substance that contributes to the development of birth defects.

tertiary prevention Active intervention into and treatment of disease; see *secondary* and *primary prevention.*

test battery A series of *psychological tests* administered to a subject to get a broader picture for *diagnostic* purposes or for planning *psychotherapy* than could be obtained by the administration of a single test.

testosterone Male sex *hormone.*

test reliability See *reliability.*

test-retest reliability A method of estimating the consistency with which a test measures what it is supposed to measure (*reliability*) that requires the test to be administered twice to see if it yields the same results.

thalamus A structure of the brain that is a relay center for *sensory* impulses to and from higher and lower nerve centers.

thanatology A discipline that focuses on the study of people's attitudes and feelings about death and dying.

therapy, therapeutic Any form of treatment; see *psychotherapy.*

thought broadcasting A *delusion* that one's thoughts are known to others.

thought control A *delusion* that one's thoughts are under the influence of, or are determined by, outside factors.

thought disorder A general term for *pathological mental* processes that include *irrational* thinking, peculiar language, and bizarre *cognitions.*

thought insertion A *delusion* that specific ideas and notions are being placed into one's thinking by an outside force.

thyroid The gland whose secretions determine the rate of *metabolism* and body growth.

time-out An *aversive* method of *behavior therapy* that, as a consequence for an undesirable act, deprives individuals of *reinforcement* by removing them from their usual environments (for example, by placing them in an empty room for a few minutes).

time sampling A technique used in behavior therapy, in which a subject's behavior is observed and assessed during representative units of time, in order to get a true picture of his or her behavior.

token economy The creation of a social environment in which *reinforcements* and rewards are given to individuals living in a social group (for example, a hospital ward), in order to *shape* the behaviors of individuals into more socially desirable patterns.

token reinforcement In a *token economy,* the use of tokens (for example, plastic chips) as positive *reinforcement* for desirable behavior, which can later be exchanged for material things, such as candy or food.

tolerance The body's tendency to be less responsive to the actions of some drugs, under continued use; one of the signs of physical *dependence,* as in *heroin addiction.*

tonic phase In a *grand mal seizure,* the phase that involves muscle tension and contraction.

torque A special term for the tendency of some people to draw circles in a clockwise direction, in contrast to the more usual counterclockwise direction.

torticollus (wryneck) An abnormal position of the head resulting from a spasm of certain neck muscles.

Tourette syndrome (Gilles de la Tourette disease) A nondegenerative *neurological* disorder characterized by involuntary movements of the face and arms, poor coordination, and sometimes grunts, barks, and obscene utterances.

toxic, toxicity Pertaining to poisonous drugs or fluids.

toxic state The behavioral, *mental,* or *physiological* consequences of consuming a noxious drug or fluid that has either temporary or permanent adverse effects on the *CNS.*

trait A more-or-less enduring, distinguishing, personal characteristic of an individual.

trait anxiety *Anxiety*-proneness, an individual's tendency to experience anxiety in various situations; contrast with *state anxiety.*

transactional analysis A type of *group therapy* that uses highly structured methods.

transference neurosis In *psychoanalysis,* the stage during treatment in which the form of the interpersonal *conflicts* between patient and therapist are more significant than the *symptoms* with which the patient entered analysis.

transsexualism See *gender identity disorder.*

transvestism, transvestite A sexual variation that involves the repeated practice of dressing like a person of the opposite sex in order to obtain sexual arousal and discharge.

trauma Any blow or injury to the body; also, can refer to social or psychological *stressor.*

traumatic organic syndrome Behavioral conditions, which can range from confusion and disorientation to persistent concentration and *attention* difficulties and impairment of coordination, that can arise from physical blows to the head.

traumatic war neurosis See *post-traumatic stress disorder.*

tremors Involuntary shaking of the body or limbs.

trepanation, trephination The drilling of a small circular hole in a person's skull, a method used in some ancient societies to "let evil spirits escape."

tricyclic A class of chemicals used to treat some *depressive* disorders.

tuberous sclerosis An *inherited* disease of the *CNS* associated with *mental retardation.*

Type A A general term for a pattern of *traits* that is presumably found in individuals susceptible to coronary (heart) disease; Type A people are tense, anxious people who worry habitually, have a great need to control people and events impinging on them, and are under constant pressure to achieve.

Type B A general term for a pattern of *traits* found in people who handle stressful situations in a relaxed way and who are more easygoing than Type A individuals.

unconditional positive regard In *client-centered therapy,* the requirement that the therapist show complete, unreserved acceptance of the client.

unconditioned response A natural *response* to a *stimulus.*

unconditioned stimulus In *classical conditioning,* the natural stimulus that evokes the *unconditioned response.*

unconscious Pertaining to *mental* content and *motivation* of which the individual is not aware.

undoing A *defense mechanism* that involves the repetition of a shameful wish, *fantasy,* or *impulse* in ritual and ceremonies in order to atone for and reduce *anxiety* in connection with it.

unilateral Pertaining to one side of the body.

unipolar depression A form of *major affective disorder* in which recurrent depressions (but no manic episodes) occur.

validity The degree to which a rating, test score, or *diagnosis* measures or reflects that which it claims to measure or reflect; its truth or correctness is usually determined *empirically.*

variable A behavior, *trait,* or characteristic that can have several degrees of intensity or strength.

vascular Pertaining to blood vessels and the circulatory system.

vasoconstriction Narrowing of the blood vessels.

vasodilation The opening or widening of the blood vessels.

verbal psychotherapy Any one of dozens of psychological treatment methods that rely primarily on talking, in contrast to the physical *therapies.*

vicarious desensitization A variation of *systematic desensitization* in which the therapist has the client watch someone else being treated for the same fear he or she has.

vicarious reinforcement The introduction of a *reinforcement* for a desired behavior to a *model* that imparts information to the subject about the probable consequences of an act.

vigilance Over-watchfulness, over-attentiveness, and over-alertness to situations and other people.

visceral Pertaining to the insides of the body, especially the abdominal area.

voyeurism The repeated need to observe unsuspecting people in the act of disrobing or in sexual activity, in order to achieve sexual arousal and discharge.

waxy flexibility In the *catatonic subtype of schizophrenia,* the tendency of patients to remain in a position in which they are placed for an unusually long time, despite discomfort and awkwardness.

Wernicke's disease A *CNS* disorder due primarily to thiamine deficiency, often associated with chronic *alcoholism* and *Korsakoff's disease.*

wish-fulfilling, wish-fulfillment An easing of anxiety by solutions to conflict or the achievement of goals in *fantasy* rather than reality.

withdrawal, withdrawal syndrome See *abstinence syndrome.*

work through The stage in *psychoanalysis* in which the analyst actively helps the patient to review the same conflicts, symptoms, and problems again and again until their origins in *unconscious* processes are clear.

X chromosome A sex *chromosome* that carries the *genes* for femaleness; the union of two X chromosomes, one from each parent, produces a female offspring.

XYY syndrome A rare *chromosomal* condition in males that has controversially been linked to extreme aggression and criminality.

Y chromosome A sex *chromosome* that carries the *genes* for maleness; the union of an X chromosome and a Y chromosome produces a male offspring.

zygote The cell resulting from the union of a maternal and paternal germ cell.

zoophilia The pleasurable act or *fantasy* of engaging in sexual activities with animals.

References

Abel, E. L. The relationship between cannabis and violence: A review. *Psychological Bulletin,* 1977, *84,* 193–211.

Abel, E. L. Fetal alcohol syndrome: Behavioral teratology. *Psychological Bulletin,* 1980, *87,* 29–50.

Abel, G. G., Barlow, D. H., Blanchard, E. B., and Guild, D. The components of rapists' sexual arousal. *Archives of General Psychiatry,* 1977, *34,* 895–903.

Abel, G. G., Blanchard, E. B., and Becker, J. V. An integrated treatment program for rapists. In R. T. Rada (Ed.), *Clinical aspects of the rapist.* New York: Grune & Stratton, 1978.

Abelson, H. I., Fishburne, P. M., and Cisin, I. *National survey on drug abuse: 1977. A nationwide study—youth, young adults, and older people (vol. 1): Main findings.* National Institute on Drug Abuse, 1977.

Abramowicz, H. K., and Richardson, S. A. Epidemiology of severe mental retardation in children. Community studies. *American Journal of Mental Deficiency,* 1975, *80,* 18–39.

Abramowitz, C. V., and Dokecki, P. R. The politics of clinical judgment: Early empirical returns. *Psychological Bulletin,* 1977, *84,* 460–76.

Abramowitz, S. I. Splitting data from theory on the black patient-white therapist relationship. *American Psychologist,* 1978, *33,* 957–58.

Achenbach, T. M. The classification of children's psychiatric symptoms: A factor-analytic study. *Psychological Monographs,* 1966, *80,* Whole No. 615.

Achenbach, T. M., and Edelbrock, C. S. The classification of child psychopathology: A review and analysis of empirical efforts. *Psychological Bulletin,* 1978, *85,* 1275–1301.

Ackerman, N. W. *Treating the troubled family.* New York: Basic Books, 1966.

Adams, H. B. "Mental illness" or interpersonal behavior? *American Psychologist,* 1964, *19,* 191–97.

Adams, H. E., Feuerstein, M., and Fowler, J. Migraine headache: Reviews of parameters, etiology, and intervention. *Psychological Bulletin,* 1980, *87,* 217–37.

Adams, H. E., and Sturgis, E. T. Status of behavioral reorientation techniques in the modification of homosexuality: A review. *Psychological Bulletin,* 1977, *84,* 1171–88.

Adams, V. Researchers say battered parent is new victim of home violence. *New York Times,* July 2, 1979, p. B9.

Adams, V. Sex therapies in perspective. *Psychology Today,* August, 1980, 35–36.

Adler, A. *The practice and theory of individual psychology.* New York: Harcourt, 1927.

Adler, S. A., Gottesman, I. I., Orsulak, P. J., Kizuka, P. P., and Schildkraut, J. J. Platelet MAO activity: Relationships to clinical and psychometric variables. *Schizophrenia Bulletin,* 1980, *6,* 226–31.

Aged live better in poorer nations. *New York Times,* July 21, 1974, p. 4.

Agee, V. L. *Treatment of the violent incorrigible adolescent.* Lexington, Mass.: Lexington Books, 1979.

A genetic link is identified for some ulcers. *New York Times,* January 14, 1979, p. 22E.

Aichorn, A. *Wayward youth.* New York: Viking, 1935.

Ainsworth, M. D. S., Blehar, M. C., Waters, E., and Wall, S. *Patterns of attachment: A psychological study of the strange situation.* Hillsdale, N.J.: Erlbaum, 1978.

Akiskal, H. S., and McKinney, W. T., Jr. Depressive disorders: Toward a unified hypothesis. *Science,* 1973, *182,* 20–29.

Akiskal, H. S., and McKinney, W. T., Jr. Overview of recent research in depression: Integration of ten conceptual models into a comprehensive clinical frame. *Archives of General Psychiatry,* 1975, *32,* 285–305.

Akiskal, H. S., Rosenthal, R. H., Rosenthal, T. L., Kashgarian, M., Khani, M. K., and Puzantian, V. R. Differentiation of primary affective illness from situational, symptomatic, and secondary depressions. *Archives of General Psychiatry,* 1979, *36,* 635–43.

Albee, G. W. Problems in living are not sicknesses: Psychotherapy should not be covered under National Health Insurance. *Clinical Psychologist,* 1977, *30,* 3–6.

Albee, G. W., and Joffe, J. M. (Eds.) *Primary prevention of psychopathology, Vol. 1: The issues.* Hanover, New Hampshire: University Press of New England, 1977.

Albin, R. Therapy research: Still a way to go. *APA Monitor,* 1977, *8,* Nos. 9 and 10, 11–12.

Alexander, F. Emotional factors in essential hypertension. *Psychosomatic Medicine,* 1939, *1,* 173–79.

Alexander, F. *Psychosomatic medicine: Its principles and applications.* New York: Norton, 1950.

Al-Issa, I. Social and cultural aspects of hallucinations. *Psychological Bulletin,* 1977, *84,* 570–87.

Allen, R. P., Safer, D., and Covi, L. Effects of psychostimulants on aggression. *Journal of Nervous and Mental Disease,* 1975, *160,* 138–45.

Allport, G. W. *Pattern and growth in personality.* New York: Holt, Rinehart & Winston, 1961.

Alpert, M., and Friedhoff, A. J. An un-dopamine hypothesis of schizophrenia. *Schizophrenia Bulletin,* 1980, *6,* 387–90.

Alpert, R. (Baba Ram Dass) *Be here now.* San Cristobal, New Mexico: Lama Foundation, 1971.

Altman, L. K. Senility is not always what it seems to be. *New York Times,* May 8, 1977, p. E9.

Altman, L. K. Clues to fetus found in mother's blood. *New York Times,* April 10, 1979, p. C1. (a)

Altman, L. K. Release of mentally ill spurring doubts. *New York Times,* November 20, 1979, pp. B1, 4. (b)

Altman, L. K. Blinding disease arouses fears after it spreads widely in Africa. *New York Times,* March 2, 1980, pp. 1, 24.

Amenson, C. S., and Lewinsohn, P. M. An investigation into the observed sex difference in prevalence of unipolar depression. *Journal of Abnormal Psychology,* 1981, *90,* 1–13.

A mental patient's rights to adequate care upheld. *New York Times,* November 9, 1974, p. 34.

American Psychiatric Association. *DSM-II. Diagnostic and statistical manual of mental disorders* (2nd ed.). Washington, D.C.: American Psychiatric Association, 1968.

American Psychiatric Association. *A psychiatric glossary* (5th ed.). Washington, D.C.: American Psychiatric Association, 1980.

American Psychiatric Association. *DSM-III. Diagnostic and statistical manual of mental disorders* (3rd ed.). Washington, D.C.: American Psychiatric Association, 1980.

Amir, M. *Patterns in forcible rape.* Chicago: University of Chicago Press, 1971.

Andre, J. M. Uniqueness of alcoholism among American Indians with some thoughts on prevention, treatment and rehabilitation. Indian Health Service, Albuquerque, N.M., 1979.

Angst, J. Genetic aspects of depression. In N. S. Kline (Ed.), *Factors in depression.* New York: Raven Press, 1974.

Angst, J., Feider, W., and Lohmeyer, B. Course of schizoaffective psychoses: Results of a followup study. *Schizophrenia Bulletin,* 1980, *6,* 579–85.

Angyal, A. *Foundations for a science of personality.* Cambridge: Harvard University Press, 1941.

Antelman, S. M., and Caggiula, A. R. Norepinephrine-dopamine interactions and behavior. *Science,* 1977, *195,* 653.

Anthony, E. J. A risk-vulnerability intervention model for children of psychotic parents. In E. J. Anthony and C. Koupernik (Eds.), *The child in his family: Children at psychiatric risk.* New York: Wiley, 1974.

Anthony, W. A. Psychological rehabilitation: A concept in need of a method. *American Psychologist,* 1977, *32,* 658–62.

Arieti, S. *Interpretation of schizophrenia* (2nd ed.). New York: Basic Books, 1974.

Aronson, H., and Overall, B. Treatment expectations of patients in two social classes. *Social Work,* 1966, *11,* 35–41.

Arthur, A. Z. Diagnostic testing and the new alternatives. *Psychological Bulletin,* 1969, *72,* 183–92.

Åsberg, M., Thorén, P., and Träskman, L. "Serotonin depression"—a biochemical subgroup within the affective disorders? *Science,* 1976, *191,* 478–80.

Asher, J. 'Behavior mod' defiled. *APA Monitor,* 1974, *5,* Nos. 9 and 10, 3.

Auerbach, S. M., and Kilmann, P. R. Crisis intervention: A review of outcome research. *Psychological Bulletin,* 1977, *84,* 1189–217.

Axline, V. M. *Play therapy: The inner dynamics of childhood.* Boston: Houghton Mifflin, 1947.

Ayllon, T., and Azrin, N. H. The measurement and reinforcement of behavior of psychotics. *Journal of Experimental Analysis of Behavior,* 1965, *8,* 357–83.

Ayllon, T., and Azrin, N. H. *The token economy: A motivational system for therapy and rehabilitation.* New York: Appleton-Century-Crofts, 1968.

Baekeland, F., and Lundwall, L. Dropping out of treatment: A critical review. *Psychological Bulletin,* 1975, *82,* 738–83.

Baekeland, F., Lundwall, L., and Kissin, B. Methods for the treatment of chronic alcoholism: A critical appraisal. In R. J. Gibbins, Y. Israel, H. Kalant, R. E. Popham, W. Schmidt, and R. G. Smart (Eds.), *Research advances in alcohol and drug problems* (vol. 2). New York: Wiley, 1975.

Baer, D. M., Wolf, M. M., and Risley, T. R. Some current dimensions of applied behavior analysis. *Journal of Applied Behavior Analysis,* 1968, *1,* 91–97.

Bakal, D. A. Headache: A biopsychological perspective. *Psychological Bulletin,* 1975, *82,* 369–82.

Bakan, P. Hypnotizability, laterality of eye movement and functional brain asymmetry. *Perceptual and Motor Skills,* 1969, *28,* 927–32.

Bandura, A. Psychotherapy as a learning process. *Psychological Bulletin,* 1961, *58,* 143–59.

Bandura, A. Behavioral modifications through modeling procedures. In L. Krasner and L. P. Ullmann (Eds.), *Research in behavior modification: New developments and implications.* New York: Holt, Rinehart & Winston, 1965.

Bandura, A. Psychotherapy based upon modeling principles. In A. E. Bergin and S. L. Garfield (Eds.), *Handbook of psychotherapy and behavior change: An empirical analysis.* New York: Wiley, 1971.

Bandura, A. *Aggression: A social learning analysis.* Englewood Cliffs, N.J.: Prentice-Hall, 1973.

Bandura, A. Self-efficacy: Toward a unifying theory of behavioral change. *Psychological Review,* 1977, *84,* 191–215. (a)

Bandura, A. *Social learning theory.* Englewood Cliffs, N.J.: Prentice-Hall, 1977. (b)

Bandura, A. The self system in reciprocal determinism. *American Psychologist,* 1978, *33,* 344–58.

Bandura, A., Blanchard, E. B., and Ritter, B. Relative efficacy of desensitization and modeling approaches for inducing behavioral, effective, and attitudinal changes. *Journal of Personality and Social Psychology,* 1969, *13,* 173–99.

Bandura, A., Jeffery, R. W., and Gajdos, E. Generalizing change through participant modeling with self-directed mastery. *Behaviour Research and Therapy,* 1975, *13,* 141–52.

Bandura, A., Jeffery, R. W., and Wright, C. L. Efficacy of participant modeling as a function of response induction aids. *Journal of Abnormal Psychology,* 1974, *83,* 56–64.

Bandura, A., Ross, D., and Ross, S. A. Imitation of film-mediated aggressive models. *Journal of Abnormal and Social Psychology,* 1963, *66,* 3–11.

Bandura, A., and Simon, K. M. The role of proximal intentions in self-regulation of retractory behavior. *Cognitive Therapy and Research,* 1977, *1,* 177–93.

Bandura, A., and Walters, R. H. *Social learning and personality development.* New York: Holt, Rinehart & Winston, 1963.

Banks, G., Berenson, B. H., and Carkhuff, R. R. The effects of counselor race and training upon counseling process with Negro clients in initial interviews. *Journal of Clinical Psychology,* 1967, *23,* 70–72.

Barber, T. X., Spanos, N. P., and Chaves, J. F. *Hypnosis, imagination, and human potentialities.* New York: Pergamon Press, 1974.

Barchas, J. D., Akil, H., Elliott, G. R., Holman, R. B., and Watson, S. J. Behavioral neurochemistry: Neuroregulators and behavioral states. *Science,* 1978, *200,* 964–73.

Barlow, D. H., Leitenberg, H., Agras, W. S., and Wincze, J. P. The transfer gap in systematic desensitization: An analogue study. *Behaviour Research and Therapy,* 1969, *7,* 191–96.

Barlow, D. H., and Wolfe, B. E. Behavioral approaches to anxiety disorders: A report on the NIMH-SUNY, Albany, Research Conference. *Journal of Consulting and Clinical Psychology,* 1981, *49,* 448–54.

Barr, H. L., Langs, R. J., Holt, R. R., Goldberger, L., and Klein, G. S. *LSD: Personality and experience.* New York: Wiley, 1972.

Barrett, C. L., Hampe, I. E., and Miller, L. C. Research on child psychotherapy. In A. E. Bergin and S. L. Garfield (Eds.), *Handbook of psychotherapy and behavior change: An empirical analysis* (2nd ed.). New York: Wiley, 1978.

Barry, H. III. Cross-cultural evidence that dependency conflict motivates drunkenness. In M. W. Everett, J. O. Waddell, and D. B. Heath (Eds.), *Cross-cultural approaches to the study of alcohol.* The Hague: Moulton, 1976.

Bassin, A., Bratter, T. E., and Rachin, R. L. (Eds.) *The reality therapy reader: A survey of the work of William Glasser, M.D.* New York: Harper & Row, 1976.

Bassuk, E. L., and Gerson, S. Deinstitutionalization and mental health care. *Scientific American,* 1978, *238,* 46–58.

Batchelor, I. R. C. *Henderson and Gillespie's textbook of psychiatry* (10th ed.). London: Oxford University Press, 1969.

Bateson, G., Jackson, D. D., Haley, J., and Weakland, J. H. Toward a theory of schizophrenia. *Behavioral Science,* 1956, *1,* 251–64.

Bateson, G., Jackson, D. D., Haley, J., and Weakland, J. H. A note on the double bind—1962. *Family Process,* 1963, *2,* 154–61.

Bauer, R., and Stein, J. Sex counseling on campus: Short-term treatment techniques. *American Journal of Orthopsychiatry,* 1973, *43,* 824–39.

Bazar, J. Psychology: Making a comeback. *APA Monitor,* 1979, *10,* Nos. 9 and 10, 17–19.

Beck, A. T. *Depression: Clinical, experimental, and theoretical aspects.* New York: Harper & Row, 1967.

Beck, A. T. The development of depression: A cognitive model. In R. J. Friedman and M. M. Katz (Eds.), *The psychology of depression: Contemporary theory and research.* Washington, D.C.: Winston, 1974.

Beck, A. T. *Cognitive therapy and the emotional disorders.* New York: International Universities Press, 1976.

Beck, A. T., Kovacs, M., and Weissman, A. Assessment of suicidal ideation: The Scale for Suicide Ideation. *Journal of Consulting and Clinical Psychology,* 1979, *47,* 343–52.

Beck, A. T., Laude, R., and Bohnert, M. Ideational components of anxiety neurosis. *Archives of General Psychiatry,* 1974, *31,* 319–25.

Beck, A. T., Rush, A. J., Shaw, B. F., and Emery, G. *Cognitive therapy of depression.* New York: Guilford Press, 1979.

Beck, A. T., Ward, C. H., Mendelson, M., Mock, J. E., and Erbaugh, J. An inventory for measuring depression. *Archives of General Psychiatry,* 1961, *4,* 561–71.

Beck, A. T., Weissman, A., Lester, D., and Trexler, L. The measurement of pessimism: The Hopelessness Scale. *Journal of Consulting and Clinical Psychology,* 1974, *42,* 861–65.

Becker, E. *The denial of death.* New York: Free Press, 1973.

Becker, J. *Depression: Theory and research.* New York: Wiley, 1974.

Becker, J. V., Abel, G. G., and Skinner, L. J. The impact of a sexual assault on the victim's sexual life. *Victimology: An International Journal,* 1979, *4,* 229–35.

Becker, R. L. Job training placement for retarded youth: A survey. *Mental Retardation,* 1976, *14,* 7–11.

Begab, M. J., and Richardson, S. A. (Eds.) *The mentally retarded and society: A social science perspective.* Baltimore: University Park Press, 1975.

Bejerot, N. *Addiction: An artificially induced drive.* Springfield, Ill.: Thomas, 1972.

Bell, A. P., and Weinberg, M. S. *Homosexualities.* New York: Simon & Schuster, 1978.

Bell, H. M. *The Adjustment Inventory: Manual for adult form.* Stanford, Calif.: Stanford University Press, 1938.

Bem, S. L. The measurement of psychological androgyny. *Journal of Consulting and Clinical Psychology,* 1974, *42,* 155–62.

Bem, S. L. Androgyny vs. the tight little lives of fluffy women and chesty men. *Psychology Today,* 1975, *9,* 58–62.

Bem, D. J., and Allen, A. On predicting some of the people some of the time: The search for cross-situational consistencies in behavior. *Psychological Review,* 1974, *81,* 506–20.

Bem, D. J., and Funder, D. C. Predicting more of the people more of the time: Assessing the personality of situations. *Psychological Review,* 1978, *85,* 485–501.

Bemis, K. M. Current approaches to the etiology and treatment of anorexia nervosa. *Psychological Bulletin,* 1978, *85,* 593–617.

Bender, L. A. A visual motor Gestalt test and its clinical use. *American Orthopsychiatric Association Research Monographs,* 1938, No. 3.

Benjamin, R. Rural black folk and alcohol. In F. D. Harper (Ed.), *Alcohol abuse and black America.* Alexandria, Va.: Douglass, 1976.

Benson, H. *The relaxation response.* New York: Morrow, 1975.

Benton, A. L. *The Revised Visual Retention Test: Clinical and experimental applications.* New York: Psychological Corporation, 1955.

Berg, I. A. The unimportance of test item content. In B. M. Bass and I. A. Berg (Eds.), *Objective approaches to personality assessment.* Princeton: Van Nostrand, 1959.

Berg, I. A. The deviation hypothesis: A broad statement of its assumptions and postulates. In I. A. Berg (Ed.), *Response set in personality assessment.* Chicago: Aldine-Atherton, 1967.

Berger, P. A. Medical treatment of mental illness. *Science,* 1978, *200,* 974–81.

Bergin, A. E. The evaluation of therapeutic outcomes. In A. E. Bergin and S. L. Garfield (Eds.), *Handbook of psychotherapy and behavior change: An empirical analysis.* New York: Wiley, 1971.

Bergin, A. E., and Lambert, M. J. The evaluation of therapeutic outcomes. In S. L. Garfield and A. E. Bergin (Eds.), *Handbook of psychotherapy and behavior change: An empirical analysis* (2nd ed.). New York: Wiley, 1978.

Berne, E. *Transactional analysis in psychotherapy.* New York: Grove, 1961.

Berne, E. *Games people play: The psychology of human relationships.* New York: Grove, 1964.

Berne, E. *Principles of group treatment.* New York: Oxford, 1966.

Bernreuter, R. G. *The Personality Inventory: Manual.* Stanford, Calif.: Stanford University Press, 1935.

Bernstein, B. Social class, speech systems and psychotherapy. *British Journal of Sociology,* 1964, *15,* 54–64.

Bernstein, N. A. *The construction of movements.* Moscow: Medgiz, 1947.

Bettelheim, B. *Love is not enough: The treatment of emotionally disturbed children.* New York: Free Press, 1950.

Betz, B. J. Experiences in research in psychotherapy with schizophrenic patients. In H. H. Strupp and L. Luborsky (Eds.), *Research in psychotherapy* (vol. 2). Washington, D.C.: American Psychological Association, 1962.

Betz, B. J. Childhood status and adult schizophrenia. *American Journal of Psychotherapy,* 1973, *27,* 27–33.

Bieber, I. A discussion of "Homosexuality: The ethical challenge." *Journal of Consulting and Clinical Psychology,* 1976, *44,* 163–66.

Bieliauskas, V. J. Mental health care in the USSR. *American Psychologist,* 1977, *32,* 376–79.

Binet, A., and Simon, T. Application des méthodes nouvelles au diagnostic du niveau intellectual chez des enfants normaux et anormaux d'hospice et d'école primaire. *Année Psychologie,* 1905, *11,* 245–336.

Binitie, A. A factor-analytic study of depression across cultures (African and European). *British Journal of Psychiatry,* 1975, *127,* 559–63.

Birch, H. G., and Gussow, J. D. *Disadvantaged children: Health, nutrition, and school failure.* New York: Grune & Stratton, 1970.

Bissell. L. The treatment of alcoholism: What do we do about longterm sedatives? *Annals of the New York Academy of Sciences,* 1975, *252,* 396–99.

Bizarre outbursts of Tourette's disease victims linked to chemical disorder in brain. *New York Times,* May 29, 1975, p. 70.

Blachly, P. H. Management of the opiate abstinence syndrome. *American Journal of Psychiatry,* 1966, *122,* 742–44.

Blackburn, M. R., and Zeiner, A. R. Change in subjective behavioral assessment with preference for alcohol. National Council on Alcoholism Conference, Washington, D.C. 1979.

Blakiston's Gould medical dictionary (3rd ed.). New York: McGraw-Hill, 1972.

Blanchard, E. B., and Young, L. D. Clinical applications of biofeedback training: A review of the evidence. *Archives of General Psychiatry,* 1974, *30,* 573–89.

Blaney, P. H. Contemporary theories of depression: Critique and comparison. *Journal of Abnormal Psychology,* 1977, *86,* 203–23.

Blasdell, K. The effects of transcendental meditation upon a complex perceptual-motor task. In D. Orme-Johnson, L. Domash, and J. Farrow (Eds.), *Scientific research on transcendental meditation: Collected papers.* Los Angeles: M.I.U. Press, 1974.

Blashfield, R. An evaluation of the DSM-II classification of schizophrenia as a nomenclature. *Journal of Abnormal Psychology,* 1973, *82,* 382–89.

Blau, E. Crime report finds Manhattan ranks as most dangerous county in the state. *New York Times,* October 3, 1977, p. 34.

Blau, T. H. Torque and schizophrenic vulnerability: As the world turns. *American Psychologist,* 1977, *32,* 997–1005.

Bleuler, E. *Dementia praecox, or the group of schizophrenias.* New York: International Universities Press, 1950. (1911)

Bleuler, M. The long-term course of the schizophrenic psychoses. *Psychological Medicine,* 1974, *4,* 244–54.

Bleuler, M. *The schizophrenic disorders: Long-term patient and family studies.* New Haven: Yale University Press, 1978.

Bloom, F., Segal, O., Ling, N., and Guillemin, R. Endorphins: Profound behavioral effects in rats suggest new etiological factors in mental illness. *Science,* 1976, *194,* 630–32.

Blum, J. D. On changes in psychiatric diagnosis over time. *American Psychologist,* 1978, *33,* 1017–31.

Bootzin, R. R. A stimulus control treatment for insomnia. *Proceedings of the American Psychological Association,* 1972, *1,* 395–96.

Bootzin, R. R. Personal communication, 1978.

Borgaonkar, D. S., and Shah, S. A. The XYY chromosome male—or syndrome? In A. G. Steinberg and A. G. Bearn (Eds.), *Progress in medical genetics* (vol. 10). New York: Grune & Stratton, 1974.

Boring, E. G. *A history of experimental psychology.* New York: Century, 1929.

Boss, M. *Psychoanalysis and daseininsanalysis.* New York: Basic Books, 1963.

Bosse, J. J., Croghan, L. M., Greenstein, M. B., Katz, N. W., Oliver, J. M., Powell, D. A., and Smith, W. R. Frequency of depression in the freshman year as measured in a random sample by a retrospective version of the Beck Depression Inventory. *Journal of Consulting and Clinical Psychology*, 1975, *43*, 746–47.

Boswell, P. C., and Murray, E. J. Effects of meditation on psychological and physiological measures of anxiety. *Journal of Consulting and Clinical Psychology*, 1979, *47*, 606–7.

Bourne, P. Alcoholism in the urban black population. In F. D. Harper (Ed.), *Alcohol abuse and black America*. Alexandria, Va.: Douglass, 1976.

Bowers, P. Hypnosis and creativity: The search for the missing link. *Journal of Abnormal Psychology*, 1979, *88*, 564–72.

Bowers, M. B., Jr. Biochemical processes in schizophrenia: An update. *Schizophrenia Bulletin*, 1980, *6*, 393–403.

Bowlby, J. *Attachment and loss. Vol. I: Attachment*. New York: Basic Books, 1969.

Bowlby, J. *Attachment and loss. Vol. II: Separation*. New York: Basic Books, 1973.

Brant, R. S. T., and Tisza, V. B. The sexually misused child. *American Journal of Orthopsychiatry*, 1977, *47*, 80–90.

Braucht, G. N. Interactional analysis of suicidal behavior. *Journal of Consulting and Clinical Psychology*, 1979, *47*, 653–69.

Breakey, A. S., Wilson, J. J., and Wilson, B. C. Sensory and perceptual functions in the cerebral palsied. III. Some visual perceptual relationships. *Journal of Nervous and Mental Disease*, 1974, *158*, 70–77.

Breggin, P. R. *Electroshock: Its brain-disabling effects*. New York: Springer, 1979.

Brener, J. Learned control of cardiovascular processes: Feedback mechanisms and therapeutic applications. In K. S. Calhoun, H. E. Adams, and K. M. Mitchell (Eds.), *Innovative treatment methods in psychopathology*. New York: Wiley, 1974.

Briddell, D. W., and Wilson, G. T. Effects of alcohol and expectancy set on male sexual arousal. *Journal of Abnormal Psychology*, 1976, *85*, 225–34.

British Medical Journal. The fetal alcohol syndrome. 1976, *2*, 1404–5.

Broadbent, D. E. *Perception and communication*. Oxford: Pergamon Press, 1958.

Brock, T. C., and Del Giudice, C. Stealing and temporal orientation. *Journal of Abnormal and Social Psychology*, 1963, *66*, 91–94.

Brody, J. E. Alcohol's effects linked to chemical. *New York Times*, February 23, 1975, p. 44.

Brody, J. E. Marriage is good for health and longevity, studies say. *New York Times*, May 8, 1979, pp. C1–2. (a)

Brody, J. E. Personal health: The incidence of incest is far more common than most people believe. *New York Times*, June 13, 1979, p. C8. (b)

Broen, W. E., Jr. *Schizophrenia: Research and theory*. New York: Academic Press, 1968.

Broen, W. E., Jr., and Nakamura, C. Y. Reduced range of sensory sensitivity in chronic nonparanoid schizophrenics. *Journal of Abnormal Psychology*, 1972, *79*, 106–11.

Broen, W. E., Jr., and Storms, L. H. Lawful disorganization: The process underlying a schizophrenic syndrome. *Psychological Review*, 1966, *73*, 265–79.

Bromet, E., Alto, P., Harrow, M., and Kasl, S. Premorbid functioning and outcome in schizophrenics and nonschizophrenics. *Archives of General Psychiatry*, 1974, *30*, 203–7.

Broverman, I. K., Broverman, D. M., Clarkson, F. E., Rosenkrantz, P. S., and Vogel, S. R. Sex-role stereotypes and clinical judgments of mental health. *Journal of Consulting and Clinical Psychology*, 1970, *34*, 1–7.

Brown, B. B. Recognition of aspects of consciousness through association with EEG alpha activity represented by a light signal. *Psychophysiology*, 1970, *6*, 442–52.

Brown, B. B. *New mind, new body—biofeedback: New directions for the mind*. New York: Harper & Row, 1974.

Brown, J. K. Migraine and migraine equivalents in children. *Developmental Medicine and Child Neurology*, 1977, *19*, 683–92.

Brown, R. A., and Cutter, H. S. G. Alcohol, customary drinking behavior, and pain. *Journal of Abnormal Psychology*, 1977, *86*, 179–88.

Brown, S. A., Goldman, M. S., Inn, A., and Anderson, L. R. Expectations of reinforcement from alcohol: Their domain and relation to drinking patterns. *Journal of Consulting and Clinical Psychology*, 1980, *48*, 419–26.

Brownmiller, S. *Against our will: Men, women and rape*. New York: Simon & Schuster, 1975.

Bruch, H. Transformation of oral impulses in eating disorders: A conceptual approach. *Psychiatric Quarterly*, 1961, *35*, 458–81.

Bruch, H. *Eating disorders: Obesity, anorexia nervosa, and the person within*. New York: Basic Books, 1973.

Buber, M. *I and thou*. New York: Scribner, 1958.

Bucher, B., and Lovaas, O. I. Use of aversive stimulation in behavior modification. In M. R. Jones (Ed.), *Miami Symposium on the prediction of behavior, 1967: Aversive stimulation*. Coral Gables, Fla.: University of Miami Press, 1968.

Buchsbaum, M. S. Psychophysiology and schizophrenia. *Schizophrenia Bulletin*, 1977, *3*, No. 1, 7–14.

Buchwald, A. M., Coyne, J. C., and Cole, C. S. A critical evaluation of the learned helplessness model of depression. *Journal of Abnormal Psychology*, 1978, *87*, 180–93.

Buell, S. J., and Coleman, P. D. Dendritic growth in the aged human brain and failure of growth in senile dementia. *Science*, 1979, *206*, 854–55.

Bunney, W. E. Psychobiological studies of manic-depressive illness. In R. R. Fieve (Ed.), *Depression in the 1970s: Modern theory and research*. The Hague: Excerpta Medica, 1971.

Burdock, E. I., and Hardesty, A. S. *Structured Clinical Interview and Inventory*. New York: Copyright, Eugene I. Burdock, 1962.

Burgess, A. W., and Holmstrom, L. L. Rape: Sexual disruption and recovery. *American Journal of Orthopsychiatry*, 1979, *49*, 648–57.

Burgess, R. L., and Akers, R. L. A differential association-reinforcement theory of criminal behavior. *Social Problems*, 1966, *14*, 128–47.

Buss, A. H. *Psychopathology.* New York: Wiley, 1966.

Buss, A. H., and Lang, P. J. Psychological deficit in schizophrenia: I. Affect, reinforcement, and concept attainment. *Journal of Abnormal Psychology,* 1965, *70,* 2–24.

Bybee, R. W. Violence toward youth: A new perspective. *Journal of Social Issues,* 1979, *35,* 1–14.

Byck, R. (Ed.) *Cocaine papers: Sigmund Freud (Notes on the Freud papers by Anna Freud).* New York: New American Library, 1975.

Byck, R., and Van Dyke, C. What are the effects of cocaine in man? In R. C. Petersen and R. C. Stillman (Eds.), *Cocaine: 1977.* National Institute on Drug Abuse Research Monograph, No. 13, 1977.

Cade, J. F. J. Lithium salts in the treatment of psychotic excitement. *Medical Journal of Australia,* 1949, *2,* 349–52.

Cadoret, R. J., and Winokur, G. X-linkage in manic-depressive illness. *Annual Review of Medicine,* 1975, *26,* 21–25.

Cahalan, D. *Problem drinkers: A national survey.* San Francisco: Jossey-Bass, 1970.

Callner, D. A. Behavioral treatment approaches to drug abuse: A critical review of the research. *Psychological Bulletin,* 1975, *82,* 143–64.

Cameron, N. Deterioration and regression in schizophrenic thinking. *Journal of Abnormal and Social Psychology,* 1939, *34,* 265–70.

Campbell, D. E., and Beets, J. L. Lunacy and the moon. *Psychological Bulletin,* 1978, *85,* 1123–29.

Cancro, R. Genetic evidence for the existence of subgroups of the schizophrenic syndrome. *Schizophrenia Bulletin,* 1979, *5,* No. 3, 453–59.

Cannon, W. B. *Bodily changes in pain, hunger, fear and rage.* New York: Appleton, 1929.

Cantor, N., Smith, E. E., French, R. de S., and Mezzich, J. Psychiatric diagnosis as a prototype categorization. *Journal of Abnormal Psychology,* 1980, *89,* 181–93.

Caplan. H. W., and Black, R. A. Unrealistic sexual expectations. *Medical Aspects of Human Sexuality,* 1974, *8,* 8–36.

Cappell, H. An evaluation of tension models of alcohol consumption. In R. J. Gibbins, Y. Israel, H. Kalant, R. E. Popham, W. Schmidt, and R. G. Smart (Eds.), *Research advances in alcohol and drug problems* (vol. 2). New York: Wiley, 1975.

Carlin, A. S., Bakker, C. B., Halpern, L., and Post, R. D. Social facilitation of marijuana intoxication: Impact of social set and pharmacological activity. *Journal of Abnormal Psychology,* 1972, *80,* 132–40.

Carlin, A. S., and Strauss, F. F. Descriptive and functional classifications of drug abusers. *Journal of Consulting and Clinical Psychology,* 1977, *45,* 222–27.

Carpenter, M. D. Sensitivity to syntactic structure: Good versus poor premorbid schizophrenics. *Journal of Abnormal Psychology,* 1976, *85,* 41–50.

Carpenter, M. D. Residential placement for the chronic psychiatric patient: A review and evaluation of the literature. *Schizophrenia Bulletin,* 1978, *4,* No. 3, 384–98.

Carpenter, W. T., Jr., Bartko, J. J., Carpenter, C. L., and Strauss, J. S. Another view of schizophrenia subtypes: A report from the International Pilot Study of Schizophrenia. *Archives of General Psychiatry,* 1976, *33,* 508–16.

Carpenter, W. T., Jr., and Strauss, J. S. Cross-cultural evaluation of Schneider's first-rank symptoms of schizophrenia: A report from the International Pilot Study of Schizophrenia. *American Journal of Psychiatry,* 1974, *131,* 682–87.

Carpenter, W. T., Jr., Strauss, J. S., and Bartko, J. J. Flexible system for the diagnosis of schizophrenia: Report from the WHO International Pilot Study of Schizophrenia. *Science,* 1973, *182,* 1275–78.

Carpenter, W. T., Jr., Strauss, J. S., and Bartko, J. J. The diagnosis and understanding of schizophrenia. Part I. Use of signs and symptoms for the identification of schizophrenic patients. *Schizophrenia Bulletin,* 1974, No. 11, 37–49.

Carter, E. N., Rice, A. P., and De Julio, S. Role of the therapist in the self-control of obesity. *Journal of Consulting and Clinical Psychology,* 1977, *45,* 503.

Cartwright, R. D. Happy endings for our dreams. *Psychology Today,* December, 1978, 66–76. (a)

Cartwright, R. D. *A primer on sleep and dreaming.* Reading, Mass.: Addison-Wesley, 1978. (b)

Cashdan, S. *Interactional psychotherapy: Stages and strategies in behavior change.* New York: Grune & Stratton, 1973.

Cattell, R. B., and Kline, P. (Eds.) *The scientific analysis of personality and motivation.* New York: Academic Press, 1977.

Caudill, B. D., and Marlatt, G. A. Modeling influences in social drinking: An experimental analogue. *Journal of Consulting and Clinical Psychology,* 1975, *43,* 405–15.

Caulfield, J. B., and Martin, R. B. Establishment of praise as a reinforcer in chronic schizophrenics. *Journal of Consulting and Clinical Psychology,* 1976, *44,* 61–67.

Cautela, J. R. Treatment of compulsive behavior by covert sensitization. *Psychological Record,* 1966, *16,* 33–41.

Cautela, J. R. Covert sensitization. *Psychological Reports,* 1967, *20,* 459–68.

Cautela, J. R. Covert modeling. Paper presented at the meeting of the Association for the Advancement of Behavior Therapy, Washington, D.C., September, 1971.

Cavior, N., and Deutsch, A. Single case study: Systematic desensitization to reduce dream-induced anxiety. *Journal of Nervous and Mental Disease,* 1975, *161,* 433–35.

Chafetz, M. *Why drinking can be good for you.* New York: Stein & Day, 1976.

Chambers, C. D., and Griffey, M. S. Use of legal substances within the general population: The sex and age variables. *Addictive Diseases,* 1975, *2,* 7–19.

Chambless, D. L., and Goldstein, A. The treatment of agoraphobia. In A. Goldstein and E. Foa (Eds.), *Handbook of behavioral interventions.* New York: Wiley, 1980.

Chapman, L. J., and Chapman, J. P. *Disordered thought in schizophrenia.* New York: Appleton, 1973.

Chapman, L. J., Chapman, J. P., and Miller, G. A. A theory of verbal behavior in schizophrenia. In B. A. Maher (Ed.), *Prog-*

ress in experimental personality research (vol. 1). New York: Academic Press, 1964.

Chesler, P. *Women and madness.* Garden City, New York: Doubleday, 1972.

Chesno, F. A., and Kilmann, P. R. Effects of stimulation intensity on sociopathic avoidance learning. *Journal of Abnormal Psychology,* 1975, *84,* 144–50.

Chess, S., Thomas, A., and Cameron, M. Sexual attitudes and behavior patterns in a middle-class adolescent population. *American Journal of Orthopsychiatry,* 1976, *46,* 689–701.

Child, I. L., Bacon, M. K., and Barry, H. III. A cross-cultural study of drinking: I. Descriptive measurements of drinking customs. *Quarterly Journal of Studies on Alcohol Supplement,* 1965, *3,* 1–28.

Child, I. L., Barry, H. III, and Bacon, M. K. A cross-cultural study of drinking: III. Sex differences. *Quarterly Journal of Studies on Alcohol Supplement,* 1965, *3,* 49–61.

Ching, C. C. Psychology in the People's Republic of China. *American Psychologist,* 1980, *35,* 1084–89.

Chiodo, L. A., and Antelman, S. H. Electroconvulsive shock: Progressive dopamine autoreceptor subsensitivity independent of repeated treatment. *Science,* 1980, *210,* 799–801.

Chorover, S. L. *From genesis to genocide: The meaning of human nature and the power of behavior control.* Cambridge, Mass.: MIT Press, 1979.

Church, R. M. The varied effects of punishment on behavior. *Psychological Review,* 1963, *70,* 369–402.

Claridge, G. *Drugs and human behaviour.* London: Allen Lane The Penguin Press, 1970.

Clarke, A. M., and Clarke, A. D. B. *Mental deficiency: The changing outlook.* New York: Macmillan, 1974.

Cleary, T. A., Humphreys, L. G., Kendrick, S. A., and Wesman, A. Educational uses of tests with disadvantaged students. *American Psychologist,* 1975, *30,* 15–41.

Cleckley, H. *The mask of sanity: An attempt to clarify some issues about the so-called psychopathic personality.* St. Louis: Mosby, 1964.

Cleveland, S. I., and Fisher, S. A comparison of psychological characteristics and physiological reactivity in ulcer and rheumatoid arthritis groups: I. Psychological measures. *Psychosomatic Medicine,* 1960, *22,* 283–89.

Cloward, R. A., and Ohlin, L. E. *Delinquency and opportunity: A theory of delinquent gangs.* Glencoe, Ill.: Free Press, 1960.

Cohen, A. K. *Delinquent boys: The culture of the gang:* New York: Free Press, 1955.

Cohen, D. B. Dysphoric affect and REM sleep. *Journal of Abnormal Psychology,* 1979, *88,* 73–77.

Cohen, J. Social work and the culture of poverty. *Social Work,* 1964, *9,* 3–11.

Cohen, S. Teenage drinking: The bottle babies. *Drug Abuse and Alcoholism Newsletter,* 1975, *4,* 1–4.

Cohen, S. Oriental syndrome. *Drug Abuse and Alcoholism Newsletter,* 1979, *8,* 1–3. (a)

Cohen, S. Inhalants. In R. L. DuPont, A. Goldstein, and J. O'Donnell (Eds.), *Handbook on drug abuse.* National Institute on Drug Abuse, 1979. (b)

Cohen, B. D., and Camhi, J. Schizophrenic performance in a word-communication task. *Journal of Abnormal Psychology,* 1967, *72,* 240–46.

Cole, J. O. Antidepressant drug treatment. In A. DiMascio and R. I. Shader (Eds.), *Clinical handbook of psychopharmacology.* New York: Science House, 1970.

Cole, C. S., and Coyne, J. C. Situational specificity of laboratory-induced learned helplessness. *Journal of Abnormal Psychology,* 1977, *86,* 615–23.

Cole, J., and Pilisuk, M. Differences in the provision of mental health services by race. *American Journal of Orthopsychiatry,* 1976, *46,* 510–25.

Coleman, L. S. Perspectives on the medical research of violence. *American Journal of Orthopsychiatry,* 1974, *44,* 675–87.

Coleman, R. E. Cognitive-behavioral treatment of agoraphobia. In G. Emery, S. D. Hollon, and R. C. Bedrosian (Eds.), *New directions in cognitive therapy.* New York: Guilford Press, 1981.

Conger, J. J. Alcoholism: Theory, problem and challenge. II. Reinforcement theory and the dynamics of alcoholism. *Quarterly Journal of Studies on Alcohol,* 1956, *17,* 296–305.

Connecticut allows marijuana cigarettes as medicine. *New York Times,* July 8, 1981, p. B1.

Conway, J. B. Behavioral self-control of smoking through aversive conditioning and self-management. *Journal of Consulting and Clinical Psychology,* 1977, *45,* 348–57.

Coombs, O. Three faces of Harlem. *New York Times Magazine,* November 3, 1974, pp. 32–34, 36, 38, 40, 44, 47, 49.

Cooper, S., and Wanerman, L. *Children in treatment: A primer for beginning psychotherapists.* New York: Brunner/Mazel, 1977.

Coppen, A. The biochemistry of affective disorders. *British Journal of Psychiatry,* 1967, *113,* 1237–64.

Costello, C. G. Depression: Loss of reinforcers or loss of reinforcer effectiveness? *Behavior Therapy,* 1972, *3,* 240–47.

Costello, C. G. A critical review of Seligman's laboratory experiments on learned helplessness and depression in humans. *Journal of Abnormal Psychology,* 1978, *87,* 21–31.

Cox, V. A distracting hypothesis. Review of: S. Schachter and J. Rodin, *Obese humans and rats.* New York: Wiley, 1974. In *Contemporary Psychology,* 1976, *21,* 3.

Cox, G., Costanzo, P. R., and Coie, J. D. A survey instrument for the assessment of popular conceptions of mental illness. *Journal of Consulting and Clinical Psychology,* 1976, *44,* 901–9.

Coyne, J. C. Depression and the response of others. *Journal of Abnormal Psychology,* 1976, *85,* 186–93.

Crimes by women found on rise, with fraud favored over violence. *New York Times,* July 25, 1978, p. 12.

Crissey, M. S. Mental retardation: Past, present, and future. *American Psychologist,* 1975, *30,* 800–8.

Cromwell, R. L., and Dokecki, P. R. Schizophrenic language: A disattention interpretation. In S. Rosenberg and J. H. Koplin (Eds.), *Developments in applied psycholinguistics research.* New York: Macmillan, 1968.

Cronbach, L. J. Five decades of public controversy over mental testing. *American Psychologist,* 1975, *30,* 1–14.

Crook, T., and Eliot, J. Parental death during childhood and adult depression: A critical review of the literature. *Psychological Bulletin,* 1980, *87,* 252–59.

Crowe, R. R. The adopted offspring of women criminal offenders: A study of their arrest records. *Archives of General Psychiatry,* 1972, *27,* 600–3.

Crowe, R. R. An adoption study of antisocial personality. *Archives of General Psychiatry,* 1974, *31,* 785–91.

Culliton, B. J. XYY: Harvard researcher under fire stops newborn screening. *Science,* 1975, *188,* 1284–85.

Cummings, N. A. Turning bread into stones: Our modern antimiracle. *American Psychologist,* 1979, *34,* 1119–29.

Darlington, R. B., Royce, J. M., Snipper, A. S., Murray, H. W., and Lazar, I. Preschool programs and later school competence of children from low-income families. *Science,* 1980, *208,* 202–4.

David, H. P., and David, T. S. Soviet mental health facilities and psychology. In R. A. Bauer (Ed.), *Some views on Soviet psychology.* Washington, D.C.: American Psychological Association, 1962.

Davids, A. Therapeutic approaches to children in residential treatment: Changes from the mid-1950s to the mid-1970s. *American Psychologist,* 1975, *30,* 809–14.

Davids, A., Kidder, C., and Reich, M. Time orientation in male and female juvenile delinquents. *Journal of Abnormal and Social Psychology,* 1962, *64,* 239–40.

Davidson, G. S., and Neale, J. M. The effects of signal-noise similarity on visual information processing of schizophrenics. *Journal of Abnormal Psychology,* 1974, *83,* 683–86.

Davis, A. E., Dinitz, S., and Pasamanick, B. *Schizophrenics in the new custodial community: Five years after the experiment.* Columbus: Ohio State University Press, 1974.

Davis, F. H., Malmo, R. B., and Shagass, C. Electromyographic reaction to strong auditory stimulation in psychiatric patients. *Canadian Journal of Psychology,* 1954, *8,* 177–86.

Davis, J. M., Gosenfeld, L., and Tsai, C. C. Maintenance antipsychotic drugs do prevent relapse: A reply to Tobias and MacDonald. *Psychological Bulletin,* 1976, *83,* 431–47.

Davis, K. M., and Blaney, P. H. Overinclusion and self-editing in schizophrenia. *Journal of Abnormal Psychology,* 1976, *85,* 51–60.

Davison, G. C. Elimination of a sadistic fantasy by a client-controlled counter-conditioning technique: A case study. *Journal of Abnormal Psychology,* 1968, *73,* 84–90.

Davison, G. C. Homosexuality: The ethical challenge. *Journal of Consulting and Clinical Psychology,* 1976, *44,* 157–62.

Davison, G. C. Not can but ought: The treatment of homosexuality. *Journal of Consulting and Clinical Psychology,* 1978, *46,* 170–72.

Davison, G. C., and Wilson, G. T. Critique of "Desensitization: Social and cognitive factors underlying the effectiveness of Wolpe's procedure." *Psychological Bulletin,* 1972, *78,* 28–31.

Dawson, J. Urbanization and mental health in a West African community. In A. Kiev (Ed.), *Magic, faith, and healing: Studies in primitive psychiatry today.* New York: Free Press, 1964.

DeFries, J. C., and Plomin, R. Behavioral genetics. *Annual Review of Psychology,* 1978, *29,* 473–515.

De Leon, G., and Rosenthal, M. S. Therapeutic communities. In R. L. Dupont, A. Goldstein, and J. O'Donnell (Eds.), *Handbook on drug abuse.* National Institute on Drug Abuse, 1979.

Dement, W. C. An essay on dreams: The role of physiology in understanding their nature. *In new directions in psychology* (vol. 2). New York: Holt, Rinehart and Winston, 1965.

Dement, W. C. Sleep and dreams. In A. M. Freedman, H. I. Kaplan, and H. S. Kaplan (Eds.), *Comprehensive textbook of psychiatry.* Baltimore: Williams & Wilkins, 1967.

Dement, W. C., and Kleitman, N. The relation of eye movements during sleep to dream activity: An objective method for the study of dreaming. *Journal of Experimental Psychology,* 1957, *53,* 339–46.

DeMyer, M. K., Churchill, D. W., Pontius, W., and Gilkey, K. M. A comparison of five diagnostic systems for childhood schizophrenia and infantile autism. *Journal of Autism and Childhood Schizophrenia,* 1971, *1,* 175–89.

De Piano, F. A., and Salzberg, H. C. Clinical applications of hypnosis to three psychosomatic disorders. *Psychological Bulletin,* 1979, *86,* 1223–35.

Depue, R. A., and Dubicki, M. D. Hospitalization and premorbid characteristics in withdrawn and active schizophrenics. *Journal of Consulting and Clinical Psychology,* 1974, *42,* 628–32.

Depue, R. A., and Monroe, S. M. Learned helplessness in the perspective of the depressive disorders: Conceptual and definitional issues. *Journal of Abnormal Psychology,* 1978, *87,* 3–20. (a)

Depue, R. A., and Monroe, S. M. The unipolar-bipolar distinction in the depressive disorders. *Psychological Bulletin,* 1978, *85,* 1001–29. (b)

Derdyn, A. P. Child abuse and neglect: The rights of parents and the needs of their children. *American Journal of Orthopsychiatry,* 1977, *47,* 377–87.

de Reuck, A. V. S., and Porter, R. (Eds.) *Transcultural psychiatry.* Boston: Little, Brown, 1965.

Derogatis, L. R., Yevzeroff, H., and Wittelsberger, B. Social class, psychological disorder, and the nature of the psychopathologic disorder. *Journal of Consulting and Clinical Psychology,* 1975, *43,* 183–91.

Deutsch, A. *The mentally ill in America: A history of their care and treatment from colonial times.* New York: Columbia University Press, 1949.

Deutsch, C. P. Social class and child development. In B. M. Caldwell and H. M. Ricciuti (Eds.), *Review of child development research* (vol. 3). Chicago: University of Chicago Press, 1973.

Deutsch, C. P., and Schumer, F. *Brain-damaged children: A mo-*

dality-oriented exploration of performance. New York: Brunner/Mazel, 1970.

Deutsch, M. The disadvantaged child and the learning process. In A. H. Passow (Ed.), *Education in depressed areas.* New York: Bureau of Publications, Teachers College, Columbia University, 1963.

DeWolfe, A. S. Are there two kinds of thinking in process and reactive schizophrenics? *Journal of Abnormal Psychology,* 1974, *83,* 285–90.

Di Chiro, G., and Brooks, R. A. The 1979 Nobel Prize in Physiology or Medicine. *Science,* 1979, *206,* 1060–62.

Diefendorf, A. R., and Dodge, R. An experimental study of the ocular reactions of the insane from photographic records. *Brain,* 1908, *31,* 451–89.

Dimijian, G. G. Contemporary drug abuse. In A. Goth, *Medical Pharmacology: Principles and concepts* (9th ed.) Saint Louis: Mosby, 1978.

Dinges, D. F., Davis, M. M., and Glass, P. Fetal exposure to narcotics: Neonatal sleep as a measure of nervous system disturbance. *Science,* 1980, *209,* 619–21.

Dishotsky, N. I., Loughman, W. D., Mogar, R. E., and Lipscomb, W. R. J. LSD and genetic damage. *Science,* 1971, *172,* 431–40.

Dohrenwend, B. P., and Dohrenwend, B. S. *Social status and psychological disorder: A causal inquiry.* New York: Wiley, 1969.

Dohrenwend, B. P., and Dohrenwend, B. S. Social and cultural influences on psychopathology. *Annual Review of Psychology,* 1974, *25,* 417–52.

Dohrenwend, B. S., and Dohrenwend, B. P. Class and race as status-related sources of stress. In S. Levine and N. A. Scotch (Eds.), *Social stress.* Chicago: Aldine, 1970.

Dohrenwend, B. S., and Dohrenwend, B. P. An approach to the problem of valid comparison of psychiatric disorders in contrasting class and ethnic groups from the general population. In M. Hammer, K. Salzinger, and S. Sutton (Eds.), *Psychopathology: Contributions from the social, behavioral, and biological sciences.* New York: Wiley, 1973.

Dohrenwend, B. S., and Dohrenwend, B. P. (Eds.) *Stressful life events: Their nature and effects.* New York: Wiley, 1974.

Dohrenwend, B. P., and Egri, G. Recent stressful life events and episodes of schizophrenia. *Schizophrenia Bulletin,* 1981, *7,* 12–24.

Do kids and alcohol mix? *New York Times,* July 17, 1977, p. E11.

Dole, V. P. Addictive behavior. *Scientific American, December, 1980, 243,* 138–54.

Dole, V. P., Nyswander, M. E., and Warner, A. Successful treatment of 750 criminal addicts. *Journal of the American Medical Association,* 1968, *206,* 2708–11.

Doll, E. A. The essentials of an inclusive concept of mental deficiency. *American Journal of Mental Deficiency,* 1941, *46,* 214–19.

Doll, E. A. *The measurement of social competence: A manual for the Vineland Social Maturity Scale.* Minneapolis, Minn.: Educational Testing Bureau, 1953.

Doll, E. A. *The Vineland Scale of Social Maturity.* Minneapolis: American Guidance Service, 1964.

Dollard, J., Doob, L. W., Miller, N. E., Mowrer, O. H., and Sears, R. R. *Frustration and aggression.* New Haven: Yale University Press, 1939.

Dollard, J., and Miller, N. E. *Personality and psychotherapy: An analysis in terms of learning, thinking, and culture.* New York: McGraw-Hill, 1950.

Domino, E. F., and Luby, E. D. Abnormal mental states induced by phencyclidine as a model of schizophrenia. In J. O. Cole, A. M. Freedman, and A. J. Friedhaff (Eds.), *Psychopathology and psychopharmacology.* Baltimore: Johns Hopkins University Press, 1973.

Dorfman, D. D. The Cyril Burt question: New findings. *Science,* 1978, *201,* 1177–86.

Douglass, F. M. IV, Khavari, K. A., and Farber, P. D. Three types of extreme drug users identified by a replicated cluster analysis. *Journal of Abnormal Psychology,* 1980, *89,* 240–49.

Dragstedt, L. R. A concept of the etiology of duodenal ulcer. *American Journal of Radiology,* 1956, *75,* 219–29.

Drug use in America: Problem in perspective. Washington, D.C.: National Commission on Marijuana and Drug Abuse, 1973.

Dubey, D. R. Organic factors in hyperkinesis: A critical evaluation. *American Journal of Orthopsychiatry,* 1976, *46,* 353–66.

Dublin, L. I. *Suicide: A sociological and statistical study.* New York: Ronald Press, 1963.

Dullea, G. Child prostitution: Causes are sought. *New York Times,* September 4, 1979, p. C11.

Dunbar, F. *Emotions and bodily changes.* New York: Columbia University Press, 1954.

Dunham, H. W. *Community and schizophrenia, An epidemiological analysis.* Detroit: Wayne State University Press, 1965.

Dunham, H. W. Epidemiology of psychiatric disorders as a contribution to medical ecology. *Archives of General Psychiatry,* 1966, *14,* 1–19.

Dunn, L. M. (Ed.) *Exceptional children in the schools: Special education in transition.* New York: Holt, Rinehart & Winston, 1973.

Dunner, D. L. Recent research on classification, genetics, and treatment of depression. *Journal of Clinical Issues in Psychology,* 1975, *6,* 14–16.

Dunner, D. L., Gershon, E. S., and Goodwin, F. K. Heritable factors in the severity of affective illness. *Biological Psychiatry,* 1976, *11,* 31–42.

DuPont, R. L. The future of the federal drug abuse program. Paper presented at Drug Dependence Conference, Mexico City, 1974.

DuPont, R. L. Foreword. In R. C. Petersen and R. C. Stillman (Eds.), *Cocaine: 1977.* National Institute on Drug Abuse Research Monograph No. 13, 1977.

Durkheim, E. *Rules of sociological method.* Glencoe, Ill.: Free Press, 1938.

Durkheim, E. *Suicide: A study in sociology.* New York: Free Press, 1951. (1897)

Dykes, M., and McGhie, A. A comparative study of attentional strategies of schizophrenic and highly creative normal subjects. *British Journal of Psychiatry,* 1976, *128,* 50–56.

Eastman, C. Behavioral formulations of depression. *Psychological Review,* 1976, *83,* 277–91.

Eaton, J. W., and Weil, R. J. *Culture and mental disorders.* Glencoe, Ill.: Free Press, 1955.

Eberhard, G. The personality at peptic ulcer: Preliminary report of a twin study. *Acta Psychiatrica Scandinavica Supplementum,* 1968, *203,* 131–33.

Edgerton, R. B. Some socio-cultural research considerations. In F. F. de la Cruz and G. D. LaVeck (Eds.), *Human sexuality and the mentally retarded.* New York: Brunner/Mazel, 1973.

Edwards Personal Preference Schedule. New York: Psychological Corporation, 1953.

Egeland, B., Breitenbucher, M., and Rosenberg, D. Prospective study of the significance of life stress in the etiology of child abuse. *Journal of Consulting and Clinical Psychology,* 1980, *48,* 195–205.

Eisenberg, L., and Kanner, L. Early infantile autism, 1943–1955. *American Journal of Orthopsychiatry,* 1956, *26,* 556–66.

Ellingson, R. J. The incidence of EEG abnormality among patients with mental disorders of apparently nonorganic origin: A critical review. *American Journal of Psychiatry,* 1954, *111,* 263–75.

Ellinwood, E. H., Jr. The epidemiology of stimulant abuse. In E. Josephson and E. E. Carroll (Eds.), *Drug use: Epidemiological and sociological approaches.* New York: Wiley, 1974.

Ellinwood, E. H., Jr. Amphetamines/anorectics. In R. L. DuPont, A. Goldstein, and J. O'Donnell (Eds.), *Handbook on drug abuse.* National Institute on Drug Abuse, 1979.

Ellis, A. *Reason and emotion in psychotherapy.* New York: Lyle Stuart, 1962.

Ellis, A., Rational-emotive therapy. In R. Corsini (Ed.), *Current psychotherapies.* Itasca, Ill.: Peacock, 1973.

Ellis, A., and Grieger, R, with contributors. *Handbook of rational-emotive therapy.* New York: Springer, 1977.

Elmer, E., and Gregg, G. S. Developmental characteristics of abused children. *Pediatrics,* 1967, *40,* 596–602.

Eme, R. F. Sex differences in childhood psychopathology: A review. *Psychological Bulletin,* 1979, *86,* 574–95.

Engel, G. L. A life setting conducive to illness. The giving-up—given up complex. *Annals of Internal Medicine,* 1968, *69,* 293–300.

English, H. B., and English, A. C. *A comprehensive dictionary of psychological and psychoanalytical terms.* New York: McKay, 1958.

Erikson, E. H. *Identity: Youth and crisis.* New York: Norton, 1968.

Eron, L. D. Symposium: The application of role and learning theories to the study of the development of aggression in children. *Proceedings of the Rip Van Winkle Clinic,* 1959, *10,* 3–61.

Eron, L. D. Prescription for reduction of aggression. *American Psychologist,* 1980, *35,* 244–52.

Erwin, E. Psychoanalytic therapy: The Eysenck argument. *American Psychologist,* 1980, *35,* 435–43.

Essen-Möller, E. A current field study in the mental disorders in Sweden. In P. H. Hoch and J. Zubin (Eds.), *Comparative epidemiology of the mental disorders.* New York: Grune & Stratton, 1961.

Everstine, L., Everstine, D. S., Heymann, G. M., True, R. H., Frey, D. H., Johnson, H. G., and Seiden, R. H. Privacy and confidentiality in psychotherapy. *American Psychologist,* 1980, *35,* 828–40.

Eysenck, H. J. *Dimensions of personality.* London: Routledge & Kegan Paul, 1947.

Eysenck, H. J. *The scientific study of personality.* London: Routledge & Kegan Paul, 1952. (a)

Eysenck, H. J. The effects of psychotherapy: An evaluation. *Journal of Consulting Psychology,* 1952, *16,* 319–24. (b)

Eysenck, H. J. *Sense and nonsense in psychology.* Baltimore, Md.: Penguin, 1957.

Eysenck, H. J. *Experiments in personality.* London: Routledge & Kegan Paul, 1960. (a)

Eysenck, H. J. *Behavior therapy and the neuroses: Readings in modern methods of treatment derived from learning theory.* London: Pergamon, 1960. (b)

Eysenck, H. J. *The effects of psychotherapy.* New York: Inter-Science Press, 1966.

Eysenck, H. J. *The biological basis of personality.* Springfield, Ill.: Thomas, 1967.

Eysenck, H. J. The learning theory model of neurosis—a new approach. *Behavior Research and Therapy,* 1976, *14,* 251–67.

Eysenck, H. J., and Beech, R. Counterconditioning and related methods. In A. E. Bergin and S. L. Garfield (Eds.), *Handbook of psychotherapy and behavior change: An empirical analysis.* New York: Wiley, 1971.

Eysenck, H. J., and Rachman, S. *The causes and cures of neurosis.* London: Routledge & Kegan Paul, 1965.

Facts on alcoholism. National Council on Alcoholism, 1979.

Fagan, T. J., and Lira, F. T. The primary and secondary sociopathic personality: Differences in frequency and severity of antisocial behaviors. *Journal of Abnormal Psychology,* 1980, *89,* 493–96.

Fagan, J., and Shepherd, I. L. *Gestalt therapy now: Theory, techniques, applications.* Palo Alto, Calif.: Science and Behavior Books, 1970.

Fairweather, G. W., Sanders, D. H., Maynard, H., and Cressler, D. L. *Community life for the mentally ill: An alternative to institutional care.* Chicago: Aldine, 1969.

Farber, B. *Mental retardation: Its social context and social consequences.* Boston: Houghton Mifflin, 1968.

Farberow, N. L. Suicide: Doesn't everybody? *Clinical Psychologist,* Fall, 1977, *31,* 16–17.

Farberow, N. L., Heilig, S. M., and Litman, R. E. *Techniques in crisis intervention: A training manual.* Los Angeles: Suicide Prevention Center, Inc., 1968.

Farberow, N. L., and Shneidman, E. S. (Eds.) *The cry for help.* New York: McGraw-Hill, 1961.

Farina, A., Fisher, J. D., Getter, H., and Fischer, E. H. Some consequences of changing people's views regarding the nature of mental illness. *Journal of Abnormal Psychology,* 1978, *87,* 272–79.

Farina, A., and Ring, K. The influence of perceived mental illness in interpersonal relations. *Journal of Abnormal Psychology,* 1965, *70,* 47–51.

Faris, R. E. L., and Dunham, H. W. *Mental disorders in urban areas: An ecological study of schizophrenia and other psychoses.* Chicago: University of Chicago Press, 1939.

Federal Bureau of Investigation. *Uniform Crime Reports—1978; 1980.* U.S. Government Printing Office.

Fenichel, O. *The psychoanalytic theory of neurosis.* New York: Norton, 1945.

Feinsilver, D. B., and Gunderson, J. G. Psychotherapy for schizophrenics—is it indicated? A review of the relevant literature. *Schizophrenia Bulletin,* 1972, No. 6, 11–23.

Feldman, H. W., Agar, M. H., and Beschner, G. M. (Eds.) *Angel dust: An ethnographic study of PCP users.* Lexington, Mass.: Lexington Books, 1979.

Feldman-Summers, S., Gordon, P. E., and Meagher, J. R. The impact of rape on sexual satisfaction. *Journal of Abnormal Psychology,* 1979, *88,* 101–5.

Fenwick, S. *Getting it: The psychology of est.* Philadelphia: Lippincott, 1976.

Ferrell, T. More choose to live outside marriage. *New York Times,* July 1, 1979, p. E7.

Ferrell, T., and Adams, V. The changing patterns of life. *New York Times,* February 20, 1977, p. 16E.

Feshbach, S. Aggression. In P. H. Mussen (Ed.), *Carmichael's Manual of Child Psychology* (3rd ed.). New York: Wiley, 1970.

Feshbach, N., and Feshbach, S. Alternatives to corporal punishment: Implications for training and control. *Journal of Clinical Child Psychology,* 1973, *2,* 46–49.

Fieve, R. R. *Moodswing: The third revolution in psychiatry.* New York: Morrow, 1975.

Fieve, R. R., and Dunner, D. L. Unipolar and bipolar affective states. In F. F. Flach and S. C. Draghi (Eds.), *The nature and treatment of depression.* New York: Wiley, 1975.

Figley, C. R. (Ed.) *Stress disorders among Vietnam veterans: Theory, research, and treatment.* New York: Brunner/Mazel, 1978.

Finger, F. W. Changes in sex practices and beliefs of male college students: Over 30 years. *Journal of Sex Research,* 1975, *11,* 304–17.

Finkelhor, D. *Sexually victimized children.* New York: Free Press, 1979.

Finney, J. C., Brandsma, J. M., Tondow, M., and LeMaistre, G. A study of transsexuals seeking gender reassignment. *American Journal of Psychiatry,* 1975, *132,* 962–64.

Fischer, H. K. Faces and masks of depression: The psychodynamic side. *Psychosomatics,* 1979, *20,* 254–68.

Fischer, M. Genetic and environmental factors in schizophrenia. *Acta Psychiatrica Scandinavica,* Supplement 238, 1973.

Fischman, M. W., Schuster, C. R., Resnekov, L., Shick, J. F. E., Krasnegor, N. A., Fennel, W., and Freedman, D. X. Cardiovascular and subjective effects of intravenous cocaine administration in humans. *Archives of General Psychiatry,* 1976, *33,* 983–89.

Fisher, S. *Body experience in fantasy and behavior.* New York: Appleton-Century-Crofts, 1970.

Fisher, S., and Cleveland, S. E. *Body image and personality.* Princeton, N.J.: Van Nostrand, 1958.

Fisher, S., and Greenberg, R. P. *The scientific credibility of Freud's theories and therapy.* New York: Basic Books, 1977.

Foltz, D. Judgment withheld on DSM-III, new child classification pushed. *APA Monitor,* 1980, *11,* No. 1, 1, 33.

Ford, C. S., and Beach, F. A. *Patterns of sexual behavior.* New York, Harper, 1951.

Fordyce, W. E. *Behavioral methods for chronic pain and illness.* St. Louis: Mosby, 1976.

For parents only: What you need to know about marijuana. U.S. Department of Health and Human Services, Alcohol, Drug Abuse, and Mental Health Administration, 1980.

Fowles, D. C., and Gersh, F. Neurotic depression: The endogenous-neurotic distinction. In R. A. Depue (Ed.), *The psychobiology of the depressive disorders: Implications for the effects of stress.* New York: Academic Press, 1979.

Frank, J. D. The present status of outcome studies. *Journal of Consulting and Clinical Psychology,* 1979, *47,* 310–16.

Frank, L. K. Projective methods for the study of personality. *Journal of Psychology,* 1939, *8,* 389–413.

Frank, L. K. *Projective methods.* Springfield, Ill.: Thomas, 1948.

Franks, C. M., and Wilson, G. T. (Eds.) *Annual review of behavior therapy: Theory and practice.* New York: Brunner/Mazel, 1976.

Freed, E. X. Alcohol and mood: An updated review. *International Journal of the Addictions,* 1978, *13,* 173–200.

Freedman, A. M., Kaplan, H. I., and Sadock, B. J. *Modern synposis of Comprehensive Textbook of Psychiatry.* Baltimore: Williams & Wilkins, 1972.

Freeman, W., and Watts, J. W. *Psychosurgery in the treatment of mental disorders and intractable pain* (2nd ed.). Springfield, Ill.: Thomas, 1950.

Freud, A. *The ego and the mechanisms of defense.* New York: International Universities Press, 1946. (a)

Freud, A. *The psycho-analytical treatment of children: Technical lectures and essays.* London: Imago, 1946. (b)

Freud, S. *The psychopathology of everyday life.* New York: Random House, 1938. (1904)

Freud, S. *An outline of psychoanalysis.* New York: Norton, 1949. (1940)

Freud, S. *Collected papers (5 vols.). London: Hogarth Press and the Institute of Psychoanalysis, 1950. (1924)*

Freud, S. Introductory lectures on psycho-analysis. In *Standard edition* (vols. 15 and 16). London: Hogarth Press, 1963.

Freud, S. *New introductory lectures on psychoanalysis.* New York: Norton, 1965. (1933)

Freudenheim, B. Chicago hospitals using new kit to help rape victims collect evidence. *New York Times,* December 2, 1978, p. 48.

Friar, L. R., and Beatty, J. Migraine: Management by trained control of vasoconstriction. *Journal of Consulting and Clinical Psychology,* 1976, *44,* 46–53.

Fried, J. Acculturation and mental health among Indian migrants in Peru. In M. K. Opler (Ed.), *Culture and mental health: Cross-*

cultural studies. New York: Macmillan, 1959.

Friedman, M., and Rosenman, R. H. *Type A behavior and your heart.* New York: Knopf, 1974.

Friedman, P. R. Legal regulation of applied behavior analysis in mental institutions and prisons. *Arizona Law Review,* 1975, *17,* 39–104.

Friedrich, W. M. and Boriskin, J. A. The role of the child in abuse: A review of the literature. *American Journal of Orthopsychiatry,* 1976, *46,* 580–90.

Frodi, A., Macaulay, J., and Thome, P. R. Are women always less aggressive than men? *Psychological Bulletin,* 1977, *84,* 634–60.

Fromm, E. *Escape from freedom.* New York: Holt, Rinehart & Winston, 1941.

Fromm, E. *Man for himself: An inquiry into the psychology of ethics.* New York: Holt, Rinehart & Winston, 1947.

Fuchs, F. Genetic amniocentesis. *Scientific American,* 1980, *242,* 47–53.

Fuller, G. D. Current status of biofeedback in clinical practice. *American Psychologist,* 1978, *33,* 39–48.

Gagnon, J. H. *Human sexualities.* Glenville, Ill.: Scott, Foresman, 1977.

Gagnon, J. H., Simon, W., and Berger, A. J. Some aspects of sexual adjustment in early and late adolescence. In J. Zubin and A. N. Freedman (Eds.), *Psychopathology of adolescence.* New York: Grune & Stratton, 1970.

Galaburda, A. M., LeMay, M., Kemper, T. L., and Geschwind, N. Right-left asymmetries in the brain. *Science,* 1978, *199,* 852–56.

Galdston, I. A. Existentialism and psychiatry. *Bulletin of the New York Academy of Medicine,* 1961, *37,* 835–47.

Garai, J. E. Sex differences in mental health. *Genetic Psychology Monographs,* 1970, *81,* 123–42.

Garfield, S. L. Research on client variables in psychotherapy. In A. E. Bergin and S. L. Garfield (Eds.), *Handbook of psychotherapy and behavior change: An empirical analysis.* New York: Wiley, 1971.

Garfield, S. L. Further comments on "Dropping out of treatment": Reply to Baekeland and Lundwall. *Psychological Bulletin,* 1977, *84,* 306–8.

Garfield, S. L. Research problems in clinical diagnosis. *Journal of Consulting and Clinical Psychology,* 1978, *46,* 596–607.

Garfield, S. L. Psychotherapy: A 40-year appraisal. *American Psychologist,* 1981, *36,* 174–83.

Garmezy, N. Intervention with children at risk for behavior pathology. *Clinical Psychologist,* 1975, *28,* 13–15.

Garmezy, N. The psychology and psychopathology of attention. *Schizophrenia Bulletin,* 1977, *3,* No. 3, 360–69.

Garmezy, N. Never mind the psychologists: Is it good for the children? *Clinical Psychologist,* 1978, *31,* 1, 4–6.

Garmezy, N., Farrarese, M., Masten, A., and Nordstrom, A. The nature of competence in normal and deviant children. Paper presented at the Vermont Conference on the Primary Prevention of Psychopathology. University of Vermont, Burlington, 1977.

Garmezy, N., and Streitman, S. Children at risk: The search for the antecedents of schizophrenia. Part I. Conceptual models and research methods. *Schizophrenia Bulletin,* 1974, No. 8, 14–90.

Garrett, G. R., and Bahr, H. M. Women on skid row. *Quarterly Journal of Studies on Alcohol,* 1973, *34,* 1228–43.

Gastaut, H. Clinical and electroencephalographical classification of epileptic seizures. *Epilepsia,* 1970, *11,* 102–13.

Gazzaniga, M. S. The split brain in man. *Scientific American,* 1967, *217,* 24–29.

Gebhard, P. H. Sexual behavior of the mentally retarded. In F. F. de la Cruz and G. D. LaVeck (Eds.), *Human sexuality and the mentally retarded.* New York: Brunner/Mazel, 1973.

Gelfand, M. Psychiatric disorders as recognized by the Shona. In A. Kiev (Ed.), *Magic, faith, and healing: Studies in primitive psychiatry today.* New York: Free Press, 1964.

Gelles, R. J. Child abuse as psychopathology: A sociological critique and reformulation. *American Journal of Orthopsychiatry,* 1973, *43,* 611–21.

Gelles, R. J. Violence toward children in the United States. Paper presented at the meetings of the American Association for the Advancement of Science, Denver, February, 1977.

Gelles, R. J., and Straus, M. A. Violence in the American family. *Journal of Social Issues,* 1979, *35,* 15–39.

Gersh, F. S., and Fowles, D. C. Neurotic depression: The concept of anxious depression. In R. A. Depue (Ed.), *The psychobiology of the depressive disorders: Implications for the effects of stress.* New York: Academic Press, 1979.

Gersten, J. C., Langner, T. S., Eisenberg, J. G., and Orzeck, L. Child behavior and life events: Undesirable change or change per se? In B. S. Dohrenwend and B. P. Dohrenwend (Eds.), *Stressful life events: Their nature and effects.* New York: Wiley, 1974.

Geschwind, N. Specializations of the human brain. *Scientific American,* September, 1979, *241,* 180–99.

Ghose, K., and Coppen, A. Noradrenaline, depressive illness, and the action of amitriptyline. *Psychopharmacology,* 1977, *54,* 57–60.

Gibbs, J. P. *Crime, punishment, and deterrence.* N. Y.: Elsevier, 1975.

Glass, D. C. Stress, competition and heart attacks. *Psychology Today,* December, 1976, 54–57, 134.

Glass, D. C. *Behavior patterns, stress, and coronary disease.* Hillsdale, N.J.: Erlbaum, 1977.

Glasser, W., and Zunin, L. M. Reality therapy. In R. Corsini (Ed.), *Current psychotherapies.* Itasca, Ill.: Peacock, 1973.

Glick, B. S. Desensitization therapy in impotence and frigidity: Review of the literature and report of a case. *American Journal of Psychiatry,* 1975, *132,* 169–71.

Glueck, S., and Glueck, E. *Unraveling juvenile delinquency.* New York: The Commonwealth Fund, 1950.

Glueck, S., and Glueck, E. *Physique and delinquency.* New York: Harper, 1956.

Goddard, H. H. *The Kallikak family: A study in the heredity of feeble-mindedness.* New York: Macmillan, 1912.

Goffman, E. *Asylums: Essays on the social situation of mental patients and other inmates.* Chicago: Aldine, 1961.

Goforth, E. G. Gilles de la Tourette's syndrome: a 25-year follow-up—single case study. *Journal of Nervous and Mental Disease,* 1974, *158,* 306–9.

Goldberg, L. Behavioral and physiological effects of alcohol on man. *Psychosomatic Medicine,* 1966, *28,* 570–95.

Goldblatt, P. B., Moore, M. E., and Stunkard, A. J. Social factors in obesity. *Journal of the American Medical Association,* 1965, *192,* 97–102.

Golden, C. J., Hammeke, T. A., and Purisch, A. D. Diagnostic validity of a standardized neuropsychological battery derived from Luria's neuropsychological tests. *Journal of Consulting and Clinical Psychology,* 1978, *46,* 1258–65.

Golden, C. J., Hammeke, T. A., and Purisch, A. D. *The Luria-Nebraska Neuropsychological Battery: Manual.* Los Angeles, Calif.: Western Psychological Services, 1980.

Golden, C. J., Strider, F. D., Strider, M. A., Moore, G. F., and Gust, W. F. Neuropsychological effects of acute syphilitic involvement of the central nervous system: A case report. *Clinical Neuropsychology,* 1979, *1,* No. 3, 24–28.

Goldfarb, W. Childhood psychosis. In P. H. Mussen (Ed.), *Carmichael's Manual of Child Psychology* (3rd ed.). New York: Wiley, 1970.

Goldfarb, W. *Growth and change of schizophrenic children: A longitudinal study.* New York: Wiley, 1974.

Goldfried, M. R. Behavior assessment. In I. B. Weiner (Ed.), *Clinical methods in psychology.* New York: Wiley, 1976.

Goldfried, M. R., and Kent, R. N. Traditional versus behavioral personality assessment: A comparison of methodological and theoretical assumptions. *Psychological Bulletin,* 1972, *77,* 409–20.

Goldman, A. L. Shift in supply increasing use of heroin here. *New York Times,* May 15, 1980, pp. 1, B16.

Goldsmith, J. M. Residential treatment today: The paradox of new premises. *American Journal of Orthopsychiatry,* 1976, *46,* 425–33.

Goldstein, A. P. *Structured learning therapy: Toward a psychotherapy for the poor.* New York: Academic Press, 1973.

Goldstein, A. J., and Chambless, D. L. A reanalysis of agoraphobia. *Behavior Therapy,* 1978, *9,* 47–59.

Goldstein, K. *The organism.* New York: American Book Co., 1939.

Goldstein, K. *After-effects of brain injuries in war.* New York: Grune & Stratton, 1942.

Goldstein, K. Methodological approach to the study of schizophrenic thought disorder. In J. Kasanin (Ed.), *Language and thought in schizophrenia.* Berkeley: University of California Press, 1944.

Goldstein, K., and Scheerer, M. Abstract and concrete behavior: An experimental study with special tests. *Psychological Monographs,* 1941, *53,* No. 2.

Goldstein, M. Brain research and violent behavior. *Archives of Neurology,* 1974, *30,* 1–35.

Goldstein, M. H., Held, J. M., and Cromwell, R. L. Premorbid adjustment and paranoid-nonparanoid status in schizophrenia. *Psychological Bulletin,* 1968, *70,* 382–86.

Goleman, D. J., and Schwartz, G. E. Meditation as an intervention in stress reactivity. *Journal of Consulting and Clinical Psychology,* 1976, *44,* 456–66.

Gomberg, E. S. Etiology of alcoholism. *Journal of Consulting and Clinical Psychology,* 1968, *32,* 18–20.

Gomberg, E. S. Women and alcoholism. In V. Franks and V. Burtle (Eds.), *Women in therapy.* New York: Brunner/Mazel, 1974.

Gomberg, E. S. Problems with alcohol and other drugs. In E. S. Gomberg and V. Franks (Eds.), *Gender and disordered behavior: Sex differences in psychopathology.* New York: Brunner/Mazel, 1979.

Gomes-Schwartz, B., Hadley, S. W., and Strupp, H. H. Individual psychotherapy and behavior therapy. *Annual Review of Psychology,* 1978, *29,* 435–71.

Goode, W. Violence among intimates. U.S. National Commission on the Causes and Prevention of Violence. Task Force on Individual Acts of Violence. *Crimes of Violence,* 1969, *13,* 941–77.

Goodenough, F. L. *Measurement of intelligence by drawings.* New York: World Book, 1926.

Goodwin, D. W., Davis, D. H., and Robins, L. N. Drinking amid abundant illicit drugs: The Vietnam case. *Archives of General Psychiatry,* 1975, *32,* 230–33.

Goodwin, D. W., Schulsinger, F., Moller, N., Hernansen, L., Winokur, G., and Guze, S. B. Drinking problems in adopted and nonadopted sons of alcoholics. *Archives of General Psychiatry,* 1974, *31,* 164–69.

Gorodetzky, C. W., and Christian, S. T. *What you should know about drugs.* New York: Harcourt Brace Jovanovich, 1970.

Gottesman, I. I., and Shields, J. *Schizophrenia and genetics: A twin study vantage point.* New York: Academic Press, 1972.

Gottesman, I. I., and Shields, J. A critical review of recent adoption, twin, and family studies of schizophrenia: Behavioral genetics perspectives. *Schizophrenia Bulletin,* 1976, *2,* No. 3, 360–98.

Gottesman, I. I., Shields, J., and Hanson, D. R. *Schizophrenia: The epigenetic puzzle.* New York: Cambridge University Press, 1982.

Gould, R. E. What we don't know about homosexuality. *New York Times Magazine,* February 24, 1974, pp. 13, 51, 54, 56, 58, 60, 62–63.

Gove, W. R., and Tudor, J. F. Adult sex roles and mental illness. *American Journal of Sociology,* 1973, *78,* 812–35.

Graham, F. K., and Kendall, B. S. Memory-For-Designs Test: Revised general manual. *Perceptual and Motor Skills Monograph Supplement,* 1960, *11,* 147–88.

Graham, J. Auditory discrimination in meditators. In D. Orme-Johnson, L. Domash, and J. Farrow (Eds.), *Scientific research on transcendental meditation: Collected papers.* Los Angeles: M.I.U. Press, 1974.

Graham, P. J., Rutter, M. L., Yule, W., and Pless, I. B. Childhood asthma: A psychosomatic disorder? Some epidemiological considerations. *British Journal of Preventive and Social Medicine,* 1967, *21,* 78–85.

Grand, S., Freedman, N., Steingart, I., and Buchwald, C. Communicative behavior in schizophrenia: The relation of adaptive styles to kinetic and linguistic aspects of interview behavior. *Journal of Nervous and Mental Disease,* 1975, *161,* 293–306.

Granville-Grossman, K. L. The early environment in affective disorder. In A. Coppen and A. Walk (Eds.), *Recent developments in affective disorders: A symposium.* Ashford, Kent, England: Royal Medico-Psychological Association, 1968.

Green, R. Patterns of sexual identity in childhood: Relationship to subsequent sexual partner preference. In J. Marmor (Ed.), *Homosexual behavior: A modern reappraisal.* New York: Basic Books, 1980.

Greenberg, S. W. The relationships between crime and amphetamine abuse: An empirical review of the literature. *Contemporary Drug Problems,* 1976, *5,* 101–30.

Greene, M. H., DuPont, R. L., and Rubenstein, R. M. Amphetamines in the District of Columbia. II. Patterns of abuse in an arrestee population. *Archives of General Psychiatry,* 1973, *29,* 773–76.

Griffin, J. I. *Statistics: Methods and applications.* New York: Holt, Rinehart & Winston, 1962.

Griffin, S. Rape: The all-American crime. In E. Goode and R. R. Troiden (Eds.), *Sexual deviance and sexual deviants.* New York: Morrow, 1974.

Grinker, R. R. *Psychosomatic concepts.* New York: Aronson, 1973.

Grinker, R. R. Diagnosis of borderlines: A discussion. *Schizophrenia Bulletin,* 1979, *5,* No. 1, 47–53.

Grinker, R. R., and Spiegel, J. P. *Men under stress.* Philadelphia: Blakiston, 1945.

Grinspoon, L., and Bakalar, J. B. *Cocaine: A drug and its social evolution.* New York: Basic Books, 1976.

Grinspoon, L., and Bakalar, J. B. Cocaine: A social history. *Psychology Today,* March, 1977, 37–39, 77–78. (a)

Grinspoon, L., and Bakalar, J. B. A kick from cocaine. *Psychology Today,* March, 1977, 41–42, 78. (b)

Grinspoon, L., and Bakalar, J. B. Marijuana: Six years of reconsideration. In L. Grinspoon, *Marijuana reconsidered* (2nd ed.). Cambridge, Mass.: Harvard University Press, 1977. (c)

Grinspoon, L., and Bakalar, J. B. Cocaine. In R. L. DuPont, A. Goldstein, and J. O'Donnell (Eds.), *Handbook on drug abuse.* National Institute on Drug Abuse, 1979. (a)

Grinspoon, L., and Bakalar, J. B. *Psychedelic drugs reconsidered.* New York: Basic Books, 1979. (b)

Grinspoon, L., and Hedblom, P. *The speed culture: Amphetamine use and abuse in America.* Cambridge, Mass.: Harvard University Press, 1975.

Grossman, H. J. (Ed.) *Manual on terminology and classification in mental retardation.* Washington, D.C.: American Association on Mental Deficiency, Special Publication Series No. 2, 1973.

Grosz, H., and Zimmerman, J. Experimental analysis of hysterical blindness. *Archives of General Psychiatry,* 1965, *13,* 255–60.

Groth, A. N., and Birnbaum, H. J. *Men who rape: The psychology of the offender.* New York: Plenum Press, 1979.

Guidelines for therapy with women. Task Force on Sex Bias and Sex Role Stereotyping in Psychotherapeutic Practice. *American Psychologist,* December, 1978, *33,* 1122–23.

Guilford, J. P. *Personality.* New York: McGraw-Hill, 1959.

Guilford, J. P., and Martin, H. G. *Guilford-Martin Inventory of Factors GAMIN: Manual.* Beverly Hills, Calif.: Sheridan Supply Co., 1948.

Gunderson, J. G. The relatedness of borderline and schizophrenic disorders. *Schizophrenia Bulletin,* 1979, *5,* No. 1, 17–22.

Gunderson, J. G., Autry, J. H. III, Mosher, L. R., and Buchsbaum, S. Special report: Schizophrenia, 1974. *Schizophrenia Bulletin,* 1974, No. 9, 16–54.

Gunderson, J. G., and Singer, M. T. Defining borderline patients: An overview. *American Journal of Psychiatry,* 1975, *132,* 1–10.

Gur, R. C., and Gur, R. E. Handedness, sex, and eyedness as moderating variables in the relation between hypnotic susceptibility and functional brain asymmetry. *Journal of Abnormal Psychology,* 1974, *83,* 635–43.

Gur, R. E., and Gur, R. C. Defense mechanisms, psychosomatic symptomatology, and conjugate lateral eye movements. *Journal of Consulting and Clinical Psychology,* 1975, *43,* 416–20.

Gur, R. E., and Reyher, J. Relationship between style of hypnotic induction and direction of lateral eye movements. *Journal of Abnormal Psychology,* 1973, *82,* 499–505.

Gurman, A. S., and Kniskern, D. P. Research on marital and family therapy: Progress, perspective, and prospect. In S. L. Garfield and A. E. Bergin (Eds.), *Handbook of psychotherapy and behavior change: An empirical analysis* (2nd ed.). New York: Wiley, 1978.

Gurland, B. J., Sharpe, L., Simon, R. J., Kuriansky, J., and Stiller, P. On the use of psychiatric diagnosis for comparing psychiatric population. *Psychiatric Quarterly,* 1972, *46,* 461–73.

Guze, S. B. *Criminality and psychiatric disorders.* New York: Oxford University Press, 1976.

Hackett, G., and Horan, J. J. Behavioral control of cigarette smoking: A comprehensive program. Paper presented at the Annual Meeting of the American Educational Research Association, San Francisco, April, 1976.

Haertzen, C. A., Eisenberg, H. A., Hooks, N. T., Jr., Ross, F. E., and Pross, M. Estimating specificity of drug and alcohol subcultural groups with slang names for drugs. *Journal of Consulting and Clinical Psychology,* 1979, *47,* 592–94.

Haley, J., and Hoffman, L. *Techniques of family therapy.* New York: Basic Books, 1967.

Haley, S. A. Treatment implications of post-combat stress response syndromes for mental health professionals. In C. R. Figley (Ed.), *Stress disorders among Vietnam veterans: Theory, research and treatment.* New York: Brunner/Mazel, 1978.

Half of 1976 murder victims had police records. *New York Times,* August 28, 1977, pp. 1, 34.

Hall, S. M. The abstinence phobia. In N. A. Krasnegor (Ed.), *Behavioral analysis and treatment of substance abuse.* National Institute on Drug Abuse Research Monograph No. 25, 1979.

Hall, S. M., Hall, R. G., Hanson, R. W., and Borden, B. L. Permanence of two self-managed treatments of overweight in university and community populations. *Journal of Consulting and Clinical Psychology,* 1974, *42,* 781–86.

Hammen, C. L., and Glass, D. R., Jr. Depression, activity, and evaluation of reinforcement. *Journal of Abnormal Psychology,* 1975, *84,* 718–21.

Hammen, C. L., and Peters, S. D. Differential responses to male and female depressive reactions. *Journal of Consulting and Clinical Psychology,* 1977, *45,* 994–1001.

Hammer, M., and Zubin, J. Culture and psychopathology. Mimeographed paper, 1968.

Hanna, J. M. Metabolic responses of Chinese, Japanese and Europeans to alcohol. *Alcoholism: Clinical and Experimental Research,* 1978, *2,* 89–92.

Hansen, H., Belmont, L., and Stein, Z. Epidemiology. In J. Wortis (Ed.), *Mental retardation and developmental disabilities: An annual review* (vol. 11). New York: Brunner/Mazel, 1980.

Hanson, D. R., and Gottesman, I. I. The genetics, if any, of infantile autism and childhood schizophrenia. *Journal of Autism and Childhood Schizophrenia,* 1976, *6,* 209–34.

Hanson, D. R., Gottesman, I. I., and Heston, L. L. Some possible childhood indicators of adult schizophrenia inferred from children of schizophrenics. *British Journal of Psychiatry,* 1976, *129,* 142–54.

Hanson, D. R., Gottesman, I. I., and Meehl, P. E. Genetic theories and the validation of psychiatric diagnoses: Implications for the study of children of schizophrenics. *Journal of Abnormal Psychology,* 1977, *86,* 575–88.

Hare, E. H., and Wing, J. K. (Eds.) *Psychiatric epidemiology: Proceedings of the International Symposium held at Aberdeen University. 22-5 July, 1969.* London: Oxford University Press, 1970.

Hare, R. D. *Psychopathy: Theory and research.* New York: Wiley, 1970.

Harlow's lecture on love in relation to aggression. *New York State Psychologist,* December 1975, *27,* 3.

Harlow, H. F., and Harlow, M. K. Social deprivation in monkeys. *Scientific American,* 1962, *207,* 136–46.

Harlow, H. F., and Harlow, M. K. Learning to love. *American Scientist,* 1966, *54,* 244–72.

Harlow, H. F., and Zimmermann, R. R. Affectional responses in the infant monkey. *Science,* 1959, *130,* 421–32.

Harper, F. D. Alcohol and crime in black America. In F. D. Harper (Ed.), *Alcohol abuse and black America.* Alexandria, Va.: Douglass Publishers, 1976.

Harper, F. D. *Alcoholism treatment and black Americans.* U.S. Department of Health, Education, and Welfare, National Institute on Alcohol Abuse and Alcoholism, 1979.

Harper, R. A. *The new psychotherapies.* Englewood Cliffs, N.J.: Prentice-Hall, 1975.

Harrington, M. *The other America: Poverty in the United States.* New York: Macmillan, 1962.

Harris, A. J. *Harris Tests of Lateral Dominance.* New York: Psychological Corporation, 1956.

Harris, J. G., Jr. An abbreviated form of the Phillips Rating Scale of Premorbid Adjustment in Schizophrenia. *Journal of Abnormal Psychology,* 1975, *84,* 129–37.

Harrow, M., Himmelhoch, J., Tucker, G., Hersh, J., and Quinlan, D. Overinclusive thinking in acute schizophrenic patients. *Journal of Abnormal Psychology,* 1972, *79,* 161–68.

Hartley, D., Roback, H. B., and Abramowitz, S. I. Deterioration effects in encounter groups. *American Psychologist,* 1976, *31,* 247–55.

Haslam, M. T. *Psychosexual disorders: A review.* Springfield, Ill.: Thomas, 1979.

Hathaway, S. R., and McKinley, J. C. *Manual for the Minnesota Multiphasic Personality Inventory.* New York: Psychological Corporation. 1943.

Heath, D. B. A critical review of ethnographic studies of alcohol use. In R. J. Gibbins, Y. Israel, H. Kalant, R. E. Popham, W. Schmidt, and R. G. Smart (Eds.), *Research advances in alcohol and drug problems* (vol. 2). New York: Wiley, 1975.

Heaton, R. K., and Victor, R. G. Personality characteristics associated with psychedelic flashbacks in natural and experimental settings. *Journal of Abnormal Psychology,* 1976, *85,* 83–90.

Heber, R. *Epidemiology of mental retardation.* Springfield, Ill.: Thomas, 1970.

Heber, R. Rehabilitation of families at risk for mental retardation: A progress report. *Rehabilitation Research and Training Center in Mental Retardation.* Madison: University of Wisconsin, 1971.

Heber, R., and Garber, H. The Milwaukee Project: A study of the use of family intervention to prevent cultural-familial mental retardation. In B. Z. Friedlander, G. M. Sterritt, and G. E. Kirk (Eds.), *Exceptional infant* (vol. 3). New York: Brunner/Mazel, 1975.

Heffner, P. A., Strauss, M. E., and Grisell, J. Rehospitalization of schizophrenics as a function of intelligence. *Journal of Abnormal Psychology,* 1975, *84,* 735–36.

Heilbrun, A. B. *Aversive maternal control: A theory of schizophrenic development.* New York: Wiley, 1973.

Heilbrun, A. B. Psychopathy and violent crime. *Journal of Consulting and Clinical Psychology,* 1979, *47,* 509–16.

Heilbrun, A. B., and Heilbrun, K. S. Content analysis of delusions in reactive and process schizophrenics. *Journal of Abnormal Psychology,* 1977, *86,* 597–608.

Heilbrun, A. B., and Norbert, N. Sensitivity to maternal censure in paranoid and nonparanoid schizophrenics. *Journal of Nervous and Mental Disease,* 1971, *152,* 45–49.

Helpern, M., and Rho, Y. M. Deaths from narcotism in New

York City: Incidence, circumstances, and postmortem findings. *International Journal of the Addictions,* 1967, *2,* 53–84.

Hendin, H. Black suicide. *Archives of General Psychiatry,* 1969, *21,* 407–22.

Henn, F. A., Herjanic, M., and Vanderpearl, R. H. Forensic psychiatry; Diagnosis and criminal responsibility. *Journal of Nervous and Mental Disease,* 1976, *162,* 423–29.

Henryk-Gutt, R., and Rees, W. L. Psychological aspects of migraine. *Journal of Psychosomatic Research,* 1973, *17,* 141–53.

Herman, C. P., and Polivy, J. Anxiety, restraint, and eating behavior. *Journal of Abnormal Psychology,* 1975, *84,* 666–72.

Hernández-Péon, R. Attention, sleep, motivation and behavior. In P. Bakan (Ed.), *Attention: An enduring problem in psychology.* Princeton: Van Nostrand, 1966.

Hes, J. Ph. The changing social role of the Yemenite Mori. In A. Kiev (Ed.), *Magic, faith, and healing: Studies in primitive psychiatry today.* New York: Free Press, 1964.

Heston, L. L. Psychiatric disorders in foster home-reared children of schizophrenic mothers. *British Journal of Psychiatry,* 1966, *112,* 819–25.

Heston, L. L. Alzheimer's disease, trisomy 21, and myeloproliferative disorders: Associations suggesting a genetic diathesis. *Science,* 1976, *196,* 322–23.

Hewett, F. M. Teaching speech to an autistic child through operant conditioning. *American Journal of Orthopsychiatry,* 1965, *35,* 927–36.

Hilgard, E. R. A neodissociation interpretation of pain reduction in hypnosis. *Psychological Review,* 1973, *80,* 396–411.

Hilgard, E. R. *Divided consciousness: Multiple controls in human thought and action.* New York: Wiley, 1977.

Hilgard, E. R., and Hilgard, J. R. *Hypnosis in the relief of pain.* Los Altos, Calif.: William Kaufmann, 1975.

Hilgard, J. R. *Personality and hypnosis: A study of imaginative involvement.* Chicago: University of Chicago Press, 1970.

Hill, D., and Pond, D. A. Reflections on 100 capital cases submitted to EEG. *Journal of Mental Science,* 1952, *98,* 23–43.

Hill, D., and Watterson, D. Electroencephalographic studies of the psychopathic personality. *Journal of Neurology and Psychiatry,* 1942, *5,* 47–64.

Hinkle, L. E., Jr. The effect of exposure to culture change, social change, and changes in interpersonal relationships on health. In B. S. Dohrenwend and B. P. Dohrenwend (Eds.), *Stressful life events: Their nature and effects.* New York: Wiley, 1974.

Hirsch, S. R., and Leff, J. P. *Abnormalities in parents of schizophrenics.* New York: Oxford University Press, 1975.

Hobson, J. A., and McCarley, R. W. The brain as a dream state generator: An activator-synthesis hypothesis of the dream process. *American Journal of Psychiatry,* 1977, *134,* 1335–48.

Hogan, R. A. The implosive technique. *Behaviour Research and Therapy,* 1968, *6,* 423–31.

Hohman, L. B. Diagnosis of schizophrenia. Paper presented at the Annual Meeting of the American Psychopathological Association, 1964.

Holden, C. Going beyond pain. *Psychology* (trial issue). Washington, D.C.: American Psychological Association, April, 1977, pp. 10–15.

Hollender, M. H. *The practice of psychoanalytic psychotherapy.* New York: Grune & Stratton, 1965.

Hollingshead, A. B., and Redlich, F. C. Schizophrenia and social structure. *American Journal of Psychiatry,* 1954, *110,* 695–701.

Hollingshead, A. B., and Redlich, F. C. *Social class and mental illness: A community study.* New York: Wiley, 1958.

Hollon, S. D. Cognitive-behavioral treatment of drug-induced pansituational anxiety states. In G. Emery, S. D. Hollon, and R. C. Bedrosian (Eds.), *New directions in cognitive therapy.* New York: Guilford Press, 1981.

Hollon, S. D., and Beck, A. T. Psychotherapy and drug therapy: Comparisons and combinations. In S. L. Garfield and A. E. Bergin (Eds.), *Handbook of psychotherapy and behavior change* (2nd ed.). New York: Wiley, 1978.

Holman, R. B., Barchas, J. D., and Elliott, G. R. Perspectives in behavioral neurochemistry. Mimeographed paper, Laboratory of Behavioral Neurochemistry, Stanford University School of Medicine, 1976.

Holman, R. B., Elliott, G. R., and Barchas, J. D. Neuroregulators and sleep mechanisms. *Annual Review of Medicine,* 1975, *26,* 499–519.

Holmes, L. B., Mack, C., Moser, H. W., Pant, S. S., Halldorsson, S., and Matzilevich, B. *Mental retardation: An atlas of diseases with associated physical abnormalities.* New York: Macmillan, 1972.

Holmes, T., and Masuda, M. Life changes and illness susceptibility. In B. S. Dohrenwend and B. P. Dohrenwend (Eds.), *Stressful life events: Their nature and effects.* New York: Wiley, 1974.

Holmes, T. H., and Rahe, R. H. The Social Readjustment Rating Scale. *Journal of Psychosomatic Research,* 1967, *11,* 213–18.

Holroyd, J. C., and Brodsky, A. M. Psychologists' attitudes and practices regarding erotic and nonerotic physical contact with patients. *American Psychologist,* 1977, *32,* 850–55.

Holzman, P. S., and Levy, D. L. Smooth pursuit eye movements and functional psychoses: A review. *Schizophrenia Bulletin,* 1977, *3,* No. 1, 15–27.

Hooker, E. The adjustment of the male overt homosexual. *Journal of Projective Techniques,* 1957, *21,* 18–31.

Hooker, E. What is a criterion? *Journal of Projective Techniques,* 1959, *23,* 278–81.

Hoon, P. W., and Lindsley, O. R. A comparison of behavior and traditional therapy publication activity. *American Psychologist,* 1974, *29,* 694–97.

Hooton, E. *Crime and the man.* Cambridge, Mass.: Harvard University Press, 1939.

Horan, J. J., Hackett, G., Nicholas, W. C., Linberg, S. E., Stone, C. I., and Lukaski, H. C. Rapid smoking: A cautionary note. *Journal of Consulting and Clinical Psychology,* 1977, *45,* 341–43.

Horan, J. J., Linberg, S. E., and Hackett, G. Reply to Russell and associates on the rapid smoking-nicotine level issue. *Journal of Consulting and Clinical Psychology,* 1980, *48,* 113–14.

Horney, K. *The neurotic personality of our time.* N.Y.: Norton, 1937.

Horney, K. *Our inner conflicts: A constructive theory of neurosis.* New York: Norton, 1945.

Horney, K. *Neurosis and human growth.* New York: Norton, 1950.

Horowitz, L. M., Post, D. L., French, R. de S., Wallis, K. D., and Siegelman, E. Y. The prototype as a construct in abnormal psychology: 2. Clarifying disagreement in psychiatric judgments. *Journal of Abnormal Psychology,* 1981, *90,* 575–85.

Horowitz, L. M., Wright, J. C., Lowenstein, E., and Parad, H. W. The prototype as a construct in abnormal psychology: 1. A method for deriving prototypes. *Journal of Abnormal Psychology,* 1981, *90,* 568–74.

Horowitz, M. J., and Solomon, G. F. Delayed stress response syndromes in Vietnam veterans. In C. R. Figley (Ed.), *Stress disorders among Vietnam veterans: Theory, research and treatment.* New York: Brunner/Mazel, 1978.

Horton, D. J. The functions of alcohol in primitive societies: A cross-cultural study, *Quarterly Journal of Studies on Alcohol,* 1943, *4,* 199–320.

Hosford, R. E., and Moss. C. S. (Eds.) *The crumbling walls: Treatment and counseling of prisoners.* Urbana: University of Illinois Press, 1975.

Houts, M. *They asked for death.* New York: Cowles, 1970.

Hsiao, S. Psychology in China. *American Psychologist,* 1977, *32,* 374–76.

Hudgens, R. W. Personal catastrophe and depression: A consideration of the subject with respect to medically ill adolescents, and a requiem for retrospective life-event studies. In B. S. Dohrenwend and B. P. Dohrenwend (Eds.), *Stressful life events: Their nature and effects.* New York: Wiley, 1974.

Huesman, L. R. Cognitive processes and models of depression. *Journal of Abnormal Psychology,* 1978, *87,* 194–98.

Hunt, W. A., and Matarazzo, J. D. Three years later: Recent developments in the experimental modification of smoking behavior. *Journal of Abnormal Psychology,* 1973, *81,* 107–14.

Hurley, R. L. *Poverty and mental retardation: A causal relationship.* New York: Random House, 1969.

Hutchings, B., and Mednick, S. A. Registered criminality in the adoptive and biological parents of registered male criminal adoptees. In R. R. Fieve, D. Rosenthal, and H. Brill (Eds.), *Genetic research in psychiatry.* Baltimore: Johns Hopkins University Press, 1975.

Huxley, A. *The doors of perception and heaven and hell.* New York: Harper & Row, 1954.

Indeterminate sentences may be yielding to fixed terms as faith in the prison system wanes. *New York Times,* October 12, 1976, p. 17.

Ingalls, R. P. *Mental retardation: The changing outlook.* New York: Wiley, 1978.

Itil, T. M. Qualitative and quantitative EEG findings in schizophrenia. *Schizophrenia Bulletin,* 1977, *3,* No. 1, 61–79.

Itil, T. M., Hsu, W., Saletu, B., and Mednick, S. Computer EEG and auditory evoked potential investigations in children at high risk for schizophrenia. *American Journal of Psychiatry,* 1974, *131,* 892–900.

Itil, T. M., Saletu, B., and Davis, S. EEG findings in chronic schizophrenics based on digital computer period analysis and analog power spectra. *Biological Psychiatry,* 1972, *5,* 1–13.

Iversen, L. L. Dopamine receptors in the brain. *Science,* 1975, *188,* 1084–89.

Iversen, L. L. The chemistry of the brain. *Scientific American,* 1979, *241,* 134–49.

Jackson, D. D. Family interaction, family homeostasis and some implications for conjoint family psychotherapy. In J. H. Masserman (Ed.), *Individual and familial dynamics.* New York: Grune & Stratton, 1959.

Jacob, T. Family interaction in disturbed and normal families: A methodological and substantive review. *Psychological Bulletin,* 1975, *82,* 33–65.

Jacobs, J. *Adolescent suicide.* New York: Wiley, 1971.

Jacobs, P. A., Brunton, M., Melville, M. M., Brittain, R. P., and McClemont, W. F. Aggressive behavior, mental subnormality and the XYY male. *Nature,* 1965, *208,* 1351–52.

Jacobson, E. *Progressive relaxation.* Chicago: University of Chicago Press, 1929.

Jacobson, E. *Depression: Comparative studies of normal, neurotic, and psychotic conditions.* New York: International Universities Press, 1971.

Jacobziner, H. Attempted suicides in children. *Journal of Pediatrics,* 1960, *56,* 519–25.

Jahoda, M. *Current concepts of positive mental health.* New York: Basic Books, 1958.

James, J., and Meyerding, J. Early sexual experience as a factor in prostitution. *Archives of Sexual Behavior,* 1977, *7,* 31–42.

Janov, A. *The primal scream—primal therapy: The cure for neurosis.* New York: Dell, 1970.

Jaspers, K. *General psychopathology.* Chicago: University of Chicago Press, 1963.

Jeans, R. F. The three faces of Evelyn: A case report. I. An independently validated case of multiple personality. *Journal of Abnormal Psychology,* 1976, *85,* 249–55.

Jellinek, E. M. *The disease concept of alcoholism.* Highland Park, N.J.: Hillhouse Press, 1960.

Jessor, R. Marijuana: A review of recent psychosocial research. In R. L. DuPont, A. Goldstein, and J. O'Donnell (Eds.), *Handbook on drug abuse.* National Institute on Drug Abuse, 1979.

Jilek-Aall, L. Alcohol and the Indian-white relationship: A study of the function of Alcoholics Anonymous among coast Salish Indians. *Confinia Psychiatrica,* 1978, *21,* 195–233.

Joesting, H., Jones, N., and Joesting, R. Male and female prison inmates' differences on MMPI scales and revised beta IQ. *Psychological Reports,* 1975, *37,* 471–74.

Johnson, A. M. Sanctions for superego lacunae of adolescents. Paper presented at the Chicago Psychoanalytic Society, 1947.

Johnson, L. D., Bachman, J. G., and O'Malley, P. M. *Highlights from: Drug use among American high school students: 1975–1977.* National Institute on Drug Abuse, 1977.

Jones, A., and Seagull, A. A. Dimensions of the relationship between the black client and the white therapist: A theoretical overview. *American Psychologist,* 1977, *10,* 850–55.

Jones, E. *The Life and work of Sigmund Freud (3 vols.).* New York: Basic Books, 1953–57.

Jones, M. C. The elimination of children's fears. *Journal of Experimental Psychology,* 1924, *7,* 382–90.

Jung, C. G. *Analytical psychology: Its theory and practice.* New York: Moffat, Yard, 1916.

Kafka, F. *Meditation: Unhappiness.* Leipsig: Ernst Rowohlt Verlag, 1913.

Kagan, J. Reflection-impulsivity: The generality and dynamics of conceptual tempo. *Journal of Abnormal Psychology,* 1966, *71,* 17–24.

Kaij, L. *Alcoholism in twins: Studies on the etiology and sequels of abuse of alcohol.* Stockholm: Almquist and Wiksell, 1960.

Kaij, L., and Dock, J. Grandsons of alcoholics: A test of sex-linked transmission of alcohol abuse. *Archives of General Psychiatry,* 1975, *32,* 1379–81.

Kales, A., Scharf, M. B., and Kales, J. D. Rebound insomnia: A new clinical syndrome. *Science,* 1978, *201,* 1039–40.

Kallmann, F. J. The genetic theory of schizophrenia: An analysis of 691 schizophrenic twin index families. *American Journal of Psychiatry,* 1946, *103,* 309–22.

Kallmann, F. J. Genetic principles of manic-depressive psychosis. *Proceedings of the 42nd Annual Meeting of the American Psychopathological Association,* 1952.

Kamin, L. J. *The science and politics of I.Q.* New York: Wiley, 1974.

Kamiya, J. Operant control of the EEG alpha rhythm and some of its reported effects on consciousness. In D. T. Tart (Ed.), *Altered states of consciousness: A book of readings.* New York: Wiley, 1969.

Kandel, D. Interpersonal influences on adolescent illegal drug use. In E. Josephson and E. E. Carroll (Eds.), *Drug use: Epidemiological and sociological approaches.* New York: Wiley, 1974.

Kandel, D. Stages in adolescent involvement in drug use. *Science,* 1975, *190,* 912–14.

Kane, F. J., and Lachenbruch, P. A. Adolescent pregnancy: A study of aborters and nonaborters. *American Journal of Orthopsychiatry,* 1973, *43,* 796–803.

Kanfer, F. H., and Saslow, G. Behavioral diagnosis. In C. M. Franks (Ed.), *Behavior therapy: Appraisal and status.* New York: McGraw-Hill, 1969.

Kanner, L. Autistic disturbances of affective contact. *Nervous Child,* 1943, *2,* 217–50.

Kaplan, H. S. *The new sex therapy: Active treatment of sexual dysfunctions.* New York: Brunner/Mazel, 1974.

Kaplan, H. S. *The new sex therapy (vol. 2). Disorders of sexual desire and other new concepts and techniques in sex therapy.* New York: Brunner/Mazel, 1979.

Kardiner, A. The neuroses of war. In S. S. Tomkins (Ed.), *Contemporary psychopathology.* Cambridge: Harvard University Press, 1943.

Karlin, R. A. Hypnotizability and attention. *Journal of Abnormal Psychology,* 1979, *88,* 92–95.

Kasanin, J., and Hanfmann, E. An experimental study of concept formation in schizophrenia. I. Quantitative analysis of the results. *American Journal of Psychiatry,* 1938, *95,* 35–48.

Kastenbaum, R., and Costa, P. T., Jr. Psychological perspectives on death. *Annual Review of Psychology,* 1977, *28,* 225–49.

Katzman, R., Terry, R. D., and Bick, K. L. (Eds.) *Alzheimer's disease: Senile dementia and related disorders.* (*Aging:* vol. 7) New York: Raven Press, 1978.

Kaufman, E., and Kaufmann, P. (Eds.) *Family therapy of drug and alcohol abuse.* New York: Gardner Press, 1979.

Kazdin, A. E., and Bootzin, R. R. The token economy: An evaluative review. *Journal of Applied Behavior Analysis,* 1972, *5,* 343–72.

Kazdin, A. E., and Wilcoxon, L. A. Systematic desensitization and nonspecific treatment effects: A methodological evaluation. *Psychological Bulletin,* 1976, *83,* 729–58.

Keane, T. M., and Lisman, S. A. Alcohol and social anxiety in males: Behavioral, cognitive, and physiological effects. *Journal of Abnormal Psychology,* 1980, *89,* 213–23.

Kelly, D. H. W., and Walter, C. J. S. The relationship between clinical diagnosis and anxiety, assessed by forearm blood flow and other measurements. *British Journal of Psychiatry,* 1968, *114,* 611–26.

Kempe, C. H., and Helfer, R. E. *Helping the battered child and his family.* Philadelphia: Lippincott, 1972.

Kempe, C. H., Silverman, F. N., Steele, B. F., Droegmueller, W., and Silver, H. K. The battered child syndrome. *Journal of the American Medical Association,* 1962, *181,* 17–24.

Kempe, C. H. Approaches to preventing child abuse. The health visitors concept. *American Journal of Diseases of Children,* 1976, *130,* 941–47.

Kendall, P. C. Anxiety: States, traits—situations? *Journal of Consulting and Clinical Psychology,* 1978, *46,* 280–87.

Kendall, P. C., and Finch, A. J., Jr. A cognitive-behavioral treatment for impulsivity: A group comparison study. *Journal of Consulting and Clinical Psychology,* 1978, *46,* 110–18.

Kernberg, O. F. Two reviews of the literature on borderlines: An assessment. *Schizophrenia Bulletin,* 1979, *5,* No. 1, 53–58.

Kety, S. S. Disorders of the human brain. *Scientific American,* 1979, *241,* No. 3, 202–14.

Kety, S. S., Rosenthal, D., Wender, P. H., Schulsinger, F., and Jacobsen, B. Mental illness in the biological and adoptive families of adopted individuals who have become schizophrenic: A preliminary report based on psychiatric interviews. In R. R. Fieve, R. Rosenthal, and H. Brill (Eds.), *Genetic research in psychiatry.* Baltimore: Johns Hopkins University Press, 1975.

Khanna, J. L. (Ed.) *New treatment approaches to juvenile delinquency.* Springfield, Ill.: Thomas, 1975.

Kiev, A. (Ed.) *Magic, faith, and healing: Studies in primitive psychiatry today.* New York: Free Press, 1964.

Kiev, A. Cultural perspectives on the range of normal human behavior. In J. H. Masserman (Ed.), *Social psychiatry, vol. 2: The range of normal in human behavior.* New York: Grune & Stratton, 1976.

Kihlstrom, J. F. Hypnosis and psychopathology: Retrospect and prospect. *Journal of Abnormal Psychology,* 1979, *88,* 459–73.

Kilmann, P. R., and Sotile, W. M. The marathon encounter group: A review of the outcome literature. *Psychological Bulletin,* 1976, *83,* 827–50.

Kilpatrick, D. G., Veronen, L. J., and Resick, P. A. The aftermath of rape: Recent empirical findings. *American Journal of Orthopsychiatry,* 1979, *49,* 658–69.

King, L. M. Social and cultural influences on psychopathology. *Annual Review of Psychology,* 1978, *29,* 405–33.

King, N. J., and Montgomery, R. B. Biofeedback-induced control of human peripheral temperature: A critical review of the literature. *Psychological Bulletin,* 1980, *88,* 738–52.

Kingsley, R. G., and Wilson, G. T. Behavior therapy for obesity: A comparative investigation of long-term efficacy. *Journal of Consulting and Clinical Psychology,* 1977, *45,* 288–98.

Kinney, J. M., and Sachs, L. B. Increasing hypnotic susceptibility. *Journal of Abnormal Psychology,* 1974, *83,* 145–50.

Kinsey, A. C., Pomeroy, W. B., and Martin, C. E. *Sexual behavior in the human male.* Philadelphia: Saunders, 1948.

Kinsey, A. C., Pomeroy, W. B., Martin, C. E., and Gebhard, P. H. *Sexual behavior in the human female.* Philadelphia: Saunders, 1953.

Kintz, B. L., Delprato, D. J., Metee, D. R., Persons, C. E., and Schappe, R. H. The experimenter effect. *Psychological Bulletin,* 1965, *63,* 223–32.

Kirman, B. H. Clinical aspects. In J. Wortis (Ed.), *Mental retardation and developmental disabilities: An annual review* (vol. 10). New York: Brunner/Mazel, 1978.

Kittrie, N. *The right to be different.* Baltimore: Johns Hopkins Press, 1971.

Kleber, H. D., and Slobetz, F. Outpatient drug-free treatment. In R. L. Dupont, A. Goldstein, and J. O'Donnell (Eds.), *Handbook on drug abuse.* National Institute on Drug Abuse, 1979.

Klein, D. C., and Seligman, M. E. P. Reversal of performance deficits and perceptual deficits in learned helplessness and depression. *Journal of Abnormal Psychology,* 1976, *85,* 11–26.

Klein, M. *The psycho-analysis of children.* New York: Grove, 1960.

Kline, N. S. *From sad to glad: Kline on depression.* New York: Putnam, 1974.

Kleitman, N. *Sleep and wakefulness* (2nd ed.). Chicago: University of Chicago Press, 1963.

Klerman, G. L. Depression and adaptation. In R. J. Friedman and M. M. Katz (Eds.), *The psychology of depression: Contemporary theory and research.* New York: Wiley, 1974.

Kline, P. *Fact and fantasy in Freudian theory.* London: Methuen, 1974.

Klonoff, H., McDougall, G., Clark, C., Kramer, P., and Horgan, J. The neuropsychological, psychiatric, and physical effects of prolonged and severe stress: 30 years later. *Journal of Nervous and Mental Disease,* 1976, *163,* 246–52.

Klorman, R., Strauss, J. S., and Kokes, R. F. Premorbid adjustment in schizophrenia—Part III. The relationship of demographic and diagnostic factors to measures of premorbid adjustment in schizophrenia. *Schizophrenia Bulletin,* 1977, *3,* No. 2, 214–25.

Kluckhohn, F., and Spiegel, J. P. *Integration and conflict in family behavior.* Report No. 27, Group for the Advancement of Psychiatry, August, 1954.

Knight, B. J., and West, D. J. Temporary and continuing delinquency. *British Journal of Criminology,* 1975, *15,* 43–50.

Kohn, M. L. The interaction of social class and other factors in the etiology of schizophrenia. *American Journal of Psychiatry,* 1976, *133,* 177–80.

Kokes, R. F., Strauss, J. S., and Klorman, R. Premorbid adjustment in schizophrenia—Part II. Measuring premorbid adjustment: The instruments and their development. *Schizophrenia Bulletin,* 1977, *3,* No. 2, 186–213.

Kolata, G. B. Gonorrhea: More of a problem but less of a mystery. *Science,* 1976, *192,* 244–47.

Kolata, G. B. Obesity: A growing problem. *Science,* 1977, *198,* 905–6.

Kolata, G. B. Behavioral teratology: Birth defects of the mind. *Science,* 1978, *202,* 732–34. (a)

Kolata, G. B. Childhood hyperactivity: A new look at treatments and causes. *Science,* 1978, *199,* 515–17. (b)

Kolata, G. B. Food additives and hyperactivity. *Science,* 1978, *199,* 516. (c)

Kolata, G. B. Mental disorders: A new approach to treatment? *Science,* 1979, *203,* 36–38. (a)

Kolata, G. B. New drugs and the brain. *Science,* 1979, *205,* 774–77. (b)

Kolata, G. B. Sex hormones and brain development. *Science,* 1979, *205,* 985–87. (c)

Kolata, G. B. Clues to the cause of senile dementia. *Science,* 1981, *211,* 1032–33.

Kolb, L. C. *Modern clinical psychiatry* (8th ed.). Philadelphia: Saunders, 1973.

Kopfstein, J. M., and Neale, J. M. A multivariate study of attention dysfunction in schizophrenia. *Journal of Abnormal Psychology,* 1972, *80,* 294–98.

Kora, T. Morita therapy. *International Journal of Psychiatry,* 1965, *1,* 611–45.

Korchin, S. *Modern clinical psychology: Principles of intervention in the clinic and community.* New York: Basic Books, 1976.

Kornetsky, C. *Pharmacology: Drugs affecting behavior.* New York: Wiley, 1976.

Kovel, J. *Complete guide to therapy: From psychoanalysis to behavior modification.* New York: Pantheon, 1976.

Kraepelin, E. *Lectures on clinical psychiatry* (3rd English ed.). Translated, revised, and edited by T. Johnstone. New York: William Wood, 1913.

Kraepelin, E. *Manic-depressive insanity and paranoia.* Edinburgh: Livingstone, 1921.

Kraepelin, E. *Textbook of psychiatry* (8th ed.). New York: Macmillan, 1923. (1883)

Krasner, L. The operant approach in behavior therapy. In A. E. Bergin and S. L. Garfield (Eds.), *Handbook of psychotherapy and behavior change: An empirical analysis.* New York: Wiley, 1971.

Kretschmer, E. *Physique and character.* Translated by W. J. H.

Sprott from *Korperbau und Charakter* (2nd ed.). New York: Harcourt, Brace, 1925. (1921)

Kringlen, E. *Heredity and environment in the functional psychoses.* London: Heinemann, 1967.

Kripke, D. F., and Simons, R. N. Average sleep, insomnia, and sleeping pill use. *Sleep Research,* 1976, *5,* 110.

Kubie, L. S. The fundamental nature of the distinction between normality and neurosis. *Psychoanalytic Quarterly,* 1954, *23,* 167–204.

Kubler-Ross, E. *On death and dying.* New York: Macmillan, 1969.

Kuhn, T. S. *The structure of scientific revolutions.* Chicago: University of Chicago Press, 1962.

Kuriansky, J. B., Deming, W. E., and Gurland, B. J. On trends in the diagnosis of schizophrenia. *American Journal of Psychiatry,* 1974, *131,* 402–8.

Kurtz, R. A. *Social aspects of mental retardation.* Lexington, Mass.: D.C. Heath, 1977.

Lachman, S. J. *Psychosomatic disorders: A behavioristic interpretation.* New York: Wiley, 1972.

Lader, M. H. Palmar skin conductance measures in anxiety and phobic states. *Journal of Psychosomatic Research,* 1967, *11,* 271–81.

Lader, M. *The psychophysiology of mental illness.* London: Routledge & Kegan Paul, 1975.

Lader, M. H., and Wing. L. Habituation of the psycho-galvanic reflex in patients with anxiety states and in normal subjects. *Journal of Neurology, Neurosurgery and Psychiatry,* 1964, *27,* 210–18.

Lader, M. H., and Wing. L. *Physiological measures, sedative drugs, and morbid anxiety.* London: Oxford University Press, 1966.

Lader, M., and Wing, L. Physiological measures in agitated and retarded depressed patients. *Journal of Psychiatric Research,* 1969, *7,* 89–100.

Laing, R. D. *The divided self.* London: Tavistock Publications, 1960.

Laing, R. D. *The politics of experience.* New York: Pantheon, 1967.

Laing, R. D. *Knots.* London: Tavistock, 1970.

Laing, R. D., and Esterson, A. *Sanity, madness and the family.* New York: Basic Books, 1964.

Lake, C. R., Sternberg, D. E., Van Kammen, D. P., Ballenger, J. C., Ziegler, M. G., Post, R. M., Kopin, I. J., and Bunney, W. E. Schizophrenia: Elevated cerebrospinal fluid norepinephrine. *Science,* 1980, *207,* 331–33.

Lambert, M. J., DeJulio, S. S., and Stein, D. M. Therapist interpersonal skills: Process, outcome, methodological considerations, and recommendations for future research. *Psychological Bulletin,* 1978, *85,* 467–89.

Lambert, N. M., Windmiller, M., Sandoval, J., and Moore, B. Hyperactive children and the efficacy of psychoactive drugs as a treatment intervention. *American Journal of Orthopsychiatry,* 1976, *46,* 335–52.

Lancaster, E., and Poling, J. *The final face of Eve.* New York: McGraw-Hill, 1958.

Landis, C., and Mettler, F. A. (Eds.) *Varieties of psychopathological experience.* New York: Holt, Rinehart & Winston, 1964.

Lando, H. A. Successful treatment of smokers with a broad-spectrum behavioral approach. *Journal of Consulting and Clinical Psychology,* 1977, *45,* 361–66.

Lang, P. J., and Buss, A. H. Psychological deficit in schizophrenia. II. Interference and activation. *Journal of Abnormal Psychology,* 1965, *70,* 77–106.

Lang, A. R., Goeckner, D. J., Adesso, V. J., and Marlatt, G. A. Effects of alcohol on aggression in male social drinkers. *Journal of Abnormal Psychology,* 1975, *84,* 508–18.

Lang, P. J., and Melamed, B. G. Case report: Avoidance conditioning therapy of an infant with chronic ruminative vomiting. *Journal of Abnormal Psychology,* 1969, *74,* 1–8.

Lang, A. R., Searles, J., Lauerman, R., and Adesso, V. Expectancy, alcohol, and sex guilt as determinants of interest in and reaction to sexual stimuli. *Journal of Abnormal Psychology,* 1980, *89,* 644–53.

Langer, D. H., Brown, G. L., and Docherty, J. P. Dopamine receptor supersensitivity and schizophrenia: A review. *Schizophrenia Bulletin,* 1981, *7,* 209–24.

Langer, E. J., and Abelson, R. P. A patient by any other name . . . : Clinical group differences in labeling bias. *Journal of Consulting and Clinical Psychology,* 1974, *42,* 4–9.

Langner, T. S., Herson, J. H., Greene, E. L., Jameson, J. D., and Goff, J. A. Children of the city: Affluence, poverty, and mental health. In V. L. Allen (Ed.), *Psychological factors in poverty.* Chicago: Markham, 1970.

Lansky, M. R., and Davenport, A. E. Difficulties in brief conjoint treatment of sexual dysfunction. *American Journal of Psychiatry,* 1975, *132,* 177–79.

Larson, C. A., and Nyman, G. E. Schizophrenia: Outcome in a birth year cohort. *Psychiatrica Clinica,* 1974, *7,* 50–55.

Lashley, K. S. *Brain mechanisms and intelligence.* Chicago: University of Chicago Press, 1929.

Lazarus, A. A. (Ed.) *Multimodal behavior therapy* (vol. 1). New York: Springer, 1976.

Lazarus, A. A. Has behavior therapy outlived its usefulness? *American Psychologist,* 1977, *32,* 550–54.

Lazarus, A. P. Learning theory and treatment of depression. *Behavior Research & Therapy,* 1968, *6,* 83–89.

Lazarus, R. S. A cognitively oriented psychologist looks at biofeedback. In T. X. Barber, L. V. DiCara, J. Kamiya, N. E. Miller, D. Shapiro, and J. Stoyva (Eds.), *Biofeedback and self-control: 1975/76.* Chicago: Aldine, 1976.

Ledwidge, B. Cognitive behavior modification: A step in the wrong direction? *Psychological Bulletin,* 1978, *85,* 353–75.

Lee, L. C. Mental health: A people's project. *APA Monitor,* 1979, *10,* Nos. 9 and 10, 20–21.

Leff, J. P. Culture and the differentiation of emotional states. *British Journal of Psychiatry,* 1973, *123,* 299–306.

Lefkowitz, M. M., Eron, L. D., Walder, L. O., and Huesmann, R. L. *Growing up to be violent: A longitudinal study of the development of aggression.* New York: Pergamon Press, 1977.

Lehmann, H. E. Epidemiology of depressive disorders. In R. R. Fieve (Ed.), *Depression in the 70's: Modern theory and research.* The Hague: Excerpta Medica, 1971.

Lehmann, H. E. Psychopharmacological treatment of schizophrenia. *Schizophrenia Bulletin,* 1975, No. 13, 25–45.
Leighton, A. H., and Murphy, J. M. Cross-cultural psychiatry. In J. M. Murphy and A. H. Leighton (Eds.), *Approaches to cross-cultural psychiatry.* Ithaca, N.Y.: Cornell University Press, 1965.
Lejeune, J., Gautier, M., and Turpin, R. Etudes des chromosomes somatiques de neuf enfants mongoliens. *Comptes Rendus de l'Académie des Sciences,* 1959, *248,* 1721–22.
Lelbach, W. K. Organic pathology related to volume and pattern of alcohol use. In R. J. Gibbons, Y. Israel, H. Kalant, R. E. Popham, W. Schmidt, and R. G. Smart (Eds.), *Research advances in alcohol and drug problems* (vol. 1). New York: Wiley, 1974.
Lentz, R. J., Paul, G. L., and Calhoun, J. F. Reliability and validity of three measures of functioning with "hardcore" chronic mental patients. *Journal of Abnormal Psychology,* 1971, *78,* 69–76.
Leon, G. R. Current directions in the treatment of obesity. *Psychological Bulletin,* 1976, *83,* 557–78.
Leon, G. R., and Roth, L. Obesity: Psychological causes, correlations, and speculation. *Psychological Bulletin,* 1977, *84,* 117–39.
Leopold, R. L., and Dillon, H. Psycho-anatomy of a disaster: A long term study of post-traumatic neuroses in survivors of a marine explosion. *American Journal of Psychiatry,* 1963, *119,* 913–21.
Lesse, S. (Ed.) *Masked depression.* New York: Aronson, 1974.
Leukel, F. *Introduction to physiological psychology* (3rd ed.). St. Louis: Mosby, 1976.
Levenson, R. W., Sher, K. J., Grossman, L. M., Newman, J., and Newlin, D. B. Alcohol and stress response dampening: Pharmacological effects, expectancy, and tension reduction. *Journal of Abnormal Psychology,* 1980, *89,* 528–38.
Levy, D. "Release therapy" in young children. *Psychiatry,* 1938, *1,* 387–90.
Levy, L., and Rowitz, L. *The ecology of mental disorder.* New York: Behavioral Publications, 1973.
Lewine, R. R. J. Sex differences in schizophrenia: A commentary. *Schizophrenia Bulletin,* 1979, *5,* No. 1, 4–7.
Lewine, R. R. J. Sex differences in age of symptom onset and first hospitalization in schizophrenia. *American Journal of Orthopsychiatry,* 1980, *50,* 316–22.
Lewinsohn, P. M. A behavioral approach to depression. In R. J. Friedman and M. M. Katz (Eds.), *The psychology of depression: Contemporary theory and research.* New York: Wiley, 1974.
Lewinsohn, P. M., and Libet, J. Pleasant events, activity schedules, and depressions. *Journal of Abnormal Psychology,* 1972, *79,* 291–95.
Lewis, D. O., Shanok, S. S., and Balla, D. A. Parental criminality and medical histories of delinquent children. *American Journal of Psychiatry,* 1979, *136,* 288–92. (a)
Lewis, D. O., Shanok, S. S., and Balla, D. A. Perinatal difficulties, head and face trauma, and child abuse in the medical histories of seriously delinquent children. *American Journal of Psychiatry,* 1979, *136,* 419–23. (b)
Lewis, G. P., Golden, C. J., Moses, J. A., Jr., Osmon, D. C., Purisch, A. D., and Hammeke, T. A. Localization of cerebral dysfunction with a standardized version of Luria's neuropsychological battery. *Journal of Consulting and Clinical Psychology,* 1979, *47,* 1003–19.
Lick, J., and Bootzin, R. Expectancy factors in the treatment of fear: Methodological and theoretical issues. *Psychological Bulletin,* 1975, *82,* 917–31.
Lidz, R. W., and Lidz, T. The family environment of schizophrenic patients. *American Journal of Psychiatry,* 1949, *106,* 332–45.
Lidz, T. Schizophrenia and the family. *Psychiatry,* 1958, *21,* 21–27.
Lidz, T. *The origin and treatment of schizophrenic disorders.* New York: Basic Books, 1973.
Lieberman, M. A., Yalom, I. D., and Miles, M. B. *Encounter groups: First facts.* New York: Basic Books, 1973.
Liebeskind, J. D., and Paul, L. A. Psychological and physiological mechanisms of pain. *Annual Review of Psychology* 1977, *28,* 41–60.
Liebowitz, M. R. Is borderline a distinct entity? *Schizophrenia Bulletin,* 1979, *5,* No. 1, 23–58.
Lindsey, D. T., Holzman, P. S., Haberman, S., and Yasillo, N. J. Smooth-pursuit eye movements: A comparison of two measurement techniques for studying schizophrenia. *Journal of Abnormal Psychology,* 1978, *87,* 491–96.
Lindsley, O. R. Can deficiency produce specific superiority: The challenge of the idiot savant. *Exceptional Children,* 1965, *31,* 225–32.
Lindsley, O. R., and Skinner, B. F. A method for the experimental analysis of the behavior of psychotic patients. *American Psychologist,* 1954, *9,* 419–20.
Lisansky, E. S. The etiology of alcoholism: The role of psychological predisposition. *Quarterly Journal of Studies on Alcohol,* 1960, *21,* 314–43.
Little, V. L., and Kendall, P. C. Note on locus of control and academic achievement in institutionalized juvenile delinquents. *Journal of Abnormal Child Psychology,* 1978, *6,* 281–83.
Lloyd, G. G. and Lishman, W. A. Effect of depression on the speed of recall of pleasant and unpleasant experiences. *Psychological Medicine,* 1975, *5,* 173–80.
Lloyd, R. W., Jr., and Salzberg, H. C. Controlled social drinking: An alternative to abstinence as a treatment goal for some alcohol abusers. *Psychological Bulletin,* 1975, *82,* 815–42.
Lobitz, W. C., and Post, R. D. Parameters of self-reinforcement and depression. *Journal of Abnormal Psychology,* 1979, *88,* 33–41.
Loftus, E. F. Alcohol, marijuana, and memory. *Psychology Today,* March, 1980, 42–56, 92.
Lombroso, C. *Crime, its causes and remedies.* Boston: Little Brown, 1911.
Lorand, S. A survey of psychoanalytical literature on problems of alcohol: Bibliography. *Yearbook of Psychoanalysis,* 1945, *1,* 359–70.
Lorand, S., and Schneer, H. I. Sexual deviations. III: Fetishism,

transvestitism, masochism, sadism, exhibitionism, voyeurism, incest, pedophilia, and bestiality. In A. M. Freedman, H. I. Kaplan, and H. S. Kaplan (Eds.), *Comprehensive textbook of psychiatry.* Baltimore: Williams & Wilkins, 1967.

Lorenz, K. *On aggression.* New York: Harcourt, Brace & World, 1966.

Lorr, M., McNair, D. M., Michaux, W. W., and Raskin, A. Frequency of treatment and change in psychotherapy. *Journal of Abnormal and Social Psychology,* 1962, *64,* 281–92.

Lovaas, O. I. Parents as therapists. Paper presented at the meeting of the International Symposium on Autism, St. Galen, Switzerland, 1976.

Lovaas, O. I., Freitas, L., Nelson, K., and Whalen, C. The establishment of imitation and its use for the development of complex behavior in schizophrenic children. *Behaviour Research and Therapy,* 1967, *5,* 171–81.

Lovaas, O. I., Koegel, R. L., and Schreibman, L. Stimulus overselectivity in autism: A review of research. *Psychological Bulletin,* 1979, *86,* 1236–54.

Luborsky, L. The patient's personality and psychotherapeutic change. In H. H. Strupp and L. Luborsky (Eds.), *Research in psychotherapy* (vol. 2). Washington, D.C.: American Psychological Association, 1962.

Luborsky, L., Chandler, M., Auerbach, A. H., Cohen, J., and Bachrach, H. M. Factors influencing the outcome of psycotherapy: A review of quantitative research. *Psychological Bulletin,* 1971, *75,* 145–85.

Luborsky, L., Mintz, J., and Christoph, P. Are psychotherapeutic changes predictable? Comparison of a Chicago counseling center project with a Penn psychotherapy project. *Journal of Consulting and Clinical Psychology,* 1979, *47,* 469–73.

Luborsky, L., Singer, B., and Luborsky, L. Comparative studies of psychotherapy. *Archives of General Psychiatry,* 1975, *32,* 995–1008.

Luborsky, L., and Spence, D. P. Quantitative research on psychoanalytic therapy. In A. E. Bergin and S. L. Garfield (Eds.), *Handbook of psychotherapy and behavior change: An empirical analysis.* New York: Wiley, 1971.

Ludwig, A. M. On and off the wagon: Reasons for drinking and abstaining by alcoholics. *Quarterly Journal of Studies on Alcohol, 1972, 33,* 91–96.

Luparello, T. J., McFadden, E. R., Jr., Lyons, H. A., and Bleeker, E. R. Psychologic factors and bronchial asthma. *New York State Journal of Medicine,* 1971, *71,* 2161–65.

Luria, A. R. *The working brain: An introduction to neuropsychology.* New York: Basic Books, 1973.

Lykken, D. T. A study of anxiety in the sociopathic personality. *Journal of Abnormal and Social Psychology,* 1957, *55,* 6–10.

Lykken, D. T. The detection of deception. *Psychological Bulletin,* 1979, *86,* 47–53.

Lyle, O. E., and Gottesman, I. I. Psychometric indicators of the gene for Huntington's disease: Clues to "ontopathogenesis." *Clinical Psychologist,* 1979, *3,* No. 2, 14–15.

Lynn, E. J. Treatment for alcoholism: Psychotherapy is still alive and well. *Hospital and Community Psychiatry,* 1976, *27,* 282–83.

Lyons, R. 20 million people or more need mental care, U.S. Panel asserts. *New York Times,* September 16, 1977, p. 16.

Lyons, R. Beneficial Valium can also prove to be bad medicine. *New York Times,* September 16, 1979, p. 20E.

Lystad, M. *An annotated bibliography: Violence at home.* Department of Health, Education and Welfare Publication No. (ADM) 75–136, 1974.

Lystad, M. Violence at home: A review of the literature. *American Journal of Orthopsychiatry,* 1975, *45,* 328–45.

MacAndrew, C., and Edgerton, R. B. *Drunken comportment: A social explanation.* Chicago: Aldine, 1969.

MacDonald, J. M. *Rape: Offenders and their victims.* Springfield, Ill.: Thomas, 1971.

MacDonald, M. L., and Tobias, L. L. Withdrawal causes relapse? Our response. *Psychological Bulletin,* 1976, *83,* 448–51.

MacDonald, N. Living with schizophrenia. *Canadian Medical Association Journal,* 1960, *82,* 218–21.

Machover, K. *Personality projection in the drawing of the human figure.* Springfield, Ill.: Thomas, 1949.

MacPhillamy, D. J., and Lewinsohn, P. M. Depression as a function of levels of desired and obtained pleasure. *Journal of Abnormal Psychology,* 1974, *83,* 651–57.

Maddi, S. R. The existential neurosis. *Journal of Abnormal Psychology,* 1967, *72,* 311–25.

Maher, B. A. *Principles of psychopathology: An experimental approach.* New York: McGraw-Hill, 1966.

Mahl, G. F. Anxiety, HC1 secretion and peptic ulcer etiology. *Psychosomatic Medicine,* 1950, *12,* 158–69.

Mahoney, M. J., and Hobbins, J. C. Prenatal diagnosis by fetoscopy and fetal blood sampling including initial attempts to diagnose Duchenne muscular dystrophy. In T. L. Sadick and S. M. Pueschel (Eds.), *Genetic diseases and developmental disabilities: Aspects of detection and prevention.* Washington, D.C.: American Association for the Advancement of Science, 1979.

Maliver, B. L. *The encounter game.* New York: Stein & Day, 1973.

Malmo, R. B. *On emotions, needs, and our archaic brain.* New York: Holt, Rinehart & Winston, 1975.

Malmo, R. B., and Shagass, C. Studies of blood pressure in psychiatric patients under stress. *Psychosomatic Medicine,* 1952, *14,* 82–93.

Malmo, R. B., Shagass, C., and Davis, J. F. A method for the investigation of somatic response mechanisms in psychoneurosis. *Science,* 1950, *112,* 325–28.

Malmo, R. B., Shagass, C., and Heslam, R. M. Blood pressure response to repeated brief stress in psychoneurosis: A study of adaptation. *Canadian Journal of Psychology,* 1951, *5,* 167–79.

Mandler, G. Helplessness: Theory and research in anxiety. In C. D. Spielberger (Ed.), *Anxiety: Current trends in theory and research* (vol. 2). New York: Academic Press, 1972.

Mann, J. J., Stanley, M., Gershon, S., and Rossor, M. Mental symptoms in Huntington's disease and a possible primary aminergic neuron lesion. *Science,* 1980, *210,* 1369–71.

Margolies, P. J. Behavioral approaches to the treatment of early infantile autism: A review. *Psychological Bulletin,* 1977, *84,* 249–64.

Marijuana and health. Eighth Annual Report to the United States Congress from the Secretary of Health and Human Services. National Institute on Drug Abuse, 1980.

Mark, V. H., and Ervin, F. R. *Violence and the brain.* New York: Harper & Row, 1970.

Marlatt, G. A. A cognitive-behavioral model of the relapse process. In N. A. Krasnegor (Ed.), *Behavioral analysis and treatment of substance abuse.* Rockville, Md.: National Institute on Drug Abuse, 1979.

Marlatt, G. A., and Gordon, J. R. Determinants of relapse: Implications for the maintenance of behavior change. Paper, Tenth International Conference on Behavior Modification, Banff, Alberta, Canada, 1978.

Marlatt, G. A., Kosturn, C. F., and Lang, A. R. Provocation to anger and opportunity for retaliation as determinants of alcohol consumption in social drinkers. *Journal of Abnormal Psychology,* 1975, *84,* 652–59.

Marmor, J. (Ed.) *Homosexual behavior: A modern reappraisal.* New York: Basic Books, 1980.

Marshall, E. Psychotherapy works, but for whom? *Science,* 1980, *207,* 506–8.

Marshall, G. R. Toilet training of an autistic eight-year-old through operant conditioning therapy: A case report. *Behaviour Research and Therapy,* 1966, *4,* 242–45.

Martin, B. *Anxiety and neurotic disorders.* New York: Wiley, 1971.

Martin, D. *Battered wives.* San Francisco: Glide, 1976.

Martin, G., and Pear, J. *Behavior modification: What it is and how to do it.* Englewood Cliffs, N.J.: Prentice-Hall, 1978.

Martin, H. P. Beezley, P., Conway, E. F., and Kempe, C. H. The development of abused children. In I. Schulman (Ed.), *Advances in pediatrics* (vol. 21). Chicago: Year Book Medical Publishers, 1974.

Marx, J. L. Stress: Role in hypertension debated. *Science,* 1977, *198,* 905–7.

Maslow, A. H. *Motivation and personality.* New York: Harper, 1954.

Massie, H. N., and Beels, C. C. The outcome of the family treatment of schizophrenia. *Schizophrenia Bulletin,* 1972, No. 6, 24–36.

Masters, W. H., and Johnson, V. E. *Human sexual response.* Boston: Little, Brown, 1966.

Masters, W. H., and Johnson, V. E. *Human sexual inadequacy.* Boston: Little, Brown, 1970.

Masters, W. H., and Johnson, V. E. *Homosexuality in perspective.* Boston: Little, Brown, 1979.

Matefy, R. E. Role-play theory of psychedelic drug flashbacks. *Journal of Consulting and Clinical Psychology,* 1980, *48,* 551–53.

Mathotra, H. K., and Wig, N. N. Dhat syndrome: A culture-bound sex neurosis of the Orient. *Archives of Sexual Behavior,* 1975, *4,* 519–28.

Matthysse, S. Overview: Biological research on schizophrenia. In R. Cancro (Ed.), *Annual review of the schizophrenic syndrome* (vol. 4, 1974–75). New York: Brunner/Mazel, 1976.

Mattinson, J., Marriage and mental handicap. In F. F. de la Cruz and G. D. LaVeck (Eds.), *Human sexuality and the mentally retarded.* New York: Brunner/Mazel, 1973.

Maugh, T. H. II. Chemicals: How many are there? *Science,* 1978, *199,* 162.

Maugh, T. H. II. Marijuana "justifies serious concern." *Science,* 1982, *215,* 1488–89.

May, P. R. A. *Treatment of schizophrenia: A comparative study of five treatment methods.* New York: Science House, 1968.

May, P. R. A., Tuma, A. H., Yale, C., Potepan, P., and Dixon, W. J. Schizophrenia: A follow-up study of results of treatment. II. Hospital stay over two to five years. *Archives of General Psychiatry,* 1976, *33,* 481–86.

May, R. (Ed.) *Existential psychology.* New York: Random House, 1961.

May, R. *Power and innocence: A search for sources of violence.* New York: Norton, 1972.

May, R., Angel, E., and Ellenberger, H. F. (Eds.) *Existence: A new dimension in psychiatry and psychology.* New York: Basic Books, 1958.

Mayfield, D. Alcoholism, alcohol, intoxication and assaultive behavior. *Diseases of the Nervous System,* 1976, *37,* 288–91.

McCarley, R. W., and Hobson, J. A. The neurobiological origins of psychoanalytic dream theory. *American Journal of Psychiatry,* 1977, *134,* 1211–21.

McClelland, D. C. Testing for competence rather than for "intelligence." *American Psychologist,* 1973, *28,* 1–14.

McClelland, D. C. Inhibited power motivation and high blood pressure in men. *Journal of Abnormal Psychology,* 1979, *88,* 182–90.

McClelland, D. C., Davis, W. N., Kalin, R., and Wanner, E. *The drinking man.* New York: Free Press, 1972.

McCollam, J. B., Burish, T. G., Maisto, S. A., and Sobell, M. B. Alcohol's effects on physiological arousal and self-reported affect and sensations. *Journal of Abnormal Psychology,* 1980, *89,* 224–33.

McCord, J. A thirty-year follow-up of treatment effects. *American Psychologist,* 1978, *33,* 284–89.

McCord, W., and McCord, J. *The psychopath: An essay on the criminal mind.* Princeton: Van Nostrand, 1964.

McDowell, D., Reynolds, B., and Magaro, P. The integration defect in paranoid and nonparanoid schizophrenia. *Journal of Abnormal Psychology,* 1975, *84,* 629–36.

McGeer, P. L., and McGeer, E. G. Chemistry of mood and emotion. *Annual Review of Psychology,* 1980, *31,* 273–307.

McGhie, A., and Chapman, J. Disorders of attention and perception in early schizophrenia. *British Journal of Medical Psychology,* 1961, *34,* 103–16.

McGlothlin, W. H. Drug use and abuse. *Annual Review of Psychology,* 1975, *26,* 45–64.

McGlothlin, W. H. Drugs and crime. In R. L. DuPont, A. Goldstein, and J. O'Donnell (Eds.), *Handbook on drug abuse.* Rockville, Md.: National Institute on Drug Abuse, 1979.

McGrath, M. J., and Cohen, D. B. REM sleep facilitation of adaptive waking behavior: A review of the literature. *Psychological Bulletin,* 1978, *85,* 24–57.

McKusick, V. A., and Ruddle, F. H. The status of the gene map of the human chromosomes. *Science,* 1977, *196,* 390–405.

McLeish, J. *Soviet psychology: History, theory, content.* London: Methuen, 1975.

Mednick, S. A. A learning theory approach to research in schizophrenia. *Psychological Bulletin,* 1958, *55,* 316–27.

Mednick, S. A. Breakdown in individuals at high risk for schizophrenia: Possible predispositional perinatal factors. *Mental Hygiene,* 1970, *54,* 50–63.

Mednick, S. A., and Christiansen, K. O. *Biosocial bases of criminal behavior.* New York: Gardner Press, 1977.

Mednick, S. A., and McNeil, T. F. Current methodology in research on the etiology of schizophrenia: Serious difficulties which suggest the use of the high-risk-group method. *Psychological Bulletin,* 1968, *70,* 681–93.

Mednick, S. A., and Schulsinger, F. Some premorbid characteristics related to breakdown in children with schizophrenic mothers. In D. Rosenthal and S. S. Kety (Eds.), *The transmission of schizophrenia.* London: Pergamon Press, 1968.

Mednick, S. A., Mura, E., Schulsinger, F., and Mednick, B. R. Perinatal conditions and infant development in children with schizophrenic parents. *Social Biology,* 1971, *18,* (suppl.), S103–S113.

Meehl, P. E. *Clinical versus statistical prediction.* Minneapolis: University of Minnesota Press, 1954.

Meehl, P. E. Schizotaxia, schizotypy, schizophrenia. *American Psychologist,* 1962, *17,* 827–38.

Mehl, L. E., and Peterson, G. H. Spontaneous peer psychotherapy in a day care setting. *American Journal of Orthopsychiatry,* 1981, *51,* 346–50.

Meichenbaum, D. Cognitive factors in biofeedback therapy. In J. Kamiya, T. X. Barber, N. E. Miller, D. Shapiro, and J. Stoyva (Eds.), *Biofeedback and self-control: 1976/77.* Chicago: Aldine, 1977.

Meichenbaum, D., and Turk, D. The cognitive-behavioral management of anxiety, anger, and pain. In P. Davidson (Ed.), *Behavioral management of anxiety, depression, and pain.* New York: Brunner/Mazel, 1976.

Melamed, B. G., and Siegel, L. J. Reduction of anxiety in children facing hospitalization and surgery by use of filmed modeling. *Journal of Consulting and Clinical Psychology,* 1975, *43,* 511–21.

Mellinger, G. D., Balter, M. B., Parry, H. J., Manheimer, D. I., and Cisin, I. H. An overview of psychotherapeutic drug use in the United States. In E. Josephson and E. E. Carroll (Eds.), *Drug use: Epidemiological and sociological approaches.* Washington, D.C.: Hemisphere, 1974.

Mellinger, G. D., Somers, R. H., Bazell, S., and Manheimer, D. I. Drug use, academic performance, and career indecision: Longitudinal data in search of a model. In D. B. Kandel (Ed.), *Longitudinal research on drug use: Empirical findings and methodological issues.* Washington, D.C.: Hemisphere, 1978.

Mellinger, G. D., Somers, R. H., Davidson, S. T., and Manheimer, D. I. The amotivational syndrome and the college student. *Annals of New York Academy of Sciences,* 1976, *282,* 37–55.

Mellor, C. S. First rank symptoms of schizophrenia. *British Journal of Psychiatry,* 1970, *117,* 15–23.

Mellstrom, M., Jr., Zuckerman, M., and Cicala, G. A. General versus specific traits in the assessment of anxiety. *Journal of Consulting and Clinical Psychology,* 1978, *46,* 423–31.

Meltzer, H. Y. Biology of schizophrenia subtypes: A review and proposal for method of study. *Schizophrenia Bulletin,* 1979, *5,* No. 3, 460–79. (a)

Meltzer, H. Y. Biochemical studies in schizophrenia. In L. Bellak (Ed.), *Disorders of the schizophrenic syndrome.* New York: Basic Books, 1979. (b)

Meltzer, H. Y., and Stahl, S. M. The dopamine hypothesis of schizophrenia: A review. *Schizophrenia Bulletin,* 1976, *2,* No. 1, 19–76.

Meltzoff, J., and Kornreich, M. *Research in psychotherapy.* New York: Atherton, 1970.

Mendels, J. *Concepts of depression.* New York: Wiley, 1970.

Menninger, K. *Man against himself.* New York: Harcourt, Brace, 1938.

Menninger, K. *Theory of psychoanalytic technique.* New York: Basic Books, 1958.

Menninger, K. *The crime of punishment.* New York: Viking Press, 1968.

Menninger, R. W. The history of psychiatry. *Diseases of the Nervous System,* 1944, *5,* 52–55.

Mercer, G. W., and Smart, R. G. The epidemiology of psychoactive and hallucinogenic drug use. In R. J. Gibbins, Y. Israel, H. Kalant, R. E. Popham, W. Schmidt, and R. B. Smart (Eds.), *Research advances in alcohol and drug problems* (vol. 1). New York: Wiley, 1974.

Mercer, J. R. *Labeling the mentally retarded.* Berkeley: University of California Press, 1973.

Mercer, J. R. SOMPA: System of Multicultural Pluralistic Assessment—technical manual. New York: Psychological Corporation, 1979.

Merlis, J. K. Proposal for an international classification of the epilepsies. *Epilepsia,* 1970, *11,* 114–19.

Merton, R. K. Social structure and anomie. *American Sociological Review,* 1938, *3,* 672–82.

Merton, R. K. The self-fulfilling prophecy. *Antioch Review,* 1948, *8,* 193–210.

Merton, R. K. *Social theory and social structure.* Glencoe, Ill.: Free Press, 1957.

Mettler, F. A. (Ed.), Columbia-Greystone Associates. *Selective partial ablation of the frontal cortex: A correlative study of its effects on human psychotic subjects.* New York: Hoeber, 1949.

Meyer, J. K., and Reter, D. J. Sex reassignment. *Archives of General Psychiatry,* 1979, *36,* 1010–15.

Milich, R. S. A critical analysis of Schachter's externality theory of obesity. *Journal of Abnormal Psychology,* 1975, *84,* 586–88.

Milkovich, L., and van den Berg, B. J. Effects of prenatal meprobamate and chlordiazepoxide hydrochloride on human embryonic and fetal development. *New England Journal of Medicine,* 1974, *291,* 1268–71.

Miller, G. A., and Chapman, L. J. Response bias and schizophrenic beliefs. *Journal of Abnormal Psychology,* 1968, *73,* 252–55.

Miller, J. Insanity defense: Mad or bad? Congress considers reforms. *APA Monitor,* 1975, *6,* 6, 14.

Miller, N. E. Theory and experiment relating psychoanalytic displacement to stimulus-response generalization. *Journal of Abnormal and Social Psychology,* 1948, *43,* 155–78.

Miller, N. E. Learning of visceral and glandular responses. *Science,* 1969, *163,* 434–45.

Miller, N. E. Biofeedback and visceral learning. *Annual Review of Psychology,* 1978, *29,* 373–404.

Miller, W. R. Psychological deficit in depression. *Psychological Bulletin,* 1975, *82,* 238–60.

Miller, W. R. Alcoholism scales and objective assessment methods: A review. *Psychological Bulletin,* 1976, *83,* 649–74.

Miller, W. R. Behavioral treatment of problem drinkers: A comparative outcome study of three controlled drinking therapies. *Journal of Consulting and Clinical Psychology,* 1978, *46,* 74–86.

Miller, W. R., and Seligman, M. E. P. Depression and the perception of reinforcement. *Journal of Abnormal Psychology,* 1973, *82,* 62–73.

Miller, W. R., and Seligman, M. E. P. Depression and learned helplessness in man. *Journal of Abnormal Psychology,* 1975, *84,* 228–38.

Miller, W. R., Taylor, C. A., and West, J. C. Focused versus broad-spectrum behavior therapy for problem drinkers. *Journal of Consulting and Clinical Psychology,* 1980, *48,* 590–601.

Millon, T. Reflections on Rosenhan's "On Being Sane in Insane Places." *Journal of Abnormal Psychology,* 1975, *84,* 456–61.

Mills, K. C., Sobell, M. B., and Schaeffer, H. Training social drinking as an alternative to abstinence for alcoholics. *Behavior Therapy,* 1971, *2,* 18–27.

Mineka, S., and Kihlstrom, J. F. Unpredictable and uncontrollable events: A new perspective on experimental neurosis. *Journal of Abnormal Psychology,* 1978, *87,* 256–71.

Mintz, E. E. *Marathon groups: Reality and symbol.* New York: Appleton, 1971.

Mintz, J., Luborsky, L., and Christoph, P. Measuring the outcomes of psychotherapy: Findings of the Penn psychotherapy project. *Journal of Consulting and Clinical Psychology,* 1979, *47,* 319–34.

Minuchin, S. *Families and family therapy.* Cambridge, Mass.: Harvard University Press, 1974.

Minuchin, S., Montalvo, B., Guerney, B. G., Jr., Rosman, B. L., and Schumer, F. *Families of the slums: An exploration of their structure and treatment.* New York: Basic Books, 1967.

Minuchin, S., Rosman, B. L., and Baker, L. *Psychosomatic families: Anorexia nervosa in context.* Cambridge, Mass.: Harvard University Press, 1978.

Mirsky, I. A. Physiologic, psychologic and social determinants in the etiology of duodenal ulcer. *American Journal of Digestive Disorders,* 1958, *3,* 285–314.

Mischel, W. Toward a cognitive social learning reconceptualization of personality. *Psychological Review,* 1973, *80,* 252–83.

Mischel, W. *Introduction to personality* (2nd ed.). New York: Holt, Rinehart & Winston, 1976.

Miss Nelson, 103, dies; confined for a century. *New York Times,* February 1, 1975, 1975, p. 30.

Mitchell, L., Doctor, R. M., and Butler, D. C. Attitudes of caretakers toward the sexual behavior of mentally retarded persons. *American Journal of Mental Deficieny,* 1978, *83,* 289–96.

Mitler, M. M., Guilleminault, C., Orem, J., Zarcone, V. P., and Dement, W. C. Sleeplessness, sleep attacks and things that go wrong in the night. *Psychology Today,* December, 1975, 45–50.

Mittelmann, B., Wolff, H. G., and Scharf, M. Emotions and gastroduodenal function. *Psychosomatic Medicine,* 1942, *4,* 5–61.

Mlott, S. R., and Mlott, Y. D. Dogmatism and locus of control in individuals who smoke, stopped smoking and never smoked. *Journal of Community Psychology,* 1975, *3,* 53–57.

Molotsky, I. L.I. finds a 'tremendous' increase in its youngsters' abuse of drugs. *New York Times,* December 1, 1978, p. B2.

Monahan, J. Prisons: A wary verdict on rehabilitation. *APA Monitor,* June, 1977, *8,* 13.

Money, J. *Sex errors of the body: Dilemmas, education, counseling.* Baltimore: Johns Hopkins University Press, 1968.

Money, J., and Gaskin, R. Sex reassignment. *International Journal of Psychiatry,* 1971, *9,* 249–69.

Monk, M. Epidemiology. In S. Perlin (Ed.), *A handbook for the study of suicide.* New York: Oxford University Press, 1975.

Morey, L. C., and Blashfield, R. K. A symptom analysis of the DSM-III definition of schizophrenia. *Schizophrenia Bulletin,* 1981, *7,* No. 2, 258–68.

Morgan, C. D., and Murray, H. A. A method for investigating fantasies: The Thematic Apperception Test. *Archives of Neurology and Psychiatry,* 1935, *34,* 289–306.

Mori, A. A., and Masters, L. F. *Teaching the severely mentally retarded: Adaptive skills training.* Germantown, Md.: Aspen, 1980.

Morris, G. O., and Wynne, L. C. Schizophrenic offspring and parental styles of communication. *Psychiatry,* 1965, *28,* 19–44.

Morris, J. B., and Beck, A. T. The efficacy of antidepressant drugs: A review of research (1958-1972). *Archives of General Psychiatry,* 1974, *30,* 667–74.

Mosher, L. R., Gunderson, J. G., and Buchsbaum, S. Special report: Schizophrenia, 1972. *Schizophrenia Bulletin,* 1973, No. 7, 12–52.

Moskalenko, V. D. A comparative study of families with one or both schizophrenic parents (translated from Russian). *Zhur-*

nal Nevropatoloii Psikhiatrii imeni S. S. Korsakova, 1972, *72,* 86–92.

Moss, C. S. Recovery from brain injury. *Clinical Psychologist,* 1980, *33,* No. 2, 5–6.

Most in poll say suicide is wrong. *New York Times,* May 4, 1975, p. 14.

Mostofsky, D. I., and Balaschak, B. A. Psychobiological control of seizures. *Psychological Bulletin,* 1977, *84,* 723–50.

Mowrer, O. H. An experimental analogue of "regression" with incidental observations on "reaction formation." *Journal of Abnormal and Social Psychology,* 1940, *35,* 56–87.

Mowrer, O. H., and Mowrer, W. M. Enuresis: A method for its study and treatment. *American Journal of Orthopsychiatry,* 1938, *8,* 436–59.

Moyer, K. E. *The psychobiology of aggression.* New York: Harper & Row, 1976.

Munro Ford, R. The causes of childhood asthma: An assessment of the relative importance of the allergic, infective and emotional factors in childhood asthma. *Medical Journal of Australia,* 1963, *2,* 128–30.

Murakami, M. Mental health in Japan. *APA Monitor,* 1979, *10,* Nos. 9 and 10.

Murphy, D. L., and Wyatt, R. J. Reduced monoamine oxidase activity in blood platelets from schizophrenic patients. *Nature,* 1972, *238,* 225–26.

Murphy, H. B. M. The epidemiological approach to transcultural psychiatric research. In A. V. S. de Reuck and R. Porter (Eds.), *Transcultural psychiatry,* Boston: Little, Brown, 1965.

Murphy, H. B. M. Sociocultural factors in schizophrenia: A compromise theory. In J. Zubin and F. A. Freyhan (Eds.), *Social psychiatry.* New York: Grune & Stratton, 1968.

Murphy, H. B. M. History and the evolution of syndromes: The striking case of *latah* and *amok.* In M. Hammer, K. Salzinger, and S. Sutton (Eds.), *Psychopathology: Contributions from the social, behavioral, and biological sciences,* New York: Wiley, 1973.

Murphy, J. M. Psychotherapeutic aspects of shamanism on St. Lawrence Island, Alaska. In A. Kiev (Ed.), *Magic, faith, and healing: Studies in primitive psychiatry today.* New York: Free Press, 1964.

Murphy, J. M. Psychiatric labeling in cross-cultural perspective. *Science,* 1976, *191,* 1019–28.

Murphy, W. D., Abel, G. G., and Becker, J. V. Future research issues. In D. Cox (Ed.), *Exhibitionism: Description, assessment and treatment.* New York: Garlinger, 1980.

Murray, H. A. *Thematic Apperception Test.* Cambridge: Harvard University Press, 1943.

Murstein, B. I. (Ed.) *Exploring intimate life styles.* New York: Springer, 1978.

Naditch, M. P. Ego functioning and acute adverse reactions to psychoactive drugs. *Journal of Personality,* 1975, *43,* 314–29. (a)

Naditch, M. P. Relation of motives for drug use and psychopathology in the development of acute adverse reactions to psychoactive drugs. *Journal of Abnormal Psychology,* 1975, *84,* 374–85. (b)

Naditch, M. P. Locus of control and drinking behavior in a sample of men in army basic training. *Journal of Consulting and Clinical Psychology,* 1975, *43,* 96. (c)

Naditch, M. P., and Fenwick, S. LSD flashbacks and ego functioning. *Journal of Abnormal Psychology,* 1977, *86,* 352–59.

Naficy, A., and Willerman, L. Excessive yielding to normal biases is not a distinctive sign of schizophrenia. *Journal of Abnormal Psychology,* 1980, *89,* 697–703.

Nash, M. R., Johnson, L. S., and Tipton, R. D. Hypnotic age regression and the occurrence of transitional object relationships. *Journal of Abnormal Psychology,* 1979, *88,* 547–55.

Nasrallah, H. A. Methodological issues in tardive dyskinesia research. *Schizophrenia Bulletin,* 1979, *5,* No. 1, 1–3.

Nassi, A. J., and Abramowitz, S. I. From phrenology to psychosurgery and back again: Biological studies of criminality. *American Journal of Orthopsychiatry,* 1976, *46,* 591–607.

Nathan, P. E., and Harris, S. L. *Psychopathology and society.* New York: McGraw-Hill, 1975.

Nathan, P. E., and Jackson, A. D. Behavior modification. In I. B. Weiner (Ed.), *Clinical methods in psychology.* New York: Wiley, 1976.

National Council on Alcoholism. Criteria for diagnosis of alcoholism. *American Journal of Psychiatry,* 1972, *129,* 127–35.

National Institute on Drug Abuse. *Phencyclidine use among youth in drug abuse treatment. Services research report.* National Institute on Drug Abuse, 1978.

Neale, J. M., and Cromwell, R. L. Attention and schizophrenia. In B. H. Maher (Ed.), *Progress in experimental personality research* (vol. 5). New York: Academic Press, 1970.

Neff, L. Traumatic neurosis. Paper presented at the annual meeting of the American Psychological Association, San Francisco, 1975.

Nemy, E. Suicide now no. 2 cause of deaths among young. *New York Times,* April 16, 1973, p. 1.

Nerviano, V. J. Common personality patterns among alcoholic males: A multivariate study. *Journal of Consulting and Clinical Psychology,* 1976, *44,* 104–10.

Nerviano, V. J., and Gross, W. R. A multivariate delineation of two alcoholic profile types on the 16 PF. *Journal of Clinical Psychology,* 1973, *29,* 371–74.

Newberger, E. H. Child abuse and neglect: Toward a firmer foundation for practice and policy. *American Journal of Orthopsychiatry,* 1977, *47,* 274–76.

Newmark, C. S., Falk, R., Johns, N., Boren, R., and Forehand, R. Comparing traditional clinical procedures with four systems to diagnose schizophrenia. *Journal of Abnormal Psychology,* 1976, *85,* 66–72.

Nisbett, R. E. Hunger, obesity, and the ventromedial hypothalamus. *Psychological Review,* 1972, *79,* 433–53.

Noble, P., and Lader, M. A physiological comparison of 'endogenous' and 'reactive' depression. *British Journal of Psychiatry,* 1972, *120,* 541–42.

Novaco, R. W. Stress inoculation: A cognitive therapy for anger and its application to a case of depression. *Journal of Consulting and Clinical Psychology,* 1977, *45,* 600–8.

Nowicki, S., Jr., and Hopper, A. E. Locus of control correlates in an alcoholic population. *Journal of Consulting and Clinical Psychology*, 1974, 735.

No worse. *APA Monitor*, 1976, *7*, 11.

Nuechterlein, K. H. Reaction time and attention in schizophrenia: A critical evaluation of the data and theories. *Schizophrenia Bulletin*, 1977, *3*, No. 3, 373–428.

Nurco, D. N. Etiological aspects of drug abuse. In R. L. DuPont, A. Goldstein, and J. O'Donnell (Eds.), *Handbook on drug abuse*. National Institute on Drug Abuse, 1979.

Nurco, D. N., Bonito, A. J., Lerner, M., and Balter, M. B. Studying addicts over time: Methodology and preliminary findings. *American Journal of Drug and Alcohol Abuse*, 1975, *2*, 183–96.

O'Brien, C. P. Group therapy for schizophrenia: A practical approach. *Schizophrenia Bulletin*, 1975, No. 13, 119–30.

O'Donnell, J. A., Voss, H. L., Clayton, R. R., Slatin, G. T., and Room, R. *Young men and drugs—a nationwide survey*. National Institute on Drug Abuse Research Monograph No. 5, 1976.

Offer, D., and Sabshin, M. *Normality: Theoretical and clinical concepts of mental health* (rev. ed.). New York: Basic Books, 1974.

Ogden, H. D. Headache studies. Statistical data. I. Procedure and sample distribution. *Journal of Allergy*, 1952, *23*, 58–75.

O'Gorman, P. A., and Lacks, H. *Aspects of youthful drinking*. National Council on Alcoholism, 1979.

O'Leary, M. R., Donovan, D. M., Freeman, C. W., and Chaney, E. F. Relationship between psychopathology, experienced control and perceived locus of control: In search of alcoholic subtypes. *Journal of Clinical Psychology*, 1976, *32*, 899–904.

Oles, M. N. The transsexual client: A discussion of transsexualism and issues in psychotherapy. *American Journal of Orthopsychiatry*, 1977, *47*, 66–74.

Omenn, G. S. Prenatal diagnosis of genetic disorders. *Science*, 1978, *200*, 958.

Opler, M. K. (Ed.) *Culture and mental health: Cross-cultural studies*. New York: Macmillan, 1959.

Orne, M. T. On the social psychology of the psychological experiment: With particular reference to demand characteristics and their implications. *American Psychologist*, 1962, *17*, 776–83.

Orne, M. T. The efficacy of biofeedback therapy. *Annual Review of Medicine*. 1979, *30*, 489–503.

Orton, S. T. *Reading, writing and speech problems in children*. New York: Norton, 1937.

Osgood, C. E., and Luria, Z. A blind analysis of a case of multiple personality using the semantic differential. *Journal of Abnormal and Social Psychology*, 1954, *49*, 579–91.

Osgood, C. E., Luria, A., and Smith, S. W. The three faces of Evelyn: A case report. II. A blind analysis of another case of multiple personality using the semantic differential. *Journal of Abnormal Psychology*, 1976, *85*, 256–70.

Osgood, C. E., Suci, G. J., and Tannenbaum, P. H. *The measurement of meaning*. Urbana: University of Illinois Press, 1957.

Osmond, H., and Smythies, J. Schizophrenia: A new approach. *Journal of Mental Science*, 1952, *98*, 309–15.

Ostow, M. *The psychology of melancholy*. New York: Harper, 1970.

Oswalt, R. M. Sexual and contraceptive behavior of college females. *Journal of the American College Health Association*, 1974, *22*, 392–94.

Otis, L. S. The facts on transcendental meditation: Part III. If well-integrated but anxious, try T.M. *Psychology Today*, 1974, *7*, No. 11, 45–46.

Ouellette, E. M., and Rosett, H. L. A pilot prospective study of the fetal alcohol syndrome at the Boston City Hospital. Part II: The infants. *Annals of the New York Academy of Sciences*, 1976, *273*, 123–29.

Ouellette, E. M., Rosett, H. L., Rosman, N. P., and Weiner, L. Adverse effects on offspring of maternal alcohol abuse during pregnancy. *New England Journal of Medicine*, 1977, *297*, 528–30.

Oztürk, D. M. Folk treatment of mental illness in Turkey. In A. Kiev (Ed.), *Magic, faith, and healing: Studies in primitive psychiatry today*. New York: Free Press, 1964.

Pagano, R. R., Rose, R. M., Stivers, R. M., and Warrenburg, S. Sleep during transcendental meditation. *Science*, 1976, *191*, 308–9.

Pankratz, L., Fausti, S. A., and Peed, S. A forced-choice technique to evaluate deafness in the hysterical or malingering patient. *Journal of Consulting and Clinical Psychology*, 1975, *43*, 421–22.

Pasamanick, B. Epidemiologic investigations of some prenatal factors in the production of neuropsychiatric disorder. In P. H. Hoch and J. Zubin (Eds.), *Comparative epidemiology of the mental disorders*. New York: Grune & Stratton, 1961.

Pasamanick, B., Scarpitti, F. R., and Dinitz, S. *Schizophrenics in the community: An experimental study in the prevention of hospitalization*. New York: Appleton, 1967.

Pattison, E. M. Nonabstinent drinking goals in the treatment of alcoholism: A clinical typology. *Archives of General Psychiatry*, 1976, *33*, 923–30.

Pattison, E. M., Sobell, M. B., and Sobell, L. C. *Emerging concepts of alcohol dependence*. New York: Springer, 1977.

Pavlov, I. P. *Conditioned reflexes: An investigation of the physiological activity of the cerebral cortex*. London: Oxford University Press, 1927.

Paykel, E. S. Life events and acute depression. In J. P. Scott and E. C. Senay (Eds.), *Separation and depression: Clinical and research aspects*. Washington, D.C.: American Association for the Advancement of Science, 1973.

Paykel, E. S., and Prusoff, B. A. Relationships between personality dimensions: Neuroticism and extraversion against obsessive, hysterical and oral personality. *British Journal of Social and Clinical Psychology*, 1973, *12*, 309–18.

Payne, P. and Shean, G. Autonomic responses of paranoid, nonparanoid schizophrenic, and normal subjects to affective visual stimulation. *Journal of Nervous and Mental Disease*, 1975, *161*, 123–29.

Payne, R. W. Cognitive abnormalities. In H. J. Eysenck (Ed.), *Handbook of abnormal psychology*. New York: Basic Books, 1961.

Payne, R. W., Caird, W. K., and Laverty, S. G. Overinclusive thinking and delusions in schizophrenic patients. *Journal of Abnormal and Social Psychology,* 1964, *68,* 562–66.

Payne, R. W., and Friedlander, D. A short battery of simple tests for measuring overinclusive thinking. *Journal of Mental Science,* 1962, *108,* 362–67.

Pearson, R. S. B. Asthma-allergy and prognosis. *Proceedings of the Royal Society of Medicine,* 1968, *61,* 467–70.

Pederson, L. L., Scrimgeour, W. G., and Lefcoe, N. M. Comparisons of hypnosis plus counseling, counseling alone, and hypnosis alone in a community service smoking withdrawal program. *Journal of Consulting and Clinical Psychology,* 1975, *43,* 920.

Pendery, M. L., Maltzman, I. M., and West, L. J. Controlled drinking by alcoholics? New findings and a reevaluation of a major affirmative study. *Science,* 1982, *217,* 169–75.

Penk, W. E., Woodward, W. A., Robinowitz, R., and Parr, W. C. An MMPI comparison of polydrug and heroin abusers. *Journal of Abnormal Psychology,* 1980, *89,* 299–302.

Perera, H. V. Two cases of Gilles de la Tourette's syndrome treated with haloperidol. *British Journal of Psychiatry,* 1975, *127,* 324–26.

Perls, F. S. *Gestalt therapy verbatim.* Moab, Utah: Real People Press, 1971.

Perls, F. S. *The Gestalt approach and Eye witness to therapy.* Ben Lomond, Calif.: Science and Behavior Books, 1973.

Persky, H., Korchin, S. J., Basowitz, H., Board, F. A., Sabshin, M., Hamburg, D. A., and Grinker, R. R. Effect of two psychological stresses on adrenocortical function. *AMA Archives of Neurology and Psychiatry,* 1959, *81,* 103–10.

Peterson, I. Stress can cause work "epidemics." *New York Times,* May 29, 1979, pp. C1–2.

Petersen, R. C., and Stillman, R. C. (Eds.) *Cocaine: 1977.* National Institute on Drug Abuse Research Monograph No. 13, 1977.

Pettigrew, T. F. *A profile of the Negro American.* Princeton, N.J.: D. Van Nostrand, 1964.

Phillips, D. L., and Segal, B. E. Sexual status and psychiatric symptoms. *American Sociological Review,* 1969, *34,* 58–72.

Phillips, L. Case history data and prognosis in schizophrenia. *Journal of Nervous and Mental Disease,* 1953, *117,* 515–25.

Phillips, L. Social competence and the process-reactive distinction in schizophrenia. Paper presented at the annual meeting of the American Psychopathological Association, 1964.

Pincus, J. H., and Tucker, G. J. *Behavioral neurology.* New York: Oxford University Press, 1978.

Pittel, S. M., and Oppedahl, N. C. The enigma of PCP. In R. L. DuPont, A. Goldstein, and J. O'Donnell (Eds.), *Handbook on drug abuse.* National Institute on Drug Abuse, 1979.

Pitts, F. N., Jr., and McClure, J. N., Jr. Lactate metabolism in anxiety neurosis. *New England Journal of Medicine,* 1967, *277,* 1329–36.

Platt, J. J., and Labate, C. *Heroin addiction: Theory, research, and treatment.* New York: Wiley, 1976.

Plotkin, W. B., and Rice, K. M. Biofeedback as a placebo: Anxiety reduction facilitated by training in either suppression or enhancement of alpha brainwaves. *Journal of Consulting and Clinical Psychology,* 1981, *49,* 590–96.

Pollack, J. M. Obsessive-compulsive personality: A review. *Psychological Bulletin,* 1979, *86,* 225–41.

Pollin, W., Allen, M. G., Hoffer, A., Stabenau, J. R., and Hrubec, Z. Psychopathology in 15,909 pairs of veteran twins: Evidence for a genetic factor in the pathogenesis of schizophrenia and its relative absence in psychoneurosis. *American Journal of Psychiatry,* 1969, *126,* 597–609.

Pollin, W., and Stabenau, J. R. Biological, psychological, and historical differences in a series of monozygotic twins discordant for schizophrenia. In D. Rosenthal and S. S. Kety (Eds.), *The transmission of schizophrenia.* New York: Pergamon Press, 1968.

Polster, E., and Polster, M. *Gestalt therapy integrated: Contours of theory and practice.* New York: Vintage Books, 1973.

Porteus, S. D. *The maze test and mental differences.* Vineland, N.J.: Smith, 1933.

Prange, A. J., and Vitols, M. M. Cultural aspects of the relatively low incidence of depression in southern Negroes. *International Journal of Social Psychiatry,* 1962, *8,* 104–12.

Prince, R. Indigenous Yoruba psychiatry. In A. Kiev (Ed.), *Magic, faith, and healing: Studies in primitive psychiatry today.* New York: Free Press, 1964.

Prinz, R. J., Roberts, W. A., and Hantman, E. Dietary correlates of hyperactive behavior in children. *Journal of Consulting and Clinical Psychology,* 1980, *48,* 760–69.

Prison official's revisionism. *New York Times,* June 6, 1976, p. E7.

Professional Staff of the United States-United Kingdom Cross-National Project. The diagnosis and psychopathology of schizophrenia in New York and London. *Schizophrenia Bulletin,* 1974, No. 11, 80–102.

Provence, S., and Lipton, R. *Infants in institutions.* New York: International Universities Press, 1963.

Purisch, A. D., Golden, C. J., and Hammeke, T. A. Discrimination of schizophrenic and brain-injured patients by a standardized version of Luria's neuropsychological tests. *Journal of Consulting and Clinical Psychology,* 1978, *46,* 1266–73.

Quadagno, D. M., Briscoe, R., and Quadagno, J. S. Effect of perinatal gonadal hormones on selected nonsexual behavior patterns: A critical assessment of the nonhuman and human literature. *Psychological Bulletin,* 1977, *84,* 62–80.

Quay, H. C. Psychopathic personality as pathological stimulation-seeking. *American Journal of Psychiatry,* 1965, *122,* 180–83.

Rabkin, J. G. The epidemiology of forcible rape. *American Journal of Orthopsychiatry,* 1979, *49,* 634–47.

Rabkin, J. G. Stressful life events and schizophrenia: A review of the research literature. *Psychological Bulletin,* 1980, *87,* 408–25.

Rabkin, J. G., and Struening, E. L. Life events, stress, and illness. *Science,* 1976, *194,* 1013–20.

Rachin, R. L. Reality therapy: Helping people help themselves. *Crime and Delinquency,* 1974, *20,* 45–53.

Rachman, S. Sexual fetishism: An experimental analogue. *Psycho-*

logical Record, 1966, *16,* 293–96.

Rachman, S., and Teasdale, J. *Aversion therapy and behaviour disorders: An analysis.* London: Routledge & Kegan Paul, 1969.

Rada, R. T. Alcoholism and forcible rape. *American Journal of Psychiatry,* 1975, *132,* 444–46.

Radloff, L. S., and Rae, D. S. Susceptibility and precipitating factors in depression: Sex differences and similarities. *Journal of Abnormal Psychology,* 1979, *88,* 174–81.

Rank, O. *Will therapy: An analysis of the therapeutic process in terms of relationship.* New York: Knopf, 1936.

Rapoport, J. L., Buchsbaum, M. S., Zahn, T. P., Weingartner, H., Ludlow, C., and Mikkelsen, E. J. Dextroamphetamine: Cognitive and behavioral effects in normal prepubertal boys. *Science.* 1978, *199,* 560–63.

Raskin, D. C., and Podlesny, J. A. Truth and deception: A reply to Lykken. *Psychological Bulletin,* 1979, *86,* 54–59.

Raw, M. Persuading people to stop smoking. *Behaviour Research and Therapy,* 1976, *14,* 97–101.

Razran, G. The observable unconsious and the inferable conscious in current Soviet psychophysiology: Interoceptive conditioning, semantic conditioning, and the orienting reflex. *Psychological Review,* 1961, *68,* 81–147.

Redfield, J., and Stone, A. Individual viewpoints of stressful life events. *Journal of Consulting and Clinical Psychology,* 1979, *47,* 147–54.

Reed, S. C. and Anderson, V. E. Effects of changing sexuality on the gene pool. In F. F. de la Cruz and G. D. LaVeck (Eds.), *Human sexuality and the mentally retarded.* New York: Brunner/Mazel, 1973.

Rees, L. Psychosomatic aspects of asthma in elderly patients. *Journal of Psychosomatic Research,* 1956, *1,* 212–18.

Rees, L. The importance of psychological, allergic and infective factors in childhood asthma. *Journal of Psychosomatic Research,* 1964, *7,* 253–62.

Rees, L. A controlled epidemiological study of the role of psychological factors in migraine. *Archivos de Neurobiologica,* 1974, *37,* 243–51.

Rehm, L. P. A self-control model of depression. *Behavior Therapy,* 1977, *8,* 787–804.

Reich, W. *Selected writings: An introduction to orgonomy.* New York: Farrar, Straus & Giroux, 1960.

Reinhold, R. Some unfortunate verdicts on writing science into the law. *New York Times,* March 9, 1980, p. 8E.

Reinhold, R. Leveling off of drug use found among students. *New York Times,* February 19, 1981, pp. A1, A19.

Reinhold, R. Panel reaffirms general doubts over marijuana. *New York Times,* February 27, 1982, pp. 1, 9.

Reinisch, J. M. Prenatal exposure to synthetic progestins increases potential for aggression in humans. *Science,* 1981, *211,* 1171–73.

Reiser, M. F. Cardiovascular disorders. In A. M. Freedman and H. I. Kaplan (Eds.), *Comprehensive textbook of psychiatry.* Baltimore: Williams & Wilkins, 1967.

Reitan, R. M., and Davison, L. A. (Eds.) *Clinical neuropsychology: Current status and applications.* New York: Wiley, 1974.

Rendon, M. Transcultural aspects of Puerto Rican mental illness in New York. *International Journal of Social Psychiatry,* 1974, *20,* 18–24.

Rensberger, B. Language ability found in right side of the brain. *New York Times,* July 1, 1975, p. 14.

Resnick, H. L. P., and Hathorne, B. C. (Eds.) *Suicide prevention in the 70's.* Washington, D.C., USGPO, 1973. DHEW Pub. No. (HSM) 72-9054.

Resnick, R. B., Kestenbaum, R. S., and Schwartz, L. K. Acute systematic effects of cocaine in man: A controlled study of intranasal and intravenous routes of administration. In E. H. Ellinwood, Jr. and M. M. Kilbey (Eds.), *Cocaine and other stimulants.* New York: Plenum, 1977.

Ricks, D., Umbarger, C., and Mack, R. A measure of increased temporal perspective in successfully treated adolescent delinquent boys. *Journal of Abnormal and Social Psychology,* 1964, *69,* 685–89.

Riddle, M., and Roberts, A. H. Delinquency, delay of gratification, recidivism, and the Porteus Maze Tests. *Psychological Bulletin,* 1977, *84,* 417–25.

Rieder, R. O. Borderline schizophrenia: Evidence of its validity. *Schizophrenia Bulletin,* 1979, *5,* No. 1, 39–46.

Rieder, R. O., Rosenthal, D., Wender, P., and Blumenthal, H. The offspring of schizophrenics—fetal and neonatal deaths. *Archives of General Psychiatry,* 1975, *32,* 200–11.

Riessman, F. *The culturally deprived child.* New York: Harper & Row, 1962.

Rife, D. C., and Snyder, L. H. Studies in human inheritance VI. A genetic refutation of the principles of "behavioristic" psychology. *Human Biology,* 1931, *3,* 547–59.

Rimland, B. Savant capabilities of autistic children and their cognitive implications. In G. Serban (Ed.), *Cognitive defects in the development of mental illness.* New York: Brunner/Mazel, 1978.

Rist, K. Incest: Theoretical and clinical views. *American Journal of Orthopsychiatry,* 1979, *49,* 680–91.

Rizzo, N. D. Dyslexia and delinquency: A new dyslexia screening test. *International Journal of Offender Therapy and Comparative Criminology,* 1975, *19,* 164–77.

Roback, H. B., McKee, E., Webb, W., Abramowitz, C. B., and Abramowitz, S. I. Psychopathology in female sex-change applications and two help-seeking controls. *Journal of Abnormal Psychology,* 1976, *85,* 430–32.

Roberts, S. V. And another: What about the halfway home idea? *New York Times,* March 19, 1978, p. E10.

Robins, E., Gassner, S., Kayes, J., Wilkinson, R. H., Jr., and Murphy, G. E. The communication of suicidal intent: A study of 134 consecutive cases of successful (completed) suicide. *American Journal of Psychiatry,* 1959, *115,* 724–33.

Robins, L. N. *Deviant children grown up.* Baltimore: Williams & Wilkins, 1966.

Robins, L. N. A follow-up of Vietnam drug users. *Special Action Office Monograph,* 1973, Ser. A, 1–23.

Robins, L. N. Addict careers. In R. L. DuPont, A. Goldstein, and J. O'Donnell (Eds.), *Handbook on drug abuse.* National Institute on Drug Abuse, 1979.

Robinson, N. M., and Robinson, H. B. *The mentally retarded child* (2nd ed.). New York: McGraw-Hill, 1976.

Rochester, S. R., Harris, B., and Seeman, M. V. Sentence processing in schizophrenic listeners. *Journal of Abnormal Psychology,* 1973, *82,* 350–56.

Rodin, J. Obesity and external responsiveness. Paper presented at the meetings of the Eastern Psychological Association, Philadelphia, April, 1974.

Rodin, J. Current status of the internal-external hypothesis for obesity: What went wrong? *American Psychologist,* 1981, *36,* 361–72.

Rodnick, E. H., and Garmezy, N. An experimental approach to the study of motivation in schizophrenia. In M. R. Jones (Ed.), *Nebraska symposium on motivation.* Lincoln, Nebraska: University of Nebraska Press, 1957.

Rodnick, E. H., and Shakow, D. Set in the schizophrenic as measured by a composite reaction time index. *American Journal of Psychiatry,* 1940, *97,* 214–25.

Roff, J. D. Adolescent schizophrenia: Variables related to differences in long-term adult outcome. *Journal of Consulting and Clinical Psychology,* 1974, *42,* 180–83.

Rogers, C. R. *Counseling and psychotherapy: Newer concepts in practice.* Boston: Houghton Mifflin, 1942.

Rogers, C. R. *Client-centered therapy: Its current practice, implications, and theory.* Boston: Houghton Mifflin, 1951.

Rogers, C. R. *On becoming a person: A therapist's view of psychotherapy.* Boston: Houghton Mifflin, 1961.

Rogers, C. R. The increasing involvement of the psychologist in social problems: Some comments, positive and negative. *California State Psychologist,* 1968, *9,* 29–31.

Roget's International Thesaurus (3rd ed.) New York: Crowell, 1962.

Rohsenow, D. J., and O'Leary, M. R. Locus of control research on alcoholic populations: A review. I. Development, scales, and treatment. *International Journal of the Addictions,* 1978, *13,* 55–78.

Rolf, J. E., and Harig, P. T. Etiological research in schizophrenia and the rationale for primary intervention. *American Journal of Orthopsychiatry,* 1974, *44,* 538–54.

Rorschach, H. *Psychodiagnostics,* Berne: Verlag Hans Huber, 1942.

Rosen, G. History. In S. Perlin (Ed.), *A handbook for the study of suicide.* New York: Oxford University Press, 1975.

Rosenbaum, M. Peptic ulcer. In A. M. Freedman and H. I. Kaplan (Eds.), *Comprehensive textbook of psychiatry.* Baltimore: Williams & Wilkins, 1967.

Rosenbaum, M., and Berger, M. M. (Eds.) *Group psychotherapy and group function* (2nd ed.). New York: Basic Books, 1975.

Rosenblatt, A. Providing custodial care for mental patients: An affirmative view. *Psychiatric Quarterly,* 1974, *48,* 14–25.

Rosengarten, H. and Friedhoff, A. J. A review of recent studies of the biosynthesis and excretion of hallucinogens formed by methylation of neurotransmitters or related substances. *Schizophrenia Bulletin,* 1976, *2,* No. 1, 90–105.

Rosenhan, D. L. On being sane in insane places. *Science,* 1973, *179,* 250–58.

Rosenthal, D. Some factors associated with concordance and discordance with respect to schizophrenia in monozygotic twins. *Journal of Nervous and Mental Disease,* 1959, *129,* 1–10.

Rosenthal, D. The offspring of schizophrenic couples. *Journal of Psychiatric Research,* 1966, *4,* 169–88.

Rosenthal, D. *Genetic theory and abnormal behavior.* New York: McGraw-Hill, 1970.

Rosenthal, D. *Genetics of psychopathology.* New York: McGraw-Hill, 1971.

Rosenthal, D., and Frank, J. D. Psychotherapy and the placebo effect. *Psychological Bulletin,* 1956, *53,* 294–302.

Rosenthal, D., and Kety, S. S. (Eds.) *The transmission of schizophrenia.* Oxford: Pergamon Press, 1968.

Rosenthal, D., Wender, P. H., Kety, S. S., Welner, J., and Schulsinger, F. The adopted-away offspring of schizophrenics. *American Journal of Psychiatry,* 1971, *128,* 307–11.

Rosenthal, D. Discussion: The concept of subschizophrenic disorders. In R. R. Fieve, D. Rosenthal, and H. Brill (Eds.), *Genetic research in psychiatry.* Baltimore: Johns Hopkins University Press, 1975. (a)

Rosenthal, D. Heredity in criminality. *Criminal Justice and Behavior,* 1975, *2,* 3–21. (b)

Rosenthal, D. Searches for the mode of genetic transmission in schizophrenia: Reflections and loose ends. *Schizophrenia Bulletin,* 1977, *3,* No. 2, 268–76.

Rosenthal, R. On the social psychology of the psychological experiment: The experimenter's hypothesis as unintended determinant of experimental results. *American Scientist,* 1963, *51,* 268–83.

Rosenthal, R. *Experimenter effects in behavioral research.* New York: Appleton-Century-Crofts, 1966.

Rosenthal, R. Covert communication in the psychological experiment. *Psychological Bulletin,* 1967, *67,* 356–67.

Rosenthal, R., and Jacobson, L. *Pygmalion in the classroom.* New York: Holt, 1968.

Rosenthal, R. How often are our numbers wrong? *American Psychologist,* 1978, *33,* 1005–08.

Rosenthal, R., and Fode, K. L. Psychology of the scientist: V. Three experiments in experimenter bias. *Psychological Reports,* 1963, *12,* 491–511.

Rosenthal, R., and Jacobson, L. Teachers' expectancies: Determinants of pupils' IQ gains. *Psychological Reports,* 1966, *19,* 115–18.

Rosenthal, R., and Rosnow, R. L. *The volunteer subject.* New York: Wiley, 1975.

Rosman, B. L., Minuchin, S., and Liebman, R. Family lunch session: An introduction to family therapy in anorexia nervosa. *American Journal of Orthopsychiatry,* 1975, *45,* 846–53.

Rosman, N. P. Neurological and muscular aspects of thyroid dysfunction in childhood. *Pediatric Clinics of North America,* 1976, *23,* 575–94.

Ross, M., Berger, P. A., and Goldstein, A. Plasma β-endorphin immunoreactivity in schizophrenia. *Science,* 1979, *205,* 1163–64.

Ross, R. R., and McKay, H. B. *Self-mutilation.* Lexington, Mass.: Lexington Books, 1979.

Roth, P. *Portnoy's complaint.* New York: Random House, 1967.

Rotter, J. B. Generalized expectancies for internal versus external control of reinforcement. *Psychological Monographs,* 1966, *80,* No. 1 (Whole No. 609).

Rowland, N. E., and Antelman, S. M. Stress-induced hyperphagia and obesity in rats: A possible model for understanding human obesity. *Science,* 1976, *191,* 310–12.

Rozensky, R. H., Rehm, L. P., Pry, G., and Roth, D. Depression and self-reinforcement behavior in hospitalized patients. *Journal of Behavior Therapy and Experimental Psychiatry,* 1977, *8,* 35–38.

Rubenstein, E. Disease caused by impaired communication among cells. *Scientific American,* 1980, *242,* No. 3, 102–21.

Rule, S. 7% of former mental patients should be readmitted, team finds. *New York Times,* February 23, 1978, p. 35.

Ruppenthal, G. C., Arling, G. L., Harlow, H. F., Sackett, G. P., and Suomi, S. J. A ten-year perspective of motherless-mother monkey behavior. *Journal of Abnormal Psychology,* 1976, *85,* 341–49.

Ruskin, A. P. Mystical or physiological? Letter to *New York Times Magazine,* February 23, 1975, p. 72.

Rutter, M. Infantile autism and other child psychoses. In M. Rutter and L. Hersov (Eds.), *Child psychiatry: Modern approaches.* Oxford: Blackwell Scientific Publications, 1977.

Rutter, M. Diagnosis and definition of childhood autism. *Journal of Autism and Childhood Schizophrenia,* 1978, *8,* 139–61.

Ryback, R. S. Psychological aspects of alcohol and alcoholism. *Massachusetts Journal of Mental Health,* 1974, *5,* 19–44.

Sabshin, M. Psychiatric perspectives on normality. *Archives of General Psychiatry,* 1967, *17,* 258–64.

Sachar, E. J. (Ed.) *Hormones, behavior, and psychopathology.* New York: Raven Press, 1976.

Sackeim, H. A., Gur, R. C., and Saucy, M. C. Emotions are expressed more intensely on the left side of the face. *Science,* 1978, *202,* 434–36.

Sainsbury, P. Suicide and depression. In A. Coppen and A. Walk (Eds.), *Recent developments in affective disorders: A symposium.* Ashford, Kent, England: Royal Medico-Psychological Association, 1968.

Salter, A. *Conditioned reflex therapy: The direct approach to the reconstruction of personality.* New York: Creative Age Press, 1949.

Saltman, J. *The new alcoholics: Teenagers.* Public Affairs Pamphlet No. 499, 1973.

Salzinger, K. The immediacy hypothesis of schizophrenia. In H. M. Yaker, H. Osmond, and F. Cheek (Eds.), *The future of time: Man's temporal environment.* New York: Doubleday, 1971. (a)

Salzinger, K. An hypothesis about schizophrenic behavior. *American Journal of Psychotherapy,* 1971, *25,* 601–14. (b)

Salzinger, K. Schizophrenia and the immediacy hypothesis: A reply to Radomisli. *American Journal of Psychotherapy,* 1972, *26,* 567–70.

Salzinger, K. *Schizophrenia: Behavioral aspects.* New York: Wiley, 1973.

Salzinger, K. But is it good for the patients? Paper presented at the American Psychological Association meetings, San Francisco, August, 1977.

Salzinger, K. A behavioral analysis of diagnosis. In R. L. Spitzer and D. F. Klein (Eds.), *Critical issues in psychiatric diagnosis.* New York: Raven Press, 1978.

Salzinger, K., Portnoy, S., and Feldman, R. S. Experimental manipulation of continuous speech in schizophrenic patients. *Journal of Abnormal and Social Psychology,* 1964, *68,* 508–16. (a)

Salzinger, K., Portnoy, S., and Feldman, R. S. Verbal behavior of schizophrenic and normal subjects. *Annals of New York Academy of Sciences,* 1964, *105,* 845–60. (b)

Salzman, L. Sexual problems in adolescence. *Contemporary Psychoanalysis,* 1974, *10,* 189–207.

Sameroff, A., and Zax, M. Schizotaxia revisited: Model issues in the etiology of schizophrenia. *American Journal of Orthopsychiatry,* 1973, *43,* 744–54.

Samuels, L. Sex differences in concordance rates for schizophrenia: Finding or artifact? *Schizophrenia Bulletin,* 1978, *4,* No. 1, 14–15.

Samuels, L. Reply to Lewine. *Schizophrenia Bulletin,* 1979, *5,* No. 1, 8–10.

Sappington, J. Psychometric correlates of defensive style in process and reactive schizophrenics. *Journal of Consulting and Clinical Psychology,* 1975, *43,* 154–56.

Sarason, I. G., Johnson, J. H., and Siegel, J. M. Assessing the impact of life changes: Development of the Life Experiences Survey. *Journal of Consulting and Clinical Psychology,* 1978, *46,* 932–46.

Sarason, S. B., and Doris, J. *Psychological problems in mental deficiency* (4th ed.). New York: Harper & Row, 1969.

Sarason, S. B., Zitnay, G., and Grossman, F. K. *The creation of a community setting.* Syracuse: Syracuse University Division of Special Education and Rehabilitation, 1971.

Sarbin, T. R. The concept of hallucination. *Journal of Personality,* 1967, *35,* 359–80.

Sarbin, T. R., and Coe, W. C. *Hypnosis: A social psychological analysis of influence communication.* New York: Holt, Rinehart & Winston, 1972.

Sargent, J. D., Green, E. E., and Walters, E. D. The use of autogenic feedback training in a pilot study of migraine and tension headaches. *Headache,* 1972, *12,* 120–25.

Sartorius, N., Shapiro, R., and Jablensky, A. The international pilot study of schizophrenia. *Schizophrenia Bulletin,* 1974, No. 11, 21–34.

Satir, V. *Conjoint family therapy: A guide to theory and technique* (rev. ed.). Palo Alto, Calif.: Science and Behavior Books, 1967.

Sauer, L. Epileptics aided by new research. *New York Times,* August 28, 1979, p. C3.

Schaar, K. House measure raises issue of learning problems and crime. *APA Monitor,* 1977, *8,* No. 4, 11.

Schacht, T., and Nathan, P. E. But is it good for the psychologists? Appraisal and status of DSM-III. *American Psychologist,* 1977, *32,* 1017–25.

Schachter, S., and Gross, L. P. Manipulated time and eating behavior. *Journal of Personality and Social Psychology,* 1968, *10,* 98–106.

Schachter, S., and Latané, B. Crime, cognition and the autonomic nervous system. In D. Levine (Ed.), *Nebraska symposium on motivation.* Lincoln: University of Nebraska Press, 1964.

Schachter, S., and Rodin, J. *Obese humans and rats.* New York: Wiley, 1974.

Schachter, S., and Singer, J. E. Cognitive, social, and physiological determinants of emotional states. *Psychological Review,* 1962, *69,* 379–99.

Scheff, T. J. *Being mentally ill: A sociological theory.* Chicago: Aldine, 1966.

Schildkraut, J. J. The catecholamine hypothesis of affective disorders: A review of supporting evidence. *American Journal of Psychiatry,* 1965, *122,* 509–22.

Schildkraut, J. J., and Kety, S. S. Biogenic amines and emotion. *Science,* 1967, *156,* 21–30.

Schildkraut, J. J., Orsulak, P. J., Gudeman, J. E., Schatzberg, A. F., Rohde, W. A., LaBrie, R. A., Cahill, J. F., Cole, J. O., and Frazier, S. H. Norepinephrine metabolism in subtypes of depressive disorders. In C. Shagass, S. Gershon, and A. J. Friedhoff (Eds.), *Psychopathology and brain dysfunction.* New York: Raven, 1977.

Schildkraut, J. J., Orsulak, P. J., Schatzberg, A. F., Gudeman, J. E., Cole, J. O., Rohde, W. A., and LaBrie, R. A. Toward a biochemical classification of depressive disorders. 1. Differences in urinary excretion of MHPG and other catecholamine metabolites in clinically defined subtypes of depressions. *Archives of General Psychiatry,* 1978, *35,* 1427–33.

Schizophrenia: Is there an answer? U.S. Department of Health, Education, and Welfare, Public Health Service: Publication No. (HSM) 73-9086, 1974.

Schmale, A. J., Jr. Relation of separation and depression to disease. I. A report on a hospitalized medical population. *Psychosomatic Medicine,* 1958, *20,* 259–77.

Schmauk, F. J. Punishment, arousal, and avoidance learning in sociopaths. *Journal of Abnormal Psychology,* 1970, *76,* 325–35.

Schmeck, H. M., Jr. Chemistry of pain begins to emerge. *New York Times,* May 1, 1979, pp. C1–2.

Schmeck, H. M., Jr. Therapy in the womb rescues unborn lives. *New York Times,* May 26, 1981, pp. C1–2.

Schmideberg, M. Some basic principles of offender therapy: II. *International Journal of Offender Therapy and Comparative Criminology,* 1975, *19,* 22–32.

Schmidt, H. O., and Fonda, C. P. The reliability of psychiatric diagnosis: A new look. *Journal of Abnormal and Social Psychology,* 1956, *52,* 262–67.

Schneider, J. W. Deviant drinking as disease: Alcoholism as a social accomplishment. *Social Problems,* 1978, *2,* 361–72.

Schneider, K. *Clinical psychopathology.* New York: Grune & Stratton, 1959.

Schofield, L. J., and Reyher, J. Thematic productions under hypnotically aroused conflict in age regressed and waking states using the real-simulator design. *Journal of Abnormal Psychology,* 1974, *83,* 130–39.

Schofield, M. *The sexual behavior of young adults: A follow-up study to The Sexual Behavior of Young People.* London: Penguin, 1973.

Schopler, E., and Reichler, R. J. How well do parents understand their own psychotic child? *Journal of Autism and Childhood Schizophrenia,* 1972, *2,* 387–400.

Schrag, P., and Divoky, D. *The myth of the hyperactive child: And other means of child control.* New York: Pantheon, 1975.

Schuckit, M. A., Goodwin, D. A., and Winokur, G. A study of alcoholism in half siblings. *American Journal of Psychiatry,* 1972, *128,* 1132–36.

Schuckit, M. A., and Rayses, V. Ethanol ingestion: Differences in blood acetaldehyde concentrations in relatives of alcoholics and controls. *Science,* 1979, *203,* 54–55.

Schulsinger, F. Psychopathy: Heredity and environment. *International Journal of Mental Health,* 1972, *1,* 190–206.

Schulsinger, F. Biological psychopathology. *Annual Review of Psychology,* 1980, *31,* 583–606.

Schulz, B. Kinder manisch-depressiver und anderer affektivpsychotischer Elternpaare. *Zeitschrift für die gesamte Neurologie und Psychiatrie,* 1940, *169,* 311–412.

Schumer, F. Gender and schizophrenia. In E. Gomberg and V. Franks (Eds.), *Gender and disordered behavior.* New York: Brunner/Mazel, 1979.

Schumer, F., and Deutsch, C. P. A study of familial, background, and cognitive style characteristics of relatively successful and unsuccessful learners (determined longitudinally) in a Harlem enrichment program. Final report, OEO Contract No. B89-4590, 1968–69.

Schumer, F., and Zubin, J. Projective techniques. In H. J. Eysenck (Ed.), *Encyclopedia of Psychology.* Zurich, Switzerland: Herder & Herder, 1972.

Schur, E. *The awareness trap: Self-absorption instead of social change.* New York: Quadrangle, 1976.

Schutz, W. C. *Elements of encounter.* Big Sur, Calif.: Joy Press, 1973.

Schuyler, D. *The depressive spectrum.* New York: Aronson, 1974.

Schwartz, G. E. Biofeedback as therapy: Some theoretical and practical issues. *American Psychologist,* 1973, *28,* 666–73.

Schwartz, G. E., Davidson, R. J., and Maer, F. Right hemisphere lateralization for emotion in the human brain: Interactions with cognition. *Science,* 1975, *190,* 286–88.

Schwitzgebel, R. K. A contractual model for the protection of the rights of institutionalized mental patients. *American Psychologist,* 1975, *30,* 815–20.

Scobie, A., and Taylor, A. J. W. Perversions ancient and modern: I. Agalmatophilia, the statue syndrome. *Journal of the History of the Behavioral Sciences,* 1975, *11,* 49–54.

Scott, J. P. and Senay, E. D. (Eds.) *Separation and depression: Clinical and research aspects.* Washington, D.C.: American Association for the Advancement of Science, 1973.

Scovern, A. W., and Kilmann, P. R. Status of electroconvulsive therapy: Review of the outcome literature. *Psychological Bulletin,* 1980, *87,* 260–303.

Selby, G., and Lance, J. W. Observations of 500 cases of migraine and allied vascular headache. *Journal of Neurology, Neurosurgery and Psychiatry,* 1960, *23,* 23–32.

Seligman, M. E. P. Learned helplessness. *Annual Review of Medicine,* 1972, *23,* 407–12.

Seligman, M. E. P. Fall into helplessness. *Psychology Today,* June, 1973, 43–48.

Seligman, M. E. P. Depression and learned helplessness. In R. J. Friedman and M. M. Katz (Eds.), *The psychology of depression: Contemporary theory and research.* New York: Wiley, 1974.

Seligman, M. E. P. *Helplessness: On depression, development, and death.* San Francisco: Freeman, 1975.

Seligman, M. E. P., Klein, D. C., and Miller, W. R. Depression. In H. Leitenberg (Ed.), *Handbook of behavior modification and behavior therapy.* Englewood Cliffs, N.J.: Prentice-Hall, 1976.

Seligman, M. E. P., and Maier, S. F. Failure to escape traumatic shock. *Journal of Experimental Psychology,* 1967, *74,* 1–9.

Selye, H. *The stress of life* (rev. ed.). New York: McGraw-Hill, 1978.

Serban, G. The process of neurotic thinking. *American Journal of Psychotherapy,* 1974, *18,* 418–29.

Serban, G. The cognitive origin of neurotic thinking. In G. Serban (Ed.), *Cognitive defects in the development of mental illness.* New York: Brunner/Mazel, 1978.

Sexton, P. C. *Spanish Harlem: Anatomy of poverty.* New York: Harper & Row, 1965.

Shagass, C., and Jones, A. L. A neurophysiological test for psychiatric diagnosis: Results in 750 patients. *American Journal of Psychiatry,* 1958, *114,* 1002–9.

Shah, S. A. Dangerousness: A paradigm for exploring some issues in law and psychology. *American Psychologist,* 1978, *33,* 224–38.

Shakow, D. Psychological deficit in schizophrenia. *Behavioural Science,* 1963, *8,* 275–305.

Shakow, D. Understanding normal psychological function. *Archives of General Psychiatry,* 1967, *17,* 306–19.

Shakow, D. Segmental set—the adaptive process in schizophrenia. *American Psychologist,* 1977, *32,* 129–39.

Shapiro, A. K. Placebo effects in medicine, psychotherapy, and psychoanalysis. In A. E. Bergin and S. L. Garfield (Eds.), *Handbook of psychotherapy and behavior change: An empirical analysis.* New York: Wiley, 1971.

Shapiro, D. *Neurotic styles.* New York: Basic Books, 1965.

Shapiro, D. H., Jr., and Zifferblatt, S. M. Zen meditation and behavioral self-control: Similarities, differences, and clinical applications. *American Psychologist,* 1976, *31,* 519–32.

Shatan, C. F. Stress disorders among Vietnam veterans: The emotional content of combat continues. In C. R. Figley (Ed.), *Stress disorders among Vietnam veterans: Theory, research and treatment.* New York: Brunner/Mazel, 1978.

Sheehy, G. The economics of prostitution: Who profits? who pays? In E. Goode and R. R. Troiden (Eds.), *Sexual deviance and sexual deviants.* New York: Morrow, 1974.

Sheldon, W. *Varieties of delinquent youth.* New York: Harper, 1949.

Sheldon, W. H., and Stevens, S. S. *The varieties of temperament: A psychology of constitutional differences.* New York: Harper, 1942.

Shields, J. *Monozygotic twins, brought up apart and brought up together.* London: Oxford University Press, 1962.

Shields, J., and Slater, E. Heredity and psychological abnormality. In H. J. Eysenck (Ed.), *Handbook of abnormal psychology,* New York: Basic Books, 1961.

Shneidman, E. S. (Ed.) *Death and the college student.* New York: Behavioral Publications, 1972.

Shneidman, E. S., and Farberow, N. L. (Eds.) *Clues to suicide.* New York: McGraw-Hill, 1957.

Shoben, E. J., Jr. Toward a concept of the normal personality. *American Psychologist,* 1957, *12,* 183–89.

Sidel, R. The role of revolutionary optimism in the treatment of mental illness in the People's Republic of China. *American Journal of Orthopsychiatry,* 1973, *43,* 732–36.

Siegel, R. K. Cocaine: Recreational use and intoxication. In R. C. Petersen and R. C. Stillman (Eds.), *Cocaine: 1977.* National Institute on Drug Abuse Research Monograph No. 13, 1977.

Siever, L. J., and Gunderson, J. G. Genetic determinants of borderline conditions. *Schizophrenia Bulletin,* 1979, *5,* No. 1, 59–85.

Silber, D. E. Controversy concerning the criminal justice system and its implications for the role of mental health workers. *American Psychologist,* 1974, *29,* 239–44.

Silverman, C. *The epidemiology of depression.* Baltimore: Johns Hopkins Press, 1968.

Silverman, J. The problem of attention in research and theory in schizophrenia. *Psychological Review,* 1964, *71,* 352–79.

Simmel, E. Incendiarism. In K. R. Eissler (Ed.), *Searchlights on delinquency.* New York: International Universities Press, 1949.

Skinner, B. F. *The behavior of organisms: An experimental analysis.* New York: Appleton, 1938.

Skinner, B. F. *Contingencies of reinforcement: A theoretical analysis* New York: Appleton-Century-Crofts, 1969.

Skinner, B. F. *Beyond freedom and dignity.* New York: Knopf, 1971.

Skopkova, H. Psychotic complications after tetraethylthiuramdisulfide used in the treatment of alcoholism. *Ceskoslovenskia Psychiatrie,* 1973, *69,* 102–11.

Slater, E. A review of earlier evidence on genetic factors in schizophrenia. In D. Rosenthal and S. S. Kety (Eds.), *The transmission of schizophrenia.* New York: Pergamon Press, 1968.

Slater, E., and Shields, J. *Psychotic and neurotic illnesses in twins.* London: Her Majesty's Stationary Office, 1953.

Slater, E., and Shields, J. Genetical aspects of anxiety. In M. H. Lader (Ed.), *Studies of anxiety.* Ashford, Kent, England: Headley Bros., 1969.

Slavson, S. R. *An introduction to group therapy.* New York: Commonwealth Fund, 1943.

Sloane, R. B., Staples, F. R., Cristol, A. H., Yorkston, N. J., and Whipple, K. *Psychotherapy versus behavior therapy.* Cambridge, Mass.: Harvard University Press, 1975. (a)

Sloane, R. B., Staples, F. R., Cristol, A. H., Yorkston, N. J., and Whipple, K. Short-term analytically oriented psychotherapy versus behavior therapy. *American Journal of Psychiatry,* 1975, *132,* 373–77. (b)

Slutsky, J. M., and Allen, G. J. Influence of contextual cues on the efficacy of desensitization and a credible placebo in alleviating public speaking anxiety. *Journal of Consulting and Clinical Psychology,* 1978, *46,* 119–25.

Smith, D. E. Changing drug patterns in the Haight-Ashbury. *California Medicine,* 1969, *110,* 151–57.

Smith, J. C. Yoga and stress. In S. Ajaya (Ed.), *Meditational therapy.* Glenview, Ill.: Himalayan International Institute of Yoga Science and Philosophy of USA, 1977.

Smith, M. L. Sex bias in counseling and psychotherapy. *Psychological Bulletin,* 1980, *87,* 392–407.

Smith, M. L., and Glass, G. V. Meta-analysis of psychotherapy outcome studies. *American Psychologist,* 1977, *32,* 752–61.

Smith, R. J. The criminal insanity defense is placed on trial in New York. *Science,* 1978, *199,* 1048–52.

Smith, R. J. Study finds sleeping pills overprescribed. *Science,* 1979, *204,* 287–89.

Sobel, D. Smoking: Clearing away the haze. *New York Times,* January 15, 1980, pp. C1–2.

Sobel, D. Dialysis for schizophrenia? Doctors debate effects. *New York Times,* March 7, 1981, pp. 1, 12.

Sobell, L. C., Sobell, M. B., and Ward, E. (Eds.) *Evaluating alcohol and drug abuse treatment effectiveness: Recent advances.* New York: Pergamon Press, 1980.

Sobell, M. B., and Sobell, L. C. *Behavioral treatment of alcohol problems: Individualized therapy and controlled drinking.* New York: Plenum Press, 1978.

Socarides, C. W. Homosexuality and medicine. *Journal of the American Medical Association,* 1970, *212,* 1199–202.

Solomon, P., Kubzansky, P. E., Leiderman, P. H., Mendelson, J. H., Trumbull, R., and Wexler, D. (Eds.) *Sensory deprivation.* Cambridge, Mass.: Harvard University Press, 1961.

Solomon, R. L., and Wynne, L. C. Traumatic avoidance learning: The principles of anxiety conservation and partial irreversibility. *Psychological Review,* 1954, *61,* 353–85.

Solursh, L. P. Psychoactive drugs, crime and violence. *Psychological Reports,* 1975, *37,* 1177–78.

Some violence statistics. *APA Monitor,* 1978, *9,* No. 2, 3.

Sourkes, T. L. Biochemistry of mental depression. *Canadian Psychiatric Association Journal,* 1977, *22,* 467–81.

Sotile, W. M., and Kilmann, P. R. Treatments of psychogenic female sexual dysfunctions. *Psychological Bulletin,* 1977, *84,* 619–33.

Spanos, N. P., and Barber, T. X. Toward a convergence in hypnosis research. *American Psychologist,* 1974, *29,* 500–11.

Spence, J. T., Helmreich, R., and Stapp, J. Ratings of self and peers on sex role attributes and their relation to self-esteem and conceptions of masculinity and femininity. *Journal of Personality and Social Psychology,* 1975, *32,* 29–39.

Spicker, H. H. Intellectual development through early childhood education. *Exceptional Children,* 1971, *37,* 629–40.

Spiegel, H. An eye-roll test for hypnotizability. *American Journal of Clinical Hypnosis,* 1972, *15,* 25–28.

Spiegel, H. *Manual for Hypnotic Induction Profile: Eye-roll levitation method (Rev. ed.). New York: Soni Medica, 1974. (a)*

Spiegel, H. The grade 5 syndrome: The highly hypnotizable person. International Journal of Clinical and Experimental Hypnosis, 1974, *22,* 303–19. (b)

Spiegel, H., Aronson, M., Fleiss, J. L., and Haber, J. Psychometric analysis of the hypnotic induction profile. *International Journal of Clinical and Experimental Hypnosis,* 1976, *24,* 300–15.

Spiegel, H. Personal communication, 1982.

Spiegel, H., and Spiegel, D. *Trance and treatment: Clinical uses of hypnosis.* New York: Basic Books, 1978.

Spiegel, J. P. The resolution of role conflict within the family. In M. Greenblatt, D. J. Levinson, and R. H. Williams (Eds.), *The patient and the mental hospital.* Glencoe, Ill.: The Free Press, 1957.

Spiegel, J. P. Homeostatic mechanisms within the family. In I. Galdston (Ed.), *The family in contemporary society.* New York: International Universities Press, 1958.

Spiegel, J. P., and Machotka, P. *Messages of the body.* New York: Free Press, 1974.

Spielberger, C. D. Conceptual and methodological issues in anxiety research. In C. D. Spielberger (Ed.), *Anxiety: Current trends in theory and research* (vol. 2). New York: Academic Press, 1972.

Spinetta, J. J., and Rigler, D. The child-abusing parent: A psychological review. *Psychological Bulletin,* 1972, *77,* 296–304.

Spiro, M. On meaning and expression in other cultures. In R. J. Friedman and M. M. Katz (Eds.), *The psychology of depression: Contemporary theory and research.* New York: Wiley, 1974.

Spitz, R. A. Hospitalism: An inquiry into the genesis of psychiatric conditions in early childhood. *Psychoanalytic Study of the Child,* 1945, *1,* 53–74.

Spitz, R. A. Anaclitic depression. *Psychoanalytic Study of the Child,* 1946, *2,* 313–42.

Spitzer, R. L. On pseudoscience in science, logic in remission, and psychiatric diagnosis: A critique of Rosenhan's "On Being Sane in Insane Places." *Journal of Abnormal Psychology,* 1975, *84,* 442–52.

Spitzer, R. L., Burdock, E. I., and Hardesty, A. S. *Mental Status Schedule.* New York: Biometrics Research, Research Foundation for Mental Hygiene, Inc., and Robert L. Spitzer, 1963.

Spitzer, R. L., and Endicott, J. DIAGNO: A computer program for psychiatric diagnosis utilizing the differential diagnostic procedure. *Archives of General Psychiatry,* 1968, *18,* 746–56.

Spitzer, R. L., and Endicott, J. The value of the interview for the evaluation of psychopathology. In M. Hammer, K. Salzinger, and S. Sutton (Eds.), *Psychopathology: Contributions from the social, behavioral, and biological sciences.* New York: Wiley, 1973.

Spitzer, R. L., and Endicott, J. Justification for separating schizotypal and borderline personality disorders. *Schizophrenia*

Bulletin, 1979, *5,* No. 1, 95–104.

Spitzer, R. L., Endicott, J., and Fleiss, J. L. Instruments and recording forms for evaluating psychiatric status and history: Rationale, method of development, and description. *Comprehensive Psychiatry,* 1967, *8,* 321–43.

Spitzer, R. L., Endicott, J., Fleiss, J. L., and Cohen, J. The psychiatric status schedule: A technique for evaluating psychopathology and impairment in role functioning. *Archives of General Psychiatry,* 1970, *23,* 41–55.

Spitzer, R. L., and Fleiss, J. L. A re-analysis of the reliability of psychiatric diagnosis. *British Journal of Psychiatry,* 1974, *125,* 341–47.

Spitzer, R. L., Fleiss, J. L., Burdock, E. I., and Hardesty, A. The mental status schedule: Rationale, reliability and validity. *Comprehensive Psychiatry,* 1964, *5,* 384–95.

Spitzer, R. L., Sheehy, M., and Endicott, J. DSM-III. Guiding principles. In V. M. Rakoff, H. C. Stancer, and H. B. Kedward (Eds.), *Psychiatric diagnosis.* New York: Brunner/Mazel, 1977.

Spring, B. Stress and schizophrenia: Some definitional issues. *Schizophrenia Bulletin,* 1981, *7,* 24–33.

Srole, L., Langner, T. S., Michael, S. T., Opler, M. K., and Rennie, T. A. C. *Mental health in the metropolis: The Midtown Manhattan study.* New York: McGraw-Hill, 1962.

Stafford, Clark, D., and Taylor, F. H. Clinical and electroencephalographic studies of prisoners charged with murder. *Journal of Neurology, Neurosurgery, and Psychiatry,* 1949, *12,* 325–30.

Stam, H. J., and Spanos, N. P. Experimental designs, expectancy effects, and hypnotic analgesia. *Journal of Abnormal Psychology,* 1980, *89,* 751–62.

Starká, L., Sipová, I., and Hynie, J. Plasma testosterone in male transsexuals and homosexuals. *Journal of Sex Research,* 1975, *11,* 134–38.

Stearns, B. C., Penner, L. A., and Kimmel, E. Sexism among psychotherapists: A case not yet proven. *Journal of Consulting and Clinical Psychology,* 1980, *48,* 548–50.

Stein, M., and Schiavi, R. Respiratory disorders. In A. M. Freedman and H. I. Kaplan (Eds.), *Comprehensive textbook of psychiatry.* Baltimore: Williams & Wilkins, 1967.

Sternbach, R. A. *Pain patients: Traits and treatments.* New York: Academic Press, 1974.

Stoller, R. J. Sexual deviations. In F. A. Beach (Ed.), *Human sexuality in four perspectives.* Baltimore, Md.: Johns Hopkins University Press, 1976.

Stolz, S. B. Why no guidelines for behavior modification? In C. M. Franks and G. T. Wilson (Eds.), *Annual review of behavior therapy: Theory and practice.* New York: Brunner/Mazel, 1978.

Stolz, S. B., Wienckowski, L. A., and Brown, B. S. Behavior modification: A perspective on critical issues. *American Psychologist,* 1975, *30,* 1027–48.

Stone, A. A. Mentally ill: To commit or not, that is the question. *New York Times,* March 19, 1978, p. E10.

Storms, L. H., Broen, W. E., Jr., and Levin, I. P. Verbal associative stability and commonality as a function of stress in schizophrenics, neurotics, and normals. *Journal of Consulting Psychology,* 1967, *31,* 181–87.

Strauss, J. S. Social and cultural influences on psychopathology. *Annual Review of Psychology,* 1979, *30,* 397–415.

Strauss, J. S., and Carpenter, W. T., Jr. Characteristic symptoms and outcome in schizophrenia. *Archives of General Psychiatry,* 1974, *30,* 429–34. (a)

Strauss, J. S., and Carpenter, W. T., Jr. The prediction of outcome in schizophrenia—II. *Archives of General Psychiatry,* 1974, *31,* 37–42. (b)

Strauss, J. S., Carpenter, W. T., Jr., and Bartko, J. J. The diagnosis and understanding of schizophrenia. Part III. Speculations on the processes that underlie schizophrenic symptoms and signs. *Schizophrenia Bulletin,* 1974, No. 11, 61–69.

Strauss, M. E. Behavioral differences between acute and chronic schizophrenics: Course of psychosis, effects of institutionalization, or sampling biases? *Psychological Bulletin,* 1973, *79,* 271–79.

Stricker, G. Implications of research for psychotherapeutic treatment of women. *American Psychologist,* 1977, *32,* 14–22.

Strupp, H. H. On the basic ingredients of psychotherapy. *Journal of Consulting and Clinical Psychology,* 1973, *41,* 1–8.

Strupp, H. H. Psychotherapy: Assessing methods. *Science,* 1980, *207,* 590.

Stuart, R. B. A three-dimensional program for the treatment of obesity. *Behaviour Research and Therapy,* 1971, *9,* 177–86.

Study finds female Ph.D.'s lag behind male counterparts in pay and job opportunities. *New York Times,* January 6, 1975, p. 16.

Stunkard, A. Obesity and the denial of hunger. *Psychosomatic Medicine,* 1959, *21,* 281–89.

Sturgis, E. T., and Adams, H. E. Right to treatment: Issues in the treatment of homosexuality. *Journal of Consulting and Clinical Psychology,* 1978, *46,* 165–69.

Suffet, F., and Brotman, R. Female drug use: Some observations. *International Journal of the Addictions,* 1976, *11,* 19–33.

Sullivan, H. S. *The interpersonal theory of psychiatry.* New York: Norton, 1953.

Sullivan, H. S. *Schizophrenia as a human process.* New York: Norton, 1962.

Sullivan, R. Disgrace of the state mental hospitals. *New York Times,* October 9, 1977, p. E5.

Sun, M. Cancer patients: Joints or THC. *Science,* 1980, *209,* 999.

Sundberg, N. D., Snowden, L. R., and Reynolds, W. M. Toward assessment of personal competence and incompetence in life situations. *Annual Review of Psychology,* 1978, *29,* 179–221.

Suomi, S. J., Eisele, C. D., Grady, S. A., and Harlow, H. F. Depressive behavior in adult monkeys following separation from family environment. *Journal of Abnormal Psychology,* 1975, *84,* 576–78.

Sutherland, E. H. Book reviews. *Journal of Criminal Law and Crimi-*

nology, 1939, *29,* 911–14.

Sutherland, E. H., and Cressey, D. R. *Principles of criminology* (7th ed.), Philadelphia: Lippincott, 1966.

Sutton, S., Hakerem, G., Zubin, J., and Portnoy, M. The effect of shift of sensory modality on serial reaction time: A comparison of schizophrenics and normals. *American Journal of Psychology,* 1961, *74,* 224–32.

Sweet, J. J., and Resick, P. A. The maltreatment of children: A review of theories and research. *Journal of Social Issues,* 1979, *35,* 40–59.

Szász, T. S. The myth of mental illness. *American Psychologist,* 1960, *15,* 113–18.

Szasz, T. S. *The myth of mental illness: Foundations of a theory of personal conduct.* New York: Hoeber-Harper, 1961.

Szasz, T. S. *Law, liberty, and psychiatry: An inquiry into the social uses of mental health practices.* New York: Macmillan, 1963.

Szasz, T. S. The moral dilemma of psychiatry: Autonomy or heteronomy? *American Journal of Psychiatry,* 1964, *121,* 521–28.

Szasz, T. S. *The ethics of psychoanalysis: The theory and method of autonomous psychotherapy.* New York: Basic Books, 1965.

Szasz, T. S. *The second sin.* Garden City, N.Y.: Anchor Press/Doubleday, 1973. (a)

Szasz, T. S. *The age of madness: The history of involuntary mental hospitalization presented in selected texts.* Garden City, N.Y.: Anchor Press/Doubleday, 1973. (b)

Szasz, T. *Ceremonial chemistry: The ritual persecution of drugs, addicts, and pushers.* Garden City, New York: Anchor Press/Doubleday, 1974.

Tallman, J. F., Paul, S. M., Skolnick, P., and Gallagher, D. W. Receptors for the age of anxiety: Pharmacology of the benzodiazepines. *Science,* 1980, *207,* 274–82.

Tarshis, M. S. *The LSD controversy: An overview.* Springfield, Ill.: Thomas, 1972.

Taylor, M. A., Gaztanaga, P., and Abrams, R. Manic-depressive illness and acute schizophrenia: A clinical, family history, and treatment-response study. *American Journal of Psychiatry,* 1974, *131,* 678–82.

Taylor, W. L. "Cloze procedure": A new tool for measuring readability. *Journalism Quarterly,* 1953, *30,* 415–33.

Terman, L. M., and Merrill, M. A. *Stanford-Binet Intelligence Scale: 1972 norms edition.* Boston: Houghton Mifflin, 1973.

The course of alcoholism: Four years after treatment. Santa Monica, Calif.: Rand Corporation, 1980.

Thigpen, C. H., and Cleckley, H. M. A case of multiple personality. *Journal of Abnormal and Social Psychology,* 1954, *49,* 135–51.

Thigpen, C. H., and Cleckley, H. M. *The three faces of Eve.* New York: McGraw-Hill, 1957.

Thomas, A., and Sillen, S. *Racism and psychiatry.* New York: Brunner/Mazel, 1972.

Thomas, E., and Dewald, L. Experimental neurosis: Neuropsychological analysis. In J. D. Maser and M. E. P. Seligman (Eds.), *Psychopathology: Experimental models.* San Francisco: Freeman, 1977.

Thompson, R. F. *Introduction to physiological psychology.* New York: Harper, 1975.

Thompson, R. J., Jr., and O'Quinn, A. M. *Developmental disabilities: Etiologies, manifestations, diagnoses, and treatments.* New York: Oxford University Press, 1979.

Thomson, K. C., and Hendrie, H. C. Environmental stress in primary depressive illness. *Archives of General Psychiatry,* 1972, *26,* 130–32.

Thorpe, T. J. Effects of hatha yoga and meditation on anxiety and body image. In S. Ajaya (Ed.), *Meditational therapy.* Glenview, Ill.: Himalayan International Institute of Yoga Science and Philosophy of USA, 1977.

Tienari, P. Schizophrenia in monozygotic male twins. In D. Rosenthal and S. S. Kety (Eds.), *The transmission of schizophrenia.* New York: Pergamon Press, 1968.

Tienari, P. Schizophrenia and monozygotic twins. *Psychiatrica Fennica,* 1971, 97–104.

Tiger, L. *Optimism: The biology of hope.* New York: Simon & Schuster, 1979.

Tobias, L. L., and MacDonald, M. L. Withdrawal of maintenance drugs with longterm hospitalized patients: A critical review. *Psychological Bulletin,* 1974, *81,* 107–25.

Torrey, E. F. Is schizophrenia universal? An open question. *Schizophrenia Bulletin,* 1973, No. 7, 53–59.

Tosteson, D. C. Lithium and mania. *Scientific American,* 1981, *244,* 164–74.

Tourney, G. A history of therapeutic fashions in psychiatry, 1800–1966. *American Journal of Psychiatry,* 1967, *124,* 784–96.

Tourney, G., Petrilli, A. J., and Hatfield, L. M. Hormonal relationships in homosexual men. *American Journal of Psychiatry,* 1975, *132,* 288–90.

Tramontana, M. G. Critical review of research on psychotherapy outcome with adolescents: 1967–1977. *Psychological Bulletin,* 1980, *88,* 429–50.

Tripp, C. A. *The homosexual matrix.* New York: McGraw-Hill, 1975.

Trotter, S. Psychosurgery—psychology enters the fray. *APA Monitor,* 1974, *5,* 1027.

Trunca, C. The chromosome syndromes. In J. Wortis (Eds.), *Mental retardation and developmental disabilities: An annual review* (vol. 11). New York: Brunner/Mazel, 1980.

Trzebiatowska-Trzeciak, O. Genetical analysis of unipolar and bipolar endogenous affective psychoses. *British Journal of Psychiatry,* 1977, *131,* 478–85.

Tsuang, M. T., and Winokur, G. Criteria for subtyping schizophrenia. *Archives of General Psychiatry,* 1974, *31,* 43–47.

Tucker, G. J., Harrow, M., Detre, T., and Hoffman, B. Perceptual experiences in schizophrenic and nonschizophrenic patients. *Archives of General Psychiatry,* 1969, *20,* 159–66.

Tucker, G. J., and Rosenberg, S. D. Computer content analysis of schizophrenic speech: Preliminary report. *American Journal of Psychiatry,* 1975, *132,* 611–16.

Tuckman, J., Kleiner, R. J., and Lavell, M. Credibility of suicide notes. *American Journal of Psychiatry,* 1960, *116,* 1104–06.

Turk, C. D., Meichenbaum, D. H., and Berman, W. H. Application of biofeedback for the regulation of pain: A critical review. *Psychological Bulletin,* 1979, *86,* 1322–38.

Turner, J. C., and TenHoor, W. J. The NIMH community support program: Pilot approach to a needed social reform. *Schizophrenia Bulletin,* 1978, *4,* No. 3, 319–48.

Ullmann, L. P., and Krasner, L. *A psychological approach to abnormal behavior.* Englewood Cliffs, N.J.: Prentice Hall, 1969.

Valenstein, E. S. *Brain control: A critical examination of brain stimulation and psychosurgery.* New York: Wiley, 1973.

Valenstein, E. S. *Psychosurgery debate: Scientific, legal and ethical perspectives.* San Francisco: Freeman, 1980.

Van Buskirk, S. S. A two-phase perspective on the treatment of anorexia nervosa. *Psychological Bulletin,* 1977, *84,* 529–38.

Van Dyke, C., and Byck, R. Cocaine. *Scientific American,* 1982, *246,* No. 3, 128–41.

Van Praag, H. M. *Depression and schizophrenia: A contribution on their chemical pathologies.* New York: Spectrum, 1977.

Van Putten, T. Why do schizophrenic patients refuse to take their drugs? *Archives of General Psychiatry,* 1974, *31,* 67–72.

Van Putten, T., and Fawzy, F. I. Sex conversion surgery in a man with severe dysphoria—a tragic outcome. *Archives of General Psychiatry,* 1976, *33,* 751–53.

Venables, P. H. The effect of auditory and visual stimulation on the skin potential response of schizophrenics. *Brain,* 1960, *83,* 77–92.

Venables, P. H. Input dysfunction in schizophrenia. In B. A. Maher (Ed.), *Progress in experimental personality research* (vol. 1). New York: Academic Press, 1964.

Venables, P. H. The electrodermal psychophysiology of schizophrenics and children at risk for schizophrenia: Controversies and developments. *Schizophrenia Bulletin,* 1977, *3,* No. 1, 28–48.

Violence is occurring in the best of families. *New York Times,* March 20, 1977, Section IV, p. 1.

Voeller, B. Society and the gay movement. In J. Marmor (Ed.), *Homosexual behavior: A modern reappraisal.* New York: Basic Books, 1980.

Volavka, J., Davis, L. G., and Ehrlich, Y. H. Endorphins, dopamine, and schizophrenia. *Schizophrenia Bulletin,* 1979, *5,* No. 2, 227–39.

Vuchinich, R. W., Tucker, J. A., and Sobell, M. B. Alcohol, expectancy, cognitive labeling, and mirth. *Journal of Abnormal Psychology,* 1979, *88,* 641–51.

Wagemaker, H., Jr. and Cade, R. The use of hemodialysis in chronic schizophrenia. *American Journal of Psychiatry,* 1977, *134,* 684–85.

Wahl, O. F. Monozygotic twins discordant for schizophrenia: A review. *Psychological Bulletin,* 1976, *83,* 91–106.

Wahl, O. F. Sex bias in schizophrenia research: A short report. *Journal of Abnormal Psychology,* 1977, *86,* 195–98.

Waldron, M. Teen-agers' visits to prisons criticized. *New York Times,* April 26, 1979, p. B3.

Walker, L. E. *The battered woman.* New York: Harper & Row, 1979.

Walker, M. J., and Brodsky, S. L. *Sexual assault: The victim and the rapist.* Lexington, Mass.: Lexington Books, 1976.

Wallace, A. F. C. Cultural determinants of response to hallucinatory experience. *Archives of General Psychiatry,* 1959, *1,* 58–69.

Wallace, J., Burger, D., Neal, H. C., van Brero, M., and Davis, D. E. Aversive conditioning use in public facilities for the mentally retarded. *Mental Retardation,* 1976, *14,* 17–19.

Walters, J. M. "Buzzin' ": PCP use in Philadelphia. In H. W. Feldman, M. H. Agar, and G. M. Beschner (Eds.), *Angel dust: An ethnographic study of PCP users.* Lexington, Mass.: Lexington Books, 1979.

Wallace, R. K. Physiological effects of transcendental meditation. *Science,* 1970, *167,* 1751–54.

Warheit, G. J., Holzer, C. E. III, and Arey, S. A. Race and mental illness: An epidemiologic update. *Journal of Health and Social Behavior,* 1975, *16,* 243–56.

Watkins, H. H. Hypnosis and smoking: A five-session approach. *International Journal of Clinical and Experimental Hypnosis,* 1976, *24,* 381–90.

Watson, J. B., and Rayner, R. Conditioned emotional reactions. *Journal of Experimental Psychology,* 1920, *3,* 1–14.

Watson, S. J., and Akil, H. "Endorphins, dopamine, and schizophrenia": Two discussions. *Schizophrenia Bulletin,* 1979, *5,* No. 2, 240–42.

Watt, N. F., Stolorow, R. D., Lubensky, A. W., and McClelland, D. C. School adjustment and behavior of children hospitalized for schizophrenia as adults. *American Journal of Orthopsychiatry,* 1970, *40,* 637–57.

Watts, A. W. *Psychotherapy East and West.* New York: Pantheon, 1961.

Webb, W. B., and Cartwright, R. C. Sleep and dreams. *Annual Review of Psychology,* 1978, *29,* 223–52.

Webster, B. Classification is more than a matter of fish or fowl. *New York Times,* February 14, 1982, p. 8E.

Wechsler, D. A standardized memory scale for clinical use. *Journal of Psychology,* 1945, *19,* 87–95.

Wechsler, D. *The Wechsler Ingelligence Scale for Children (WISC).* New York: Psychological Corporation, 1949.

Wechsler, D. *The Wechsler Adult Intelligence Scale (WAIS).* New York: Psychological Corporation, 1955.

Wechsler, D. *The Wechsler Preschool and Primary Scale of Intelligence (WPPSI).* New York: Psychological Corporation, 1967.

Wechsler, D. *The Wechsler Intelligence Scale for Children (WISC-R).* New York: Psychological Corporation, 1974.

Wechsler, H. Epidemiology of male/female drinking over the last half century. In *Alcoholism and alcohol abuse and women: Research Issues.* Research Monograph No. 1. National Institute on Alcohol Abuse and Alcoholism, U.S. Department of Health, Education, and Welfare, 1980.

Wechsler, H., and Thum, D. Alcohol and drug use among teenagers: A questionnaire study. In M. E. Chafetz (Ed.), *Proceedings of the Second Annual Alcoholism Conference of the National Institute on Alcohol Abuse and Alcoholism.* National Institute on Alcohol Abuse and Alcoholism, 1973.

Weckowicz, T. E., Fedora, O., Mason, J., Radstaak, D., Bay, K. S., and Yonge, K. A. Effect of marijuana on divergent and convergent production cognitive tests. *Journal of Abnormal Psychology,* 1975, *84,* 386–98.

Weinberg, M. S., and Williams, C. J. Sexual embourgeoisement? Social class and sexual activity: 1938–70. *American Sociological Review*, 1980, *45*, 33–48.

Weiner, B. "On being sane in insane places": A process (attributional) analysis and critique. *Journal of Abnormal Psychology*, 1975, *84*, 433–41.

Weiner, H. *Psychobiology and human disease*. New York: Elsevier, 1977.

Weiner, I. B. *Principles of psychotherapy*. New York: Wiley, 1975.

Weinraub, B. A fog and a furor over G.I. drug use. *New York Times*, July 30, 1978, Section IV, p. 4.

Weiss, B., Williams, J. H., Margen, S., Abrams, B., Caan, B., Citron, L. J., Cox, C., McKibben, J., Ogar, D., and Schultz, S. Behavioral responses to artificial food colors. *Science*, 1980, *207*, 1487–89.

Weiss, G., and Hechtman, L. The hyperactive child syndrome. *Science*, 1979, *205*, 1348–54.

Weiss, J. Ulcers. In J. D. Maser and M. E. P. Seligman (Eds.), *Psychopathology: Experimental models*. San Francisco: Freeman, 1977.

Weissman, J., and Paykel, E. *The depressed woman: A study of social relationships*. Chicago: University of Chicago Press, 1974.

Weissman, M., and Klerman, G. L. Sex differences and epidemiology of depression. In E. S. Gomberg and V. Franks (Eds.), *Gender and disordered behavior*. New York: Brunner/Mazel, 1979.

Welkowitz, J., Cohen, J., and Ortmeyer, D. Value system similarity: Investigation of patient-therapist dyads. *Journal of Consulting Psychology*, 1967, *31*, 48–55.

Wesson, D. R., and Smith, D. E. Treatment of the polydrug abuser. In R. L. DuPont, A. Goldstein, and J. O'Donnell (Eds.), *Handbook on drug abuse*, National Institute on Drug Abuse, 1979.

Weithorn, C. J., and Ross, R. Stimulant drugs for hyperactivity: Some additional disturbing questions. *American Journal of Orthopsychiatry*, 1976, *46*, 168–73.

Weitzenhoffer, A. M., and Hilgard, E. R. *Stanford Profile Scales of Hypnotic Susceptibility Scale, Forms A and B*. Palo Alto, Calif.: Consulting Psychologists Press, 1959.

Weizenbaum, J. *Computer power and human reason: From judgment to calculation*. San Francisco: Freeman, 1976.

Wender, P. H., Rosenthal, D., Kety, S. S., Schulsinger, F., and Welner, J. Cross-fostering: A research strategy for clarifying the role of genetic and experiential factors in the etiology of schizophrenia. *Archives of General Psychiatry*, 1974, *30*, 121–28.

Wener, A. E., and Rehm, L. P. Depressive affect: A test of behavioral hypotheses. *Journal of Abnormal Psychology*, 1975, *84*, 221–27.

Wenrich, W. W., Dawley, H. H., and General, D. A. *Self-directed systematic desensitization: A guide for the student, client, and therapist*. Kalamazoo, Mich.: Behaviordelia, 1976.

Wesson, D. R., and Smith, D. E. *Barbiturates: Their use, misuse, and abuse*. New York: Human Sciences Press, 1977.

Westinghouse Learning Corporation/Ohio University. *The impact of Head Start: An evaluation of Head Start on children's cognitive and affective development*. Springfield, Va.: National Technical Information Service, 1969.

Whitehill, M., DeMyer-Gapin, S., and Scott, T. J. Stimulation seeking in antisocial preadolescent children. *Journal of Abnormal Psychology*, 1976, *85*, 101–4.

Whitehorn, J. C., and Betz, B. J. A study of psychotherapeutic relationships between physicians and schizophrenic patients. *American Journal of Psychiatry*, 1954, *111*, 321–31.

Whitehorn, J. C., and Betz, B. J. Further studies of the doctor as a crucial variable in the outcome of treatment with schizophrenics. *American Journal of Psychiatry*, 1960, *117*, 215–23.

Whitely, B. E., Jr. Sex roles and psychotherapy: A current appraisal. *Psychological Bulletin*, 1979, *86*, 1309–21.

Whitlock, F. A. The aetiology of hysteria. *Acta Psychiatrica Scandinavica*, 1967, *43*, 144–62.

Widom, C. S. A methodology for studying noninstitutionalized psychopaths. *Journal of Consulting and Clinical Psychology*, 1977, *45*, 674–83.

Wikler, A. Dynamics of drug dependence: Implications of a conditioning theory for research and treatment. *Archives of General Psychiatry*, 1973, *28*, 611–16.

Wilkins, W. Self-fulfilling prophecy: Is there a phenomenon to explain? *Psychological Bulletin*, 1977, *84*, 55–56.

Williams, D. A., Lewis-Faning, E., Rees, L., Jacobs, J., and Thomas, A. Assessment of the relative importance of the allergic, infective and psychological factors in asthma. *Acta Allergolica*, 1958, *12*, 376–95.

Wilson, E. O. *Sociobiology: The new synthesis*. Cambridge, Mass.: Harvard University Press, 1975.

Wilson, E. O. *On human nature*. Cambridge, Mass.: Harvard University Press, 1978.

Wilson, G. T., and Evans, I. M. Adult behavior therapy and the therapist-client relationship. In C. M. Franks and G. T. Wilson (Eds.), *Annual review of behavior therapy: Theory and practice*. New York: Brunner/Mazel, 1976.

Wilson, G. T., and Lawson, D. M. Effects of alcohol on sexual arousal in women. *Journal of Abnormal Psychology*, 1976, *85*, 485–97. (a)

Wilson, G. T., and Lawson, D. M. Expectancies, alcohol, and sexual arousal in male social drinkers. *Journal of Abnormal Psychology*, 1976, *85*, 587–94. (b)

Wilson, G. T., and Lawson, D. M. Expectancies, alcohol, and sexual arousal in women. *Journal of Abnormal Psychology*, 1978, *87*, 358–67.

Wilson, G. T., Lawson, D. M., and Abrams, D. C. Effects of alcohol on sexual arousal in male alcoholics. *Journal of Abnormal Psychology*, 1978, *87*, 609–16.

Winer, L. R. Biofeedback: A guide to the clinical literature. *American Journal of Orthopsychiatry*, 1977, *47*, 626–38.

Winick, C. Some aspects of careers of chronic heroin users. In E. Josephson and E. E. Carroll (Eds.), *Drug use: Epidemiological and sociological approaches*. New York: Wiley, 1974.

Winn, R. B. (Ed.) *Psychotherapy in the Soviet Union.* New York: Grove Press, 1961.

Winokur, G. The genetics of manic-depressive illness. In R. R. Fieve (Ed.), *Depression in the 1970's: Modern theory and research.* The Hague: Excerpta Medica, 1971.

Winokur, G. Unipolar depression: Is it divisible into autonomous subtypes? *Archives of General Psychiatry,* 1979, *36,* 47–52.

Winokur, G., Cadoret, R., Baker, M., and Dorzab, J. Depression spectrum disease versus pure depressive disease: Some further data. *British Journal of Psychiatry,* 1975, *127,* 75–77.

Winokur, G., Clayton, P. J., and Reich, T. *Manic depressive illness.* St. Louis: Mosby, 1969.

Wishner, J. The concept of efficiency in psychological health and in psychopathology. *Psychological Review,* 1955, *62,* 69–80.

Wishner, J., and Wahl, O. Dichotic listening in schizophrenia. *Journal of Consulting and Clinical Psychology,* 1974, *42,* 538–46.

Witelson, S. F. Developmental dyslexia: Two right hemispheres and none left. *Science,* 1977, *195,* 309–11.

Witkin, H. A., Mednick, S. A., Schulsinger, F., Bakkestrøm, E., Christiansen, K. O., Goodenough, D. R., Hirschhorn, K., Lundsteen, C., Owen, D. R., Phillip, J., Rubin, D. B., and Stocking, M. Criminality in XYY and XXY men. *Science,* 1976, *193,* 547–55.

Wittkower, E. D., and Dubreuil, G. Cultural factors in mental illness. In E. Norbeck, D. Price-Williams, and W. M. McCord (Eds.), *The study of personality: An interdisciplinary appraisal.* New York: Holt, Rinehart and Winston, 1968.

Wittkower, E. D., and Rin, H. Recent developments in transcultural psychiatry. In A. V. S. de Reuck and R. Porter (Eds.), *Transcultural psychiatry.* Boston: Little, Brown, 1965.

Wolfensberger, W. The origin and nature of our institutional models. In R. B. Kugel & W. Wolfensberger (Eds.), *Changing patterns in residential services for the mentally retarded.* Washington: President's Committee on Mental Retardation, 1969.

Wolfgang, M. E. Husband-wife homicides. *Corrective Psychiatry and Journal of Social Therapy,* 1956, *2,* 263–71.

Wolpe, J. An approach to the problem of neurosis based on the conditioned response. Unpublished M. D. thesis, Witwatersrand Medical School, 1948.

Wolpe, J. The systematic desensitization treatment of neuroses. *Journal of Nervous and Mental Disease,* 1961, *132,* 189–203.

World Health Organization Expert Committee on Drug Dependence. *WHO Technical Report Series,* No. 407, 1969.

World Health Organization Expert Committee on Drug Dependence. *WHO Technical Report Series,* No. 618, 1978.

Wolberg, A. Patterns of interaction in families of borderline patients. In B. F. Reiss (Ed.), *New directions in mental health.* New York: Grune & Stratton, 1968.

Wright, G. L. T. Asthma and the emotions: Aetiology and treatment. *Medical Journal of Australia,* 1965, *1,* 961–67.

Wurtman, R. J., and Wurtman, J. J. (Eds.) *Nutrition and the brain* (vols. 1 and 2). New York: Raven, 1977.

Wyatt, R. J., and Murphy, D. L. Low platelet monoamine oxidase activity and schizophrenia. *Schizophrenia Eulletin,* 1976, *2,* No. 1, 77–89.

Wyatt, R. J., Potkin, S. G., Bridge, T. P., Phelps, B. H., and Wise, C. D. Monoamine oxidase in schizophrenia: An overview. *Schizophrenia Bulletin,* 1980, *6,* 199–207.

Wyatt, R. J., Termini, B. A., and Davis, J. Biochemical and sleep studies of schizophrenia: A review of the literature—1960–1970. *Schizophrenia Bulletin,* 1971, No. 4, 10–66.

Wyatt v. *Stickney,* 344 F. Supp. 373 (M.D. Ala. 1972).

Wynne, L. C., Ryckoff, I. M., Day, J., and Hirsch, S. I. Pseudomutuality in the family relations of schizophrenics. *Psychiatry,* 1958, *21,* 205–20.

Wynne, L. C., and Singer, M. T. Thinking disorders and family transactions. Paper presented at joint meeting of the American Psychiatric Association and the American Psychoanalytic Association, 1964.

Yalom, I. D. *The theory and practice of group psychotherapy* (2nd ed.). New York: Basic Books, 1975.

Yalom, I. D., and Lieberman, M. A. A study of encounter group casualties. *Archives of General Psychiatry,* 1971, *25,* 16–30.

Yates, A. J. Psychological deficit. *Annual Review of Psychology,* 1966, *17,* 111–44.

Yates, A. J. *Theory and practice in behavior therapy.* New York: Wiley, 1975.

Yates, A. J. *Biofeedback and the modification of behavior.* New York: Plenum Press, 1980.

Yochelson, S., and Samenow, S. E. *The criminal personality* (vol. 1): *A profile for change.* New York: Aronson, 1976.

Yochelson, S., and Samenow, S. E. *The criminal personality* (vol. 2): *The change process.* New York: Aronson, 1977.

Youkilis, H. D., and DeWolfe, A. S. The regression hypothesis and subclassifications of schizophrenia. *Journal of Abnormal Psychology,* 1975, *84,* 36–40.

Zahn, T. P. Comments on "reaction time and attention in schizophrenia." *Schizophrenia Bulletin,* 1977, *3,* No. 3, 452–56.

Zax, M., Sameroff, A. J., and Babigian, H. M. Birth outcomes in the offspring of mentally disordered women. *American Journal of Orthopsychiatry,* 1977, *47,* 218–30.

Zeiner, A. R., Blackburn, M., Stratton, R., and Paredes, A. Tarahumara revisited. *Biological Psychology Bulletin,* 1978, *5,* 113–19.

Zeiner, A. R., and Paredes, A. Differential biological sensitivity as a predictor of alcohol abuse. In D. E. Smith (Ed.), *Multicultural view of drug abuse.* Cambridge, Mass.: Schenkman, 1978.

Ziferstein, I. Psychotherapy in the USSR. In S. A. Corson and E. O. Corson (Eds.), *Psychiatry and psychology in the USSR.* New York: Plenum, 1976.

Zigler, E. F. Research on personality structure in the retardate. In N. R. Ellis (Ed.), *International review of research in mental retardation* (vol. 1). New York: Academic Press, 1966.

Zigler, E. F. Developmental versus difference theories of mental retardation and the problem of motivation. *American Journal of Mental Deficiency,* 1969, *73,* 536–56.

Zigler, E. F. The retarded child as a whole person. In D. K. Routh (Ed.), *The experimental psychology of mental retardation.* Chicago: Aldine, 1973.

Zigler, E. F., and Balla, D. Personality factors in the performance of the retarded: Implications for clinical assessment. *Journal of Child Psychiatry,* 1977, *16,* 19–37.

Zigler, E. F., and DeLabry, J. Concept switching in middle class, lower class, and retarded children. *Journal of Abnormal and Social Psychology,* 1962, *65,* 267–73.

Zigler, E. F., Hodgden, L., and Stevenson, H. W. The effect of support and nonsupport on the performance of normal and feebleminded children. *Journal of Personality,* 1958, *26,* 106–22.

Zigler, E., and Levine, J. Premorbid adjustment and paranoid-nonparanoid status in schizophrenia: A further investigation. *Journal of Abnormal Psychology,* 1973, *82,* 189–99.

Zigler, E., Levine, J., and Zigler, B. The relation between premorbid competence and paranoid-nonparanoid status in schizophrenia: A methodological and theoretical critique. *Psychological Bulletin,* 1976, *83,* 303–13.

Zigler, E., and Phillips, L. Psychiatric diagnosis: A critique. *Journal of Abnormal and Social Psychology,* 1961, *63,* 607–18.

Zigler, E. F., and Trickett, P. The concept of competence and national social policy in the child and family life area. Paper presented at the Vermont Conference on the Primary Prevention of Psychopathology, University of Vermont, Burlington, 1977.

Zilbergeld, B., and Evans, M. The inadequacy of Masters and Johnson. *Psychology Today,* August, 1980, 29–34, 37–43.

Zilboorg, G., and Henry, G. W. *A history of medical psychology.* New York: Norton, 1941.

Zimmerman, E., and George, R. (Eds.) *Narcotics and the hypothalamus.* New York: Raven Press, 1974.

Zinberg, N. E. Nonaddictive opiate use. In R. L. DuPont, A. Goldstein, and J. O'Donnell, (Eds.), *Handbook on drug abuse.* National Institute on Drug Abuse, 1979.

Zubin, J. Classification of the behavior disorders. *Annual Review of Psychology,* 1967, *18,* 373–406.

Zubin, J. Cross-national study of diagnosis of the mental disorders: Methodology and planning. *American Journal of Psychiatry* (Supplement), 1969, *125,* 12–20.

Zubin, J. Scientific models for psychopathology in the 1970's. *Seminars in Psychiatry,* 1972, *4,* 283–96.

Zubin, J. But is it good for science? *Clinical Psychologist,* 1977–1978, *31,* 1, 5–7.

Zubin, J. Chronic schizophrenia from the standpoint of vulnerability. In C. Baxter and T. Melnechuk (Eds.), *Perspectives in schizophrenia research.* New York: Raven Press, 1980.

Zubin, J., Eron, L. D., and Schumer, F. *An experimental approach to projective techniques.* New York: Wiley, 1965.

Zubin, J., Salzinger, K., Fleiss, J. L., Gurland, B., Spitzer, R. L., Endicott, J., and Sutton, S. Biometric approach to psychopathology: Abnormal and clinical psychology—statistical, epidemiological, and diagnostic approaches. *Annual Review of Psychology,* 1975, *26,* 621–71.

Zubin, J., and Spring. B. Vulnerability—a new view of schizophrenia. *Journal of Abnormal Psychology,* 1977, *86,* 103–26.

Zung, W. W. K. The depression status inventory: An adjunct to the self-rating depression scale. *Journal of Clinical Psychology,* 1972, *28,* 539–43.

Zuroff, D. C., and Schwarz, J. C. Effects of transcendental meditation and muscle relaxation on trait anxiety, maladjustment, locus of control, and drug use. *Journal of Consulting and Clinical Psychology,* 1978, *46,* 264–71.

Index of Names

Index of Concepts

1 2 3 4 5 6 7 8 9 0